THE CAMBRIDGE
WORLD HISTORY OF MEDICAL ETHICS

The Cambridge World History of Medical Ethics is the first comprehensive scholarly account of the global history of medical ethics. Offering original interpretations of the field by leading bioethicists and historians of medicine, it will serve as the essential point of departure for future scholarship in the field. The book reconceptualizes the history of medical ethics through the creation of new categories, including the life cycle; discourses of religion, philosophy, and bioethics; and the relationship between medical ethics and the state, which includes a historical reexamination of the ethics of apartheid, colonialism, Communism, health policy, imperialism, militarism, Nazi medicine, Nazi "medical ethics," and research ethics. Also included are the first global chronology of persons and texts; the first concise biographies of major figures in medical ethics; and the first comprehensive bibliography of the history of medical ethics. An extensive index will guide readers to topics, texts, and proper names.

Robert B. Baker is William D. Williams Professor of Philosophy at Union College and Director of the Union Graduate College–Mount Sinai School of Medicine Bioethics Program. The author and editor of numerous articles and books, including the award-winning *American Medical Ethics Revolution*, he has received grants from the National Endowment for the Humanities and is codirector of a grant from the National Institutes of Health Fogarty International Center.

Laurence B. McCullough holds the Dalton Tomlin Chair in Medical Ethics and Health Policy in the Center for Medical Ethics and Health Policy, Baylor College of Medicine, Houston, Texas, where he is also Professor of Medicine and Medical Ethics and Associate Director for Education and Faculty Associate of the Huffington Center on Aging. He has published extensively on aspects of the history of medical ethics, conceptual issues in medical ethics, clinical ethics of various medical specialties, and research ethics, as well as the philosophy of Leibniz. His scholarly research has been supported by fellowships and grants from the National Endowment for the Humanities and the American Council of Learned Societies.

Editorial Board

THE CAMBRIDGE WORLD HISTORY OF MEDICAL ETHICS

EDITED BY

ROBERT B. BAKER
Union College, Union Graduate College

LAURENCE B. MCCULLOUGH
Baylor College of Medicine

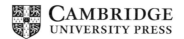

CAMBRIDGE
UNIVERSITY PRESS

CAMBRIDGE UNIVERSITY PRESS
Cambridge, New York, Melbourne, Madrid, Cape Town, Singapore, São Paulo, Delhi

Cambridge University Press
32 Avenue of the Americas, New York, NY 10013-2473, USA

www.cambridge.org
Information on this title: www.cambridge.org/9780521888790

First published 2009

Printed in the United States of America

A catalog record for this publication is available from the British Library.

Library of Congress Cataloging in Publication Data

The Cambridge world history of medical ethics / edited by Robert B. Baker, Laurence B. McCullough.
    p. ; cm.
Includes bibliographical references and index.
ISBN 978-0-521-88879-0 (hardback)
1. Medical ethics – History.   I. Baker, Robert B., 1937–   II. McCullough, Laurence B.
III. Title: World history of medical ethics.
[DNLM: 1. Ethics, Medical – history. W 50 C178 2008]
R724.C3274   2008
174.2–dc22   2007037915

ISBN   978-0-521-88879-0 hardback

To Our Wives
Arlene Baker and Linda Quintanilla
Sine Quibus Non

CONTENTS

ix

Part IV

The Discourses of Religion on Medical Ethics

Part V

The Discourses of Philosophy on Medical Ethics

Part VI

The Discourses of Practitioners on Medical Ethics

Part VII

The Discourses of Bioethics

Part VIII

Discourses on Medical Ethics and Society

A. Ethical and Legal Regulation of Medical Practice and Research

B. Medical Ethics, Imperialism, and the Nation-State

C. Medical Ethics and Health Policy

PREFACE

Once upon a time, not so very long ago, books on the history of medicine were about doctors. They were tales of heroic struggle, of well-intentioned failures, and, ultimately, of doctors' triumphs over disease. These triumphal images permeated the literature from popular books on microbe hunters to massive volumes published by distinguished university presses. Few noticed what was missing. Triumphal images employed the historian's chiaroscuro to put physicians and researchers in the bright foreground, relegating ethics and economics, and intellectual, gender, political, racial, religious, and socio-cultural factors to broad brushstrokes fading into dull background. For several decades, historians of medicine have been repainting this canvas, highlighting much that was previously obscure. *The Cambridge World History of Medical Ethics* contributes to that project. In its original design it sought to repaint the history of medical ethics on a larger canvas, limning broad intellectual, political, religious, and socioeconomic movements, and placing patients and nonprofessionals next to physicians in the foreground.

The Cambridge World History of Medical Ethics also aims to make its subject accessible not only to scholars but to the public, to students, to practicing health care professionals, and, of course, to bioethicists. For several decades, bioethicists have assisted pluralistic societies to negotiate the hazardous moral shoals surrounding fundamental

ethical and policy questions posed by medicine and the biomedical sciences. Founding and first-generation bioethicists were well prepared for this task. They were an interdisciplinary group with a broad humanistic education in history, law, philosophy, and theology, as well as medicine and nursing. Yet, the drama of the issues they confronted – the war crimes trials of the Nazi doctors at Nuremberg, turning off Karen Ann Quinlan's respirator, ending the abuse of African American research subjects in the Tuskegee syphilis experiment, and so forth – riveted their attention on the present. A pragmatic, problem-oriented focus became characteristic of bioethics teaching and scholarship. Initially, this orientation was balanced by the broad humanistic orientation of bioethicists themselves. As bioethics has "professionalized," however, the broad knowledge base integral to bioethics' initial success is atrophying. The editors hope that bioethicists will use *The Cambridge World History of Medical Ethics* to gain historical perspective on their own endeavors, to bring long-term social forces into focus, and to contemplate alternatives to currently accepted viewpoints. The editors also hope that the global sweep of *The Cambridge World History of Medical Ethics* will assist readers in understanding the deeper cultural and historical background of medical ethics.

Generally speaking, medical ethics is understood to comprise diverse discourses on the responsibilities of healers to the sick and the well, to society, to each other, and to the gods or God. We use the term "discourse" in the sense given prominence by the German philosopher, Jürgen Habermas, who extended the meaning of "discourse" to include a wide range of discussion and writing in the public sphere. The editors have adopted this sense of the term because it is broad enough to embrace oral conversations and traditions, epithets, pamphlets, letters, discursive texts of various sorts, statutes, court rulings, and trial transcripts – as well as the formal oaths and codes that have often taken center stage in traditional histories of medical ethics. Our aim in using the term discourse is to expand the scope of what should be considered primary sources for the history of medical ethics.

The editors faced several challenges in developing *The Cambridge World History of Medical Ethics*: how to put nonprofessionals and patients into the picture without ignoring practitioners; how to weigh the more abundant scholarly literature in certain areas and eras of medical ethics against sparser literature in other areas and eras; how to balance newer against more traditional conceptions of the history of medicine and the history of medical ethics; how to represent the bioethics revolution within the broader context of medical ethics; how to demarcate the point at which the present becomes the past, transforming current events into "history"; how to balance our present conception of ethical issues in the biomedical sciences and medicine against past conceptions of medical ethics; and how best to characterize "medical ethics" itself.

The editors' responses to these questions are evident throughout the volume. Part of the response involved dividing *The Cambridge World History of Medical Ethics* into eight parts. Part I provides an introduction to the history of medical ethics, addressing the history of the concept of "medical ethics," the historiography of the subject, and the interrelationship between bioethics and the history of medical ethics.

Chronology is the backbone of history. To situate major figures and texts in the context of world history and the history of medicine, we have created a chronology and made it Part II of the volume, rather than an appendix, as customary. A cursory perusal of the chronology readily reveals a robust history of medical ethics stretching across eras and cultures. We intend the chronology as an aid to the reader in subsequent chapters and to situate each chapter's content and figures in the larger context of the history of medical ethics.

Culture is the focus of Part III. Nature dictates a life cycle – conception, birth, growth, maturity, aging, dying, and death – but culture shapes and interprets it. Part III presents diverse cultural interpretations of the life cycle, serving as an interpretive framework and background to the discourses on medical ethics that are explored in subsequent chapters.

Parts IV to VII, which encompass more than half of the volume, address the discourses of religion (Part IV), the discourses of philosophy (Part V), the discourses of practitioners (Part VI), and the discourses of bioethics (Part VII). The order of these four parts is intended to reflect, in a rough but serviceable fashion, the sequence in which discourses unfolded; thus religious concepts come first and bioethical conceptions last.

Medical ethics is often discussed apart from culture and society, as if it were autonomous. Seeking to situate medical ethics in its socio-cultural context, we devote Part VIII to discourses on medical ethics and society. Ethics is but one of the mechanisms of social control that societies use to regulate medical practitioners and researchers. The first section explores the marketplace, law, and formal codes as mechanisms of social control that are rich in ethical content. Another aspect of culture, often overlooked or underemphasized in traditional approaches to the history of medical ethics, is the emergence and impact of the strong nation-state. This history was pivotal to the development of both contemporary medical ethics and bioethics, and thus the second section addresses Japanese imperialism, Nazism, Communism, the Cold War, and Apartheid. The final section of Part VIII deals with health policy, including eugenics, public health ethics, organ transplantation, and the determination of death.

The appendices are designed to assist readers by providing them with brief biographies of major figures in the history of medical ethics and a comprehensive bibliography of the subject. Before the publication of these appendices there was no single place to turn to find brief biographies of Hippocrates, or Thomas Percival (the inventor of the expression "medical ethics"), or André Hellegers (founder of the Kennedy Institute of Ethics), not to mention such less-well-known figures as Leopold (Leo) Alexander, John Cotta, Kaibara Ekiken, Isaac Hays, Friedrich Hoffmann, Christoph Wilhelm Hufeland, Henri de Mondeville, or Gabriele Zerbi. There was, moreover, no place to turn for a comprehensive bibliography of the primary and secondary sources for the global history of medical ethics. A comprehensive index completes the volume. We have prepared these to provide the reader detailed guidance to discussions of major historical figures and texts, concepts, and topics in the discourses on medical ethics addressed in the chapters and chronology. Information on contributors can be found immediately following this preface.

By design, *The Cambridge World History of Medical Ethics* does not offer the familiar geocultural chronological account of medical ethics. Our intent is to open the field to a variety of conceptions of and approaches to the subject. Readers will find some authors taking fairly traditional scholarly approaches to a now distant past. Others provide case studies, or, lacking the perspective of distance because they are addressing recent history, tend to preserve memory and to bear witness. We encouraged these different styles of history – chronologically arrayed histories of various discourses, case studies, participant accounts – because they capture the scope of the global history of medical ethics from ancient times to the end of the twentieth century.

Practical constraints inevitably fetter good intentions. Despite the editors' intention to represent the history of medical ethics as broadly as possible, the limits of the present scholarly literature tended to shape the contours of the volume. Inevitably, sections on such traditional areas as practitioners' discourses – oaths, codes, and the like – tend to draw on more robust scholarly resources than innovative attempts to capture a sense of medical ethics from the perspective of the sick and the well. There is thus more detail in some chapters than in others and some areas and eras are unfortunately underrepresented. Moreover, many of the concerns of historians of the late twentieth century – gender, race, social class – were not concerns in the texts and oaths of earlier eras, which were often more concerned about issues of competence, conscience, religion, and society. Rather than imposing our current concerns inappropriately on the past, we urged contributors to present the concerns of earlier eras to readers. Finally, we should note that, for a variety of reasons, some of those authors originally invited to contribute were unable to complete their chapters; as a consequence, some sections are less robust than we originally intended.

Practical constraints led to the editors' decision to end this history in 2000, the last year of the twentieth century. A further challenge was how to treat the emergence of the new discourse of bioethics: a discourse that evolved in the second half of the twentieth century as humanists, social scientists, lawyers, philosophers, and theologians began to collaborate with nurses, physicians, policy makers, and researchers on addressing challenges created by new advances in biomedicine. The "bioethics revolution" and its attendant preoccupations and discourses became an international phenomenon, and its concerns about autonomy, patients' rights, and informed consent could easily have dominated the pages of this volume. Yet, in the context of the long history of medical ethics, bioethics is but a recent and not wholly original development. We compromised by restricting a direct history of the discourse to eight chapters. Other chapters, of course, touch on topics integral to contemporary bioethics, such as truth telling and care of the dying, but we treated these topics as we did other contemporary preoccupations, by asking contributors to focus on the central concerns of eras past, rather than the present.

One could cast the development of this volume as an academic melodrama, playing up the aspects of courtship, and the redemptive achievement of actually producing a comprehensive volume on the global history of medical ethics. Terence Moore (1953–2004), late Humanities Editor for Cambridge University Press in New York

City, conceived of the project and courted potential editors. Spurned by at least one famous name, he rebounded, on the advice of Tom Beauchamp and Raymond Frey, by courting the two of us by e-mail. At the time, 1996, we were mere acquaintances. Both of us had been active in bioethics, both of us published on the history of medical ethics, and one of us had contributed a paper to a conference and a volume edited by the other. Beyond that we were almost strangers. So, two bespectacled, bearded, balding, middle-aged scholars of distinctly different temperaments began a mutual courtship. We found that we had both majored in some form of history as undergraduates, that we loved art and ballet, that we had a common middle name and a common taste for archival scholarship, and that we both believed, as we were to write in a grant proposal, that "a historically uninformed, crisis-centered mind-set will rob bioethics of critical perspective, rendering its intellectual footing precarious." On this basis we built a fertile partnership and an enduring friendship.

Once we accepted Terry Moore's invitation to submit a proposal to him, the burdens of courtship were reversed. We found ourselves courting Terry, Cambridge University Press, and its Syndicate at Cambridge University, even as Terry, a coy but brazen suitor, urged us to continue the suit and to make a formal proposal. Before we could propose, however, we had to be certain of our own motives. In 1995, the second edition of the *Encyclopedia of Bioethics* was published. As the *Encyclopedia's* Editor-in-Chief, Warren T. Reich, wrote in his introduction, he had recruited the world's leading scholars to write a "monumental" thirty-four-article, "book-length set of articles on the history of medical ethics" for the *Encyclopedia* (Reich 1995, 1: xxx). After rereading the history of medical ethics section of the *Encyclopedia*, we were profoundly impressed by the breadth and solidity of the scholarship. Nonetheless, we found ourselves restive with the geocultural-chronological approach that the articles offered. We had a vision of an alternative approach to the construction of the history of medical ethics. As we were to write in our prospectus to Cambridge University Press, we wanted to offer readers a sense of the different voices, or discourses, that contribute to the history of medical ethics: "religious medical ethics, philosophical medical ethics, practitioner-generated medical ethics, the connections between medical ethics and social ethics, public policy, medical police, and medical jurisprudence," so that readers will understand the diversity and conflicts that have historically informed what has come to be called "medical ethics."

We sent the earliest drafts of our prospectus to Warren Reich, hoping to draw on his editorial acumen and experience. We profited enormously from his generous advice and perceptive comments. He, in turn, commended our "design" for *The Cambridge World History of Medical Ethics*, which, as he wrote in a supporting letter, "takes the field well beyond anything the *Encyclopedia of Bioethics* accomplished" because we had "constructed a new framework for the history of medical ethics . . . provid[ing] a broader-than-usual historical and cultural setting . . . [and] developing major themes ingredient in this history that have never before been worked out in the way they propose." Having assured ourselves that our proposed volume would offer something different, we recruited an editorial advisory board, including Warren, and submitted our prospectus, first to them, and then to Terry Moore – who circulated it to commentators from around the globe. We spent an additional 6 months revising the prospectus in response to comments. Especially perceptive and helpful were the critical comments and suggestions by Onora O'Neill and her colleagues at the Syndicate.

Once the contract was approved, we were again cast in the role of suitors, seeking contributors and funding. Our application to the Collaborative Research Program in the Division of Research of the National Endowment for the Humanities, an agency of the U.S. government, was approved and provided major support for this project in the form of a 3-year grant. Our program officers at the NEH, Daniel Jones and Kathy Toavs, were exceptionally supportive during the application process and throughout the duration of this project. Crucial matching funding for the collaborative editorial conference in Houston, Texas, in September 2000, was generously provided by the Earhart, Greenwall, and Lucius N. Littauer Foundations and the Milbank Memorial Fund. We especially want to thank Daniel Fox, then-president of the Milbank Memorial Fund, and William Stubing, president of the Greenwall Foundation.

At Baylor College of Medicine, Baruch Brody, the director of the Center for Medical Ethics, saw the importance of this project from its conception and offered ongoing and substantial institutional support and guidance. Thomas Moore, then of Baylor's Office of Development, helped in crucial ways to secure funding from the private foundations mentioned previously, as did Dr. Ralph Feigin (1938–2008), then-president of the college. At Union College, the Humanities Faculty Research Fund was generous in its support. Pam Simmons, then of the Development Office, assisted in the drafting of the proposal to the NEH, Felmon Davis of the Philosophy Department was a superlative critical reader of the proposal, Judy Manchester assisted with the financial details, and Deans Christina Sorum and Linda Cool provided encouragement and institutional support. Both institutions provided secretarial and research staff support. We wish to thank Gloria Johnson, Andrew Laccett, Ann Marie Nolte, Anjlee Patel, Anna Louise Penner, Fariha Ramay, Emily De Santis, Erika Selli, Jason Shames, Delores Smith, Kristel Tomlinson, Marianne Snowden, and Andrew Yerkes for their assistance. We especially thank Terrence McEachern for his many excellent contributions to the preparation of the volume's

bibliography and Lisa Angotti and Ian Dempsey for assistance with indexing. We are also indebted to Warren Reich, who reviewed the final draft of the manuscript for Cambridge University Press and who, in the process, helped us to clarify pivotal aspects of the volume's preface, introduction, and table of contents.

A sixty-three-chapter book is, of necessity, an extensive collaboration. We are deeply indebted to the authors of the chapters in this volume and to the international team of scholars on the Editorial Board. Authors and Editorial Board members set aside time from their other projects to participate in this volume. Many took the risk of exploring previously uncharted areas. All have risen to the numerous challenges of interdisciplinary collaboration, working, often by e-mail, with partners from other parts of the globe. They have done so with grace and humor. Finally, this book could never have been prepared and edited without the patience, understanding, tolerance, and support of our wives, Arlene Baker and Linda Quintanilla, who sacrificed innumerable weekends and evenings so that the two of us could collaborate on the editing of this volume. We dedicate the volume to them.

Sadly, three of the contributors to this volume, Dorothy Nelkin (1933–2003), Chester Burns (1937–2006), and Mikhail Yarovinsky (1933–2007) died while *The Cambridge World History of Medical Ethics* was being completed. Dot Nelkin's collaborator, David Rosner, graciously and expertly completed the final editing of their chapter. Chester Burns and Mikhail Yarovinsky died as the book entered production. Chester's scholarship pioneered the field of the history of medical ethics and has had a lasting influence of both of us, making this volume possible. We mourn their deaths. The scholarly world will be less interesting and less lively in their absence.

As we noted earlier, Terry Moore conceived the idea for this volume; unfortunately, he died before this book was published. We would like to acknowledge our debt to him for his encouragement, for his editorial acumen, and for his support during the 8 years in which he guided us. We are honored to add to the many volumes prepared under Terry's editorial direction that have contributed so significantly to the world of scholarship. He was an inspiring editor with a wonderful and wonderfully dry sense of humor. His abiding and deep commitment to scholarship, his wit, and his insight will be sorely missed. We are extremely grateful to Beatrice Rehl of Cambridge University Press for ably assuming the editorship role for the volume and shepherding it through its last stages, and to Peggy Rote and her colleagues at Aptara for seeing it into print.

Robert B. Baker, Schenectady, New York
Laurence B. McCullough, Houston, Texas
July 2008

CONTRIBUTORS

DARREL W. AMUNDSEN, PH.D., is Professor Emeritus and former chair of Classics in the Department of Modern and Classical Languages at Western Washington University in Bellingham, Washington. His books include *Medicine, Society, and Faith in the Ancient and Medieval Worlds* (1996); *Different Death: Euthanasia and the Christian Tradition* (with Edward Larson 1998); and *Caring and Curing: Health and Medicine in the Western Religious Traditions* (coedited with Ronald Numbers 1998, first edition 1986). He also prepared the entries on the history of medical ethics in Europe and in the ancient near and Middle East for the *Encyclopedia of Bioethics*.

ROBERT B. BAKER, PH.D., is William D. Williams Professor of Philosophy at Union College, Professor of Bioethics and Director of the Center for Bioethics at Union Graduate College, Director of the Union Graduate College–Mount Sinai School of Medicine Bioethics Program, and a Visiting Fellow at the Center for Bioethics at the University of Pennsylvania. He has authored, coauthored, edited, or coedited several books and government reports including the award-winning *American Medical Ethics Revolution* (with A. Caplan, L. Emanuel, and S. Latham 1999). A four-time National Endowment for the Humanities awardee, Baker is currently codirector of a grant from the National Institutes of Health Fogarty International Center. He coedits the Advances in Bioethics and the Classics in the History of Medical Ethics book series, is founding chair of the Affinity group on the History of Medical Ethics of the American Society of Bioethics, and serves on the American Philosophical Association's Committee on Philosophy and Medicine. He has been a Fellow of the American Philosophical Society and of the Institute for Health and Human Values, a visiting scholar at the former Wellcome Institute for the History of Medicine (London), and a Wood Institute Fellow of the College of Physicians of Philadelphia. In 2002, he was Hyderabad/Sind National Collegiate Board Visiting Professor at the University of Mumbai.

RONALD BAYER, PH.D., is a professor at the Center for the History and Ethics of Public Health, Mailman School of Public Health, Columbia University. Prior to coming to Columbia he was at The Hastings Center. Bayer's research has examined ethical and policy issues in public health. His empirical work has focused especially on AIDS, tuberculosis, illicit drugs, and tobacco. His broader project is to develop an ethics of public health. He is an elected member of the Institute of Medicine (IOM), National Academy of Sciences, is on the IOM Board on Health Promotion and Disease Prevention, and has served on IOM committees dealing with the social impact of AIDS, tuberculosis elimination, vaccine safety, smallpox immunization and the Ryan White Care Act. His books include *Homosexuality and American Psychiatry: The Politics of Diagnosis* (1981); *Private Acts, Social Consequences: AIDS and the Politics of Public Health* (1989); *AIDS in the Industrialized Democracies: Passions, Politics and Policies* (edited with David Kirp 1991); *Confronting Drug Policy: Illicit Drugs in a Free Society* (edited with Gerald Oppenheimer 1993); *Blood Feuds: Blood, AIDS and the Politics of Medical Disaster* (edited with Eric Feldman 1999); *AIDS Doctors: Voices from the Epidemic* (written with Gerald Oppenheimer 2000); *Mortal Secrets: Truth and Lies in the Age of AIDS* (written with Robert Klitzman 2003); and *Unfiltered: Conflicts over Tobacco Policy and Public Health* (edited with Eric Feldman 2004).

KLAUS BERGDOLT, M.D., PH.D., is head of the Institute of the History of Medicine and Bioethics at Cologne University in Germany. He took his M.D. specializing in ophthalmology at Heidelberg University Hospital and his Ph.D. in the History of Fine Arts at Heidelberg University. From 1990 to 1995, he was the director of the German Institute in Venice. His main research and teaching interests are the history of health and of the plague, the links of arts and medicine, the history of medical ethics, and the history of medicine and science with a particular focus on the Italian Renaissance.

BELA BLASSZAUER is a lawyer and candidate of medical sciences. He worked as a teacher of medical ethics for more than 25 years at the Medical University of Pecs, Institute of Behavioral Sciences. At present – as a retired bioethicist – he is a scientific advisor for the Institute of Family Medicine at the University of Pecs, Faculty of Medicine. He has attended more than fifty international conferences as an invited lecturer and has been an invited scholar at such places as The Hastings Center, Creighton University, and Thomas Jefferson University in Philadelphia. He is the author of seven books, twelve book chapters in English-language publications, and more than one hundred articles (more than two dozen in English) on issues of medical ethics. He has translated Elisabeth Kübler-Ross's *On Death and Dying* into Hungarian. His textbook on medical ethics is now in its second edition and is used by most Hungarian medical universities and health colleges. Most recently, he published two articles (on informed consent and euthanasia) in the

"Ethical Eye" series of the European Council's publisher. For his life's work in the field of medical ethics, Dr. Blasszauer received the Gold Cross of Merit of the Hungarian Republic on the National Day, March 15, 2004.

KENNETH BOYD, PH.D., FRCPED, holds a personal chair in Medical Ethics in the College of Medicine and Veterinary Medicine, University of Edinburgh, Scotland. He is also general secretary of the UK Institute of Medical Ethics, chair of the Boyd Group on the use of animals in medical research, and a deputy editor of the *Journal of Medical Ethics*. His research interests include both clinical and public policy issues in medical ethics, the ethics of research with animals, and the historical development and current curriculum of medical ethics and medical humanities in medical education.

BARUCH A. BRODY, PH.D., is Leon Jaworski Professor of Biomedical Ethics, Distinguished Service Professor, and Director of the Center for Medical Ethics and Health and Policy at Baylor College of Medicine in Houston, Texas. He is also Andrew W. Mellon Professor of the Humanities in the Department of Philosophy at Rice University in Houston, Texas. He is widely published in philosophy and bioethics. His *The Ethics of Biomedical Research: An International Perspective* was published in 1998 and *Taking Issue: Pluralism and Casuistry in Bioethics* in 2003.

CHESTER R. BURNS, M.D., PH.D. (1937–2006), was the James Wade Rockwell Professor of Medical History Emeritus at the Institute for the Medical Humanities at the University of Texas Medical Branch in Galveston, where he taught for 36 years. Dr. Burns was the author of more than 100 publications dealing with the history of medical ethics in the United States, the history of health care in Texas, and the history of humanities education in American medical schools.

H. TRISTRAM ENGELHARDT, JR., PH.D., M.D., is a professor in the Department of Philosophy, Rice University, and Professor Emeritus, Departments of Internal Medicine and Community Medicine and Center for Medical Ethics and Health Policy, Baylor College of Medicine, Houston, Texas. He is Senior Editor of the *Journal of Medicine and Philosophy*, Senior Editor of the journal *Christian Bioethics*, editor of the book series Philosophy and Medicine, and senior editor of the book series Philosophical Studies in Contemporary Culture. Engelhardt has authored more than 300 articles, coedited more than twenty-five volumes, and his most widely translated work is *The Foundations of Bioethics*, 2nd ed. (1996). His most recent book,

The Foundations of Christian Bioethics (2000), has also appeared in Portuguese.

RUIPING FAN, M.B., PH.D., is Associate Professor of the Department of Public and Social Administration at City University of Hong Kong. He received a Bachelor of Medicine from Baotou College of Medicine in Inner Mongolia and a Ph.D. in philosophy from Rice University in Houston, Texas. His research focuses on East–West comparative studies in bioethics and the philosophy of medicine. He edited *Confucian Bioethics* (1999) and authored more than forty scholarly papers, which appeared in journals such as *Philosophy East & West*, *Journal of Chinese Philosophy*, *Journal of Medicine and Philosophy*, *Bioethics*, *HEC Forum*, and *Journal of Law, Medicine & Ethics*. Currently, he serves as Associate Editor of the *Journal of Medicine and Philosophy* and coeditor of *International Journal of Chinese and Comparative Philosophy of Medicine*. He is also on the editorial board of the *Dao: A Journal of Comparative Philosophy*.

GARY B. FERNGREN, PH.D., is Professor of History at Oregon State University. He specializes in the social history of ancient medicine and the historical relationship of religion to medicine and science. His publications include *The History of Science and Religion in the Western Tradition: An Encyclopedia* (2000) and *Science and Religion: A Historical Introduction* (2002).

MARY E. FISSELL, PH.D., teaches in the Department of the History of Medicine at the Johns Hopkins University. Her research focuses on the patient/practitioner relationship, gender, and popular medicine in early-modern England. She is the author of *Patients, Power and the Poor in Eighteenth-Century Bristol* (1991) and *Vernacular Bodies: the Politics of Reproduction in Early Modern England* (2005).

DANIEL M. FOX, PH.D., is President Emeritus, Milbank Memorial Fund, an endowed foundation that works with decision makers in the public and private sectors to use the best available evidence to improve policy for health care and population health. Prior to joining the Fund in 1990, he served in federal and state government and as a faculty member and administrator at two universities. He has published books and articles about the politics of policy making for health and the intellectual history of health policy.

RENÉE C. FOX, PH.D., is the Annenberg Professor Emerita of the Social Sciences in the Department of Sociology at the University of Pennsylvania, Senior Fellow at the Center for Bioethics, and an associated faculty member of the Solomon Asch Center for the Study of Ethnopolitical Conflict. In addition, she is a research associate at Queen Elizabeth House, Centre for Refugee Studies, University of Oxford, in the United Kingdom. Professor Fox is currently working on a coauthored book with Judith P. Swazey about the genesis, evolution, and significance of U.S. bioethics. She is also in the midst of an ongoing, first-hand, field research study of some of the practical and moral dilemmas associated with medical humanitarianism and human rights witnessing action. Médecins Sans Frontières (Doctors Without Borders) is the "case study" around which this research turns.

EUGENIJUS GEFENAS, PH.D., is Associate Professor and Director of the Department of Medical History and Ethics at the Medical Faculty of Vilnius University. He is also chairman of the Lithuanian Bioethics Committee as well as a Senior Research Fellow at the Institute of Culture, Philosophy and Arts. His international activities include membership in the Council of Europe Bioethics Committee (CDBI), the International Bioethics Committee (IBC) of UNESCO, as well as the European Society for Philosophy of Medicine and Health Care. During the period 2000–2004, he was a member of the European Committee for the Prevention of Torture and Inhuman or Degrading Treatment or Punishment. He graduated from the Medical Faculty of Vilnius University and obtained his Ph.D. from the Institute of Philosophy, Sociology and Law. His professional interests include such issues as teaching and developing bioethics infrastructure in transition societies, ethical and philosophical problems of biomedical research, ethical aspects of health care reform, and resource allocation.

DIEGO GRACIA, M.D., PH.D., is Professor of History of Medicine and Bioethics in the Department of Public Health and History of Science of the School of Medicine of Complutense University in Madrid, Spain. His main areas of research are the history of medical ethics, deliberation, and the ethics of responsibility. His books include *Fundamentos de bioética* (Fundamentals of Bioethics) (1986), *"Primum non nocere"* (First Do No Harm) (1990), *Procedimientos de Decisión en Ética Clínica (Decision Making Procedures in Clinical Ethics)* (1991), *Ética y Vida* (Ethics and Life) (4 vols., 1998), *Como Arqueros al Blanco: Estudios de bioética* (As Archers to White: Studies in Bioethics) (2004), and *"Medice, cura te ipsum"* (Physician Heal Thyself) (2004).

ILHAN ILKILIC, M.D., PH.D, has studied medicine, philosophy and Islamic sciences in Istanbul, Bochum, and Tübingen. He has worked as a researcher on project "Health Literacy" as a member of the research group "Culture-Transcending Bioethics" funded by the

German Research Council. He is currently coordinator of project "Public Health Genetics" at the Institute for History, Philosophy and Ethics of Medicine, University of Mainz. His special interests include Islamic bioethics, transcultural bioethics, health literacy, and public health genetics. His books include *Der muslimische Patient* (The Muslim Patient) (2002), *Begegnung und Umgang mit muslimischen Patienten* (Clinical Encounters with the Muslim Patient) (2003), and *Gesundheitsverstaendnis und Gesundheitsmuendigkeit in der islamischen Tradition* (Conceptions of Health and Healthcare Literacy in Muslim Culture) (2005); articles include "Bioethical Conflicts between Muslim Patients and German Physicians and the Principles of Biomedical Ethics" (*Medicine and Law* 2002) and "New Bioethical Problems as Challenge for Muslims" (*Chennai Journal of Intercultural Philosophy*, 2005).

ALBERT R. JONSEN, PH.D., is Codirector of the Program in Medicine and Human Values, California Pacific Medical Center, San Francisco. He is professor of Ethics in Medicine Emeritus and past Chairman, Department of Medical History and Ethics, School of Medicine, University of Washington. He is a member of the Institute of Medicine, National Academy of Sciences. He is the author of *The Birth of Bioethics* (1998), *A Short History of Medical Ethics* (2000), and *The Abuse of Casuistry: A History of Moral Reasoning* (with Stephen Toulmim 1987).

RIHITO KIMURA, PH.D., is President of Keisen University in Tokyo and professor emeritus of Bioethics, Waseda University in Japan. His main area of research is cross-cultural bioethics. His two most recent works are *Bioethics Handbook* (2003) and "Medical Ethics, History of South and East Asia IV: Contemporary Japan" in *Encyclopedia of Bioethics*, 3rd ed., edited by Stephen G. Post (2004).

RUDOLF KLEIN is Emeritus Professor of Social Policy at Bath University and visiting professor at the London School of Economics and at the London School of Hygiene. His publications include *The New Politics of the NHS* (2006) and books and monographs about rationing, accountability, and regulation. In 2004, he published a study (with Patricia Day) of the Commission for Health Improvement, the NHS's inspectorate. He is currently working on various aspects of the politics of health policy making.

STEPHEN R. LATHAM, J.D., PH.D., is Deputy Director of Yale University's Interdisciplinary Center on Bioethics. His writings on professional ethics, bioethics and health policy have appeared in a wide variety of law, medical, and bioethics journals. Latham is a former Graduate Fellow of Harvard's Safra Foundation Center on Ethics and a former Research Fellow of the University of Edinburgh's Institute for Advanced Studies in the Humanities. He currently serves on the board of the American Society for Bioethics and Humanities, and on Connecticut's Stem Cell Research Advisory Committee. He is working on two books, one on the ideas of moral authority and expertise, and another on the medical ethics of American Puritans.

SUSAN E. LEDERER, PH.D., is Robert Turell Professor and Chair of the Department of Medical History and Bioethics at the University of Wisconsin, Madison. Formerly associate professor in the Section of the History of Medicine at Yale University School of Medicine, and in the Departments of History and African American Studies at Yale University, she is the author of *Subjected to Science: Human Experimentation in America Before the Second World War* (1995), *Frankenstein: Penetrating the Secrets of Nature* (2002), and *Flesh and Blood: A Cultural History of Blood Transfusion and Organ Transplantation* (2008). Her research focuses on the history of American medical ethics, especially research ethics, and medical culture in twentieth-century America.

BARRON H. LERNER, M.D., PH.D., is the Angelica Berrie–Arnold P. Gold Foundation Associate Professor of Medicine and Public Health in the Department of Medicine and the Mailman School of Public Health at the Columbia University Medical Center in New York City. Dr. Lerner is the author of three books on the history of medicine, *Contagion and Confinement* (1998), *The Breast Cancer Wars* (2001), and *When Illness Goes Public: Celebrity Patients and How We Look at Medicine* (2006), as well as numerous articles in scientific journals. He also writes regularly for the Science Times section of *The New York Times*. Dr. Lerner teaches medical ethics and the history of medicine at Columbia's Center for the History and Ethics of Public Health.

LUN LI, PH.D., is Professor at the Institute of Ethics, Hunan Normal University, China, and was a Research Ethics Fellow of Harvard School of Public Health from 2002 to 2005. He is the author of *Virtues behind the Mouse* (2002). His current interests include bioethics and cyberethics. He is doing a research project titled "Influence of Japanese Criminal Human Experiments in China 1932–1945 and the American Cover-up on Postwar Research Ethics in China."

BOLESLAV L. LICHTERMAN, M.D., PH.D., graduated from Gorky State Medical Institute in 1982, specialized in neurosurgery, and defended his doctoral thesis on calculated outcome prediction of traumatic cerebral compression in 1988. From 1988 to 2001, he served as chair of Pediatric Neurosurgery at the Russian Postgraduate Medical Academy in Moscow, combining clinical work with historical research. Since 1997, he has been a scientific editor of a Russian National medical periodical "Meditsynskaya Gazeta." Currently, he is a senior researcher at The Centre for the History of Medicine of Russian Academy of Medical Sciences in Moscow. He is completing his habilitation thesis about an early history of neurosurgery (1920s–1930s). His current research is focused on a history of clinical neuroscience, the history of Russian/Soviet medicine, and the history of medical ethics.

MARY LINDEMANN, PH.D., is Professor in the Department of History, University of Miami. She has written a new book titled *Liaisons Dangereuses: Sex, Law, and Diplomacy in the Age of Frederick the Great* (2006). In addition, she is working on a project exploring the medical and biological determinants of civil competency and criminal responsibility in the period 1648 to circa 1800 and on a study of political culture in three early modern cities: Amsterdam, Antwerp, and Hamburg. She has recently edited a collection of articles on early modern German history titled *Ways of Knowing: Ten Interdisciplinary Essays* (2004).

ANDREAS-HOLGER MAEHLE, DR.MED.HABIL., PH.D., is Professor of History of Medicine and Medical Ethics and head of the Department of Philosophy at Durham University, where he also directs the Centre for the History of Medicine and Disease. His present major research areas are the development of medical professional ethics and the history of pharmacology. His recent publications include *Drugs on Trial: Experimental Pharmacology and Therapeutic Innovation in the Eighteenth Century* (1999) and *Historical and Philosophical Perspectives on Biomedical Ethics: From Paternalism to Autonomy?* (coedited with Johanna Geyer-Kordesch 2002). He is currently writing a book on medical ethics in Imperial Germany.

JOSÉ ALBERTO MAINETTI, M.D., PH.D., holds a doctorate in Medicine and a doctorate in Philosophy from the Universidad Nacional de La Plata, Argentina. He is cofounder of the Mainetti Foundation (1969) and director of its Institute for Bioethics and Medical Humanities (1972), which publishes the journal *Quirón* and many books on the field. He is commonly acknowledged as the man who started bioethics in Latin America by developing the history of medicine, medical anthropology, and medical ethics of Pedro

Laín Entralgo's school of thought in Argentina and the surrounding regions.

LAURENCE B. MCCULLOUGH, PH.D., holds the Dalton Tomlin Chair in Medical Ethics and Health Policy and is Associate Director for Education of the Center for Medical Ethics and Health Policy at Baylor College of Medicine in Houston, Texas. He is also Adjunct Professor of Philosophy at Rice University in Houston and Adjunct Professor of Ethics in Obstetrics and Gynecology and of Public Health at Weill Medical College of Cornell University in New York City. He has worked in the history of medical ethics for 30 years. His *John Gregory and the Invention of Professional Medical Ethics and the Profession of Medicine* and, as editor, *John Gregory's Writings on Medical Ethics and Philosophy of Medicine* were published in 1998, with preparation of both supported by an American Council of Learned Societies fellowship.

JAMES C. MOHR, PH.D., is College of Arts and Sciences Distinguished Professor of History at the University of Oregon, where he teaches and writes about many aspects of life in the United States during the nineteenth century. Among his several books are *Abortion in America: Origins and Evolution of National Policy, 1800–1900* (1978); *Doctors and the Law: Medical Jurisprudence in Nineteenth-Century America* (1993); and *Plague and Fire: Battling Black Death and the 1900 Burning of Honolulu's Chinatown* (2005). He has held Guggenheim, Rockefeller-Ford, and NEH fellowships and has twice testified before the U.S. Senate on the history of medical policy. Among his many articles are "The Paradoxical Advance and Embattled Retreat of the 'Unsound Mind': Evidence of Insanity and the Adjudication of Wills in Nineteenth-Century America," *Historical Reflections/Reflexions Historiques* (1998) and "American Medical Malpractice Litigation in Historical Perspective," *Journal of the American Medical Association* (2000).

JONATHAN D. MORENO, PH.D., is David and Lyn Silfen University Professor in the Center for Bioethics and a Penn Integrates Knowledge Professor in the Schools of Medicine and Arts and Sciences at the University of Pennsylvania. He was the Emily Davie and Joseph S. Kornfeld Professor of Biomedical Ethics and director of the Center for Biomedical Ethics at the University of Virginia. His interests include the history of clinical research ethics, especially in the context of experiments related to national security, and the role of moral consensus in bioethics. He was senior staff for two presidential advisory committees and is a member of the Institute of Medicine Board on Health Sciences Policy. Among his books are

Deciding Together: Bioethics and Moral Consensus (1995), *Undue Risk: Secret State Experiments on Humans* (2001), *In the Wake of Terror: Medicine and Morality in a Time of Crisis* (2003), *Ethical and Regulatory Aspects of Clinical Research* (2003), *Is There an Ethicist in the House? On the Cutting Edge of Bioethics* (2005), and *Mind Wars: Brain Research and National Defense* (2006).

MAURIZIO MORI, M.A., PH.D., teaches bioethics at the University of Turin, Italy. After graduating in Philosophy from the State University of Milan (1974), he was Fulbright scholar at the University of Arizona (Tucson), receiving an M.A. in philosophy; and then a Ph.D. from the University of Milan. He has contributed to bioethics since the late 1970s; in 1985, he started a bioethical group working within the Center "Politeia" in Milan; in 1989, he was a cofounder of the "Consulta di Bioetica," an association devoted to promoting pluralistic bioethics. Since 1993, he has been the editor of *Bioetica Rivista Interdisciplinare*, the only Italian journal of bioethics open to ethical pluralism. He has written five books (one defending a utilitarian view, two on artificial insemination, one on abortion, the last one, in 2002, a textbook). He is the author of more than 250 papers published in Italian in international journals. His major interests are in reproductive issues and those concerning the end of life. He has also written on the history and nature of bioethics, on truth telling, the role of Ethics Committees, resource allocation, and ethics of transplants, among other subjects. He has also contributed to ethical issues about the environment and nonhuman animals, as well as to business ethics. He was a member of the board of directors of the International Association of Bioethics from 1992 to 2001; vice-president of the Ethics Committee of Glaxo-Wellcome from 1993 to 1996; and president of the Ethics Committee of the S. Paolo Hospital in Milan from May 1998 to October 2000; member of the "Dulbecco Commission," which was nominated by the Italian minister of health to report on stem cells in the fall of 2000. Currently he is a member of the Ethics Committee at the Fondazione Floriani, Milan, Italy.

DOROTHY NELKIN (1933–2003) was university professor at New York University and among the most prolific and renowned sociologists of science in the world. Her groundbreaking research examined the interplay between science, technology, and society, as well as how science is perceived – and, often, misperceived – by the public. Her work often involved calling attention to the implications of unchecked scientific advances, and she considered the commercialization of the human body, as scientists seek patents for genes and tissues, a valid concern. She was skeptical that science could live up to the hopes of its promoters, many of whom stood to make a lot of money. She was also concerned about civil liberties issues raised by efforts to amass databases of people's DNA for crime-fighting purposes. Nelkin earned her bachelor's degree at Cornell University. She was a prolific author who wrote or cowrote twenty-six books including *Controversy: Politics of Technical Decisions* (1979); *The DNA Mystique*, (with M. Susan Lindee 1995): *The Gene as a Cultural Icon* (2003); *The Language of Risk* (1985); *The Body Bizarre* (with Lori Andrews 2001); *Creation Controversy* (1981); *Dangerous Diagnostics* (with Laurence Tancredi 1981); *Selling Science* (1995); and *The Molecular Gaze: Art in the Genetic Age* (2003).

JING-BAO NIE, B.MED., M.MED., M.A., PH.D., is Senior Lecturer at the Bioethics Centre, University of Otago, New Zealand, and an adjunct or visiting professor at several Chinese universities. He has published more than sixty journal articles and book chapters and is the author of *Behind the Silence: Chinese Voices on Abortion* (2005) and *Medical Ethics in China: Major Traditions and Contemporary Issues* (2006). Areas of his current research are Japanese wartime medical atrocities in China and aftermath, the Chinese birth control program, and Chinese–Western cross-cultural comparative bioethics.

JIRO NUDESHIMA, PH.D. (Sociology), is Senior Researcher in the Center of Life Science and Society, Kawasaki, Japan. He graduated from the School of Sociology of Tokyo University in 1988. He is the author of *Bioethics, Religious Culture, and Public Policy in Japan and the West: Echoes of Peace* (2006) and "Human Cloning Legislation in Japan," *Eubios Journal of Asian and International Bioethics* (2001).

VIVIAN NUTTON, D.PHIL., is Professor of the History of Medicine at the Wellcome Trust Centre for the History of Medicine, University College London. He has written extensively on all aspects of medicine from the Greeks to the seventeenth century, and particularly on Galen and the Galenic tradition. His *editio princeps* of Galen's *On My Own Opinions* was published in 1999, and he is preparing the first modern edition of Galen's *On Movements Hard to Explain*. His most recent book, *Ancient Medicine*, which covers the history of Greek and Roman medicine from Homer to Paul of Aegina, appeared in 2004. He is a Fellow of the Academia Europaea, an Honorary Fellow of the Royal College of Physicians, and a member of the Deutsche Akademie der Naturforscher Leopoldina.

ROBERT A. NYE, PH.D., is Thomas Hart and Mary Jones Horning Professor of the Humanities and Professor of History at Oregon State University. He has published books in French history, the history of the social sciences, and, most recently, an Oxford Reader, *Sexuality* (1999), a documentary history of sexuality from the Greeks to the present. His present project is a history of masculinity in the professions in the United States and Western Europe from 1800 to the present.

WENDY ORR, M.D., qualified as a medical doctor at the University of Cape Town, South Africa, in 1983. In 1985, while working in the medical examiner's office in Port Elizabeth, she became the first and only doctor in government employment to reveal police torture and abuse of political detainees, when she successfully obtained a court order to protect detainees from police assault. After leaving Port Elizabeth, she worked in a number of health care settings, including the private sector, nonprofit sector, and tertiary education. In 1995, she was appointed by then-President Mandela as a Commissioner on the Truth and Reconciliation Commission of South Africa. She served on the TRC until its closure in 1998. She was responsible for organizing the TRC hearing into the role of health professionals in human rights abuses, and she assisted with the investigation into the military doctors who participated in South Africa's Chemical and Biological Warfare program. Since August 1999, she has been employed as director of Transformation and Employment Equity at the University of the Witwatersrand, Johannesburg.

MARTIN S. PERNICK, PH.D., is Professor of History and Associate Director of the Program in Society and Medicine at the University of Michigan, where he studies the history of value issues in medicine and the relationship between medicine and mass culture. He received a Ph.D. in American history from Columbia University and has taught at Harvard University and at Pennsylvania State University's Hershey Medical Center. He has published two books: *A Calculus of Suffering* (1985), on professional and cultural attitudes toward pain and anesthesia in nineteenth-century America, and *The Black Stork* (1996), on eugenics and euthanasia in American medicine and motion pictures. He is currently completing a book tentatively titled, *When Are You Dead?* on the history of uncertainty about the definition of death, from the 1740's fear of premature burial to current debates over brain death. He is the author of many historical articles on eugenics, medical professionalism, informed consent, medicine in motion pictures, definitions of death and disability, and the cultural politics of epidemics.

VARDIT RISPLER-CHAIM, PH.D., teaches Islamic studies at the Department of Arabic Language and Literature at the University of Haifa, Haifa, Israel. Her main fields of research and publication are Islamic law, Islamic medical ethics, and human rights in Islam. She has published several articles on the position of Islamic ethics on topics such as abortion, genetic engineering, postmortem examinations, the beginning of life, selecting the sex of the embryo, and more. She is the author of the book *Islamic Medical Ethics in the Twentieth Century* (1993). She is also the editor of a 2002 issue of *Medicine and Law*, dedicated to topics on Islamic medical law and ethics, published by the International Center for Health, Law and Ethics, at the University of Haifa, Law Faculty.

DAVID ROSNER, PH.D., is Professor of History and Public Health at Columbia University and director of the Center for the History of Public Health at Columbia's Mailman School of Public Health. He and Gerald Markowitz have recently authored *Deceit and Denial: The Deadly Politics of Industrial Pollution* (2002). He was University Distinguished Professor of History at the City University of New York. He has been a Guggenheim Fellow, a National Endowment for the Humanities Fellow, and a Josiah Macy Fellow. Presently, he is the recipient of a Robert Wood Johnson Investigator Award. He has been awarded the Distinguished Scholar's Prize from the City University, the Viseltear Prize for Outstanding Work in the History of Public Health from the APHA, and the Distinguished Alumnus Award from the University of Massachusetts. He is author of *A Once Charitable Enterprise* (1982, 1987) and editor of *"Hives of Sickness," Epidemics and Public Health in New York City* (1995) and *Health Care in America: Essays in Social History* (with Susan Reverby 1979). In addition, he has coauthored and coedited, with Gerald Markowitz, numerous books and articles, including *Deadly Dust: Silicosis and the Politics of Occupational Disease in Twentieth Century America*, (1991, 1994); *Children, Race, and Power: Kenneth and Mamie Clarks' Northside Center* (1996, 2000); *Dying for Work* (1987); and *"Slaves of the Depression": Workers' Letters About Life on the Job* (1987).

SHIZU SAKAI, M.D., PH.D., is Professor of Medical History at Teikyoheisei University and visiting professor at Juntendo University in Japan. Her major area of scholarship and teaching is the history of medicine. She has recently published "Perspectives on the Evolution of Japanese Medicine" in the *Journal of the Japan Society of Medical History*. Her *An Illustrated History of*

Diseases and Health in Edo Period was published in 2003, and *A History of Diseases in Japan Viewed from Historical Points* was published in 2002.

ULF SCHMIDT, D.PHIL., is Professor of Modern History at the University of Kent, Canterbury, and a Fellow of the Royal Historical Society. He was previously Wellcome Trust Post-Doctoral Research Fellow; senior associate member of St. Antony's College, Oxford; and research associate at the Wellcome Unit for the History of Medicine at the University of Oxford. His research interests are in the area of the history of modern medical ethics and policy in twentieth-century Europe and America. He has published on the history of Weimar and Nazi Germany; the history of human experimental abuse; the history of the Nuremberg Doctors' Trial and the Nuremberg Code; the history of eugenics, euthanasia, and racial policy; and the history of medical film. His books include *Medical Films, Ethics and Euthanasia in Germany, 1933–1945* (2002), *Justice at Nuremberg: Leo Alexander and the Nazi Doctors' Trial* (2004); *History and Theory of Human Experimentation* (with Andreas Frewer 2007); and *Karl Brand: The Nazi Doctor: Medicine and Power in the Third Reich* (2007). Dr. Schmidt has begun a 3-year Wellcome Trust-funded research project on "Cold War at Porton Down: Medical Ethics and the Legal Dimension of Britain's Biological and Chemical Warfare Programme, 1945–1989."

JUDITH P. SWAZEY, PH.D., is an independent scholar and adjunct professor of Socio-Medical Sciences, Boston University Schools of Medicine and Public Health. Her major areas of research are social, ethical, and policy aspects of biomedical research and therapeutic innovation, graduate and professional education, and bioethics. She is coauthor with Renée C. Fox of *Spare Parts: Organs Replacement in American Society* (1992).

JUAN CARLOS TEALDI, M.D., is the Director of the Program on Bioethics at the Hospital de Clínicas of Buenos Aires University, the president of BIO&SUR (the Association of Bioethics and Human Rights), and the coordinator of the National Council on Ethics and Human Rights for Biomedical Research. He is especially interested on the field of health, ethics, and human rights in Latin America. He has a new book forthcoming, *An Introduction to a Bioethics of Human Rights*.

ULRICH TRÖHLER, M.D., received his M.D. and Ph.D. (History of Science) from the Universities of Zurich (1972) and London (1979), respectively. He is Emeritus Professor of the History of Medicine, Institute of Social and Preventive Medicine, University of Berne, Switzerland. He was professor and director

of the Institutes for the History of Medicine at the Universities of Göttingen (1983–1994) and Freiburg, Germany (since 1994). He was the founding president (1991–1995) of the European Association for the History of Medicine and Health. Following his book *"To Improve the Evidence of Medicine": The 18th Century British Origins of a Critical Approach* (2000), he is now expanding this field under the working title *"Methods, Numbers, Obligations": New Alliances and Procedures in Medical Statistics, Pharmacology and Drug Regulation in Germany 1930–1985.*

TAKASHI TSUCHIYA, M. A., is Associate Professor of the Department of Philosophy, Faculty of Literature and Human Sciences, Osaka City University, Japan. He teaches philosophical and biomedical ethics. One of his major research areas is ethics of human experimentation, including comparative historical study of research abuses in Nazi Germany, Japan, and the United States.

ROBERT M. VEATCH, PH.D., is Professor of Medical Ethics and former director of the Kennedy Institute of Ethics, Georgetown University. He was a consultant to the President's Commission on the Study of Ethical Problems in Medicine and Biomedical and Behavioral Research in their work on the definition of death. The authority of the patient to make clinical decisions in areas of critical and terminal care is his primary area of research. Among his many books, the most recent are the second edition of *The Basics of Bioethics* (1999) and *Disrupted Dialogue: Medical Ethics and the Collapse of Physician-Humanist Communication (1770–1980)* (2005).

HEINRICH VON STADEN, PH.D., is Professor of Classics and History of Science in the School of Historical Studies at the Institute for Advanced Study in Princeton, New Jersey. He previously served as the William Lampson Professor of Classics and Comparative Literature at Yale University. Von Staden's research covers a broad range of topics in classical philosophy and literature. His most recent book is *Herophilus: The Art of Medicine in Ancient Alexandria*, published by Cambridge University Press in 2004. His current research projects include the preparation of a book-length work on Erasistratos (the Hellenistic pioneer of human dissection), a study of the relation between "nature" and "art" (techné) in ancient science, and a study of medical ethics in ancient Greece and Rome.

ANGELA AMONDI WASUNNA, L.L.B., L.L.M., is Director, Corporate Affairs and Policy, Pfizer, Inc. Previously, she was Associate for International Programs at The Hastings Center, New York. She is a lawyer by training and an Advocate of the High Court of Kenya. She received a Bachelor of Laws degree from the University of Nairobi Kenya in 1996, a Master of Laws degree with a bioethics specialization from McGill University, Montreal, Canada, and a Master of Laws degree from Harvard Law School in 2000. She is a member of the Board of Directors of the International Association of Bioethics. Her research and writing interests include international health law, health and human rights issues, reproductive law and policy, financing of health care in developing countries, ethical issues raised by international research, as well as ethical-legal issues arising from HIV/AIDS. She currently manages bioethics research projects in Africa and the Caribbean. She is the author of several articles on developing world bioethics and she has just completed a book, *Medicine and the Market: Equity v Choice* (2006), with Daniel Callahan Ph.D. on the effect of market mechanisms on global health care systems. The book was selected as an "Outstanding Title for 2007," by *Choice*, the journal of academic libraries.

ANDREW WEAR, D. PHIL., is Reader in the History of Medicine at the Wellcome Trust Centre for the History of Medicine at UCL. He is the coeditor of *Doctors and Ethics: The Earlier Historical Setting of Professional Ethics* (1993). His other books include, *Medicine in Society* (1992), *The Western Medical Tradition*, with Lawrence Conrade, Michael Neve, Vivian Nutton and Roy Porter (1995), and *Knowledge and Practice in English Medicine, 1550–1680* (2000). He is currently writing a book on colonial settlement, medicine, and the environment.

URSULA WEISSER, PH.D., retired professor of the History of Medicine, has taught at the Universities of Erlangen and Mainz and was director of the Institute of the History of Medicine at Hamburg University from 1987 to 2000. She has undertaken research in several areas of science and medicine in medieval Islam with emphasis on the reception and adaptation of the ancient tradition by Arab-speaking doctors and the transmission of Arabic medicine to the medieval West. Her special fields of interest are Arabic deontological texts and theories of reproduction and embryology. Her publications include *Zeugung: Vererbung und pränatale Entwicklung in der Medizin des arabisch-islamischen Mittelalters* (Belief, Heredity and Development in Prenatal Medicine in the Arab-Islamic Middle Ages) (1983), *Iparchus Minutientis alias Hipparchus Metapontinus. Untersuchungen zu einer hochmittelalterlichen lateinischen Übersetzung von Nemesios von Emesa, De natura hominis, Kapitel 5* (Iparchus Minutientis alias Metapontinus Hipparchus: Investigations into a high medieval Latin translation of Nemesios of Emesa's, *De natura hominis*, Chapter 5: *De elementis* with an interlinear edition of the text and the Greek-

Arabic translation template) (1997, coauthored by H. Grensemann); an edition of *Kitāb Sirr al-khalīqa* by Balīnūs (The Book of the Secret of Creation) (1979), and a commentary on this cosmological encyclopedia titled *Das "Buch über das Geheimnis der Schöpfung" von Pseudo-Apollonios von Tyana (The Book of the Secret of Creation by Pseudo-Apollonious of Tyana)* (1980).

MIKHAIL YAROVINSKY, M.D., PH.D., (1933–2007), taught a course on medical ethics and held a chair of medical history and cultural studies at the Sechenov Moscow Medical Academy. He graduated in 1961 from sanitary and hygiene faculty at Tashkent State Medical Institute in Uzbekistan. In 1967 he also graduated from the All-Union State Institute of Cinematography and for several years ran a popular medical program at Uzbek Television. In 1974 Dr. Yarovinsky organized a Museum of Healthcare of Uzbekistan in Tashkent and was a director of this museum until he moved to Moscow in 1976. From 1976 to 1991, he was a head of the division of medical museums at a department of medical history at The Semashko Institute of Social Hygiene and Healthcare Organization (now National Institute for Public Health). He has published on sanitary education, medical history, medical museums, and medical ethics.

KATHERINE K. YOUNG, PH.D., is James McGill Professor, professor of Hinduism in the Faculty of Religious Studies, and member of the Centre of Medicine, Ethics, and Law at McGill University. She publishes in the areas of Hindu and Buddhist ethics, comparative ethics, gender and religion, and South Indian Hinduism. With H. C. Coward and Julius J. Lipner, she has written *Hindu Ethics: Purity, Abortion and Euthanasia* (1989). In addition, she has written "Hindu Bioethics," in *Religious Methods and Resources in Bioethics* (1994); "A Cross-cultural Historical Case Against Planned Self-Willed Death and Assisted Suicide" in *McGill Law Journal* (1994); "Death: Eastern Thought" in the *Encyclopaedia of Bioethics* (1995). "The Status of the Fetus in Scriptural Hinduism" (the Nationaler Ethikrat, Berlin, (2004); "Health" in *The Blackwell Companion to Religious Ethics* (2005); and a chapter on altruism and religion in the context of planetary stress in *Bioethics for a Small Planet: Responding to Health Needs as a Test Case* (forthcoming). Her current project in bioethics is a book based on a comparative and historical study of the interface of religion, medicine, and ethics. She teaches a graduate course on Bioethics and World Religions in the interdisciplinary Bioethics M.A.

NOAM J. ZOHAR, PH.D. (Hebrew University 1991), is a member of the Philosophy department at Bar Ilan University, where he teaches Rabbinic Thought and

Moral and Political Philosophy, and is director of
the Graduate Program in Bioethics. He is Senior
Research Fellow at the Shalom Hartman Institute
in Jerusalem, board member of the Academic Coalition for Jewish Bioethics, and member of the steering
committee for Bar Ilan's Graduate Program in Gender Studies. Dr. Zohar has published extensively in
these various fields; his publications include *Alternatives in Jewish Bioethics* (1997) and (with Michael
Walzer and others), *The Jewish Political Tradition* (Volume 1: Authority, 2000; Volume 2: Membership,
2003, volumes 3 and 4, forthcoming), and "Cooperation Despite Disagreement: From Politics to Healthcare," *Bioethics* (2003).

Part I

An Introduction to the History of Medical Ethics

CHAPTER 1

WHAT IS THE HISTORY OF MEDICAL ETHICS?

Robert B. Baker and Laurence B. McCullough

I. INTRODUCTION

This chapter's title is an interrogative: "What is the history of medical ethics?" Readers perusing the table of contents might be prompted to ask precisely this question. The expected chronological account seems hidden behind a façade of unfamiliar rhetoric about discourses, life cycles, and society. Our approach reflects a new era of scholarship on the history of medical ethics. Because readers may not be cognizant of the new scholarship, we introduce this volume with a chapter exploring the history of the history of medical ethics and the reasons why scholars have begun to take new approaches to the subject.

II. HOW OLD IS "MEDICAL ETHICS"?

Histories have to begin somewhere. The expression "medical ethics" was not coined until 1803, when Thomas Percival (1740–1804), a physician from Manchester, England, introduced it in his eponymous book *Medical Ethics* (Percival 1803b) as a description of the professional duties of physicians and surgeons to their patients, to their fellow practitioners, and to the public (see Chapters 18 and 36). As Percival was the first person to use the expression medical ethics, there is a sense in which the history of something designated medical ethics cannot predate

1803. Most historians, however, treat the history of medical ethics as coextensive with the history of medicine. They presume that it does not matter when the expression medical ethics was coined. As Juliet famously remarked, "What's in a name? A rose by any other name would smell as sweet." Yet Juliet continues, lamenting, "Romeo, Romeo, wherefore art thou Romeo! Deny thy father and refuse thy name!" Names matter. Words matter. They articulate conceptual frameworks, that is, the way in which people think about things. Juliet and Romeo would die because her family name was Capulet and his family name was Montague. In their world, one family was conceived as in opposition to the other. As the philosopher Ludwig Wittgenstein observed, *"the limits of my language* mean the limits of our world"* (Wittgenstein [1922] 1961, 115, Proposition 5.6). It is thus an open question whether a subject like "medical ethics" existed before it had a designation. Could medical ethics really have existed before 1803, if no one had used an expression designating this concept? Surely, anyone who wishes to extend the concept of medical ethics to eras earlier than 1803 needs to demonstrate that this extension makes sense.

Historians wishing to argue that the history of medical ethics predates Percival's invention of the expression could argue that equivalent terminology existed well before Percival invented his neologism in 1803. In 1563, for example, John Caius (1510–1573) inserted the term *moralibus* ("moral") into the title of the penal rules of the Royal College of Physicians of London (established 1518). These rules set penalties for members found guilty of publicly squabbling with fellow members, "stealing" their patients, or publicly accusing them of malpractice. Caius apparently inserted the term *moralibus* "out of respect for doctoral dignity" (Clark 1964–1966, 1:95). The English translation of Cauis's new title is "Ethical and Penal Rules." After 1563, therefore, medical practitioners sometimes characterized these rules as "ethical rules."

As it happens, however, we have no evidence of any earlier use of *moralibus* or its cognates in the context of Western medicine (Schleiner 1995, ix). One finds a variety of different terms in Latin and other languages that seem to play a role similar to medical ethics: *de cautelis medicorum* ("on rules of caution for physicians"), *decorum medici* ("the physician's decorum"), *déontologie médicale* ("medical deontology"), "gentlemanly honor," *jurispruden-tia medica* ("medical jurisprudence"), *medicus politicus* ("the politic physician"), "religious duty," *savoir faire* ("know-how"), and so forth. Yet each of these terms seems to reflect concepts – prudence, decorum, duty, honor, jurisprudence, and know-how – that differ significantly from what Percival meant, and what we today mean, by medical ethics. One could thus legitimately construct a history of medical ethics that traced the ascendancy of the concept from 1803 to the present, with some reflections on its sixteenth-century antecedents, its sporadic evolution in nineteenth- and early twentieth-century America and Europe, and its mid-twentieth-century globalization. Such a history could relate how one particular conception evolved to provide the dominant conceptual framework and discourse for articulating the intersection of self-regulation, morality, custom, and medical conduct.

Some historians have explored this approach (Amundsen 2001, 126–27; see Chapter 28). More radically, some historians have even probed the notion that the concept of medical ethics and related notions such as informed consent are post-Holocaust phenomena, that is, concepts that gained currency in response to the 1947 Nazi doctors trial at Nuremberg. On this interpretation, the concept of medical ethics was valorized to distance and to distinguish "traditional," and presumably "ethical," medical practice from the "deviant and unethical" practices of Nazi physicians and medical researchers (Weindling 2001). For the most part, however, historians of medical ethics tend to hold that, although names may come in or out of fashion, the history of medical ethics dates back to the oaths of Caraka and Hippocrates and other ancient texts. They presume, without methodological reflection, an ancient lineage dating back to Babylonian, Chinese, Egyptian, Greek, Hebrew, and/or Sanskrit texts. How do historians justify this claim?

III. Constructing Histories of Medical Ethics: Some Strategies and Their Problems

1. Presentist Constructions of the History of Medical Ethics

Many historians of medical ethics make the "presentist presumption," that is, they assume that because we today have the concept medical ethics, people in other places and earlier eras must also have had a similar conception, and they construct their histories accordingly. Historian Martin Pernick characterizes this presumption as *presentism*, which he defines as "the anachronistic application of present assumptions to the past," which is problematic because it "obscures both change and continuity" (see Chapter 2). Presentism is anachronistic with respect to medical ethics because earlier medical practitioners who thought about matters we would deem medical ethics thought about them in terms of other concepts – decorum, honor, jurisprudence, prudence – that we no longer take to be directly applicable (Fissell 1993; see Chapters 18, 36, and 46). So the question remains: How can one extend the history of medical ethics to eras before 1803 or 1563?

2. Bioethicists' Pragmatic Constructions of the History of Medical Ethics

Bioethicists often brush off such methodological concerns by taking a pragmatic approach to history. Bioethics is a future-oriented and policy-driven field whose practitioners prefer to think in terms of historical narratives that serve to contextualize problems or "issues." These narratives engender a plot line that centers on problems and potential solutions. As Todd Chambers astutely remarks, this methodology permits bioethicists to frame the past to reflect their approach to the future (Chambers 1998, 20). This pragmatic problem-solving approach to history also serves as a typical framework for bioethicist-authored histories and historical anthologies (see, e.g., Reiser, Dyck, and Curran 1977).

Such pragmatic approaches seem to circumvent methodological questions generated by differences in linguistic and conceptual frameworks. Issues seem to endure, even if the conceptual frameworks and the language used to address them change. Yet, as several historians have pointed out, bioethicists' pragmatic issue-oriented constructions of history are rife with presentist presumptions (Amundsen 2001; Rütten 1996c). They presume that issues deemed "problematic" today would have been seen as problematic issues in earlier eras. They also presume that norms that we today accept as "solutions" to these problems were actually thought to address and/or to resolve these problems in the past. It is not obvious, however, that some issue, say trust in the patient–physician relationship – an issue that came to be seen as problematic in an era of large-scale medical research, national health systems, and managed care – was considered equally problematic in earlier eras.

It is often claimed, for example, that the Hippocratic Oath addressed issues of trust in the physician–patient relationship (Pellegrino and Thomasma 1993; Veatch 1981). As it turns out, during the Roman era at least one first-century Greek physician, Scribonius Largus (fl. 14–54), a court physician to the emperor Claudius, adduced a line in the Hippocratic Oath as evidence of the trustworthiness of the medicines that Greek physicians prescribed for Romans. Romans distrusted Greek physicians not because they were *physicians*, but because they were *Greeks*, that is, aliens, who might use their Roman patients as human guinea pigs to test new drugs for potentially harmful side effects (Hamilton 1986; Temkin 1991, 59–61). Scribonius reassured Romans that the Hippocratic Oath prohibited killing, even killing the unborn. Thus, no Greek physician would prescribe a medication that might prove deadly to any patient.

Scribonius appealed to the oath to reassure Romans who suspected that Greek physicians might be untrustworthy; however, we have no evidence that Greeks distrusted their fellow Hellenes or that they used the oath to address this or some comparable problem of trust. In the absence of such evidence, one wonders whether bioethicists who portray the Hippocratic Oath as a solution to problems of distrust in Greek medicine are really reporting on a problem with an ancient pedigree or simply projecting a problem of the present day onto the past. To construct a history around a problem or issue, one needs evidence that it was a problem or issue in some earlier era and not one that appears real to us from our perspective but that never actually vexed those who lived in earlier eras. Absent such evidence, one has no justifiable grounds for interpreting norms, conventions, and texts from earlier eras as responses to particular problems.

To construct a history of medical ethics in terms of the continuity of issues or problems, one needs evidence that these problems were thought to exist in earlier eras, that they continued to exist, and that they are, in some sense, the ancestors of the issues and problems that we face today. In what is perhaps the first essay devoted to historiographic reflections on the construction of histories of medical ethics, historian Darrel Amundsen addresses the question of how best to establish a tradition with respect to some problem or issue. In doing so, he warns against two vices: presentism and essentialism. He defines the latter as "the tendency to see ideas . . . as free-floating in time and space . . . without reference to any temporal context other than the present, and . . . idea[s] . . . as essentially the same everywhere and at all times" (Amundsen 2001, 134). Amundsen puts the following questions to anyone who would claim that a tradition has arisen to address an issue:

Is there a discrete tradition in [a culture's] history regarding these issues? Is there evidence for counter-traditions plentiful enough to discard the concept of "tradition" in these areas? . . . When the behavior of [practitioners] seems to have been at variance with tradition, does that represent a counter-tradition or simply the reality of the inconsistency between ideals and practice? (Amundsen 2001, 140)

Few of those who have attempted to delineate the history of medical ethics in terms of so-called core issues, such as abortion, euthanasia, and trust have attempted to answer Amundsen's questions. Given the paucity of our knowledge on these subjects, it remains unclear whether any issue or tradition can truly be said to define the substantive core of the history of medical ethics from the beginnings of medicine to the present day.

3. Traditionalist Constructions of the History of Medical Ethics

No one conception of the intersection of medicine and morality clearly traces back to the beginnings of medicine. No common set of issues, problems, or traditions involving medicine and morality demonstrably forms one or more continuing threads that can be traced back to the earliest days of medicine. Why, then, is it commonly assumed that the history of medical ethics is coincident with the history of medicine itself? Perhaps the most compelling reason is precedent: This is how histories of medical ethics have traditionally been constructed. Evocations of precedent, however, merely recapitulate the question in a different form: Why have histories of medical ethics been constructed in just this way? Part of the answer lies in proclivities toward essentialism and presentism; another part lies in the third leg of this triad – traditionalism.

Traditionalism arises from the penchant to legitimate something by wrapping it in the mantle of ancient authority. In tradition-oriented eras and cultures, ancient lineage elevates the social status of ideas and practices. The more ancient and noble a heritage, the stronger is its claim to legitimacy. The past is thus appropriated to lay claim to the legitimating mantle of *tradition* for policies affecting the future. Just as contemporary bioethicists' historical frames reflect the pragmatic problem-solving orientation of the late twentieth-century society that nurtured the bioethics movement, earlier historical frames reflect the preoccupations of cultures that venerated tradition.

The objective of "traditionalist" histories and historical frames is to appropriate the authority of some tradition or of some revered figure – or some figure valorized to induce reverence – in an attempt to legitimate, or to delegitimate, policies or practices. Confucius, Galen, Hippocrates, Jesus, Maimonides, Muhammad, and numerous other cultural icons, as well as innumerable ancient or sacred or revered texts, traditions, or sayings associated with them, have been pressed into service in historical frames designed to legitimate or to delegitimate a practice or policy (see, e.g., Cantor, 2002). In tradition-oriented societies, debates over new initiatives can focus more intently on the need to appropriate the legitimating authority of the past than on the future consequences of implementing the initiative. Thus, in nineteenth-century Spain the debate over whether to introduce new "French-style" empirical approaches to clinical medicine took the form of a dispute over whether or not these new approaches to clinical practice were more properly "Hippocratic" than then-current practices (see Chapter 33).

It is difficult to overestimate the role of traditionalist frames in the history of medical ethics. Before the twentieth century the *only* body of literature that might reasonably be characterized as histories of medical ethics or some presumptively kindred concept (*de cautelis medicourm*, *déontologie médicale*, *medicus politicus*, medical jurisprudence, etc.) was the literature of traditionalist frames. To make the same point more emphatically: Except for traditionalist historical frames and sundry traditionalist comments, there is no history of medical ethics or of any kindred concept before the early nineteenth century.

IV. CONSTRUCTIONS OF THE HISTORY OF MEDICAL ETHICS: A HISTORICAL PERSPECTIVE

1. Michael Ryan's Traditionalist Archetype

The first known text specifically to address itself to the history of something explicitly called medical ethics was written by Michael Ryan (1800–1841), a Dublin- and Edinburgh-educated, London-based Irish obstetrician, who was also the first person to style himself a "professor of medical ethics" (Ryan 1831a, 1832). From the 1820s through the early 1830s, Ryan began to offer lectures on medical jurisprudence, which included a set of lectures on medical ethics and its history. He published them in a monograph titled *A Manual of Medical Jurisprudence* (Ryan 1831b, 1832). Ryan held that medical ethics was properly a preliminary to medical jurisprudence. He asked his audience of medical students, "Is it not a matter of astonishment that medical students in every part of this empire never hear a single observation during their education on the ethical duties they owe the profession and the public?" He continued, "A man who obtains the degree of M.D. is . . . ignorant of medical ethics . . . he is ushered into practice without the slightest acquaintance with the moral and delicate duties which he has to perform." "Hence," he concludes, "the dishonourable conduct for which the profession in this age is so remarkably distinguished, and . . . the chief cause of the humiliation and degradation of the noblest of human sciences in the

estimation of the public." If only "students [were] duly informed o[f] the duties and responsibilities they owe the profession and the public, those disgraceful private disputes, and those disreputable blunders made in our courts, would be of rare occurrence" (Ryan 1831b, 2).

Ryan taught that knowledge of medical ethics was properly preliminary to understanding medical jurisprudence because ignorance of medical ethics was a leading cause of the sort of dishonorable practitioner conduct that ended up in courts of law. As to the subject matter of medical ethics, "the only essays we have on medical ethics are those of Drs. Gregory and Percival" (Ryan 1831b, 2–3). Yet, instead of commending Gregory and Percival as innovators, Ryan insinuated an ancient pedigree for the new concept of medical ethics:

> There never was a period in medical history in which ethics was so neglected and violated as in this present "age of intellect". . . . It is, therefore, necessary, to inform rising members of the profession, of those virtuous and noble principles which regulated the professional conduct of their predecessors, and procured that unbounded confidence and universal esteem bestowed on them by society *in every age and country*. (Ryan 1832, 12, emphasis added)

Notice that medical ethics is portrayed as a source of professional esteem and "in every age and country" – except for the present age.

Instead of claiming that Gregory and Percival had invented a new but sadly neglected conception, Ryan projected their ideas onto the past. He laid out a plot line that would have been familiar to his audience: the fall from grace and the path to redemption – at least for those adhering to the "traditional wisdom" propounded by Gregory and Percival. To mute the conflict between this traditionalist claim and his earlier observation that "the only essays we have on medical ethics" are those of Gregory and Percival, Ryan broadens his characterization of medical ethics. The subject now extends to "virtuous and noble principles which regulate professional conduct," a conception that enables Ryan to find a common thread tying Gregory and Percival to Hippocrates. "The duties and qualifications of medical men were never more fully exemplified," Ryan continues, "than by the conduct of Hippocrates or more eloquently described than by his own pen" (Ryan 1832, 12). Having made this connection, Ryan discusses the character of Hippocrates and the Hippocratic texts, tracing medical ethics through the "Middle Ages" until he reaches a chapter on "Ethics of the Present Period." Ryan's chronological narrative thus portrays Gregory and Percival as heirs to cumulative wisdom of the ages and casts their writings as the apex of traditional wisdom on professional character and conduct. The precedent for presuming that the history of medical ethics is coextensive with the history of medicine itself was thus set in the very first work on the history of the subject.

We do not know what motivated Ryan's recourse to traditionalism: a felt need to cope with the waning influence of Gregory and Percival in Britain; the social aspirations of the young medical professionals to whom he was lecturing; a propensity toward traditionalism widespread in the culture of the period; or, perhaps, a desire to seek the unity of ideas in their origins? His traditionalist framework set the precedent for future histories of medical ethics. The standard history of medical ethics would thereafter emphasize oaths, codes, rules, principles, and other formalizations of medical self-regulation, underlining that they were founded on ancient traditions that are continuous and influential to the present day.

2. Traditionalism and Modernism: Differing Approaches to Constructing History in Medical Ethics and in Science

To appreciate the influence of the traditionalist archetype on our understanding of the history of medical ethics, compare the construction of histories of science with the construction of histories of medical ethics. Like medicine and medical ethics, science can produce an ancient pedigree. Yet, modern science, including modern medical science, tends to be presented as an artifact of the Enlightenment. None of the major figures in what has been denominated "the scientific revolution" – Galileo, Harvey, Newton, and their colleagues – is represented as perpetuating the wisdom of the past. As Roy Porter (1946–2002) put it, in their hands, "The Enlightenment secured a radical new rendering of the constitution of Nature" (Porter 2000, 138).

John Gregory and Thomas Percival were Enlightenment thinkers; neither sought to wrap himself in the legitimating mantle of ancient Hippocratic authority. Although clearly aware of the Hippocratic corpus, they seldom mentioned it and never treated it as authoritative. Gregory, in particular, scorned physicians who approached medicine with a "warm admiration of antiquity which . . . attached physicians to the ancient writers in their own profession" including the "blind and stupid admiration of Hippocrates" (Gregory [1772b] 1998b, 146). Gregory and Percival believed themselves to be creating a new ethics for a new medicine that was appropriate to a new and more enlightened age. Had the history of medical ethics been constructed following the pattern of histories of science, the plot line of the narratives about these eighteenth-century figures would center on the "invention of professional medical ethics" (McCullough 1998a) or "the medical ethics revolution" (Baker 1999, 2002a). Certainly, Gregory and Percival would have wished their work remembered in this way. Yet, ironically, the traditionalist archetype presents them, not as founders of the new,

but as conservers of the old, and, in striking contrast to the history of science, the history of medical ethics is typically narrated as the story of the conservation of ancient traditions.

3. Inverting the Ryan Archetype: The History of Medical Ethics as Delegitimation

In one of those odd pranks of history, professional historians have tended to portray Gregory and, especially, Percival not as innovators, or even as purveyors of a tradition, but as conservative defenders of the status quo. The tradition of constructing delegitimating histories, that is, histories that invert Ryan's intent but otherwise hew to his traditionalist construction, originates in the 1880s in the context of a debate over the legitimacy of the American Medical Association's (AMA's) Code of Ethics (Post 1883). Nathan Smith Davis (1817–1904), sometimes called "the father of the American Medical Association" and a former president of the organization, defended the organization and its code of ethics by writing a history of medicine that made the AMA's Code of Ethics an apical achievement of modern medicine (Davis [1903] 1907).

Davis had the "last word" for only two decades. His views on the significance of the AMA's Code of Ethics were challenged by Chauncey Leake (1896–1978), president, at different points in his life, of four influential institutions: the American Pharmacology Society; the American Association for the Advancement of Science; the American Association for the History of Medicine; and the History of Science Society. Leake's scholarly voice was one of the most influential of his era, especially among historians of medicine and science.

Motivated by animus against the AMA, which, in his view, was abdicating its moral and social responsibilities by successfully disguising "trade union rules" as a code of ethics, Leake tried to demonstrate that codes of professional medical ethics typically serve to mask professional avarice and privilege. Correctly tracing the origin of the AMA's Code of Ethics back to Percival's *Medical Ethics*, Leake laid blame for this semantic charade at Percival's feet. "The term 'medical ethics' introduced by Percival," Leake charged, "is really a misnomer, it refers chiefly to the rules of etiquette developed in the profession to regulate professional contacts of its members with each other" (Leake 1927, 2). Worse yet, Leake charged, "subsequent systems of general professional advice, whether official or not, have received the same title. As a result, confusion has developed in the minds of many physicians between what may be really a matter of ethics and what may be concerned with etiquette" (Leake 1927, 2).

Genuine ethics, according to Leake, is "concerned with ultimate consequences of the conduct of physicians toward their individual patients and toward society as a whole"; it should also include "a consideration of the will and motive behind this conduct" and should be predicated on "analyses of ethical theory made by recognized ethical scholars" (Leake 1927, 2–3). Insofar as practitioners' self-regulatory schemes are not applications of a recognized ethical theory, insofar as they deal with intrapractitioner relationships, and insofar as they eschew discussions of motive and consequences, they are mere "medical etiquette." Leake thus concluded that Percival's *Medical Ethics*, the paradigm for all professional medical ethics and the model for the AMA's Code of Ethics, was really etiquette, "trade union rules," parading as ethics. The history of medical ethics, he held, is really the history of this charade, and the medical historian's mission was to unmask it.

Leake's conception of the professional historian as unmasker of professional medical ethics was well received by later generations of medical historians, in part because it was congruent with the social history of medicine paradigm that emerged in the 1940s. This movement (Porter D, 1995) was pioneered by such figures as the Swiss-American medical historian Henry Sigerist (1891–1957; see Sigerist 1940). Following Sigerist, social historians of medicine strove to bring social science perspectives to bear on the history of medicine and to broaden both the sources and the scope of the history of medicine so that it embraced perspectives other than those of elite practitioners. Social historians of medicine were thus inclined to be sympathetic toward Leake's views and sought to advance his project through a social scientific unmasking of medical ethics. This became the received approach to the history of medical ethics among professional social historians of medicine (see, e.g., Konold 1962).

In 1975, two sociologists, Jeffrey Berlant (1975) and Ivan Waddington (1975), updated Leake's analysis. Although their positions differ (see Waddington 1984), both took aim at the then-dominant functionalist theories of professionalism championed by such sociologists as Talcott Parsons (1902–1979). Functionalists justify the prerogatives of professions as necessary requisites and suitable rewards for the services that they offer to society. Berlant and Waddington attempted to deconstruct this scenario by arguing that professions asserted ethical claims as fig leaves to disguise assertions of monopolistic privileges "to the powers that be and to the public." Berlant's formulation of the theory treats Percival as "a naively saintly man" (Berlant 1975, 56) whose "ethics were . . . the organizational tool . . . for monopolistic traditions for all professions, [and] an important device for suppressing competition between different types of professions" (Berlant 1975, 59).

Many social historians embraced this analysis. It fit their conception of the medical historian's role as "demystifying rhetorics, representations, and power relations in medicine . . . defrocking doctors, and 'unmasking' medicine as a 'political enterprise' . . . exposing the cultural relativity of truth, rationality, ethics and morals" (Cooter 1995, 260). The fig leaf thesis also attracted American physicians disillusioned with the AMA's lobbying efforts against Medicaid and Medicare programs (which provide health insurance for the medically indigent, the disabled, and citizens older than the age of 65 years) and its efforts to stymie plans for a national health insurance plan for the United States. Disgusted, one of America's leading physicians, Carleton B. Chapman (1915–2000), wrote a comprehensive delegitimating global history of medical ethics.

Like Leake, Chapman had been dean of a medical school (Dartmouth), and president of a national organization (The Commonwealth Fund). His book, *Physicians, Law and Ethics* (Chapman 1984), began in Mesopotamia and ended with the ethics of the AMA as of 1980. Throughout, Chapman hewed to an inverted Ryan archetype, emphasizing that principles or norms of practitioner self-regulation were founded on ancient traditions continuous and influential to his day. In era after era, however, Chapman found that professional medical ethics was self-serving and monopolistic. As to the book that started it all, *Medical Ethics*, its "chief aim . . . is to enhance the honor and dignity and security of the profession itself" (Chapman 1984, 85).

4. Challenging Delegitimating Histories of Medical Ethics

Even as the fig leaf/monopolization theory gained advocates among dissident physicians and social historians of medicine, medical humanists and nascent bioethicists were developing a different reading of Percival and of codes of professional ethics. In the 1970s the medical humanities movement – an international interdisciplinary effort to broaden the scope of medical education by including the humanities and social sciences – began to take concrete form in medical humanities institutes and programs established at medical schools in the United Kingdom, the United States, and South America (see Chapters 39 and 42). These institutes were located in medical schools, and their faculty was charged with discussing the history and morality of medicine. Approaching Percival from this perspective, Chester Burns (1937–2006) of the Institute for Medical Humanities (Galveston) and Edmund Pellegrino of Georgetown University found the then-current Leake-influenced delegitimating reading of *Medical Ethics* unsustainable. Their groundbreaking commentaries undermined the fig leaf/monopolization theory by showing that the text of *Medical Ethics* satisfies all of Leake's criteria for "genuine medical ethics" (Burns 1977b; Pellegrino 1985).

Scholars associated with the nascent bioethics movement also read Percival differently. As one historian tells the tale (Rothman 1991), the movement began with a 1966 whistle-blowing article by Harvard Medical School professor Henry Beecher (1904–1976) that indicted twenty-two experiments for violating the rights of the individuals subjected to the research (Beecher 1966). Four years later, Beecher constructed a traditionalist historical frame for his proposed reform of human subjects research by reprinting sections from historic documents on the regulation of experiments on human subjects (Beecher 1970). A section from *Medical Ethics* was reprinted as a pioneering work in research ethics:

> It was evident [to Percival] 166 years ago that [experiments] must take place only when "scrupulously and conscientiously governed by sound reason, just analogy, and well authenticated facts" [Percival 1803, Chap. I, Art. XII] . . . and that the innovator must, prior to the study, consult with his peers. Echoes of all of these points are present in most up-to-date codes. (Beecher 1970, 218)

The leading figure in the movement to reform human subjects research ethics was aptly citing a 166-year-old passage from Percival's *Medical Ethics* as anticipating the ethical safeguards found in "the most up-to-date codes." In this context, the dismissal of *Medical Ethics* as mere "etiquette" or a "fig leaf" was dubious.

Other scholars associated with the nascent bioethics movement also read *Medical Ethics* as real ethics. Another reformer, Jay Katz, wrote "*Medical Ethics* set forth principles of broad ethical significance to society and humanity. . . . Percival urged his colleagues to be solicitous of their patients' welfare and to provide good custody: 'Every case, committed to the charge of a physician or surgeon should be treated with attention, steadiness and humanity' [Percival 1803, Chap. II, Art. I]" (Katz 2002, 17). Like Beecher, Burns, and Pellegrino, Katz found in Percival, not an apologist for the status quo, but a fellow reformer (Katz 1969, 486–87; 1972, 321). An interpretational cleavage was thus forming: On one side were bioethicists and medical humanists who found in Percival a kindred moral spirit; on the other were professional social historians of medicine who continued to hew to Leake's agenda of "unmasking" medical ethics, especially Percival's and the AMA's.

5. Evolving Patterns in the Construction of Histories of Medical Ethics 1970s to 1990s

In the late 1970s, as the medical humanities and bioethics movements began to merge, collections of historical materials were compiled to "use in the classroom" (Burns 1977a, 1) and for "teaching medical ethics to undergraduate and graduate students at Harvard University" (Reiser, Dyck, and Curran 1977, xiii). Two major collections were published to support the new pedagogy: Chester Burns' *Legacies in Ethics and Medicine* (1977a) and the collaboration by Stanley Reiser, Arthur Dyck, and William Curran, *Ethics*

in Medicine (1977). Both anthologies used traditionalist constructions, treating the history of medical ethics as "the history of . . . professional ideals and their associated values as they have been discovered and claimed from antiquity to the present day" (Burns 1977a, 1) and as "the development of medical ethics as a form of professional self-regulation [that] has a history as long and as venerable as the history of medicine itself from the Hippocratic Oath" (Reiser, Dyck, and Curran 1977, 1).

Ethics in Medicine focuses on primary sources and constructs its history around such enduring "issues as abortion, euthanasia, triage, eugenics and the cost-effectiveness of medical procedures" (Reiser, Dyck, and Curran 1977, 1). *Legacies* reprints historical studies of professional self-regulation. These articles represent an important scholarly tradition in which materials dealing with the normative dimensions of medicine – particularly oaths and codes – are analyzed for the insights that they offer into practitioners' belief systems and standards of conduct. This tradition traces back to critical debates among such German-trained scholars as Karl Deichgräber (1903–1984), Ludwig Edelstein (1902–1965), and Hans Diller (1905–1977), who debated the authenticity, date, and significance of the Hippocratic Oath (Deichgräber 1955; Diller 1962; Edelstein 1967; Jones 1924). Some major scholars working in this tradition, although not necessarily on the Hippocratic corpus, include Darrel Amundsen (Amundsen 1996; see Chapters 7 and 12), Lester King (King 1958), Owsei Temkin (1902–2002) (Temkin 1991), Vivian Nutton (see Chapter 23), Heinrich von Staden (see Chapter 24), and Chester Burns (see Chapter 31).

In 1978, a year after these trail-blazing anthologies were published, the field of the history of medical ethics was transformed by the publication of a 97,000-word section on "Medical Ethics: History of," edited by the eminent bioethicist Albert Jonsen for Warren Reich's *Encyclopedia of Bioethics*. Within this section were twenty-nine commissioned articles (Reich 1978, 1995; Post 2004). Like *Ethics in Medicine*, Jonsen's section of the *Encyclopedia of Bioethics* was constructed in terms of "issues." The *Encyclopedia's* extensive treatment of the history of medical ethics centers on a chronologically ordered, geographical account of the history of medical ethics in "Primitive Societies," "Near and Middle East and Africa," "South and East Asia," and "Europe and the Americas."

The sheer bulk of the "Medical Ethics: History of" served a traditionalist legitimating function, not only for the field of bioethics, but also for the encyclopedia itself. The four-volume work was published before bioethics was a recognized field and before the neologism "bioethics" (coined in 1971) was recognized in standard dictionaries (Reich 1994, 1995b). Reich thus had to justify creating an encyclopedia for a field in the earliest stages of its formation. The "long history" of medical ethics provided a perfect justification: "Although it is unusual, perhaps unprecedented, for a special encyclopedia to be produced almost simultaneously with the emergence of its field... many of the issues... are not new; they were waiting to be gleaned from centuries of literature in the fields of philosophy, medical ethics, history of medicine and other fields" (Reich 1978, xvi). Thus Ryan's notion of the long history of medical ethics, reconfigured in Jonsen's issues-based geochronological construction of the history for medical ethics, helped Reich to justify the "perhaps unprecedented" coemergence of an encyclopedia with its field.

The Jonsen–Reich view that "a central concern of bioethics is the entire history of medical ethics" (Reich 1978, 876) was unusual in the problem-driven, future-oriented field of bioethics (and remains so to this day: see Baker 2002a; McCullough 1998b, 2–3), but it was fortunate for the history of medical ethics. The historical entries in the encyclopedia served as a catalyst for the career interests of a significant subset of the scholars who wrote them. It is noteworthy that several of the contributors to this volume, including both editors, wrote historical articles for the first edition of *Encyclopedia of Bioethics* (Amundsen 1996, viii; Baker 2002b, 376–77; McCullough 2002, 362–63).

Historical scholarship during this period was not exclusively Anglo-American. As the medical humanities and bioethics movements spread, they promoted early compilations and histories of medical ethics in various scholarly traditions (see, e.g., Unshuld 1979). One of the most important of these was Pedro Laín Entralgo's *El Médico y el Enfermo* (Laín Entralgo 1969a) [translated as *Doctor and Patient* (Laín Entralgo 1969b)], perhaps the first attempt to explore the history of the physician–patient relationship.

6. Beyond Traditionalism: The Scholarly Explosion of the 1990s

In the 1990s, research and publication on the history of medical ethics and bioethics expanded exponentially. More articles, commentaries, and monographs were published in this decade than in the 166 years since Ryan first lectured on the subject. Much of the impetus for histories of medical ethics can be traced to a newfound interest in the history of bioethics itself. The first historical case-based textbook of bioethics began publication in the 1990s (Pence 1990, 1995, 2000, 2004). Two major monographs on the history of bioethics and the first monograph on the global history of medical ethics were published in this decade (Jonsen 1998, 2000; Rothman 1991). These accounts of the birth of bioethics tend to focus on its conception, growth, and success, first in the United States (see Chapter 38) and then elsewhere (Chapters 39–45).

Although they differ in detail, the initial histories of bioethics tend to portray it as a response to the research scandals of 1970s and to the problems associated with such new medical technologies as assisted reproduction, cardiopulmonary resuscitation, dialysis, organ transplantation, ventilators, xenografts, and so forth. They also underline the role of an interdisciplinary mix of clinicians, lawyers, philosophers, scientists, social scientists, and theologians in pronouncing on these issues and take note of the ultimate displacement of these multidisciplinary discourses by a common "bioethical" discourse, a pidgin that draws on aspects of all these fields but depends heavily on argument forms and discourse styles derived from analytic philosophy (see Chapter 36; Evans 2002).

For the most part, the narrative line around which these histories are constructed is that of a morality tale. They open with portrayals of the excesses of the mandarins of an exponentially expanding biomedicine running amuck in self-importance. Unelected, unaccountable, and unresponsive, these elites treat the institutions of biomedicine as private fiefdoms – resisting calls for accountability by either religious authorities or public funding sources. Patrons, politicians, and the public react by championing a new field, bioethics, whose mission was essentially democratic: holding the biomedical elite accountable to broader cultural and religious values and to the interests of patients and the public. Some accounts theorize that the recruits for the new discipline were drawn from elements of the liberal intelligentsia energized by the American civil rights and anti–Vietnam war movements and by the democratizing antiauthoritarian forces of the 1960s. As these intellectuals critiqued medicine, they naturally transposed the moralizing language of the 1960s movements into the clinic and onto government commissions, moving, as it were, from civil rights to patients' rights.

As soon as these initial histories of bioethics were published, however, dissent arose over their tenor and content. Bioethicists from other countries objected to the emphasis on the American roots of bioethics (see Chapter 39; Campbell 2000) and their failure to recognize that, as bioethics became internationalized, Asian, European, and Latin American bioethicists began to develop alternatives to the autonomy-based conception of bioethics prevalent in America (see Chapters 39–45). Closer to home, anthropologists, sociologists, and historians trained in the Leakean tradition of "unmasking" medical ethics began to challenge the morality-tale structure of these narratives. Instead of serving as watchdogs policing the moral bounds of biomedicine, these critics proclaimed bioethicists "lapdogs," legitimating the cultural authority of medicine, medical technologies, and dominant ideals of (White Anglo-Saxon Protestant male) American culture (Cooter 1995; DeVries and Subedi 1998; Evans 2001; Stevens 2000). The debate over the unmasking of medical ethics that had preoccupied commentators in the 1970s and 1980s was thus recast as the unmasking of bioethics.

Scholarship on the history of traditional medical ethics also expanded exponentially in the 1990s. Three volumes based on conferences supported by the Wellcome Trust were pivotal. *Doctors and Ethics: The Earlier Historical Settings of Professional Ethics*, a collection of papers by professional historians of medicine, opens with the astute observation that "perceptions of the 'ethical' have changed greatly in the past" (Wear, Geyer-Kordesch, and French 1993, 1). The volume's editors and contributors touch on the complexity of constructing the history of medical ethics. In his chapter on philosopher-physician Gabriel de Zerbi (1445–1505), for example, editor Roger French (1938–2002) observes that it is not "unproblematic, that medical ethics have a history." He also remarks that "one must ... address problems that looked ethical to [earlier ages], but not necessarily to us" (French 1993, 72). It is thus a testament to the enduring power of traditionalism that the editors nonetheless pay deference to the idea of a "long tradition" of medical ethics in their prefatory remarks. "Medical ethics," they remark, "were a constant part of the history of medicine." Their volume merely "tackles the gap on the subject that exists between" the Hippocratic Oath and Percival's *Medical Ethics* (Wear, Geyer-Kordesch, and French 1993, 1).

A more concerted challenge to traditionalist readings of the history of medical ethics was mounted in other Wellcome conferences. The organizers were Robert Baker and Dorothy and Roy Porter – longtime friends and sometime colleagues – who had worked at the Wellcome Institute for the History of Medicine in London (Baker, Porter, and Porter 1993; Baker 1995). The volumes open with the observation that "medical [ethical] issues ... have never been timeless" (Baker, Porter, and Porter 1993, 2). Mary Fissell – Baker's carrel mate at Wellcome – challenged traditionalist presumptions of continuity:

> While the shade of Hippocrates looms large in our current assumptions about the roots of medical ethics, early modern medical practitioners rarely looked to antiquity for guidance. Indeed, no ethics particular to their profession or vocation governed conduct. Rather, appropriate behavior was inculcated through the institution of apprenticeship, shaped by general norms of master/servant and client/patron interactions. It was only in the 1770s that a medical ethics became possible or desirable, following changes in the structure of medical practice and shifts in more general cultural assumptions. (Fissell 1993, 19)

In an introductory section, Baker's editorial comments draw out some implications of Fissell's claims:

> The dominant myth in the history of medical ethics is that of the Hippocratic footnote, the idea that the foundations of Western medical ethics were laid down in the Hippocratic Oath ... and ... the history of medical ethics from that time to the present is a series of comments ... on premises laid down in the Oath ... It is ... difficult, as Mary Fissell points out ... to reconcile the purported dominance of Hippocratic morality with the absence of any specific mention of the Oath or the aphorisms [in eighteenth century cases and texts]. (Baker 1993b, 16)

Focusing on specific cases and texts, contributor after contributor to the *Codification* volumes (Baker, Porter, and Porter 1993; Baker 1995) emphasize the diversity of alternative conceptions of standards of practitioner conduct, including *casus conscientiae* (cases of conscience), decorum, dispute behavior, medical jurisprudence, *theologia moralis*/moral theology, requisites of patronage, unwritten juridically enforced standards of "infamous conduct," and, of course, medical ethics. Joining Baker and Fissell in raising questions about presumptions of continuity in the history of medical ethics are bioethicists Laurence McCullough and Robert Veatch and medical historians Peter Bartrap, Johanna Geyer-Kordesch, David Harley, John Pickstone, and Russell Smith. The *Codification* volumes thus challenged the prevailing presumption that the history of medical ethics could be constructed in terms of some one continuous conceptualization or some standard set of issues internal to medicine and descended intact from the Hippocratic era.

Around the same time, Winfried Schleiner also began to reflect on the discontinuous nature of the history of "medical ethics." As a preliminary to constructing a history of Renaissance "medical ethics," Schleiner consulted the "catalogue of the ... Herzog August Biblitothek ... generally an indispensable tool for a thematic access to the field of Renaissance medicine," only to discover that "it has no entry for 'Ethik' [Ethics]" (Schleiner 1995, ix). Schleiner thus had to construct a concept of medical ethics for an era that lacked one. The earliest treatises that he found on something akin to medical ethics had been written by nominally Christianized Jewish physicians from Portugal known as "Lusitani." Needing to function in an adamantly Christian and openly anti-Semitic world, these Lusitani physicians turned to secular humanism as an alternative to religiously based ideals of morality in relation to medical conduct. Schleiner quotes a passage from *Medicus-Politicus: Sive, De Officiis Medico-Politicis Tractatus* (*The Politic Physician: Or A Treatise on Medico-Political Duties*) (de Castro 1614) by Rodrigo de Castro (1564–1627; pseudonym Amatus Lusitanus) as an example of the Lusitani search for a nonreligious humanistic basis for medical conduct: "[W]hoever is requesting individual medical care, the physician should take that person up and attempt to cure that person with all diligence, whether Christian, Jew, Turk, or heathen; for all are linked by the law of *humanitas*, and *humanitas* requires that they all be treated equally by the physician" (Schleiner 1995, 77).

For these Lusitani physicians, therefore, the law of humanity – Ciceronian Stoic humanism – and not religion or tradition, served as the true guide for medical conduct. Out of their need for a nonreligious basis for medical morality, Schleiner argues, the seeds for what would become modern medical ethics were planted. Schleiner's intriguing hypothesis is thus that what would later be called "medical ethics" was initially developed by physicians from a persecuted religious minority seeking secular alternatives to religious ethics.

Schleiner's hypothesis can be extended to later eras. Many voices prominent in the creation of both modern medical ethics and contemporary bioethics belonged to comparatively empowered persons from persecuted or powerless religious minorities. Gregory was a Presbyterian in Anglican-dominated Scotland; Percival was a dissenting Unitarian in Anglican England.; Ryan was probably a dissenting Roman Catholic in Protestant London – although he may have been reared as a minority Protestant in Catholic Ireland. Continuing on to the nineteenth century: an Irishman and a Sephardic Jew in Anglo-Saxon Protestant America, John Bell (1796–1872) and Isaac Hays (1796–1879), respectively, wrote the AMA's Code of Ethics (American Medical Association [1847] 1999a). In the twentieth century, a Jew in anti-Semitic interwar Germany, Albert Moll (1862–1939), wrote the first German monograph on medical ethics. Many of the key figures who founded American bioethics and its leading institutions – Daniel Callahan, H. Tristram Engelhardt, Jr., André Hellegers (1911–1979), Albert Jonsen, Edmund Pellegrino, David Thomasma (1939–2002), Warren Reich, and the Kennedy family through its foundations – were Roman Catholics seeking a nonreligious moral voice, or at least a religiously pluralistic voice, in Protestant America.

As Schleiner was advancing his secular-voice-for-religious-minorities hypothesis about the origins of medical ethics, other scholars were also probing the relationship between religion and the origins of medical ethics. In *Medicine and Morals in the Enlightenment*, Lisbeth Haakonssen (1945–1999) challenged received views of both the traditionalist and the Enlightenment origins of modern medical ethics (Haakonssen 1997). She advanced the thesis that what came to be called modern medical ethics was largely an artifact of a dissenting Protestant sensibility disseminated by three fatherless, Edinburgh-educated, philosophically trained physicians: John Gregory, Thomas Percival, and Benjamin Rush (1745–1813).

Almost simultaneously, Laurence McCullough gave the scholarly community the opportunity to read Gregory by publishing the first edition of Gregory's work available in English in almost two centuries (McCullough 1998b). In a companion monograph, McCullough analyzed Gregory's medical ethics, and, in contrast to Haakonssen, portrayed Gregory as a paragon of Enlightenment secularism and the inventor of a new English-language medical ethics (McCullough 1998a). McCullough argued that Gregory did *not* inherit a philosophical or religious account of

medical ethics, but rather invented a secular field by analyzing the norms of medical propriety in terms of a theoretical account of ethics grounded in philosophical theory, specifically, David Hume's (1711–1776) account of sympathy. McCullough also argued that Gregory's Humean medical ethics involved the insertion of a feminine ethics of care – predicated on such feminine virtues of sympathy as steadiness and tenderness – into the ultramasculine domain of eighteenth-century medicine (see Chapters 18 and 30).

A 1997 conference celebrating the sesquicentennial of the AMA's code of medical ethics continued the debate over the origins of modern medical ethics. "Few things seem less radical than the successful revolutions of yesteryear," the editors remarked, asserting the concept of moral revolutions (Baker et al. 1999, xiii). The bioethics revolution of the 1970s drew on the cultural patrimony of an earlier ethics revolution, the American medical ethics revolution of 1847, that is, the revolution that led to the world's first national code of medical ethics, the AMA's Code of Ethics (see Chapter 36). Contributors to that volume emphasized the innovative aspects of American medical ethics and – drawing on groundbreaking research by historian John Harley Warner – discussed a backlash that led to an antiethics counterrevolution (Warner 1999; see also Warner 1991).

By the late 1990s, historians were actively reinterpreting the history of medical ethics. Three events that unfolded in 1997 reinforced these ever-broadening conceptions of the history of medical ethics: the birth of Dolly the sheep (1997–2003), President Clinton's historic apologies for the radiation experiments and for the Tuskegee syphilis experiment (Clinton 1997; Reverby, 2000), and the semicentennial of the Nuremberg Code of research ethics.

It might seem odd to suggest that Scottish scientist Ian Wilmut's announcement that he had cloned a sheep, Dolly, helped to broaden our conception of the history of medical ethics. The announcement, however, galvanized media attention and stimulated speculation about potential abuses of genomics (i.e., the science of human and animal genomes), renewing interest in the history of eugenics. The lingering shade of eugenics' dark past had always cast a shadow over the glowing picture of future genomics. From its inception in 1990, the Human Genome Project had funded an Ethical, Legal, and Social Implications (ELSI) Project, whose purview included the history of eugenics. As four influential American bioethicists wrote in one ELSI-supported volume, "anything reminiscent of eugenics is bound to be suspect... but... if we are to avoid the errors of the past we must know what they were... in our own consideration of eugenics [we] benefited... from superb reconsiderations of the movement by historians in the last decade" (Buchanan et al. 2000, 28–29). Bioethicists were thus turning to historians to provide the material basis for their assessment of ethical issues in genomic ethics (genethics) and biomedicine.

President Clinton's apologies also prompted the expansion of the scope of the history of medical ethics. Events precipitating two of Clinton's presidential apologies began to unfold in 1993 when the *Albuquerque Tribune* (New Mexico) published a series of articles about people who had been intentionally injected with plutonium by researchers during the Cold War years – without any subject's knowledge or consent. In response to the exposé, President Clinton formed the Advisory Committee on Human Radiation Experiments (ACHRE). Led by bioethicist Ruth Faden, ACHRE's objective was to determine the U.S. government's role in the human radiation experiments and to explore the "lessons learned from studying past . . . research standards and practices [that] should be applied to the future" (Advisory Committee on Human Radiation Experiments, 1996, xxiv; see also Chapter 36).

Bioethicists were thus mandated to work with historians to fashion a history of Cold War research and research ethics that justified both a presidential apology and compensation for victims (Advisory Committee on Human Radiation Experiments 1996; see also Chapter 57). In doing so, they challenged the received view that modern research ethics is attributable to the Nuremberg Code. Although bioethicists were later to valorize the Nuremberg Code as a foundational document, the ACHRE found that it was initially dismissed as "a good code for barbarians but an unnecessary code for ordinary physicians" (Advisory Committee on Human Radiation Experiments 1996, 86). This view was not restricted to moral troglodytes; it was even held by future heroes of bioethics. Henry Beecher had *opposed* the Nuremberg Code, believing that informed consent was unnecessary because "the character, wisdom, experience, honesty, imaginativeness and sense of responsibility of the investigator in all cases of doubt or where serious consequences might remotely occur, will [prompt him to] call in his peers and get the benefit of their counsel" (Advisory Committee on Human Radiation Experiments 1996, 91).

Beecher famously changed his mind in his 1966 whistleblowing article that publicized, among other morally problematic experiments, the Tuskegee syphilis study. Tuskegee was the subject of another Clinton presidential apology. The Tuskegee study of untreated syphilis had been conducted by the U.S. Public Health Service center at Tuskegee Alabama, on 399 male African-American subjects. For 40 years, from 1932 to 1972, the subjects' diagnosis was kept a secret from them, even in the postwar era when effective and relatively inexpensive treatments for syphilis became readily available. In 1972, more than half a decade after Beecher had alerted the medical world to the morally problematic nature of the study, the Associated Press broke the story to the public. Congressional hearings soon led to the creation of the National Commission for the Protection of Human Subjects of Biomedical and Behavioral Research (1974–1978), which proposed regulations and policies to prevent future research scandals. The National Commission's mandate was to deal with issues of human subjects protection generally, and the issue of apologies never arose. Once President Clinton had apologized to the predominantly White victims of the radiation experiments, however, questions naturally arose about offering a comparable apology – and comparable compensation – for the African-Americans exploited in the Tuskegee experiment. The ensuing debate culminated in both the sought-after apology and a compensation agreement with the victims.

Clinton's Tuskegee apology prompted a scholarly reanalysis of the case. This time, less emphasis was placed on scandal, scoundrels, and heroic whistle-blowing doctors than on the practices of institutional racism in medicine and related issues of class and gender (Rhodes 1999). Historian James Jones' now-classic study of the Tuskegee syphilis experiment (Jones 1981) was reissued with a new introduction (Jones 1993), and historian Susan Reverby published a collection of essays and materials on the Tuskegee experiment and the presidential apology (Reverby 2000). Renewed interest in the history of human subjects research also provided a fertile environment for historian Susan Lederer's history of human subjects research in America to the Second World War (Lederer 1995; see also Chapter 49), the first monograph on the subject. Lederer's account of research ethics underlined such overlooked themes as the role played by antivivisectionism – a popular movement concerned with protecting nonhuman animals – in the evolution of research ethics. Lederer suggested that a humane concern for the welfare of nonhuman animal research subjects paved the way for later protections for human research subjects. All of these subjects – popular movements, animal–human relationships, and even biomedical research – lay well beyond the purview of the Ryan archetype.

Eugenics, unconscionable research, and racial, religious, and ethnic prejudice had, of course, inspired many foundational documents of bioethics, including the Nuremberg Code. Yet, bioethicists had been curiously reluctant to explore their Holocaust patrimony or the role of eugenics, institutional racism, and religious prejudice. A 1989 conference, "When Medicine Went Mad: Bioethics and the Holocaust," hosted by prominent bioethicist Arthur Caplan, marked a change in attitude (Caplan 1992). Among the many important results of the conference was the realization that historians were challenging the pathological model implicit in the title of the conference, that is, the presumption that Nazi medicine was an insane artifact of a society gone mad. By the 1980s, historians in Germany and the United States were probing connections between Nazi medical theory and the eugenics movement in the United States (Proctor, 1988, 1999; see also Chapters 54 and 59). To quote historian Robert Proctor, they were discovering that "Nazi doctors looked to America to defend their policies of racial sterilization, racial segregation, and the abusive experimentation . . . [and that] the threads [of Nazi medicine] stretch before 1933 . . . east into the communist block and Asia, and west into the rest of Europe and the Americas" (Proctor 1999, 277).

Historians argued that the Nazi euthanasia program had its roots in liberal debates during the Weimar Republic, well before the Nazis came to power in 1933 (Burleigh 1994; see also Chapters 18, 34, and 54). They also observed that Japanese physicians had conducted brutal experiments using conquered Chinese as involuntary subjects (Harris 1994; see Chapter 53). Perhaps the most disturbing question raised by historians touched on connections between the National Socialist concept of *Rassenhygiene* (racial hygiene) and models of public health. Proctor was able to show that *Rassenhygiene* had serious public health aspirations, including promoting exercise, natural organic foods, whole grain breads, teetotalism, vegetarianism (Hitler was a vegetarian), and animal welfare and campaigning against smoking tobacco. Indeed, Nazi scientists found some of the first evidence implicating smoking as a cause of cancer and launched one of the first public health campaigns against smoking (Proctor 1999). Historians were thus questioning the inclination to dismiss Nazi medicine as madness, and asking whether, in some sense, Nazis subscribed to an alternative ethics-like ethos that embraced different conceptions of the right and the good in medicine, and even a new concept of "care" (Reich 2001). They explored the notion that the expression "Nazi medical ethics" might not be an oxymoron.

Pursuing these issues further, in 1992 health lawyer and human rights advocate George Annas and physician Michael Grodin published the *Nazi Doctors and the Nuremberg Code* (Annas and Grodin 1992). In 1996 and 1997, medical historian Ulrich Tröhler and bioethicist-philosopher-psychologist Stella Reiter-Theil organized a series of workshops and conferences to commemorate the semicentennial of the Nuremberg Code (Tröhler and Reiter-Theil 1997, 1998). Their workshops, conferences, and volumes further expanded the scope of the history of medical ethics by raising questions about medical ethical conduct during periods of war and the ethical standards for the military use of biomedical knowledge. They also explored the irony that, unlike the German doctors, the Japanese doctors who used unconsenting Chinese as their research subjects had never been tried for war crimes (see Chapter 53).

The scholarly ferment of the 1990s – the radical expansion of the literature on the history of medical ethics, the cross-disciplinary historiographic debates, the internationalization of the field – opened the field of the history of medical ethics to a remarkable variety of narratives. At the end of the decade a leading scholar, Albert Jonsen, boldly attempted to synthesize these newer approaches in one concise but comprehensive volume, *A Short History of Medical Ethics* (Jonsen 2000), perhaps the first monograph on the global history of medical ethics. Jonsen recognized three different discourses of medical morality: decorum, deontology, and politic ethics. By using the expression "medical morality," Jonsen addressed a subject "much wider [than medical ethics, as traditionally understood]. It includes the responses of other individuals [besides physicians] and institutions [besides medical ones] to medical activities" (Jonsen 2000, ix–xi). By "decorum" Jonsen means "outward behaviors that manifest inner virtue," which can be characterized as "politeness" (Jonsen 2000, x). This expanded notion of decorum gives Jonsen conceptual room to include Renaissance and early modern commentaries on *de cautelis medicorum* and savoir faire (know-how) In addition, Jonsen held that medical morality encompasses "politic ethics," which is meant to capture the idea of a just relationship between physicians and their community and the political economy. The concept enabled Jonsen to discuss Castro's *medicus politicus*. Finally, Jonsen's concept of medical morality included "deontology," or "the long tradition . . . created by physicians writing about how physicians ought to behave" (Jonsen 2000, xi), that is, it incorporates the traditional medical ethics as understood in the Ryan archetype.

A Short History of Medical Ethics is an extraordinary work whose conceptual foundations liberalize the scope of what can be treated in a scholarly work on the history of medical ethics. Yet, some strands of contemporary scholarship lie outside the scope of even Jonsen's conception of medical ethics. The primary emphasis on "medical activities" makes it difficult to include topics like eugenics, which is only mentioned in passing in *A Short History of Medical Ethics*. Moreover, the emphasis on continuity within the "long tradition" is at odds with constructions emphasizing conceptual and normative change. Thus, although Jonsen's innovative reconceptualization of the subject broadened the scope of the history of medical ethics significantly, it was not broad enough to capture the full range of historical issues explored in the 1990s

V. CONSTRUCTING *THE WORLD HISTORY OF MEDICAL ETHICS*

It is something of an exaggeration to claim that we initially planned this book around a new conception of medical ethics that was broad enough to accommodate the full range of scholarship on the history of medical ethics that emerged in the 1990s. This volume, its content, its structure, and our conception of the subject matter of the history of medical ethics evolved over time in the context of an intensely collaborative project.

Influenced by Jürgen Habermas, a leading proponent of "discourse ethics," we borrowed his term "discourses" to operationalize our experientially rooted concept of many voices articulating norms and values related to health and health care. We planned the first part of the volume around discourses that address the intersection of health care and morality: the discourses of medical ethics through the life cycle; the discourses of religious figures; the discourses of philosophers; the discourses of practitioners; the discourses of bioethicists; and the discourse on medical ethics and society. We believed that the concept of discourses would render moot any questions about the appropriateness of characterizing pre–1803 Western writings, and writings from various non-Western cultures, as "medical ethics." We also hoped to present the rich history of religious and practitioner discourses addressing the intersection of health care and morality without unduly imposing post–nineteenth-century Western conceptions on the materials presented. Finally, out of respect for tradition, we included a large section on the discourses of practitioners to capture the traditional core of the history of medical ethics – practitioner writings on self-regulation – within a broader framework that accommodated recent scholarly inquiry.

Our aim was to construct a history of medical ethics whose structure would eschew essentialism, presentism, traditionalism, and Eurocentrism and that would, as much as current scholarship will permit, be responsive to the subordinate as well as the dominant voices with cultures. We also sought an organizational structure broad enough to accommodate the full range of work in the history of medical ethics and cosmopolitan enough to embrace a variety of perspectives on the nature of this history. The conceptual and organizational framework provided by "discourses" seemed to play that role well, and we sent all contributors to this volume the following characterization of "discourses" to guide them in their work:

> A discourse is a written or oral communication about a subject over time. Until recently, the history of medical ethics has focused on formalizations of medical morality, such as oaths and codes. The expression 'discourses' indicates a broader conception of this history, embracing the perspectives of religious figures, philosophers, the public and patients, as well as practitioners. 'Discourses' include oral forms of expression as well as texts on medicine, religion, philosophy, and bioethics. It also includes various forms of patient and public expression and social commentary. Sources may include not only published texts but cartoons, graffiti, inscriptions, letters, pamphlets and other vehicles that the general public, patients, practitioners, and religious and social figures have used to express moral values, ideals, standards and norms for healthcare and sickness care, and for practitioners and medical practice.

Perceptive readers of this introduction might, at this point, be puzzled about our choice of title for the volume. If this is really a history of discourses about the intersection of biomedicine and morality, should not the volume have been titled "A History of Discourses of Medicine and Morality" or something similar? Such a title would not only capture the intent of the volume more accurately, it would also avoid some of the awkward connotations of the expression "medical ethics," which, as we noted at the beginning of this chapter, originally referred to the moral obligations of physicians and surgeons to the exclusion of apothecaries, nurses, and other health care professionals. Innovators, however, are all too often hostage to convention, and, in a sense, prisoners of the past. We envision our reader as someone – a student, a patient, a policy maker, a health care professional, a scientific researcher, a scholar, a bioethicist – seeking historical perspective on some current controversy or some aspect of biomedical or health care ethics. A volume titled "Discourses" is likely to seem too abstruse and academic to be of practical value; however, a volume with the title "The Cambridge World History of Medical Ethics" might seem exactly right. Bowing to convention, we titled this volume to suit the understanding of prospective readers rather than to capture our reformist intent. Moreover, as this historical survey of the meaning of the expression "medical ethics" indicates, the expression is elastic enough to encompass the range of issues encompassed in the volume. At a deeper level, we would hope that, after reading this introduction and perusing the volume, the reader will agree that the book might have been more aptly titled "A History of the Discourses at the Intersection of (Bio) Medicine and Morality."

ACKNOWLEDGMENTS

This chapter has benefited from the careful reading and critical comments by Albert Jonsen, Martin Pernick, and Warren Reich. The authors gratefully acknowledge their astute, careful, critical, and learned commentaries.

Chapter 2

Bioethics and History

Martin S. Pernick

I. Introduction

Medical historians helped create the field that became bioethics, and medical ethicists contributed to medical history, even before the word bioethics existed (Jonsen 1993; Jonsen 1998; see also Chapter 38). Both bioethics and the social and cultural history of medicine developed as academic fields at roughly the same time and for similar reasons. Each professed a break with pre-1960s doctor-dominated approaches to their subjects, yet each also drew crucial support from reformers within medicine (Burnham 1999). Despite their similarities, however, the vast potential for interdisciplinary interchange has not been achieved.

This chapter sketches one historian's view of the relationship between medical history and bioethics. It does not survey all that has been done but rather emphasizes unrealized potentials. Disciplinary differences and mis-understandings are mapped as necessary, but the goal is to find new opportunities for cooperation, not to berate those who "got it wrong."

II. What History can do for Bioethics

Perhaps the greatest potential contribution of history to bioethics is that studying the past can help to reveal otherwise unnoticed value issues at stake in the nondramatic daily events of modern health care. Ethical and other value issues pervade all aspects of medicine. Medical values are not limited to high-profile controversies such as abortion or euthanasia; the question "Is my sore throat bad enough to see a doctor?" is as value-laden as the question "Should the doctor pull the plug?"

But bioethicists rarely study uncontroversial, routine medicine, in part because the values involved are so widely shared in modern Western cultures that they are almost invisible. Medical history can make visible these otherwise-overlooked quotidian value judgments. Because past values often differed from current values, past values are easier to recognize and can be used to help to illuminate the hidden evaluations in ordinary medicine today. The ease of seeing past values can be mistaken for proof that past medicine was less objective than medicine now (Kevles 1993), but historical comparisons should problematize rather than assume modern objectivity (Kuhn 1962; Proctor 1991).

Other comparative disciplines – cultural anthropology or comparative literature, for example – can provide similar insights. Combining international, cross-cultural, and historical comparisons gives bioethics both inclusiveness and self-awareness. The use of history to reveal hidden values in medicine has been particularly fruitful in studying

16

concepts of disease. Early bioethicist H. Tristram Engel-hardt's classic essay on the nineteenth-century patholo-gizing of masturbation used history to argue that disease has always been a value-based concept (Engelhardt 1974; Engelhardt 1986b). Defining disease may seem removed from the core issues of bioethics, but it directly affects a vast range of canonical bioethics problems, from allocat-ing health care resources (Daniels 1985) to defining death (Veatch 1976).

Some of the most exciting work in medical history today focuses on the changing cultural construction or framing of disease (e.g., Rosenberg and Golden 1992; Aronowitz 1998). Feminist historians and historians of mental illness pioneered such studies (e.g., Showalter 1985), but many others now argue that history reveals the value-laden nature of all disease categories (Rosenberg 1999b, 32; Lerner 2000; Pernick 1996; Proctor 1988). Historians also examine how values shaped concepts of disease causation, tracing the intertwined histories of eti-ology, responsibility, blame, and guilt (Tesh 1988; Leavitt 1996; Rosenberg 1962).

Since the 1970s, however, few bioethicists have uti-lized this rich vein of historical scholarship, which may be because bioethicists have a stake in dividing science and values (an early exception is Engelhardt and Callahan 1980). Professional turf would be easier to defend if we could draw a sharp line and say "these are the objective parts for the doctors to decide, and these are the eval-uative parts for the ethicist to determine." Good fences make good specialties. Bioethicists also may have feared becoming caught in the crossfire of the "science wars," the recent round of recriminations in the United States between extreme advocates and critics of scientific claims to objective truth. In addition, philosophers usually assign questions like defining disease to epistemology rather than to ethics. Even if medical knowledge is value laden, not all values are derived from ethics and not all philosophy of medicine is bioethics. Indeed, some bioethicists and his-torians promote value-free definitions of disease, such as the claim that disease is a deviation from "species-typical functioning" (Boorse 1975; Daniels 1985; Lennox 1995; Shorter 1997).

History, however, helps to reveal problems with such definitions. If "typical" means simply statistically average, then the historically unique, high life expectancies in the modern Western world would have to be called a disease. If typical means not the actual average, but rather the way the average ought to be, the normative ideal, then values have been imported back, in a classic example of the nineteenth-century naturalistic fallacy.

A brief thought experiment using a historical compar-ison can illustrate the point. Suppose we could transport Alfred Kinsey back to the nineteenth century to confront a medical establishment that considered masturbation a serious disease. Kinsey presents surveys claiming that more than 90 percent of postpubescents have masturbated and concludes that masturbation could not be a disease because it is "species-typical" behavior. The nineteenth-century doctors gasp in horror: "It is even worse than we thought. It is not just a disease, it is an epidemic!" To dis-tinguish species-typical from epidemic (or hyperendemic) requires value judgments about whether the condition is bad and whether it ought to exist.

History reveals hidden values in all aspects of health care, not just in defining disease. For example, changes in the history of therapeutics resulted from changes in which outcomes were evaluated as beneficial, not just from changes in the technical ability to produce the desired effects (Pernick 1985; Rosenberg 1979; Rothman 1997). Of course, historical examples alone do not prove that modern medicine contains hidden values, but they suggest new places that bioethics might usefully question modern assumptions of objectivity.

History thus expands the focus of bioethics, from a handful of canonical, hot-button but relatively rare cases like euthanasia, to the role of values in every aspect of rou-tine health care. This does not mean that every medical decision needs an ethics consult, much less that every-thing in medicine will be as intractably controversial as abortion. The values that require history to make them vis-ible are hard to see precisely because they are presently so uncontroversial. Because most modern Americans agree that dying young in great pain is a bad thing, they agree that conditions such as cystic fibrosis are diseases, but the badness of such deaths is still a value judgment. Such val-ues may be mundane, but they are not trivial. Their very pervasiveness makes them important. By using the past to help to understand the value consensuses that make routine medical practice routine, modern bioethics might even learn something about how to find some consen-sus on the handful of visibly contentious disputes that comprise the current agenda of bioethics (Bayertz 1994; Rosenblatt 1992).

Conversely, recent historical studies of diversity and multiplicity in past values offer examples that might aid bioethicists' efforts to build on diverse gender, race, and cultural perspectives today (Leavitt 1996). History also can expand the menu of currently recognized choices by recovering forgotten alternatives, such as less-negative past evaluations of aging.

Bioethics also benefits from history's societal as opposed to individual focus (Rosenberg 1999b, 30). Distributive justice and discrimination, the social power of the pro-fession, and the social causes of disease were concerns of medical ethics for centuries (Jonsen 2000, x), but modern bioethics concentrates on individuals. This volume (espe-cially Part VIII) demonstrates how history may promote socially oriented bioethics.

Like medicine, bioethics shared and promoted mod-ern culture's fascination with novelty and its indifference toward the past. By taking history seriously, bioethics can evaluate the ethical consequences of modernity's amnesia.

In addition to contributing substantive content, history may foster cognitive and methodological skills vital to both bioethics and medicine. To document that historical study actually produces such results would require empirical studies not yet possible to conduct; however, my own 30 years of experience using history to teach bioethics suggests at least five valuable ways of thinking that may be fostered by studying change and continuity over time.

First, understanding past changes may help to prepare for future change. Modern medicine changes rapidly, and change can be threatening. Dogmatism or nihilism offers some comfort, but neither is favorable to ethical deliberation. Using history to make change more familiar and comprehensible may diminish the appeal of such antiintellectual defenses and may thereby promote openness to bioethical reasoning.

Second, history constitutes a crucial methodology for testing assumptions of biological or cultural inevitability. Many medical phenomena are assumed to be dictated by either biology or tradition because it is hard to imagine them being other than they are today – until they are examined historically and found to have changed considerably over time.

Third, history tests assumptions of novelty. Many ethical dilemmas assumed to be unprecedented effects of new technologies actually have long histories. Disproving incorrect assumptions of newness can help to avoid blaming new technology as the sole cause of ethical problems or expecting technical magic bullets to solve them (Brandt 1985). For example, the supposedly modern problem of allocating scarce health resources actually arose whenever past practitioners had a rare or complex therapy they considered effective. Deciding who gets the gold amulet or the intricate sandpainting is not inherently different from allocating organs for transplantation (Pernick 1996, 13).

Fourth, history helps us to understand and reason correctly about the causes of medical change. For example, health policies and clinical decisions in response to the serious problem of antibiotic resistance too often incorporate the erroneous presumption that antibiotics were responsible for the dramatic twentieth-century decline in infectious disease deaths (Lerner 1998; Leavitt and Numbers 1978).

Fifth, and perhaps most important, history can help bioethicists and healers to empathize with others who do not share their professional knowledge. The effort required to understand past doctors and patients, whose beliefs often differed sharply from modern concepts, trains historians to suspend their own preconceptions and listen to a different viewpoint, a skill vital to communicating with modern patients as well (Lerner 2000, 279).

Although all aspects of medical history thus can contribute to bioethics, collaboration long has focused on the history of medical ethics itself (e.g., Burns 1977a), the subject of this volume. These histories of medical ethics reflect several conflicting perspectives; however, such divisions are not unique to that subject. They arise in many areas of history, including medical history, and recent medical historians offer useful examples of how the history of medical ethics might bridge such multiple perspectives.

For example, histories of medical ethics by bioethicists and by historians often reflect the divergent perspectives of practitioners and "outsiders" toward the history of any field, including the internalist–externalist split among recent historians of medicine.[1] Practitioners' histories of bioethics promote and display the maturation of the field as an autonomous, self-defining, self-reflective discipline (McCullough 2000, 6), whereas nonpractitioners emphasize that the discipline was shaped by larger social forces (Cooter 2000, 454; Martensen 2001, 172–73) and that it often ironically depended on medical power (Rosenberg 1999b, 36–41).

Modern bioethicists use history to demonstrate the newness of their approach to medical ethics in contrast with the "long tradition" of doctor-dominated medical ethics before 1960 (Jonsen 2000; Rothman 1991). Nonpractitioners often emphasize continuities between past and present, while pointing out that bioethicists have a stake in constructing themselves as newer than they are (Pernick 1999, especially 22–24).

Even more fundamental than the internal–external distinction is the difference between past and present goals for studying the history of medical ethics. Some histories seek to re-create past ways of seeing the world ("emic"); others attempt to explain past events by using modern concepts ("etic"). These different goals result in very different ways of defining which past activities count as "medical ethics."

Some emic histories study what past authors meant when they wrote about "medical ethics," focusing on the handful of formal codes and other texts so titled (e.g., Baker, Porter, and Porter 1993; Baker 1995a). Wider-ranging emic histories examine what past writers meant when they used terms like "good," "virtuous," or "professional" to describe healers (Burnham 1998).

By contrast, etic histories seek past examples of topics that current bioethics considers important, whether or not anyone in the past saw them as ethics: Were there antecedents of informed consent or brain death? Did past doctors perform human experimentation or euthanasia (e.g., Boyd 1995)?

Etic history can lead to anachronistic criticisms of the past for failing to live up to modern values, what historians denounce as ahistorical or presentist judgments.[2] For example, past physicians often combined medical authoritarianism with patient choice, based on their belief in the interdependence of morality, enlightenment, self-discipline, and health. Such reasoning simply cannot be translated into the language of modern bioethics, with its sharp dichotomy between the principles of autonomy and beneficence. In the struggle to establish bioethics as new and liberatory, however, some pioneers of informed consent condemned the past for not fitting their new categories. That strategy may have gained support for the new discipline, but at the expense of distorting the past (Pernick 1982; Powderly 2000; Belkin 1998; vs. Katz 1984; see also Faden and Beauchamp 1986). Even my claim that early-twentieth–century medicine was value laden can be criticized as anachronistically imposing modern perceptions on people who deeply believed that medicine was objective.

Emic history may strike modern physicians and ethicists as limited to reproducing the irrelevant or harmful medical and moral "mistakes" of the past. Especially when dealing with past horrors, such as racist eugenics, emic efforts to understand the perspectives of the perpetrators may be read as preserving, excusing, or even promoting their actions (Pernick 1996).

These differences, between internal and external and between emic and etic, are not unique to the history of medical ethics, and recent historians of other aspects of medicine have successfully bridged them (e.g., Leavitt 1996). For example, historians of disease often use both emic and etic perspectives. They want to recover what it was like to live in a world that blamed epidemics on witches, but they also want to know how modern medicine explains those epidemics. Both perspectives are valuable and cannot be fully separated, but historians should carefully distinguish when their intention is to re-create the past and when their goal is to provide modern explanations.

Likewise, both internal and external approaches can be used to uncover past alternatives to the conceptual categories of modern bioethics and to examine how bioethical categories themselves were created. Such histories would be useful to modern bioethics, not as a source of specimens to be cataloged according to the latest taxonomy or as a series of object lessons in the superiority of current conceptual categories, but as a way of recapturing alternative ways of thinking outside the boxes of today's medical and ethical classifications, and thus of learning how the boxes were built (Belkin 1998; DeVries and Subedi 1998; Rosenberg 1999b; Stevens 2000). Problematizing the category "medical ethics" is important not just because historians value complexity (though many do), but because awareness of how bioethics was constructed helps us to understand the content and shape of the discipline today. History not only can expand the boundaries of bioethics, but it also can reveal the interplay of internal and external forces that drew the current borders of the field ("Talking Across Disciplines" 1999).

III. WHAT BIOETHICS CAN DO FOR HISTORY

Comparison between past and present is a two-way street. Just as history can make visible hidden values in today's medicine, familiarity with modern bioethics can reveal values in past medicine that might otherwise be missed. Modern bioethics can help historians to avoid becoming so immersed in re-creating past perspectives that the value assumptions and unmentioned subjects taken for granted in the past remain unexamined.

Such comparisons are essential if history is to study the motion picture of change and continuity over time, rather than simply re-creating static snapshots of separate moments in the past. In studying how past medical values have changed, modern bioethics can provide a vital benchmark.

Occasionally, modern bioethics can even make intelligible aspects of the past that would otherwise be inaccessible today because key information was lost or suppressed in the intervening years. Thus, the debate over the 1980s' Baby Doe cases first enabled me to understand that a 1927 motion picture I had discovered in the 1970s was about selectively withholding treatment from impaired infants, an issue whose history had been so thoroughly forgotten that by itself the old film was no longer comprehensible (Pernick 1996).

In addition, bioethics can do for medical history what it has done for philosophy: make a seemingly arcane academic discipline appear more relevant, exciting, and socially useful. Furthermore, just as history makes bioethicists aware that their own concepts and identities have been historically constructed, bioethics can make historians more precise and rigorous in their analysis of past values. History and bioethics also share methodologies such as narrative.

Perhaps not surprisingly, as a historian I have more to say about how history can help bioethics than vice versa. Because the past is filled with unintended outcomes, bioethics probably will have many additional currently unpredictable effects on future historians.

IV. CONCLUSION: REMAINING DIFFERENCES BETWEEN THE DISCIPLINES

Although I have emphasized how medical history and bioethics can enrich each other and the practice of medicine, important differences remain. Like medicine, bioethics is much more focused on the present than on the past and more interested in solving problems (McCullough 2000), whereas historians discourage expectations that the past holds ready-made answers to today's problems. Bioethicists, like physicians, rarely share historians' relish for ambiguity, irony, and particularities. They usually value permanent truths over historical contingencies.

Historians and doctors use empirical data more than bioethicists do. Many historians and physicians are also uncomfortable with ethics because they associate it with the now-unprofessional moralizing of their nineteenth-century predecessors (Sheehan 1985).

Historians also like to keep some distance from their sources, and they resist identifying too closely with current decision makers. Thus, historians of medical ethics may see bioethicists as their objects of study rather than their partners, as the sources of "primary" data to be interpreted but not as legitimate participants in the interpreting.

Despite such differences, medical history and bioethics often find themselves allied. Both are seen as applying the "humanities" to healing, as opposed to purely "scientific" medicine. History and bioethics sometimes do compete for the increasingly inadequate resources provided to medical education, but medical humanities programs can minimize such conflicts while nurturing the synergies. Finally, history reminds us that current differences in disciplinary cultures are not immutable. Future relations between history and bioethics will be shaped by contingencies we can only dimly imagine.

ACKNOWLEDGMENTS

I am grateful for comments and suggestions from Allan Brandt, Robert Aronowitz, Susan Lindee, Tom Tomlinson, Barron Lerner, Rob Martensen, Rebecca Walker, Susan Goold, Joel Howell, Nick Steneck, John Burnham, and the audiences at the American Society for Bioethics and Humanities October 29, 1999, and the University of Michigan Program in Society and Medicine October 30 and November 17, 2000.

NOTES

1. Twentieth-century historians frequently divided over whether scientific knowledge resulted from methods and ideas developed within the sciences themselves ("internalism") or whether such knowledge was shaped by wider social, cultural, and material contexts ("externalism"). Influential early externalists in the 1930s included Soviet physicist Boris Hessen, American social theorist Robert K. Merton, and German-American medical historian Henry Sigerist (Bynum, Browne, and Porter 1981, 145, 211).

Medical practitioners often favored internalist histories, and nonphysician historians frequently emphasized externalism, but the debate crossed disciplinary boundaries. Sigerist and other early externalists were physicians, whereas nonphysician intellectual historians often were internalists. Prominent early externalists utilized Marxian concepts to link science and society, and, during the Cold War, critics equated the social history of sci-

ence with socialism, but externalism drew on many non-Marxist sources as well (Reverby and Rosner 1979). Conflict resumed during the so-called science wars of the 1990s in the United States (Ross 1996), exemplified by a hoax in which the cultural studies journal *Social Text* accepted physicist Alan Sokal's parody of postmodern science studies (Editors of *Lingua Franca* 2000).

Among medical historians, such disputes were less polarized than in the "hard" sciences. Even most internalists viewed medicine as an application of science to people within cultures. Few externalists claimed pain, disease, and death to be completely culturally malleable. Charles Rosenberg's view that disease was "framed" by the intersection of internal and external forces exemplified a theoretical approach in which each factor bounded but neither fully determined the other (Rosenberg 1992).

Tensions did remain. The concerns, assumptions, and jargons of each approach continued to be difficult to comprehend for those who followed the other. By the 1980s, however, many medical historians treated internal and external influences as competing but complementary topics for study or as endpoints on a spectrum of variably interacting factors, not as mutually exclusive methods or as incompatible world views.

2. Historians define presentism as the anachronistic application of present assumptions to the past. One type of presentism measures the past by modern standards, judging past doctors ignorant for not knowing modern science or condemning them as evil for not following modern ethics. Another form of presentism studies only those parts of the past that fit present preconceptions, especially what Herbert Butterfield in 1931 labeled "Whig" history: selectively emphasizing events that seemingly led to modern progress (Butterfield 1931). A history of infection focused on ideas that anticipated modern bacteriology would exemplify Whig presentism.

Presentism produces a twisted picture of the past, obscures both change and continuity, and even misrepresents the historical nature of the present. Although presentism is often intended to make history useful, its distortion of the past undermines history's distinctive utility (Fischer 1970, 132–44).

Recognizing and avoiding presentism defined twentieth-century historians' claims to professional expertise. Presentism marked the untrained amateur; shunning it was essential to thinking like a historian. Medical historians particularly made presentism a defining issue. History written by and for doctors often glorified a linear march of progress that academically trained historians considered the worst kind of Whig presentism.

However, historians disagree about the scope of presentism and what methods if any can avoid it. Some consider any use of present concepts an impermissible imposition on the past. Others dismiss as illusory the belief that historians can ever escape their own times.

Greater clarity about the goals of historical inquiry may help to mediate such disputes. This approach would not consider it inherently ahistorical to ask which specific microbe caused the Black Death or what led to modern concepts of autonomy. However, it would condemn conflating such present concerns with the goal of understanding what people in the past meant by freedom or what life was like during the 1348 pandemic. The essence of presentism thus becomes unclear intent, not simply current content.

PART II

A CHRONOLOGY OF MEDICAL ETHICS

Robert B. Baker and Laurence B. McCullough

Chronology is the backbone of history, the spine along which historical accounts are constructed. To structure the historical events, biographies, and publications discussed in the various chapters of this volume, and to set them in a global historical perspective, we have constructed a chronological timeline presented in four columns: Dates, Events, Persons, and Texts. The dates, events, persons, and texts cited in the chronology are, for the most part, those mentioned in this volume. Perusing the timeline should assist readers by offering a broad sense of comparative historical developments in their temporal relationship to each other.

Our format for the timeline was adopted from Werner Stein's *Kulturfahrplan* (Stein 1982). Our selection of medical events was influenced by the chronology of medical events listed in *The Cambridge Illustrated History of Medicine* (Porter 1996). As should be evident from the outset this chronology, unlike Stein's or Porter's, does not attempt to chronicle every major historical event in the history of the world, or even of the world of medicine. It chronicles the history and historiography of medical ethics through the end of the twentieth century, using a few noteworthy events in world and medical history as chronological signposts. Following Porter, the chronology opens circa 4000 BCE: the dates of the earliest known urban centers. The first person mentioned is the Hebrew prophet, Moses,

the second Kong Qiu, known in the West as Confucius. The earliest medical entry is circa 650 BCE, a description of epilepsy in a Babylonian text; the Hippocratic corpus, several centuries younger, constitute the first texts cited. The chronology ends in 2000, closing with an act prohibiting cloning and a book by Albert Jonsen (2000), on the history of medical ethics.

Any chronology is, by nature, selective. In selecting persons, events, and texts for inclusion we no doubt inadvertently overlooked some that should qualify for inclusion. We also made a number of decisions that may appear arbitrary. In selecting which events, persons, and texts to include in the chronology, we initially focused on those mentioned in the various chapters of this book. Our editorial board and the chapter authors then reviewed the draft chronology and made extensive corrections and recommendations. We revised the chronology accordingly. For reasons of economy, and because of the difficulty of putting the present into historical perspective, we restricted entries in the Persons column to those who are deceased. We also listed persons by their birth dates to reflect generational cohorts. Unfortunately, a person's achievements are never correlated with her or his birth date, and seldom with his or her death date. The Persons column is thus not synchronized with the Events and Texts columns. One advantage of listing persons by their birth dates, however, is that they are introduced to readers in advance of their accomplishments, so to speak. Themes emphasized by the contributors to this volume are naturally followed and emphasized in the chronology. Readers might question some of these themes, some of the information included in the chronology, or some of the material included or omitted from it. History, including chronologies, is constantly reconstructed. We therefore welcome reader's corrections, comments and suggestions. Feel free to contact us at bioethics@union.edu.

Acknowledgments

We would like to thank Jason Tucciarone, Kristel Tomlinson, and Erika Selli for their assistance in developing the chronology, and Robert Veatch for his careful research into the seemingly simple question, "When did the Common Rule become the common rule?" We would also like to express our gratitude to the chapter authors and to the editorial board for the numerous invaluable suggestions for improving this chronology.

Dates	Events	Persons	Texts
Before Common Era (BCE)			
c. 4000	First Urban Centers (Mesopotamia)		
c. 3000	Writing invented		
c. 1200		Moses, Hebrew prophet	
c. 650	Epilepsy described in Babylonian text		
551		Kong Qiu, the Master Kong (Kong-fu zi or Kongzi), whose writings on "the way of the gentleman," transform Chinese life; known as the philosopher "Confucius" in the West (551–479)	
563		Gautama Buddha, Prince Siddhartha, Indian religious teacher; founder of Buddhism (c. 563–c. 482)	
c. 470		Socrates, Athenian philosopher; best known for a method of questioning; immortalized by his student, Plato (c. 470–399)	
428		Plato, Athenian philosopher; student of Socrates; earliest known Western philosopher of medicine; his argument that some lives are unworthy of being lived used to valorize eugenic–euthanasia movement in Weimar and Nazi Germany (428–347)	
c. 460		Hippocrates of Cos (460–c. 375–353) credited with founding the tradition of empirically based, secular Western medicine and until recent times, credited with being the author of the Hippocratic Oath	
c. 400			Hippocratic Corpus, remains of a library containing 34 books attributed to Hippocrates and his followers including *Ancient Medicine, the Art, On the Sacred Disease,* the *Oath* and other medical texts (late fifth early–fourth century BCE)

Dates	Events	Persons	Texts
384		Aristotle of Stagira, philosopher and scientist; Plato's student at the Academy; founder of the Lyceum; tutor and advisor to Philip and Alexander of Macedon; considered "the greatest biologist before Linnaeus" by Charles Darwin because Aristotle's biology was based on careful observation (384–322 BCE)	
356		Alexandros III Philippou of Macedon, "the Great," world conqueror and Hellenizer (356–323 BCE)	
300	Alexandrian museum and library founded		
103		Marcus Tullius Cicero (called "Tully" by eighteenth-century English admirers), Stoic philosopher; Roman Senator and defender of the Republic. Coined the term "humanitas" – humanism, humanitarian (103–43 BCE)	
c. 25 BCE–c. 50		Celsus, encyclopedist, catalogued arguments for and against performing medical experiments on prisoners (fl. 14–37)	
Common Era (CE)			
4		Jesus Christ, religious teacher and founder of Christianity (c. 8–4 BCE– c. 29–33 CE)	
14		Scribonious Largus, Greek court physician during reign of Roman Emperor Claudius; commentator on Hippocratic Oath (fl. 14–54)	
129		Galen (Claudius Galenus of Pergamum), Greek physician to Roman Emperor Marcus Aurelius (121–180); commentator on Hippocratic corpus whose views influenced European medicine through the Renaissance; practitioner of vivisection – experiments on living animals (129–c. 200),	
313	Christianity legalized in the Roman Empire		
330	Constantinople founded as Eastern capital of the Roman Empire		

(*continued*)

Dates	Events	Persons	Texts
354		St. Augustine, Bishop of Hippo (born Tagaste, North Africa, now in Algeria) educated in Carthage (Tunisia); baptized in Milan (Italy); Church Father; philosopher, accepts concept of original sin and divine predestination; believed that the Diaspora of the Jews was just punishment for their rejection of Jesus, but was against killing Jews; argued that commandment against murder encompasses suicide (354–430)	
413			*De Civitate Dei*, (City of God), St. Augustine; first thorough Christian theological analysis, includes discussion of the morality of suicide – condemns it as a violation of the commandment prohibiting murder
570		Muhammed, Arab prophet and founder of Islam (570–632)	
538		Gregory of Tours, Bishop of Tours, historian and theologian (538 or 539–593 or 594)	
581		Sun Simiao, Chinese physician; author of earliest known Chinese text to deal explicitly with moral aspects of medical conduct (c. 581–681)	
610	Byzantine Empire established		
618	Tang Dynasty founded in China		
711–713	Berber governor of Tangier, Tariq ibn Ziyad (?–720) defeats the Visigothic Empire in Spain beginning nearly eight centuries of Islamic domination of Spain		
800	Charlemagne crowned Holy Roman Emperor		
c. 850–c. 899		Ishaq ibn Ali ar-Ruhawi, Iraqi Christian or Jewish commentator on Arabic medical morality	*More Questions and Answers*, Hunain ibn Ishaq; *The Ethos of the Doctor*, Ali ar-Ruhawi
865		Abu Bakr Ar-Razi (Rhazes) Persian physician and medical writer (c. 865–c. 925)	
c. 900		Ishaq al-Israili (Issac Iudaeus) Tunisian–Jewish physician, probable author of *The Physician's Guide* (c. 900–955)	
929	Caliphate established in Cordoba		

Dates	Events	Persons	Texts
c. 936–c. 940		Al-Zahrawi (Abulcases, Albucasis, Bulcasis, Bulcasim, Bulcari, etc.). Andalusian surgeon and medical encyclopedist, born near Cordoba; wrote on physician–patient relationship, medical morality (c. 936–1013)	
960	Song Dynasty in China (960–1279)		
973		Abu-Rayan Al-Biruni, Islamic historian and scientist (973–1048)	
980		Ibn Sina (Avicenna), Islamic physician; philosopher; author of *Canon of Medicine* (980–1037)	
984			*Ishimpo* (Medicine's Heart and Method), oldest extant Japanese medical encyclopedia. Compiled by Yasuyori Tanba (912–995) from Chinese texts; frames medical ethics in relation to religion; combines Buddhism and Confucianism
988	Russians adopt Orthodox Christianity		
1058		Abu Hamid Al-Ghazali Islamic philosopher, theologian, and legal scholar (1058–1111)	
1066	Norman Conquest of England		
1072			*Mirror for the Physician* by Iraqi Christian physician, Said ibn al-Hasan
1095	Christian Crusades for Jerusalem		
1114		Gerard of Cremona, translator of Ibn Sina's *Canon* (1114–1187)	
1126		Ibn Rushd (Averroes), Andalusian–Arab astronomer, legal scholar, philosopher, and physician; born in Cordoba, Spain; wrote commentaries on Aristotle, highly influential on Christian, Islamic, and Jewish thought (1126–1198)	
1135		Rabbi Moish (Moses) ben Maimon (Maimonides), sometimes called Rambam (רמב״ם): Cordoba-born Jewish physician and philosopher; physician to the Sultan of Egypt; wrote extensive commentaries on Jewish law (1135–1204)	
1136	Pantokrator Hospital founded in Constantinople		

(*continued*)

Dates	Events	Persons	Texts
1140			*Concordia Discordantium Canonum* (A Harmony of Discordant Canons), later known as *Decretum*, first major systematization of Christian canon law
1187			*Ad Aures* (1.14.7), c. 1187–1191, first Christian canon law on medical morality, addresses guilt for medical error
1193		Albertus Magnus (Doctor universalis), German (Bavarian) Dominican philosopher, theologian, and scientist argued for the peaceful coexistence of science and religion (1193?–1280)	
1198		Ibn Jumay, Jewish physician to Sultan Saladin; author of medical ethics manual (?–1198)	
1204	Crusaders sack Constantinople		
1214		Roger Bacon (see 1219)	
1215	Pope Innocent III's Fourth Lateran Council mandates annual confession for all Christians; physicians required to summon a confessor for their patients		
1219		Roger Bacon, Oxford/Paris-educated English Franciscan Friar, logician, theologian, scientist; Professor at Oxford; exiled, censured, censored, and imprisoned during various decades of his life for radical writings (c. 1214–1292)	
1225		St. Thomas Aquinas, Dominican Italian Catholic theologian and philosopher; presented a comprehensive systematic treatment of Catholic theology, including proofs of the existence of God (1225?–1274)	
1234			*Decretales*, Gregory IX, replaces earlier formulation of canon law
1240		Arnold of Villanova, French, Professor of Medicine, Montpellier; Physician to King of Spain (c. 1260–1311)	
1258	Mongols sack Baghdad; end of Abbasid caliphate		
c. 1260–1270		Henri de Mondeville, French surgeon (c. 1260–after 1325)	*Opus Maius*, c. 1265, *De erroribus. medicorum*, c. 1270? Roger Bacon, decries lack of standard formulary. "Bad (*maledicta*) drugs are more frequent that good ones (*benedicta*)" Physicians are complacent, ignorant, shirk responsibility for their failures

Dates	Events	Persons	Texts
1265		Dante Alighieri, Italian (Florence) poet, author of *La Divina Commedia* (The Divine Comedy), completed in parts: Inferno (finished before 1316); Purgatorio (finished before 1320); Paradiso (finished before 1321); one of Europe's most important poets (1265–1321)	
1275	Marco Polo arrives in China		
Second half of thirteenth century		Nicholas of Poland, Dominican priest and medical educator,; author of *Anti Hippocras* (c. 1270), diatribe against orthodox medicine	
c. 1305			*Chirurgia* (Surgery) Henry of Mondeville, French, urges elevated standards of conduct to improve the reputation of surgery (fl. 1306–1320)
1315	First documented public dissection in modern Europe, conducted in Bologna (Italy) by Mondino de' Luzzi (c. 1270–1326)		
1337	Hundred Years War between England and France begins (ends 1453)		
1347	Black Death begins (ends 1352)		
1352			*Invectiva contra medicum quondam,* (Invective Against Any Physician), Francesco Petrarca (Petrarch) (1304–1374) argues that medicine is a sinful attempt to penetrate God's secrets. He ridicules physicians as greedy but unworldly theoreticians who use Latin-scholastic terminology to cheat patients; charges that physicians are the only occupational group who can kill people and go unpunished
1368	Ming dynasty founded in China		
1424	First recorded European regulations for midwives, Brussels		
1445		Gabriele de Zerbi, Italian physician and professor of medicine at Padua, wrote rules for physician conduct (1445–1505)	
1452		Leonardo da Vinci, artist, inventor, anatomist, Renaissance man (1452–1519)	

(continued)

Dates	Events	Persons	Texts
1453	Ottoman Turks capture Constantinople; end of Byzantine Empire		
c. 1455			Gutenberg's Bible printed at Mainz
1460		Thomas Linacre, English physician and classical scholar; founder of the College of Physicians of London (1460?–1524)	
1477	*Protomedicato* (Protomedical Council) first institution charged with regulating medicine and public health established in Spain (to 1822)		
1483		Martin Luther, leader of Protestant Reformation (1483–1546)	
1492	Christopher Columbus crosses the Atlantic. Fall of Granada – Edicts of Expulsion; Monarchs Ferdinand and Isabella of Castile, Argon, Sicily, Granada, Toledo, Valencia, Seville, Barcelona, etc., expel all Moslems and all Jews from their kingdoms (Spain and Sicily)		
1493		Paracelsus (Theophrastus von Hohenheim) Swiss alchemist and physician (1493–1541)	
1495			*De Cautelis Medicorum*, Gabriele de Zerbi, one of the first comprehensive books on medical conduct in the Renaissance, references the Hippocratic Oath; physicians are to value integrity over fame and fortune
1498	Vasco da Gama (1460–1524) sails to India via the Cape of Good Hope		
1510		John (Keys) Caius (1510–1573), English physician; cofounder of Gonville and Caius College, Cambridge. As President College of Physicians of London, in 1563 changed the name of its penal code to *De Statutis Moralibus seu Penalibus*, or "Ethical or Penal Statutes" Ambroise Paré, French Surgeon (1510–1590)	

Dates	Events	Persons	Texts
1511	Parliamentary act requires that anyone practicing physic in London be examined by Bishop of London or Dean of St. Paul's	Michael Servetus (Miguel Serveto), Spanish physician and theologian; burned alive at the stake in Geneva on the order of John Calvin (1511–1553)	
1514		Andreas Vesalius, Italian anatomist; publicly dissected living animals and corpses of executed criminals (1514–1564)	
1516		Realdo Colombo, Italian anatomist; publicly dissected human and animal corpses, discovered pulmonary circulation (1516–1559)	
1517	Martin Luther (1483–1546) nails 95 theses against the practice of selling indulgences to the door of Castle Church Wittenberg, signaling the start of the Protestant Reformation		
1518	College of Physicians of London (later Royal College of Physicians) founded as purely secular examining body to protect populace from "ignorant persons . . . [who] hurt, damage . . . many of the King's liege people"		
1519	Ferdinand de Magellan, Portuguese (1480–1521) begins circumnavigation of the globe (to 1522)		Thomas Linacre's translation of Galen's *Method and Healing*
1521	Hernando Cortez (1485–1547) completes Spanish conquest of Aztec Empire in Mexico; Mexico City built on top of the ruins of Aztec city Tenochtitlan	Pieter van Foreest, Dutch physician, critic of uroscopists as charlatans (1521–1597)	
1525			*Hippocratis Octoginta volumina, quibus maxima ex parte, annorum circiter duo millia Latina caruit lingua. Graeci vero, Arabes, et prisci nostri medici, plurimis tamen utilibus praetermissis, scripta sua illustrarunt, nunc tandem per M. Fabium Calvum Latinitate donata ac nunc primum in lucem aedita*

(continued)

Dates	Events	Persons	Texts
			(Hippocrates Works in eight Volumes . . . translated into Latin by M. Fabium Calvum); first printed edition of the Hippocratic Corpus, published in Rome, edited and translated by Francisci Minitii Calvi (Marco Fabio Calvo fl. 1526), includes the Hippocratic Oath, sets the stage for use of Hippocrates as a valorizing figure throughout the sixteenth century
1526	Henry VIII of England breaks with Rome – Church of England founded

Mughal Dynasty founded in India | | |
1530			"Syphilis sive morbus Gallicus" (Syphilis or the French Disease), a poem by Hieronymus Fracastorius (Girolamo Fracastoro) (1478–1553), gives an account and names the disease "syphilis"
1540	The companies of Barbers (surgeons) unite in London		
1541		Rodrigo à Castro (Lusitanus), Portuguese–Jewish Converso physician; educated in Spain, emigrates to Germany, Professor of Medicine, Hamburg; writer on the politic physician, uses a casuistic approach to specific questions of medical conduct, for example, are physicians obligated to tell patients the truth about their prognosis (1541?–1627)	First known occurrence of the expression "the medicynall profession" in English
1543			De Humani Corporis Fabrica (On the Fabric of the Human Body) Adreas Vesalius, revolutionary anatomy text beautifully illustrated with clever woodcuts; transformed the teaching of anatomy and medicine and set the precedent for medical illustration

De revolutionibus orbium coelestium (Polish: O obrotach sfer niebieskich; On the Revolutions of the Heavenly Spheres) written 1506–1530 by Nicholaus Copernicus, but not published until the year of his death, 1543; challenges the Ptolemaic "common sense" position that the sun rises and sets around the earth for a heliocentric conception of the earth rotating around the sun – cornerstone of the scientific revolution; |

Dates	Events	Persons	Texts
			De Statuis Penalibus (Penal Statutes), College of Physicians of London
1544	Council of Trent, Catholic response to Protestant Reformation, standardizes Roman Catholic ritual and articles of faith, ends medieval Catholicism (to 1563)		
1546			
			De Contagione et Contagiosis Morbis (On Contagion and Contagious Disease), Hieronymus Fracastorius (Girolamo Fracastoro) (1478–1533), early version of the germ theory of disease
1548		Giodarno Bruno (Nola, Campania, now in Italy), astronomer/astrologer, Dominican friar, philosopher; defender of Copernicus; critic of Aristotlean physics, believed stars were suns and that the universe was infinite. Tried and convicted of heresy by the Roman Inquisition and burned at the stake in the Campo de Fiori, Rome, after refusing to recant (1548–1600)	
1553	Michael Servetus burnt at the stake in Geneva on the order of John Calvin (1509–1564) founder of Calvinism		
1555			John Caius reorganizes the penal statues of the College of London to include a section on *De Conservatione Morali et Statutis Poenalibus* (Concerning Ethical or Penal Statutes)
1556			*Enchiridion sive Manuale Confessariorum et Poenitentium* (Enchiridion or Manual of Confession and Penitence), Martin Azpilcueta (Navarrus) (1493–1586) develops casuistry as a method of dealing with moral questions
1558	Hippocratic Oath introduced at University at Heidelberg		
1561		Francis Bacon, English philosopher, statesmen, and proponent of empirical science. Under King James I of Britain, Bacon was Baron Verulam, Viscount St. Albans, and became Lord	

(*continued*)

Dates	Events	Persons	Texts
1561		Chancellor of England. Bacon's defense of experimental science encompassed "putting nature to the rack" by experiments, including animal vivisection; Bacon argued that research was a moral imperative and he redefined the term "euthanasia" to encompass both a physically painless and easy death, and a good spiritual passage (1561–1626)	
1563			John Caius dubs the penal rules of the College of Physicians of London *De Statutis Penalibus et Moralibus* (Moral and Penal Statutes) adding the term "Moralibus" to "Penalibus," to preserve dignity
1564		Galileo Galilei, Pisa-born Florentine (Italian) astronomer, mathematician, and physicist, accused of heresy by the Italian Inquisition and forced to recant view that earth rotates around the sun (1564–1642). William Shakespeare (1564–1616), English playwright and poet, wrote of seven ages of man	
1566	Pope Pius V mandates physicians to discontinue treatment unless patients certify that they have confessed; candidates for medical or surgical degrees to take oath swearing to obey this requirement; physicians/surgeons who violate it to be declared "infamous," to be denied privilege of practicing, and to be ejected from their university or medical/surgical associations		*A Detection and Querimonie of the Daily Enormities and Abuses Committed in Physic*, John Securis (fl 1566); plea for an ethics of competence in medicine, including standards of malpractice; contains early Latin and English translations of the Hippocratic Oath, offered as a statement of consumer rights; enjoins physicians not to be greedy and to treat the poor without collecting a fee
1573		John Donne, English poet and divine, Dean of St. Paul's, London, author of *Biathanatos* (Self-killing) the first defense of suicide in English (1573–1631)	
1575		John Cotta, English physician: wrote on medical conduct (c.1575–c.1650). Abraham Zacuto (Zacutus Lusitanus): Converso Jewish physician, wrote on medical conduct (1575–1642)	In commentary on Thomas Aquinas' *Summa Theologica* (Theological Summation) Spanish Dominican theologian Bartholomew Medina (1527–1581) develops "probabilism," a method of weighing plausible opinions to determine which is probably correct

Dates	Events	Persons	Texts
1578		William Harvey, Cambridge- and Padua-educated English physician and anatomist; physician to Kings James I and Charles I of England; dissected human cadavers and living animals to demonstrate the circulation of the blood, using experiments to challenge the theories and authority of Galen. His theories were controversial in his time because they undermined the theoretical reasons for the popular practice of blood letting (1578–1657)	
1579		Johannes Baptista van Helmont, Flemish chemist and physician (1579–1644)	
1584		Paulus Zacchias (Paolo Zacchia), Spanish medical casuist and physician to Popes Innocent X, Alexander VII; author *Quaestiones Medico-Legales* (Medico-Legal Questions) and *Protomedico* (1584–1659)	
1588	Spanish Armada defeated by English fleet	Thomas Hobbes, English philosopher, classicist, teacher, social contract theorist, materialist, proponent of Galileo's view of the universe. As a Royalist Hobbes sought refuge in France (1640–1651) during British Civil War; corresponded with Descartes; published major work *Leviathan* (1651); proposed social contract theory involving natural rights of all humans. In 1666, the British House of Commons empowered a committee "to receive information touching such books as tend to atheism, blasphemy and profaneness . . . in particular . . . the book of Mr. Hobbes called the *Leviathan.*" Censors then silenced Hobbes, who thereafter wrote in Latin and translated Homer's *Odyssey* into English (1588 –1679)	
1586			*The Olde mans Dietarie*, Cleric Thomas Newton (1542?–1607) includes English translation of the Hippocratic Oath, which contains the very Christian line, "That I shall not be squeamish to bestow my skill in the Art upon the poor and needy, freely, without either fee or other covenant certainly agreed upon," which does not appear in the original Oath

(*continued*)

Dates	Events	Persons	Texts
1588			*A most excellent and compendious method of curing woundes in the head, and in other partes of the body, with other precepts of the same arte . . . translated into English by John Read . . . Whereunto is added the exact cure of the carbuncle, never before set foorth in the English toung. With a treatise of the fistulae in the fundament, and other places of the body, translated out of Johannes Ardern. And also the discription of the emplaister called dia chalciteos, with his use and vertue,* John Read (fl. 1588). Contains an English translation of "The oath of Hippocratus which he gave unto his disciples and scholars which professing Physic and Chirurgerie, is very worthy to be observed and kept faithfully, of every true and honest Artist, though he himself were but a heathen man, and without the true knowledge of the living God, yet for his noble and excellent skill in Physic and Chirurgerie, he ought not to be forgotten of us his posterity, but to be had in an honorable remembrance for ever"
1590	English and Dutch East Indies Companies founded		
1591			*De Christina, ac tuta medenidi rationae* (Christian and Certain Healing), Giovanni Battista Condronchi (1547–1621)
1596		René Descartes, French, exceptionally influential philosopher and mathematician, inventor of analytic geometry; author of the famous line "cogito, sum" (I think, I am), Descartes believed that the mind and body were separate but interacting substances; "Cartesian medicine" thus came to mean a medicine that treats the body as if it were a machine independent of the mind. Descartes was a proud vivisectionist who held that animals may be conscious but could not be self-conscious and thus were comparable to automata (1596–1650)	

Dates	Events	Persons	Texts
1597			*A discourse of the whole art of chyrurgerie. Wherein is exactly set downe the definition, causes, accidents, prognostications, and cures of all sorts of diseases ... Whereunto is added the rule of making remedies which chyurgions doe commonly use: with The Presages of divine Hippocrates.* Peter Lowe (1550?–1612?), surgical text with English translation of "The protestation and oath of divine Hippocrates" (later editions in 1612, 1634, 1654)
1600	Giordano Bruno convicted of heresy by Roman Inquisitor Cardinal Robert Bellarmine and burned at the stake at the Campo de Fiori, Rome		
1602	Tokugawa shoguns begin rule in Japan (to 1868)		First systematic treatises on medical conduct published in Japan
1603	Dutch East Indies Company founded Girolamo Fabrizio's study of veins		
1605			*The Proficience and Advancement of Learning,* Francis Bacon, offers plan to advance human knowledge through the interrogation of experience by experiment; envisions self-regulated scientific medicine committed to preventing and curing illness, extending human longevity, and relieving suffering in sickness and death. Calls the latter "outward *Euthanasia,* or the easy dying of the body"
1607	First permanent English settlement in America – Jamestown, Virginia		
1608	French colonists found Quebec		
1610	First well-documented Caesarian section (in Germany)		
1611			*THE HOLY BIBLE, Conteyning the Old Testament, and the New: Newly Translated out of the Originall tongues: & with the former Translations diligently compared and revised, by his Majesties Special*

(continued)

Dates	Events	Persons	Texts
			Commandment. Appointed to be read in Churches: later known as the Authorized King James' version of the Bible: English translation and compilation of holy scripture by a committee appointed by King James I of Britain; committee met from 1604 to 1611
1612			*A Short Discoverie of the Unobserved Dangers of Several Sorts of Ignorant and Unconsiderate Practisers of Physike in England, profitable not onely for the deceived multitude, and easie for their meane capacities, but raising reformed and more advised thought*, John Cotta argues for a medicine based on learning, urges a medicine of virtue and competence
1614			*Medicus Politicus; sive, De officiis medico-politicis tractatus, quatuor distinctus libris: in quibus non solum bonorum medicorum mores ac virtutes exprimuntur, malorum vero fraudes & imposturae deteguntur* (The Politic Physician: or A Treatise on Medico-Political Duties . . . distinguishing the virtues of true doctors from frauds), Roderigo de Castro: applied casuistic methods to questions of medical conduct; affirms Stoic ideals of medical humanism, which embraces all suffering humanity
1615		Richard Baxter (1615–1691), Puritan theologian and physician	
1618	Pilgrims leave from England for the New World on the *Mayflower*		
1619	First slaves brought to a British colony, Jamestown, Virginia		
1621			*The anatomy of melancholy, what it is. With all the kindes, causes, symptomes, prognostickes, and severall cures of it. In three maine partitions . . . Philosophically, medicinally, historically, opened and cut up. By Democritus Iunior . . .* Robert Burton (1577–1640)
			Quaestiones Medico-Legales (Medico-Legal Questions), Paolo Zacchia

Dates	Events	Persons	Texts
1623		Blaise Pascal, French mathematician and physicist (demonstrated the existence of vacuums), develops foundations of mathematical theory of probability; critic of Jesuits, of casuistry, and of probablism; popularly known for argument described as Pascal's Wager: "If God does not exist, one will lose nothing by believing in him, while if he does exist, one will lose everything by not believing" (1623–1662)	
1624		Thomas Sydenham, Oxford-educated English physician and military surgeon who reconceptualized illnesses in terms of diseases (discrete entities with a history over time, e.g., typhus) rather as than as symptoms (so that physicians would think of a patient as having "typhus" rather than as having "fever"); known as the "English Hippocrates" because of his insistence on observation rather than of speculation in describing and treating diseases; credited with inventing a practical form of laudanum, that is, liquid opium. "Among the remedies which it has pleased Almighty God to give to man to relieve his sufferings, none is so universal and so efficacious as opium" (1624–1689)	
1628			*Exercitatio Anatomica de Motu Cordis et Sanguinis in Animalibus* (Anatomical Exercise on the Motion of the Heart and Blood in Animals), William Harvey writes on the circulation of the blood challenging Galen
c. 1630	Obstetrical forceps invented by Peter Chamberlen	Kaibara Ekiken, Japanese physician, Neo-Confucian scholar, and philosopher, wrote on medical morality (1630–1714)	
1632		John Locke, Oxford-educated English Puritan, administrator, philosopher, political theorist, and physician, empiricist, egalitarian, social contractarian, and rights theorist – author of *An Essay Concerning Human Understanding, A Letter Concerning Toleration, Two Treatises of Government*; all published in 1689–1690, the latter two anonymously (1632–1704).	*Dialogo dei due massimi sistemi del mondo* (Dialogue Concerning the Two Chief Systems of the World), Galileo Galilei, supports Copernicus' counterintuitive theory that the earth rotates around the sun

(continued)

Dates	Events	Persons	Texts
		Samuel von Pufendorf, German natural law philosopher, argued that animals lack rights because they lack a sense of duty (1632–1694)	
		Baruch Spinoza, (Bento d'Espiñoza) Dutch–Jewish of Portuguese descent; oculist and philosopher, founder of modern biblical criticism; defender of freedom of thought and political liberty; excommunicated from Portuguese Jewish Synagogue in 1656. Throughout the seventeenth and eighteenth centuries "Spinozist" was a term of condemnation widely applied to free thinkers including many physicians (1632–1677)	
1633	Inquisition places Galileo's *Dialogue Concerning the Two Chief Systems of the World* on the *Index Librorum Prohibitorum,* (Index of Banned Books), Inquisitor Cardinal Robert Bellarmine calls Galileo before the Inquisition in Rome		*Statement of Abjuration*, Galileo Galilei: "I have been judged vehemently suspected of heresy, that is, of having held and believed that the Sun is the center of the universe and immoveable, and that the Earth is not the centre of the same, and that it does move . . . I abjure with sincere heart and unfeigned faith, I curse and detest the said errors and heresies." Tradition has it that Galileo said under his breath *"E pur si muove!"* (But it does move!)
1636	Harvard College, first American College, founded		
1638			*Discorsi e Dimostrazioni Matematiche, intorno á due nuoue scienze* (Discourses and mathematical demonstrations concerning the two new sciences) Galileo Galilei, challenges Aristotelian physics establishing laws of motion and inertia
1641			*Meditationes de Prima Philosophie* (Meditations on First Philosophy), Renee Descartes' foundational work in modern philosophy, contains famous line *cogito sum*, (I think, I am)
			Second edition of *De Officiis Medico-Polticis Tractatus* (The Politic Physician: Or A Treatise on Medico-Political Duties), Roderigo de Castro Lusitanus, secular medical ethics based on Stoic humanism, by Jewish physician converted to Christianity

Dates	Events	Persons	Texts
1642	Three British Civil Wars begin: Parliamentarians against Royalists (1642–1651); supporters of King Charles I against Long Parliamentarians (1648–1649), Charles II against the Rump Parliament (1649–1651) ends with the establishment of a parliamentary democracy in Britain; an estimated 10 percent of the population of England, Ireland, and Scotland died because of the wars		
1644	End of Ming dynasty in China, and founding of Qing dynasty by the Manchus First recorded New World epidemic of yellow fever begins in Barbados		*Ortus medicinae; id est, Initia physicae inaudita. Progressus medicinae novus, in morborum ultionem ad vitam longam* (Oriatrike; or, Physic refined ... Being a new rise and progress of philosophy and medicine, for the ... prolongation of life), Johannes Baptiste van Helmont (Baron Franciscus Mercurius van Helmont 1618–1699). *Biathanatos* (Self-killing) John Donne, the first defense of suicide in English, probably composed in 1607 or 1608, published c. 1644–1647
1649		Francis Hutcheson, Scottish moral sense philosopher (1649–1746)	
1653	Aurangzeb Alamgir (1618–1707), Moghul Emperor, begins rule in India		
1656			*Lettres Provinciales* (Provincial Letters), Blaise Pascal a scathingly hilarious attack upon probabilism, eroded the influence of casuistry; book banned and ordered burned by King Louis XIV of France
1660	Royal Society of London founded	Friedrich Hoffman, German physician (Halle), author of *Medicus Politicus* (The politic physician), envisions living things in purely physio-mechanical terms (1660–1742)	

(continued)

Dates	Events	Persons	Texts
1663		Cotton Mather, American, Harvard-educated Puritan minister and health care reformer. His *Memorable Providences Relating to Witchcraft and Possessions* (1689) set the stage for the 1692 Salem Witchcraft Trials (1663–1728). The first native-born American to be a fellow of the Royal Society of London; Mather persuaded Boston physician Zabdiel Boylston (1679–1766) to inoculate against smallpox during the epidemic of 1721; 240 people were inoculated, all but 6 survived	
1665	Great Plague of London		
1666	*Académie des Sciences* founded in Paris by Jean Baptiste Colbert (1619–1683) *contrôleur général* (minister of finance) under King Louis XIV of France		*Ventilabrum medico-theologicum quo omnes casus, tum medicos, cum aegros, aliosque concernentes eventilantur*, Michiel Boudewyns (1601–1681) early work on Catholic medical morality
1670		Bernard Mandeville, Dutch physician–philosopher who emigrated to London after participating in an uprising in Rotterdam; in two poems, *The Grumbling Hive: or, Knaves Turn'd Honest* (1705) and *The Fable of the Bees, or: Private Vices, Publick Benefits* (1714), argues for the public benefits of pursing selfish private interests (1670–1733)	
1672	*Cinchona* bark included in the *London Pharmacopoeia* as a fever treatment		*An Essay Concerning Human Understanding*, a defense of empiricism, John Locke
1687			*Philosophiæ Naturalis Principia Mathematica* (The Mathematical Principles of Natural Philosophy), commonly referred to as "The Principia," Isaac Newton; capstone work of the scientific revolution, sets out the laws or motion (classical mechanics) and the law of universal gravitation presenting a comprehensive unified theory of the physical universe
1688	"Glorious Revolution" in Britain, William of Orange and wife Mary assume the English throne	Herman Boerhaave, Dutch Calvinist physician and chemist; denied a religious career because of charges of "Spinozism;" he became a physician and instituted bedside teaching, postmortem autopsy to establish clinicopathological correlations, taught using clinicopathological conferences and lectured on ethical precepts, for example, "our best patients are the poor because the Lord has taken	

Dates	Events	Persons	Texts
		it upon himself to pay us for them;" memorialized by Samuel Johnson (1649–1703) in *The Gentleman's Magazine* (1668–1738)	
1689			*An Essay Concerning Human Understanding*, John Locke (probably written at various times between 1671 and 1689), critique of the concept of innate ideas, views the mind as a *tabula rasa* or blank slate, on which experience writes, strong defense of empiricism
			Two Treatises of Government, John Locke (written 1679–1682, published anonymously): the first treatise is a critique of the divine right of kings to rule; the second treatise, often cited as a manifesto for liberal democracy and as the intellectual basis of the American Revolution, argues that all men are created equal and endowed with certain inalienable rights, specifically the rights to life, liberty, health, and property; when governments fail to protect these rights citizens have a right to revolt and set up a representative government
1695		John Rutherford, Edinburgh physician and medical educator (1695–1779), gives short lectures on medical ethics at medical school in Edinburgh as early as 1750	
1696		Alphonsus Liguori, Italia (Marianella, near Naples) Roman Catholic moral theologian (1696–1787)	
1700	Bourbons replace Hapsburgs as rulers of Spain		
1701	Small pox inoculation introduced in Constantinople		
1703		Antonio Jose Rodriguez, Spanish writer on medical morality (1703–1777)	
1704			*Opticks*, Sir Isaac Newton (1642–1727) popularizes physical science, making its concepts accessible to intellectuals throughout Europe
1707	Death of Aurangzeb, decline of Moghul power in India		
	Act of Union; England and Scotland become United Kingdom		

(*continued*)

Dates	Events	Persons	Texts
1708			*Institutiones Medicae, aphorismi de cognoscendis et curandis morbis.* Herman Boerhaave, recommends fluids rather than surgery for the treatment of kidney and gall stones, considers surgery "an act of faith"
1709	Great Plague in Russia		
1710		William Cullen, Scottish physician, medical educator, nosologist, Professor Edinburgh University (1710–1790) Thomas Reid, Scottish moral sense theorist, cousin to John Gregory, held contractarian view of physician–patient relationship, believed morality based on both sympathy and reason (1710–1796)	*Bonifacius, Or Essays to Do Good,* Cotton Mather (more than 15 editions, latest 2003). The first North American guide for Puritans who want to connect Christian ideals with occupational roles; provided specific imperatives for ministers, teachers, lawyers, and physicians *Onania; or, The Heinous Sin of Self-Pollution, and all its Frightful Consequences in Both Sexes, Considered,* Anonymous text published in London asserts masturbation has deleterious medical effects
1711		David Hume, Scottish philosopher, historian, statesman, moral sense/sympathy theorist, and atheist (1711–1776) Jean Jacques Rousseau, French philosopher and autobiographer; characterizes childhood as an age of innocence in the life cycle (1712–1778)	
1713			*Yojokun* "Teaching on the Care of Life," Ekiken Kaibara (1630–1714), popular Japanese book on health care
1714	Gabriel David Fahrenheit constructs the mercury thermometer	Étienne Condillac, French empiricist philosopher and logician (1714–1780)	*Midwife's Oath,* New York City
1717	Lady Mary Wortley Montagu (1689–1762), wife of the British consul in Constantinople, brings Turkish practice of smallpox inoculation to England; "the *smallpox,* so fatal and so general among us, is here entirely harmless by the invention of *engrafting* . . . the old woman comes with a nutshell full of the best matter of smallpox . . . and puts into the vein as much matter as can lie on the head of a needle"		

Dates	Events	Persons	Texts
1718		William Hunter, Glasgow and Edinburgh-educated Scottish anatomist and obstetrician, founder Great Windmill Street school of medicine in London; his collection became basis of Hunterian museum in Glasgow; offered psychiatric defense of mothers who committed infanticide on newborns (1718–1793)	
1723		Adam Smith, Scottish professor of logic and moral philosophy, Glasgow University, and customs inspector, Edinburgh, political economist, moral sense theorist, philosopher (1723–1790)	
1724		John Gregory, deist Scottish physician, philosopher and medical educator, First Physician to His Majesty, the King in Scotland, taught at Edinburgh medical school, lectured in English to medical students on their moral duties and character as physicians before they began their clinical training at the Royal Infirmary of Edinburgh (1724–1773)	
		Immanuel Kant, Prussian Pietist philosopher and ethical theorist, defender of the Enlightenment (*Aufklärung*), believed in morality based on rational principles, held that humans' duty to cultivate compassion required sensitivity to animals; lectures and publications on religion banned from 1792 to 1797 by King Frederick William II of Prussia (1724–1804)	
1726	Edinburgh University Medical School founded		
1728	Pierre Fauchard describes how to fill a tooth	John Hunter, Scottish anatomist and surgeon, and teacher; a founder of modern surgery (1728–1793)	
1730	First tracheotomy for treatment of diphtheria performed		
1731			Edinburgh University version of the Hippocratic Oath, in Latin; translates precepts of classical oath into the language of gentlemanly virtue and honor (1731–1867)
1733	Measurement of blood pressure	Joseph Priestly, English Unitarian minister, chemist, discoverer of oxygen, Fellow of the Royal Society, teacher at Warrington Academy, friend and teacher of Percival; fled to America after burning of his church,	William Cheselden's *Osteographia Systema Naturae* published by Linnaeus

(*continued*)

Dates	Events	Persons	Texts
		his laboratory, and his expulsion from the Royal Society; cofounder of the American Unitarian Church, honored by American Philosophical Society (1733–1804)	
1735		Martha Ballard, American midwife (1735–1812)	
1736	Discovery that citrus fruits cure scurvy First successful appendectomy performed in France		*Primae Lineae Physiologiae*, Albrecht von Haller
1739			*Treatise of Human Nature*, David Hume, develops sympathy-based account of morality that influences physician John Gregory
1740		Thomas Percival, Warrington-, Edinburgh-, and Leiden-educated English Unitarian physician, antislavery activist, hospital and public health reformer; writer of morality tales for children, author of first code of medical ethics and inventor of the modern concepts of *medical ethics*, *profession*, *professional ethics*, and *professional etiquette* (1740–1804)	
1741		William Withering, English physician; distills digitalis for treatment of angina; involved in infamous flyte and pamphlet war with Robert Darwin – son of Erasmus, father of Charles (1741–1799)	
1742		Samuel Bard, Edinburgh-educated American physician and medical educator; physician to U.S. President George Washington, a founder of Kings College Medical School (1767, second in the United States – renamed Columbia after American Revolution), and first President of Columbia College of Physicians and Surgeons (1807); published first English-language work on modern "medical ethics" (1742–1821)	*Nuevo aspecto de theologia medico-moral y ambos derechos o paradoxas physico-theologico legales . . .* (New Aspects of Medical-Moral Theology), Antonio Rodriquez
1743		Antoine Lavoisier, French chemist, discovered law of conservation of mass; set up major European chemistry laboratory, repeated Priestly's experiments and called the substance detected "oxygen;" beheaded during French Revolution. Mathematician, Joseph-Louis Lagrange, remarked, "It took them only an instant to cut off that head, and a hundred years may not produce another like it" (1743–1794)	

Dates	Events	Persons	Texts
1745	The Company of Surgeons splits from the Barbers in London	Johann Peter Frank, Bavarian physician from French family; Professor of Medicine at Göttingen, Pavia, Vienna, and St. Petersburg; public health reformer, believed in public hygiene, invented concept of "medical police" (1745–1821)	
		Philippe Pinel, French physician and psychiatrist, disciple of Condillac, together with asylum manager Jean-Baptiste Pussin (1745–1811) reformed mental health system in post-Revolutionary France by removing shackles from the insane and replacing physical with moral or psychological therapy (1745–1826)	
		Benjamin Rush, Edinburgh-educated American physician, student of John Gregory, signer of Declaration of Independence, physician to Continental Army, physician at Pennsylvania Hospital (founded by Benjamin Franklin and Thomas Bond in 1751, oldest in the United States), Professor of Medicine/Materia Medica University of Pennsylvania, a founder of Dickenson College, medical educator and lecturer on "medical ethics" (1745–1813)	
1747		John Aikin, Warrington-educated, dissenting English physician and writer (1747–1822)	*Primitive Physick or An Easy and Natural Method of Curing Most Diseases*, published anonymously by John Wesley (1703–1791), founder of Methodism. Called "the most important book in medicine of the eighteenth century," it is hostile to orthodox practitioners, offers an alternative to professional medicine
1748	Royal College of Surgeons founded in Cadiz	Jeremy Bentham, English utilitarian philosopher, coined the term "deontology;" defender of moral status of animals; had his corpse dissected publicly to challenge taboo against dissection (1748–1832)	*Account of the Putrid Sore Throat*, John Fothergil – describes diphtheria. *Theologia Moralis* (1st edition 1748, 9th 1785), by Catholic theologian Alphonsus Liguori (1696–1781), developed philosophy of equiprobabalism; argued that physicians are morally obligated to provide gratuitous treatment to the indigent
1749		Edward Jenner, English surgeon, military surgeon, student of John Hunter; discovered vaccination with cow pox as a way of immunizing against small pox, used his own son, other children, and servants as his experimental subjects (1749–1823)	

(continued)

Dates	Events	Persons	Texts
1751			*The Four Stages of Cruelty* – William Hogarth print series, condemns animal torture
1752			*Theory and Practice or Treatise on Midwifery*, William Smellie (1697–1763) – first scientific approach to obstetrics
1753			*Treatise of the Scurvy*, James Lind (1716–1794)
1754	First female medical doctor graduates from the University of Halle		
1755		Christian Friedrich Samuel Hahnemann, German physician (Saxony) and founder of homeopathy (medical practice based on assisting the body to produce effects similar to the symptoms of disease; known as the law of similars), critic of conventional medicine's belief in symptom relief and of blood-letting; introduced practice of quarantine to Prussia (1755–1843)	*Dictionary of the English Language*, Samuel Johnson (1709–1784), the standard dictionary of the English language for more than 150 years. Prepublication circulation of "Of Suicide" – a defense of the morality of suicide – promotes controversy Withdrawn by publisher but clandestine copies appear anonymously in French (1770) and English (1777). David Hume's name is attached to the publication in 1783; the original essay, as revised by Hume, first published in the twentieth century
1757	Warrington Academy (Britain): Dissenting academy founded by Quakers and Unitarians to provide education free of state or Church of England control. John Aiken Sr., John Seddon, Joseph Priestly were the faculty; Thomas Percival was the first student to enroll (to 1786)	Pierre-Jean-Georges Cabanis, French physician, medical educator, a founder of *Idéologues* movement (1757–1808)	
1758		Thomas Gisborne (1758–1846) Anglican minister, antislavery activist and follower of John Locke; in 1794, wrote a "social compact" describing the duties of physicians as moral gentleman; corresponded with Thomas Percival	*A Treatise on Madness*, William Battie (1704–1776), English physician, argues that madness is not one disorder, but many, each requiring different methods of treatment, but all requiring confinement
1759			*A Theory of Moral Sentiments*, Adam Smith, foundational work in moral sense theory
1760		Thomas Beddoes, English physician, chemist, medical reformer (1760–1808)	*Onanism: Or a Treatise Upon the Disorders produced by Masturbation: Or, the Dangerous Effects of Secret and Excessive Venery*, by Simon-Auguste-Andre-David Tissot (1728–1797), medicalizes masturbation

Dates	Events	Persons	Texts
1762		Christoph Wilheim Hufeland, internationally renowned German physician (practiced in Weimar and Berlin), invented a theory of macrobiotics to prolong life; medical moralist, developed an approach to medical morality based on Kantian moral philosophy (1762–1836)	
		Felix Pascalis, American physician, coeditor of the first American medical journal, *The Medical Repository*; coauthor Medical Society of New York's *System of Medical Ethics* (1762?–1833)	
1763	First American medical society founded in New London, Connecticut		
1765	First American medical school at the College of Pennsylvania, Philadelphia (later part of the University of Pennsylvania)		*A Comparative View of the State and Faculties of Man with those of the Animal World*, John Gregory.
			Anweisung zur Kenntniss und Cur der Kinderkrankheiten (The Diseases of Children and Their Remedies) Nils Rosen von Rosenstein (1706–1773), first modern pediatrics textbook
1766			*San-Ron* (Thesis on Obstetrics), Gen'etsu Kagawa (1700–1777), confirms that the normal position of the fetus in utero is upside down, challenging traditional Japanese understanding of the position of fetal development
1768		Baron Dominique-Jean Larrey, Surgeon-in-Chief to Napoleon's Army; inventor of concept and practices of ambulance to transport patients to field hospitals and triage to sort patients into treatment categories according to medical need rather than status or rank (1768–1841)	*Observations on the Dropsy of* the Brain, Robert Whytt (1714–1766), first description of tuberculosis meningitis in children
1769		Samuel Thomson, American, founder of eponymous anti-elitist populist school of medicine based on botanical cures (1769–1843)	*Discourse on the Duties of A Physician* (1769), Samuel Bard, first published English-language work on "medical ethics," introduces the concept of the sympathetic physician
1770		Georg Wilhelm Friedrich Hegel, German (born Stuttgart) philosopher; one of the influential thinkers in the modern world; held "idealist" view of history as the unfolding of the logic of ideas and movements (1770–1831)	*Observations on the Duties and Offices of a Physician, and on the Method of Prosecuting Enquiries in Philosophy*, student anonymous version of John Gregory's lectures.
			Of Suicide, David Hume (French edition)

(*continued*)

Dates	Events	Persons	Texts
1771		Marie-Francoise-Xavier Bichat, French physician, medical reformer, developed concept of tissue that underlies modern pathology, believed in establishing clinicopathological correlation through autopsy (1771–1802)	*The Natural History of the Human Teeth*, John Hunter
		Félix Janner, Spanish, author of *Moral Médica*, introduces John Gregory's thought to Spain (1771–1865)	
1772	James Cook circumnavigates the southern oceans (to 1775)		*Lectures on the Duties and Qualifications of a Physician*, John Gregory, applied moral sense theory to medicine promulgating the ideal of the sympathetic and humane physician
1774	Oxygen named by Lavoisier. Hypnosis introduced as medical treatment	Gaspard-Laurent Bayle, French physician and encyclopedist (1774–1816)	*Anatomy of the Human Gravid Uterus*, William Hunter
			A Father's Legacy to his Daughters, posthumous publication of John Gregory letters to his daughters, whom he considers men's "companions and equals; as designed to soften our hearts and polish our manners"
1776	American Declaration of Independence. Demonstration that the sweetness of diabetic's urine is caused by sugar		*An Inquiry into the Nature and Causes of The Wealth of Nations*, Adam Smith, foundational work in modern economic theory
1780		Nathanial Chapman, American physician, medical educator, teacher/mentor to John Bell and Isaac Hays; President of the American Philosophical Society, first President of the American Medical Association (AMA) (1780–1853)	
1781	Massachusetts Medical Society founded (oldest continuously operating medical society in the United States)	Rene-Théophile-Hyacinthe Laennec, French physician, inventor of stethoscope (1781–1826)	
1782		James R. Manley, American physician, founding coeditor *The Medical Repository*; coauthor Medical Society of New York's *System of Medical Ethics* (1782?–1851)	
1783			*Of Suicide*, David Hume (English edition)
1786		Jacob Bigelow, author of first American textbook on botany and medical botany (1786–1879)	

Dates	Events	Persons	Texts
1788	"Doctors Riot," New York City, large scale riot to protest grave robbing of corpses used to teach anatomy	Arthur Schopenhauer, Polish-born (Gdansk) German philosopher from Dutch family, who urged universal compassion – for animals as well as humans – as basis of morality (1788–1860). Southwood Smith, English physician, medical reformer and disciple of Bentham (1788–1861)	
1789	Edward Jenner begins experimenting with swine pox inoculations against small pox, using his 10-month-old son, Edward Jenner, Jr. as a subject French Revolution begins (to 1799) George Washington becomes the first president of the United States of America		*Traite elementaire de Chimie* (Treatise on the Elements of Chemistry), Laruent Lavoisier, foundational text in modern chemistry
1790		Marshall Hall, English physiologist, proposed a code of ethics for experiments on animals (1790–1857)	
1791	Edward Jenner continues experiments on his son, Edward Jr. (1798–1819), inoculating him with small pox – Edward Jr.'s arm swells in response Edward Jr. becomes a sickly child and shows signs of arrested mental development	Granville Sharp Pattison, Scottish–American anatomist, medical educator, duelist (1791–1851) Theodric Romeyn Beck, American (Schenectadian, Union College alumnus); physician and lawyer his treatise *On the Elements of Medical Jurisprudence* established framework for American medico-legal doctrines (1791–1851)	
1792	Thomas Percival chairs committee drafting new rules for Manchester Infirmary		
1794	France abolishes slavery in its territories; Lavoisier guillotined	John Conolly, Irish born British physician, mental health reformer (1794–1866) Charles Hastings, founder of British Medical Association (BMA), proponent of codes of medical ethics (1794–1866)	*An Enquiry into the Duties of Men in the Higher and Middle Classes of Society in Great Britain Resulting from their Respective Stations, Professions and Employment,* Thomas Gisborne (Social contract formatted as gentleman's manual) *Essay on the Principles of Population,* Thomas Malthus (1766–1834) propounds thesis that nature produces more offspring than can survive; influenced Darwin *Macrobiotics, or the Art to Prolong One's Life,* C. W. Hufeland, early work on prevention of aging

(continued)

Dates	Events	Persons	Texts
			Medical Jurisprudence; or A Code of Ethics and Institutes, Adapted to the Professions of Physic and Surgery, Thomas Percival, small edition of precursor to his *Medical Ethics*; no conception of medical ethics or professional ethics in this edition
1795	Scottish physician Alexander Gordon reports that puerperal fever is caused by putrid matter introduced into the uterus by hands of physician or midwife; hand washing recommended as preventative; advice ignored		
1796	Edward Jenner (1749–1823) tests his theory that inoculation with cowpox pus will immunize against small pox using children and servants as subjects; asks permission of their parents and masters; calls his procedure vaccination; challenges his theory by inoculating vaccinated and nonvaccinated subjects with smallpox pus; "To convince myself . . . I at the same time inoculated a patient with [small pox pus] who never had gone through the cow-pox, and it produced the smallpox in the usual regular manner"	Carl Friedrich Heinrich Marx, German professor of medicine, advocate of Baconian euthanasia in the original sense of palliative care (1796–1877) John Bell, physician, journal editor, and lecturer, University of Pennsylvania, nominal chair of committee that drafted 1847 AMA Code of Ethics (1796–1872) Isaac Hays Sephardic Jewish physician, anonymous editor of the *American Journal of the Medical Sciences*; initiated proposal to found AMA, organized founding convention, secretary to committee that drafted the 1847 AMA Code of Ethics, apparently edited the Code of Ethics (1796–1879)	
1797			*Die Kunst das menschliche Leben zu verlängern* (The Art Prolonging Life), Christian Wilhelm Hufeland, classic work on preventing unhealthy old age *The Medical Repository*, first American medical journal; originally edited by Samuel Latham Mitchill (1764–1831), Elihu Hubbard Smith (1771–1798), and Edward Miller (1760–1812), published until 1824

Dates	Events	Persons	Texts
1798			*An Inquiry into the Causes and Effects of the Variolae Vaccinae, a Disease Known by the Name of Cow Pox*, Edward Jenner; theory of vaccination initially provokes ridicule, but no one comments on his experiments on vulnerable subjects; theory validated and accepted within 2 years
1799		Eli Geddings, physician, medical educator, editor, *Baltimore Medical and Surgical Journal and Review* (1831–1837), chaired committee that wrote Medico-Chirurgical Society of Baltimore's *System of Ethics* (1799–1878)	
1800	Chlorine used to purify water. Francoise Bichat studies postmortem changes in human organs Phillippe Pinel advocates a more humane treatment of the insane	Sir Edwin Chadwick, English utilitarian, disciple of Jeremy Bentham, and sanitarian reformer (1800–1890). Michael Ryan, Dublin- and Edinburgh-educated Irish (probably Catholic) obstetrician and medical educator; first professor of medical ethics, first to propose the informed consent of research subjects as a principle of research ethics; first historian of medical ethics (1800–1841)	*Traité des membranes en général et diverses membranes en particulier* (Treatise on membranes in general and certain membranes in particular), Marie-Francoise-Xavier Bichat, fundamentally transformed the conception of the body by visualizing organs as made from different types of tissues and membranes
1801			*Anatomie générale à la physiologie et à la médecine* (General anatomy applied to physiology and medicine), Marie-Francoise-Xavier Bichat, argues that disease is localized to certain tissues within an organ and thus within the body; conceptual foundation of modern approach to autopsy. *Traité medico-philosophicqeu sur l'alienation mentale ou la manie* (Medico-Philosophical treatise on mental alienation), Philippe Pinel urges humane treatment of mentally ill, including unshackling them
1802	British Parliament awards Edward Jenner £10,000 to acknowledge his discovery of vaccination Consul Napoleon Bonaparte legalizes slavery in French territories		

(continued)

Dates	Events	Persons	Texts
1803	Performing or receiving an abortion becomes a criminal offense in Great Britain		*Medical Ethics; Or, A Code of Institutes and Precepts, Adopted to the Professional Conduct of Physicians and Surgeons*, by Thomas Percival, introduces expressions "medical ethics" and "professional ethics" to the world, except in the United States, world ignores the book and the concepts
1804	Hippocratic Oath swearing introduced at Montpellier University (France). Napoleon Bonaparte crowned Emperor of France		
1805			*Observations on the Duties of a Physician, and the Methods of Improving Medicine. Accommodated to the Present State of Society and Manners in the United States*, Benjamin Rush, early American essay on medical ethics by student of John Gregory
1806	Medical Society of the State of New York founded	Worthington Hooker, American physician (Connecticut); critic of homeopathy; critic of paternalism; defender of truth telling in patient–physician relationship (1806–1867)	Oath of the Medical Society of the State of New York, English-language version of Edinburgh virtue ethics version of Hippocratic Oath
1807	Bavaria becomes the first country to make vaccination against small pox compulsory, setting a precedent followed by most European governments. Slave trade abolished within the British Empire	Maxmilien Isidore Amand Simon introduced concept of medical deontology into French and European medicine; addressed physicians' moral responsibilities during epidemics (1807, fl. 1845–1865)	
1808	Association of Boston Physicians founded. Importation of slaves banned in the United States		*Boston Medical Police*: minimalist Percivalean code of medical ethics drafted by John Warren (1753–1815), Lemuel Hayward (1749–1821) and John Fleet (1766–1813) for the Association of Boston Physicians
1809		Charles Darwin, British biologist, inventor of modern evolutionary theory, revolutionizes biology (1809–1882) Oliver Wendell Holmes, Sr., American physician and writer (1809–1894)	
1810			*Organon der Heilkunst* (Principles of Medicine), Samuel Hahnemann introduces the theory of homeopathy

Dates	Events	Persons	Texts
1811			*Sixteen Introductory Lectures* Benjamin Rush, lectures delivered at the University of Pennsylvania, introduces students to the ideal of the virtuous, sympathetic, and humane physician
1812			*Medical Inquires and Observations upon the Diseases of the Mind,* Benjamin Rush
1813		Claude Bernard, French experimental physiologist, introduces concept of homeostasis; defends experimentation on animals; urges restricting experiments on humans to therapeutic interventions (1813–1878) John Snow, British anesthesiologist and epidemiologist (1813–1858) Richard Wagner, German composer, links antivivisectionism with anti-Semitism (1813–1883)	
1815	Battle of Waterloo	Chancellor Otto von Bismarck of Germany (1815–1898), founder of modern Germany and creator of state social insurance pensions and "sickness" funds to provide health insurance	*Elements of the Practice of Medicine,* Thomas Addison (1793–1860) and Richard Bright ((1789–1858), first description of the etiology of appendicitis
1816	Alphonsus Liguori beatified by Roman Catholic church		
1817	Global cholera pandemic begins	Nathan Smith Davis, American medical education reformer, "father of the AMA," defender of 1847 AMA Code of Ethics (1817–1904)	
1818		Karl Marx, German, (born in Trier) initially Jewish later atheist, philosopher, political economist; critic of capitalism; communist theorist and revolutionary; together with fellow German Friedrich Engels (1820–1895) developed a materialist economic theory of history stated most famously in the first line of their 1848 *Communist Manifesto,* "the history of all previous ages is the history of the class struggle" (1818–1883) Ignaz Phillip Semmelweis, Hungarian obstetrician, identifies child birth fever as iatrogenic, introduces antisepsis; proposals ridiculed (1818–1865)	*Frankenstein; or The Modern Prometheus* Mary Wollstonecraft (Godwin) Shelley (1797–1851) dramatized idea of organ transplantation, resuscitation/reanimation, and concept of danger in irresponsible scientific innovation *System der praktischen Heilkunde,* (System of Practical Medicine), Christoph Wilhelm Hufeland, revised editions by the author to 1828; translated into many languages including Japanese; drawing on precepts of Immanuel Kant argues, "the fundamental law for . . . physician is: Regulate all your actions in a manner, consistent with the highest end of your vocation: saving life, restoring health, and relieving the sufferings of humanity"

(continued)

Dates	Events	Persons	Texts
1819		Queen Victoria of Britain (Victorian era, 1837–1901)	*De l'auscultation mediate* (Mediated Auscultation), René Théophile Hyacinthe Laennec (1781–1826) introduces the stethoscope and its use
1820	Lexington, Kentucky, chapter of the Kappa Lambda Society of Hippocrates formed by Dr. Samuel Brown (1769–1830)	Florence Nightingale, English nurse, hospital reformer, author of *Notes on Nursing* (1820–1910). Herbert Spencer, English philosopher of Social Darwinism, coined the expression "survival of the fittest" (1820–1903)	
1821		Elizabeth Blackwell, first American woman physician (1821–1910). Mary Baker Eddy, American founder of Christian Science Church (1821–1910). Rudolf Virchow, Prussian (born Schivelbein, Pomerania, now part of Poland), politician, public health activist, physician, a founder of three fields (anthropology, cellular pathology, comparative pathology) founded Deutsche Gesellschaft für Anthropologie, Ethnologie und Urgeschichte (German Society for Anthropology, Ethnology and Pre-History); developed standard autopsy procedure; defender of animal experimentation; role model for physician as social activist (influenced Abraham Jacobi), "physicians are the natural attorneys of the poor and the social problems should largely be solved by them" (1821–1902)	*Extracts from the Medical Ethics or A Code of Institutes and Precepts, Adapted to the Professional Conduct of Physicians & Surgeons in Private or General Practice by Thomas Percival, MD.*, Anonymous [Lexington, Kentucky, Chapter of the Kappa Lambda Society of Hippocrates] first U.S. edition of Percival's Code, deletes discussion of hospital ethics, and chapter on law; Americanizes the text *The Lancet*, reform medical journal begins publication in London
1822	British Cruelty to Animals Act enacted. Philadelphia branch of Kappa Lambda Society of Hippocrates founded by Dr. Samuel Jackson (1787–1872), enrolls medical reformers (to 1835). Roman Catholic church removes Galileo's writings from the *Index Librorum Prohibitorum* (Index of banned books)	Sir Francis Galton, English polymath, cousin to Charles Darwin, inventor of social Darwinism and of the term "eugenics" (1822–1911). Louis Pasteur, French chemist and microbiologist, elected to French Academy of Medicine even though not a physician or a surgeon; along with Robert Koch develops bacteriological model of disease and several important vaccines (1822–1895)	
1823			*Elements of Medical Jurisprudence*, Theodric Romeyn Beck, establishes basic framework for American medical jurisprudence *System of Ethics*, Medical Society of the State of the New York – authors, James Manley (1752?–1851),

Dates	Events	Persons	Texts
			Felix A. Ouvière Pascalis (1750?–1833), John Steele (1764–1815) – the most comprehensive code of ethics published by any medical society to this date
			Extracts from the Medical Ethics of Dr. Percival, Kappa Lambda Society of Hippocrates Kappa Lambda Society, Philadelphia chapter (edited by John Bell and Isaac Hays) became the underlying text for the 1847 AMA's Code of Ethics
1824	Society for the Prevention of Cruelty to Animals founded in London		
1825		Jean-Martin Charcot, French pathologist and neurologist (1825–1893)	
1827	New York State bans slavery within its borders		*Reports on Medical Cases, Selected with a View to Illustrate the Symptoms and Cure of Diseases by a Reference to Morbid Anatomy* by Richard Bright (1789–1858): volume correlates clinical picture during life with the pathology of the internal organs; Brights' insightful characterization of the symptoms of "dropsy" subsequently earns him the accolade of having the condition renamed *Morbus Brightii* or "Bright's disease"
			Use of the Dead to the Living, Thomas Southwood Smith (1788–1861): argument for the permissibility of dissecting voluntarily donated cadavers by a Benthamite physician and sanitary reformer
1828	Edinburgh trial of itinerant construction workers William Burke (1792–1829) and William Hare (1792–1870) for serial murders committed to sell corpses to anatomist Dr. Robert Knox (1791–1862) of Edinburgh University, whose students dissected the bodies		

(*continued*)

Dates	Events	Persons	Texts
1829	Pope Leo XII declares whomever is vaccinated ceases to be child of God; smallpox is a judgment of God William Burke convicted of murder and hung; Profession Alexander Monro, III (1773–1859) dissected Burke's body with his medical students, who skinned sections of it; patches of Burke's skin were later displayed at Edinburgh University museum		
1830		Abraham Jacobi, German–American (born Hartum Westphalia), emigrates to the United States after exiled from Germany for participation in revolution of 1848; founding editor *American Journal of Obstetrics*; founder of American pediatrics; sanitarian reformer;leader of revolt against AMA's 1847 Code of Ethics; advocated return to Hippocratic Oath (1830–1919)	
1831	Chloroform discovered Nat Turner (1800–1831) leads slave insurrection in Virginia; caught, executed, and skinned On a close vote, Virginia legislature declines to abolish slavery		*A Critical and Experimental Essay on the Circulation of the Blood*, Marshall Hall (1790–1857) proposes ethics code for experiments on animals *A Manual of Medical Jurisprudence*, Michael Ryan, chapters on medical ethics provide first history of the subject, identifies Gregory and Percival as heirs to Hippocrates; Ryan argues that research on humans requires prior animal experiments and the consent of the research subject *Frankenstein; or The Modern Prometheus*, 3rd and most popular edition, Mary Wollstonecraft (Godwin) Shelley (1797–1851)
1832	As directed in his will, Jeremy Bentham's corpse is publicly dissected by his friend and disciple, Dr. Thomas Southwood Smith, in the Anatomy Theatre of University College London to dispel superstitious dread of dissection; as he directed,		*System of Medical Ethics*, Medico-Chirurgical Society of Baltimore, Eli Geddings (1799–1878), Henry Willis Baxley (1803–1876), Thomas H. Wright, John Fonderden (1804–1869), and John Graves advanced concept of professional code of ethics, model for 1847 AMA Code of Ethics

Dates	Events	Persons	Texts
	Bentham's body is still preserved as an auto-icon – a wax replica molded around his skeleton – in the library of University College London		
	Parliament passes Anatomy Act legalizing donation of bodies for dissection in England		
	Provincial Medical and Surgical Association founded (precursor to BMA)		
1833		Carlos Juan Finlay (nee Juan Carlos Finlay), Cuban of Franco–Scottish descent, Chief Health Officer and President of the Board of Health of Cuba, identified the *Aëdes aegypti* mosquito as the transmitter of Yellow Fever; Finlay's hypothesis was confirmed by work of the Walter Reed Commission; General Leonard Wood, U.S. military governor of Cuba in 1900, a physician, proclaimed "The confirmation of Dr. Finlay's doctrine is the greatest step forward . . . in medical science since Jenner's discovery of the vaccination"	
1834	Emancipation of all slaves in the British Empire	Ernst Haeckel, German zoologist and Social Darwinist, advocate of voluntary mercy killing for the terminally ill, and involuntary killing of the incurably mentally ill, and of all handicapped newborns (1834–1919)	*Experiments and observations on the gastric juice, and the physiology of digestion*, William Beaumont (1785–1853): contains contract with research subject Alexis St. Martin (1794–1880) "to serve, abide, and continue with said William Beaumont, wherever he shall go or travel or reside in any part of the world his covenant servant and diligently and faithfully . . . submit to assist and promote by all means in his power such . . . medical experiments as the said William shall direct or cause to be made on or in the stomach of him, the said Alexis;" considered by some to be the first example of written consent by a U.S. research subject
1836			*Enchiridion Medicum* (Medical Handbook), Christoph Wilhelm Hufeland, classic palliative care text; praises opium and uses Kantian moral theory as basis of medical morality
1837	Queen Victoria ascends to the British throne		

(continued)

Dates	Events	Persons	Texts
1839	Alphonsus Liguori canonized by Roman Catholic Church as "St. Alphonsus"		*Mikroskopische Untersuchungen über die Übereinstimmung in der Struktur und dem Wachstum der Tiere und Pflanzen* (Microscopical Researches into the Accordance in the Structure and Growth of Plants and Animals), Theodor Schwann (1810–1832) characterizes the cell as the basic unit of life
1840	First Opium War between China and Britain Institute of Nursing founded in London		
1841		Karl Binding, German law professor, advocate of involuntary mercy killing of the mentally ill (1841–1920) V. A. Manassein, Russian, professor, editor of *Vrach* (Doctor), and champion of medical ethics (1841–1901)	
1842		Mary Corinna Putnam Jacobi (nee Mary Putnam), Anglo-American physician and pharmacist: first woman to graduate New York College of Pharmacy; first woman graduate of the *École de Médecine* (Paris); founding president of the Association for the Advancement of the Medical Education of Women, first woman member of the Academy of Medicine (1842–1906) William James, American psychologist and philosopher (1842–1910)	*Report on the Sanitary Conditions of the Labouring Population of Great Britain*, major work by Benthamite Edwin Chadwick, assembles empirical data promoting sanitary reform, leads to Britain's first public health act (to prevent cholera)
1843	McNaughton Rule introduced to clarify criminal responsibility of the insane	Ernst Haeckel, "Darwin's German apostle," fused *euthanasie* with eugenics, championing killing and infanticide of those burdensome to society (1843–1919) Robert Koch, German physician and bacteriologist, together with Louis Pasteur develops bacteriological theory of disease, including three postulates for detecting microorganic origins of a disease (1843–1910)	"The Contagiousness of Puerperal Fever." Oliver Wendell Holmes, Sr., claims that puerperal fever caused by putrid matter on physician's hands; report and author ridiculed
1844	Nitrous oxide used to pull teeth painlessly	Friedrich Wilhelm Nietzsche, German, classicist, critic, philosopher, "cultural physician" who strove to cure Europe of its cultural diseases; his statement, "the sick man is a parasite of society" was used to valorize eugenic euthanasia movement in Weimar and Nazi Germany (1844–1900)	*Manual of the Practice of Medicine*, English translation of Christoph Hufeland's *Enchiridion Medicum*, major text for Baconian euthanasia as palliative care movement

Dates	Events	Persons	Texts
1845	First failure of Irish potato crop, leads to mass starvation		*Déontologie médicale; ou, Des devoires et des droits* (Medical Deontology, or Some Rights and Responsibilities), Maxmilien Isidore Amand Simon, French physician, appropriates and introduces Bentham's concept of deontology as the core concept underlying medical morality; deontology becomes the dominant French correlate of what in English became known as medical ethics
1846	Medical Society of State of New York holds national convention on medical education standards, launching call for new national medical association		
	Smithsonian Institution established in Washington DC (opened in 1855)		
	William Thomas Green Morton (1819–1868) uses inhaler device to successfully demonstrate the effectiveness of ether as a general anesthetic during surgery at the Massachusetts General Hospital, Boston; successful demonstrations soon follow in Paris, London, Berlin, Edinburgh, St. Petersburg; newspaper headlines "Happy Hour! We Have Conquered Pain!"		
1847	Ignaz Philipp Semmelweiss demonstrates that "putrid matter" clinging to the hands of physicians and medical students after cadaveric dissections causes puerperal fever; report and reporter ridiculed despite confirming cross-over study		*Code of Ethics*, AMA, first national code of ethics, drafted by committee nominally chaired by John Bell and led by Isaac Hays

(*continued*)

Dates	Events	Persons	Texts
1848	AMA endorses use of anesthesia in surgery. Ignaz Semmelweis introduces antiseptic methods into hospital in Vienna decreasing puerperal fever Liberal democratic revolutions in France, Germany, Romania, Poland, Sicily and other countries (suppressed) Second Republic of France abolishes slavery in French territories		
1849	Elizabeth Blackwell, English-born American abolitionist (1821–1910) becomes first woman to qualify as a doctor in a regular medical college, Geneva Medical College (Geneva, New York)	William Osler, Canadian, born Bond Head, Tecumseh County, Upper Canada (after 1864, the province of Ontario): first Physician-in-Chief, Johns Hopkins University Hospital; designed revolutionary curriculum for Johns Hopkins University Medical School; Regis Professor of Medicine, Oxford University, inventor of concept of *aequanimitas* (1849–1919) Robert Saundby, British, first chair of BMA's Central Ethics Committee, author of British codes of medical ethics, BMA never officially adopts codes (1849–1918)	*Ikai* (Medical Admonition). Seikyo Sugita (1817–1859), Japanese translation of Hufeland's *System der praktischen Heilkunde*, discusses the responsibilities of Physicians, asserts that physicians have a duty to care for all patients regardless of their social or economic status; widely read and accepted by Japanese physicians "On The Mode of Communication of Cholera," John Snow argues that cholera must be transmitted through contaminated water
1850	John Snow uses chlorine in an attempt to disinfect the water supply (Broad Street pump, London) during a cholera epidemic: first use of chlorine to prevent water-borne cholera		
1851		Julius Pagel, German medical historian, author of a medical deontology, historian of medical ethics (1851–1912) Henry Salt, teacher at Eton, Benthamite and founder of the Humanitarian League (1851–1939)	
1852			*Deontología médica; treinta lecciones sobre los deberes de los médicos en el estado actual de la civilización, con un breve resumen de sus derechos. Arreglada al castellano por Francisco Ramos y Borguella.* Spanish edition of Maximilien Isidore Amand's *Déontologie médicale; ou, Des devoires et des droits*, introduces concept of *medical deontology* into Spanish culture

Dates	Events	Persons	Texts
1853	John Snow administers chloroform to Queen Victoria to ease the pain of the birth of Prince Leopold of Britain Smallpox vaccination made compulsory in England		
1854	Crimean War begins – anesthesia in surgery used extensively by both sides (war ends 1856) John Snow has handle removed from a contaminated well on Broad Street (London), ending a cholera epidemic and demonstrating that cholera is spread by water	Paul Ehrlich, German, inventor of Salvarsan, antisyphilitic, first disease-specific chemotherapeutic agent (1854–1915)	
1855	AMA Code of Ethics becomes binding on members and on all affiliated organizations (every regular asylum, dispensary, hospital, and medical school in the United States)	Walter Reed, American military physician, directed campaign against yellow fever; required consenting volunteers for experiments (1855–1902)	
1856	Provincial Medical and Surgical Association (founded 1832) reconstituted as BMA	Sigmund Freud, Austrian Jewish neurologist, emigrates to London after *Anschluss*, the 1938 annexation of Austria by Nazi Germany; founder of psychoanalytic movement in psychiatry (1856–1939) George Bernard Shaw, Anglo-Irish playwright, Fabian Socialist; protested imprisonment of Oscar Wilde; peace activist, 1925 Nobel prize for literature; antivivisectionist, critic of the medical profession, opponent of vaccination; credited with inventing expression "human guinea pig" (1856–1950)	
1857	AMA launches campaign to outlaw prequickening abortion		
1858	French physicians form *Association Génerale des Médicins de France.* Medical Reform Act sets up Medical Register and General Medical Council (GMC) in Britain		*Die Cellularpathologie*, Rudolf Virchow, foundational work of cellular pathology, popularizes dictum, *"Omnis cellula e cellula"* ("every cell originates from another cell")

(*continued*)

Dates	Events	Persons	Texts
1859		Pierre Curie, French physical chemist, professor at Sorbonne, pioneer in studying crystallography, magnetism, and radioactivity, with wife Marie Curie isolated radium and coined term "radioactivity," in 1903; Marie and Pierre jointly awarded Nobel Prize (1859–1906)	*Notes on Nursing*, Florence Nightingale, basis of modern professional "sanitary" nursing *On Liberty*, John Stuart Mill, philosophical essay on the limits of the state's right to intervene in the lives of its citizens *Origin of Species*, Charles Darwin introduces modern theory of evolution of species
1860	Nightingale Nursing School founded at St. Thomas's Hospital, London	Willem Einthoven, Dutch physiologist, inventor of closed chest cardiac message, better known as cardiopulmonary resuscitation or "CPR" (1860–1927)	
1861	American Civil War begins (to 1865) Louis Pasteur discovers anaerobic bacteria		*The Etiology, the Concept and Prophylaxis of Childbed Fever*, Ignaz Semmelweis offers iatrogenic explanation of puerperal fever
1862		Albert Moll, German–Protestant neurologist, and sexologist, author of the first German monograph on medical ethics; subjected to Nazi anti-Semitic measures by virtue of Jewish ancestry despite early conversion to Christianity (1862–1939)	
1863	First modern campaign against an animal researcher in Britain. President Abraham Lincoln signs the Emancipation Proclamation, freeing slaves in rebellious Confederate States Sphygmograph invented to measure blood pressure	Ignatz Nascher, Hungarian-American physician, founder of the field of geriatric medicine (1863–1945)	
1864	International Red Cross founded	Max Weber, German, founder of modern sociological theory (1864–1920),	
1865	General Robert E. Lee surrenders Confederate Army to General Ulysses S. Grant, Appomattox Court House, Virginia, ending U.S. Civil War (estimated 600,000 deaths) Joseph Lister begins aseptic surgery, introducing phenol as a disinfectant	Alfred Hoche, German psychiatrist, advocate of the involuntary mercy killing of the mentally ill (1865–1943) Hungarian physician Ignaz Semmelweiss beaten to death by medical attendants in Viennese insane asylum	*Versuche über Pflanzen-Hybride* (Treatise on Plant Hybrids), Abbot Gregor Mendel (1822–1884) introduces laws of inheritance and modern genetics *Introduction à l'Etude de la Médecine Expérimentale* (Introduction to Experimental Medicine) founder of modern physiology, Claude Bernard, drawing on Christian morality, states "never perform an experiment on man which might be harmful to him,

Dates	Events	Persons	Texts
	13th Amendment to U.S. Constitution ends slavery in the United States		even though the result might be highly advantageous to science;" urges animal experiments instead
1866	Clinical thermometer invented	Muhammad Rashid Rida, founder of the Salafiyya movement and fundamentalism in Islam (1865–1935) Abraham Flexner, American medical education reformer (1866–1958)	*Why Not? A Book for Every Woman* Horatio Robinson Storer, MD (1830–1922), popular pamphlet, makes the argument against abortion in terms of the need to protect women's health
1867	First international medical congress in Paris	Marie Curie (nee Marya Sklodowska), born in Warsaw (currently Poland, then Russia), French physicist; denied education in Russia as a Pole and a woman; emigrated to Paris to study physics and chemistry, first woman to teach at Sorbonne; codiscoverer of radium, awarded Nobel Prizes in 1903 (physics) and 1911 (chemistry); although a Catholic, was target of anti-Semitic campaign, died of radiation-induced leukemia (1867–1934)	
1868	AMA's Committee on Ethics rules that 1847 Code of Ethics does not exclude women from membership AMA expels leading ophthalmologist for advertising Meiji Emperor resumes rule, Japan modernizes	Richard Clarke Cabot, American physician, Professor of Medicine and Chair of Department of Social Ethics, Harvard University; founder Social Services department Massachusetts General Hospital; initiates Clinical-Pathological conferences at Massachusetts General Hospital; defends telling terminal patients the truth about their diagnosis (1868–1939)	
1869	Pope Pius IX's Vatican Council I (1869–1870) rejects distinction between "fetus animatus" (animated fetus, postquickening) and "fetus inanimatus" (prequickened inanimate fetus), making abortion at any stage of pregnancy an excommunicable offense. Sophia Jex-Blake (1840–1912) becomes first woman to matriculate in medicine at Edinburgh University; after university reverses this decision in 1873, Blake graduates as a physician from Irish College of Medicine Suez Canal opens		

(*continued*)

Dates	Events	Persons	Texts
1870	Franco–Prussian War 1870–1871 Pope Pius IX's Vatican Council I (1869–1870) announces doctrine of Papal Infallibility in moral teachings	Dr. Charles Killick Millard founder of first mercy- killing, voluntary euthanasia, advocacy group (1870–1952)	"Euthanasia," Samuel Williams published in *Essays of the Birmingham Speculative Club*, argues for mercy killing, which he calls "euthanasia"; earliest known use of term in this non-Baconian sense
1871	AMA votes to admit women members	Walter Bradford Cannon, American physician physiologist, research ethics reformer (1871–1945)	*Descent of Man*, Charles Darwin argues for the descent of man from earlier hominid mammals
1873	BMA admits first woman member, Elizabeth Garret Anderson (1836–1917), first British woman physician	Alexis Carrel, French-born American surgeon, botanist and eugenicist (1873–1944)	
1874	American Humane Society established AMA issues first censure of researcher for inhumane treatment of subjects London School of Medicine for Women (later the Royal Free Hospital) opens Louis Pasteur suggests placing instruments in boiling water to sterilize them		
1875	Public Health Act passes in Britain Victoria Street Society founded (later, National Anti-Vivisectionist society and British Union for the Abolition of Vivisection)		Munich medical society adopts AMA-style Code of Ethics
1876	Alexander Graham Bell patents the telephone Association of American Medical Colleges (AAMC) formed as Provisional Association of American Medical Colleges British parliament legalizes medical education for women. Cruelty to Animals Act enacted in Britain Robert Koch identifies the anthrax bacillus		*Karlsruhe* Code of Medical Ethics (Germany)

Dates	Events	Persons	Texts
1877			*Pastoral-Medcin* Carl Capellmann, influential work on Roman Catholic medical ethics (English translation as Pastoral Medicine, 1879)
1880	Blood parasite that causes malaria isolated	Abraham Jacobi (1830–1919), public health reformer, founder of the AMA specialty section on Diseases of Children (1880), leading figure in founding American pediatrics; President of AMA and leading opponent of AMA's Code of Ethics	
1881	Institute of Midwives established in London		
	Louis Pasteur devises a vaccine for anthrax		
1882	Robert Koch isolates tubercle bacillus		Amédée Dechambre, "Déontologie Médicale," *Dictionnaire Encyclopédique des Scienes* (Medical Deontology, published in Encyclopedic Dictionary of Science)
	Medical Society of New York adopts "New Code of Ethics:" permits association with irregulars, silent on physician–patient relations		Royal College of Physicians, *Of the Duties and Conduct of Fellows, Members and Licentiates*, title no longer contains reference to "ethics"
1883	Chancellor Otto von Bismarck introduces compulsory national health insurance in Germany	Margaret Louise Sanger, American social reformer and birth-control pioneer (1883–1966)	
	Robert Koch discovers cholera bacillus		
	Francis Galton coins the term "eugenics"		
1884		Eleanor Roosevelt, First Lady of the United States, first American Ambassador to the United Nations (UN), Chair, Committee that drafted UN's Universal Declaration of Human Rights (1884–1962)	*Archives of Pediatrics* began to be published, term "pediatrics" first appears in print
1885	Louis Pasteur develops rabies vaccine		
	Prussian ministerial decree regulating animal experiments		
1886	Association of American Physicians founded as "ethics free" alternative to the AMA for researchers and specialists		*The Relation of Hospitals to Medical Education*, Charles Francis Withington (1852–1917) proposes Bill of Rights for subjects of experiments "to secure patients against any injustice from the votaries of science"

(continued)

Dates	Events	Persons	Texts
1887			*Euthanasia; or Medical Treatment in Aid of An Easy Death*, William Munk, major palliative care text, "euthanasia" used in original Baconian sense
1888			*Götzen-Dämmerung, oder Wie man mit dem Hammer philosophiert (The Twilight of the Idols: Or, How to Philosophize with a Hammer)* Friedrich Nietzsche, characterizes the sick as "parasites of society"
1889	Johns Hopkins Hospital opens in Baltimore Germany's 74-year-old Chancellor Otto von Bismarck designs and implements the first state-funded pension for those "disabled from work by age (65) and disability" and a national health insurance plan		
1890	Vaccines against tetanus and diphtheria developed Surgical gloves introduced	Hasanayn Muhammad Makhluf, known as the "*Mufti* of the Egyptian Lands," was appointed *mufti* of Egypt in 1945 (1890–1990)	
1891	Humanitarian League founded in London to campaign for animal protections	Henry Sigerist, Swiss-American medical historian, founder of the social history of medicine movement (1891–1957)	
1892			*The Principles and Practice of Medicine: Designed for the Use of Practitioners and Students of Medicine*, William Osler, standard textbook of medicine in English-speaking world for approximately 40 years
1893	Johns Hopkins Medical School opens, curriculum designed by William Osler First open-heart surgery	Herman Göring, German, Nazi leader and antivivisectionist (1893–1946) Andrew C. Ivy, American physician, AMA representative at Nuremberg War Crime trials, proposed human rights–based code of research ethics to AMA, testifies on universal ethical principles of "civilized research" at Nuremberg trials, influenced Nuremberg Code of research ethics (1893–1978) Mahmud Shaltut, reformist Muslim religious scholar (1893–1963)	*Nightingale Pledge*, attributed to Lystra Gretter, a version of the Hippocratic oath adapted for nurses in an effort to elevate nursing to professional status, originally sworn by nursing graduates in Detroit, Michigan
1894	Nicholas II becomes last Czar of Russia		*On The Care of the Dying: A Lecture to Nurses*, Oswald Brown, one of last palliative care texts to use "euthanasia" in original Baconian sense

Dates	Events	Persons	Texts
1895	X-rays discovered by Wilhelm Roentgen (1845–1923)		*Das Recht Auf den Tod* (The Right to Die), Dr. Adolf Jost, first German monograph defending euthanasie (mercy killing, not Baconian palliation) for those who are a burden to themselves or to others
1896		Chauncey Leake, president American Pharmacology Society, American Association for Advancement of Science, American Association for History of Medicine, History of Science Society; initiated tradition of historical critiques of professional codes of ethics (1896–1978)	
1897	Malaria parasite located in the Anopheles mosquito		*Medicinische Deontologie* (Medical Deontology), Julius Pagel
	Bleach solution used to sanitize drinking water during typhoid epidemic in Maidenstone England, leads to water treatment throughout Britain and dramatic decrease in typhoid		*Studies in the Psychology of Sex*, Havelock Ellis, first of revolutionary 7-volume series in the psychology of sex
1899	Aspirin introduced		
	Boer War begins (ends 1902); British introduce "concentration camps" for noncombatant population, first use of the expression		
	London School of Hygiene and Tropical Medicine founded		
	Prussian disciplinary board condemns Albert Neisser for experimenting on patients without their consent		
1900	Association of German Doctors founded	Hans-Georg Gadamer German philosopher (1900–2002)	
	Bill to license researchers who use human subjects proposed in U.S. Congress		
	Human blood groups (A, O, B, identified)		
	Prussian Ministry for Medical Affairs issues directive requiring consent before any		

(continued)

Dates	Events	Persons	Texts
	patient can be used as a research subject		
	U.S. Army Yellow Fever Commission headed by Walter Reed confirms Finlay's hypothesis that Yellow fever is a mosquito-borne disease; Reed uses written consent forms from his human subjects		
1901	First Nobel Prizes; Emil von Behring, Germany, wins prize in medicine for serum therapy	Death of Queen Victoria (end of Victorian age)	
1902	Central Ethics Committee (CEC) of British Medical Association founded Registration of Midwives Act, Britain		*Ärztliche Ethik: Die Pflichten des Arztes in allen Beziehungen seiner Thätigkeit* (Physicians Ethics: Physicians Duties on all their Occupational Relationships), Albert Moll (1862–1939), discusses physician–patient relationships, criticizes unethical experiments in detail
1903	Anti-ethics rebels take control of AMA Electrocardiograph invented First appearance of term "pediatrician" in print U.S. Marine Hospital Service becomes "U.S. Public Health Service" Wright Brothers fly powered aircraft	Hans Jonas, German–Jewish theologian and philosopher taught at the New School for Social Research in New York City; introduced the Precautionary Principle; influenced development of environmental and research ethics (1903–1993)	First Russian translation of Moll's *Ärztliche Ethik* *Principles of Medical Ethics*, AMA, revision of 1847 Code of Ethics, construed as statement of advisory principles "The Use of Truth and Falsehood in Medicine," *British Medical Journal*, Richard Cabot, draws on "experimental method" to argue for telling terminal patients truth about their prognosis (essay revised and reprinted in various versions through 1938)
1904	Rockefeller Institute for Medical Research opens in New York City	Henry Beecher, American, Harvard anesthesiologist, headed committee that defined brain death, exposed abuses on human subject research (1904–1976) Karl Brandt, German, Hitler's personal physician, director of eugenic–euthanasia program (1904–1948) Georges Canguilhem, French physician, historian and philosopher of science; physician to the anti-German resistance during German occupation of France; professor at the Sorbonne; role model to a generation of French intellectuals and philosophers,	Second Russian translation of Moll's *Ärztliche Ethik*

Dates	Events	Persons	Texts
		including Michel Foucault (1904–1995)	
		Werner Theodore Otto Forssmann, German Physician, auto-experimenter, inventor of angiography (1904–1979)	
		Mustafa Al- Zarqa', Islamic legal scholar (1904–1998)	
1905	Alfred Ploetz founds Society for Racial Hygiene in Germany	Joseph Fletcher, American, Protestant Theologian, inventor of Situation Ethics (1905–1991).	
	First artificial hip joints	Leo (nee Leopold) Alexander, Austrian-born America–Jewish neurologist and psychologist, investigator for Nuremberg War Crimes Trial, contributed to Nuremberg Code (1905–1985)	
	First direct blood transfusion		
	U.S. Food and Drug Administration (FDA) founded		
	U.S. Supreme Court rules mandatory smallpox vaccination constitutional (*Jacobson v. Massachusetts*)		
1906	Accessory food factors (vitamins) discovered		
	Initiative by Charles Eliot Norton, founder the *Nation* magazine, to legalize euthanasia/ mercy killing in the state of Ohio, defeated by a vote of 79 to 23		
1907	"Typhoid Mary" (Mary Mallon, cook 1869–1938) first identified typhoid carrier, quarantined 1915–1938		
1908	AMA's Council for the Defense of Medical Research (CDMR) founded in response to antivivisectionist movement		*Canons of Professional Ethics,* American Bar Association
	Sulphanilamide first synthesized		
1909	Chinese Nursing Association established		"Doctor's Dilemma," play by George Bernard Shaw, "the medical profession [is] a conspiracy to hide its own shortcomings"

(*continued*)

Dates	Events	Persons	Texts
			"Longevity and Rejuvenescence," *New York Medical Journal*, Ignatz Nascher calls for a field of geriatrics modeled on pediatrics, first use of the term "geriatrics"
1910	Discovery of Salvarsan for syphilis, beginning of chemotherapy Swedish branch of Society for Racial Hygiene founded	Abd al Halim Mahmud, Sufi Muslim theologian and philosopher (1910–1978)	*Medical Education in the United States and Canada; A Report to the Carnegie Foundation*, Abraham Flexner (1866–1959) sets standards for science-clinic–based medical education that catalyze education reform movements in the United States and Canada
1911	National Insurance Act sets Bismarckian state medical insurance plan for Britain Massachusetts Society of Examining Physicians founded (later became American Society of Law, Ethics and Medicine, ASLME)	André Hellegers, Dutch-born, Edinburgh-educated physician, advisor to the Vatican, founder Joseph and Rose Kennedy Institute of Ethics (1911–1979) Muhammad Mutawalli Al-Muhammad Mutawalli al-Sha'rawi, commentator on the Qur'an (1911–1998)	
1912	AMA's Presidential Committee on Ethics, becomes the Judicial Council (later, the Council on Ethics and Judicial Affairs or CEJA); empowered to enforce AMA's Code of Ethics Term "vitamin'" coined Titanic sinks on maiden voyage	'Abd al-'Aziz B. 'Abd Allah Ibn Baz, a reformer who issued a collection entitled, *Fatwa Islamiyya* (1988, 1995) (1912–1999)	First Chinese translation of AMA's Code of Ethics *Principles of Medical Ethics*, AMA reasserts responsibility of physicians to obey profession's ethical standards
1913	First extracorporeal artificial kidney Medical Research Committee (Council from 1920) established in Britain	Paul Ramsey, American, Protestant theologian, wrote on death and dying, definition of death, transplant, genetics, and abortion; author of *Patient as Person* (1913–1988)	*Das monistische Jahrhundert* (The Monist Journal), edited by Ernst Haeckel, publishes open letter from a dying patient calling for a law to legalize *euthanasie*
1914	AMA's Council on Defense of Medical Research proposes research ethics principles – never implemented Outbreak of World War I (WWI) (ends 1918) Panama Canal opens		
1915	Chinese Medical Association established		

Dates	Events	Persons	Texts
1916	Margaret Sanger founds first American birth-control clinic Proposal to require consent of human subjects of experiments debated in AMA but considered unnecessary		"General Theory of Relativity," Albert Einstein (1879–1955) "The Black Stork," film shown in U.S. movie theaters until the 1940s based on eugenicist practices of Chicago physician Harry Haiselden, who withheld surgery from infants born with major but operable anomalies and who may have "speeded their deaths"
1917	Czar Nicholas II abdicates Russian throne Russia declared democratic republic; Bolsheviks seize power	Ali Jad al-Haqq Jad al-Haqq, appointed *Mufti Al-Diyar Al-Misriyya* (prime *mufti* of Egypt) in 1978, served as Minister of Religious Endowments in 1983, and was Sheikh Al-Azhar from 1982 until his death; his *fatwas* were published in *Al-Fatawa Al-Islamiyya* (1917–1997)	
1918	Armistice ends World War I Influenza pandemic kills 20 to 40 million people, exceeding death toll from WWI	Dame Cicely Saunders, British lady almoner (medical social worker) who qualified as a physician to found St. Christopher's Hospice (London) and the modern hospice movement (1918–2005)	
1919	Ernest Rutherford splits the atom, opening nuclear age Kaiser Wilhelm Institute for Genealogy founded in Munich, propounds theory of racial hygiene Weimar Republic in Germany (to 1933)		
1920	Abortion legalized in Russian Soviet Republic (first legalization in Western country) League of Nations formed Medical Research Council founded in Britain to fund research		*Die Freigabe der Vernichtung lebensunwerten Leben.* (Permission for the Destruction of Life Unworthy of Life), Karl Binding and Alfred Hoche: legal and medical arguments rejecting traditional medical morality and proclaiming "Life unworthy of life," declaring "ballast existence" and "useless eaters" subject to *euthanasie*
1921	Marie Stopes opens birth-control clinic in London	Immanuel Jakobovits, Chief Rabbi for the United Kingdom, wrote first book on Jewish medical ethics (1921–1999),	
1922	Physician-assisted suicide legalized and recriminalized in Russian Soviet Republic Union of Soviet Socialist Republics (USSR) formed	Richard McCormick, American, Roman Catholic Jesuit moral theologian, wrote "Notes on Moral Theology" for *Theological Studies* from 1965 to 1984, championing a liberal interpretation of the Catholic moral tradition (1922–2000)	

(continued)

Dates	Events	Persons	Texts
1923	Turkish republic formed – end of Ottoman Empire		
1924	AMA gives Council on Ethical and Judicial Affairs investigatory powers		
1925	Geneva Convention banning biological and chemical warfare		*Das Problem der Abküzung 'lebensunwerten' Lebens* (The Problem of the Curtailment of Life 'Unworthy' of Life) response to Binding and Hoche by Ewald Meltzer, director of the Katharinenhof Asylum at Grosshennersdorf, Saxony
1926	First enzyme (urease) crystallized	Michel Foucault, French philosopher, psychiatrist, philosopher of sex, postmodern theorist and historian of social institutions, including medicine: open homosexual and prisoners' rights activist; founder *Groupe d'information sur les prisons* (Information on Prisons Group), AIDS activist, died of AIDS (1926–1984) Ivan Illich, Viennese-born philosopher, priest, critic of technology, introduced concept of *iatrogenesis* in 1976 book *Medical Nemesis* (1926–2002) Elisabeth Kübler-Ross (1926–2004) Swiss-American psychiatrist and author of works on the psychology of dying André Hellegers (1926–1979), the "Pope's biologist," Roman Catholic lay theologian, founder and founding Director of the Kennedy Institute of Ethics at Georgetown University Muhammad B. Salih al-Uthaymin, one of the great muftis of Saudi Arabia, author of books on Islamic law and theology (1926–2001)	*Mein Kampf* (My Struggle), Adolf Hitler (1889–1945), envisions medical campaign to cleanse Germany on degenerates and defectives
1926	League of Nations *Slavery Convention* bans slavery globally		
1927	Iron lung invented Kaiser Wilhelm Institute for Anthropology, Human Heredity and Eugenics founded in Berlin Citing compulsory vaccination precedent, U.S. Supreme Court upholds eugenic		"The Care of the Patient," *Journal of the American Medical Association*, Francis Peabody (1881–1927) discusses patient care from the perspective of a physician who is also a terminal cancer patient; "One of the essential qualities of the clinician is interest in humanity, for the secret of the care of the patient is in caring for the patient"

Dates	Events	Persons	Texts
	sterilization of the "mentally unfit" (*Buck v. Bell*)		*Medical Ethics*, by Thomas Percival, ed. Chauncey Leake; editor's introduction offers delegitimating "etiquette" interpretation of Percival and of AMA's Code of Ethics
1928	Penicillin discovered		
	Vitamin C isolated		
1929	*Confédération des Syndicates Médicales Francais* (CSMF) formed		*Racial Hygiene: A Practical Discussion of Eugenics and Race Culture*, Thurman B. Rice (1888–2001); American eugenics tract
	Wall Street crash, heralds onset of world-wide economic depression		
	Werner Forssmann develops cardiac catheter using himself as first subject		
1930	First test to measure the clotting ability of blood		
	First sulfa drug		
1931	Japanese invasion and occupation of China begins with invasion and annexation of Manchuria (to 1945)	John C. Fletcher, American, Episcopal theologian and the first bioethicist for the U.S. National Institutes of Health (1931–2004)	*Guidelines for Innovative Therapies and Performing Scientific Experiments on Humans*, Germany Ministry of Interior: strengthens control on human subjects research, requiring prior animal experiments as well as consent of patient
1932	U.S. Public Health Service initiates Tuskegee study of untreated syphilis in African American males (to 1972), participants misinformed of nature of the experiment	Maurice Pappworth, British, qualified for Royal College of Physicians 1936 – awarded membership 57 years later, 1993; denied hospital consultancy because "no Jew could ever be a gentleman;" tutor to future consultants; wrote exposés of unethical human subjects research (1932–1994)	
	U.S. Secretary of the Navy orders experiments on human subjects to be limited to "informed volunteers"		
1933	National Socialists (Nazis) come to power in Germany		*The Professional Ethics of Medicine*, Song Guobin, first monograph on medical ethics in modern China
	Nazis enact laws to protect animals used in research, license animal researchers, and ban Kosher butchering		

(continued)

Dates	Events	Persons	Texts
	Law to Prevent Hereditarily Ill Offspring (Sterilization Law) enacted in Germany		
1935	Development of prefrontal lobotomy		*Rats, Lice, and History: being a study in biography, which, after twelve preliminary chapters indispensable for the preparation of the lay reader, deals with the life history of typhus fever*, Hans Zinsser (1878–1940) influential popular history of epidemic diseases
	Hitler pledges to introduce eugenic–euthanasia program should war break out		
	Social Security, a national old-age retirement fund, implemented in the United States		
	Voluntary Euthanasia Legislation Society formed in Britain to legalize mercy killing		
1936	Abortion criminalized in USSR		*Code de Déontologie* (Code of Ethics) *Confédération des Syndicats Médicales Français*
	Bill to legalize voluntary euthanasia defeated in British Parliament by combined medical and religious opposition 35 to 14		
	Electroconvulsive therapy (ECT) described		
1937	Cadavers become public property in USSR – consent of relatives not needed for autopsy or to harvest organs		
	Estrogen synthesized.		
	First antihistamine		
	Half of all physicians in USSR are women (first in any Western country)		
	Japanese invasion of China; Nanking atrocities commence ("Rape of Nanking"): Japanese military kills approximately 400,000 Chinese civilians, raping approximately 80,000 women (to 1938)		
	Vaccine against yellow fever		

Dates	Events	Persons	Texts
1938	Euthanasia Society of America founded by Reverend Charles Francis Potter		
	First total artificial hip replacement		
	New Zealand Social Security Act pioneers national health service		
1939	Aktion T-4 program granting *euthanasie* to children with disabilities commences in Nazi Germany (to 1941, more than 70,000 killed)	David Thomasma, American, founding bioethicist, bioethics educator, journal editor (1939–2002)	
	World War II (to 1945)		
1940	First gassing of mental patients in Nazi Germany		
	Penicillin developed		
	Rhesus factor in blood discovered		
	Vichy régime rules France (dissolves *Confédération des Syndicats Médicales Français*)		
1941	Rubella (German measles) in pregnancy linked to abnormalities in children		
	Swiss courts rule that assisting suicide is not a criminal offense		
1942	U.S. Supreme Court reverses itself on the legality of eugenic sterilization (*Skinner v. Oklahoma*)		*Social Insurance and Allied Services* (William) Beveridge Commission report paves way for British National Health Service
1943	First kidney dialysis machine		
	Streptomycin discovered		
1944	First blue-baby operation performed		
	Pope Pius XII addresses Italian Medical-Biological Union of St. Luke, summarizing Catholic medical ethics		

(*continued*)

Dates	Events	Persons	Texts
1945	First Spanish Medical Deontology Germany surrenders ending WWII in Europe (May 8) Hiroshima and Nagasaki Japan A-bombed (August 6, 9) Japan surrenders unconditionally ending WW II in Asia (August 15) London Agreement on the Punishment of the Major War Criminals of the European Axis	Lisbeth Haakonssen, Australian-American philosopher-historian, author of early monograph on history of modern medical ethics (1945–1999)	
1946	British Parliament passes legislation replacing Bismarck-style national health insurance plan with a government-run National Health Service First meeting of United Nations (UN) General Assembly in New York First randomized clinical trials of streptomycin for tuberculosis International War Crimes Tribunal for Far East (to 1948 – NB: no medical trials) Nuremberg Medical War Crimes Trials open (December 23), defendants accused of criminal experiments and crimes against humanity (*U.S. v Karl Brandt et al.*)	Roy Porter, English, prolific and influential historian of medicine, science, and the Enlightenment, coorganizer of early bioethicist-historian conferences on the history of medical ethics (1946–2002)	"Principles of Research Ethics," AMA, require medical supervision, subject consent, prior animal experimentation for experiments on human subjects "Sinews of Peace" speech, Sir Winston Churchill (1874–1965) declares Cold War in "Iron Curtain" speech delivered at Westminster College (Missouri): "From Stettin in the Baltic to Trieste in the Adriatic an *iron curtain* has descended across the Continent. Behind that line lie all the capitals of the ancient states of Central and Eastern Europe. Warsaw, Berlin, Prague, Vienna, Budapest, Belgrade, Bucharest and Sofia . . . in what I must call the Soviet sphere, and all are subject in one form or another, not only to Soviet influence but to a very high and, in some cases, increasing measure of control from Moscow"
1947	Nuremberg Medical War Crimes Trial end (October): 15 defendants found guilty of crimes against humanity, 7 sentenced to death World Medical Association (WMA) founded in London		*Nuremberg Code*: in passing judgment on Nazi researchers and doctors, Nuremberg War Crimes Tribunal cites 10 Principles of Research Ethics as universally accepted by all civilized societies – including the principle of informed voluntary consent of the subject

Dates	Events	Persons	Texts
1948	British National Health Service opens U.S. National Institutes of Health (NIH) founded World Health Organization (WHO) formed within the UN		*Declaration of Geneva*, WMA: modernized version of the Hippocratic Oath, promulgated in reaction to Nuremberg Trials *Sexual Behavior in the Human Male*, Alfred Kinsey (1894–1956), first major empirical study of male sexual conduct *Universal Declaration of Human Rights*, UN General Assembly, written by committee headed by Eleanor Roosevelt; inspired, in part, by revelations at Nuremberg Trials; bans slavery; lays foundation for international bioethics
1949	Council for International Organizations of Medical Science (CIOMS) established by UNESCO and WHO Soviet Khabarovsk war crimes trial of Japanese physicians for chemical and biological experiments on humans		*International Code of Medical Ethics*, WMA "Medical Science Under Dictatorship," Leo Alexander: influential analysis of medical atrocities: attributes problem to medical "ethical" principles valuing group/state over individual/patient; praises Dutch for resisting Nazi medical "ethics," Nazi medicine
1950	Pius XII declares Alphonsus, Patron Saint of Confessors and of Moral theologians		
1951	First heart–lung machine Japan Medical Association issues its first code of medical ethics		
1952	Amniocentesis developed Jonas Salk (1914–1995) develops a killed virus vaccine against polio; Open-heart surgery begins Polio epidemic in Copenhagen leads to the invention of the first practical artificial ventilator by anesthesiologist Bjorn Ibsen; mortality rate lowered from 87 percent to 26 percent		

(*continued*)

Dates	Events	Persons	Texts
	Pope Pius XII addresses 1st International Congress of Histopathology of Nervous System, endorses scientific research for human good, subject to moral constraints, announces Principle of Totality – that the good of the part is subordinate to the good of the whole		
	U.S. Army adopts Nuremberg Principles for human subjects research		
1953	At 26th Congress of Urology Pius XII endorses organ transplants declaring that the Totality Principle, that every part of the human body "exists for the sake of the whole" (St. Thomas Aquinas, *Summa Theologica* II, Question 65, Article 1), permits sacrifice of a part of the human body for the continued survival for the person		*Sexual Behavior in the Human Female*, Alfred Kinsey, first major empirical study of female sexual conduct
	Experiments demonstrate that tobacco tars cause cancer in mice		
	First Intensive Care Unit (ICU) opened in Copenhagen by Bjorn Ibsen		
	James Watson and Francis Crick describe the double-helical structure of DNA		
	Joseph Stalin dies, paving the way for reform of the USSR		
1954	Albert Sabin (1906–1993) develops oral polio vaccine by using weakened live virus		*Morals and Medicine, The Moral Problems of the Patient's Right to Know the Truth, Contraception, Artificial Insemination, Sterilization, and Euthanasia*, Joseph F. Fletcher applies philosophical ethics (Situational Ethics) to medical ethical dilemmas, affirms patients' rights to know the truth and to euthanasia – written before the creation of bioethics discourse
	First successful kidney transplant		
	Jonas Salk's vaccine successful in large scale clinical trials		

Dates	Events	Persons	Texts
	Pope Pius XII addresses the 8th Congress WMA, endorses consent-based research on humans, and organ donation (corneas)		*Principles for Those in Research and Experimentation*, WMA, introduces concept of surrogate consent – absent from Nuremberg code and earlier research ethics
	Universities Federation for Animal Welfare (UFAW) initiates project to define humane principles for research on animals (project produces Three Rs Principles of 1959)		
1956	Abortion legalized in USSR		*Vprosy Khirurgichesko Deontologii* (Problems of Surgical Deontology) introduces concept of "deontology" into Russia medical discourse
	Pope Pius XII informs Italian Society of the Science of Anesthetics that analgesia intended to remove of pain and consciousness is permitted "even if one foresees that the use of drugs will shorten life . . . provided that no other means exist"		
	UN adopts International Covenant on Civil and Political Rights (reiterates ban on slavery, including child slavery)		
1957	Bruno Haid, Austrian anesthesiologist, petitions Pope Pius XII for permission to disconnect mechanical ventilator for patients with no hope of recovery; Pope states that it is permissible to disconnect a ventilator provided the patient or a surrogate consents, because the ventilator represents an "extraordinary means,'" of preserving life; Pius XII also recognizes brain death but forbids euthanasia		
	Treaty of Rome, lays foundation for European Union (EU)		

(*continued*)

Dates	Events	Persons	Texts
	WHO-supported large-scale tests establish safety and efficacy of Sabin oral polio vaccine		
1958	European Economic Communitys (precursor of EU) founded		
	Ultrasound diagnosis of fetal disorders		
1959			*Jewish Medical Ethics*, Immanuel Jakobovits, first book on the subject, defines the concept of "Jewish medical ethics"
			"Le Coma Dépassé" Revue Neurologique, Pierre Mollaret, M. Coulon – first identification of brain death. The Principles of Humane Experimental Technique, W. M. S. Russell and R. L. Burch, first statement of Three Rs Principles for humane research on animals: Reduction (of numbers of animals used in research), Refinement (to decrease experiments involving pain and suffering), Replacement (of experiments involving animals with those that do not)
1961	21st Congress of Communist Party of USSR initiates moral rebuilding initiative		*Torzhestvennogo Obeshanija Vracha* (Solemn Oath of a Medical Doctor), Sechenov Moscow Medical Institute Number 1; part of moral rebuilding initiative
	Belding Scribner, Seattle physician, invents arteriovenous shunt, makes prolonged renal dialysis possible		
	Harvard Medical School issues research ethics guidelines that weaken informed consent requirements for "therapeutic" experiments		
1962	Cuban missile crisis		*A History of American Medical Ethics, 1847–1912*. Donald Konold, first monograph on the history of American medical ethics
	Pope John XXIII convenes Vatican Council II (1962–1965): urges Roman Catholic church to modernize, to engage other faiths in ecumenical dialogue and to engage with secular world; mass delivered in vernacular		"They Decide Who Lives Who Dies," *Life Magazine*, Shana Alexander – questions Belding Scribner's "God Committee's" right to determine access to renal dialysis

Dates	Events	Persons	Texts
	Research guidelines, BMA, British Medical Research Council		Maurice Pappworth publishes 14 examples of research in violation of the Nuremberg Code
	Thalidomide no longer prescribed for pregnant women: birth defects resulting from administration of the drug fuel an international debate over therapeutic abortions		
1963	First human liver transplant		*Naissance del la Clinique: une archéologie du regard medical* (Birth of the Clinic: An Archaeology of Medical Perception), Michel Foucault analyzes clinical relationships in terms of power and dominance
	London Medical Group (LMG) founded by Edward Shotter, Anglican priest, to organize lectures and symposia on medical ethics at London medical schools – publishes *Journal of Medical Ethics* (from 1975)		*Responsibility in Investigations on Human Subjects*, British Medical Research Council
	Measles vaccine licensed for general use in the United States		
	Tranquilizer "Valium" (diazepam) introduced		
1964	Gulf of Tonkin resolution authorizes Pres. Lyndon Johnson to initiate U.S. participation in Vietnam civil war (to 1975)		*Declaration of Helsinki*, WMA statement on the ethics of research on human subjects
	Home dialysis initiated		*La Relación Médico-Enfermo: Historia y Teoría* (The Physician–Patient Relationship: History and Theory) Pedro Laín Entralgo (1908–2001) groundbreaking history of physician–patient relationship
			U.S. *Surgeon General's Report on Smoking*, declares smoking likely cause of lung cancer
1965	U.S. national health insurance programs initiated for those over 65 (Medicare) and, jointly with states and counties, for the medically indigent (Medicaid)		

(*continued*)

Dates	Events	Persons	Texts
1966	Great Proletarian Cultural Revolution begins in Mao Zedong's China, intellectuals and physicians persecuted, Confucius' tomb and temple vandalized (to 1976) U.S. Laboratory Animal Welfare Act		"Ethics and Clinical Research," *New England Journal of Medicine*, Henry Beecher – influential exposé of the abuse of human research subjects in the United States "Concentration Camps for Dogs" photo-essay in *Life Magazine*, prompts U.S. congress to pass Animal Welfare Act UN code of research ethics
1967	Abortion liberalized in Great Britain, no longer criminal offense First aortocoronary bypass operation (CABG) for blocked arteries performed at Cleveland Clinic by Argentine surgeon Rene Favaloro (1923–2000) First human heart transplant operation performed in South Africa by South African surgeon Christiaan Barnard (1922–2001) Mammography for detecting breast cancer introduced		*Human Guinea Pigs*, Maurice Pappworth – exposé of research abuse; 205 experiments cited in institutions and prisons; 78 in British National Health Service hospitals
1968	Uniform Anatomical Gift Act, (U.S.) National Conference of Commissioners on Uniform State Laws – permits competent adults to donate organs and tissues after death		"A Definition of Irreversible Coma: Report of the Ad Hoc Committee at Harvard University to Examine the Definition of Brain Death," *Journal of the American Medical Association*; Committee chaired by Henry Beecher introduces concept of "brain death," creates basis for transplantation from cadaveric donors *Humane Vitae*, Pope Paul VI, rejects recommendations for reform and reaffirms Catholic church's traditional teaching prohibiting birth control and artificial means of reproduction
1969	Hastings Center founded under the title "The Institute of Society, Ethics and the Life Sciences" in Hastings-on-Hudson, New York by philosopher Daniel Callahan and psychiatrist Willard Gaylin		*Daedalus: Journal of the American Academy of Arts and Sciences*, Special Issue on Research on Human Subjects *Doctor and Patient*, Pedro Laìn Entralgo, influential English translation of *La Relación Médico-Enfermo: Historia y Teoría El Médico y el Enfermo*, a history of the physician–patient relationship

Dates	Events	Persons	Texts
	Institute for Medical Humanities of the José Maria Mainetti Foundation founded in La Palta, Argentina		*Medische Macht en Medische Ethiek* (Medical Power and Medical Ethics) by Dutch psychiatrist Jan van den Berg argues that physicians' duty "to protect save and prolong human life" is limited to contexts "where and when this is meaningful"
	Neil Armstrong lands on the Moon		
	Patrick Steptoe and Robert Edwards of the British National Health Service announce the fertilization of human eggs outside the body (In Vitro Fertilization, IVF)		*On Death and Dying*, Elisabeth Kübler-Ross presents a 5-stage analysis of the psychology of dying based on interviews with terminal patients
	Society for Health and Human Values (SHHV) founded in the United States		
1970	First U.S. state (Kansas) legally recognizes brain death		*Asia-Jewish Medical Ethics* in Hebrew
	Hastings Center taskforces founded in four areas –Death and Dying; Behavior Control; Genetics, Population – would later issue influential reports		*The Patient as Person*, Protestant theologian Paul Ramsey develops theory of research subjects' rights
1971	Abortion and forced sterilization legalized in India		*Bioethics: Bridge to the Future*, Van Rensselaer Potter (1911–2001); first use of "bioethics" in print; Potter's usage is broader than Sargent Shriver's, who used the term in naming Center for Bioethics (Kennedy Institute) in the same year; Potter's usage emphasizes what later became known as "environmental ethics," which Potter characterized as the "science of survival;" Shriver's usage, which became dominant, emphasizes ethics in biotechnology and medicine
	Eunice Kennedy Shriver produces film "Who Shall Survive" about decision made at Johns Hopkins University Hospital (Baltimore, U.S.) by an infant's parents to allow it to die, refusing to consent to a surgical repair of a blockage to its stomach because the infant was "Mongoloid" (had Down syndrome, trisomy 21)		
	Joseph and Rose Kennedy Institute of Ethics founded as the Center for Bioethics in the Joseph and Rose Kennedy Center for the		

(*continued*)

Dates	Events	Persons	Texts
	Study of Human Reproduction and Bioethics at Georgetown University in Washington DC by Dutch biologist Andres Hellegers – NB term "bioethics" in title coined by cofounder Sargent Shriver, during a party he gave with his wife and cofounder, Eunice		
	Solemn Oath of a Medical Doctor mandatory at all medical schools in the Soviet Union (to 1990)		
1972	Computerized axial tomography (CAT scan) introduced commercially		*The Angel of Bethesda An Essay Upon the Common Maladies of Mankind*, Cotton Mather, a self-help medical guide for Puritans completed in 1724, first published in 1972, discusses medical ethics
	End-stage renal disease incorporated into U.S. Medicare Program; provides national health insurance coverage for all citizens for dialysis and kidney transplants		*Bibliography of Bioethics* edited by Le Roy Walters
			Code of Medical Ethics, Medical Council of India
	Total hip arthroplasty technique developed by British surgeon John Chamley provides effective practical method of hip replacement		*Euthanasie* (Euthanasia) by Dutch physician P. Muntendam, initiates debate over euthanasia in the sense of mercy killing in the Netherlands
	Professional Standards Review Organizations (PSROs) introduced in the United States		*Experimentation with Human Beings*, Jay Katz, groundbreaking compendium on history of ethical and legal regulation of human subjects research
			Modern Medicine and Jewish Law, Fred Rosner
			Moral Dilemmas in Medicine, A. V. Campbell book based on a course for nurses, by philosopher and lecturer in Christian Ethics at Edinburgh University, and later founding editor of the *Journal of Medical Ethics*, Professor of Biomedical Ethics at Otago Medical School, New Zealand, and of Ethics in Medicine at Bristol University, England)
			First British publication to interpret modern medical ethics in terms of moral philosophical theory
			Washington Star article by Jean Heller of the Associated Press blows the whistle on U.S. Public Health Service's (USPHS) Tuskegee Syphilis Study (source of story was former USPHS employee Peter Buxtun)

Dates	Events	Persons	Texts
1973	Dutch physician Geetruda Postma found guilty of mercy killing her 78-year-old mother; given suspended sentence of 1 week		*Ética en medicina*, A. León Cecchini, transitional work bridges Spanish medical deontology and bioethics
	KNMG (Royal Dutch Medical Association) negotiates arrangement with Dutch prosecutors: physicians will not face prosecution if mercy killing restricted to informed, suffering, competent patients who voluntarily and explicitly make reiterated requests for euthanasia, provided no alternative routes to relieve suffering available and second physician confirms these conditions satisfied		English translation of Michel Foucault's *Naissance del la Clinique: une archéologie du regard medical* as *Birth of the Clinic: An Archaeology of Medical Perception*
			The Final Report of the Tuskegee Syphilis Study Ad Hoc Advisory Committee reviews Tuskegee Syphilis study, which was formally terminated
			Patient's Bill of Rights, *American Hospital Association*
	P. Mutendam, leading member of KNMG, founds *Nederlandse Vereniging voor een Vrijwillig Levenseinde* (NVVE, Netherlands Society for the Right to Die)		
	Roe v Wade, U.S. Supreme Court decriminalizes abortion		
	Soviet-style medical oaths introduced into East European countries		
1974	U.S. National Research Act, requires institutional review boards (IRBs) to review, approve, and monitor research on humans; also establishes National Commission for the Protection of Human Subject of Biomedical and Behavioral Research (to 1978)		*Medical Nemesis*, Ivan Illich introduces concept of medically induced illness, in article in *Lancet* (has not yet coined "iatrogenic")
			New Catholic Encyclopedia, first Roman Catholic encyclopedia to have section on "Medical Ethics," earlier encyclopedias of 1967 and 1911 do not contain such an entry

(continued)

Dates	Events	Persons	Texts
1975	Generalissimo Francisco Franco dies, Juan Carlos Borbón assumes throne; democratization of Spain begins		*Animal Liberation*, Peter Singer introduces concept of *speciesism* – unethical bias toward one's own species – intellectual basis of modern antianimal experimentation movement
	Research Center for Bioethics founded in Barcelona, Spain		*Journal of Medical Ethics* published by London Medical Group
	Society for the Study of Medical Ethics formed in UK (later, Institute for Medical Ethics)		*On Dying Well*, Board of Social Responsibility, Church of England, working report (included moral theologian G. R. Dunstan, and hospice pioneer, Dame Cicely Saunders) endorsing palliative and hospice care at the end of life, while condemning euthanasia
	Thirty-Five nations sign Helsinki accords on cooperation and human rights		
	Tokyo amendment to *Declaration of Helsinki* requires peer review via ethics committees or IRBs		
1976	Ebola virus epidemic in Sudan and Zaire		*Death, Dying and the Biological Revolution*, Robert Veatch, philosophical analysis of concept of brain death
	In Re Quinlan, NJ Supreme Court decides that Karen Ann Quinlan's right to privacy encompasses the right to disconnect a ventilator, and that her parents may act as her surrogates in making this decision		*Medical Nemesis*, Ivan Illich introduces concept of iatrogenic illness, that is, medically induced illness
	Natural Death Act of California establishes right to refuse certain life-sustaining treatments		*Resolution on the Rights of the Sick and the Dying*, Council of Europe
	Tarasoff v Regents of the University of California establishes psychiatrists' duty to breach confidentiality and warn specific persons likely to be endangered by a patient		
1977	Criminalization of amniocentesis for sex selection in India		*Dictionary of Medical Ethics*, edited by A. S. Duncan, G. R. Dunstan, and R. B. Wellbourn, many contributors from the London Medical Group
	Popular protest leads to repeal of India's forced sterilization policy		*Ethics in Medicine: Historical Perspectives and Contemporary Concerns*, Stanley Reiser, Arthur Dyck, William Curran:

Dates	Events	Persons	Texts
			groundbreaking anthology distinctive for its emphasis on the history of medical ethics
			Legacies in Ethic and Medicine, Chester Burns, early collection of papers by historians on history of medical ethics
			Professional Conduct and Discipline, General Medical Council (Britain)
1978	Louise Joy Brown, first human baby born using IVF "test tube" born in England, dubbed "test tube" baby by the press		*Encyclopedia of Bioethics,* edited by Warren Reich, presents the subject matter of the new field of *bioethics* – one of the earliest uses of the term "bioethics" – contains 97,000-word entry, "Medical Ethics: History of" edited by Albert Jonsen, with an appendix of historical texts edited by Robert Veatch
	U.S. National Commission for the Protection of Human Subjects of Biomedical and Behavioral Research recommends that "institutions receiving federal support for the conduct of research involving human subjects should be governed by uniform federal regulations applicable to the review of all such research;" this policy, later known as "the common rule," is not implemented until 1991		*Alternatives to Animal Experiments,* David Smyth, survey of known Three R humane alternatives to standard treatment of animals in research laboratories
1979	People's Republic of China introduces mandatory "one child policy," limiting families to one child, to deal with overpopulation		*Belmont Report,* U.S. National Commission for the Protection of Human Subjects stipulates three ethical principles governing research: beneficence, respect for persons, and justice – provides first comprehensive ethical rationale for research ethics
	WHO declares the eradication of smallpox, although cultures of the virus are kept by the Centers for Disease Control and Prevention (CDC) in the U.S. and at the Institute of Virus Preparations in Siberia, Russia		*Das Prinzip Veramtwortung: Versuch einer Ethik für die technologische Zivilisation,* (The Imperative of Responsibility: In Search of an Ethics for the Technological Age) Hans Jonas: introduces *Vorsorgeprinzip* (Precautionary Principle), a core moral principle of the European "Green" or environmental movement

(continued)

Dates	Events	Persons	Texts
			Principles of Biomedical Ethics, Tom Beauchamp and James Childress stipulate four principles for both clinical and research ethics – beneficence, nonmaleficence, autonomy, and justice – exceedingly influential comprehensive theory of bioethics
1980	Experimental vaccine against hepatitis B developed Center for Bioethics founded in Paris. Hemlock Society founded in the United States by Derek Humphrey to champion assisted suicide U.S. President's Commission for the Study of Ethical Problems in Medicine and Biomedical and Behavioral Research formed (to 1983)		*Declaration on Euthanasia*, Pope John Paul II forbids euthanasia but permits disconnection of ventilators for terminal patients with patient or surrogate's consent *Universal Islamic Declaration of Human Rights* (UIDHR), issued in Paris
1981	AIDS recognized by CDC Brain death recognized by Canada Center for Alternatives to Animal Research founded at the Johns Hopkins University School of Public Health Hastings Center Working Group on AIDS and Ethics formed		*A Theory of Medical Ethics*, Robert Veatch criticizes Hippocratic ethics as paternalistic and offers a contractarian theory of bioethics in its place *Bad Blood: The Tuskegee Syphilis Experiment*, Jones, James, definitive study of the USPHS's Tuskegee syphilis experiment *Defining Death*, U.S. President's Commission, recognizes "brain death" *Familiaris Consortio*, "On the Role of the Christian Family in the Modern World," Pope John Paul II denounces abortion and condemns as corrupt the ideal of an "autonomous power of self-affirmation . . . for one's own selfish well-being" *Unmasking of Medicine*, by British legal reformer, Ian Kennedy: a critique of British medicine and medical paternalism inspired, in part, by Ivan Illich's *Medical Nemesis*
1982	Dr. Barney Clark, patient at University of Utah hospital receives Jarvick-7 artificial heart implant and survives for 112 days		*Clinical Ethics*, Albert Jonsen, Mark Siegler, and William Wimslade, highly influential casuistic approach (the four box method) to clinical ethics

Dates	Events	Persons	Texts
	Hospital research ethics committees set up in People's Republic of China		International Guidelines for Biomedical Research Involving Human Subjects, *Council of International Organizations of Medical Science (CIOMS)*
	Swiss charity, Exit, offers assistance in suicide to terminally ill patients who are Swiss nationals		*Splicing Life*, U.S. President's Commission, coins expression "genetic engineering"
1983	*Comité National d'Etique* (French National Committee on Ethics) founded		*Deciding to Forego Life-Sustaining Treatment*, President's Commission: legitimates advance directives, and consensual withholding and withdrawing of life-sustaining treatment
	Peer Review Organizations (PROs) replace PSROs in the United States		*The Case for Animal Rights*, Tom Regan: philosophical defense of animal rights
1984	"Alkmaar Case," Dutch Supreme Court officially recognizes the agreement between Dutch prosecutors and the KNMG re: nonprosecution for mercy killing		*The Imperative of Responsibility: In Search of an Ethics for the Technological Age*, Hans Jonas, introduces the Precautionary Principle (*Vorsorgeprinzip*) into the English-language bioethics and environmental ethics literatures
	Ministry of Health, People's Republic of China, sets up advisory committee on bioethics		*Inquiry into Human Fertilisation and Embryology*, Dame Mary Warnock et al., leads to UK legislation permitting embryo research
	National Organ Donor Transplantation Act (U.S.) prohibits sale or purchase of human organs, empowers United Network for Organ Sharing (UNOS), a nonprofit agency, to allocate donated organs		*Silent World of Doctor and Patient*, Jay Katz – powerful critique of physician paternalism
1985			*International Guiding Principles for Biomedical Research Involving Animals*, WHO CIOMS
1986	Gene for Duchenne muscular dystrophy discovered		*Declaration on Chemical and Biological Weapons*, WMA
	Human Genome Project set up; funds set aside for ethical and social implications of project		*Declaration of Physician Independence and Professional Freedom*, WMA
	Instituto Colombiano de Estudios Bioéticos founded, Bogota, Columbia		*European Convention for the Protection of Vertebrate Animals Used for Experimental and Other Scientific Purposes*, Council of Europe

(continued)

Dates	Events	Persons	Texts
	Model U.S. federal policy for the protection of human subjects (the common rule) published for discussion		
	Pope John Paul II inaugurates Center for Bioethics in Rome		
	Society for Bioethics Consultation (SBC) founded in the United States		
	U.S. Congress passes Alternatives to Animal Use in Research, Testing and Education Act		
1987			*Donum Vitae* ("Instructions on Respect for Human Life"), Congregation for the Doctrine of the Faith, approved by Pope John Paul II: affirms sanctity of human life; condemns killing even for eugenic or public health reasons; condemns abortion, euthanasia, suicide; defines embryos as persons; condemns nontherapeutic genetic engineering and sex selection; legitimates consensual experiments on humans if within moral law; legitimates consent-based cadaveric and live donor organ transplantation
			The Emergence of Roman Catholic Medical Ethics in North America: An Historical Methodological–Bibliographical Study, David Kelly: major historical study of Roman Catholic medical ethics
1988	European Society for the Philosophy of Medicine and Healthcare formed, holds first annual conference		*The Abuse of Casuistry: A History of Moral Reasoning*, Albert Jonsen and Stephan Toulmin: offer an alternative to Beauchamp and Childress's principalism grounded in casuistic approach to moral reasoning
	Medical Research Councils of Germany, Sweden, and 8 other European countries, accept somatic cell gene therapy as legitimate form of clinical research		*Bioética*, Fernando Lolas, a guide to bioethics for Latin American readers
			For the Patient's Good: The Restoration of Beneficence in Health Care, Edmund Pellegrino and David Thomasma argue that the ethics of autonomy has been overemphasized, and urge a new ethics of dedication, competence and trust

Dates	Events	Persons	Texts
			La crisis de la razón médica. Introducción a la filosofía de la medicina, José Alberto Mainetti, introduces the bioethical paradigm to Latin America
			Racial Hygiene: Medicine Under the Nazis, Robert Proctor: argues that Holocaust was an expression of a eugenic-racial–public health movement
1989	*Consulta di Bioetica,* secular Italian bioethics consultant group founded		*Fundamentos de Bioética,* Diego Gracia, The first major bioethics textbook in Spanish
	Danish Council of Ethics rejects brain death		*Glover Report to the European Commission* on new reproductive technologies
	"East–West Conference on Medical Ethics," Pecs, Hungary		
	Peter Singer Affair, Germany: Australian–Jewish philosopher attacked as "Nazi" and silenced during lecture by militant Cripples Movement because Singer argues that infanticide of severely handicapped infants is morally permissible. Prominent Social Democrats push for formal government declaration that the thought of Anglo-Saxon Bioethics institutes "such as the Kennedy Institute of Ethics, the Hastings Center, or the Center for Human Bioethics (in Australia)," be declared "incompatible with the norms of the [German] Constitution"		
	Wellcome conferences on history of medical ethics commence (to 1990)		
	"When Medicine Went Mad: Bioethics and the Holocaust," conference hosted by prominent bioethicist Arthur Caplan		

(*continued*)

Dates	Events	Persons	Texts
1990	*Cruzan v Director Missouri Department of Health*, U.S. Supreme Court, upholds the patient's right to withdraw life-sustaining treatments, including artificial nutrition and hydration, and affirms the right of individual states to regulate standards of consent for such withdrawals, including "clear and convincing evidence" standard for surrogate consent ELABE, Latin American School of Bioethics founded in Argentina by Jose Alberto Mainetti France and Spain appoint research "Ethics Committees" (RECs) Human Genome project initiated: includes funding for ELSI project on the Ethical, Legal, and Social Implications of the genomics Italian National Bioethics Committee appointed Retired U.S. pathologist Jack Kevorkian assists Janet Adkins to suicide after she experiences the initial symptoms of Alzheimer's disease		*Classic Cases in Medical Ethics: Accounts of Cases that Have Shaped Medical Ethics With Philosophical, Legal and Historical Backgrounds*, Gregory Pence: major bioethics textbook centered on history of classic cases *Declaration of Inuyama*, consensus statement by representatives of 24 countries on human gene mapping, genetic screening and testing and human gene therapy
1991	Collapse of USSR "Common Rule" (currently the Office for Human Research Protections (OHRP) Federal Policy for the Protection of Human Subjects) governing research on human subjects research formally adopted by 16 U.S. government agencies		*Commissie Onderzoek Medische Praktijk inzake Euthanasie* (Remmelink Commission) finds significant underreporting of mercy killing and massive euthanizing of patients incapable of consenting: violations of the agreements tolerating mercy killing *Final Exit: The Practicalities of Self-Deliverance and Assisted Suicide for the Dying*, Derek Humphry: a popular best selling book on killing one's self

Dates	Events	Persons	Texts
	Jack Kevorkian's license to practice medicine revoked by U.S. state of Michigan		*Strangers at the Bedside: A History of How Law and Bioethics Transformed Medical Decision Making*, David Rothman, first monograph on the history of bioethics
			"On Being Silenced in Germany," Peter Singer, *New York Review of Books*, Peter Singer's reflections on academic freedom and the censorship of his speeches and writings in Germany
1992	Birth of Bioethics Conference organized by Albert Jonsen at University of Washington		*Medicine Betrayed: The Participation of Doctors in Human Rights Abuses*, Working Party, BMA
	Edict of Inquisition lifted against Galileo Galilei by Pope John Paul II "Galileo, a sincere believer, showed himself to be more perceptive . . . regard[ing] the relationship between religion and science than the theologians who opposed him"		*Nazi Doctors and the Nuremberg Code: Human Rights in Human Experimentation*, eds. George Annas and Michael Grodin: ground-breaking reassessment of Nuremberg Code
			Patients' Bill of Rights revised, American Hospital Association
	International Association of Bioethics (IAB) founded in Amsterdam; Peter Singer elected first president		*When Medicine Went Mad: Bioethics and the Holocaust*, ed., Arthur Caplan
	"Presumed consent" model organ donation adopted in Russia authorizes use of organs without donor's consent unless donor or relatives explicitly opt out of donation		
1993	Advisory Committee on Human Radiation Experiments (ACHRE), led by bioethicist Ruth Faden, established by U.S. President William Clinton to investigate unethical radiation research (to 1996)		*Doctors and Ethics: The Earlier Historical Settings of Professional Ethics*, Andrew Wear, Johanna Geyer-Kordesch, trailblazing collection of papers by professional historians of medicine
	First World Congress on Alternatives and Animal Use in the Life		*The Codification of Medical Morality*, Volume I, Robert Baker, Dorothy and Roy Porter: papers by bioethicists and historians challenge traditional construction of history of medical ethics

(*continued*)

Dates	Events	Persons	Texts
	Sciences were held in (Baltimore, U.S.) Michigan bans assisted suicide in response to Kevorkian's assistance in suicides U.S. NIH Revitalization Act requires inclusion of minorities and women in clinical research (called "new paradigm")		*International Guidelines for Biomedical Research Involving Human Subjects* (revised) CIOMS
1994	American Association of Bioethics (AAB) founded The Americas declared polio free British House of Lords, rejects legalization of euthanasia Pan-American Health Organization (PAHO) forms Regional Program in Bioethics, Santiago de Chile		*Dakar Declaration*, Inter-Country Consultation of the African Network on Ethics, Law and HIV: statement of ethical principles, legal and human rights of individuals affected with AIDS *Death and Deliverance: 'Euthanasia' in Germany c. 1900–1945*, Michael Burleigh traces origins of Nazi euthanasia program to pre–Nazi Weimar Germany *Factories of Death: Japanese Biological Warfare, 1932–1945, and the American Cover-up*, Sheldon Harris documents Japanese scientists use of prisoners of war as subjects in biological warfare research during the Japanese occupation of Manchuria and subsequent U.S. cover-up in exchange for Japanese expertise on biological warfare *Growing Up Tobacco Free*, Institute of Medicine – urges restraints on tobacco advertising
1995	WHO licensed to develop and to distribute malaria vaccine		*Codification of Medical Morality*, Volume II, ed., Robert Baker challenges delegitimating histories of medical ethics *Encyclopedia of Bioethics*, 2nd edition, edited by Warren Reich *Evangelicum Vitae*, Pope John Paul II, statement on the dignity and value of the human being condemns current "culture of death" as "conspiracy against life" that undermines the life of the most vulnerable and "betrays a completely individualistic concept of freedom, which ends up by becoming the freedom of 'the strong' against the weak who have no choice but to submit"

Dates	Events	Persons	Texts
			International Guidelines for Biomedical Research Involving Human Subjects, revised, CIOMS. *Medical Ethics in the Renaissance*, Winfried Schleiner, theorizes on the converso Jewish origins of secular medical ethics
			Peter Singer in Deutschland: Zur Gefährdung der Diskussionsfreiheit in der Wissenschaft, (Peter Singer in Germany: Threats to Freedom of Scientific Discussion) ed. Hartmut Kliemt: a collection of papers on the Peter Singer affair
			Subjected to Science: Human Experimentation in America before the Second World War, Susan Lederer, first history of American research ethics
1996	*Zentrum für Ethik und Recht in der Medizin der Albert-Ludwigs-Universität Freiburg* (ZERM – the Center for Ethics and Law in Medicine of Albert Ludwig's University, Freiburg) Workshop on Nuremberg Code		*The Human Radiation Experiments: Final Report of the President's Advisory Commission*, edited by Ruth Faden
1997	50th anniversary of the Nuremberg Tribunals and Nuremberg code of research ethics	Sheep, "Dolly," cloned from mammary tissue extracted from a ewe – named after singer with famous mammaries (1997–2003)	*Convention on Human Rights and Biomedicine* commits European Union to a human dignity and human rights approach to bioethics
	AMA conference celebrating the 150th anniversary of its founding and its Code of Ethics		*Medicine and Morals in the Enlightenment: John Gregory, Thomas Percival and Benjamin Rush*, Lisbeth Haakonssen argues for Protestant origins of modern medical ethics
	International Conference On Codes of Ethics in Medicine since 1945; *Zentrum für Ethik und Recht in der Medizin der Albert-Ludwigs-Universität Freiburg*: first bioethics conference in Germany since Peter Singer affair		*Submission to Truth and Reconciliation*, Truth and Reconciliation Commission of South Africa condemns physician complicity in torture
	Japan accepts limited concept of brain death		*Ethik und Medizin 1947–1997 Was leistet de Kodification von Ethik?* (Ethics and Medicine: What is the Meaning of the Codification of Ethics?), collection of papers based on Freiburg conference on Nuremberg Code, edited by historian Ulrich Tröhler and bioethicist-psychiatrist Stella Reiter-Theil
	Oregon becomes first U.S. state to legalize physician-assisted suicide.		

(continued)

Dates	Events	Persons	Texts
	President William Clinton apologizes for the Tuskegee Syphilis Experiment		
	Scottish scientist Ian Wilmut announces birth of a sheep, Dolly, cloned from adult mammary tissue		
1998	American Society for Bioethics and Humanities (ASBH) founded consolidating, the Society for Health and Human Values (SHHV), the Society for Bioethics Consultation (SBC), and the American Association of Bioethics (AAB)		*The Birth of Bioethics*, Albert Jonsen, semi-autobiographical, comprehensive history of bioethics
	Jack Kevorkian announces that he has assisted in the 100th suicide, defying legal authorities, CBS TV show "60 Minutes" shows him administering a lethal injection to 52-year-old suffering from amyotrophic lateral sclerosis (ALS, Lou Gehrigs disease)		*John Gregory and the Invention of Professional Medical Ethics and the Profession of Medicine*, Laurence McCullough, first monograph on a founder of modern medical ethics
			Ethics Codes in Medicine: Foundations and achievements of codification since 1947, eds., Ulrich Tröhler and Stella Reiter-Theil
	Swiss charity, *Dignitas* offers assistance in suicide to terminally ill patients irrespective of nationality, prompting assisted-suicide tourism		
1999	Peter Singer appointed to a chair at Princeton University Center for Human Values		*The American Medical Ethics Revolution*, R. Baker, A. Caplan, L. Emanuel, and S. Latham, eds., bioethicists-historians debate over history of American medical ethics and impact of AMA's Code of Ethics
	Jack Kevorkian convicted of second degree murder for giving lethal injection to ALS patient		*Declaration of Bologna: On Reduction, Refinement and Replacement Alternatives and Laboratory Animal Procedures*, Third World Congress on Alternatives and Animal Use in the Life Sciences: affirmation and updating of the 1959 Three Rs principles for animal experimentation

Dates	Events	Persons	Texts
			The Nazi War on Cancer, Robert Proctor situates Nazi racial hygiene in public health ethics; argues that "Nazi medical ethics" is not an oxymoron
			"Princeton's New Philosopher Draws a Stir," Sylvia Nasar, *New York Times*, on controversy over the appointment of Peter Singer at Princeton
2000	*Human Cloning Regulation Act* (Japan), prohibits reproductive human cloning, but not therapeutic cloning (cloning embryo for embryonic stem cell research) Japan Medical Association issues revised code of medical ethics		*Compendio Bioético*, José A Mainetti, existential and phenomenological conception of bioethics. *A Short History of Medical Ethics*, Albert Jonsen, first concise global history of medical ethics

Part III

Discourses of Medical Ethics
through the Life Cycle

CHAPTER 3

MEDICAL ETHICS THROUGH THE LIFE CYCLE IN HINDU INDIA

Katherine K. Young

I. INTRODUCTION

All human lives go through physical changes from birth to death. This is the biological base line of the life cycle. How these changes are defined and marked as stages, however, has been religiously based in most societies. Birth and death, in turn, frame the life cycle and pose the fundamental religious questions of human meaning and destiny. Because the life cycle is intertwined with the reproductive and intergenerational cycles, on which species and group survival are based, religions have used their highest authority to complement biology with culture to create order in the form of norms. Because human life has its phases and moments of vulnerability (birth, illness, old age, and dying), religions have also used their authority to protect the vulnerable through an ethics of care, if not inviolable sanctity ascribed to life itself.

II. STAGES AND RITUAL MARKINGS OF THE LIFE CYCLE

There are different views on the number of stages in the Hindu life cycle (Tilak 1989, 70–71), some late accounts numbering forty (an indication of the extensive ritualism of the religion). For the three upper castes (*brāhmaṇas*, *kṣatriyas*, and *vaiśyas*) stages are marked by rituals called

*saṃskāra*s, performed by *brāhmaṇa*s (Brahmin priests). One set of rituals exists at the beginning of life (conception to early childhood). This cluster can be attributed to the religion's family orientation, its recognition that conception and a stable pregnancy resulting in birth are never guaranteed, and its awareness that pregnancy, infancy, and early childhood are times of great vulnerability.

Hinduism has been a pronatal religion for several reasons. It has been an ethnically defined religion in the sense that one is born a Hindu, some currents of universalism notwithstanding. Its beginnings harken back to the prehistory of small-scale societies, when life spans were short because of death in war, childbirth, and epidemics, with pronatal values being the antidote. When the contours of its worldview were being classically formulated, its economy was largely agricultural, which encouraged large families for labor. Its pronatal policy contributed to population pressure in core areas and subsequent migrations to other parts of the subcontinent, new minorities then wanting security through increasing their own numbers.

In Hinduism, the immediate, human life cycle belongs to a larger concept of cyclic time called *saṃsāra*: the cycle of life, death, and rebirth. Entry into the human realm (*manuṣyaloka*) occurs at the beginning of a *kalpa*, a particular cycle in the cosmic scheme. Entry could be as a plant, animal, god, or demon, such ontic status being determined by the individual's karma (the impressions or coded information, not unlike DNA, of past action that might be activated in this life).

The right moment for conception refers to a woman's fertile period called *ṛtu* (defined as the fourth through the twelfth day after menses). After her 4 days of menses, she ritually bathes, dresses well with ornaments, utters a *mantra*, and then has intercourse with her husband (*Suśruta-saṃhitā, Śārīrasthānam* II.25). [In the Dharmaśāstras, the ritual for conception is called the gift of an embryo (*garbhadāna*).] Reproduction in the context of marriage is a universally required and sacred act, although several exceptions to marriage are made: spiritually evolved, male ascetics intent on the pursuit of liberation and women outside of the formal marriage system (some female bhakti saints, performers, courtesans, and so forth).

One ritual (*saṃskāra*) at the time of the fetus' first movement aims to prevent miscarriage and ensure that the fetus will be male. A ritual at 6 months marks the fact that birth might occur any time but this time should be extended as long as possible. Further rituals upon birth include one called *jātakarma*. Before the umbilical cord is cut, the father passes his debt for life from the ancestors onto his son and prays for the intellect of the infant to open to the world, the body to be strong, and life to be long. Subsequent rituals in the first 2 years of life include naming the child (*nāmakaraṇa*), viewing the sun for vision and future erotic pleasure (*niṣkarmaṇa*), eating the first solid food (*annaprāsana*), and cutting the hair for the first time to symbolize the end of infancy (*cāḍākaraṇa*).

After childhood, the life cycle is marked by initiation into education with several nonscriptural rituals, and *upanayana* for twice-born males. The latter begins the stage called *brahmacarya* of scriptural (Vedic) and philosophical study under a guru. As a kind of puberty ritual taking place between 8 and 13 years, depending on the caste, it marks the end of childhood and rebirth as a man with caste, educational, and ritual duties. (Circumcision has not been a Hindu practice. It has shared this absence with other Indo-European groups.) Girls lost out on this education by the Classical period when it was no longer done in the home, and so their *upanayana* was said to be marriage. Between 16 and 20, the boy returns to society to marry, pay his debt to the ancestors with offspring, and support his family, a stage called *gārhastya*.

The turning point from growth to decay for a man is said to be the moment when his first son is born or when his hair turns gray, his physical body weakens, and he escapes into past memories. Cross-culturally, there are different contexts of aging, but they all involve some form of disengagement (Tilak 1989, 3–5). For Hindu men, this has generally involved pursuit of the spiritual path of asceticism or renunciation: withdrawing to the forest (*vānaprastha*), with or without the wife, and/or male renunciation of fam-

ily and society (*saṃnyāsa*) and wandering alone, with the former wife remaining in the extended family (solitary asceticism of these last two stages being a male prerogative). Even for those who remain as householders, there is an increasing importance of disengagement and religious acts such as fasting, *mantras*, and pilgrimage along with rejuvenation therapies to supplement the tension created by the desire not to die and the inevitability of the aging process, often accompanied by chronic or incurable diseases. Sometimes the dying man takes *saṃnyāsa* (involving tonsure, donning of ochre robes, and initiation) even though he is bed-ridden. This is called *ātura saṃnyāsa*. The more common brahmanical death rituals begin with the person's sense of approaching death, calling relatives to the bedside, and making gifts to *brāhmaṇas*, which symbolize the after-death journey. Those gathered at the bedside watch attentively the stages of the dying process.

Some of these life cycle rituals are still practiced in modern, Vedically influenced Hinduism, although they are often attenuated and simplified. Women now study Sanskrit, the Vedas, and other religious topics in universities and some religious institutions, if they so desire. Public, secular education has replaced religious education for both sexes, although accessibility to education is often minimal in rural areas, especially for girls.

III. ETHICAL ISSUES IN THE HINDU LIFE CYCLE

1. Exposure, Infanticide, Miscarriage, and Abortion

Infanticide and exposure have been viewed as moral wrongs in Hinduism. This does not mean that both were never done; practice, after all, does not always follow precept. Infanticide was practiced for two main reasons: to eliminate an infant born, according to astrology, at an inauspicious moment (Dubois and Beauchamp [1906] 1959, 500) and to eliminate female infants who were sometimes rejected because they were economic liabilities (see later discussion of sex selection).

One famous story about abandonment occurs in the great epic *Mahābhārata*, The Book of the Beginning. Queen Kuntī was given the boon of being favored by a son by whichever god she named. She called out the name of the Sun god and subsequently gave birth to Karṇa, who was to be a mighty hero, after which her virginity was restored to her. "To hide her misconduct and out of fear for her relations, Kuntī then threw the boy, who bore the marks of greatness, into the river. Adhiratha, Rādhā's renowned husband who was born a *sūta*, saved the abandoned child, and he and his wife adopted him as their own son" (van Buitenen 1973, 241).

To discuss abortion, it is necessary to analyze the Hindu view of conception. The nature of conception is elaborated in the Āyurvedic texts (literally the texts on "life," i.e., longevity; see Chapters 9 and 20), notably, the *Caraka-saṃhitā* and *Suśruta-saṃhitā*, composed some time from the third century BCE.[1] The *Suśruta* bases its analysis of the human body and birth on Sāṃkhya philosophy, a dualism consisting of self/soul (*puruṣa*) and matter (*prakṛti*), including the psyche or subtle body that contains the karmically coded information from previous lives (*Suśruta-saṃhitā, Śārīrasthānam* I.1–17) (see Chapter 9).

One's past karma will determine what kind of body one will assume. Just as the equilibrium of a seed is disturbed when placed in an appropriate environment – the conditions of soil, water, and sun, thereby initiating the process of growth or manifestation – so the equilibrium of the unmanifest embodied soul is disturbed when the proper conditions or environment are present. The *Suśruta* states that these consist of (1) the father's fluid (*śukra*: translated as semen by modern authors), which contributes bone, hair, nerves, arteries, and so forth; (2) the mother's fluid (*artavam*: literally blood, but translated as ovum by modern authors), which contributes flesh, blood, fat, and so forth; (3) the nutritional serum (*rasa*), provided by the mother, which serves as food and contributes to strength and growth; and (4) the *ātmaja*, defined by the *Suśruta* as that which arises from the self, "the sensual organs, consciousness, knowledge, wisdom, duration of life (longevity), pleasure and pain" (*Suśruta-saṃhitā Śārīrasthānam* III.19), in other words, that which arises from the unmanifest life principle or *jīva*. Two other factors are mentioned in this passage: *sattvaja* and *sātmyaja*. These last two terms have caused a great deal of scholarly confusion, which is apparent in the translations of both the *Suśruta* and the *Caraka*. I will define *sattva* as the karma that chooses the appropriate conditions for a particular type of body and then links the subtle body with these conditions to form the gross body. *Sātmya* is the healthy condition or wholesomeness of the reproductive organs that makes reproduction possible.

The moment of conjunction (see the *Caraka-saṃhitā Śārīrasthāna* III.5) is the *moment of conception*. It begins the change from the subtle body to the gross body, that is, the arising of the conditions of name and form (*nāma-rūpa*), also called the process of manifestation. The mainstream Hindu position is that personhood exists from the *moment* of conception because the fetus at that time has soul and subtle body, including the karmic inheritance that defines individuality. Hindu views of conception and human person follow this general scheme, although some other schools of thought replace Sāṃkhya's basic dualism with nondualistic (*advaita*) or qualified nondualistic (*viśiṣṭadvaita*) ontologies. An alternative view, found only in the *Garbha-upaniṣad*, a very minor text of the second or third century, claims that the descent of the soul into matter occurs only after the seventh month (Lipner 1989, 54).

The medical texts describe the growth of the fetus, noting stages of physical development from a being in the form of a gelatinous lump (*kalala*) to one with organ differentiation (*peśī*) to one with movement and dream-like consciousness (*garbha*). The *Suśruta* says that in the fifth month the fetus is endowed with mind (*manas*) and wakes up from the sleep of its subconscious existence (*Suśruta-saṃhitā Śārīrasthānam* III.16) to manifest consciousness (expressed through the desires of the mother) (*Suśruta-saṃhitā Śārīrasthānam* III.14). In the sixth month, the subtle body (*buddhi*) develops. Although stages are described, there is no categorical change from one to the other.

In the scriptures, abortion is contrasted with miscarriage described by ethically neutral terms such as flow or emission of the fetus (*garbhāsrava*); falling, fall (*śraṃsana; pata*); issue (*prasuti*); and generation (*sutaka*) – terms that correspond to phases in the pregnancy (Lipner 1989, 43). A seventh-century text, *Kaśyapa's Compendium* (Wujastyk 1998, 208–24), attributes miscarriage to attack by the goddess *Jātahārinī* (a "child snatcher" in the form of a jealous, infertile witch or woman forced into asceticism because of infertility) on those fetuses that are demons in disguise or the fetuses of evil, selfish, and promiscuous women who ignore their feminine duties (*strīdharma*). The misogynist text then describes how *brāhmaṇa* priests or midwives provide amulets or *mantras* to prevent miscarriage.

By contrast, terms for abortion denote some kind of active killing (*hatyā; vadha*) of the fetus (*garbha; bhrūṇa*) (Lipner 1989, 42–43). The one who performs abortion (*bhrūṇaghni*) or kills a pregnant woman is described as reprehensible: a thief, beefeater, drunkard, outcaste, murderer of parents, fornicator with the guru's wife, or *brāhmaṇa*-killer. Punishment includes loss of caste (and therefore occupation, status, and ritual eligibility) or large fines. All fetuses of whatever status – slaves, low caste, mixed caste, and illegitimate – are not to be aborted.

The *Suśruta* says that removing a fetus from the womb when there is a medical problem is extremely difficult and may result in the death of fetus or mother. For this reason, the king should be informed (to avoid subsequent charges of homicide). The physician is advised to make every effort to save the fetus if it is alive, proceeding with great care and with the chanting of mantras to save both it and the mother. If the physician is certain the fetus is dead in the womb, it should be extracted utilizing surgery for dismemberment. If a live fetus cannot be removed safely, then the mother's life must be protected (an exception to the general or *sāmānya* rule of *ahiṃsā* is self-defense, this being a case in point) (*Suśruta-saṃhitā Cikitsasthānam* XV.1–11 ff).

Because a human life is the opportunity for the stored (*prārabdha*) karma to come to fruition and thereby be eliminated – a necessary antecedent for liberation – it has been considered wrong to interfere with this precious opportunity by causing an untimely death. As for arguing that abortion is to be condoned because the law of karma acknowledges the freedom to act, it has been said that freedom can lead to either good or bad karma. Because killing (*himsā*), with few exceptions, is *adharma* or unrighteous, abortion is wrong. Finally, the modern argument that a woman should have reproductive privacy is countered by the concept of public duty to marry and have children (Lipner 1989, 10–11).

Abortion was legalized in India in 1971 (The Medical Termination of Pregnancy Act). Abortion on request can occur during the first 20 weeks of pregnancy in government hospitals free of charge. India's abortion policy allows abortion to save the woman's life, to preserve physical health, to preserve mental health, for rape, for incest, and for fetal impairment but not for economic or social reasons and not on request (Simon 1998, 40). (It is striking that Nepāl, a country that has Hinduism as the state religion, does not allow abortion for any reason.)

From the 1950s, the Indian government encouraged family planning through information on birth control. By the mid-1960s, it began to look on family planning as a way to reduce the population, and in the mid-seventies, Indira Gandhi, under emergency powers, introduced forced sterilization (numbers went to 2.5 million in 1976, before her government lost power in 1977 in part due to public reaction against forced sterilizations). "The most recent data on abortion rates have them at 3.3 per 1000 women 15 to 44 years of age, as of 1989 [which is the second lowest rate in the world] according to 1988–1991 statistics" (Simon 1998, 22, 52).

Be that as it may, it is curious that there was initially little discussion of the conflict between the traditional Hindu prohibition of abortion (except when the mother's life was at stake) and its modern legalization (Lipner 1989, 61 note 1). It is also curious that a survey reveals that the Indian public supports abortion at a high rate:

> While not indicating as high an approval rating for abortion as the Chinese, at least 60 percent of the 2500 respondents said they approved of abortion on each of the four grounds... Demographic characteristics do not significantly differentiate on any of the criteria – mother's health, child handicapped, mother unmarried, couple does not want more children, save the Muslims were somewhat less likely to approve of abortion than Hindus. (Simon 1998, 94)

When Catholic, Protestant, Fundamentalist Protestant, Jewish, Muslim, Hindu, and Buddhist religions are compared, 89.6 percent of Hindus compared with 96 percent of Buddhists and 83.9 percent of Catholics approve of abortion to protect the mother's health; the percentage of approval for abortion of a handicapped child – 68.7 percent of Hindus – is about the same as that of Catholics, 68 percent, and Muslims, 68.6 percent; of all the religions, Hindus have the highest approval rating if the mother is unmarried – for example, Hindus 64.1 percent, Catholics 22.3 percent – and they rank third highest for abortion if no more children are wanted (see chart, Simon 1998, 64). In May 2000, India's population reached 1 billion, the second largest in the world. Hindus seem to approve of abortion but do not practice it. This could be explained in one of two ways. Either they practice contraception (including sterilization), and so the need does not arise (although theoretically they want the option for themselves or others), or the abortion statistics are not representative because the sample does not include rural, illiterate people or because most abortions are illegal. The rate of illegal abortions, for instance, has remained high because many rural and poor women do not have access to appropriate medical facilities; 20 percent of maternal deaths are due to unsafe abortions (Simon 1998, 21).

In light of this survey it is striking that the popular magazine *Hinduism Today* devoted an article to the subject of abortion and proclaimed in no uncertain terms, "Across the board, Hindu religious leaders perceive abortion at any stage of fetal development as killing (some say murder)... and as an act that has serious karmic repercussions" (March 1986; cited by Murti and Deer 1998, paragraph 7). It might not be incidental that this magazine is published in the United States, where abortion has caused so much controversy. Interest in Hinduism's perspective might also be brewing in India itself with the renewal and politicization of Hindu identity. On a more academic note, Veena Das wrote "Without a discussion of the responsibility of society (either through the State or other agencies) towards the embryo, the foetus, and the infant as also towards those who are charged with caring for them, a discussion of the morality of abortion is incomplete" (Lipner 1989, 69, note 74).

There are several hermeneutical principles within Hinduism that conceivably could be used to justify abortion today. One is the principle of *āpaddharma* (literally, *dharma* in distress, *āpad*). According to this, normative behavior may be changed in times of crisis when survival and well-being are at stake. Applying this to the topic at hand, if the population crisis has caused extreme poverty, environmental destruction, and unprecedented misery, then the norm of being antiabortion might be temporarily abandoned until the escalating population is brought under control (but then there must be a ritualized return to the normative practice), or it could be argued that norms have changed in this period, the *kaliyuga*, a time characterized by much unrighteousness (*adharma*), and people are no longer accountable to a higher standard because at this *yuga* level fate is involved. The world will automatically be three-quarters evil in this age. Alternatively, it could be argued that in the *kaliyuga*, the order (*krama*) of the four authorities (*śruti*, *smṛti*, *sadācāra*, and *ātmatuṣṭi*) is changed so that the latter (personal experience and conscience) is now first. Gandhi had used such logic – although in another context (he was categorically against abortion) – to argue for change. By and large, it seems, urban, educated Hindus have preferred to prevent the problem of abortion and the karmic effects of killing altogether by the practice of contraception (for which there are no scriptural prohibitions) to limit family size, which enhances well-being in urban, industrialized societies. Practice of contraception has lagged, however, in rural areas because of illiteracy and poverty (Ramu 1988, 83, 120–21).

2. The Ethics of New Reproductive Technologies

It might seem odd on first glance that India, a country with such a large population, is so sympathetic to problems of infertility and their technological solutions. This can be explained in part by its traditional, pronatal orientation: men repaying their debt of life to the ancestors, good rebirth being premised on parenting, and upper-caste female identity being almost exclusively centered on the role of good wife and mother.

The *Suśruta* has remedies for male and female impotency, dealing with seminal defects and menstrual irregularities (*Suśruta-saṃhitā Śārīrasthāna* II.1–16). The longer conception took, with its corollary of growing fear of infertility, the greater was the resort to religion. If this was to no avail, there were other solutions. From other texts, we know that polygamy was allowed: The problem of an infertile wife could be solved by the husband's taking another wife. If the problem was the husband's (or if he had died before she conceived), the elders of the family could solve the problem by levirate marriage (*niyoga*). Ideally, according to the Dharmaśāstras, this was to be done with a brother-in-law. To prevent sexual chaos within the extended family, *niyoga* was highly ritualized to constrain sex for sexual pleasure. The number of children to be conceived in this manner was also limited to one or two (Kane [1941] 1974, 600).

The plight of royal lineages in need of offspring to ensure orderly succession is posed poignantly as the central event of the *Mahābhārata*, a epic from the Classical period (c. 600 BCE to 600) that has been relived by each generation of Hindus. Its first book describes the crisis of succession in the ruling Bhārata dynasty because of lack of offspring on account of widowhood (Ambikā, Ambālikā, Śaradaṇóāyinī, and the widows of Vicitravīrya) or male infertility (Pāṇḍu, Kalmāṣapāda Saudāsa, and Balin). The choice of a male partner for *niyoga* includes *brāhmaṇa* sages (Vyāsa, Vasiṣṭha, Dīrghatamus) or, in a more supernatural vein, deities. The *Mahābhārata* even turns a blind eye to single women seducing men – sometimes described as a temporary marriage – to try to become pregnant (Sarmiṣṭhā, Hiḍimbā, Ulupī, and Citrāṅgadā) (Dhand 2000). This was not quite the same as today's (Western) concept of single motherhood by choice, because, at least according to the

male authority of the Dharmaśāstras, it was viewed as a last resort in cases in which opportunity for marriage had been problematic, and it therefore was an *exception* to the general rule of children within marriage (Dhand 2000).

Closely related to the context of *niyoga* is that of surrogacy. One famous story of surrogacy is found in *Mahābhārata*:

> The princess of the Kāśis decked a slave woman, as beautiful as an Apsara, with her own jewelry and sent her to Kṛṣṇa. When the seer came, the woman rose to meet him and greeted him; and with his consent she lay with him and served him with all honor. The seer waxed content with the pleasure of love he found with her, and he spent all night with her as she pleasured him. When he rose, he said to her, 'You shall cease to be a slave. There is a child come to your belly, my lovely.'... Thus was born Vidura. (van Buitenen 1973, 236)

Before leaving this topic of insemination by donor, three observations must be made. One is that when donors were chosen beyond the family (as in the *Mahābhārata*), first *brāhmaṇa* sages and second *brāhmaṇa* priests were most desired by the *kṣatriya* caste. Because the epics and the Dharmaśāstras were either redacted or authored by *brāhmaṇa*s, the privileging of *brāhmaṇa* semen, a privileging accepted by others who viewed them at the top of caste hierarchy, is understandable. There might, however, also be a perceived hereditary component (*brāhmaṇa*s, especially sages, were considered highly intelligent and the semen of ascetics especially powerful), and there was an especially close relation between *brāmaṇa*s and *kṣatriya*s in the epic (which might indicate groups that intermarried in the particular region where the epic was written). The second observation is that *brāhmaṇa* men were allowed to take perpetual studentship (*brahmacarya*) in cases of impotency, blindness, and other deformities (Kane [1941] 1974, 351 note 852; 376). The third observation is that surrogacy was largely a nonissue because of the tradition of polygamy. Even though monogamy was promoted, multiple marriages were allowed for men, although polygamy was common only if the wife was barren (Kane [1941] 1974, 553). Authors of the Dharmaśāstras hold minor differences on how long (generally 8 to 10 years) a husband should wait if infertility, repeated miscarriages, or birth of daughters appeared to be a problem (*Āpastamba-dharmaśāstra* II.5.11.12–13; *Kauṭilya-arthaśāstra* III.2; *Manu* V.80 and *Yājñavalkya* I.80). Even colonial legislation recognized the right for a second wife if the first was barren (*Madras Act* XXI of 1933). Finally, it could be argued that Hindus, at least traditionally, would have been concerned with the idea of anonymous donors of sperm (and therefore sperm banks) because this would lead to caste mixtures, anathema in the eyes of the upper castes. To the degree that caste consciousness is receding, this would be less of an issue in the modern period. According to one contemporary source, "The idea of surrogate motherhood is foreign to Indian mothers . . . However, it is interesting to note that Indian society considers that a child born of a surrogate mother is a normal child" (Bhardwaj and Azariah 1999, 72).

Because the Hindu practice of *niyoga* is analogous to artificial insemination by donor (except that the means differ: intercourse rather than syringe), it could be argued that the latter should be legally allowed in modern India to solve problems of infertility. But this would be to ignore the fact that there was considerable debate by the authors of the Dharmaśāstras over the morality of the practice of *niyoga*. It was to be officially stopped, according to *Āpastamba-dharmaśāstra* II.10.27.2–6 (c. 800–400 BCE) "on account of the weakness of (men's) senses;" otherwise both the wife and her husband would go to hell (Kane [1946] 1974, 644, 926–27). *Manu* IX.64–68 (c. 200 BCE–200) concluded that the practice was beastly because it was no longer practiced within restraints as in former times (Kane [1946] 1973, 602–603). Other authors said it was allowed only for *kṣatriyas* (as in the cases of the *Mahābhārata*) or poor *śūdras*. There were also debates over to whom the child belonged: the begetter (although it undercut the very purpose of *niyoga*), or the infertile husband (in which case, there had to be a formal agreement), or both the begetter and the infertile husband (Kane [1941] 1974, 605). Confusion was compounded in the colonial period when judges, who did not know Sanskrit, tried to rule on whether the offspring of a *niyoga* relationship could be adopted (Kane [1946] 1973, 682–83). Scholars of Hinduism today describe clandestine traditions of women's intercourse with *brāhmaṇa* priests at special pilgrimage centers to overcome the problem of their husband's infertility (Kinsley 1996, 60–70).

Joseph Schenker, characterizing religious views regarding treatment of infertility by assisted reproductive technologies, says of Hinduism

> The important concepts of the Hindu religion relating to the problem of infertility are as follows: (a) Marriage is considered sacred and permanent; (b) Male infertility is not a cause for divorce; (c) The emphasis in reproduction is not just on having children, but on having a male offspring; (d) It is a religious duty to provide a male offspring. Therefore, the wife of a sterile male could be authorized to have intercourse with a brother in-law or another member of the husband's family for the purpose of having a male offspring. (Schenker 1992, 4)

He argues by analogy that because *niyoga* was legitimate for Hindus, sperm donation would be legitimate if it comes from a closer relative of the husband. He then extends the analogy and says that oocyte donation would be acceptable as well and so would surrogacy, and he argues that

research on "preembryos" would be possible because the soul (*ātman*) is eternal. (This argument, however, would generally not be made by Hindus who value human life for providing the opportunity for enlightenment.)

Today the treatment of infertility is changing, thanks to *in vitro* fertilization. In 1978, Dr. Subash Mukerjee and his team reported they had successfully concluded an in vitro fertilization, claimed to be the second one to take place in the world and the first to use cryopreservation (the embryo was frozen for 53 days prior to implantation). International credit for this was lost, it has been claimed, because the physician reported it in a minor journal and had promised not to reveal the identity of the in vitro fertilization baby and its parents, thus making it impossible to verify the scientific breakthrough (Verma 1997, 67).

It can be extrapolated from the Hindu perspective on abortion that one major problem with in vitro fertilization would be selective abortion. Another is its relation to sex selection. Firuza Parikh, head of the department of assisted reproduction, Jaslok Hospital, Mumbai, warned (April 1998) that in vitro fertilization may be used for sex selection (see later discussion) in India because it tracks the pregnancy with ultrasound, making it possible to determine the sex and resort to selective abortion, although the cost of this technique would be prohibitive for most (Parikh 1998). Although Indian clinics have access to cryopreservation of embryos and other techniques, the Indian rate of in vitro fertilization may be low (less than 5 percent) because clinics do not have the latest, expensive technology. According to one critic, the government has no knowledge of the treatments, risks, rate of success, and expenses in the private clinics. Because of the proliferations of clinics, they do not know their number or their case loads. The in vitro centers, moreover, are part of international networks using technologies or procedures banned or untested in the West. According to one report

> Midland Fertility Services, in London, is planning to fly its patients to 'inexpensive' clinics in Banglore and Mumbai next month to carry out a new treatment, using immature sperms. A Government watchdog called Human Fertilization and Embryology has banned the treatment in Britain announcing that using sperms that are yet to complete the maturation process increases the risk of genetic abnormalities and deformities in the children. (The Human Body Shop 1998, paragraphs 11–14)

One of the most popular new reproductive technologies in India is sex selection because it provides a way to satisfy the desire for sons. Various late Vedic texts (*Taittirīya-saṃhitā* VI.3.10.5; *Śatapatha-brāhmaṇa* I.7.2.11; *Aitareya-brāhmaṇa* 33.1) describe three religious debts a man owes to gods, ancestors, and sages: sacrifices, birth of a son, and Vedic study, respectively. *Suśruta-saṃhitā Śārīrasthānam* (II.26–30) stipulates that if a couple wants a male child, they should abstain from sex the preceding month, ritually prepare for intercourse by anointing their bodies with oil, consume special foods, recite *mantras*, and then have intercourse on the fourth, sixth, eighth, tenth, or twelfth night after the menses.

Unwanted daughters have sometimes been subject to a slow death by malnutrition and medical neglect (thought to avoid the bad karma of active killing). In the past, they have also been given as servants to families, offered to communities of independent female dancers, singers, and prostitutes, or dedicated to Hindu temples, Buddhist monasteries, or, in the modern period, Christian orphanages. By contrast, boys were rarely killed or abandoned, because of their religious importance – a son was mandatory to perform his father's funeral rituals. If for some reason a son was not needed for this purpose in his natal family and was not wanted, he would be in high demand for adoption for the same reason. (For the extensive, technical literature on adoption see Kane 1974 3:674ff; sex, age, *niyoga* offspring, male sibling order, caste, region, and mental and physical condition were all discussed.) Along with the religious importance of sons (by birth or adoption) was the aforementioned economic importance of sons.

Son preference has led to an imbalanced sex ratio. Cross-culturally there have been 105 males to 100 females at the time of birth. Already low at the turn of the twentieth century in India, the number of females to males in India has been declining, so that in 1995 there were 106.9 males per 100 women. In other words, there is a deficit of 50 million women in India (Rajan 1996, paragraph 1).

In 1975, the Indian Council of Medical Research introduced amniocentesis for prenatal testing for suspected cases of genetic anomalies. Realizing even then that they might be used for sex selection, the government made the latter a penal offence in government hospitals and clinics, according to three circulars published between 1977 and 1985. Unfortunately, criminalization of amniocentesis (or ultrasound) for sex selection has pushed the practice underground and has led to its commercialization and unsanitary practice in rural areas, where it has fast been replacing infanticide. During the same period, only 9 million girls of the 12 million born annually lived to be 15 years old. This was also a time of escalating dowries or their introduction for status definition in communities that had never had the practice. In other words, amniocentesis has been contributing to the relative decline in numbers of women: "A report released in 1989 claimed that from 1978 to 1982, 78,000 fetuses were aborted after sex determination tests" (Patel; cited by Simon 1998). The states of Maharashtra, followed by Haryana, Punjab, and Gujarat and finally the federal government on 1 January 1996, introduced laws against the practice but with little effect. Even though the doctor, the woman, and her relatives can be punished, there have been no convictions. Moreover,

the practice has the collusion of some health care workers, government officials, and ordinary women who argue that selective abortion will help to address the population problem by satisfying the desire for a son without repeated pregnancies. The most recent approach to curb sex selection has been to educate youth. In 1999, for instance, a rally was organized by the Indian Medical Association, the National Commission for Women, nongovernmental organizations, and the United Nations Children's Fund (Health Education Library for People 1999). Education along with improvement in women's economic status through jobs and property is now considered the way to sustainable change. The fact that *Hinduism Today* has had an article on sex selection by these new methods (Rajan 1996) suggests that the link to traditional Hindu values that has favored sons is recognized.

Curiously, cloning (the creation of genetically identical human beings by asexual means) has attracted more comment from Hindus in recent years than other new reproductive technologies. This can be attributed to the 1997 request of the U.S. National Bioethics Advisory Committee on behalf of President Bill Clinton to find out whether religious communities might have objections. When contacted, the editors of *Hinduism Today* in turn contacted many Hindu swamis around the world to assess their position. They replied that science is morally neutral: Only what one *does* with new knowledge is a moral issue. They made an analogy from the Hindu concept of the four human goals (*puruṣārthas*) – *dharma*, economic gain, pleasure, and liberation – that, just as *dharma* (righteousness, morality, and so forth) comes first in the list because it morally constrains the middle two items, so *dharma* in the modern period must morally constrain the use of science. In this American context, there was no appeal to Hindu scriptures (*śruti* or *smṛti*) for authority, but rather to the behavior of the good or virtuous people (*sadācāra*) (the third source of authority in the traditional list of types of authority). Hindu religious leaders were mainly concerned with whether cloning would affect the *prārabdha* karma (the karma coming to fruition in the present life) if a body were cloned and lived on beyond the source body's death. A related problem was whether the former would have to wait in the astral plane for its clone to die so it could be released from its body ("Swami, Bill Clinton has a Question" 1997, paragraph 10). Finally, Hindus could argue that cloning would destroy the uniqueness of each life, which is a product of its karma.

One other new reproductive technology is of interest when the topic is Hindu antecedents. That is ex utero genesis (gestation outside the womb or ectogenesis). In the *Mahābhārata*, we are told how Gāndhārī, after having received a boon to have 100 sons from Vyāsa, became pregnant. But after 2 years the sons had still not been born; she became worried and tried to get out what was in her belly; she was caught in the act by Vyāsa because this was like abortion. To fulfill the boon as he had promised, he told her to douse the "aborted" ball of flesh with water. When it fell apart into 100 pieces, Vyāsa placed them in pots filled with clarified butter (a sacred substance) and had them guarded. After a month, the full 100 sons were born (van Buitenen 1973, 244–45). This story could be used to justify ex utero pregnancy and multiple pregnancies generated in this way. It could also be used to justify preventing abortion by transferring the unwanted fetuses to ex utero "pots" for gestation. Of course, this is an epic tall story, which might not make it worthy of ethical precedent by way of analogy today.

A survey of fifty Indian academics in the sciences showed that they accepted in vitro fertilization, gamete intrafallopian transfer, intracytoplasmic sperm injection, and surrogacy as natural but that 75 percent rejected cloning as unnatural. When asked whether it could be a technique to counter the imbalanced sex ratio by cloning more females, 45 percent disagreed (and 30 percent said they did not know.) The majority did not want to prevent modification to the human genome until there was more knowledge (Bhardwaj and Azariah 1999, 71). They also rejected creation of encephalic fetuses to generate organs or changes to the human genome. There were virtually no Hindu references in their arguments.

It can be argued that there is a basic human right to have children and that the state should interfere with this basic right only in extreme cases. But because new reproductive technologies involve *creating* a possibility for having children, there are more ethical issues involved than when the process is natural (Somerville 2000, 22–54; 76). If the new reproductive technologies lead to commercialization of reproduction – buying and selling sperm and eggs and the objectification of human nature, then it would interfere with the Hindu view of what it means to be human – a strong presumption for the sacrality and unique individuality of life. Because of the precedent of *niyoga* in Hinduism, it could be argued that artificial insemination by donor would be acceptable to Hindus and that brothers-in-law would be suitable donors (especially now that there can be artificial insemination, which eliminates the problem of adultery). In cases in which the husband is infertile (and not dead), there is the danger of two men within the family assuming the role of father (but only one being the biological father). This problem might have been one reason many of the authors of the Dharmaśāstras spoke out against the very practice of *niyoga*, and there was an attempt to prohibit it by the tenth century (a Kalivarjya prohibition).

3. The Ethics of Risk Assessment, Truth Telling, and Terminal Care

Risk assessment and the balance of benefits and risks were rare in premodern Hindu medical ethics for two main

reasons: (1) risk is a largely a modern concept related to rapid technological change (and the need to assess and prevent "new" harms) and (2) conflicts in traditional Hindu ethics were generally resolved not by quantification but rather by ranking them according to their merits or by acknowledging an irresolvable moral dilemma. Nevertheless, there are some examples of risk assessment in the Āyurvedic texts. An important one assesses the patient's prognosis from the perspective of the physician: What are the risks to his professional reputation if the patient is dies while under his care? In an age of quacks, physicians wanted success stories, which was the best kind of advertisement for their expertise (and to protect themselves against charges of homicide). To determine if a disease were incurable, there is a detailed analysis of the signs of death. In *Caraka-saṃhitā Indriyasthānam* (XII.43–61), for instance, there are twelve chapters devoted to a discussion of the signs (*ariṣṭas*) of imminent death consisting of physical changes ["affliction of *prāṇa* (vital breath); clouding of understanding; drainage of strength from limbs; cessation of movements; destruction of sensory faculties; impairment of consciousness; restlessness in the mind; affliction of the mind with fear; deprivation of memory, intellect, *hrī* (natural modesty) and *śrī* (lustre) of the body; aggravation of *pāpmā* (diseases caused by sinful acts) . . . cruel dreams"] and omens of various kinds.

Alternatively, physicians could treat the incurable if there was public knowledge that the disease was terminal and if the news would not cause a problem for the patient or the relatives:

> A physician should not announce the imminence of death without being specially requested for that, even if he is aware of the onset of such bad prognostic signs. Even when specially requested, he should not say anything about the approaching death if such announcement is likely to result in the collapse of the patient or distress of others. The wise physician should however refrain from treating patients having signs of imminent death without making announcement of the approaching death. (*Caraka-saṃhitā Indriyasthānam* VII.43–61)

In Hinduism, words themselves have power. They can make something happen. The refusal to inform the patient about terminal illness would be against the virtue of truth telling (*satya*) with its underlying rule "tell no lie." It was usually second in the list of universal virtues (*sāmānya*) (see Chapter 9). This poses an apparent conflict between the universal duty to tell the truth and the idea that in the case of a dying person it might cause distress, and therefore harm, which is against the first universal virtue: *ahiṃsā* (literally, being without even desire to harm). A way to resolve this moral dilemma is to make the case of dying an exception to the general rule. Another way to resolve it, though, is to think about the negative rule form of the virtue: Do not lie is not the same as "tell the truth" because one always has the option to keep quiet. Still, it could be argued that it is important for Hindu patients to know the nature of their disease, its prognosis, the types of treatment, and so forth so that they can prepare for death calmly because it is such an important time to influence destiny (see subsequent discussion). Moreover, many modern Hindus as well have criticized paternalism and are trying to create a more equal society. For this reason, they would advocate a presumption in favor of full disclosure to the patient. Religions change, as do people.

4. End-of-Life Care

Most care of the terminally ill has been provided within the family context. There are few nursing facilities or long-term care institutions, and they are often looked down on as "Western creations" for the abandonment of the elderly and dying. With the current growth in nuclear families, however, the elderly now fear such "abandonment." The ideal place to die for many Hindus is Vārāṇasī (Banaras), on the banks of the Gaṅgā:

> They spend their final days in a hospice where spiritual help but no medicine is provided. Hearing the names of the gods chanted continually, they eat sacred *tulsī* leaves and drink Ganges water, focusing their thoughts exclusively on God. Śiva, Lord of Death, whispers the ferryboat *mantra* into their ears. After they die, their corpses are taken to the cremation ground.... If dying by the Ganges is impossible, dying at some other *tīrtha* in India may be a substitute.... And if even that is impossible, simply thinking about the Ganges at the moment of death may influence destiny. (Young 1995, 1:490)

According to one text, at the moment of dying, the person is laid on the solid ground to keep in contact with "objective reality." Sacred substances – Gaṅgā water, seeds, kuśa grass, and flowers – are spread on the person as the smell of incense fills the air. Sacred texts are chanted – Vedas for *brāhmaṇas* and the *Bhagavadgītā* and *Rāmāyaṇa* for others (*Garuḍa-purāṇa* II.2.6–8; cited by Filippi 1996, 116–17).

This shows that the time of dying is ritualized: Time and space become sacred.

5. Religion and the Ethics of Pain Relief

A good death has meant a peaceful death for Hindus. This was one of the reasons that physicians were reluctant to tell patients and their families that death was impending. The implication of this view for modern medicine is that pain relief provided by a physician might make the dying process peaceful and therefore auspicious in Hindu terms. Chanting sacred texts at the moment of death helps to focus the person's mind on religion.

Hindus believe that uttering the name of their chosen deity at the moment of death will influence their destiny, and so they must remain completely alert. This implies that in the context of modern medicine, pain relief should not be allowed to cloud consciousness (Young 1995, 490). But does this mean that if hospital staff knows that a patient is Hindu, the patient should automatically not be given pain relief? Pain relief has been called a human right, and so the presumption for all patients should be that adequate pain relief should be available, even if it shortens life (Somerville 2000, 139). Moreover, there is enormous diversity within religions and often dramatic differences between historical and modern forms of religion, and there is likely diversity between religious practices within the homeland and its practice in the diaspora. Therefore, it would be impossible to know modern Hindu views on this topic without directly requesting them from the individual patient.

This does not make knowledge of textual forms of the religion superfluous, however. It can be used to raise questions for living wills, about what the patient might want done at the time of dying in a hospital setting. Because consciousness is the issue, it is assumed that in any case patients will be able to change their mind at any time and request pain relief. When they lose consciousness, presumably relief can and should be given because being alert is no longer an issue, and Hindus believe in a peaceful death.

6. Ethical Treatment of the Comatose

According to the *Caraka*, "Even if somebody has lost some of his sense organs – vocal and motor faculties, in a dream he does experience the various objects of sense happiness, miseries, and so forth. He cannot, therefore, be treated as a creature devoid of consciousness" (*Caraka-saṃhitā Śārīrasthānam* III.22–24). There are three "Hindu" arguments against withdrawal of treatment when the mind withdraws into breath (*prāṇa*) – the situation of deep sleep or coma: (1) the *jīva* or embodied soul still exists; (2) karma still comes into fruition in this state; and (3) the general premise of Hinduism is to do no harm (*ahiṃsā*). Modern bioethics generally argues the right of patients to refuse treatment (including artificial nutrition) based on their right of inviolability (not to be touched without consent) or right of privacy (Somerville 2000, 137). Physicians are to recognize the patient's will through informed consent, living wills, or what is understood to be the patient's will based on proxy (the assessment of legal representatives or family members). In this case, it would seem that if Hindus do not want withdrawal of treatment or nutrition in the case of being comatose, they should request this formally in a living will. In addition, the burden of proof should be on the physician who wants to withdraw treatment (Somerville 2000, 163–64).

7. The Ethics of Transplantation

The ethics of transplantation has involved three major issues: defining the moment of death, the nature of the body, and the scope for exploitation. Defining the moment of death has been an issue for transplantation because one has to remove the organs or tissue quickly to maintain the condition of the organ or tissue for transplantation but not so quickly that one might cause death to the donor (if there is still chance of life). Brain death, defined as the irreversible cessation of brain functions, is more conducive to transplantation than cardiopulmonary criteria of death because, when a patient is on life-support the heart continues to beat (See Chapters 62 and 63).

There are two key Hindu passages on the time of death. They both belong to the most sacred and authoritative category of scripture called *śruti*. According to *Bṛhadāraṇyaka-upaniṣad*, there is the withdrawal of the five senses followed by the mind (*manas*), touch, intellect (*buddhi*), and then the principle of consciousness together with karma (collectively known as the *jīva* or the subtle body) (see *Bṛhadāraṇyaka Upaniṣad* 1968, 35–57). The body was considered to have nine gates (openings). According to this passage, the *jīva* could depart through any of them. *Chāndogya-upaniṣad* 6.8.6 says: "When this man is about to depart, dear boy, his speech merges in the mind (*manas*), mind in breath (*prāṇa*) breath in fire (*tejas*) and fire in the supreme deity." According to Śaṅkara's commentary (eighth century),

> As the face reflected in mirror merges back into the real face when the mirror is broken, similarly, with the merging of the mind and other accessories, the 'living self' reflected therein also remains as Brahman. As the knower of Brahman has the realization of truth 'I am being,' he does not come back from that state; but a man without that knowledge, rises again from his source (Being) like a man awaking after deep sleep, and again enters into the meshes of the body. (slightly altered, Swāhānanada trans., *Chāndogya-upaniṣad* 1956, 452)

The *Caraka-saṃhitā* (c. third century BCE or following) divides death into two types – timely and untimely – and discusses them. The text concludes

> Therefore, death occurs on time and even otherwise. One cannot say that it always occurs in [*sic*] time. If there was no untimely death, then the span of every one would have been fixed and therefore the knowledge of wholesome and unwholesome objects would be of no use at all. The sources of knowledge like perception, inference and verbal testimony accepted in all scriptures would cease to be sources of knowledge because all these sources of knowledge clearly prove that there are factors

which are conducive to longevity and otherwise. (*Caraka-saṃhitā Śārīrsthāna* VI. 28)

In other words, karma from previous lives defines the life span, but its length can be affected in this life by how one lives.

In the *Caraka-saṃhitā*, a parallel is drawn between birth and death. When the *sattvam* – the karma that had selected the type of body (human, animal, or other) and connected the soul in the subtle body (*jīva*) to the conditioning factors that had given rise to the gross body at the time of birth – starts to withdraw, the sense organs become disturbed, strength diminishes, and disease attacks. When the *sattvam* disconnects, so do the sense organs and the breath (*Caraka-saṃhitā Śārīrasthāna* III.13). This suggests that death is a process, but it has a beginning point: a change in the *sattvam*, which destabilizes the person.

In 1994, India redefined "death as cessation of brain stem activity and organs can legally be removed after brain death" (Tharien 1996, 168). There seems to have been no consultation on this matter regarding Hindu precedent. (India is defined as a secular state, and legal authorities need not consult religious texts or their representatives.) As for the issue of whether the physical body is inviolable according to Hinduism or whether parts can be removed, the latter would likely be the case because shortly after death, the bodies of most Hindus are cremated (except for children and ascetics, who are buried). Although the new law on defining death as brain death has facilitated transplantation on the Western model of brain death, other problems have occurred.

According to one report, lack of law and commercialization of organs through organized networks stretch from hospital and nursing home physicians to touts who cater to rich Indians and foreigners by obtaining kidneys and other organs from poor and often desperate people in the slums and rural villages. This is eroding the ethical foundation of the medical profession. Needless to say, there is question about whether voluntary, informed consent occurs in these cases. To circumvent an Indian law that the donor should be a spouse or relative, some foreigners, especially from the Persian Gulf states, marry a girl before the operation and divorce her afterward (dubbed "kidney marriages"). Sometimes organs are illegally removed during routine operations for appendectomy or kidney stones. The racket has extended to the smuggling of organs by live carriers through foreign countries that do not have legal restrictions on such traffic. The Indian Parliament passed a bill in 1994 to curb this exploitation, based on the World Health Organization's guiding principles to restrict the purpose to therapy and make the process transparent and subject to informed consent. Violation of the laws carry heavy penalties: imprisonment from 2 to 7 years and a fine of 10,000 to 20,000 rupees for the middle man (Tharien 1996, 168–69).

The ethical permissibility of transplantation has been argued on the premise that it is to be a gift. Whereas exploitation can be prevented in many countries, it is difficult to prevent it in others, such as India, where there is extreme poverty. This raises the question of whether ethics in a global age should refer only in the place or culture of its origin. Does commercially exploitative organ transplantation with international networks count as real harm? And should this lead the international community to ban the practice altogether or take responsibility for its regulation worldwide (which in turn raises the problem of regulation within national boundaries of other countries)? There is another danger. If some countries ban certain kinds of experimentation, such as using pigs' organs for human transplantation (xenotransplantation) or altering the gene cell line, these experiments could be moved to Third World countries where there is no legislation or where surveillance is more difficult.

8. The Ethics of Self-Willed Death and Euthanasia

Ancient Vedic religion had an ideal of long life (one hundred years) with the implication of natural death upheld by *Īśa-upaniṣad* 2–3 (approximately the sixth century BCE), which warned that people who slay the self (*ātman*) go to hell (Sharma and Young 1990). Despite the Vedic view and subsequent popularity of *ahiṃsā* (analogous to the Western idea of the sanctity of life) as a common rule, self-willed death was gradually accepted (perhaps from examples of Jains and other ascetics). This occurred first as an exception for warriors and ascetics and then from about the first century BCE for the very old (older than 70 years) and very ill (*Atri* 218–19), a position reiterated by Aparāka some centuries later (cited by Kane [1941] 1974, 926).

Still, there were explicit rules of how to distinguish legitimate self-willed death from suicide and homicide (for the following history see Young 1994a). Proper funerals (*śrāddhas*) could not be held for suicides, for they were bound for hell. Legitimate self-willed death involved being without family obligations, making a public vow (*saṃkalpa*) to ensure its voluntary nature, and using a difficult means (not drugs or poison), to avoid reckless behavior in depression. In the *Mahābhārata*, for instance, some members of the royal family culminated the phase of living in the forest in old age (*vānaprastha*) by drowning, burning, fasting, jumping, or walking until dying from exhaustion. It can be argued that a slippery slope developed by the medieval period because of the popularization of faster and easier means and Puranic eulogies that self-willed death would lead directly to heaven or enlightenment. Groups of warriors, servants, and women (*satī*s who burned themselves on the funeral pyre of their husband) performed self-willed death. Some philosophers and religious leaders avoided mention of self-willed death (*Śaṅkara*);

others died in this manner, according to traditional accounts (*Abhinavagupta; Jñānadeva*). Despite general idealization of self-willed death, which contributed to enculturation, it was never associated with assistance, except when priests held down a *satī* on the burning funeral pyre. The latter was considered legitimate because her relatives had already tried by all means to dissuade her, and her free choice and her yogic resolve had been tested after she had publicly declared her intention.

More to the point here, physicians and drugs were never forms of assistance, though deadly poisons were readily available. Refusal to assist suicide was one means of distinguishing physicians from quacks. It is important to note that there was internal indictment against these forms of self-willed death in the *Kalivarjya* prohibitions (approximately the tenth century). But it was only after more criticism by Muslims and Christians that the practice was legally branded with Regulation XVII of 1829, which declared that abetting suicide was an act of homicide, and Section 309 of the Indian Penal Code of 1860 (based on the British Penal Code), which declared that the attempt to commit suicide (now understood to include the former category of self-willed death) or counsel or abet it were punishable by imprisonment. This virtually ended the practice (but reports of some isolated *satī*s in 1914, 1919, 1934, 1983, and 1987 made Indian legislators wary of decriminalizing suicide also because politically motivated self-willed death such as martyrdom had occurred) (Young 1994a). The decriminalization of suicide occurred, however, in 1994, when the Supreme Court of India gave a verdict that suicide is not a crime (Tharien 1995, 33).

Even today, it is believed dying ascetics might use their special powers to postpone death until an astrologically opportune moment or at an ideal place (such as the holy city of Vārāṇasī on the banks of the Gaṅgā) and then fast to death.

One contemporary author writing in a bioethics journal argued for euthanasia:

> Hinduism believes that living is more important than being alive. This places Hinduism squarely on the side of those who would argue for active euthanasia on the grounds of the quality of life over the claims of vital existence.... As the composite of matter, the body is impermanent and therefore to relate to it as permanent is gross ignorance. Hinduism says that agonising situations sometimes arise when the drive for self-preservation must halt, and even ahimsa must yield to the request to end it all. Hindu ethics is not passive in the face of suffering. Karma does not give us the right to keep such people alive and in pain when all they want is a peaceful death. Their karma is our dharma. We have a duty to our fellow-beings. If they are suffering because of some sin, it is no less a sin to let them suffer.

Mahatma Gandhi asked, 'God comes to a hungry man in the form of a slice of bread.' In what form does God come to a person begging to die? (Pandya 1999, 43)

Pandya ignores the fact that Hindu "law-givers" had prohibited the practice of self-willed death and shows how quickly a link can be made between the practice of self-willed death in the past and euthanasia as physician-assisted suicide today. Even if one were not to consider the *Kalivarjya* prohibitions, one would still have to admit that the past tradition had tried to maintain control by insisting on very difficult means, whereas Pandya's proposal would use drugs. It is highly questionable whether Gandhi would have endorsed self-willed death in terminal illness, even though he was greatly influenced by Jainism, and he used the threat of self-willed death with his own fasts as a way to gain power over the British.

Note

1. All citations from *Caraka-saṃhitā* follow the numbering system of Sharma and Dash (1976–1977). All quotations are from these sources unless otherwise noted. (On occasion, I have offered my own translations.) All citations of *Suśruta-saṃhitā* are from Bhishagratna (1963). I have taken the liberty of eliminating sexist language in translations when it is clear that the reference can be to both men and women.

CHAPTER 4

MEDICAL ETHICS THROUGH THE LIFE CYCLE IN BUDDHIST INDIA

Katherine K. Young

I. INTRODUCTION

Birth, development, decay, death – these form the biological base line of human existence. The idea of cycle suggests that there is something similar about the beginning and the end of the process – in this case vulnerability and dependence. To say more is to enter into the field of comparative religion and culture, for it involves cultural notions of time, cosmos, and human destiny. The concept of cycle is particularly appropriate for Buddhism (and Hinduism: see Chapter 3) become the notion of time is cyclical. The cycle of a human life is a microcosm of the cycles of the cosmos (an idea repudiated by Western religions with their linear view of time). The cycles of life are viewed ambivalently in Buddhism (and Hinduism): They are negative in the sense that they represent ignorance and bondage (which includes not only human but also animal and plant life); the human life cycle is also viewed positively, however, because it represents an opportunity for liberation, escape from the cycles of life altogether.

Just as the understanding of cycle involves cultural information about the nature of time, cosmos, and destiny, so does the understanding of the cycle's stages. Cultures divide the human life cycle in different ways; the number of stages and their length of time differ. They also ritually mark these stages in distinctive ways, and, of course, they assign different meanings to the purpose of the stages. The fact that culture (especially religion) is involved in organizing and interpreting the life cycle is not a mere epiphenomenon. Rather, nature and culture are correlatives in human existence. By removing what is instinctual in other species, human beings gain flexibility with their greater capacity for adaptation and creativity, an evolutionary asset. Because this can create chaos and self-destruction, however, human behavior has to be ordered in a definitive way. This gives rise to customs, norms, and morality with religious authority of some kind (from ancestors, spirits, or deities) so that the meaning of the cycle does not have to be reinvented with each person, a precarious proposition to be sure. In the final analysis, all this creates a storehouse of collective wisdom on human survival, testimony both to continuity (for stability) and to change (to meet new conditions of life with the development of new ecological conditions, new technologies, or new cultural insights).

II. STAGES AND RITUAL MARKINGS OF THE LIFE CYCLE

According to the Pāli Canon, both men and women should ideally renounce the world while still young and vigorous to pursue liberation (*nibbāna*; Skt. *nirvāṇa*[1]). From this perspective, sexuality is problematic because desire (taṇhā; Skt. tṛṣṇā) by which the wheel of rebirth (saṃsāra; Skt. saṃsāra) is constantly turned, is related in part to sexual desire, enlightenment being its very elimination. Because the Pāli Canon largely ignored the perspective of the laity, it did not comment on whether people have reproductive responsibilities toward society. Marriage was a secular contract and was not conducted by priests (Harvey 2000, 102). Nor did the Canon elaborate on the stages of the life cycle with their ritual markers. (The Sigālovāda Sutta (Dīghanikāya III.180–93) does, however, describe the reciprocity between parents and children and between husbands and wives.) As a result, the laity followed the prevailing stages of the life cycle in the general culture (for instance, patrilineal, extended families being the norm in India with adoption of a male child if there were no son). By the eighth century in India, however, Mahāyāna and Vajrayāna Buddhism had reinterpreted brahmanical rites of passage to create a Buddhist version (most fully developed in the Nepālese Buddhist text called the Jana-jīvan-kriyā-paddhati). Just as Hinduism had upanayana, which functioned as an upper caste male coming of age ritual connected to Vedic learning, so Nepālese Buddhism had a ritual to mark whether a boy would enter the monastery or become a householder (like Hinduism, Buddhism has had no coming of age ritual marked by circumcision).

Buddhism focuses on the nature of suffering. This is said to begin in the womb itself: According to Buddhaghosa in Visuddhi-magga (XVI.37), the suffering that results from being in the womb (a cramped, dark, hot, smelly place) is like a worm in rotting fish, dough, or cesspools (Ñānamoli trans., Visuddhi-magga 1975, 569). (Attributing all suffering to birth in a female womb is an example of misogyny by some male ascetics.)

Because there are few distinctively Buddhist rituals for birth or the middle stages of the life cycle (aside from one marking the choice of whether to become a monk or householder) and because Buddhism itself has focused on dying and death, we go to the last link in the Buddhist twelvefold formula of dependent co-arising (pratītya-samutpāda). Early Buddhism had rejected the naive and pre-reflective life affirmation of the Vedas and had focused instead on the nature of becoming, momentariness, and the inevitable process of aging as a series of unhappy moments that culminate in decrepitude, disease, and death (Tilak 1989, 62–63). According to one text, "Whichever way he takes a step, he comes closer to death" (Udāna-varga I.13–17 cited by Wayman 1982, 287). Put otherwise, "in life there is nothing more than life, and in death nothing more than death, as we are being born and dying at every moment'" (Lang 1990, 210). Even though the Nepālese text Jana-jāvan-kriyā-paddhati refers to several elaborate rituals (saüskāras) to mark divisions of old age (defined by the number of moons witnessed or age 77, 80, and 90) (Lewis

1994, 14), such ritualism was not common in other Buddhist countries.

Paradoxical though it may sound, one must, in the Theravàda Buddhist scheme, embrace suffering (dukkha; Skt. duḥpkha) because it starkly reveals impermanence as the true nature of life and may prompt the desire for renunciation more than at any preceding time in life (Majjhima-nikāya II.54–74 cited in Tilak 1989, 63). Understanding the meaning of suffering, aging, and death, in other words, is penultimate to liberation. As said in the Mahāyāna-parinirvāṇa-sūtra, "among all ideas (saññā; [Skt. samjñā]) the best are the ideas of impermanence and death. These dispel all the lust, nescience, and pride of the three worlds" (cited in Wayman 1982, 286).

Along with these doctrinal aspects of death, there are mythic ones as well that cluster around Yama, the Indian god of death. He becomes associated with the cycles of rebirth, the underworld, and hell; his messenger Mṛtyu (the personification of death) and Māra (the personification of destruction and evil); the myth of the loss of paradise; and stories about the ghosts of the departed (pretas) who inhabit the numerous hells of the cosmos but also return to earth to interact with human beings (Wayman 1982, 294), a belief that mixed with the local spirit traditions of many Buddhist cultures.

III. ETHICAL ISSUES IN THE BUDDHIST LIFE CYCLE

Because Buddhism largely ignored the laity and the life cycle, it follows that it did not discuss in detail ethical issues (such as exposure, infanticide, miscarriage), although it had more to say about abortion because of its association with killing. It also had more to say about the final stages of the life cycle because of its doctrinal focus on suffering, old age, and death. In addition, Buddhism reflected the generalization of human experience through male experience rather than female (with its focus on birth and therefore the beginning of the cycle).

1. Exposure, Infanticide, Miscarriage, and Abortion

There is little textual information on exposure or infanticide in South and Southeast Asian Buddhism, but it may be surmised from Buddhism's position on abortion that these practices were illicit. To determine the Buddhist view on abortion, it is necessary to understand its theory of conception. Conception is really reconception. This life is but one in a beginningless series of lives. According to Majjhima-nikāya I.266; II.157 of the Pāli Canon, for conception, there must be sexual intercourse with right timing; the union of sperm and blood; and the presence of a gabbha (Skt. garbha) (a living entity) (see discussion later).

It is necessary to examine these three in more detail. Sexual intercourse with right timing means the woman must be in the fertile phase of her menstrual cycle (*mātā utunī hoti*). The union of sperm and blood means that sperm and blood must assemble or come together according to *Papañcasūdanī* II.310 (this text is Buddhaghosa's commentary on the *Majjhima-nikāya* mentioned in the preceding paragraph). The commentator defines coming together as being combined as one lump. He refers to the term *gabbha* as follows: (1) the descent of the *gabbha*; (2) the fetus after fertilization (*Vinaya-piṭaka* IV.316); and (3) the womb. *Papañcasūdanī* II.310 then mentions "a being that is propelled by the mechanism of *kamma* into another birth" (Boisvert 2000, 303).

The meaning of *gabbha* has been a matter of debate. According to Buddhaghosa in *Visuddhi-magga* XVI.81,110, consciousness (*viññāna*; Skt. *vijñāna*), one of the five basic constituents (*skandhas*; Skt. skandhas) or aggregates of human beings, is of eighty-nine types in fourteen modes, the first being the rebirth-linking consciousness according to the Theravāda and other early schools. This consciousness contains the *kamma* (Skt. *karma*) from previous lives, and this karma makes it possible to select a body and hold everything together. (See also *Visuddhi-magga* XVII.165, which says: "An echo, or its like, supplies the figures here; connectedness. By continuity denies identity and otherness. And with a stream of continuity there is neither identity nor otherness" (Ñāṇamoli, trans. [1956] 1975).) In answer to the question of what transmigrates after the cessation of the aggregates (*skandhas*), Buddhaghosa replies "In continuity the fruit is neither of nor from another. Seeds' forming processes will suit to show the purport of this matter" (*Visuddhi-magga* XVII.169; Ñāṇamoli, trans. [1956] 1975). (See also XVII.133–36 and XX.29, which elaborate on *kamma*-born materiality, the many types of rebirth-linking consciousness, and so forth). In short, *kamma* defines what kind of body one enters and the very experience of entering as well (it can be traumatic or pleasant). This rebirth-linking consciousness (which contained the seeds of *kamma*) came to be understood as an intermediate being in Tibetan Buddhism following Vasubandhu's *Abhidharmakośa* (the interpretation followed by Keown (1995) and Boisvert (2000)).

But the canon, especially the *Jātakas*, also has stories of extraordinary birth in which pregnancy occurs by mere touch in the navel or elsewhere or parthenogenically. This conflict among the accounts of conception – by the rebirth-linking consciousness or touch or parthenogenesis – was resolved by Nāgasena in *Milindapañha*. He states that the three conditions for pregnancy are present even in the apparently extraordinary accounts because the *gabbha* can enter through the mouth or elsewhere (see Boisvert 2000 for references and discussion). "In the *sutta* literature, the *Yakkhasaṃyuttaṃ* classifies periods of gestation into five distinct stages, the first one being the *kalalam*, followed by

the *abduda*, *pesi*, *ghana*, and *pasākha*" (Boisvert 2000, 307). The same classification is enumerated in the *Kathāvatthu* as well. The *Mahāniddesa* mentions these five stages to highlight the insignificance of life, says Boisvert; "the body will die within 100 years at the most; it could be within any of these five stages, or at any other time after birth" (Boisvert 2000, 307). The text more likely refers to the vulnerability of life at this stage, which had to be protected by many rituals. The commentary on the *Yakkhasaṃyuttaṃ* assigns 7 days to each of these stages (Boisvert 2000, 307–8). Boisvert points to two meanings of *kalalam*. One he translates as the ovum [pointing out on page 308 that *Milindapañha* 49 "also uses the word *kalalam* to refer to what is contained within the egg (*aṇḍa*) of a hen."], which transforms itself after fertilization, and the other is the first stage of the pregnancy. I suggest, however, because the latter is the same as the Āyurvedic descriptions in the *Caraka* and *Suśruta* (see Chapters 9 and 20 for discussion of these Hindu texts), it would be the mainstream idea. The former must be a variant introduced by Nāgasena in his attempt to explain extraordinary births.

In modern debates, personhood has sometimes been defined as the development of consciousness. A controversy is reported in *Kathāvatthu* over exactly when fetal consciousness develops, all at once or gradually. This was resolved by the commentator who said that consciousness (*manāyatana*) and touch were reborn at the moment of conception, whereas the other physical sense organs took 77 days (discussed by Boisvert 2000, 307; McDermott 1999, 174). Textual scholars of scriptural Buddhism conclude that the fetus is a person from the moment of conception.

A human being, moreover, has special status because only in this form can enlightenment be achieved. According to *Dhammapāda* 130: "'Life is precious and dear for every living being,' said the Buddha. 'Judging from your own life's valuableness don't kill and don't let kill'" (cited by Young 1994a, 666). The killing of a human is a qualitative wrong (Zeyst 1961; Keown 1995; Taniguchi 1987, 1994; Young 1994a; McDermott 1999; Birnbaum 1989).

Personhood in the West has been defined by some people as rationality and freedom to choose (which presupposes maturity). Buddhists would not make these the basis of moral status, however, because personhood arises gradually in fetal and child development and rationality and choice are constantly in flux (even in mature adults) (Keown 1995, 28–29). Personhood as a psychophysical totality, moreover, is a continuous process, transcending this particular lifetime.

With this discussion of conception in mind, we turn to the topic of abortion. For Buddhists, not killing regulates human life through daily discipline and involves abstention from doing harm to or killing *living beings* (which includes the fetus). According to Buddhaghosa, killing a living being (*satta*; Skt. *sattva*) means depriving the living being of life by cutting off the life faculty in the sense of obstructing or disrupting the causal continuity of the physical life faculty, which in turn takes away the immaterial life faculty because of their mutual dependency (*Visuddhi-magga* II.438 cited by Keown 1995, 148).

The precept against killing was linked directly to the issue of abortion in the Pāli Canon's monastic rules (*Vinaya*; Skt. *Vinaya*). In *Mahāvagga* (*Vinaya-piṭaka*), a general rule is given: "whatever monk intentionally deprives a human being of life – even to the extent of causing an abortion – he becomes no longer a (true) recluse (*samaṇa* [Skt. *śramaṇa*]), not a son of the Sakyans [that is, no longer a follower of the Buddha]" (*Vinaya-piṭaka* I.97 cited by McDermott 1999, 164). In other words, the monastic has been excommunicated from the monastery. Buddhist monks face excommunication if they perform abortions, provide the means or information to do so, or if they assist in killing a person who is physically dependent or deformed, as in the case where a monk assisted a family to kill a family member whose hands and feet were "cut off" (*Vinaya-piṭaka* III.85). This means that monastics must not be involved in infanticide or killing any deformed person at any stage of life. From several specific cases in the *Vinaya*, it is clear that the morality of the act is defined by the agent's will or intention (*cetanā*) to kill but the consequence of this specific "will" (death of the one who was willed to die) is taken into consideration to determine the punishment. McDermott (1999, 164ff) summarizes these patterns as follows according to three kinds of offenses and punishments defined by the monastic rules. *Pārājika* means extraordinary offense or excommunication, often translated as "defeat." *Thullaccaya* means grave offense, and, *dukkaṭa* means ordinary offense: "(1) intended victim (only) dies – *pārājika*; (2) intended victim dies and unintended victim dies – *pārājika*; (3) unintended victim dies while intended victim survives – *thullaccaya*; (4) intent but no victim (i.e. no unintended victim; intended victim survives) *thullaccaya*; (5) unintended victim dies where no victim is intended – *dukkaṭa*" (McDermott 1999, 168).

Buddhist scholars have argued that the intention for abortion in turn is based on greed, hatred, or delusion (all aspects of selfish craving). Thus, abortion is considered unskillful or unbeneficial (*akuśala*) to self and others and creates bad karma. Because of the doctrine of coconditionality (*pratītya-samutpāda*), which frames the problem of abortion in the context of interconnectedness, the intentional killing of a fetus implicates the pregnant woman, the one who gave advice, and the one who performed the act. In short, the monastic rules were against involvement with abortion (Florida 1991). This wrong is related to intent and direct (but not indirect) consequence. Buddhism shares with Roman Catholicism the doctrine of double effect; even though the mother is killed, when this is not intended, the wrong belonged to a less serious category.

Comment must be made on a related modern controversy: Is late abortion morally more reprehensible than early abortion? Does Buddhaghosa's comment "with regard to animals it is worse to kill large ones than small" extend to the fetus? Florida, Ratanakul, Harvey, and Ling claim "yes," but Keown and McDermott claim "no" because the connection is not explicit in the text and the next sentence connects human beings with something else.

Unlike the case of Japan (see Chapter 44), it is difficult to provide a historical profile on the topic of abortion for Thailand, but we can glean some insight into the topic in modern Thailand. Although Theravāda Buddhism is the state religion, abortion is illegal except in two cases – threat to the mother's health and rape – and is punishable by a prison term or fine. Because health has been given a broad interpretation, however, and abortions for reasons of health can be procured in private clinics, doctors' offices, and even government and nongovernmental organizations' clinics, there is a high rate. As for abortions for reasons of genetic abnormalities, such as Down syndrome, or for acquired immunodeficiency syndrome, Ratanakul (1999, 59) observes that some women will have the child to avoid the bad karma of abortion (and give it a chance to use up its own bad karma which caused the problem), but if it does not die quickly will abandon it at the hospital. Others will not abort or even abandon it because they want to accumulate good karma by raising such a child.

According to one modern survey, Buddhists have the highest percentage of approval of abortion when compared with Catholic, Protestant, Fundamentalist Protestant, Jewish, Muslim, and Hindu groups on the criterion of abortion to protect the mother's health (96 percent), just behind Judaism on abortion for a handicapped child, third on abortion if the mother is unmarried (58.3 percent), and first on abortion if the couple want no more children (64.1 percent) (Simon 1998, 64).

This survey also shows that contemporary views on abortion vary considerably when Japan, Korea, Thailand, Burma, Sri Lanka, and Vietnam are compared. (The statistics give some suggestion of how Buddhists might view abortion because the countries officially have Buddhism as the state religion or have a sizeable Buddhist population. China has not been included in this survey because of its modern secular history, its distinctive policy, and its unique enforcement.) Vietnam's rate of abortion is the seventh highest in the world. According to statistics for 1988–1991, Korea is ninth in the top ten countries with the lowest abortion rate (1988–1991) (Simon 1998, 52). In addition, we learn that motivations differ from one Buddhist country to another. Japan, Republic of Korea, Cambodia, Myanmar, Thailand, Vietnam, and Sri Lanka all accept abortion to save the mother's life; Japan, Republic of Korea, Thailand, and Vietnam to preserve the mother's physical health; Japan, Republic of Korea,

Vietnam to preserve mental health; Japan, Korea, Thailand, and Vietnam for rape or incest; Republic of Korea, Thailand, or Vietnam for fetal impairment; Japan and Vietnam for economic or social reasons; and Republic of Korea and Vietnam on request (Simon 1998, 39–41).

Several observations are in order. First, there is enormous difference between what Buddhist texts have held on the topic of abortion and modern views. There are also differences in modern views, which may or may not align with official law and government policy. Even though a country may have Buddhism as a state religion, monastics often do not interfere with government policy because of a long-time tradition of preventing friction by keeping the affairs of monastery and state separate. A country's position on abortion has as much to do with its public policy of modernization as it has to do with whether Buddhism is officially a state religion or not. Thailand being officially Buddhist but promodernization has a relatively liberal abortion policy; Myanmar being officially Buddhist but anti-Western and often antimodernization has been categorically antiabortion (except to save the mother's life, a position articulated by Buddhist scripture). To underscore the range, Myanmar and Sri Lanka allow abortion only to save the mother's life whereas Vietnam and Korea allow abortion on demand.

Today, the Buddhist view on abortion is being hotly debated because a variety of prochoice arguments are emerging in Buddhist circles. In Thailand, although monks have avoided the controversy over abortion, a wide range of opinion exists among physicians (Florida 1999). Pinit Ratanakul (1999) presents the following arguments for a prochoice position, even though he wants to avoid the language of rights on account of the Buddhist doctrine of coconditionality (*paṭicca-samuppāda*; Skt. *pratītya-samutpāda*): "abortion could be a skilful act" depending on the intention; Buddhist precepts are ideals, not commands; it is not necessary to deal with problems of poverty, education, and abortion confrontationally; abortion may be the lesser of two evils; and Thai women are embracing ideas of human rights, reproductive choice, and family planning and so abortion is permissible."

Many Western Buddhists are also developing a Buddhist prochoice position. Robert Aitken (cited by Florida 1991, 46–47), an American Roshi, has said, for instance, that if a woman approaches him, he acts with compassion, exploring with her the options. If she is committed to having an abortion, he encourages her to do it with loving nurture and awareness of the sadness that pervades the universe. James Hughes (1999) states that Buddhist scriptures provide no specific guidance on abortion; there are conflicting views over when conception occurs and its embryology is prescientific and full of error (he provides no textual documentation for this assessment). In any case, he continues, authentic Buddhism need not be textual and historically based. There is room for criticism

and contextualization of the religion in a new situation. He suggests, for instance, that because utilitarianism is the dominant interpretation of Buddhist ethics in the West (a debatable point), it should seek the greatest happiness for the greatest number and work to lessen the suffering of all beings. As long as the woman and her collaborators have good intentions for the abortion, it relieves suffering and is not wrong.

On the topic of abortion, Peter Harvey makes a distinction between ethics and law. He cites several authorities who make this distinction (Philip Leso, Roshi Jiyu Kennett, and Helen Tworkov) but points out that traditionally there was a fluid relationship between Buddhist ethics and law. Arguing that the "anti-abortion/pro-choice" position (that is, it is morally wrong but legally available) is not supported by a number of Buddhist texts and suggesting that this desire to have it both ways is particularly characteristic of American Buddhists, he concludes that "Buddhist principles suggest that the state should do what it can to persuade people to give up evil. It is true that Buddhism has never advocated making all immoral actions illegal, as doing so might itself threaten social order, as well as removing genuine moral choice from people. . . . Should protecting innocent humans be outweighed by the fact that this would upset some people and reduce their choice? On Buddhist grounds, the answer is surely 'no'" (Harvey 2000, 349). He opens the door to one exception, however: abortion of a badly impaired fetus on grounds of compassion for the mother and argues that other cases should be reduced by encouraging the use of contraception.

Sometimes the debate over the Buddhist view of abortion becomes heated. George Tanabe, for instance, has suggested that William LaFleur has imputed to Buddhism a proabortion position (even though the texts are antiabortion). LaFleur has responded (1995) by arguing that Japanese Buddhists (see Chapter 44) prefer to use the language of suffering (*ku*) rather than sin (*tsumi*), that the Buddhist virtue of compassion is a "mechanism" that can be used to deal with the "dilemma," and that there is a need to recognize folk and popular religions rather than just the classical form defined by the Pāli Canon as well as the voices of ordinary women rather than monks, or, for that matter, any voices rather than the silence of monks.

Keown (1995, 1999a, 1999b) has provided the most extensive analysis of Buddhist views on abortion. He argues that an adequate interpretation must be based on the Buddhist scriptures and be faithful to traditional Buddhist interpretive principles (according to Buddhaghosa, these include scripture, that which conforms to it, commentaries, and personal opinion in that order). He thinks that any claim to represent Buddhism must represent the most broad-based Buddhist view possible and finds this in the *Vinaya* (monastic rule) sections of the various canons, which have remarkable consistency. On this basis, he concludes that Buddhism is categorically antiabortion, that the case of Japan is a cultural exception that has deviated from the Buddhist textual tradition, and that modern Buddhists, especially Japanese and Western Buddhists, have taken liberties with the textual tradition in their hermeneutical strategies.

Likewise, Shoyo Taniguchi (1987, 1994) says that the Pāli Canon is categorically against abortion, and that it belongs to the category of unskillful (akusala; Skt. akuśala) action (see Chapter 10) because not only the fetus but also the woman could experience physical and mental harms. Buddhism would reject the argument that a woman has a right to control her own body because the very idea of having a body as something substantial is only a convention of speech. Extrapolating from ideas on the importance of human life (which includes the fetus) and nonviolence, she says that the fetus should not be killed in cases of rape, incest, or contraceptive failure.

James McDermott, another textually oriented scholar, states, somewhat more cautiously, that: "the philosophical foundation for objection to abortion can in principle be derived from these texts" (1999, 177), even though the issue has been framed differently (punishments for monastics and karmic consequences for the laity) than in the modern West. (See McDermott 1999, 158–61 for discussion of Jātaka stories about lay women performing abortions.) He points out that abortion involves the person in a cycle of karmic retribution such as rebirth as ghosts. He also observes that there is no difference in the retribution based on the stage of the pregnancy; this includes destroying the kalala, the original lump, which would rule out research on human fetuses.

In short, Westerners have been major contributors to the abortion discussion, either through being Buddhists themselves with a bent for socially engaged Buddhism, or scholars of Buddhism who are concerned that the textual record be presented accurately. Mediating these two groups are Western ethicists who look to the Buddhist texts from a comparative angle or an exegetical one informed by commitment to a particular Western school of ethics.

2. The Ethics of New Reproductive Technologies

A few people have discussed the new reproductive technologies from a Buddhist perspective. One is Taniguchi (1994, 52), who observes briefly that as long as new technologies, such as in vitro fertilization, do not cause suffering to any of the parties involved and bring benefits, they would be acceptable to Buddhism.

A more extensive discussion is offered by Keown (1995, 132–37). He has extrapolated what the Buddhist position on several new reproductive technologies should be, given its traditional prohibition of abortion. In vitro fertilization,

he suggests, could be allowed if there is no freezing of embryos (because about half are lost in the process or later eliminated if not needed), and no selective abortion of fetuses (when more than desired are introduced into the uterus because of the usually low rate of implantation but more than expected actually implant). In addition, in vitro fertilization would be acceptable as long as the fetus is not used for research to benefit others or without its consent (which, of course, is impossible). As for artificial insemination by donor, he deduces that it might infringe on the spirit but not the letter of the third precept against sexual misconduct because a third party would be involved, but there would be no problem with artificial insemination by husband. He finds no reason to forbid obtaining semen by masturbation, unlike Roman Catholicism. Keown gives no specific Buddhist passages to support all this aside from the first and third precepts (on not killing and no sexual misconduct respectively). Unlike Roman Catholicism's rejection of contraception, however, Keown finds Buddhism has no clear position, and so it has been allowed (ancient techniques, for instance, have included pharmacopoeia and magic).

Joseph Schenker (1992) has also briefly discussed Buddhist views on new reproductive technologies but comes to very different conclusions. He begins, in good postmodern fashion, by observing that Buddhism has a broad array of positions because of its decentralized organization, its presence in different countries with varying cultures, its lack of scriptural consistency, and its differing precepts for monastics and laity, the latter being far more lenient. He argues that lay people have license to act in any way as long as no concrete harm is done. As a result, they can resort to treatment for infertility, and it can be given to both unmarried and married couples. He gives no proof texts from Buddhist scriptures for these claims nor does he give argumentation. He observes that the Japanese have had in vitro fertilization since 1982 (see Chapter 44) and alludes to the fact that destruction of unwanted frozen embryos might be problematic from a Buddhist perspective on abortion. The freezing of preembryos would be permissible as would be research on them because there are always other rebirths. (He ignores the Buddhist doctrine that this human life is viewed as extremely valuable because it is an opportunity to try to achieve enlightenment and get out of the cycle of rebirths altogether.) There would be no prohibition against the donation of sperm or eggs, but this should be done as little as possible. As for surrogacy, there is no prohibition, although it is recognized that the practice could create moral and legal problems for families. (Once again no reasons are given.) In his conclusion, Schenker remarks that individuals should have the freedom to choose how they wish to reproduce, which is in line with universal human rights. Then he throws down the gauntlet.

Religious authorities, despite the powerful influence they exercise on public minds, should not prohibit a therapeutic approach to infertility, which would limit the area within which individuals are free to decide. Religious authorities, in order to maintain their strength, power, and efficiency, should undergo continual development, and change in the same way that science does. While religious principles may be unchangeable, they may, nevertheless, undergo significant changes in their implementation. (Schenker 1992, 8)

It comes as no surprise to find that he writes for the *Journal of Assisted Reproduction and Genetics*. This journal along with other scientific and professional journals on this topic, have generally promoted libertarian views, that is, anything can be done and one should have free choice as long as no specific and concrete harms can be demonstrated.

Cloning has yet to be discussed (to my knowledge) in the Buddhist literature. If animals are to be used as a source for cloning organs for transplantation, Buddhists might be against it (because of the monastic rule not to kill living beings and the tradition of vegetarianism in some forms of Buddhism).

3. The Ethics of Terminal Care

Traditional texts have recognized transitions to dying and ritually marked them. The Nepālese text *Jana-jīvan-kriyā-paddhati* notes, for instance, that the idea of a final illness will arise if the physician (*baidya*) has given appropriate medicines and the patient has performed a ritual to pacify malevolent spirits and deities, heard the curing *mantras*, consulted the astrologer to determine what planets are causing the affliction, and ritually neutralized these negative influences – all to no avail (Lewis 1994, 15). In general, there has been an unwillingness to tell the patient that death is imminent as reports from Japan, Cambodia, and Thailand indicate (Hardacre 1994; Nudeshima 1989; Nakayama 1976–1977; Lang 1990; Lindbeck 1984). This is attributed to the need to provide hope but also might be related to the traditional refusal to treat terminal cases or to paternalism and avoidance of discussing death by physicians (for discussion of the ethics of risk assessment and truth telling, see Chapter 44).

The treatment of the very old and dying is closely related to the meaning of death. It can easily be argued that the chronic disability accompanying aging and dying, in fact, is the point at which medicine and religion converge) (see Chapter 44 for Japanese Buddhism). American Buddhists have become active in the hospice movement. The Zen Hospice Project (San Francisco), the hospice Maitri (San Francisco), the Rigpa Fellowship: Spiritual Care Education and Training Program (San Francisco), the

Living/Dying Project (Fairfax, CA), Upaya (Santa Fe), and Naropa Institute (Boulder) provide spiritually assisted and long-term care for cancer, acquired immunodeficiency syndrome, and other patients. They train volunteers to help people to die without fear through the practice of mindfulness and body awareness. Naropa even offers a Master of Arts in Gerontology and Long-Term Care Management.

4. Buddhism and the Ethics of Pain Relief

In Buddhism, how one handles the moment of dying is the culmination of one's spiritual preparation throughout life. This involves understanding the nature of death and controlling consciousness at this transitional event to avoid fear. The *Majjhima-nikāya* in the Pāli Canon, using the analogy of untamed and tamed elephants, says that a monk who has not exhausted the fluxes (ideas that intoxicate the mind) (*āsava*; Skt. *āśrava*) has an untamed death whereas one who has, experiences a tamed death. Asaṅga (fifth century) comments on this text to the effect that the heedful person will guard life, strength, the mind, and action. This will lead, through mindfulness on breathing, eating, and so forth and by meditating daily on the fact that death could occur at any moment, to *enlightenment*, the deathless state (*Aṅguttara-nikāya*, the First and Second *Maraṇasati-sutta*, cited in Wayman 1982, 284). In short, the untamed will die (and be reborn), the tamed will not (having achieved liberation).

According to the *Bhaddaka-sutta* in the *Aṅguttara-nikāya* of the Pāli Canon, a disciple of the Buddha called Sariputta described how the death-time act (*kālakiriya*; Skt. *kālakiriyā*) determines an unfortunate or fortunate death. Asaṅga comments on this passage by calling the experience "a vision of form ... comparable to a dream, especially due to the causal karma" (*Yogācārabhūmi*, Part I, p. 17.4–6; cited by Wayman 1982, 281). Buddhaghosa, in his *Visuddhi-magga* (VIII.8ff) gives eight meditations on death to create mindfulness of it. For Theravādins, dying should be a time for mindfulness and emptying the mind of all visions and thoughts (*vipassanā*; Skt. *vipaśyanā*): As one modern Buddhist puts it "The more exhausted you feel, the more subtle and focused your concentration must be, so that you can cope with the painful sensations that arise ... Don't go grasping at thoughts of your children and relatives, don't grasp at anything whatsoever. Let go" (Subatto 1997, 25).

Śāntideva in his *Śikṣāsamuccaya*, a Mahāyāna text, cites the *Pitāputrasamāgama-sūtra* to the effect that the moment of death has two conditions, the death consciousness or death-time act (the last consciousness, *vijñāna*), which is the most important factor, and the secondary or supporting factor of karma, which gives rise to the form of death-time, that is, a death vision. The next life is determined by these two conditions (Wayman 1982, 281).

In Tibet, during the time of a person's death, short texts have been read aloud to the person or sermons on the topic given by monks. One of the most popular books has been the *Tibetan Book of the Dead* (*Bardo Thodol*) by Padmasambhava (eighth century). Basically, it identifies the progressive states of the visions over a period of 49 days in the realm between death and rebirth (the intermediate state called *bardo*), and exhorts the dead person to recognize all dying experiences as but a projection of the mind because this defines enlightenment. Those who have prepared for death through years of meditation will experience at the moment of death a brilliant clear light, which is none other than realization of the void, the *dharmakāya* body of the Buddha. If this moment of enlightenment is missed, it becomes progressively more difficult each day of the *bardo*.

Because of the relation of consciousness to destiny at the time of death and during the *bardo*, according to Tibetan medicine, no strong painkillers or other mind altering drugs should be used because consciousness could be decreased (Clifford 1984, 110–11). Buddhists in other countries make the same point. Chaicharoen and Ratanakul (1998, 39) writing about Thailand say, for instance, that Buddhist hospices can help patients die "in a calm, conscious state, so that possible good rebirth is obtained. The hospice specialists have successfully demonstrated not only that no one needs to suffer from unbearable pain toward the end of life, but that most people can be maintained at a level of pain-relief which does not impair their faculties or cloud consciousness, but permits them to have meaningful lives at the end." In addition, Buddhists argue that painkillers should not be used because pain is punishment for bad karma (Lang 1990, 210). In other words, the experience of pain is a kind of expiation. In Cambodia, family and friends distract the patient from pain by prayers, songs, Buddha stories, or having the patient repeat the words "*poot-tho*" (Lang 1990, 210). (For a discussion of Buddhism and palliative care in Japan, see Chapter 44.)

Rick Fields, an American (Tibetan) Buddhist, has said in an interview when he was dying of cancer: "I want to be as conscious as possible at the end . . . I asked Lama Tharchin this question, about painkillers, and he laughed and said that they aren't a problem. For one thing, if you are feeling a lot of bodily pain it's harder to practice and concentrate. And when the body and mind separate there is so much general confusion and chaos at that moment that it would be very difficult and not even very useful to keep your consciousness. And anyhow, your Buddhanature has survived through countless lifetimes – the fires of hell, of drowning. God knows what. Buddha knows what. It's survived. So a little morphine isn't really going to affect your Buddha-nature, don't worry about it" (Fields in Tworkov 1997, 100).

What does all this mean for the practice of modern medicine? It could be argued that the following should be present: attentiveness to the immediate desire of the patient while still conscious and good palliative care (including adequate pain relief) when consciousness disappears. Pain can be considered torture. If pain is not treated and people are being tortured, then they might become so stressed, they might die sooner. Thus, it is a fundamental right to relieve pain (Somerville 2000, 137).

5. Ethical Treatment of the Comatose

Keown reflects on what the Buddhist perspective might be for end of life decisions related to patients in a coma (persistent vegetable state). He bases his analysis on Buddhism's definition of the person as the combination of the five factors (*skandha*s) and the concept of the good as involving the whole person. "Since life is a good intrinsic to each individual the loss of higher faculties does not mean that human life ceases to be good. Human existence is embodied existence and no distinction of any moral significance should be drawn between the organic life of an individual and their [sic] psychological experiences" (Keown 1995, 161). Keown concludes that from a Buddhist perspective, people in a persistent vegetable state deserve the same care as other patients.

As for whether there is a duty to feed a comatose patient or whether there can be the moral withdrawal of nourishment, Keown finds some grounds for viewing feeding as a medical treatment (based on the fact that the Buddha had sanctioned butter, oil, honey, and molasses as medicines and the fact that food can be inserted through a tube) but argues that food is not necessarily a treatment and the tube is just a device, hardly a technological one, for introducing nutrition to the body. For these two reasons, he concludes, nutrition is not medical treatment. Moreover, there is the issue of whether it is a futile treatment, which takes one back to fundamental issues of what it means to be a person. As a result, there is a duty to maintain nutrition. He concludes that "what is prohibited by Buddhist precepts is the deliberate attempt to destroy life: (omission such as with-holding nutrition with the intent of killing the person, would be as morally wrong as the intent to kill)" (Keown 1995, 167). Keown thinks that it is not necessary to respond to secondary complications such as pneumonia (for which there is a medical treatment) if there is not a serious possibility of improvement in the patient's condition. The issue of maintaining nutrition, he argues, is different from the use of life-support systems. The latter is a technological aid, an extraordinary means of keeping a person alive. Many other ethicists, however, regard nutrition as treatment and accept the idea of withdrawal of treatment, if the patient (or the patient's proxy) requests this. If nutrition or life support systems make it possible for a person to live, these systems cannot be called futile; withdrawal of nutrition can be understood as respecting a person's right to inviolability (not to be touched) or right to privacy and to be the judge through a living will or proxy, when fully informed of the options (Somerville 2000, 163–64).

6. The Ethics of Transplantation

To remove organs to be used for transplants from individuals at the time of death, it is necessary to have a definition of death that facilitates the transplantation process while protecting the donor against premature removal. Defining death as brain death (the cessation of brain waves and therefore the irreversible end of brain functions) works better for this modern technology than cardiovascular signs of death.

Some modern Buddhists have begun to think about this issue of the time of death by looking to scriptural statements and their commentaries. Death (*marana*; Skt. *marana*), according to Buddhaghosa, is the interruption of the life faculty within one life (Ñāṇamoli trans., *Visuddhi-magga* VIII.1). According to the *Suttanipāta* III.143: "When three things leave the body – vitality (*āyu* [Skt. *āyus*]), heat (*usma* [Skt. *uṣmā*]) and consciousness (*viññāna* [Skt. *vijñāna*]), then it lies forsaken and inanimate (*acetanā* [Skt. *acetanā*]), a thing for others to feed on" (cited by Keown 1995, 145; Sanskrit terms added). The discourse on the Greater Miscellany observes that vitality and heat are the organic foundation for the five senses of sight, hearing, smell, taste, and touch (*Majjhima-nikāya* I.295–6 cited by Keown 1995, 145).

Keown suggests that the Buddhist position is basically biological. Biological death can mean cessation of vital functions such as respiration or heartbeat or unreceptivity, unresponsivity, or reflexivity (the 1968 criteria of the Harvard Medical School). He points out that this definition creates the problem of whether there is total or only partial brain death. The latter is defined by neocortical death or loss of self-consciousness and awareness, popularly known as the vegetative state, and called loss of personhood by some (Keown 1995, 143). From the texts, Keown concludes that, according to the Buddhist textual passages that bear on this issue, "We would define the Buddhist concept of death as follows: death is the irreversible loss of integrated organic function" (Keown 1995, 156–58), even though nails and hair of a body may still grow and the heart can still beat for some time. The key term in this context, he says, is *bhinna* (Skt. *bhinna*), which means broken asunder, death being 'the break-up of the body' (*kayassa bheda*). Because an individual is a psychophysical whole, this breakdown is the breakdown of the whole and not just the loss of consciousness or intellectual functions (Keown 1995, 154–56).

The Nepālese text *Jana-jīvan-kriyā-paddhati* suggests that death occurs when the breath (*prāṇa*) leaves the body and goes to the gate of the god of death (Yama), who reveals the amount of good and bad karma that will determine destiny. In the Tibetan tradition, a discussion of death omens developed in the medieval Buddhist Tantras. The *Gyu-zhi* describes the following signs of death: losing strength and color in the complexion; feeling dull, heavy, cold, thirsty, dry; becoming immobile; being unable to digest food; losing control of urination and defecation; having difficulty breathing; being mentally disturbed, angry, and unfocused; fading in and out of consciousness; and experiencing different kinds of visions depending on one's karma (Clifford 1984, 108–10). At this stage the person may appear to be dead, but consciousness and the life-force have not yet left the body, and so the body should not be tampered with in any way. (This can take up to a few days for a normal person or a few weeks for advanced meditators, who benefit immensely from the unusual and powerful state of expanded consciousness at the time of dying) (Clifford 1984, 110). Next, the four elements dissolve into consciousness, consciousness dissolves into the heart, and from there it leaves the body, dissolving into space. The person experiences this as falling or fainting. This defines the moment of death. With death, the breath completely stops, and the body becomes stiff and rigid with red and white fluids being discharged from the nostrils of the corpse.

According to Buddhism, death is of two types. *Timely death* occurs when good kamma is exhausted or when the time of a normal lifespan (100 years for a human) has come to an end. By contrast, *untimely death* occurs when continuity is interrupted by the individual's present kamma or (metaphorically) by "assaults with weapons" that is, the "poisoned arrows" because of previous kamma (Ñāṇamoli trans., *Visuddhi-magga* X.VIII). Asaṅga makes much the same point but expands on the nature of untimely death: consisting of nine types defined by various dietary or constitutional problems, refusal of medicine, traveling at the wrong time, or impure conduct (*Yogācārabhūmi* Part I, 15.7–16.20 cited by Wayman 1982, 279).

Buddhaghosa explains that after death has occurred (the body has withered, the faculties of sight and other senses have ceased, and body, mind, and life faculties have withdrawn into the heart-basis, then consciousness supported by the heart-basis and containing the kamma for destiny is propelled forward by craving and ignorance. Abandoning its former support like a person crossing a river by swing from a rope, it swings over to the "other shore" of a new life. "The former of these [two states of consciousness] is called 'death (*cuti*)' because of falling (*cavana*), and the latter is called 'rebirth-linking (*pati-sandhi*)' because of linking (*pati-sandha*) across the gap separating the beginning of the next becoming" (Ñāṇamoli trans., *Visuddhi-magga*

XVII.163); (see also *Samyutta-nikāya* II.2; for Asaṅga's gloss, see Wayman 1982, 277).

Debates over transplantation have included not only problems defining the moment of death but also the nature of the body, more specifically whether it is sacred and must be kept whole. S. H. J. Sugunasiri (1990, 948) argues, for instance, that the idea of a person or body, which suggests something substantial and permanent, belongs merely to conventional (*sammuti*; Skt. *samvṛtti*) language because all that consists of name and form (*nāmarūpa*; Skt. *nāmarūpa*) is impermanent. Thus, death is but "the temporary end of a temporary phenomena." Therefore, the physical body in whole or part, dead or alive, is not intrinsically sacred, though life, respect, and gratitude for the body, including the corpse, according to Buddha, were important for the social good (*attha saṃhitā*). Despite the importance of respect, Sugunasiri thinks that transplantation can be accepted by Buddhists because other central Buddhist values – generosity, skill-in-means, and compassion, which are important both for social living and enlightenment – can be used to support transplantation (Sugunasiri 1990, 948). He warns, however, that the psychological component of transplantation is worthy of consideration because the rejection of an organ might result from mental incompatibility – the body part of one whose last thought was immoral might not fit the more refined body of the moral recipient (morality being correlated with physical refinement) and so a psychologist should be part of the transplant team. (For Japanese Buddhist views on transplantation, see Chapter 44.)

Casy Frank – a Western Buddhist, a lawyer, and a student of Philip Kapleau – has developed a set of questions for living wills that would be of interest to Buddhists contemplating offering their organs for transplantation. He discusses the concern for many Buddhists that because death comes when consciousness leaves the body and with the final breath and because the circumstances of the final time can influence destiny, it is believed that "it is best not to cut into the body for three days following clinical death or risk disturbing the process... The request by many Buddhists that their bodies not be tampered with for three days following clinical death – even though clinical death is itself an imprecise term – disqualified them from donating organs and tissue, since those parts of the body must be harvested sooner than that" (Frank 1997, 76). He then discusses various ways that Buddhists can be donors and how to make their intentions clear in a living will.

7. The Ethics of Self-Willed Death and Euthanasia

Peter Harvey observes that one of the three cravings in Buddhism is craving for annihilation and elimination of unpleasant situations (Harvey 2000, 286). He argues, following the commentary on *Vinaya* III.82, that killing oneself is just as much in violation of the first precept against killing as homicide. He thinks, however, that fasting to death is permissible (1) if one is so intent on obtaining a meditative state that there is no time to collect food (although once the state is obtained one should then eat); (2) if one wishes to relieve the burden on caregivers during a severe, long illness or terminal illness; (3) if one intends to attain a meditative state and self-starvation is an unintended side-effect; (4) if it is related to a compassionate act; or (5) if death is near at hand (making further meditation possible) and further eating would be futile (Harvey 2000, 291). Harvey concurs with Keown (see later) that "Buddhism has life as an ultimate value, or 'basic good,' and that it should never be sacrificed even in the name of another such value, friendship or compassion. This means that to have compassion as a motive, but to intend death in the process, is unacceptable" (Harvey 2000, 295). He observes that Mahāyāna Buddhists, however, might use the idea of skillful means (*upāya*) (see Chapter 10) to legitimate euthanasia as an expression of compassion. Although he admits that "on Buddhist principles, euthanasia is unethical and inadvisable," he thinks that "[t]his does not entail, though, that completely self-administered euthanasia, i.e., suicide in the case of a difficult illness – should be *illegal*" (Harvey 2000, 299). To support his position, he notes that only under British influence was suicide criminalized and that occurred only in Sri Lanka. He also points to the case of Channa (who attained enlightenment while killing himself) in the Pāli Canon and concludes that "[s]uicide (if followed by rebirth) is unethical, but a person still has a right to do unethical actions" (Harvey 2000, 299). (See the discussion of Channa and others later.)

According to Keown, "Euthanasia is the intentional killing of a patient by act or omission as part of ... medical care ... Each of these two modes of euthanasia can take three forms: (i) voluntary, (ii) non-voluntary and (iii) involuntary" (Keown 1995, 168). Here Keown understands omission as withdrawal of nutrition and includes it in his definition of euthanasia. He sees the withdrawal of life support as another category altogether, which is not euthanasia. He makes a distinction between withdrawal of nutrition as natural and ordinary (nonmedical treatment), which he argues against, and withdrawal of life support as technological and extraordinary (medical treatment), which he allows. Observing that because there are no exact equivalents in Buddhist texts to modern euthanasia, Keown argues that it is necessary to proceed by way of analogy. He concludes: "What the ... cases show is a consistent pro-attitude towards life in circumstances where its value may be thought in doubt" (Keown 1995, 172–73). Before turning to the relevant Buddhist passages themselves, it is necessary to raise some questions about Keown's definition of euthanasia and his discussion. Elsewhere euthanasia has been defined as "A deliberate act that causes death and that is undertaken by one person with the primary intention of ending the life of another person in order to relieve that person's suffering . . . " physician assistance is when the physician gives patients the "means to kill themselves with the intent that patients use them" (Somerville 2000, 120). As already discussed, many ethicists do not include withdrawal of artificial nutrition as euthanasia. With withdrawal of treatment the physician's intention is not to kill the person but to respect the person's right not to be touched and let nature takes its course. In such cases, pain relief should be administered even if it shortens life (Somerville 2000, 140).

As with the issue of abortion, Buddhist reflections on assisted death arose out the general prohibition against killing in the first precept. It also arose out of events in the monastery. There are six relevant cases. (1) In the section on abortion, we have already discussed the first case about not killing the one whose "hands and feet are cut off," that is, an invalid. (2) In one case, monks who were practicing meditation on their bodies as impure (*asubha;* Skt. *aśubha*), when the Buddha was away, began to think that it would be best to eliminate their bodies altogether and so requested the monk Migalaṇḍika to kill them. Egged on by Mārā (the personified figure of evil) who said that this would help the monks cross *saṃsāra* (the cycles of rebirth) to enlightenment, Migalaṇḍika increased his killings up to sixty monks in 1 day. When the Buddha learned of what had transpired, he said that intentionally depriving a human being of life or even providing the knife for such an act, was not worthy of a recluse and leads to excommunication from the monastery. Then the Buddha replaced this meditation with one on breathing, which brought peace (Horner trans., *Book of Discipline* 1949, 117–23; see also *Majjhima-nikāya* III.269; *Suttanipāta* IV.62, V.320ff; *Vinaya* III.68ff cited by Wiltshire 1983, 129). The following incident highlights the problem of self-interest despite ostensibly compassionate motives. (3) Six monks instigated the death of a very ill man, who was the husband of a woman with whom they were infatuated, by telling him that death would be preferable to the difficulties of his present circumstances, and he would be reborn in a heaven. This inspired the man to kill himself by eating "detrimental" food and drink. After criticizing this, Buddha ruled "Whatever monk should intentionally deprive a human being of life or should look about so as to be his knife-bringer, or should praise the beauty of death, or should incite (anyone) to death . . . he also is one who is defeated [excommunicated, *pārājika*], he is not in communion" (Horner trans., *Book of Discipline* 1949, 125–26). In short, it is forbidden to instigate the death of others or provide the means for them to do it (the commentator says that "knife" stands for other means such as arrow, cudgel, stone, sword, *poison*, or rope). This would be analogous to physician-assisted suicide today by providing a lethal injection (drugs or poison) with informed consent. (4) In yet another incident, some monks, feeling compassion

for an ill monk, praised death's beauty. Because the praise was intentionally given to make the monk want to die, and led to his death, Buddha ruled that the punishment was again excommunication (*pārājika*). (5) In another case, when monks tried to cure an ill monk by a heat treatment and he died, Buddha ruled that this was only a grave offense because the death was not intended. (6) In yet another case, a monk encouraged an executioner to get on with the inevitable job of killing a criminal slated to die (and thus to shorten the latter's fear and agony). This was deemed an offense (*dukkaṭa*) (this last case is found in *Vinaya* III.85 cited by Keown 1995, 171).

Using the categories excommunication (*pārājika*), grave offense (*thullaccaya*), and offense (*dukkaṭa*), these cases can be summarized as follows: (1) Intended victim only dies – *pārājika* [though this incident serves as a general warning against any kind of assisted-killing]; (2) intended victim only dies – *pārājika*; (3) intended victim only dies – *pārājika*; (4) intended victim only dies – *pārājika*; (5) unintended victim dies – *thullaccaya*; and (6) intended victim (as defined by the State, not the monk) dies more quickly because of the monk's instigation – *dukkaṭa*.

The analysis presented here is based on monastic considerations. This does not rule out the fact that all of these cases will involve personal karmic consequences. The general principle that can be gleaned from these examples is that "For expulsion, the act must be intended by the one who gives the orders and also by the one who carries them out; if pain or injury occurs, it is a grave offence, but if death occurs, it is an offence of 'defeat' necessitating expulsion from the monastery. If an act is unintentional, but the person dies, it is a grave offence but not 'defeat'" (Young 1994a, 667). If the intended death was unavoidable (because it has been mandated by the State) and out of compassion one tries to change the timing to make it an easier death, it is simply an offense.

The cases of Vakkali, Godhika, Channa, and possibly Assaji and the lay disciples Anāthapiṇḍika and Dīghāvu, however, seem to acknowledge the acceptability of self-willed death in a very specific context: These are all cases in which (1) the person is terribly ill and in serious pain, (2) all possible help had already been extended but to no avail, and (3) the person is not clinging to the desire for rebirth (which either means the monk is enlightened or attains enlightenment at that moment). Channa, for instance, was then examined on the Buddhist doctrines of impermanence and no soul to confirm that he had no desire for rebirth (Horner trans., *"Discourse on an Exhortation to Channa [Channovādda-sutta]*, *Majjhima-nikāya*, 1959, 315–19). After he had satisfied others about his state of awareness, he killed himself. He was considered without blame. Thus, self-willed death in this very special context seems to have been an exception to the general prohibition against self-willed death at the time of the Buddha. (Besides, they no doubt recognized that there was no alternative except to restrain the monk by force.) It was rarely resorted to for some centuries. Without the Buddha himself there to pronounce the monk's enlightenment, few would make such a claim because of another rule that monastics must not proclaim they are *arhat*s (enlightened ones; Skt. *arhat*).

In this context, it is intriguing to consider the death of the Buddha himself. It was reported that when he fell ill after eating some pork, he chose the time and place and circumstance (during meditation) for his end. This was called his final enlightenment (*mahāparinibbāna*; Skt. *mahāparinirvāṇa*). The idea of choosing the time and place implies self-willed death. Does this mean Buddha was an exception to the general reluctance to allow this in early Buddhism? An alternative interpretation is that this account was really a Jain story about how Mahāvīra, the founder of Jainism, had died (Jainism had a tradition of fasting to death) and the early Buddhist community simply imitated it.

In the Pāli text, The Questions of King Milinda (*Milindapañha*), the monk Nāgasena posed a riddle: "A monk should not commit suicide because he must be a guide for others, but also that the Buddha taught that one must end life to get beyond rebirth" (cited in Young 1994a, 674). Although this suggests an ongoing ambiguity about the whole issue of self-willed death, it is significant that the Chinese Buddhist monk I-Ching (682–727), who traveled to India, reported that monks there did not practice self-willed death unlike the Mahāyāna monks in China. If so, what caused the change? One possibility is that changes were introduced by *Jātaka* tales about how *bodhisattva*s would sacrifice their bodies out of altruism (to feed a starving animal, for instance). There is a clue that self-willed death might have entered Mahāyāna circles in India, even though this had not been observed by I-Ching, because Śāntideva (c. 700) in his *Śikṣāsamuccaya* queries whether a beginning disciple should imitate the former *bodhisattva*s who had sacrificed their bodies for the welfare of others and whether it was useful to bring about universal welfare (Young 1994a, 674 citing Poussin 1922, 26 n. 20). One key passage for this change is found in the *Saddharmapuṇḍarīka*. This Mahāyāna text, which became influential in China by the fifth century CE, describes how the *bodhisattva* Bhaiṣajyarāja died by self-immolation because he was dissatisfied with his worship. The Chinese (and the Japanese) might have imitated this act (see Chapter 44). There are a few clues, moreover, that drugs might have been used to hasten death. In Tibet, Buddhist Tantras had rituals called "creating death" (*mṛtyuvañcana*) (Wayman 1982, 278 and n. 17) and the Nepálese text *Jana-jīvan-kriyā-paddhati* remarks that in the case of fatal disease a powerful medicine was given to increase respiration so that the breath could exit from one of the portals of the body (Lewis 1994, 15).

There are indications of a slippery slope for the practice of self-willed death – initial legitimation for the elite (monks and warriors) extending to the vulnerable (lepers, widows, and old people), in India, China, and Japan – although it never officially involved physicians and rarely drugs (Young 1994a, 678–80). These traditions of self-willed death (and their occasional assistance) were eventually ended by governmental decrees in the modern period (India, China, and Japan) (Young 1994a, 697 citing Westermarck, Becker, Fus, and Harada).

Keown analyzes the arguments of modern Buddhist thinkers such as Philip Kapleau and Louis van Loon on this topic. (1) Euthanasia interferes with the working of karma (Kapleau and van Loon). (2) It deprives one of a human life (Kapleau). (3) It involves drugs, which makes the person unconscious and unable to practice mindfulness (which directs destiny) (van Loon). Keown concludes that these arguments do not adequately represent the Buddhist position. He argues that it is impossible to know what might be retribution according to the law of karma and what might be considered a mindful death (some people might die peacefully in their sleep), and so the arguments of van Loon and Kapleau could be made for and against euthanasia (Keown 1995, 184–85).

Van Loon thinks that Buddhism accepts euthanasia in those cases when a person is in a coma or experiencing extreme pain with loss of quality of life. Keown points out that neocortical death has not been a criterion for death even in the West. The issue of self-willed death in the case of extreme pain, though, was the possible exception allowed by the Buddha (which Keown does not mention). Here there is an extremely important difference from the one mentioned by van Loon. In Buddhism, self-willed death must have no assistance and there must be no clinging to life (which amounts to enlightenment).

Ratanakul (1988, 310–11) argues that suffering is the expression and therefore the elimination of karmic potency. As a result, it is best to let it run its course so that it will not rise again in another life. Although Ratanakul uses this as a good reason to prohibit euthanasia and the killing of people in a persistent vegetative state from a Buddhist perspective, he argues for pain relief treatment (although he does not explain the contradiction that suffering is necessary in the former but not in the latter). In addition, he argues that physicians who perform or assist in suicide or euthanasia will accumulate bad karma because they encourage people to avoid suffering (elsewhere he says that it also violates the Buddhist first precept against killing (1998, 40), even though he does accept self-willed death by an enlightened person when terminally ill, and in extreme pain, after good palliative care had been offered (pointing to the cases of Vakkali, Godhika, Channa, and others in the Pāli Canon (based on Ratanakul 1988 in Young 1995, 494–95).

From a survey of recent articles on euthanasia by Asian authors, it is clear that a distinction between euthanasia as active killing and withdrawal of treatment based on the patients (or proxy's) decision, followed by adequate pain relief, is not clearly made, especially when the term passive euthanasia is used for the latter. When the term euthanasia is used for both these contexts, even greater confusion occurs. Chaicharoen and Ratanakul (1998, 38–40) point out that although some Thai Buddhists argue that passive euthanasia or the letting-go-of-life (that is, withdrawal of treatment) expresses a Buddhist middle way between active euthanasia and maintaining life at all costs and in all circumstances, most elderly Thais, both monks and laity, desire a natural death because Buddhists are taught to face the inevitability of death and because they acknowledge there are too many risks and uncertainties to intervene. They point to hospice care with a "holistic" approach and a "natural end" to life as a better Buddhist solution. Even so, in Thailand there have been reports of removal of life-support systems, use of lethal overdoses, and lack of informed consent by physicians (Lindbeck 1984).

IV. CONCLUSION

Buddhism by and large left reproductive and family matters to other religions, focusing instead on liberation as the ultimate telos of life. As a result, for Buddhists, each phase of life is characterized by suffering, especially the last phase of old age and dying. The more intense the experience of suffering, the more it might prompt insight and the fundamental religious experience of the true nature of reality defined by the Four Noble Truths (see Chapter 10). The subject of birth in the texts holds theoretical interest regarding how people are reborn. Images of old age and dying are of real existential interest as symbols of what is to come; they are used for meditation throughout life and as warnings not to waste this precious opportunity of human embodiment (necessary for enlightenment).

The life cycle for Buddhists is being profoundly affected by the development of modern, medical technologies. The impact of Western medicine on Asian countries has escalated in the last half of the twentieth century. There

has been transfer not only of the new reproductive technologies and transplantation technologies but also of the ethical and legal issues they have raised (the international networks are strong). This in turn has sparked discussions of religious, cultural, and regional identities. Sometimes this has encouraged a return to the scriptures to figure out what the religious response should be. This has been common in Buddhism to date, and one can only speculate on the reasons why. Much of the Buddhist debate, it seems, has developed because Buddhism now has a broad movement called Socially Engaged Buddhism (see Chapter 10), which is attentive to general ethical issues and has attracted a number of Westerners, who have been evolving their own distinctive interpretations of Buddhism in light of ethical issues faced in the West. When Socially Engaged Buddhism meets Textual Buddhism, there has been debate. One striking point in the literature is that few female ethicists are contributing to the literature on Buddhist bioethics (although their voices might exist in other feminist forums).

An insight to be gleaned from this study is that there are sometimes differences within canonical traditions, and there are even greater differences when the views of scripture are compared with those of today's law in the various countries not to mention those of public opinion studied through large-scale surveys. This makes the quest for culturally and religiously sensitive positions problematic. Because many of the countries are religiously pluralistic and some are officially secular, developing consensus for new policies is difficult. Yet, people recognize that it must be done, and done in ways that are meaningful to people.

NOTE

1. In the literature on Buddhism, Sanskrit terms are often considered standard and will be used here when discussing Buddhism as a whole. In the context of discussion on Theravāda Buddhism or the Pāli Canon, the Sanskrit equivalent for common Pāli terms will be indicated at its first occurrence. For uncommon terms, however, the Sanskrit equivalent will not be indicated.

CHAPTER 5

MEDICAL ETHICS THROUGH THE LIFE CYCLE IN CHINA

Jing-Bao Nie

I. INTRODUCTION

In the West, human life is believed to be precious and sacred mainly because the first human was created in the image and likeness of God according to the Judeo-Christian tradition. In Chinese civilization, the preciousness and even sacredness of human life is often believed to originate in nature, from which human beings come and on which human existence depends. In both Confucianism and Daoism, every individual's life from the very beginning to the end is seen to be closely and mysteriously related to nature, physically and spiritually understood. This idea has been argued and promoted in numerous medical and nonmedical works. For example, as the twenty-fifth book "Treasuring Life and Preserving Health" in *Suwen of Huangdi Neijing* (The Yellow Emperor's Classic of Medicine) puts it, "Of all things in the universe, nothing is more precious than human beings" because what is called human life "is born from the earth, depends on the heaven, and begins with the intercourse of heavenly and earthly *qi*" (Nanjing Zhongyi Xueyuan 1981, 209). Li Pengfei, a physician in the Yuan Dynasty (1271–1368), stated that the human is the most precious entity between heaven and earth, although, due to the restriction of our physical existence, few know why this is so. We human beings are precious not only because we are an organic part of nature, but also because we are in correspondence with nature. In Li's words,

> The roundness of the human head is like and corresponds with that of the heaven; the square shape of the human foot that of the earth [The most popular cosmology in ancient China holds that the heaven is round and the earth square]; human eyes the sun and the moon; the hairs, flesh and bone the mountains, forest, soil and stones; exhaling the wind; inhaling the dew; joy the virtue star and the colorful (lucky) clouds; anger the powerful thunderbolt; the flow of blood the rivers and seas; four limbs the four seasons and times [the morning, evening, day, and night]; the five *viscera* [the heart, lung, spleen, liver, and kidney] the five phrases [wood, fire, earth, metal, and water]; the six bowels [the stomach, small intestine, large intestine, bladder, gallbladder, and triple burner] the six tone of sounds. My body exists together and corresponds with the heaven and the earth. If this is so, isn't human life the most precious? (Wang 1995, 2)

In other words, human life is the most valuable because it comes from not only the loving-kindness of father and mother, but also the grace of heaven and earth.

In China, an individual life as a whole is often perceived as a pilgrimage or as a cycle. Confucius described his own life as a process of continuing growth, from setting his heart on learning at age 15, to taking his stand at age 30, to understanding the way of heaven at 50 years of age, and to giving his heart-and-mind free without overstepping any line at 70 years of age. In Chinese medical and Daoist traditions, life is often seen as a cycle, like the change of the four seasons. In the theories and practice of traditional Chinese medicine, since *The Yellow Emperor's Classic of Medicine*, human life, like that of animals, plants, and seasons, has usually been divided into five stages: birth, growth, maturing, aging, and death, corresponding to the *wuxing* (five elementary phases or elements): wood, fire, earth, metal, and water.

With this general view of the harmony of human life and nature as its basic theme, this chapter provides an account of Chinese perspectives on ethical issues through the life cycle, with focus on those at the beginning and end of life.

II. THE ABORTION DEBATE IN CHINA

Legally permissible and easily available, abortion is widely practiced in contemporary China for a number of reasons, from personal choice to national family planning policies. In striking contrast with the enduring controversy regarding abortion in the West, so far the Chinese people appear to be basically silent on this subject. It is accepted wisdom that the typical Chinese attitude toward abortion is very permissive or "liberal" and that Chinese usually do not consider abortion morally problematic because they think a human life begins at birth. According to a survey conducted in 1997 in the People's Republic of China, the majority of the sample surveyed does not agree with the view that abortion is a serious moral problem. Moreover, the majority of respondents disagreed, although a large number agreed, that aborting a fetus is equivalent to taking a life or killing a human being. The survey also showed that, in general, the Chinese very strongly (greater than 90 percent of subjects surveyed) or strongly (greater than 70 percent) believe that a woman should have an abortion under one or more of the following situations: if the fetus has a genetic disease or is malformed; if the woman might give birth to a defective baby; if the pregnancy resulted from incest or rape or extramarital sex; if the pregnant woman has a mental illness or is mentally retarded; if the pregnant woman is a prostitute; if an unmarried young college/university student is pregnant; if the woman is alcoholic or smokes heavily; if the couple do not want more children or have decided to divorce; if the pregnant woman feels that she must terminate her pregnancy; or if she has taken some medicine that might have an adverse influence on the fetal development (Nie 2002e, 2004c; see Chapter 21).

Yet, although it may exaggerate a bit to say that there is an abortion debate in China, because no genuine intellectual and public debate has yet occurred, there are certainly diverse voices behind the apparent silence. Although the official state position approves of almost any kind of abortion at any stage, except abortion for sex selection, and the better educated a person is, the more likely he or she is to have no moral concerns about abortion, there are other standpoints. Most notably, three religious groups – Roman Catholics, Protestants, and Buddhists – hold a more conservative position on the morality of abortion than urban and rural people, university and medical students, and medical ethics/humanities scholars. For the majority of these three religious communities, abortion is a serious moral problem because it is equivalent to killing an innocent human being. Furthermore, a large number of people with no particular religious commitment – for example, one-fourth of respondents in three rural samples and nearly one-fifth in two urban population groups – are also troubled by and even explicitly oppose abortion (Nie 2002e; 2004c).

The pervasive political and social acceptance of abortion and the apparent silence on the issue in contemporary China have resulted in the assumption that this was also the case in the past; however, recent studies show that the assumption that the Chinese view of abortion has always been permissive is historically unfounded (Nie 2002a, 2002d, 2004c). As in the present, there existed different and opposing views about abortion in the past. It is true that for generations Chinese physicians prescribed abortifacients, mainly herbs, and sometimes performed abortion by other means, such as acupuncture. Without raising ethical concerns about abortion as such, the sixteenth-century Confucian physician-scholar Li Shizhen listed at least seventy-two agents, derived from animals, vegetables, and minerals, under the entry of *duo shengtai yao* (drugs for dropping the living fetus) in his *Bencao Gangmu* (The Great Pharmacopoeia) (Li [1592] 1988). Actually, physicians in late imperial China prioritized the mother's health over the life of the fetus. Surviving case reports show that when the continuation of pregnancy represented an unmistakable and severe danger to the woman's health, abortion was definitely regarded as the lesser of two evils. Nevertheless, "distaste for taking life, together with the theory that the interruption of a natural process can be harmful, combined to make many orthodox physicians reluctant to terminate a pregnancy if there was a chance of saving both mother and child" (Bray 1997, 325).

Many Chinese, not only Buddhists but also Confucians, believed that deliberately terminating pregnancy destroys a human life that starts far earlier than at birth. The following story from the *Yi Shuo* (Stories about Medicine) by Zhang Gao, a Buddhist-Confucian physician in the thirteenth century, illustrates this conservative viewpoint vividly:

> In the capital city there lived a woman whose family name was Bai. She was good-looking. So people in the capital all called her "Bai Mu-dan" (The White Peony). She made a living by selling abortifacient drugs. She suddenly started to suffer from headaches. Her head became swollen and increased in size day by day. All the renowned physicians treated her, but no one was able to cure her. After many days, an ulceration developed and the offensive odor was unbearable. She cried every night and her crying could be heard near and far. One day she requested of her family members: "Burn all the prescriptions of abortion that I have kept." She also admonished her offspring: "Take an oath not to pass on such a trade." Her son asked his mother: "You have built yourself up by this. Why do you want to give it all up?" His mother answered, "I dream of hundreds of infants and small children who suck my head every night. This is why I cry out in pain. All this is the retribution for my selling poisonous drugs to damage fetuses." Immediately after saying this, she died. (Unschuld 1979, 48–49; Ma 1993, 670)

The moral of the anecdote is clear: The fetus is a human life and at least a potential child, and terminating pregnancy is thus not permissible because it is equivalent to killing a child.

Although ancient Chinese physicians and laypeople alike opposed abortion mainly due to the influence of Buddhism (which was imported) and although Confucianism (which was home grown) does not oppose abortion as explicitly and strongly as Buddhism, historically, people in the Confucian tradition seemed to tolerate, accept, and even promote the Buddhist condemnation and restriction of abortion. Moreover, a less "liberal" attitude toward abortion is more logically and theoretically consistent with Confucian moral principles and ideas (Nie 2002a, 2002d, 2004c).

Legally speaking, although related ancient Chinese laws took "a far more flexible and situational, and a far less moralistic, approach to the question of abortion" than modern Western abortion laws (Luk 1977), for centuries it was a crime to induce abortion by assaulting a pregnant woman or to deliberately procure abortion that resulted in the mother's death. Partly due to Western influence, abortion was prohibited legally from 1910 to the early 1960s in China. That is to say, even in the first decade of People's Republic of China, abortion was against law and social policy.

III. Perspectives on Fetal Life

It is assumed that most Chinese agree with the great, ancient Confucian Xun Zi (286–238 BCE) that "human life" begins at birth and ends with death. As well indicated in the policies and popularity of *yousheng* (well-birth, eugenics) and abortion in contemporary China (Aird 1990; Rigdon 1996; Dikotter 1998), the fetus until birth is of little moral significance in current Chinese official and mainstream discourses. As one sociological study shows, however, in contemporary China 70 percent of the participants in a survey believe that human life begins some time before birth. Nearly half of the respondents simply see conception as the starting point of a human life. Although the majority of respondents believe in the existence of a soul in the human being but not in the fetus, Chinese Catholics and Protestants and a large number of others strongly or very strongly believe in the existence of a soul in both. Even though most doctors who perform abortion and the majority of women who have had abortions rarely think of the aborted fetus, a few doctors and some women have very strong feelings about the fetus and see the fetus as a growing human life or even as a child (Nie 2001c, 2002d, 2004c).

In fact, ancient Chinese physicians and laypeople developed views about what happens in the womb after conception (Nie 2002d, 2004c). Conservative Chinese views on the morality of abortion find support in the ancient Chinese medical accounts of fetal life. By the time of the Sui Dynasty (581–618) Chinese medicine, as evidenced in the gynecological and obstetrical literature, already had an amazingly detailed account of fetal development. As early as the second century BCE, the Daoist classic *Huananzi* described the 10 months of pregnancy as follows: "in the first month a blob of fat is formed, in the second sinews, in the sixth bone. In the seventh month [the fetus] is fully formed, in the eighth it is active, in the ninth it is boisterous, and in the tenth it is born" (Furth 1999, 101 footnote). Physicians in traditional China proposed various schemes to explain fetal development. For example, according to *Wuzang Lun* (On Five Organs), a work that was attributed to the "saint of medicine" Zhang Zhongjing (circa second century), the fetus grows in the womb during each of 10 lunar months in this way:

1st month: Like a pearl of dew
2nd month: Like a peach flower
3rd month: Male and female differentiate
4th month: Physical form is visible
5th month: Sinews and bones are formed
6th month: Hairs grow
7th month: The *hun* soul wanders and the child moves its left hand
8th month: The *pei* soul wanders and the child moves its right hand
9th month: The thrice-turning-body moves about
10th month: *Qi* is sufficient. (Furth 1999, 104)

To summarize the accounts of the 10 months of pregnancy as understood since the second century BCE, the following points are salient. First, from early times, Chinese people and physicians in particular did not lack accounts of fetal development. Second, in these accounts the traditional Chinese medical understanding of fetal life distinguished among the embryo, the unformed fetus, and the formed fetus. Third, traditional Chinese medical understanding of fetal life is an organic part of Chinese cosmology and human physiology. Fourth, for at least some ancient physicians and laypeople, human life was regarded as beginning much earlier than at birth, at the very early stages (the first month) of pregnancy, and the human being was seen as physically formed at some time during pregnancy (Nie 2002d, 2004c; see Chapter 21).

Probably due to this medical knowledge on fetal life, *xusui* (nominal age) – considering a person 1 year old at birth and adding a year each lunar new year – is a long-rooted and still widely practiced custom in China. Chinese medicine and culture early on developed a distinctive theory of *taijiao* (fetal education). According to this theory, the fetus in the womb can perceive and be influenced by what the mother perceives. Not only the food the mother consumes during pregnancy but also the materials she listens to, sees, and reads have both direct and indirect influences on the physical, intellectual, and moral character of her fetus. Children's education should thus start as early as pregnancy. Many medical works from ancient China have detailed discussions and special sections on fetal education. Fetal education as a social practice was popularized in late imperial and modern China (Dikotter 1998); it is interesting that it has become popular again in mainland China since the 1980s. In conclusion, many Chinese, including Confucians and Confucian physicians throughout history, consider that a human being is formed at some time between conception and birth, if not at conception itself.

To a great degree, more traditional values and practices remain in Taiwan, and even Hong Kong, than in mainland China. A recent fascinating ethnographic survey reveals that, as a result of traditional Chinese ideas and Japanese influence, in modern Taiwan, belief in fetus ghosts and fetus demons is prevailing, and aborted fetuses are often "memorialized" in Buddhist temples for appeasement (Moskowitz 2001). Although obviously at odds with the dominant discourse in mainland China, Taiwanese belief and practice seem to fit perfectly into the traditional Chinese understandings of abortion and fetal life.

IV. At the End of Life

1. Truth Telling about Terminal Illness

Acting paternalistically in the name of the patient's good, many contemporary physicians in China, along with family members and friends, do not directly tell the whole truth to patients who are suffering from terminal disease. Is this practice of concealing the diagnosis of terminal illness from the patient *the* Chinese way of dealing with the issue, as is widely believed? Historically, the answer is no. Current practice is far from the standard practice in traditional China. To some degree, the dominant way of dealing with the diagnosis of terminal illness in contemporary China – not disclosing directly and fully to the patient – should be seen as following the old-fashioned Western paternalistic model that was well articulated in the influential 1847 Code of Ethics of the American Medical Association but started to change radically in the 1960s and 1970s in the West. It is simply wrong to see the contemporary standard practice in China – not always telling the truth – as an intrinsic part or logical development of traditional Chinese culture and medical moralities (Nie 2001b, 2002e).

The sixteenth-century Confucian physician Li Yan considered it a kind of deception not to be honest with gravely ill patients about their diagnosis (see Chapter 21). Ancient Chinese texts, however, seldom recommended that physicians should tell the truth to patients suffering from a terminal illness. Nevertheless, to lie for whatever reason was also seldom suggested. As a matter of fact, the biographies of famous physicians in antiquity clearly indicate that to tell patients the diagnosis and prognosis truthfully, even in the situation of terminal disease, is what a physician should do. In both classic and contemporary Chinese languages, *"bing ru gaohuang"* (the disease has attacked the vitals) has been the phrase very commonly used to refer to terminal illness. The idiom originated in the famous physician known as Yi Huan in the Spring and Autumn period (770–476 BCE). According to the *Zuozhuan* (The Chronology of the State of Lu), an early historical work, Yi Huan once treated Duke Jin. After examining the Duke, the physician directly said to him: "The disease is beyond cure. It is above *gao* and below *huang* [unknown anatomical places] . . . No medicine can reach it. So it is beyond cure." Duke Jin replied: "Good doctor indeed!" With "expensive gifts" (high payment) Yi Huan was dismissed, and Duke Jin died after some days (Chen [1723] 1962:73). The *Zuozhuan* also reports that Yi He, another medical sage living in approximately the same period as Yi Huan, told his patient of the diagnosis of terminal illness just as Yi Huan did. Yi He also was praised as a good doctor and rewarded with expensive gifts (Chen [1723] 1962:74). Yi He and Yi Huan were so well known in ancient China that the term *he-huan* became the word for "healer." According to historical records, such great doctors as Bian Que (approximately 500 BCE, called the "father of medicine" by some historians) and Hua Tuo (in the second century BCE, the "father of surgery") always told the truth to their patients when their diseases were diagnosed as terminal (in Chen [1723] 1962). The great sixteenth-century realist novel *Jingpingmei* (four-volume English translation titled *The Golden Lotus*) further reveals that in traditional China, physicians, family members, relatives, and friends rarely made efforts to conceal medical information, including the diagnosis of terminal disease, from the patient, but usually told the ill person everything directly.

2. Death and Dying, Euthanasia

In China, there are many different perspectives on death and dying. For example, Daoism as a religion has developed a tradition of pursuing longevity and even physical immortality persistently and often irrationally through such techniques as alchemy (gold elixir), breathing exercises (e.g., *taiji* and meditation), pharmacopoeia, gymnastics, the art of the bedroom (sexual techniques), and the cultivation of virtues. There is a discourse of Daoist philosophy in which death and dying is accepted and appreciated as a rest and returning to one's origin. In Confucianism, birth and death are seen as determined by the Heavenly Way. For Chinese communism, revolutionary heroism – actively sacrificing the individual's interests and even life for the great cause of revolution and socialism – is promoted and propagated as the only correct attitude toward death and dying.

In most traditional Chinese medical works, human mortality and the limits of medicine are well acknowledged. As early as in the *Huangdi Neijing* there were discussions on dying and death. There were also different definitions of death in the medical literature (Qiu 1999). One theory understands death to be the loss of *shen* (spirit) or the separation of spirit from the body. The spirit is located in various vital organs of the human body. Another theory understands death as the dispersion of *qi* (energy or vital force) away from human body. Both theories define death as not just a biological phenomenon, but also as a spiritual and social event. Death concerns the spiritual and social features of human existence as present or not. It seems that orthodox traditional Chinese medical practitioners fully acknowledged human mortality and usually opposed prolonging life at any cost (as the stories of Yi Huan and Yi He indicate). For them, a tormented life was worse than death. Once death is diagnosed as imminent, they seemed to consider it morally problematic to continue treatment and thus meddle with nature through strenuous efforts to avert death in such cases.

In contemporary China, unlike the issue of abortion, *anlesi* (mercy killing, euthanasia) has been one of the most prominent topics in Chinese medical ethics, both as an academic discipline and as a public discourse (see Sleeboom-Faulkner 2006). Since the 1980s, this topic has attracted the attention of scholars and medical professionals (e.g., many articles on euthanasia in the two premier Chinese journals in the field, *Medicine and Philosophy* and *Chinese Medical Ethics*, as well as national and local media). Although active euthanasia at the request of the patient and/or family members is illegal, withdrawing treatment

is widely accepted and practiced. Many sociocultural and intellectual forces are leading toward the legalization of active euthanasia. The major and most widely accepted reason in favor of passive as well as active euthanasia for a number of patients, including seriously impaired newborns and people suffering from late-stage cancers and other terminal diseases, is that treating and caring for these patients poses an unbearable and unjustifiable burden on the health care system and society. In the words of one textbook on medical ethics, euthanasia "will allow society to use the limited resources to meet more urgent needs and thus help the social stability and development. To save dying and meaningless cases is an enormous waste and wrongful allocation of social wealth" (Li [1592] 1988; He 1988, 194). This argument for euthanasia reflects not only the official ideology of collectivism or socialism (in which individual human life should be subjected to the interests of the state and society) and economic determinism, but also the recent revival of social Darwinism.

As the literature on euthanasia has often acknowledged, however, strong sociocultural and intellectual forces oppose euthanasia, especially active euthanasia. This resistance to what can be called the "Euthanasia Movement" in contemporary China reflects the other side of the discourse of medical ethics, in which individual life is valued as precious. As the saying in the popular culture goes, "a good death is not as good as a bad life." This is a belief still held by many Chinese. Thus, *ren yi* (humaneness/humanity and righteousness) should be ensured in dealing with matters of life, suffering, and death, and *huoren* (to save human life) is the first priority for medicine as an art of humanity.

V. CONCLUSION

In contemporary bioethics, there are some widespread misconceptions and misuses of culture. One of them is the assumption of a homogeneous or single culturally distinctive medical ethics in every society and the subsequent dichotomy between Western versus non-Western medical ethics. Another is that the present mainstream or standard viewpoint or practice in any particular society is often treated as *the* particular way in the society or culture as a whole. Materials presented in this chapter demonstrate that this is certainly not the case with medical ethics in China. The current dominant and official line on such subjects as abortion, fetal life, truth telling about terminal illness, and euthanasia does not necessarily accord with historical values and practices. Moreover, there is not now, nor has there ever been, *the* Chinese medical ethics or *the* singular Chinese perspective on any moral issue in medicine (Nie 2000; see also Chapter 21). A brief review of Chinese perspectives on ethical issues at the two ends of human life provides further evidence on the diversity, richness, flux, changeability, historical complexity, openness for new possibilities, and contradictory elements of Chinese medical morality.

The contemporary dominant Chinese views on abortion, eugenics, and euthanasia seem to support the commonly accepted view that individual human life is less respected in Chinese culture than in the West. The prominent German historian of medicine in China, Paul Unschuld, has questioned this generalization and concluded in one of his works on medical ethics in China that

> from studying the history of medicine and medical ethics in China it is obvious Chinese culture for at least two millennia has placed as much emphasis on the value of human individual life as has Western culture. Keeping in mind that in German history we have experienced only half a century ago a period where traditional cultural values were turned upside down, the findings by Dorothy Wertz [on the acceptance of eugenics by Chinese genetic professionals, see Wertz 1998] and the medical media report on human rights violations in contemporary China may lead us to conclude that the phenomena described by these findings and reports have their origin in a difficult contemporary situation; they are definitely not intrinsic elements of Chinese culture. (Unschuld 2001)

Although the validity of this bold statement obviously needs more detailed and systematic Chinese–Western comparative studies, the account in this chapter of Chinese medical ethics through the life circle, in spite of its sketchy nature, challenges the common wisdom on the value of individual life in China and the West and verifies Unschuld's general thesis (Nie 2002e, 2004c).

Acknowledgments

I am grateful to Prof. Paul Unschuld, Dr. Ole Döring, and Prof. Qingshan Yan for their helpful comments and suggestions.

CHAPTER 6

MEDICAL ETHICS THROUGH THE LIFE CYCLE IN JAPAN

Rihito Kimura and Shizu Sakai

I. INTRODUCTION

The notion of the life cycle in the human life process from birth to death is integral to Japanese culture and has been influenced by Shintoism and Buddhism. This chapter addresses four key aspects of the life cycle with reference to medical ethics in Japan.

There are four concepts that are crucial to understanding Japanese conceptions of the life cycle: *Sho, Ro, Byo,* and *Shi* (Kimura 2000). *Sho* means both life and the coming into existence of life in this world. *Ro* means aging, an inevitable phenomenon in our life cycle. *Byo* means disease or being sick. Finally, *Shi* means death and dying. This set of these four key words encompasses quite a commonly accepted notion of the life cycle among the Japanese. This reflects the idea of suffering life expressed in various Buddhist scriptures such as the *Lotus Sutra* (Murano [1974] 1991). They are well-known expressions in Japan (Robert 1998).

The underlying theme of these four concepts can be summarized as *Ku* (suffering), which is an inevitable aspect of human existence according to the teaching of Buddha. In Buddhist teachings, people have to accept the reality of transitory life, governed by this process of *Sho, Ro, Byo, Shi* (Ui 1943). In Japanese thought all of this occurs in the *Uki-Yo,* which literally means "floating world," denoting the transient secular world of people. Through these experiences of suffering in the life cycle, people have a chance to seek the final and everlasting "truth" for the sake of salvation.

Throughout Japanese history, Shintoism and some traditional folk religions, such as animism, joined with Buddhism, Taoism, and Confucianism to teach an appreciation of nature as an integrated part of human life in the Japanese environment. The notion of the cycle of life developed through analogies to nature and its constant phenomena of perpetual change. The essence of nature is explained in the framework of the embodied spirit, *rei, tama,* or *chi,* which can be transformed in the human body as a source of sacred existence and activity (Ishida 1963, 18–25).

II. *SHO* AND THE BEGINNING OF THE LIFE CYCLE: *TAIKYO* AS A PREPARATION FOR CHILDBIRTH

There are various aspects of *Sho. Tanjyo* (birth) is one of the most important. The human life cycle begins with birth; however, even before birth, life begins in the mother's body. The unborn child in the mother's body should be protected and educated so that it can be born as a healthy and happy baby, according to classic Japanese medical ethics. The word *Taikyo* (teaching for the unborn child)

132

appears in the oldest extant Japanese medical encyclopedia, titled *Ishinpo* (Tanba [984] 1991), which literally means "Medicine's Heart and Method;" it was compiled by Yasuyori Tanba, who quoted various Chinese medical sources (Tanba [984] 1991; Kimura 1987, 119–23).

Volume 22 of *Ishinpo* deals entirely with *Taikyo Syussan*, which means "teaching for the unborn child and its delivery" (Tanba [984] 1991, 1895–1942). The medical technique of acupuncture to ensure the health of the unborn baby is explained in detail according to the month, accompanied by drawings of a pregnant woman and a baby in her body. Expectant mothers are advised to look at beautiful things, to keep a peaceful mind, and to eat mild food, inasmuch as hot meals would have bad effects on the unborn baby. A sound spiritual environment for mothers leads to the birth of a healthy baby. *Taikyo* is still a widely accepted idea more than 1,000 years since the publication of this medical classic. It is worth noting here that the preface of *Ishinpo* states that "in order to heal the disease, it is important to have a mind of *Daiji-Sokuin*," which means the great mercy of Buddha and the Confucian teaching of compassion (Tanba [984] 1991, 5–7). This statement is based on the expression of Sun Ssu-mo's (581–682) *Ch'ien-ching-fang*, a work on prescribing (see Chapter 21).

III. THE BEGINNING OF LIFE AS AN END OF *SHO*. THE NOTIONS OF ABORTION AND INFANTICIDE

In addition to these positive elements of respecting the fetus' life, there are also negative aspects of *Sho*, leading immediately to *Shi* (death) of the unborn and/or born child. *Datai* (abortion), or to use another expression, *ko-oroshi*, is commonly used to characterize aborting a fetus. The latter term literally means "to let fall down (*oroshi*) the unborn child (*Ko*)." The traditional God–Buddha (*Shin–Butsu*) approach to ideas relating to the beginning of life is vague and does not exclude abortion.

The Japanese word *Mabiki* is equivalent to "infanticide" (Takahashi 1936). This commonly used term is analogous to "the thinning out" of plants to encourage growth of the good ones, which could also be referred to as *ko-gaeshi* (returning the child) to God–Buddha, that is, returning the child from this world to another one for the time being in a kind of reverse life cycle. In Shinto folk religion some people believe that during the first week of a newborn baby's life its ongoing existence is not positively established and it therefore still has a possibility of returning back to the place from where it came. Thus, both the practice of abortion (*Ko-oroshi*) and infanticide (*Ko-gaeshi*) can be interpreted in the context of Japanese society, culture, and the life cycle as shaped by religious tradition. The extreme poverty caused by large-scale famine in regions such as Hokuriku (Japan Sea side of Central Honshu Island) and the Tohoku (northeastern part of Honshu Island) region

in the years 1231, 1461, 1624, 1732, 1782, and 1833 may have encouraged the development of this belief to cope with the multiple shocks of great loss of life (Takahashi 1936).

In the sixteenth century, the practice of abortion and infanticide caught the attention of the Portuguese Jesuit priest Luis Frois (1532–1597). He came to Japan in 1563 and lived in Hirato, Sakai, and Kyoto for approximately 30 years, working as a Catholic priest. During this time he observed the Japanese and wrote a short essay comparing European and Japanese cultures (Frois [1585] 1983). Francisco Xavier arrived at Kagoshima in 1549 and traveled to Yamaguchi in 1550, where he publicly denounced the cruel practice of abortion in his preaching. Roman Catholic moral influence, however, did not take root among the Japanese. Indeed, the Catholic mission was officially banned by the Tokugawa feudal lord Hidetada Tokugawa in 1612. It lasted until 1873, when the Japanese government under the Emperor Meiji changed its policy and declared the freedom of religion.

Japan was isolated for more than two centuries (Edo era, 1603–1867). During the Edo era, clinical obstetrics was well developed by Gen'etsu Kagawa (1700–1777). For the first time, Kagawa confirmed that the normal position of the fetus was upside down. This was quite a shift from the traditional understanding of the position of the fetus in the womb, and Kagawa wrote a famous book, *San-Ron* (Thesis on Obstetrics) in 1766. Kagawa reported on his radical operative techniques, in which he used tools of his own invention to save pregnant women from extremely difficult deliveries (*kaisei-jyutsu*, or the art of restoring life) by destroying the fetus in the womb and evacuating the remains (Sakai 1999b, 2003). He justified this surgical procedure as life saving for the pregnant woman (Fujikawa [1904] 1941).

In the Edo era, there was a tendency to have abortions to avoid unwanted births. The family name of a famous physician, Chujyo, became synonymous with, and was used as an alternative expression for, "abortion" (Sakai 2003). Those who denounced the practice of abortion and/or infanticide often included calligraphic signs of *Chujyo* and associated abortion and infanticide with scenes of hell and the devil in another world. This implied that those who had abortions would sometimes be punished in front of *Emma-Daioh* (Great King of Hell). The Tokugawa government officially denounced abortion in the middle of Edo era (Fujikawa [1934] 1978).

IV. *SHO* AND HEALTH: THE CLASSIC TEACHING OF *YO JYO KUN*

To maintain wellness or health in life (*Sho*), a classic text, *Yo Jyo Kun*, recommends harmony of the self with nature, people, and other living beings. The word *Yojo* literally means "to take care (*Yo*)" of "life" (*Sho*, pronounced as *Jyo* in combination with the word *Yo*). Because the word *Kun* means teaching, the title of this book can be translated as "The Teaching of Care for Life" (Kaibara [1713a] 1961b).

There are many different kinds of "*Yojo*" stories and books. One of the most eminent contributors to this literature was Ekiken Kaibara (1630–1714) in the Edo era. He published his book *Yojokun* (Teaching for the Care of Life) in 1713 (Kaibara [1713a] 1961b). He embodied the neo-Confucius ideal of the physician as an extraordinary scholar and teacher.

Kaibara stated that moderation in work, food, drink, sleep, and exercise, as well as emotional stability (e.g., stability in feeling, as well as in mind, without having a hot temper) contribute to good health. The care for life, *Yojo*, is the result of a lifelong daily effort on the part of each person. The uniqueness of Kaibara's teaching lies in its emphasis on health, not as physical strength, speed, and power but as a moderate, integrated, and harmonious lifestyle. His detailed suggestions on how to achieve a proper balance of spirit, body, and mind were very creative and also drew on traditional Chinese and Japanese medical knowledge of the time and his own experiences as a clinician and as a Confucian ethicist. The content of his *Yojokun* is still appreciated as effective even in the context of contemporary medicine (Kimura 1987a, 124–5).

One of Kaibara's key ideas is the importance of ritual behavior in daily life, from morning until the end of day. For example, one should wash one's face each morning and evening at the proper time and eat foods that have been prepared properly, for which he provided instructions. Kaibara also advises on the need for modesty and control over excess sexual desire according to the aging process, particularly after the age of 40. He thought that the way to nourish the very basis of life is to expend one's sexual energy sparingly in youth and preserve it even more after the age of 40 by not having discharges. He had quite a positive and productive life until his death at the age of 84 years. Indeed, his *Yojokun* was published when he was 83 years old. The care of life (*Yojo*) was valued by many Japanese as a source of the most practical, ethical, and humane recommendations for maintaining healthy lives throughout the life cycle.

In his book titled *Gojokun* (Five Constant Teachings), Kaibara made several important points about the relationship between nature and humans. He observed that

> all humans (*Hito*) may be said to owe their birth to their parents, but a further inquiry into their origins reveals that the humans came into being because of the grace by the "Heaven and Earth". – Thus all humans beings in the world are children born of heaven and earth, and heaven and earth are the great parents of us all. (Kaibara [1711b] 1970, 95)

Kaibara's ideas about respecting one's body beyond feudalistic ideology and filial piety were unique in his time.

To follow the way of heaven and earth is one of his key concepts, which has been extended to the idea of enjoying a healthy life in respecting one's life and body. "One must learn the art of care for life in order to keep one's life well. This is the most important thing in life, for one's body is priceless and irreplaceable by the entire earth." The ethical approach to medicine by professionals and the teaching of health to people through these books are still regarded as effective by contemporary Japanese.

Kaibara also wrote that the practice of medicine is a humanitarian art. Physicians should be motivated by the desire to help people and should not be concerned primarily with protecting their own interests. Anyone aspiring to become a doctor should be well versed in the Confucian classics. Those who are ignorant of the *I-ching*, the Book of Changes, cannot become a doctor. He quoted the idea of the great Chinese medical authority Sun Ssu-mo, who said that "it is necessary to understand Confucian writings to become a great physician" because the basic notion of medicine was derived from the *yin-yang* principle of the *I-ching* (Kaibara [1713a] 1961b, 125; [1713b] 1974, 121).

V. APPROACHING THE GRADUAL DECAY OF LIFE: *RO* AND *BYO* AS UNAVOIDABLE PROCESSES IN THE LIFE CYCLE

Toward the end of life, we gradually become *Ro* (old and aging). Sometimes, the concept of *Byo* (disease) appears to be combined with aging. In contrast to Buddha's admonition to acquiesce in the natural cycle of *Ro* and *Byo*, Kaibara underscores the positive aspects of aging. In his "Care for the Aging (*Yo Ro*)," Chapter 8 of *Yojokun*, Kaibara noted that filial piety to elderly parents, a central Confucian moral concept, is regarded as definitive of human relationships. He explained that the elderly still have some work to do and should spend a tranquil life with compassion toward others.

In Japan, one image of happiness is a healthy and respected elderly person surrounded by family members. Longevity is seen in Japan as a positive outcome of a healthy daily lifestyle, good *Yojo*. The elderly are respected for this accomplishment, as well as for their contributions to society. Living a long and healthy life is valuable in itself, and questions of productivity, important though they are, are irrelevant to the basic ethical notion of respect for the elderly.

In contrast, there are folk tales about the practice of abandonment of old people. Even though it is difficult to confirm the existence of this kind of practice, the legend symbolically denotes a negative evaluation of the elderly and aging. The sharp, dichotomous juxtaposition of the concepts of positive respect for the elderly and the negative feeling against old people suggests contradictory attitudes in traditional Japanese culture. The impoverished and miserable conditions that resulted from a series of famines may be the source of fictional legends of abandonment of elderly people as expressed, for example, in the novel *Narayamabushi Ko* (Fukasawa 1981).

Kaibara distinguishes disease from aging. The concept of disease, *byo*, also called *Byo-Ki*, the *Chi* of disease, or *Yamai*, illness, is not necessarily associated with the life cycle of *Ro* (aging), although there may have been some interaction. In traditional Japanese medicine, *Byo-Ki* could be caused by *Chi* (*Ki*), as well as by wrongdoing or karmic consequences of acts in a previous life. People need to commission *Kaji-Kito* (incantations and prayers), to be performed by professionals called *Onyoji* (experts on the *yin* and *yang* principles), to heal disease. To avoid contracting disease, it is necessary to have a positive *Chi* constantly inside one's body and mind. Kaibara wrote about the clinical management of disease, arguing that disease coexists with humans throughout the life cycle. Disease is not unnatural. Therefore, people should not be distressed by disease but should learn to cope with it. If death becomes unavoidable, it is a destiny mandated by the rule of heaven, which we have to accept as our *Tenmei* (life given by heaven) (Kaibara [1713a] 1961b, 40).

Classical physicians vigorously debated the source of disease. One of the most radical, Todo Yoshimasu (1702–1773), developed the theory that all diseases are caused by particular poisons. Even though this is naive in a sense, it reflected a turn to pathology as essential to the concept of disease. This marked a departure in thought about the cause of disease because the traditional idea was that disease is caused by *Chi* (Sakai 1986, 243–48).

VI. THE END OF LIFE CYCLE AS *SHI* AND THE BEYOND: THE IMAGE OF POSITIVE DEATH IN CULTURAL CONTEXT

The traditional sociocultural understanding of the human life cycle admits the natural process of death as a positive event marking the end of life. Japanese Zen Buddhist phrases such as "accept death as it is" and "life-death as one phenomenon" have been a key motif that is totally integrated into the Japanese understanding of life and death as later influenced by Confucius teachings (Katsube 1978, 65–68). As a natural event, a person's death has been understood in familial, communal, and social terms for many thousands of years. Indeed, even the intentional ending of one's life has been regarded as positive if it is intended for some noble cause within a particular historical context that justifies the action. For example, *Jyunshi* (self-immolation) and *Seppuku* (disembowelment; the same as *Harakiri*) are methods of sacrificing one's life for the greater benefit of one's feudal lord or the Emperor, and in some cases for family and friends (Suyematsu 1905, 163–70). This emphasis on readiness for self-sacrifice also has its negative side. The Japanese value communal goals more than mere biological life. The Japanese have a tendency

to sacrifice individual lives for larger ideals beyond their life in this world (Suzuki 1972, 140–53).

In the Japanese cultural tradition, death is given special concern and recognition as an event. Many heroic and unique Japanese figures appear in historical documents, usually expressing their last words in the form of *Jisei*, a kind of poem composed on the occasion of one's death and consisting of thirty-one syllables (Hoffman 1986). Although death itself is abhorred, it is understood and accepted as a natural part of the life process. In this sense, *Jisei* could be interpreted as a traditional cultural expression of a dying person. For the Japanese, death disturbs the rhythm of all living things, and therefore it should not be hastened. In contrast to the concern not to prolong the dying process unnecessarily, the Japanese are far more concerned with maintaining dying rituals and not ending life prematurely.

Japanese ethical values also affect attitudes toward the dead and dying. Confucian teaching embodies the notion of ancestor worship with its implications for family relationships based on filial piety. These concepts provide strong prohibitions against harming one's own body because it is derived from one's parents (Kurihara 1986). We can see a strong repugnance against organ transplants in this Japanese cultural context.

Many Japanese, for example, believe that a gradual decrease in body warmth should be felt in the process of dying and that hastening this and removing organs from a still-warm body suggests an unnatural end to human life. Resistance to hastening death and harvesting organs also comes from the traditional Japanese image of human beings as completely integrated mind–body units rather than distinct and separate units of mind, body, and spirit. This unity continues after death, so that removing an organ from a cadaver is seen as disturbing this spiritual and corporeal unity.

History teaches that a change in public attitudes in Japan is possible. At one time, the Japanese had strong objections to blood donation. This has been overcome, and the Japanese now have one of the highest rates of blood donation in the world. The brain death controversy since the first heart organ transplants in 1968 highlights the importance, although it took quite a few years, for public discussion between the public and professionals, which led finally to the enactment of the Law for Organ Transplants in 1997. This law required organ donors explicitly to state that they agree with the criteria of death based on brain assessment as opposed to the traditional criteria of death based on cardiac arrest, cessation of breathing, and dilation of pupils. In addition, the 1997 law required family consent to the patient's wishes to donate organs. This creates a conflict between the wishes of the patient and the patient's family. Thus, this represents an ethical dilemma at the end of the life cycle for Japanese people (Kimura 1998b, 55–58).

VII. CONCLUSION

Traditional medical ethics in Japan has faced grave changes challenged by the development of modern biomedical technologies such as organ transplantation. The Japanese life cycle is becoming more similar than different to the situation in the medically advanced countries of the world. The understanding of the life cycle has been vanishing as the Japanese have applied modern biomedical technologies more frequently in well-equipped hospital settings (Kimura 2004).

The unique Japanese sociocultural elements of each life cycle of *Sho, Ro, Byo, Shi* have been generally converging toward either birth/life (*Sho*) or death (*Shi*) by disregarding the stages of *Ro* and *Byo*, very often particularly by having artificial interventions at both the beginning and end of life. Some traditional elements of the involvement of family members in the process of *Sho, Ro, Byo, Shi* continue in a variety of ways, as reflected in the newly established framework of the Law for the Care of the Elderly, which was enacted after considerable public debate.

As Japan has one of the most rapidly increasing populations of elderly in the world, Japanese medical ethics, with special reference to the Japanese notion of the life cycle, can use the wisdom of *Yojokun* and particularly the positive concept of *Ro* to establish a global multicultural context toward future humane medical care (Sakai 1999b).

CHAPTER 7

MEDICAL ETHICS THROUGH THE LIFE CYCLE IN EUROPE AND THE AMERICAS

Robert B. Baker and Laurence B. McCullough

I. INTRODUCTION

Life cycles are constructed when the seemingly natural, foreordained, biological, or social changes of an organism's life are segmented into a series of linked sequential stages, for example: conception, birth, childhood, adolescence, adulthood, old age, dying and death; or, toddler, preschooler, grade schooler, high-schooler, college student, graduate, employee, and retiree. These stages are typically infused with social meanings that, in turn, become the lenses through which biological and social changes are interpreted. Societies construct life cycles differently: some recognize adolescence/teen age as intervening between childhood and adulthood; others do not recognize any interim stage. In any society, alternative conceptions of the life cycle and its meanings are articulated in discourses that may be congruent, overlapping, competing, or conflicting.

This chapter focuses on biomedical conceptions of the life cycle in European culture and its (post–fifteenth-century) extension in the Americas, examining their complex interactions and conflicts with other conceptions of the life cycle, in particular with those informed by Judeo-Christian religious traditions (a subject dealt with in Chapters 12, 13, 14, and 17). In treating the richly diverse cultures of three continents as if they were one culture that embraced a single conception of the life cycle, and in focusing on what came to be called "allopathic medicine," we of necessity oversimplify much and ignore more. We hope, however, that the insights gained from our history of the impact of the allopathic biomedical model on social conceptions of life stages will yield insights sufficiently rich to compensate for the distortions of oversimplification.

II. THE BIOMEDICAL GAZE: HOW MEDICAL MODELS AFFECT SOCIAL CONCEPTS OF THE LIFE CYCLE

In his watershed work, *Naissance de la Clinique* (Birth of the Clinic), French philosopher, Michel Foucault (1926–1984), observed that the medical perception of the world, the medical gaze, as he called it, anatomizes persons, stripping away personhood, replacing it with a perception of biophysiological processes (Foucault [1963] 1973). Foucault never dealt with the life cycle per se, but much the same can be said of the medicalization of the life cycle. The biomedical gaze strips the life cycle of its social meanings, perceiving only biophysiological events, blinded to the nested social relationships that surround them.[1] Yet, even as the medical gaze seeks to eschew social and religious meanings in the name of science, it is never free from their influence.

Foucault's medicalizing gaze has its origins in the Hippocratic texts of ancient Greece. The authors of these texts sought causal accounts of sickness and health, healing, and wellness, positing causes in a natural order of things that did not appeal to anything beyond, or above, nature. This naturalistic focus was evident in an early (circa 400 BCE) Hippocratic text, *On the Sacred Disease*. The text's unknown author challenges magico-religious accounts of a disease characterized by episodes in which those affected foamed at the mouth and kicked – symptoms that would today be diagnosed as a grand mal seizure. The magico-religious accounts that were challenged vested this phenomenon with social meaning, envisioning it as communication with the sacred, freighting events that might otherwise appear random and meaningless with significance. *On the Sacred Disease*, insistently naturalistic account of these symptoms "com[ing] from the brain, when it is not healthy, but becomes abnormally hot, cold, moist, or dry, or suffers any other unnatural affection to which it was not accustomed. The explanation that madness comes from its moistness" (Hippocrates 1923b, 175) strips these symptoms and the disease of any meaning.

Consider the case of the ancient Greek philosopher Socrates (469–399 BCE), who reported experiencing extended trances in which he heard voices that he interpreted as communications with a personal *daimon* (spirit). Socrates recognized the abnormality of hearing voices in trance states but took pride in these trances – his communication with his *daimon* – which gave meaning and structure to his life (Plato 1968, 4). The authors of *On the Sacred Disease* and later physicians, on the other hand, treat such trances as absence seizures, symptoms of brain pathology, or epilepsy. The philosopher and the physician recognize the abnormality of involuntary trances, yet one sees them as profoundly meaningful, the other as pathological. The difference between profundity and pathology, between an exalted state and a diseased state, reflects the difference between a gaze that embraces the sacred in every day life, and one that sees only naturalistic causal chains of biophysiological events (see Fadiman 1997).

Some proponents of the medical gaze characterize it as objective and value-free (Boorse 1975). Yet medical conceptions of the life cycle often reflect social values. Socrates' life again provides an example. By the standards of Athenian society, Socrates had abnormal sexual predilections: he was a monogamous heterosexual. Normally, the sexual life cycle of upper class Athenian males commenced with same-sex relationships with older males, moving on to heterosexual relationships in adulthood, when they were expected to marry and to have reproductive relationships with females. As males aged, however, they were expected to revert to same-sex relationships

with younger males, completing their sexual life cycle. The typical sexual life cycle of upper class Athenian males thus involved bisexual maturation, evolving from same-sex to heterosexual to same-sex relationships (Dover 1989).

Unlike his contemporaries, Socrates was, abnormally, a committed heterosexual who became a faithfully monogamous married male. As an adult he had many relations with attractive young men (his students), yet, again abnormally, these relationships were consistently asexual. His fellow Athenians found Socrates' sex life odd. Nonetheless, the medical gaze was not particularly powerful in ancient Greece and, just as Socrates trances were never medicalized, neither were his "abnormal" heterosexual predilections.

In later eras, as the medical model came to dominate ever-larger swaths of the life cycle, sexuality became medicalized. In pre-Christian Europe, sexual intercourse was guiltless, reflecting the pro-erotic views of pagan culture. Medical authorities believed that regular ejaculations (spending one's seed) and intercourse were conducive to health; correlatively, that the retention of seed was unhealthy, causing headaches, lethargy, fainting, and bizarre behavior. Because the male sexual paradigm applied to females as well – as Aristotle (384–322 BCE) famously remarked, "a woman is as it were an impotent male, for it is through a certain incapacity that the female is female" (Aristotle, *On the Generation of Animals*, I, 20, 728a) – medical writers believed that females had seed or sexual fluid that needed to be expressed through orgasm. The general consensus was that retention of male seed in the testes or female seed or sexual fluids in the womb – a condition known as hysteria, from *hysterikos* the Greek term for disturbances of the uterus – would manifest itself as fainting, fits, and other physical symptoms.

The most famous Greek physician of the Roman era, Galen (Claudius Galenus of Pergamum, 131–201) recommended either regular sexual intercourse or masturbation as a form of preventive medicine. Masturbation was also recommended as the appropriate treatment for hysteria. As evidence of its therapeutic efficacy, Galen cites the case of a widow afflicted with nervous tension. Diagnosing the problem as hysteria, a midwife manipulated the widow's sexual organs until she reached orgasm. As a result, Galen reported, the woman secreted a large quantity of fluid and was cured (Galen 1976, Book 6, Chapter 5, 185).

Judeo-Christian culture offered a radically different view of sexuality, eroticism, and masturbation. It perceived masturbation through the lens of Genesis 38:8–10 – a short passage, in which God condemns and slays a man, Onan, for refusing to consummate a levirate marriage by having intercourse with his deceased brother's childless widow (so that the deceased brother will have off-spring to carry on the line). Onan's nonconsummation involved "spilling his seed on the ground." No guidance is offered about whether the act for which God condemned and slew Onan was intentional defiance, refusal to consummate a levirate marriage, or spilling his seed, as either *coitus interruptus* or masturbation.

By the Renaissance, however, Christianity and Judaism interpreted Onan's sin as masturbation (Laquer 2003). Renaissance physicians thus felt the need to discard Galen's recommendations for the treatment of hysteria because "the spiritual harm outweigh[ed] any temporal gain" (Schleiner 1995, 123). By the eighteenth century, physicians began to project the Judeo-Christian moral critique of masturbation onto the act itself and masturbation came to be viewed as *unhealthy* as well as immoral. The transformation was initiated in 1710 when an anonymous medical tract, *Onania; or, The Heinous Sin of Self-Pollution* was published in London (Anonymous [1723] 1986). Inverting the characteristics traditionally associated with retained seed or hysteria, the author claimed that the sin of masturbation carried with it such deleterious medical consequences as loss of appetite, weakness, sleeplessness, exhaustion, and fainting fits.

Circa 1760, a Swiss physician, Simon-Auguste-Andre-David Tissot (1728–1787), defended much the same thesis in *Onanism: Or a Treatise Upon the Disorders produced by Masturbation* (Tissot [1760] 1767), claiming that masturbation caused memory loss, clouded sight, and led to gout, rheumatism, weakness of the back, and consumption. Tissot had again inverted Galen's account of hysteria and its treatments, attributing to masturbation the very symptoms previously assigned to hysteria. Masturbation was thus instantly transformed from cure to cause, from therapy to pathology – not as a function of new scientific discoveries, but as an infusion of religious and social values into the seemingly objective medical gaze or model.

Conceived in the Victorian era (1819–1901), modern psychiatry assimilated Tissot's pathologizing of masturbation, taking the further step of transforming the act from a precipitating cause of various somatic or physical maladies into a psychiatric illness (Porter 1997, 203). In 1893, no less a figure than Sigmund Freud classified masturbation, not as a form of insanity per se, but rather as a leading cause of a condition known as neurasthenic neurosis (Freud 1971, I:50).

Throughout the nineteenth and early twentieth centuries, treatments for masturbatory insanity, onanism, and neurasthenia were often extreme, ranging from electroshock to sexual surgery – including clitorectomy (removal of the clitoris for female masturbators), desensitizing scarification, and castration (typically for male masturbators) and institutionalization in an asylum (Barker-Benfield 1976; Engelhardt 1981). Under one name or another, masturbation remained an active psychiatric diagnosis through the 1930s. Its epitaph was written in the Kinsey reports of 1948 and 1953, which reported that 92 percent of males and 62 percent of females practiced masturbation (Kinsey 1948, 1953). Believing that something

so common could not be unnatural, the pathologization of masturbation ceased. By the 1960s, the gynecologist–psychologist team of William Masters (1915–2001) and Virginia Johnson completed the circle, returning the medical conception of masturbation to its classic roots, as a requisite of normality. In their studies on human sexuality, they treat the capacity for masturbation as the litmus test for sexual health (Masters and Johnson 1966, 1970). Medical views of masturbation had thus come full circle: from a requisite of health, to a therapy, to a cause of disease, to a disease, and finally, once again, to a prerequisite of health – a normal part of puberty and integral aspect of maturation in the sexual life cycle.

The remarkable transformation in the medical understanding of masturbation in the sexual life cycle provides a striking example of the extent to which the seemingly objective medical gaze is prone to mirror social values. Pagan Greece and Rome celebrated sensuality and its medicine reflected these values, endorsing masturbation as both healthy and therapeutic. Judeo-Christianity, loathing eroticism and relegating sexuality to the realm of dutiful reproduction, saw masturbation as sinful. As medicine and psychiatry flourished in the eighteenth and nineteen centuries, this sin was transformed into a sickness. When the influence of religion waned in twentieth-century Europe and North America, society became less puritanical and its medicine could accept normality of masturbation, once again treating it as a sign of healthy sexuality. At every turn, including its present incarnation, social values inform the medical gaze not only with respect to masturbation and homosexuality but also with respect to the life cycle generally. Any historical account of the relationships between biomedicine and the life cycle must thus address two countervailing tendencies: the tendency of the medical model to strip social and religious meaning from its account of the life cycle, and the countervailing tendency for society to reinfuse medicine's seemingly objective, nonvalue laden accounts with the very social and religious meanings that the ideology of medicine ostensibly rejects.

III. Pregnancy and Childbirth

Until the late eighteenth century and, arguably, through much of the nineteenth century as well, childbirth was not medicalized. As late as 1900, the percentage of in-hospital births in Europe and the Americas was less than 5 percent. By the end of the twentieth century, these ratios were reversed: more than 95 percent of births in Europe (exclusive of the Netherlands) and North America were in hospitals – reflecting the comparatively rapid medicalization of pregnancy and childbirth in the twentieth century.

Premedicalization, childbirth was an exclusively female social event, presided over by female relations and neighbors, and assisted, at times, by nonmedically trained female midwives. The expectant mother was center stage. Men were off stage. The medicalization of childbirth would shift the locus of delivery from the personal domain of the woman, the household bedchamber, to the professional domain of the obstetrician, the hospital. Males – the man-midwife or *accoucheur*, as obstetricians were sometimes called, the surgeon, and the general practitioner – moved to center stage, directing the delivery, pronouncing its success or failure to the expectant parents and documenting it for society in birth certificates and hospital records.

The medicalization of childbirth, originally a middle and upper class phenomenon that originated in Europe, spread to the same classes in the Europeanized Americas, eventually becoming standard for all classes of Europeans and North Americans. Historians date the origins of medicalization to the mid-eighteenth century.

> The employment of medical men for normal childbirth occurred quite suddenly. Numerous reports confirm the story of the very capable and experienced midwife, Sarah Stone: following in the footsteps of her mother she practiced midwifery . . . When she began her career, men-midwives were unknown. [In] Bristol in 1730 . . . she found that 'every young MAN who hath served his apprenticeship to a Barber-Surgeon, immediately sets up for a man-midwife, as ignorant, or indeed much ignoranter than the meanest woman of the Profession.' What Sarah Stone reported was occurring, then or soon after, all over the country. (Loudon 1993, 1051)

Historians stress various factors to explain the medicalization and concomitant defeminization of childbirth: the prestige and fashionableness of science; the acceptance of technology in the form of forceps; assertions of social status by the woman (attendance by an *accoucheur* as conspicuous consumption); and the economic and social ambitions of medical men. One major factor was women's apprehensions about childbirth. In the absence of effective contraceptives, a married woman could expect to have between five and eight babies, often closely spaced. These high rates of pregnancy meant that the average married woman had approximately one chance in eight of dying in childbirth (Leavitt 1986). Sending for a medical man thus seemed like a reasonable form of insurance, and families who could afford it called in surgeons to assist in difficult deliveries, particularly breech births. After 1730, moreover, obstetrical forceps had become more common and surgeons were more skillful in their use.

Some physicians, such as the Scot, Alexander Gordon (1752–1799), and the American, William Shippen (1736–1808), tried to preserve birth as a feminine affair by setting up schools to teach (typically illiterate) midwives how to practice their trade scientifically. From 1818 onward,

Dutch medical regulation mandated such education for midwives, laying the foundation for the system that prevails in the Netherlands today. Nonetheless, since well into the twentieth century, surgeons were typically male, except in the Netherlands, the medicalization of childbirth resulted in the assertion of masculinity into a previously feminine domain.

Male medical practitioners tried to facilitate their intrusion into the feminine domain of birth by offering "ethical" protections prohibited to midwives. Eighteenth-century midwives were obligated to reveal infant deaths and suspected bastards. The 1716, New York City Midwives Oath, which was modeled on similar British oaths, states that a midwife

> . . . shall be diligent and ready to help any woman in labor, whether she be poor or rich; that in time of necessity, she will not forsake the poor woman and go to the rich; that she will not cause or suffer any woman to name or put any other father to the child, but only him which is the true father thereof, indeed, according to the utmost of her power; that she will not suffer any women to pretend to be delivered of a child who is not, indeed, neither to claim any other woman's child as her own; that she will not suffer any woman's child to be murdered or hurt; and as often as she shall see any peril or jeopardy, either in the mother or the child, she will call in other midwives for council; that she will not administer any medicine to produce a miscarriage; that she will not enforce a woman to give more for services than is right; that she will not collude to keep secret the birth of a child; will be of good behavior; and will not conceal the birth of bastards. (Davis [1903] 1907, 134–35)

By contrast, the new ethics for physicians and surgeons developed by John Gregory (1724–1773; see Chapter 30) and Thomas Percival (1740–1804; see Chapter 36) guaranteed confidentiality. Gregory wrote that "Secrecy is particularly requisite where women are concerned" (Gregory [1772b] 1998b, 27) and Percival echoed the sentiment: "Secrecy . . . should be strictly observed. And females should always be treated with the most scrupulous delicacy" (Percival 1803, Chap. I, Art. 5, 11; see also I).

For these and other reasons, women increasingly chose male physicians over female midwives. The male intrusion on a female domain was justified by the implicit promise that medical men could offer women less painful, safer, deliveries of healthier children. Part of that promise seemed to be actualized on 7 April 1853, when John Snow (1813–1858) administered a newly discovered analgesic, chloroform, to Queen Victoria of Britain, who delivered Prince Leopold safely and painlessly. "The effect," Her Majesty wrote of the chloroform "was soothing, quieting

& delightful beyond measure" (Porter 1997, 366). Despite objections by medical conservatives, like the Philadelphia obstetrician Charles Meigs (1792–1869), who wrote that anesthesia "contravene[s] the operations of those natural and physiological forces that Divinity has ordained us to... suffer" (Pernick 1985, 50) and the protests of religious fundamentalists – who cited Genesis 3:16, "in sorrow thou shalt bring forth children" – European and American women demanded, and soon received, similar treatment. Labor pain became dispensable and the era of analgesic medicalized and masculinized childbirth had begun.

Childbirth also became safer. Whereas in the mid-seventeenth century maternal mortality in England and Wales was approximately 15 per 1,000 (1.5 percent of births), and neonatal mortality was approximately 100 per 1,000 (10 percent), two centuries later, when Queen Victoria gave birth to Prince Leopold, maternal mortality had declined to 5.5 per 1,000 (0.55 percent). Neonatal mortality had declined to 50 per 1,000 (5 percent of all births) (Smith 1993, 1682). Still, the shadow of puerperal fever – from the Latin *puer*, child, and *parere*, to give birth – hung over masculine scientific obstetrics. As William Farr (1807–1883), a health statistician ("Compiler of Abstracts") pointed out in the 1870s, deliveries by male doctors in hospitals (approximately 8 percent of all deliveries) had unacceptably high maternal mortality rates of approximately 200 or more deaths per 10,000 births (approximately 2 percent). In contrast, home deliveries (approximately 90 percent of all deliveries) – *half* of which were still presided over by *female* midwives – enjoyed a lower maternal mortality rate of approximately 0.5 percent.

The reason for this discrepancy should not have been a mystery. Women giving birth in hospitals suffered higher rates of puerperal fever – a disease that had been associated with hospitals since it was first documented at a major Paris hospital, the Hôtel Dieu, in 1646 (Loudon 1986b). More astonishing still, by the 1870s the cause of puerperal fever had been discovered not once, but three times. As early as 1795, the Scottish physician Alexander Gordon reported that the cause was putrid matter introduced into the uterus by a physician or midwife. His remedy was hand washing. In 1843, an American physician, Oliver Wendell Holmes, Sr. (1809–1894), published a paper that came to the same conclusion. Most famously, in 1847 Ignaz Philipp Semmelweis (in Hungarian, Ignác Fülöp Semmelweis) (1818–1865) demonstrated that "putrid matter" clinging to the hands of physicians and medical students after they had performed dissections on cadavers caused puerperal fever. Observing that maternity wards serviced by medical students suffered a 29 percent rate of infection from puerperal fever whereas those served by midwives only had a 3 percent infection rate, Semmelweiss conducted a crossover trial by having medical students and midwives switch wards. High infection rates followed the medical students; low rates followed the midwives. Having the medical students wash their hands in an antiseptic solution lowered their sepsis rates to those of the midwives, demonstrating that handwashing prevented puerperal fever (von Hebra 1847, 1849).

Gordon, Holmes, and Semmelweis should have been lauded as medical innovators. Instead, the medical establishment ignored Gordon, lambasted Holmes and ostracized Semmelweis. The leading American obstetricians of the day, the Philadelphia obstetricians Charles Meigs and Hugh L. Hodge (1796–1873) – founder of the American antiabortion movement (see Chapter 36) – adamantly rejected the indictment of iatrogenesis (from the Greek *iatros*, doctor, and *genesis*, originated; that is, diseases caused by doctors). "Doctors," Meigs protested, "are gentlemen, and gentlemen's hands are clean" (Wertz and Wertz 1989, 122).

The American medical establishment's disdainful dismissal of Holmes was mild in comparison with the Austrian medical establishment's treatment of Semmelweis. Despite his impressive data and his innovative use of a prospective crossover trial to demonstrate that hand washing in a mild antiseptic solution decreased the level of puerperal fever, and despite his replication of contagion in an animal model, rabbits, the medical establishment repudiated not only Semmelweis's data and theories, but Semmelweis himself. He lost his position at the Lying-In Hospital in Vienna. When Semmelweis presented his work to the Medical Society of Vienna in 1850, such medical luminaries as the pathologist Rudolph Virchow (1821–1902) and the prominent obstetrician Friedrich Wilhelm Scanzoni (1821–1891) dismissed his views as absurd.

Returning in despair to his native Budapest, Semmelweis suffered a mental collapse and ultimately died in a Viennese insane asylum – from a beating administered by asylum attendants (Nuland 2003, 167–69).

How is one to assess over a century of persistent rejection of the demonstrated etiology and control of puerperal fever? Were the messengers inept? Some fault Semmelweis's personality, his prose style, his failure to master academic protocol and politics, Austrian xenophobia, and generational politics (Nuland 2003)? No doubt these were contributing factors, but they do not explain the similarly hostile reception accorded to the eminently respectable Oliver Wendell Holmes, Sr., the first dean of the Harvard Medical School, a consummate academic politician, a founder of the *Atlantic Monthly Magazine*, an elegant, widely published, and widely read prose stylist. Probing for a deeper explanation, some historians have given a Kantian account. Kant famously held that percepts without concepts are blind, that we cannot perceive what our minds lack the concepts to understand. Appealing to this notion historians of medicine sometimes aver that Semmelweis's studies – and, one might add, those of Gordon and Holmes – "being entirely empirical and with no theoretical foundation, were only partially recognized by the academic community" (Tröhler 1993, 987). On this analysis, the significance of Semmelweis's data could be appreciated only *after* Robert Koch (1843–1910) and Louis Pasteur (1822–1895) developed the germ theory of disease (Nuland 2003, 177–80).

Despite the intellectual elegance of this analysis, it is not supported by the data on maternal mortality. Had the absence of supporting theory been the roadblock preventing the Holmes–Semmelweis hygienic reforms, these reforms would have been implemented in the period between 1880 and 1900, that is, shortly after medical acceptance of the germ theory and Pasteur's 1879 identification of the germ that causes puerperal fever, *Streptococcus pyogenes*, now characterized as β-hemolytic streptococcus (Pasteur 1879). Yet, very few countries implemented hygienic reforms between 1880 and 1900. Those that did, the Netherlands and Scandinavia, experienced 50 percent and even 75 percent declines in maternal mortality from puerperal fever between 1870 and 1905. In England, Scotland, Wales, and the United States, however, hygienic practices and maternal mortality remained substantially unchanged. Only after 1935, when Gerhard Domagk (1895–1964) discovered the sulphonamides, an effective antibiotic treatment for puerperal fever, did these countries experience a rapid decrease in maternal mortality (Loudon 1986, 1993). Drugs, not hygiene, were responsible for the decline in maternal mortality in most of Europe and North America.

A more plausible explanation for the persistent rejection of the (Gordon)–Holmes–Semmelweis hygiene hypothesis and for the berating of the hypothesizers lies in the iatrogenic nature of their claim, that is, their insistence that puerperal fever was a disease caused by doctors' dirty hands. The (Gordon)–Holmes–Semmelweis explanation "was unpopular because it indicted medical practitioners as the transmitters of this dreadful disease" (Loudon 1993, 1060). Hodge, who taught at the most prestigious American medical school of the era, the University of Pennsylvania, instructed his students that the dirty hands hypothesis was incompatible with the ideal of the physician as a "minister of mercy" (Wertz and Wertz, 1989, 121). His colleague, Meigs, rejected the analysis as "injurious to the profession of medicine, pernicious to the people . . . filling the minds of interested parties with alarm." Unable to accept the notion that he himself could have been the agency of maternal death Meigs declared that "I have practiced midwifery for long years. I have attended thousands of women and passed through epidemics of childbirth fever . . . I certainly never was the medium of its transmission" (Wertz and Wertz 1989, 122).

Semmelweis disdained such assessments as self-serving. "As painful and depressing . . . as such an acknowledgment is the remedy does not lie in concealment . . . the truth must be made known" (Nuland 2003, 104). In the end, frustrated by their indifference to his data, Semmelweis began to castigate fellow obstetricians as "murderers" (Nuland 2003, 159–60). Holmes also condemned the continuation of traditional unsanitary childbirth practices as a "crime" (Wertz and Wertz 1989, 123), proclaiming that "if it can be shown great numbers of lives have been and are sacrificed to ignorance or blindness . . . if [physicians] can be shown to carry disease and death instead of health and safety, the common instincts of humanity will silence every attempt to explain away their responsibility" (Holmes 1942, 605). Holmes was wrong: historians and physicians seldom censured Hodge, Meigs, Scanzoni, or Virchow for silencing the data; they typically laud their accomplishments, without mentioning their rejection of hygienic measures to prevent puerperal fever.

IV. Abandonment and Infanticide

Exposure and infanticide were common practices in pre–Judeo-Christian Europe, permitted and perhaps even required by Roman law, and abetted by Roman physicians (Bouillon-Jensen 1995, 1200). As Europe and its medical practices became more Christian, the practices of abandonment, exposure, and infanticide were increasingly condemned and criminalized in law and in medical tracts. Foundling hospitals for abandoned newborns – an innovation from thirteenth-century Italy that spread, over the course of centuries, to France, England, Russia, and the Americas – were thought to provide a humane Christian alternative to abandonment and infanticide (although some scholars have suggested that mortality in foundling homes was so high that they merely served as a socially acceptable facade for infanticide). Even after the establishment of foundling hospitals, however, abandoned newborns and the corpses of infants dead from exposure were not uncommon sights in European cities (Hoffer and Hull, 1981; Bouillon-Jensen 1995; Jackson 2002; Larson 2004). Laws aimed at preventing abandonment and infanticide were enacted in France in 1556, in Britain in 1624, and later in other parts of Europe and the Americas. British and French law stipulated that any woman found to have concealed the death of a baby would be presumed to have committed infanticide – unless there was evidence that the baby was stillborn (Crawford 1993, 1625; Percival 1803, Chap. IV, Art. XI, 80–86). These laws forced women accused of concealing the death of an infant to solicit testimony from physicians declaring the infant to have been stillborn.

Testifying as an expert witness raised medical questions about how to distinguish infanticides from miscarriages and, more generally, about how physicians ought to conduct themselves in court cases. Early works on medical ethics and medical jurisprudence typically addressed these issues. The man-midwife William Hunter (1718–1783), for example, turned a medicalizing gaze on the plight of women who concealed the death of their infant children. He argued that they were in state of postpartum depression and, even if they killed their newborn children, they could not be held responsible for their acts.

> [In] the greatest number of what are called murders of bastard children ... [the mother] loses the hope ... In this situation many of these women, who are afterwards accused of murder, would destroy themselves ... In that state often they are overtaken before they expected; their schemes are frustrated; their distress of body and mind deprives them of all judgment and rational conduct ... [they] become insensible of what is passing; and when they recover a little strength, find that the child, whether still-born or not, is completely lifeless ... If the law punishes such a woman with death for concealing her shame, does it not require more from human nature than weak human nature can bear? In a case so circumstanced, surely the only crime is having been pregnant, which the law does not mean to punish with death, and the attempt to conceal it by fair means should not be punishable with death, as that attempt seems to arise from a principle of virtuous shame. (Hunter, *Medical Observations and Inquiries*, volume VI, 271ff quoted in Percival 1803b, Chap. IV, Art. XI, 82–84) (see also Percival 1794, Sec. IV, Art. IX)

Percival, who quoted from Hunter at length, rejected Hunter's medicalization of maternal infanticide, because it "exalt[s] the sense of shame into the principle of virtue" (Percival 1803b, Chap. IV, Art. XI, 84) (see also Percival 1794, Sec. IV, Art. IX). Percival, however, compassionately urged that the punishment meted out to women for concealing the death of an infant should be made more proportionate to the crime.

Percival and Hunter debated the medicalization of maternal responsibility for infanticide when faced with the illegitimate birth of normal babies. But what were the responsibilities of physicians and mothers if a woman gave birth to a legitimate but visibly abnormal infant, a "monster," as such infants were called traditionally? Seen through a religious gaze, a "monster" was a sign or portent sent by God for the punishment of sin (Walton et al. 1993). By the late nineteenth century, however, a secularizing medical gaze had reconfigured monstrous births into "anomalies" and "birth defects" – although, the term 'monster' lingers in medical discourse and is searchable in the U.S. National Library of Medicine electronic database, PUBMED. (A search using the term, "monster," in 2005 called up 4,641 articles, 287 marked as highly relevant.)

By the 1870s, some physicians in Britain advocated abandoning and directly killing infants with "incurable conditions" (Pernick 1996, 22). This medical debate came to considerable public prominence in early twentieth-century America in 1916, with the release of the film, "The Black Stork" a 'eugenic love story'" (Pernick 1996, 41). The film, which ran in movie theaters in the United States until the early 1940s, was based on the practices of Harry Haiselden, a Chicago surgeon who had withheld surgery from infants born with major but potentially operable anomalies and who may have "speeded the deaths" in some cases (Pernick 1996, 4).

> The ... film begins with Claude, who has an unnamed inherited disease. Despite repeated graphic warnings from Dr. Dickey (played by Haiselden himself), Claude marries his sweetheart, Anne. Their baby is born so severely disabled that it needs immediate surgery to save its life, but Dr. Dickey refuses to perform the operation. Anne is torn by uncertainty until God reveals a lengthy vision of the child's future, filled with pain, madness, and crime. Her doubts resolved, she accepts Dr. Dickey's judgment, and the baby's soul leaps into the arms of a waiting Jesus. (Pernick 1996, 5–6)

Haiselden appealed to scientific theories of heritable traits to provide seemingly objective eugenic justifications for non-treatment of infants with major (or minor) anomalies; however, neither the American Medical Association (AMA), nor any other medical or scientific organization ever endorsed Haiselden's activities.

Nazi eugenic infanticide policies of the 1930s, however, were approved by official organizations and integrated into the medical curriculum. Thus "the director of the Eglfinger-Haar asylum, Herman Pfannmüller ... gave tours of the eugenic-euthanasia program to young physicians" (Burleigh 1994, 45). As the following autobiographical remarks by Ludwig Lehners attest, some on those on the tour rejected Pfannmüller's medicalized public health conception of infanticide.

> Since I had studied psychology in 1934/1935 as part of my professional training ... I took part in a conducted tour ... The asylum director ... Pfannmüller, led us into a childrens' ward ... [He] explained ... "As a National Socialist, these creatures ... naturally only represent to me a burden upon the healthy body of our nation. We don't kill (he may have used a more circumlocutory expression ...) with poison, injections, etc ... No: as you see, our method is simpler and even more natural." With these words, and assisted by a nurse ... he pulled one of the children out of the bed. As he displayed the child around like a dead hare, he pointed out, with a knowing look and a cynical grin, "This one will last another two

or three days." The image of this fat, grinning man, with the whimpering skeleton in his fleshy hand is still clear before my eyes. (Burleigh 1994, 45–46)

Where Pfannmüller saw "a burden upon the healthy body of our nation," whose elimination was necessary to ensure public health, Lehners saw a child.

V. Abortion

It might be presumed that during those eras when Europe and the Americas tolerated infanticide, they would also tolerate abortion. As it turns out, there is little correlation between the social and legal status of the two practices. Abortion was as illegal in infanticidal Nazi Germany, as it was in Britain, France, and the Americas (see Chapters 32, 34, and 36). Prior to the nineteenth century, European society had tolerated prequickening abortion because of the widely held belief that the unanimated fetus was not yet alive. Secular law and Christian doctrine distinguished between the sin and crime of aborting a quickened or moving fetus and inducing the miscarriage of prequickened (first trimester) unanimated fetus, which was considered, at worst, a misdemeanor.

By the end of the eighteenth century, this distinction began to break down. Percival, for example, rejected the distinction between a prequickened and a quickened fetus, holding that inducing a miscarriage was just as reprehensible as performing an abortion: both acts should be considered equally unacceptable and criminal.

> [Traditionally it has been held that] "if a woman be quick with child, and, by a potion or otherwise, killeth it in her womb, this is a great misprision, yet no murder. But if the child be born alive, and dieth of the potion or otherwise, this is murder" ... the *foetus* being regarded as a portion of the womb of the mother, she was supposed to have an equal and full right over both. This [is a] false opinion ... since no female can be privileged to injure her own bowels, much less the foetus, which is now well known to constitute no part of them. To extinguish the first spark of life is a crime of the same nature, both against our Maker and society, as to destroy an infant, a child, or a man; these regular and successive stages of existence being the ordinances of God, subject alone to His divine will ... Hence the father of physic [Hippocrates], in the oath enjoined on his pupils, which some universities now impose on the candidates for medical degrees, obliged them solemnly to abjure the practice of administering the *pessary*.... to procure an abortion. (Percival 1794, Sec. IV, Art. 8, emphasis original) (see also Percival 1803b, Chap. IV, Art. 10, 78–79)

The elements of Percival's arguments echoed down the decades of the nineteenth century, leading first to the reconceptualization of the induction of miscarriages as abortions, then, beginning in Britain in 1803, to the criminalization of first trimester abortions (see Chapter 36) and later to the 1869 condemnation of such abortions as excommunicable offences by the Roman Catholic Church. By the end of the nineteenth century prequickening abortions – indeed, abortions at all stages of pregnancy – were officially considered unacceptable and illegal throughout Europe and the Americas and were universally condemned by European and American professional medical societies.

Percival's indictment rested on the newly emerging knowledge about pregnancy, which allowed him to reject "false opinion." The fetus, he asserted confidently, constitutes "no part" of the woman's womb, that is, the fetus is an independent life from conception. After 1819, the year in which René Laennec (1781–1826) invented the stethoscope – an instrument that enabled practitioners to hear the separate and distinct sound of the prequickened fetus' heartbeat – what had been evident to Percival in 1794 became self-evident to the entire medical profession. In an era that equated the heartbeat with life, the sound of the independent fetal heartbeat provided seemingly irrefutable medical evidence that the prequickened fetus was a living independent human being. The justification of prequickening abortion thus seemed to rest on nothing more than self-serving unenlightened ignorance.

Percival also offered what would become the standard "life-stage-argument" against elective abortion. Having established that the pre-quickened fetus is an independent organism, with a life of its own, he concluded that, "To extinguish the first spark of life is a crime of the same nature ... as to destroy an infant, a child, or a man." In other words, since the fetus, the infant, the child, and the adult are all are parts of a continuous life cycle, to extinguish any one part is to deprive the organism of the rest of its natural life cycle. Destruction at any point is criminal because it deprives living individuals of the rest of their lives.

The German physician, Johann Peter Frank (1745–1821), would later concur with Percival's position that "a child is just as much a living creature before half the pregnancy is over, as it is after the first half" (Lesky 1976, 104). Frank supplemented these considerations with an antiabortion argument that would gain resonance in the nineteenth century: the "damage which the state thereby suffers" from abortion: "thus mankind is robbed of a ... member" (Lesky 1976, 104).

Medicalization is fickle. As we have seen, by the nineteenth century medicalization seemed to favor the criminalization of abortion and until the 1960s professional medical societies throughout Western Europe and the

Americas adamantly opposed abortion, except when necessary to protect maternal life or health. The medical gaze, however, strives for neutrality: sometimes favoring one policy, and yet, a few decades later, supporting the reverse. In their struggle to decriminalize first trimester abortion, nineteenth- and twentieth-century suffragettes, feminists, and their allies in humanist and political reform movements had to resist the medicalization of abortion; after the 1960s, they found that medicalization suited their needs.

The introduction of the concept of brain death helped to change the direction of the medical gaze. After more than a decade of experience with patients in irreversibly comatose states whose hearts were kept beating by machines, the medical profession accepted an alternative to cardiopulmonary criteria for death – brain death. A person could be considered dead if his or her brain had irreversibly ceased to function, a state indicated by flat lines on an electroencephalograph, or EEG, but which required additional confirming evidence to be definitive (Harvard Medical School 1968). Once medicine had disassociated human life, the life of a human person, from the beating of the human heart, the fact that the first trimester fetus had a heartbeat no longer sufficed to establish it as a living human person. Moreover, well-known facts about neurological development of the embryo and fetus indicated that during the first trimester, and perhaps beyond, the fetus did not have sufficient neurological development to be considered "brain alive" – even though its heart was beating. The medical evidence that had supported the criminalization and prohibition of first trimester abortion now seemed to favor decriminalization. Ironically, medicalization, formerly the strongest suit of those advocating criminalizing abortion, now lay on the side of feminists and their allies. So feminists and their allies began to champion "scientific" medicine with its nonmoral gaze, and professional medical societies ceased to oppose abortion.

Opponents of decriminalization, on the other hand, began to denigrate the medical model, relying increasingly on moral arguments and emotional appeals to defend their position. By the end of the twentieth century, first trimester abortion was again legal in almost all European states and throughout the United States. Abortion policy had come full circle: first accepting the legal and moral permissibility of first trimester abortions, later considering them impermissible and illegal, and then accepting their permissibility. There is a singular exception. In countries in which the Roman Catholic Church has a strong political voice, such as Ireland, Poland, and throughout Latin America, abortion is viewed through the lenses of a Catholic moral gaze. Consequently, at the end of the twentieth century, abortion in any trimester is illegal in these countries, except for certain allowable medical reasons (which vary from country to country).

VI. CHILDHOOD AND AGING

Geriatrics and pediatrics are intriguing medical specializations in the context of this chapter because they medicalize two stages of the life cycle. Surgeons practice surgery and are defined in terms of their training and skills: So too are general practitioners, nurses, pharmacists, and radiologists. Other forms of medicine are characterized in terms of body parts: dentistry (teeth), ophthalmology (eyes), otolaryngology (ear, nose, and throat), and podiatry (feet). Still other forms of medicine are defined in terms of diseases: "infectious disease," oncology (specialists in cancer care). Pediatrics and geriatrics, however, define themselves not in terms of a skill set, organ system, or a disease, but in terms of life stages – childhood and old age. Their very names reflect this, conjoining the Greek words "paid" for child, and "geras" for old age, with the "iatros," physician, one who heals or treats. In both a superficial and deep sense, these specialties are dedicated to medicalizing the life cycle.

The *Jahrbuch für Kinderheilkunde* (*Almanac of Pediatrics*, later *Annales Paediatrici* (*Annals of Pediatrics*, today *Pediatric Research*)) was first published in 1868. The term "pediatrics" first appeared in print in 1884, the same year that the *Archives of Pediatrics* began to be published and the American Pediatric Society had its first meeting in 1889. The term, "pediatrician," referring to someone who specializes in treating childhood diseases, first appeared in print in 1903 (Mahnke 2000).

The neologism "geriatrics" was minted in the same decade, in 1909, by the Austrian-born American physician, Ignatz Nascher (1863–1945), who called for a field modeled on pediatrics. The new field was to be called

> Geriatrics, from *gera*, old age, and *iatrikos*, relating to the physician . . . to cover the same field, in old age, that is covered by the term 'paediatrics' in childhood . . . to emphasize the necessity of considering senility and its diseases apart from maturity and to assign to it a separate place in medicine. (Nascher 1909, cited in Thane 1993, 1103)

Nascher followed this appeal with a book *Geriatrics* (Nascher 1914), published – with some difficulty – a decade later. Introducing the volume was none other than the German-born American pediatrician, Abraham Jacobi (1830–1919), founder of the American Medical Association specialty section on Diseases of Children (1880), who is also credited as the founder of American pediatrics (Shulman 2004).

One American immigrant, a German-speaking founder of the first life stage–oriented medical specialty, was thus assisting a fellow German-speaking American immigrant physician to found another life stage–oriented medical specialty. Yet, as late as 1926, Nascher was the only physician in the Americas or Europe to actually refer to himself as a "geriatrician." Money and prestige in the form of a $10,000 Josiah Macy Jr. Foundation grant to the U.S. Public Health Service to support a specialist in aging began to change attitudes. In 1942, the American Geriatrics Society was founded.

By 1953, however, there were only three professors of geriatrics in the United States; Britain – because of the efforts of Marjorie Warren (1897–1960) was Europe's leading center of geriatric medicine (Evans 1997) – first appointed a professor of geriatrics in 1964. In 2000, there were approximately 35 million people older than the age of 65 in the United States; more than 4 million were older than the age of 85. The older-than-85 population was cared for by approximately 9,000 geriatricians; approximately 2.25 geriatricians per 100,000 persons. In contrast, in 2000 the approximate 60 million children aged 14 or younger in the United States were cared for by 106.2 pediatricians per 100,000 children.

Pediatrics and pediatricians were more widely accepted than geriatrics and geriatricians. Why? A number of factors appear to be in play: conceptions of childhood and old age; economics; pronatalism; tensions over the medical division of labor; and societal attitudes toward children, women, and the elderly more generally. Conceptual issues appear primary.

Childhood, some historians have claimed, is an invention of the various national Enlightenments of the seventeenth through early nineteenth centuries. As historian Roy Porter has observed, prior to the Enlightenments:

> Mainstream Christian doctrine was put in a nutshell by the leading Evangelical educator Hannah More: were not infants "beings who bring into the world a corrupt nature and evil disposition, which it should be the great end of education to rectify?" In line with such original sin tenets – the biblical spare the rod and spoil the child – brutal, indeed bloody, childrearing practices had been both preached and practiced . . . traditional upbringing was stern, and beatings were the lot of the young at home, at school and in the work place . . . Some historians have further argued that pre-industrial society scarcely even entertained a distinctive concept of children, seeing them instead as Lilliputian adults: what possible reason could there be to privilege their condition? (Porter 2000, 340)

Between them the British philosopher John Locke (1632–1704) and the French Philosopher Jean Jacques Rousseau (1712–1778) offered an answer: Children were innocents: their minds were blank slates on which experience – positive or negative – would leave its mark shaping their future and the future of society. Pediatrics thus flourished as a natural emanation of the Enlightenment's idealization of children and childhood as the pathway to the future and to progress.

Although the Enlightenment buoyed the development of pediatrics, it weighed down the development of geriatrics. Medical partisans of the Enlightenment, like Percival, wrote openly about "the commencement of that period of senescence when it becomes incumbent on a physician to decline the offices of his profession" (Percival 1804, Chap. II, Art. XXII 52). Writing movingly at the age of 63 about his own old age, Percival remarks that even those "exempt, in a considerable degree, from the privations and infirmities of age" will find that, "in the ordinary course of nature, the bodily and mental vigour must be expected to decay progressively, though perhaps slowly, after the meridian of life is past" (Percival 1803, Chap. II, Art. XXXII, 52).

Percival and other Enlightenment physicians never challenged the equation of old age with decline, decay, dependency, senescence, and death. William Shakespeare (1564–1616) anticipated what became the received view of Enlightenment European and American cultures when he wrote that all men and women evolve through seven ages, with senescence starting in the sixth age during which a man finds

> his shrunk shank; and his big manly voice,
> Turning again toward childish treble, pipes
> And whistles in his sound. Last scene of all,
> That ends this strange eventful history,
> Is second childishness and mere oblivion,
> Sans teeth, sans eyes, sans taste, sans everything.
> (Shakespeare As You Like It, II. vii. 139–66)

Old age means physical decline, loss of body mass, loss of "manly voice," loss of teeth, loss of sight, a second age of dependency, or childishness, all culminating in death.

One notable voice dissented: Shakespeare's contemporary, the philosopher Francis Bacon (1561–1626). Bacon identified three "offices" of medicine: "the first whereof is the Preservation of Health, the second the Cure of Diseases, and third the Prolongation of Life" (Bacon 1875, 383). About prolongation of life Bacon wrote:

> But this last the physicians do not seem to have recognized as the principal part of their art . . . For they imagine that if diseases be repelled before they attack the body, and cured after they have attacked it, prolongation of life necessarily follows. But . . . they have not penetration to see that . . . the lengthening of the thread of life itself, and the postponement for a time of that death which gradually steals on by natural dissolution and the decay of old age, is a subject which no physician has handled in proportion to its dignity. (Bacon 1875, 383)

The "natural" aspects of aging, usually taken as immutable givens in religious and other accounts of the life cycle, like Shakespeare's, are here portrayed as mutable. They lack "givenness" and become, instead, problems to be managed by focusing medicine on prevention and prolongation. Aging and old age thus become malleable human experiences, to be brought under the increasing supervision of physicians. Until Nascher, however, mainstream medicine in Europe and the Americas never embraced Bacon's reconceptualization of aging – and Nascher himself may not have been aware of Bacon's views. Unlike pediatrics, which was congruent with and supported by conceptions of childhood that had become widespread in European and American societies after the Enlightenments, geriatrics presumed a conception of aging incongruent and thus unsupported by the popular conceptions of old age.

Economics exacerbated the differential impact of societal conceptions of aging. Pediatrics was seen as an investment in the future. This trend became pronounced in France after the "demoralizing debacle of the Franco-Prussian War (1870–1871)... [when] politicians began to pay increased attention to their population problems [urging] physicians... to reduce [childhood] disease" (Loudon 1993, 1075). In contrast, after 1889 when Chancellor Otto von Bismarck (1815–1898) of Germany introduced state social insurance funds to cover expenses involved in accidents, sickness, and to provide old age pensions, expenditures on "old age pensioners" came to be viewed as a drain on the economy – albeit a drain necessary to prevent class warfare.

Bismarck-style social insurance programs spread throughout Europe and Canada, growing more robust after World War II. Because governments continually operated under financial constraints, the limited resources available to finance social insurance pitted generational interests against each other. These tensions were particularly strong in Britain, which, in 1948, abandoned a rickety and problematic Bismarck-style health insurance program, to implement National Health Service (NHS) – not a health insurance plan, but a medical service provided directly by the government. The British government's intent was to provide "health for all," at a high level, "universalizing the best." Within 2 years, however, the NHS had a budgetary crisis and in consequence the NHS budget was capped – exacerbating intergenerational conflict over resources. Throughout continental Europe, and especially in Britain and in countries that adopted a British-style national health service, health care for the elderly was seen as a drain on economic resources that drew down funds that could be more productively "invested" in children and in adult workers. Economic considerations thus incentivized the retention of traditional stereotypes of the elderly as hopelessly debilitated "old age pensioners," discouraging expenditures on health care for the elderly and encouraging a deaf ear to calls for a new field of "geriatrics" emanating from the United States.

Social insurance developed differently in the United States. Social Security, a retirement program funded through federal payroll taxes on employees and employers, was introduced in 1935. It took another three decades before two federally funded health insurance programs were enacted in 1965: a federal Medicare program for the persons older than 65, and a federal–state Medicaid program to finance health care for the poor. These forms of social insurance became known as "entitlement programs," because anyone who was either older than 65 or medically indigent was "entitled" to benefits. In principle, funding for entitlement programs could not be capped; in practice, to constrain costs, criteria were continually redefined to limit "entitled" populations – who counted as "poor," or as "old" (initially older than 65, but gradually creeping to 67 for Social Security).

The targeted nature of these programs – some for the elderly (who, unlike their European cousins, the "old age pensioners," were soon rechristened "senior citizens"), others for the indigent – created political constituencies directly interested in sustaining "their" programs. In the absence of a Bismarck-style national health insurance system, or a British-style national health service, with its capped budgets, there was little overt intergenerational conflict over health care resources. In this context, economics supported the development of geriatrics and the abandonment of ageist stereotypes. Geriatrics promised healthier senior citizens who would be hospitalized less frequently and less expensively and who were thus less likely to add to the cost of the Medicare program.

Additional factors inhibiting the development of geriatrics are two "isms" and an unspoken practice. The "isms" are ageism and sexism: unjustified discrimination on the basis of age, in the one case, and sex in the other. The unspoken practice is "age-rationing:" allocating resources in a way that favors some (typically younger individuals) or declining to allocate resources needed by (typically older) individuals on the grounds of (old) age. Age and sex are biological givens: all humans age and almost all come with a biologically determined sex (although some infants are born as intersexuals, with ambiguous genitalia, or with genitalia that appear not to match their chromosomes). Life stages and gender differences – the roles attributed to age and sex – are social constructs that can be assessed ethically. Those who believe that a social construction of old age or gender is unethical, inequitable, unjust, or unfair can, and often do, castigate it is "ageist" or "sexist."

Age-rationing practices in continental Europe and in Britain have been characterized as both ageist and sexist. Worldwide, life expectancy for females in the year 2000 was 4 years longer than life expectancy for males; in Europe as a whole, and in the European Union (EU), females outlive males by 8 years, on average; in Britain they outlive males by 5 years; in the Americas they outlive males by 6 years, and in the United States by 5 years. Any (old) age-based limitation on access to health care services anywhere in the world is therefore likely to have a differentially greater impact on females than on males because old women outnumber old men. Any age-rationing policy is thus open to charges of sexism; however, the question of whether age-rationing policies are motivated by a sexist bias against postreproductive females, specifically "old ladies," is underresearched. Nonetheless, dozens of treatment-specific studies strongly suggest antifemale ageist bias – discrimination against "old ladies" – in health care delivery (see, e.g., Alter, et al. 2002; Kemeny et al. 2003; Tannenbaum et al. 2005; Woodward et al. 2003).

The question of whether age rationing is ageist is similarly complex. In Britain, informal age-rationing practices were an outgrowth of the NHS's underfunding of new medical technologies that became available in the 1970s (critical care technologies, hip replacement, renal dialysis, transplantation, and so forth). By the end of the 1980s the NHS had the longest waiting lists for widely accepted innovative technologies in the developed world (Yates 1987). There were extraordinary queues even for homegrown procedures such as hip replacement surgery, which had been developed in 1972 by John Charnley (1911–1982), a surgeon at the Manchester Infirmary. The procedure was a highly successful technological advance, the efficacy of which was undeniable because it enabled the halt, the lame, and the wheelchair-bound to walk normally once again.

Studies found informal age rationing hidden behind a façade of deception. Here is one nephrologist's description of how he would deal with a hypothetical case of a 65-year-old female patient with end-stage renal disease (ESRD).

> Obviously the patient is sixty-five and therefore does not come within the regional dialysis [or transplantation] program. I would say [to the family] that mother's or aunt's kidneys have failed... and that there is very little that anybody can do about it because of her age and general physical state, and that it would be my... advice that we spare her... any further procedure and we do what we can to make her as comfortable as we can for what remains of her life. (Aaron and Schwartz 1984; see also Halper 1989)

Notice that the nephrologist did not inform this woman, or her family, that she is being denied dialysis on the grounds of old age. Instead, they are told "there is very little that anybody can do about it because of her age." This systematically ambiguous characterization will likely be heard as one of medical fact, not as a statement that, as a matter of policy, she is being denied dialysis because the regional program does not accept anyone older than the age of 55. A rationing decision is disguised as a medical

judgment; medicalized language thus masks a social policy denying the patient and her family more than access to dialysis and transplantation. They are also denied the opportunity to appeal, to protest, to take political action, and, more practically, to seek alternative sources of dialysis or transplantation.

Age-based rationing in the NHS during the 1980s had a real impact. Although younger British patients with ESRD underwent dialysis and transplantation at rates comparable to their EU counterparts, males older than the age of 65 received dialysis and/or underwent transplantation at approximately *half* the rate of their EU counterparts (excluding Spain, whose national health service also practiced age rationing) and female British ESRD patients older than the age of 65 underwent dialysis and/or transplantation at one-third the rate of their EU counterparts (exclusive of Spain). Thousands of British men and especially British women were denied years of life through age-rationing practices (Baker 1993c, 1993d).

Until as late as the 1990s, when the Blair New Labour Government infused capital into the NHS, covert age rationing effectively denied the elderly access to lifesaving and life-transforming medical technologies, including not only renal dialysis, but hip and knee replacement, critical care medicine (coronary care units, and so forth), and various forms of transplantation. Age rationing was never a formal or official practice; it was just the "done thing." In consequence, the British public never became aware of the practice. Academics, however, became cognizant of the practice, opening a decade-long debate over its propriety and, in the process, creating one of the more serious discussions of the ethics of the life cycle.

Three distinguished bioethicists took the lead in defending age rationing: John Harris in Britain (Harris 1985), and Daniel Callahan (Callahan 1987) and Norman Daniels (Daniels 1988) in the United States. All three held that age rationing is permissible because medicine's aim is to assist people to live healthily through a "natural life span." Old people, who are at the end of their life span, have had their "fair innings," according to Harris, and thus it is no misfortune for them to die at the end of their natural life span. It is, however, a misfortune for younger people to die before the end of their natural life span. Consequently, fairness requires that scarce medical resources be allocated to the younger rather than older people so that all may have as full a life as possible.

Callahan's arguments also turn on the concept of a "natural life span." Identifying the natural with the good, he argues that desire to live beyond one's natural life span (approximately 75 years) was imprudent for the individual, unreasonable for medicine, and uneconomical for society. The proper goal of medicine, Callahan claimed, ought to be living well within our natural life span, not squandering resources to extend one's life unnaturally after a normal life span had been attained.

Like Callahan's, Daniels' analysis turns on a conception of medicine's goal, which, he argued (drawing on a principle known as "fair equality of opportunity" developed by the renowned American philosopher, John Rawls [1921–2002]) ought to be providing everyone with a fair opportunity to live a normal life (Rawls [1971] 1999). Consequently, Daniels held, medical resources are more properly expended on the young than the old, because avoidable illness, disability, and death are more likely to deprive the young of the opportunity to lead a normal life than old people – who have already had this opportunity.

Critics of age rationing responded by challenging the concept of a "normal" or "natural" life span and the identification of the natural with the good. They pointed out that, in the developed world, life spans have virtually doubled: they were 38 to 40 in 1850, changing to 48 to 51 in 1900 (with less than 5 percent living beyond the age of 65), and then to 75 to 85 (with 13–15 percent living beyond 65) in 2000. Which life span was "normal" or "natural," 38 to 40 or 75 to 85? If 78 to 85 is "unnatural," does that mean that it is not good, or does it mean that the equation of the natural with the good must be flawed? Alternatively, if 78 to 85 is "natural" and 38 to 40 "unnatural," does it not that imply that a longer life span is good and that an even longer life span of 99 to 101 would be just as "natural" and perhaps even better? Perhaps, critics suggested, we merely use the term, "natural," as an accolade for whatever we presume to be good for other reasons.

Probing the fairness of age rationing, critics questioned the rationality of preferentially allocating medical services to younger populations, who had the least need for them, while denying them to older populations, who typically have the greatest need for medical care. Noting that age rationing might easily serve to rationalize stinginess, critics focused on the covert nature of age-rationing practices, pointing out that secrecy violates Rawls' publicity principle – which stipulates that it is unfair to allocate resources according to principles that are not publicly accessible to those affected by them (Rawls [1971] 1999). Critics also raised the question of whether any democratic society could publicly announce an age-rationing policy. Any such pronouncement would effectively state that a society believes that it is not worthwhile to expend resources on saving the lives of old people – thus proclaiming the lives of the old valueless, or at least not as valuable as those of younger individuals (Baker 1993c, 1993d). John Harris, who changed sides in this debate, observed that in its public pronouncements and laws society holds the lives of persons of all ages to be equally valuable – which is why the punishment for homicide is equally severe for the killing of both old persons and young persons. What all persons have in common, what society's laws protect equally for all, and what persons of all ages value, Harris holds, is "the rest of their lives" (Harris 2005).

The age-rationing debate died down in the 1990s without having much effect on health care policy. The British NHS began to invest belatedly in new technologies and age rationing thus became less of an issue. In its aftermath, the debate left behind a decade of bioethical reflection on the life cycle, its "naturalness," and the appropriateness of devoting health care resources to persons in various stages of the life cycle. Philosophical debates, however, never die. In bioethics, they are merely reincarnated in the context of new technological breakthroughs.

The ageism debate had a new incarnation 1998 after the rediscovery and cultivation of pluripotent stem cell lines by James Thomson and John Gearhart. The pluripotency and totipotency of these cells – that is, their capacity to transform into many (pluri) or all (toti) more specialized cells and tissues – seemed to hold the prospect of repairing the human organism at the cellular level, and perhaps thereby extending the "natural" human life span. Callahan, now aided by new allies (Fukuyama 2003), opposed this line of research, reasserting his old position. Harris, having switched sides, rose to the defense of the new technologies with their promise of life span extension and disease-free aging (Harris 2004). Thus the life span debate, reparsed in terms of stem cells, closed out the twentieth century and opened the twenty-first.

VII. Dying and Death

The Enlightenments transformed dying as profoundly as they had transformed birth. By the end of the twentieth century, the locus of both birth and death had moved from the patient's home to the doctor's house – the hospital. Pre-Enlightenment, dying and the deathbed were the province of the clergy. As late as 1738 Friedrich Hoffmann (1660–1742) in his widely influential text, *Medicus Politicus* (The Politic Physician), (see Chapters 28 and 30), still taught that the physician "should abstain from visiting the dying" (Hoffmann 1749, 29).

The philosopher Francis Bacon had earlier urged a redefinition of the "offices," or duties, of physicians in his influential 1605 essay *The Advancement of Learning*.

> I esteem it likewise to be clearly the office of a physician, not only to restore health, but also to mitigate the pains and torments of diseases; and not only when such mitigation of pain, as of a dangerous symptom, helps and conduces to recovery; but also when all hope of recovery is gone; it serves only to make a fair and easy passage from life.... But in our times, the physicians make a kind of scruple and religion to stay [away from] the patient after he is given up; whereas in my judgment, if they would not be wanting to their office, and indeed to humanity, they ought both to acquire the skill and to bestow the attention whereby the dying may

pass more easily and quietly out of life. This part I call the inquiry concerning *outward Euthanasia*, or the easy dying of the body (to distinguish it from that Euthanasia which regards the preparation of the soul); and set it down among the desiderata. (Bacon [1605] 1875, 387, emphasis original)

Bacon's outward euthanasia called for direct involvement of physicians in the care of the dying. Medical partisans of the Enlightenment, such as John Gregory, a close reader of Bacon's writings, answered and advanced that call, on the one hand, echoing Bacon's view that among the "offices" of medicine is the physician's obligation to "smooth the avenues of death," while, on the other hand, condemning abandoning the dying as a "barbarous custom" (Gregory [1770] 1998, 35).

> Let me here exhort you against the custom of some physicians, who leave their patients when their life is despaired of, and when it is no longer decent to put them to further expense. It is as much the business of a physician to alleviate pain, and to smooth the avenues of death, when unavoidable, as to cure diseases. (Gregory [1772b] 1998b, 35–36)

In following Bacon and holding that physicians should continue to attend the dying, Gregory had to address the problem of shared responsibility with clergy.

> Neither is it proper that he should withdraw when a clergyman is called to assist the patient in his spiritual concerns. On the contrary, it is decent and fit that they should mutually understand one another and act together. The conversation of a clergyman, of cheerful piety and good sense, in whom a sick man confides, may sometimes be of much more consequence in composing the anguish of his mind, and the agitation of his spirits, than any medicine; but a gloomy and indiscreet enthusiast may do great hurt; may terrify the patient, and may contribute to shorten a life that otherwise might be saved. (Gregory [1772b] 1998b, 36)

In the first line of this passage, Gregory claims a place for the physician at the deathbed; in the last line he asserts the priority of medicine's claim to control over the deathbed, which is justified in terms of the duty to prevent unnecessary and harmful psychological disturbance and "shorten[ing] a life that otherwise might be saved." The medical gaze has moved biopsychosocial concerns to center stage, displacing not all clergy, but those who pose medical risks to the gravely ill.

Percival, another close reader of Bacon, followed Gregory, holding that "the physician" should displace the clergyman as "minister of hope and comfort to the sick; that by such cordials to the drooping spirit, he may smooth the bed of death, revive expiring life, and counteract the depressing influence of those maladies which rob the philosopher of fortitude, and the Christian of consolation" (Percival 1803b, Chap. II, Art. III, 32) (see also Percival 1794, Sec. 2 Art. III). Like Gregory, Percival allowed religion a place in the hospital provided that "officiating clergymen" perform their "sacred offices ... with propriety and discrimination," that is, appropriately. Overly superstitious or enthusiastic clergy, however, were to be "exclu[ded] from the sick wards or the hospital" because their "effects have often been known to be not only baneful, but even fatal" (Percival 1803b, Chap. I, Art. VI) (see also Percival 1794. Sec. 1, Art. VI). Clergy were thus welcome in the hospital, the doctor's house, but only as guests, subject to their host's medical ethical judgments about the boundaries of acceptable conduct.

The writings of Gregory and Percival were influential throughout Europe and the Americas (see Chapters 30 and 36). By 1832, their views were echoed by physicians in such comparatively out-of-the-way places as the predominately Roman Catholic community of Baltimore, Maryland. There, the Medico-Chirurgical Society adopted a code of ethics that characterized the role of the physician "when the last agonizing moment approaches and the feeble doubting spirit is trembling upon the brink of eternity" as acting to "fortify resolution, [to] administer the blessed consolations of religion, [and to] smooth the descent into the tomb" (Baltimore Medico-Chirurgical Society, 1832, 6).

It is one thing for physicians to claim a role at the deathbed, it is quite another for their claims to be accepted by families. Why did the public, or, more accurately, why did nineteenth-century upper and middle class families accept the physician's role at the deathbed? The fecklessness of medicine was well known. Lord Holland wrote in 1841 that "The longer one lives the less one can place faith in the [doctors]: I think – theirs at best is a science of guess work – how often their guesses are wrong" (Jalland 1996, 78). Everyone was well aware that the physician's therapeutic armamentarium offered little that was effectively curative. Why, then, were doctors accepted at the deathbed?

The answer can be summed up in a single word, euthanasia. Bacon's concept of "outward euthanasia" had crossed over from philosophy to medicine by 1708. It appeared in the fifth edition of Blanchard's medical dictionary, in which the shortened term "euthanasia" was defined as "a soft easy Passage out of the World, without Convulsions or Pain" (Blanchard 1708, 126, cited at Fye 1978, 493). Gregory, Percival, and other Enlightenment physicians effected easy, pain-free passages out of this world through the skillful administration of opiates, such as laudanum (a potent, analgesic, sedating liquid consisting of alcohol, distilled water, and opium). In the nineteenth century the physician's analgesic armamentarium expanded to include morphine (1806), codeine (1836), and acetylsalicylic acid, better known as "aspirin" (1892) – supplemented, after mid-century, by such anesthetics (a term coined, in mid-century, 1846, by Oliver Wendell Holmes, Sr. [1809–1894]) as chloroform and ether.

Doctors were thus welcomed to the deathbed for the same reason that man-midwives/obstetricians had been welcomed to the birth bed – to minimize pain. The medical model being created by partisans of the Enlightenment such as Bacon, Gregory, Percival and innumerable nineteenth-century physicians equated the effective management of pain with progress. The sedating effects of opiates and anesthesia, the *ars medendi* or medical arts applied to dying, were, however, directly antithetical to the traditional Christian *ars moriendi*, the Christian art of dying – which emphasized awake and aware repentance and redemption through suffering. By accepting physicians at the deathbed, upper and middle class families were thus embracing Enlightenment values over the traditional *ars moriendi* and were, in effect, asking attending clergy to tolerate, not only physicians, but also the Enlightenment values embraced by modern medicine.

The classic works of the *ars medendi* of euthanasia – the art of using medicine to create a pain free and peaceful death – included *Enchiridion Medicum* (A Manual of Physick) (1836) by Christoph Wilhelm Hufeland (1762–1836), which was translated into English in 1844 as *Manual of the Practice of Medicine*; William Munk's (1816–1898) *Euthanasia; or Medical Treatment in Aid of An Easy Death* (1887); and Oswald Brown's *On The Care of the Dying* (1894). These later authors looked upon Hufeland, the most renowned German physician of his era, as a medical and moral authority.

Hufeland, Director of the Prussian Medical-Surgical Academy and a personal friend of the poet and playwright Johann Wolfgang von Goethe (1749–1832), was influenced by a fellow Prussian, the Enlightenment philosopher, Immanuel Kant (1724–1804). Hufeland expressly applied Kant's notion of moral law to medical morality. "The fundamental moral law governing a physician," Hufeland wrote, is to "Regulate all your actions in a manner, that the highest end of your vocation, which is saving life, restoring health, and relieving the sufferings of humanity, be attained as far as possible" (Hufeland [1836] 1844, 3). In practicing their vocation, moreover, physicians "must never consider the patient as a means, but always as an end; never as the object of a natural experiment or of art alone, but as a man, as the highest scope of nature itself" (Hufeland [1836] 1844, 4).

These same moral precepts served to guide the physician's conduct at the deathbed.

The office of the physician is not confined to curing diseases; it behooves him as a duty and merit also to *prolong life*, and *relieve suffering* in maladies pronounced incurable. How much, then, at fault are they who . . . neglect or forsake a patient when there

is no prospect of a cure! . . . It is an act of pity . . . in such cases to make life tolerable, to raise dying hope, and to bring consolation at least where there is no salvation. Moreover, we are too short-sighted to be capable of always deciding with certainty that help is not possible . . . I consider it as one of the most important rules of practice, never to give up hope . . . Even in the stage of the dying the physician ought not to forsake the sick; even then he may become a benefactor, and if he cannot save, may at least relieve departing life. (Hufeland [1836] 1844, 6–7)

Hufeland offered his fellow physicians clear practical advice on how best to relieve departing life: "opium . . . surpasses every narcotic . . . in alleviating sufferings and pains, soothing, raising the mind and easing the act of dying . . . like its brother, sleep, [opium is] the highest gift of God" (Hufeland [1836] 1844, 47). "Who would be physician without opium?" Hufeland asks, for without "this great drug . . . that soothes . . . in the most splendid manner" who would be "able . . . to effect the 'euthanasia,' which is the sacred duty and the highest triumph of the physician, when it is not in his power to retain the ties of life" (Hufeland [1836] 1844, 47–48). In performing euthanasia, however, it is impermissible to shorten human life.

[Some might wonder whether] when a patient is tortured by incurable evils, when he prays for death as the end of his suffering . . . would it not be permitted, be even a duty, to rid the miserable sufferer of his burden a little earlier? Though such reasoning may be plausible, be supported even by the suggestions of the heart, it is false, and the mode of action based on such principles would be a crime. It annihilates the vocation of the physician. He is bound in duty to do nothing but what tends to save life; whether existence be fortunate or unfortunate, whether life be valuable or not, is not for the physician to decide. If he once permits such considerations to influence his actions, the consequences can not be estimated, and he becomes the most dangerous person of the community. For if he once trespass his line of duty and think himself entitled to decide on the necessity of an individual's life, he may by gradual progressions apply the measure to other cases. (Hufeland [1836] 1844, 8)

Hufeland's conception of ethical euthanasia – opiate-and-analgesic-assisted dying, constrained by a strict prohibition on directly killing the patient – described accepted medical practice in nineteenth-century European (see Marx 1826) and American medicine (see Emanuel 1994, 793–95). Later medical texts provided detailed pharmacological advice on how best to practice euthanasia, and to provide nursing care for the dying, but Hufeland's writings laid out the overall parameters. The consensus view was that euthanasia, the alleviation of pain, was appropriate practice – but physicians could not administer a dose of opiates or other analgesics that threatened to shorten the patient's life. Nineteenth-century physicians' cautiousness about shortening life sometimes constrained their use of opiates, limiting their ability to deliver the "euthanasia" that they promised their patients (Kemp 2002, 43–44).

Hufeland also set the parameters of nineteenth-century end-of-life care in another respect: truth-telling.

It is [the physician's] sacred duty... to avoid all things that may have a tendency to discourage the patient and lower his spirits... The physician, therefore, must be careful to preserve hope and courage in the patient's mind, represent his case in a favorable light, conceal all danger from him, and, the more serious it becomes, show a more cheerful appearance; and least of all betray uncertainty and irresolution.... He can guard himself from the suspicion of having not fully appreciated the nature of the case by giving a true description of the patient's situation to the relative, and if they be fickle and negligent, to state it rather darker than lighter. Hence it will appear, how blamable is the conduct of those physicians who do not hesitate to announce to the sick the danger, even fatality of their situation, and how injudiciously those relatives act, who desire the physician to do so. To announce death is to give death, which is never the business of him, who is employed to save life. Even if the sick person desires to know the truth, under the pretext of arranging his affairs or the like, it is not advisable to pronounce his sentence. (Hufeland [1836] 1844, 8–10)

Hufeland's advice flies directly in the face of that offered by Gregory (Gregory [1772] 1995, 174–75) and Percival (Percival 1803, Chap. II, Art. III), who sought to *inform* the patient in a sympathetic and caring manner, by filtering information about terminal prognoses through family members. Historians of eighteenth- and nineteenth-century British medical practice are divided over whether, having been informed of a terminal diagnosis, families would actually inform the patients themselves. Roy Porter observes that after the publication of Gregory's lectures, "people were no longer allowed their own deaths; for in the name of sympathy and avoiding distress, their families and doctors were allowing them to slip away oblivious to their fate" (Porter 1989, 89, cited at Jalland 1996, 108). Jalland's study of the death in the nineteenth-century Victorian family led to the opposite conclusion, that indirect truth-telling was effective: nineteenth-century fami-

lies did inform patients that they were dying (Jalland 1996, 108–18).

Despite these problems in determining whether eighteenth- and nineteenth-century middle- and upper-class patients were actually informed of a terminal prognosis, it is clear that Anglo-American medical ethicists believed that patients should be informed of their impending death – either by physicians or by family members – differing only on the details concerning by who, when, and how this information should be imparted. The American Samuel Bard (1742–1821), advised his fellow practitioners, "never buoy up a dying Man with groundless Expectations of Recovery ... it is really cruel, as the stroke of Death is always most severely felt when unexpected" (Bard 1769, 21) and the Connecticut physician Worthington Hooker (1806–1867) also advised "strict adherence to truth in our intercourse with the sick" (Hooker 1849, 378–79). In contrast, Hufeland, speaking for a tradition that would still be followed in parts of continental Europe at the end of the twentieth century, held that it was improper for *anyone*, family member or physician, to rob patients of hope by informing them that they were dying.

Except on this one point, however, Hufeland set the parameters for euthanasia in Europe and North America through the end of the nineteenth century. By the early twentieth century, however, Hufeland's Baconian sense of "euthanasia" was displaced by a new sense, "mercy killing." This displacement raises classic historical questions: When, where, who, and, above all, why?

Thanks to the work of historian N. D. A. Kemp, who has carefully surveyed the evolution of discourse on euthanasia in nineteenth-century Britain, we have a good sense of when the displacement occurred. Kemp found that the modern sense of "euthanasia," in the sense of "mercy killing," did not appear in the British medical literature until 1896 (Kemp 2002, 42) – although the usage had crept into U.S. medical journals as early as 1873 (Emanuel 1994, 793–95). The influential displacement, however, was British. It began in 1870, when an obscure publication, the *Essays of the Birmingham Speculative Club* (Williams 1870), printed an essay, "Euthanasia," by one Samuel D. Williams, Jr. – in all likelihood a schoolteacher and definitely a nonphysician.

Williams devoted his essay on euthanasia to demonstrating the "reasonableness" of the proposition.

That in all cases of hopeless and painful illness, it should be the recognized duty of the medical attendant, whenever so desired by the patient, to administer chloroform or some other anaesthetic ... so as to destroy consciousness at once and put the sufferer to a quick and painless death; all needful precautions being adopted to prevent any possible abuse of such duty. (Williams 1810, cited at Kemp 2002, 12–13)

William's essay is noteworthy in four respects: first, in urging the reasonableness of an act – mercy killing at the patient's request – hitherto condemned by modern medical, legal, and religious authority; second, in appropriating the term "euthanasia" to characterize this act; third, because Williams was a nonphysician whose only notable accomplishment was this essay; and fourth and finally, because, in spite of the fact that the essay was written by a nonentity and published in an obscure volume, the public took notice. More specifically, the *Essays of the Birmingham Speculative Club* were reviewed in *The Saturday Review* (Anonymous, 1870, 632–34), which singled out William's essay for discussion. Within 2 years, the essay was reprinted as a small book; within 3 years, it was in its fourth edition. The article in the *Saturday Review* sparked a response: an article on "Euthanasia" in another popular publication, *The Spectator* (18 March 1871, 314). After that, the public debate – and the public usage of "euthanasia" in the sense of "mercy killing" – took off.

By 1873 the debate had spread to medical journals, which had begun to publish articles on "The Euthanasia" and "The Doctrine of Euthanasia." The prestigious *Boston Medical Surgical Journal* (known after 1928 as *The New England Journal of Medicine*) and the *Journal of the American Medical Association* joined the chorus, with articles on "Permissive Euthanasia" and "the Moral Side of Euthanasia" (Emanuel 1994, 793–94); by 1896 and 1897 the more conservative British medical press joined the fray and even the *British Medical Journal* was discussing "euthanasia" (Kemp 2002, 42–43, Reiser 1977). Without exception, the medical press condemned "euthanasia." In doing so, however, they used "euthanasia" in Williams' sense, which quickly displaced the original Baconian–Hufeland meaning in medical as well as popular parlance. By 1902 Robert Saundby's (1849–1918) medical dictionary was defining "euthanasia" in the modern sense as "the doctrine that it is permissible for a medical practitioner to give a patient suffering from a mortal disease a poisonous dose of opium or other narcotic in order to end his sufferings" (Saundby 1902, 12).

By 1902, the concept of euthanasia as mercy killing, although almost universally condemned by physicians on both sides of the Atlantic, had nonetheless displaced the Baconian–Hufeland concept of a smooth and easy pain free death. In its haste to condemn euthanasia-as-mercy-killing, the medical profession inadvertently had deprived the Baconian–Hufeland concept of a name. Although, as Juliet famously remarked, "That which we call a rose, by any other word would smell as sweet," to "doff thy name ... which is no part of thee" has consequences (Shakespeare, c. 1591, *Romeo and Juliet* Act 2, Scene 2). "The work of Dr. Munk and other Victorian pioneers of medical care of the dying was largely forgotten in the half century or so after 1920 and had to be reinvented by later twentieth-century writers who nothing of

their predecessors ... Munk was the Victorian equivalent of [Elisabeth] Kübler-Ross (1926–2004), Cicely Saunders (1918–2005), and John Hinton, and it is remarkable how much of their work he anticipated" (Jalland 1996, 95–96, 82).

The Baconian–Hufeland euthanasia would remain nameless until 1975, when Balfour Mount, a physician at Montreal's Royal Victoria Hospital, rechristened it "palliative care." In the interim, no specialists could be trained in a nameless field and no professorships allotted to it. Little place was given to a nameless subject in the medical school curriculum, and knowledge of the subject swiftly atrophied. Even the occasional article on a nameless subject could not be reliably indexed and thus could not be reliably searched. (By contrast, a 2005 search of the U.S. National Library of Medicine under the term "palliative care" found 9,981 books, videos, and related materials, and 25,020 publications in medical journals.)

Why did the modern concept of euthanasia displace the traditional concept? The answer lies in a curious combination of accident, semantics, and the interaction between realms of discourse. Williams was not a medical professional and thus, like most members of the public, was indifferent to, and perhaps even unaware of, the way euthanasia was used by medical professionals. Once his usage had entered public discourse, medical professionals were keen to condemn it, and, in condemning it, began to adopt and thus legitimate the mercy killing usage. This said, the question remains: Why did the public discuss Williams' essay and proposal so readily? Kemp (2002) has argued that the novelty of anesthesia and the emergence of a new form of death, cancer death, the pain of which was resistant to control by opium, stirred public interest in the topic. Emanuel (1994) suggests that the public was attracted to euthanasia as mercy killing because it suited ideals of individualism (later denominated "autonomy") inspired by the capitalist ethos of the period. All of these elements appear to have been factors: Williams was clearly intrigued by chloroform, then a relatively new medical innovation; cancer deaths in Williams's England had almost doubled from 274 per million living people in 1847–1850, to 445 per million in 1871–1875, the years in which Williams's essay is reprinted (Kemp 2002, 95) – and cancer deaths were specifically cited in the early euthanasia debates (e.g., Tollemache 1873, cited at Reiser 1977, 75). Cancer would become the paradigm of a painful death in many future end-of-life palliative care/euthanasia debates.

By the early twentieth century, therefore, the concept of "euthanasia" as mercy killing had entered European and American discourse about death and dying. Proponents of euthanasia, for the most part nonphysicians, often cited cases of painful deaths in their efforts to legalize mercy killing and the subject was perennially debated throughout the twentieth century. The first legalization campaign was initiated in 1905–1906, when an 88-year-old Harvard professor of art history and literature, Charles Eliot Norton (1827–1908), coeditor of the *North American Review* and founder of the *Nation* magazine, was inspired by the agonies of a cancer patient to campaign to legalize euthanasia in the state of Ohio. Strongly opposed by medical opinion on both sides of the Atlantic, the proposal was defeated.

In 1931, Dr. Charles Killick Millard (1870–1952) advocated legalizing voluntary euthanasia in an address at a British medical meeting. Four years later, with support from a terminal patient, Mr. O. W. Greene (d. 1935), Millard formed the Voluntary Euthanasia Legislation Society, the first euthanasia society. In 1936, a bill to legalize euthanasia was defeated in the House of Lords; a similar effort failed in 1950. On the other side of the Atlantic, the Reverend Charles Francis Potter (1885–1962) organized the Euthanasia Society of America in 1938 to lobby for legalizing voluntary euthanasia. Despite persistent efforts throughout the twentieth century, euthanasia was never legalized in Europe or the Americas – although the practice was officially "tolerated" in two European countries (Nazi Germany and the Netherlands) and would become legal in one European country (Netherlands 2002) and one South American country (Columbia – declared legal in the first years of the twenty-first century).

In continental Europe, the debate over euthanasia began in earnest in 1895, when Dr. Adolf Jost published *Das Recht Auf den Tod* (The Right to Die) (Jost 1895), the first German monograph defending *euthanasie*, as euthanasia was called in German. According to historian Michael Burleigh, Jost's book marks the turning point at which the German concept of *euthanasie* transitions from the earlier palliative Bacon–Hufeland conception to a more modern conception that embraces mercy killing. The twentieth-century German concept of *euthanasie* included, in addition to the concept of voluntary euthanasia, a new notion,

> The concept of negative human worth, i.e., not only the life-negating suffering of a dying person, but also the negative burden placed on relatives or the community by the incurably ill and mentally defective. (Burleigh 1995, 12)

Jost's broad concept of *euthanasie* made the concept attractive to eugenicist and social Darwinist thinkers such as the biologist Ernst Haeckel (1843–1919), popularly known as "Darwin's German apostle," who fused *euthanasie* with eugenics, championing the notion of killing those people who placed a negative burden on society. Haeckel wrote of a physically and mentally handicapped child that "a small dose of morphine or cyanide would not only free this pitiable creature itself but also its relatives from the burden of a long, worthless, and painful existence" (Haeckel cited at Weikart 2004, 147).

In 1913, Haeckel's *Monist Journal* (*Das monistische Jahrbundert*) published an open letter from a dying patient calling

for a law to legalize *euthanasie*, sparking debate throughout Germany (Burleigh 1995, 12–14). The most influential German work on the subject was, *Die Freigabe der Vernichtung lebensunwerten Leben* – in an English translation, *The Release and Destruction of Life Devoid of Value* (Binding and Hoche 1920) – a small tract by the lawyer–psychiatrist team of Karl Binding (1841–1920) and Alfred Hoche (1841–1920) that was published a year after the armistice that ended World War I. Following the precedents laid down by Jost and Haecke, the tract justified *euthanasie* both in the sense of voluntary euthanasia and in the sense of the *involuntary* killing of those living a life unworthy of being lived (see Chapters 34 and 48).

Binding and Hoche's tract had an instant and immediate impact on the German medical profession. As historian Michael Burleigh writes, the subject of *euthanasie*:

> Was no longer a matter of academic contemplation; millions of people had died in the recent war, and hard choices on resources had been made. The fact that one of those choices involved the mass starvation of mental patients not only went unmentioned, but was consciously denied. It is difficult to decide whether [Binding and Hoche's] tract was prescriptive or an uneasy and evasive rationalization of what had already taken place. Building . . . upon a series of unimpeachably liberal premises, the tract systematically rehearses a series of illiberal . . . arguments in favour of involuntary euthanasia. (Burleigh 1995, 15)

Similar ideas were circulating elsewhere in Europe and in the United States. As we noted earlier, during the war, Chicago surgeon, Harry Haiselden made a film dramatizing his infanticidal treatment of infants with disabilities. After the war, in 1936, Franco-American Nobel Laureate Alexis Carrell (1873–1944) of the Rockefeller Institute for Medical Research, proposed that the mentally ill "humanely and economically be disposed of in small euthanasia institutions supplied with the proper gases" (Carrel [1936] 1988, 180).

France, America, and Britain did not implement this proposal; Nazi Germany did. In 1939, after carefully reviewing the writings of Binding and Hoche on *euthanasie*, Nazi health authorities were contemplating legalizing both voluntary euthanasia and the involuntary termination of persons suffering from those forms of mental illness that require permanent institutionalization. When Hitler received a petition by a family to grant *euthanasie* to a child who had been born blind, Hitler approved a bureaucratic initiative to register and kill "malformed" newborns. Although never formalized as a law, the initiative was extended to apply to seriously ill mental patients under the title "Aktion T-4."

The Nazi *euthanasie* program is discussed in detail elsewhere (Chapters 18, 34, and 54). In the aftermath of the war, as details of the role physicians played in planning and executing the Nazi eugenics and *euthanasie* programs – and the Holocaust – were revealed at the 1947 Nuremberg War Crimes Tribunal, the world recoiled in horror. The newly formed World Medical Association (WMA) denounced the Nazi doctors for "ignor[ing] the sanctity and importance of human life" (World Medical Association 1949, 1). Another new organization, the United Nations (UN) passed a Universal Declaration of Human Rights, designed in large measure to ensure that no one would be treated as the Nazis had treated, not only Gypsies, homosexuals, and Jews, but also infants with disabilities and the mentally ill (Baker 2001a).

Declaring that "never again" would doctors "ignore the sanctity and importance of human life," in 1948 the WMA adopted the Declaration of Geneva, a modern adoption of the Hippocratic Oath published in three languages and designed to reassert the fundamental integrity of the medical profession to the entire world. The oath stipulated that on "being admitted as a member of the medical profession," new physicians would "solemnly pledge [themselves] to consecrate [their lives] to the service of humanity . . . [taking] the health of [their] patients [to] be [their] first consideration." The oath strongly affirms a commitment to human life. "I will maintain the utmost respect for human life, from the time of conception; even under threat, I will not use my medical knowledge contrary to the laws of humanity." The French version is even stronger, making the respect for human life "absolute" – "*Je garderai le respect absolu de la vie humaine, dès la conception.*" (I will hold absolute respect for human life from conception.) The reference to the "laws of humanity" harks back to the Nuremberg trials, where the Nazi doctors had been convicted for violating the laws of humanity, aligning the WMA's Declaration of Geneva with the contemporaneous UN Declaration of Human Rights, which specifies the laws of humanity. The strong affirmation of the sanctity of human life that emerged as a reaction to Nazi atrocities in the immediate postwar era made the rejection of euthanasia a hallmark of the European and American medical professions – except in the Netherlands, where the Dutch Medical Association broke ranks in the early 1970s.

The first incident to challenge the post-Holocaust aversion to euthanasia began to unfold in Copenhagen, Denmark, on August 26, 1952, during the last worldwide polio pandemic. Anesthesiologist Bjorn Ibsen was asked to consult on an 11-year-old polio patient. She was dying despite receiving what was at the time state-of-the-art care – negative pressure ventilation through an "iron lung." Adapting a technique occasionally used in the operating room, Ibsen performed a tracheostomy (he cut a hole or "stoma" in her trachea, or windpipe, a procedure also called a "tracheotomy") permitting nurses to clear her lungs of secretions and to provide oxygen directly to the lungs through

a small pump (positive pressure ventilation). Ibsen's hastily contrived positive-pressure apparatus would later come to be called a "ventilator."

The girl's condition improved immediately. The mortality rate associated the respiratory failure of polio patients on iron lungs was 87 percent; mortality rates for the polio epidemic in Copenhagen appeared even higher. By adopting Ibsen's innovation, however, the Copenhagen hospital was able to lower the mortality rate dramatically to 26 percent. Within a year, Ibsen had established a clinical unit around his innovation. This, in turn, became the model for what would later be called a critical care unit, or an intensive care unit (ICU). As word of Ibsen's success spread, ICUs were established in major medical centers worldwide (Lassen 1953; Trubuhovich 2004).

As these events were unfolding, Pope Pius XII was turning the attention of the Roman Catholic church toward issues in medical ethics. In a 1957 allocution (a formal statement of papal opinion, see Chapter 14), Pius XII effectively resolved a moral conundrum that had hamstrung nineteenth-century palliative care. The leader of the largest Christian church in the world officially declared that it is morally permissible to administer analgesics in as large a dose as is necessary to provide effective pain relief, even doses that risk killing the patient, "provided that the physician's intent is to relieve pain, not to kill the patient" (Pius XII 1957).

Although it is difficult to overstate the significance this allocution on palliative care for dying patients, its importance was eclipsed by an allocution issued with respect to Ibsen's "artificial respiration apparatus." An Austrian anesthesiologist, Dr. Bruno Haid, asked the Pope whether anesthesiologists were required to use the apparatus "in all cases," even in cases "of deep unconsciousness . . . considered . . . completely hopeless?" Would turning off a ventilator be considered "euthanasia?"

Drawing on the distinction between "ordinary" and "extraordinary" means or burdens, a traditional precept of Catholic moral theology, Pius XII replied that the patient or the family has the power to release the anesthesiologist from the obligation to perform "resuscitation . . . if it appears that the attempt at resuscitation constitutes in reality such a burden for the family that one cannot in all conscience impose it upon them" (Pope Pius XII 1958). Pius XII thus informed anesthesiologists, and the world at large, that nonresuscitation and turning off ventilators is *not* euthanasia, even though this means that the patient is likely to die immediately thereafter. However – and this is a pivotal caveat – the moral authority to disconnect a ventilator does *not* belong to the doctor. Moral authority to make this decision resides with patients and their families, for they are uniquely positioned to determine whether continued artificial respiration is "extraordinarily" burdensome for them.

Dr. Haid had also put to Pope Pius XII another newly vexing question: When is someone dead? By providing respiration artificially, Ibsen's ventilator had severed the historic connection between breathing and life. Sad experience had established that the ventilator could keep patients' hearts and lungs working indefinitely, even though their brains and other vital organs had ceased to function. The traditional cardiopulmonary criteria for death, absence of a pulse or heartbeat and irreversible cessation of breathing, were thus clinically inapplicable to mechanically ventilated patients. The concept of death itself – defined in Roman Catholic theology as the separation of the soul from the body – was unaffected by the ventilator; however, the device had made a shambles of the traditional *medical* criteria for determining death. Hence Haid's question: "At what time does the Catholic Church consider the patient 'dead?'"

Pius XII's stunningly simple reply would impact medical criteria for death for the last third of the twentieth century and beyond: "The answer can not be deduced from any religious and moral principle and . . . does not fall within the competence of the Church." In other words, medical criteria for determining that death has occurred is a matter best left to doctors of medicine, not doctors of theology, the conference of cardinals, or even the papacy itself (all quotations from Pope Pius XII 1958).

With these allocutions – the substance of which was reaffirmed by Pope John Paul II in his *Declaration on Euthanasia* of May 5, 1980 (Sacred Congregation for the Doctrine of the Faith, 1980) – Pius XII set the moral parameters for the ethics of death and dying for most of Europe and the Americas for the rest of the twentieth century. The Church's condemnation of euthanasia in the sense of mercy killing was reaffirmed, even as sincerely intended efforts at pain control were legitimated. Pius XII thereby prepared the moral ground for the hospice and palliative care movements that would soon be initiated. The allocutions also legitimate the discontinuation of resuscitation, ventilator support, and other "extraordinarily burdensome means" of life-prolonging treatment of dying patients, thereby laying the groundwork for terminally ill patients' and surrogates' rights to decline or discontinue a wide variety of life-prolonging technologies from antibiotics and artificial hearts to cardiopulmonary resuscitation (CPR) and hemodialysis.

Finally, in recognizing the authority of medicine to determine neurological criteria for determination of death in contexts in which the older cardiopulmonary criteria of breath and pulse were no longer applicable, Pius XII's allocutions set the stage for the redefinition of death as "brain death." Not surprisingly, given the moral authority attaching to these allocutions, the only reference cited in the entire *Report of the Ad Hoc Committee of the Harvard Medical School to Examine the Definition of Brain Death*, the report that

effected the transition from cardiopulmonary criteria for death to brain death criteria, was to Pius XII's allocation (Harvard Medical School 1968). (For further discussion of brain death, see Chapter 63.)

In 1958, the same year in which Pius XII published this allocation, a British Lady Almoner (female social worker), who had earlier qualified as a nurse, became a newly minted physician in the hope that the title would provide the status she needed in the hierarchical world of medicine to promote her theories of pain control for dying patients. To implement her ideas she took a position at St. Joseph's, a London hospice for the dying poor run by nuns. In that position she experimented with various methods of pain control and wrote a series of articles on care for the dying that were published in *Nursing Times* in 1959. In her articles, she contended that there was no such thing as intractable pain, only intractable doctors who failed to provide adequate pain control at the end of life.

That same year, with seed money from a grateful patient, she began to plan St. Christopher's, the first hospice built around the concept of comprehensive pain control for dying patients. The 54-bed nondenominational hospice opened in 1967. From this base the woman, who would later be known as Dame Cicely Saunders, launched a worldwide hospice movement whose mission was to provide patients with effective end-of-life care that would permit them to die pain-free, and, if possible, in their own beds, in their own homes.

Unbeknownst to Saunders, she had been striving to reestablish the then-nameless medical ideals and concepts the medical profession had abandoned at the beginning of the century. She was attempting to do so, moreover, in the context in which medicine – in the reductive version of the medical gaze – saw only signs and symptoms, losing sight of the patient. Here, for example is a case study published in the *British Medical Journal* around the time that Saunders was establishing St. Christopher's hospice. The article's title is "Not Allowed to Die."

A doctor aged 68 was admitted to . . . hospital [for] a large carcinoma [or cancer] of the stomach . . . The patient was told of the findings and fully understood their import. In spite of increasingly large doses of pethidine [an anti-spasmodic painkiller] and of morphine at night, he suffered constantly with severe abdominal pain . . .

On the tenth day after [his] gastrectomy [the surgical removal of part or all of his stomach], the patient collapsed with classic manifestations of massive pulmonary embolism [a blood clot in the lungs that the medical staff treated successfully]. When the patient had recovered sufficiently he expressed his appreciation of the good intentions and skill of his younger colleagues. At the same time, he asked that if he had a further cardiovascular collapse no steps should be taken to prolong his life, for the pain of his cancer was now more than he would needlessly continue to endure. He himself wrote a note to this effect in the case records, and the staff of the hospital knew his feelings.

His wish notwithstanding, when the patient collapsed again, 2 weeks [later] with acute myocardial infarction and cardiac arrest, he was revived by the hospital emergency resuscitation team. His heart stopped on four further occasions and each time was restarted artificially. The body then recovered to linger for 3 more weeks, but in a decerebrate state, punctuated by episodes of projectile vomiting accompanied by generalized convulsions. [He received innumerable treatments including intravenous feeding and a tracheotomy.] On the last day of the illness preparations were being made for the work of the failing respiratory center to be given over to an artificial respirator, but the heart finally stopped before this endeavor could be realized.

> This case is submitted for publication without commentary or conclusions, which are left for those who may read it to provide for themselves. (Symmers, W. St. C. Sr. 1968, 442, cited at Katz 1972, 709)

Although Symmers, the author of this case study, believes *res ipsa loquitur*, the case speaks for itself, it actually speaks to the historical context in which Saunders founded the hospice movement and in which Pius XII issued his allocutions. The case dramatizes the extent to which medicine of the period had become oblivious to the patient's pain, to the patient's voice, and to the patient's express wishes. Seeing only pathology and recognizing only the duty to treat it and to preserve life, the clinicians moved blindly forward. Cicely Saunders, Pius XII – and their allies in the nascent bioethics movement (asserting itself through statements like the American Hospital Association's *Patients' Bill of Rights* (American Hospital Association 1973, 71) – had to retrain the medical gaze so that it would (once again) recognize pain as well as pathology, and so that it could see a duty to recognize patient's wishes, as well as a duty to preserve life. Bioethicists would also need to work with physicians to create such innovations as a Do-Not-Resuscitate (DNR) order, to implement the patient's wishes in the form of a physician's order in the medical record, but the impetus for the Pope, for Saunders, and bioethicists was a medicine focused on signs and symptoms, and oblivious to the voice of patients and families.

By the end of the twentieth century, medical perceptions of end-of-life care had changed significantly. Some 640 hospices and palliative care institutions or units were dispersed through the United Kingdom, nurtured by NHS funding. Across the Atlantic an estimated 3,300 hospices and palliative care units in the United States.

were supported by Medicare and Medicaid funding – and a growing number of hospices were being developed throughout the EU and Latin America. United Kingdom hospices treated approximately 37,000 new patients annually, more than 95 percent had cancer. Approximately one-fifth of the estimated 155,000 or so terminally ill cancer patients who die in the United Kingdom each year received hospice care (Eve and Higginson 2000). In the United States, hospice units treated approximately 950,000 patients annually; approximately half had a diagnosis of cancer. Half of all U.S. hospice patients died in their own homes, twice as many as those not receiving hospice care (National Hospice and Palliative Care Organization 2003). In Britain, North America, and increasingly in continental Europe and South America, terminally ill patients were being a offered choice of modes of clinical care and ever larger numbers were choosing hospice and palliative care.

The old order of medical perception did not yield without a struggle. The issue of patients' rights in end-of-life care came to a head in the United States. in April 1975, when a comatose 21-year-old Roman Catholic, Karen Ann Quinlan, was admitted to St. Claire's, a Roman Catholic hospital, in Denville, New Jersey. Neurologist Julius Korein had determined that Quinlan was in what later came to be called a "permanent vegetative state" (PVS, an irreversible comatose state). After Karen Ann's parents, Joseph and Julia, consulted with their parish priest, they asked Karen's physician, Robert Morse, to turn off an incarnation of Ibsen's innovation, Karen's MA-1 ventilator. Dr. Morse refused. The matter went to the courts (Quinlan et al. 1977).

Dr. Morse presumed, correctly, that it was customarily the physician's prerogative to decide questions about continuing and discontinuing medical treatment. He also presumed, incorrectly as it turned out, that physicians were morally and legally obligated to provide ventilator support for patients in permanent vegetative states. As testimony at the trial would later confirm (Stevens 2000, 113, 137), physicians at elite academic medical centers had informal procedures for disconnecting ventilators. In the early 1970s, however, the stream of funding unleashed by the passage of Medicaid and Medicare enabled hospitals in medical backwaters, like Denville, to purchase such exotic equipment as MA-1 ventilators. At Denville, Dr. Morse was not privy to the unstated ethos of the elite, nor was he protected by their elite status nor, in fairness, was he at ease with the notion of disconnecting a ventilator – an act that appeared to kill a patient. So he resisted the Quinlans' request.

In November 1975, a New Jersey court upheld Dr. Morse (*In the Matter of Karen Quinlan: An Alleged Incompetent* 1975). Karen's parents appealed and in January 1976, the New Jersey Supreme court ruled unanimously in favor of her parents (*In Re Quinlan* 1976) holding that Karen Ann's "right to privacy" would have permitted her to refuse ventilator support and that a duly appointed surrogate could exercise this right on her behalf. The court had also conferred legal immunity on Dr. Morse, so that he would not be a legal risk for disconnecting the ventilator – provided that the case had been reviewed by an "ethics committee."

For the physicians involved, however, the issue was one of conscience. Instead of disconnecting Karen's ventilator, as the Quinlan parents had requested, they weaned Karen off the ventilator. Karen Ann Quinlan lingered in a persistent vegetative state, for more than a decade despite the court's affirmation of her right to taken off of the ventilator, and despite her parents' determination to exercise this right on her behalf. She died on June 13, 1986.

Just 4 years later, in 1990, the U.S. Supreme Court recognized the rights of capacitated patients to refuse any form of treatment, including artificial nutrition and hydration, and further recognized the right of a proxy or surrogate to exercise this right on behalf of an incapacitated patient. The decision also affirmed a state's right to set standards authorizing someone to act as a proxy or a surrogate (*Cruzan v. Director*, Missouri Department of Health, 110 S. Ct. 2841, 1990). Patients and duly authorized proxies and surrogates now had the legal authority to say "no" to any treatment, including artificial nutrition and hydration. Moreover, as Pope Pius XII had asserted over three decades earlier, physicians and other health care providers were ethically and, in the United States at least, legally bound to abide by their wishes.

Reinforcing the courts, in the same year, 1990, the U.S. Congress enacted the Patient Self Determination Act. The Act required all institutions receiving Medicare or Medicaid funding to recognize a series of patients' rights: the right to participate in health care decision making; the right to accept or to refuse treatment; and the right prepare "advance directives." These directives provide a mechanism for patients to explain their wishes "in advance" of the need for decisions about discontinuing treatments in advance of losing decision-making capacity, to inform their physicians and their family of these wishes, and they empowered patient's proxies and surrogates to act on their wishes. Curtailing the aggressive paternalism of the medical gaze in the United States thus literally took an act of congress and a Supreme Court decision – and yet, despite these initiatives, studies indicate that, as often as not, U.S. physicians still ignored patients' wishes (Baker and Strosberg 1995; SUPPORT Principal Investigators 1995).

By the end of the twentieth century, European patients had even less choice and less voice in their end-of-life care than U.S. patients. The first patients' rights legislation in the EU came out of the Netherlands in 1995 as part of its Medical Contract Law. A year earlier, the Netherlands had hosted a meeting of the European division of the World Health Organization (WHO), which proposed a new European Declaration of Patients' Rights (referred to as the Amsterdam Declaration, Sheldon 1994). These Dutch initiatives gave impetus to the passage of patients' rights legislation in Lithuania in 1996, Iceland in 1997, and Denmark in 1998. It is unclear whether, by the end of the twentieth century, this flurry of patients' rights legislation made a significant difference to end-of-life options open to European patients.

One reason is that European medicine had more modest resources at its disposal than U.S. medicine, where targeted entitlement programs (Medicare and Medicaid) guaranteed an overabundance of end-of-life facilities (nursing homes and ICUs). European physicians were thus less likely to overuse resources. Consequently, European patients' rights organizations were more concerned about *access* to treatment than about whether patients' rights to *refuse* treatment are being honored. To put the point somewhat differently, the Quinlan saga was in many ways unique to the United States: It is as much a story of a surfeit of resources as it is a tale of the aggressively narrow paternalistic focus of the medical gaze at that time. Nonetheless, European physicians too can be aggressively paternalistic: Surveys of European hospital care conducted in the early twenty-first century by patients' rights groups found that, despite a meticulously legalistic concern for getting signatures on consent forms, many hospital-based European physicians appear indifferent to the point of insensitivity to the wishes of terminal patients and their families (Lamanna, Moro, and Ross 2005).

At the dawn of the twenty-first century, some European patients, most notably those in Belgium, the Netherlands, and Switzerland, had end-of-life options unavailable to other Europeans and to most American patients: assisted suicide and euthanasia. Although euthanasia was illegal in all European countries throughout the twentieth century, two countries (Nazi Germany and the Netherlands) had at times officially tolerated the practice. A third country, Switzerland, had provided a legal exception to the law prohibiting aiding and abetting suicides since 1941. The Swiss exception states that assisting a suicide is not a criminal offense *if* the assistance is altruistically and honorably motivated, such as that offered at the express request of a patient suffering irremediable pain.

The Netherlands began to officially tolerate euthanasia in 1973. Approximately a half decade earlier euthanasia had become a subject of popular debate following the publication of a small book, *Medische Macht en Medische Ethiek* (Medical Power and Medical Ethics) by psychiatrist Jan van den Berg. Protesting the aggressiveness of medicine and urging limits on the power and authority of physicians, van den Berg argued that the physician's duty "to protect save and prolong human life" is limited to contexts "where and when this is meaningful" (van den Berg 1969, 47, cited by Kimsma and van Leeuwen 1998, 40). In 1971, Dr. P. Mutendam (1901–1986) published the first Dutch book defending *euthanasie* (Mutendam 1971) and in that same year a Dutch physician, Geertruida Postma, turned herself over to Dutch legal authorities reporting that she had intentionally injected her partially paralyzed deaf mother with morphine to induce unconsciousness, and then with curare (a paralytic agent), to kill her. At her trial, Dr. Postma testified that her mother was "a human wreck, hanging in that chair" and that she, Dr. Postma, "couldn't stand it any more" (Postma cited by Pence 2000, 88). Postma was found guilty; however, she was given a lenient sentence of 1 week's imprisonment, which was suspended (Thomasma et al. 1998, 7).

In its ruling, the court declared that had a terminally ill patient experiencing severe or interminable suffering *explicitly* requested a life-terminating intervention, physicians need not consider themselves duty-bound to maintain life. Thus, had the Postma case met these conditions the court would have excused her actions. Noting this, the Royal Dutch Medical Association (known by its Dutch initials, KNMG) negotiated an arrangement with Dutch prosecutors. Physicians would not face prosecution for murder if they performed euthanasia on fully informed competent patients who had voluntarily and explicitly made reiterated requests for euthanasia, provided that the patient was severely or unendurably suffering, that alternative routes to relieving suffering did not exist, and that a second physician confirmed that all of these conditions had been satisfied.

In the same year, Dr. P. Mutendam, who was a leading member of the KNMG, also founded the *Nederlandse Vereniging voor een Vrijwillig Levenseinde* (NVVE, Netherlands Society for the Right to Die). By the end of the twentieth century, the NVVE would claim a membership of more than 100,000.

In 1984, in a ruling on what came to be known as the "Alkmaar Case," the Dutch Supreme Court officially recognized the agreement between Dutch prosecutors and the KNMG, declaring euthanasia "excusable" for physicians under the conditions specified in the agreement. The court argued that under these conditions, physicians' duties to preserve life conflicted with their duties relieve suffering. It was thus permissible for physicians to act on either duty and if they acted to relieve suffering, they were released from their obligation to preserve life.

In setting out these legal conditions, Dutch courts, prosecutors, and the KNMG faced what Gerrit van der Wal of the KNMG and health inspector Robert Dillman, characterize as a "conceptual issue," sometimes characterized as a "definitional question" (Blijham and Tjabbes-Meijer 2002; van der Wal and Dillmann, 1994). Dutch and German use the same word for euthanasia, "*euthanasie.*" This term was linked in living memory to the Nazi *euthanasie* program, which Dutch physicians had resisted to the point of being sent to concentration camps. Their resistance had even been widely lauded as model of medical integrity under a dictatorship (Alexander 1949, see Chapter 36). To make *euthanasie* conceptually palatable and to reconcile it with their own history the Dutch redefined *euthanasie* to mean "the intentional termination of life by someone other than the person concerned, at his or her express request" (Blijham and Tjabbes-Meijer 2002, 285).

Redefinition in hand, confident in the integrity of their own medical profession because of its historic resistance to the Nazi euthanasia program, the Dutch began to explore the possibility of making humanely inspired voluntary euthanasia available to patients who requested it. After 1984, euthanasia was officially excusable and legally tolerated by Dutch prosecutors; however, as a condition for excusing euthanasia, the Dutch legal system asked physicians to report acts of euthanasia to prosecutors, who would then investigate to determine whether physician should be subject to criminal charges.

In 1990, a Dutch government commission headed by Professor J. Remmelink, attorney general of the High Council of the Netherlands, investigated Dutch euthanasia practices (*Commissie Onderzoek Medische Praktijk inzake Euthanasie* 1991; van der Wal and Dillmann 1994). The commission found that in 1990 there were approximately 5,000 requests for euthanasia. Approximately 2,300 patients, roughly 2 percent of the 130,00 people who died in the Netherlands that year, were formally euthanized. Another 400 or so received medically assisted suicide. Euthanasia was typically performed in the patient's home by a general practitioner with the family present, although patients also received euthanasia in hospitals and nursing homes. Three quarters of all euthanized patients had a diagnosis of terminal cancer. The most important reason given for euthanasia was either futile suffering (29 percent) or unbearable suffering (18 percent), that is, the reasons required by Dutch law. Pain was a factor in approximately 40 percent of all cases; fear of humiliation was a factor in one-quarter of all cases.

In more than half of all cases in which euthanasia was performed, however, it was *not* recorded on the death certificate and was *not* reported to the prosecutor's office (van der Wal and Dillmann 1994). The Remmelink commission also found that 1,040 incapacitated patients who had not requested euthanasia were nonetheless "euthanized" – a clear violation of the Dutch definition of "*euthanasie*" and of spirit and letter of the agreement negotiated between the KNMG and the prosecutor's office. These findings were repeated in later studies (van der Maas, van der Wal, and Haverkate 1996). Almost all of these cases involved terminal patients who would have died within days or weeks. Nonetheless, despite the definitional and conceptual limitations built into the Dutch conception of *euthanasia*, and despite the safeguards built into the excusing conditions accepted by the courts and the prosecutor's office, approximately one-third of all cases of euthanasia in the Netherlands were nonvoluntary and legally inexcusable.

In 1991, a new method of reporting was introduced and reports to prosecutors increased. Nonetheless, more than half of all euthanasia cases remain unreported. In all, physicians reported some 6,324 cases of euthanasia to prosecutors during the period from 1991 through 1995. In thirteen cases, the prosecutor's office formally investigated physicians. Although, in all cases, charges were dismissed, the persistent underreporting of euthanasia undermined the checks and balances negotiated to monitor excusable euthanasia (van der Maas et al. 1996a, 1996b, van der Wal, Gerrit, deGraaff and Dilmann 1994). To correct the situation, a law was passed in 2001 legalizing reported cases of euthanasia. The law removed all risk of legal prosecution, but only for physicians who formally report their acts of euthanasia (Blijham and Tjabbes-Meijer 2002).

One reason why Dutch doctors may resort to illegal nonvoluntary euthanasia in providing end-of-life care is that neither hospice care nor state-of-the-art palliative care are readily available in the Netherlands. Although, in principle, a country can embrace a wide range of end-of-life care options, including effective palliative care, hospice care, assisted suicide, and euthanasia, to date euthanasia tends to preempt other treatment modalities wherever it is available, claiming the conceptual and institutional space that they would otherwise occupy. By the end of the twentieth century, euthanasia had become *the* primary treatment modality in the Netherlands for dealing with pain and suffering at the end of life, preempting all others. Where UK and U.S. medical textbooks discuss palliative care, Dutch medical textbooks discuss the practice of euthanasia instead (Kimama and van Duin 1998). Dutch palliative care practices and hospice care have been radically underdeveloped by comparison with countries that have strongly embraced the hospice and palliative care models (Henlin 2002; Jansen and ten Have 1999; Zylicz 1993). It is perhaps not surprising therefore that Dutch physicians practiced euthanasia on incapacitated terminally ill patients who were experiencing extreme pain and suffering, Dutch physicians may not be able deliver alternative or even envision other forms of pain control.

Assisted suicide, in contrast, has not historically been at odds with palliative care or hospice in either Switzerland or in the one U.S. jurisdiction in which the practice is legal, the state of Oregon. In 1997, Oregon become the first U.S. state to decriminalize physician-assisted suicide. Despite the vigorous opposition of the AMA, the Oregon Medical Association, the Roman Catholic Church, and

Christian fundamentalists, by popular referendum on a vote of 51 percent to 49 percent in 1994, and again – after the law was repealed by the legislature – by a vote of 60 percent to 40 percent in 1997, the Oregon Death with Dignity Act became law. The law prohibits euthanasia but legalizes physician-assisted dying for capacitated terminally ill patients who are Oregon citizens. Such patients were given a legal right to request a prescription for a lethal medication from a physician, provided that they had reiterated their requests both orally and had, in a formally signed and witnessed document, been advised of palliative care and pain control options. Further requirements include a second physician consult confirming their terminal prognosis. Once the lethal medication is prescribed, patients must take the lethal medication themselves.

The Oregon Death with Dignity Act also required that all prescriptions written to assist dying and all medically assisted deaths be reported publicly. Opponents of the Act had demanded public reporting and advocates could not reject the demand because it satisfied the principle of transparency lauded by bioethicists and by good governance groups. Consequently, data on all medically assisted deaths are published annually and posted on an official Oregon Department of Health website (http://egov.oregon.gov/DHS/ph/pas).

Oregon had a population of approximately 3.5 million people in 2004. Of these approximately 31,000 died; 37 of these deaths officially involved medical assistance – approximately 1 death in 800 (0.125 percent). Between 1998, when physician-assisted dying became legally available in Oregon, and the end of 2004, a total of 208 patients had actually availed themselves of this option. Although very few patients actually exercised their right to assisted dying, many – nearly one of every five patients with a terminal diagnosis (17 percent) – had discussed assisted suicide with their families. Only 2 percent of patients with terminal diagnoses formally request information about assisted dying (Tolle et al. 2004), and only a few dozen carry out the act. One reason for the small number is that physicians only grant one request of every six for a prescription for a lethal medication, and only one lethal prescription in ten culminates in death by suicide (Ganzini et al. 2000).

Cumulative data from 1998 to 2004 portray the typical Oregon physician-assisted death as occurring in a private home (94 percent of the time) with family and friends present and with a health care practitioner in attendance (83 percent). Suicides typically occurred just over a month after the first request for assistance in committing suicide. When a patient takes a lethal prescription he or she typically becomes unconsciousness within 5 minutes and death usually occurs approximately a half hour later (although some patients have lingered as long as 4 days). Almost all deaths (95 percent) were described as "uncomplicated."

The primary reasons why patients who died from physician-assisted suicide sought suicide were "loss of autonomy" (87 percent), "inability to engage in activities that make life enjoyable" (84 percent), "loss of dignity" (80 percent), "loss of control of bodily functions" (59 percent), "burden on family, friends/caregivers" (36 percent), "inadequate pain control or concern about it" (22 percent), and "financial implications of treatment" (3 percent). The last entry is significant because approximately 18 percent of Oregon's population is without health insurance; however, 99 percent of the patients who received assisted suicide had health insurance (63 percent through private insurance, 36 percent through either Medicare or Medicaid).

The typical assisted-death patient was a married or widowed college-educated (61 percent in 2004 – by comparison only 33 percent of Oregonians are college educated) Caucasian who was dying approximately 7 years younger than most other Oregonians (at a mean age of 69 as opposed to 76). Cancer (malignant neoplasm) was the most common diagnosis (79 percent of all assisted suicides); acquired immunodeficiency syndrome (AIDS) and amyotrophic lateral sclerosis (ALS), although a small portion of the assisted suicide population, were significantly overrepresented (Oregon Department of Health Services, 2005).

As practiced in Oregon, physician-assisted dying differs markedly from euthanasia as it is practiced in the Netherlands. The percentage of physician-assisted deaths in Oregon is very low (0.125 percent) in comparison with the percentage of Dutch patients euthanized (2–3 percent). In striking contrast to the Netherlands where hospice care is for the most part unavailable, 86 percent of all patients who received a physician-assisted death in Oregon during the years 1998–2004 were receiving hospice care. Assisted death in Oregon is not a substitute for palliative and hospice care; it functions as a last resort for patients seeking a form of relief that hospice and palliative care seem unable to deliver. Perhaps as a consequence, the oft-criticized slippage from voluntary to nonvoluntary termination of life that is so evident in the practice of euthanasia in the Netherlands is not evident in Oregon. Another factor constraining slippage may be the atmosphere of openness and transparency surrounding the Oregon initiative. Data are collected and published annually and Oregon physicians, unlike their Dutch counterparts, fully report their activities (Tolle et al. 2004).

Differences between the acts themselves may also tend to keep physician-assisted death as a form of suicide: something one does to oneself. Physicians may assist by prescribing lethal medications but, whether in Oregon or in Switzerland, it is the patient's own hand that brings the lethal dose to the patient's mouth and the patient who thus takes responsibility for ending her or his life. Were a physician or anyone else to administer to a patient a lethal dose, the very nature of the act would change from assisting suicide to homicide. In euthanasia, however, it is not the patient's hand but the physician's that injects the lethal dose into the patient's body. From the physician's perspective, there is thus little inherently different in injecting a lethal dose into the arm of a capacitated patient, who voluntarily seeks death, or into that of an incapacitated patient whose family seeks death on the patient's behalf – and it is easy for the physician to believe that both are morally excusable.

VIII. CONCLUSION

For four centuries, Europe and the Americas have experimented with the medicalization of the life cycle: conception, childbirth, sexual maturation, aging, and dying. Enlightenment ideals motivated this experiment and, judged in terms of these ideals, many aspects must be considered a success. By the end of the twentieth century mother and child were much more likely to survive childbirth in good health than in any prior period. Much of the pain of delivery had been muted, and the aura and fear of death that once attended childbirth had been dissipated. Children typically survived their birth and infancy, growing into healthy adults likely to live longer than people in any previous era – the life span of the average European or North American has doubled since Bacon first envisioned a truly scientific medicine. Dying could now be made comparatively painless for most people and death could sometimes be deferred by resuscitation and other medical innovations.

Yet, even by the standards of the Enlightenments, progress came at a price. By focusing reductively on natural causal explanations of health and disease the medical gaze was blind to religious and cultural meanings depriving Europeans and Americans of much that had once made life cycle events significant. Medicalization seemed always to provoke moral questions, if not moral crises. It seldom proved as objective or as straightforwardly progressive as some partisans of the Enlightenments originally envisioned. The medicalization of sexuality transformed sins into sicknesses. The medicalization of birth allowed men to colonize a female and feminine domain. When male physicians discovered that their own dirty hands were causing the massive maternal mortality associated with puerperal fever, they elected to silence the discoverers rather than to wash their hands. After claiming the authority to monitor clergy at the deathbed, for the better part of a century, physicians lost the art of palliation at the end of life, and then regained it only after a woman, a nonphysician, led a campaign that extricated end-of-life care from the hospital, moving it to the hospice. In medicine's darkest moment, anti-Semitism, racism, homophobia, and prejudice against people with disabilities were objectified as scientific eugenics, and medicine became the hand-maiden of eugenic euthanasia, abetting the Holocaust. Despite these failings, judged by the standards of the Enlightenments, the European–American four-century-long experiment with medicalizing the life cycle might still be considered a success – albeit not an unmitigated success, and the margin of success is smaller and more precarious than one might initially imagine.

NOTE

1. Psychodynamic models of the life cycle or life stages are a notable exception. (See, e.g., Erikson 1959, 1968.)

Chapter 8

Medical Ethics through the Life Cycle in the Islamic Middle East

Ilhan Ilkilic

I. Introduction

The revelation of God in the Quran as the Holy Scriptures of Islam and the sayings of the Prophet not only contain statements about religious beliefs and duties, but also give meaning to each part of the life cycle. The content of such concepts as the beginning of life, childhood, illness, growing old, and death is constructed out of the faith and interpreted accordingly. These interpretations reveal themselves in corresponding rituals and ceremonies of everyday life, some of which go back to the time of the Prophet. This chapter discusses the interpretations of these stages of life that can be derived from Islamic sources and some medically relevant moral obligations that arise from them. To understand Islamic conceptions, one needs to comprehend certain pivotal texts and key terms. Much of this chapter therefore focuses on close readings of relevant texts (see also Chapter 17).

A sophisticated concern with the moral obligations of practitioners and patients is first found in the works of the ninth to fourteenth centuries of the Islamic Middle Ages. The main objective of medical practice in these works, in which the contribution of ancient authors is unmistakable, is to maintain and restore health. Scientific competence, medical skill, and moderation in all areas of life are the essential personal traits of practitioners. A

patient is expected to protect himself from illnesses by means of preventive measures, search for a trustworthy practitioner in case of illness, and follow the instructions of his or her doctor.

II. The Beginning of Human Life

The first verses of the Quran in the Surah (chapter) al-ʿAlaq are: "Recite in the name of thy Lord who created – created man from a clotted blood[1] [ʿalaq]. Recite, for thy Lord is the most generous, Who taught the use of the pen – taught man what he did not know" (Surah 96:1–5). The word ʿalaq, when it is used as a verb, means "hang or hold onto." Clotted blood and blood clots are called ʿalaq, as are leeches on account of their stickiness. In addition to these material meanings, the word can also refer to metaphysical attachment, love, and affection. In his interpretation of these verses, the Turkish commentator Elmalılı Hamdi Yazır (d. 1942) emphasized two dimensions of human development. The first concerns the anatomical and physiological development of the human being. The creation of a human being from a clot of blood, or an embryo, is to be considered a miracle of God. The equipping of that human being with intellectual abilities that enable him to read, write, and search for knowledge are also, according to Yazır, divine gifts of His mercy (Yazır

1971, 8:5951–3). The development of the embryo in the womb is described in other verses as follows:

> Thus, He begins the creation of man out of clay; then He causes him to be begotten out of the essence of a humble fluid; and then He forms him in accordance with what he is meant to be, and breathes into him of His spirit: and [thus, O men,] He endows you with hearing, and sight, and feelings as well as minds."[2] (Surah 32:7–9)

The following verse explains the development in the womb, birth, death after a certain period of life, and resurrection in the next world as components of a continuum with different qualities of being:

> Verily We created man from a product of wet earth; Then placed him as a drop [nutfa] (of seed) in a safe lodging; Then fashioned We the drop a clot [calaqa], then fashioned We the clot a little lump [mudga], then fashioned We the little lump bones, then clothed the bones with flesh, and then produced it as another creation. So blessed be God, the best of Creators! Then lo! After that ye surely die. Then lo! On the Day of Resurrection ye are raised (again). (Surah 23:12–6 by Pickthall 1930)

Breathing of the spirit, that is, when the embryo or fetus has a soul, was already a central topic of discussion about the beginning of human life in the early period of Islam. Although there are no explicit statements in the Quran about the precise moment at which the embryo receives a soul, in the course of the establishment of Islamic jurisprudence in the eighth and ninth centuries the following calculation begins to be accepted. For all of the stages in the above-quoted verses up to the breathing in of the soul, that is, the drop of water (nutfa), the embryo (calaqa) and the fetus (mudga), 40 days are calculated. In total, therefore, it is 120 days until animation. This calculation is based on the following Hadith:

> Each one of you collected [as nutfa] in the womb of his mother for forty days, and then turns into a clot [calaqa] for an equal period (of forty days) and turns into a piece of flesh [mudga] for similar period (of forty days) and then God sends an angel and orders him to write things, i.e., his provision, his age, and whether he will be of the wretched or the blessed (in the Hereafter). Then the soul is breathed into him . . . " (Buhari 1985, 8:387)

The determination of the point at which the breathing in of the spirit takes place, based on these Hadiths, plays a decisive role in the assessment of abortion. The complex and diverging decisions of the legal schools can be summarized as follows.[3] An abortion before the 120th day of pregnancy is allowed by the Zaidites, a portion of the Hanafites, and a portion of the Shafiites. Some Hanafites and Shafiites despise abortions; they are nevertheless allowed if there are cogent reasons. Some Malikites prohibit abortions without exception. The official opinion of the Malikites is that abortion is forbidden. The Hanbalites forbid it after 40 days. All legal schools agree that it is forbidden after the breathing of the soul into the fetus, that is, after the fourth month. After this point, an abortion can only be performed if the life of the pregnant woman is in danger. There is also wide agreement about the permissibility of temporary contraception (Gräf 1967, 228–32; Elwan 1967, 469–70; Mahmood 1977, 39–48; Khoury 1981, 7; Musallam 1983, 61–88; Omran 1992, 225–38; Lohlker 1996, 22). The fact that even within a given legal school diverging opinions about the beginning of a human life are found can be traced back to the dynamics inherent in the system by which Islamic verdicts are reached (Macdonald 1903; Schacht 1964; Schacht 1975; Rahman 1985; Motzki 1991).

Although the 120-day limit is decisive for many traditional legal scholars, Abu Hamid al-Ghazali (1058–111) – one of the most influential scholars in the Islamic Middle Ages – maintained a different opinion, one which would not be acceptable to all legal scholars. He favored contraception for a wide range of reasons. If, for example, one is afraid that a pregnancy would endanger the beauty of a woman, then, according to al-Ghazali, one has a legitimate reason for contraception (al-Ghazali [1352] 1933, 2:47); however, he takes a firmly negative position with respect to abortion. Even if the egg cell, from fertilization until birth, is equipped with different features and capabilities according to stage of development, one is still dealing with the same living being. Therefore, the fertilized egg cell possesses full rights to protection, independent of its physical development and the in-breathing of the soul. Al-Ghazali wrote the following on this:

> Contraception is not to be equated with abortion and the killing of children, for the latter are crimes against an entity which already exists. There are several stages of existence: the first stage consists of the sperm entering the uterus, mixing with the woman's water, and preparing itself for receiving life; disturbing this is a crime. If the life which has been received becomes an embryo and a fetus, then the crime becomes worse. And when the soul is breathed into the fetus and it becomes a creature, the wickedness of the crime increases. The crime is most wicked when the child, although alive, is aborted (by the mother) . . . In our opinion, the origin of existence lies in the fact that the seed is received into the womb, not in its emergence ex membro virili; for the child emerges not from the seed of the man alone, but from that of both partners together, from

his and hers [or from the semen of the man and the menstrual blood]."[4] (al-Ghazālī [1352] 1933, 2:47)

The main reason for the discussions about the beginning of human life in the Islamic Middle Ages was not the theological and philosophical questions to which this problem gave rise (cf. Musallam 1990, 32–46; Hitchcock 1990, 70–8). Rather, the discussions about abortion and contraception had a juridical background concerned with criminal or family law.

> The question of whether a foetus had a legal status as a person was important in a number of legal contexts among the Arabs as well: to questions about blood money paid if a pregnant woman was injured and miscarried; to questions about inheritance (could the foetus benefit from inheritance although yet unborn?); to questions of personal status (if a slave aborted a "formed" foetus, would she ultimately gain freedom as umm walad? [mother of a child]); and to questions of burial for the foetus if miscarried or stillborn. (Bowen 1997, 163)

To prosecute someone for abortion, it is necessary to prove that a pregnancy existed. Despite a number of uncertain tests for pregnancy, the repeated failure to menstruate and particular physical changes were certain signs of pregnancy in the Islamic Middle Ages; however, these methods took a long period of time (on pregnancy tests in the Islamic Middle Ages, see Weisser 1983, 154–9). With the methods of diagnosis then available, it was also difficult to decide whether what had been aborted was an embryo or fetus or whether one was dealing with something else. These and similar difficulties have received almost no attention in the current academic debate on Islamic law and could be the reason for the relatively long period – 120 days – that a pregnancy had to achieve before a presumed criminal act could be justly punished.

The discussion about the beginning of human life and the moral status of the embryo experienced an unmistakable upswing in the Islamic world in the second half of the twentieth century. The reasons for this were not only new scientific discoveries about the human embryo and developments in medical technology, but also sociopolitical and economic factors such as population growth, birth control, and poverty. The governments and rulers of many Islamic countries often saw birth control as the only, and a quick, solution of their socio-economic problems (Omran 1980, 147–97; Spenlen 1994, 51–8). The success of these political goals presupposes the assent of the population, which, in turn, depends on their perceived compatibility with the Islamic value systems of the people. Scholars favoring a flexible regulation of abortion often receive official support and their statements favor corresponding legislative initiatives in countries such as Tunis,

Turkey, and Pakistan (Elwan 1968, 57–71; Bowen 1997, 168).

A number of Islamic intellectuals and legal scholars, however, openly oppose these developments. They argue that prohibitions against killing of human life in the Quran include prohibition of killing children for fear of poverty. In Surah 17, verse 31, we read:

> Hence, do not kill your children for fear of poverty: it is We who shall provide sustenance for them as well as for you. Verily, killing them is a great sin. (similarly Surah 6:151, Surah 5:32, and others)

They also make clear that measures facilitating birth control serve Western ideals and interests. Instead of allowing abortion, they call for measures to oppose poverty, to distribute resources fairly, to create equal opportunity, and to oppose corruption. They often cite recent research results in embryology and genetics in support of their position, noting that human organs develop very early. Modern embryology undermines the view that human life is only worthy of protection from the 120th day of pregnancy onward. Abortion is therefore forbidden before and after the breathing of the soul. Abortion can only be justified if the continuation of pregnancy threatens the life of the mother (Abdul-Rauf 1977, 126; Šaltūt 1965, 218–37; Khoury 1981, 24–5; Ghanem 1982, 60–1; Ghanem 1989, 347–8).

III. Birth, Infancy, and Childhood

1. Birth and Religious Rituals

According to Islamic belief, the emergence of a human being from a drop is to be considered a miracle of God (Surah 35:11; Surah 41:47). The birth of a child is a unique experience and a cause of great joy in the family and among relatives. This important event is celebrated in Islamic countries with different rituals and ceremonies of traditional and religious nature. Immediately after the birth, the *adān* (call to prayer) – as a common religious ritual – is recited into the ear of the child (Juynboll 1960, 1:187–8). Either immediately after the *adān* recitation or on the seventh day after the birth, the child is named. The parents fulfill their duty to give their child a beautiful name by means of a selection of the names of the prophets, wives of prophets, friends of the prophets, or the virtuous (Schimmel 1989). Seven days after birth, the child's hair is cut and one or more sacrificial animals slaughtered (ʿaqīqa) as a sign of gratitude (Buḫārī 1985, 7:272–8). Relatives and neighbors are invited to the feast and money of the value of the weight of the hair in gold or silver is given to the poor. These rituals and ceremonies change according to time and place. Among Islamic legal scholars, various opinions are held about how religiously obligatory these rituals are (Juynboll and Pedersen, 1960, 1:337; Bilmen 1986, 395; Imam Malik 1989, 199; Gilʾadi 1992, 35–41; Ali Rıza Bey 2001, 1–7; Dessing 2001, 15–42).

The Islamic understanding of freedom from bodily harm, and specific norms for dealing with strangers of the opposite sex, and the sense of honor, lead to odd ways of treating the mother during birth. Due to these norms and their implications, the birth of a child should be presided over by a female doctor and female medical staff, unless no such women are available. Although these preferences are well integrated into the health system in Islamic countries, numerous administrative and medical-ethical conflicts in everyday practice in non-Islamic countries are not uncommon (Ilkilic 2002, 79–82).

For 40 days after the birth of her child, the mother is considered to be particularly worthy of protection and should be left in peace. She does not have to fulfill the usual religious duties during this time, such as fasting or obligatory prayer, and she is forbidden to have sex. She often receives help with housework and is spoiled by her circle of acquaintances (Ali Rıza Bey 2001, 1–5; Bainbridge 1982, 2–3; Weiner 1985, 48). There are statements about feeding an infant in the Quran and the Sayings of the Prophet that have certain implications for the obligations of the parents, social life, and not least jurisprudence (Gilʾadi 1999).

2. Circumcision

Circumcision (ḫitān) is certainly one of the most important religious rituals in the childhood of a Muslim boy and is traced by Jews and Muslims back to the Prophet Abraham (Blaschke 1998). Although circumcision is not explicitly mentioned in the Quran, there are numerous Hadiths that refer to it. In a Saying of the Prophet Muhammad we read: "Five practices are characteristic of the Fiṭra [nature]: "circumcision [of boys], shaving the pubic hair, cutting the moustaches short, clipping the nails, and depilating the hair of the armpits" (Buḫārī 1985, 7:516). Circumcision involves the removal of the foreskin (praeputium) of the penis so that the glans is fully exposed. There are different opinions in the legal schools about the extent to which circumcision is religiously binding and about when it should be performed. It can take place from the seventh day after the birth through to the attainment of majority (bulūġ). Geographical, socio-cultural and financial conditions are decisive for the date of the circumcision as well as the kinds of festivities before and afterward (Risa 1906, 589–92; Bainbridge 1982, 4–5; Canan 1988, 2:457, 7:532; Orhonlu 1993, 245–6; Ali Rıza Bey 2001, 328–32; Dessing 2001, 43–78).

Female circumcision is often discussed by medical ethicists and human rights activists in the West as an attack on freedom from bodily harm. The intense debates and massive criticism of female circumcision, as opposed to male circumcision, are probably to be explained by the familiarity of the latter in the Jewish and Islamic traditions (Szasz 1996, 143; Dessing 2001, 43–44). Through the historical sources we know that female circumcision was practiced during the lifetime of Prophet Muhammad as a pre-Islamic custom. Many contemporary Muslim intellectuals and legal scholars disapprove of female circumcision. This negative approach is based on two arguments. First, this practice cannot, in accordance with Islamic sources and decision methods, be accepted as an Islamic binding duty. Second, it is only a geographically (especially East and West Africa) conditioned custom (Rahman 1987, 120–1; Canan 1988, 7:532; Anees 1989, 57–60; and on different positions of Muslim scholars see Krawietz 1999, 13–18). Poor hygienic conditions associated with this practice, which can have fatal consequences, strengthen the negative arguments of Muslim scholars. This subject with its cross-cultural dimensions is a challenge for medical ethics. It requires some different aspects with hermeneutical reflection. In these discussions, the problem of social acceptance through being circumcised must get the attention it deserves.

3. Marriage, Children, and in vitro Fertilization

If a Muslim man or woman is in a position to fulfill the necessary prerequisites and duties of marriage, he or she is obliged to start a family. The family is the smallest community, in which the man and the woman each have their own rights and responsibilities (Siddiqi 1986, 28–122). The stability of the structure of society depends on harmonious marriages. By means of family life, Islam institutionalizes the satisfaction of sexual desire in a long-term relationship. This is because the expression of sexual drives in a nonmarital relationship is forbidden both for men and women (Surah 17:32, Surah 23:5, Surah 25:68, Surah 70:29–31, among others). The renunciation of sex, as is practiced in the monastic movement or as a part of the celibate commitment in the Catholic tradition, is frowned upon in Islamic sources (Surah 57:27, Surah 5:87; Al-Qaradawi 1984, 171–3). Alongside stable social structures and the legitimate satisfaction of sexual desires, having children is also a basic purpose of marriage. Al-Ghazālī writes:

> Its [marriage's] purpose is the preservation of the species, that the human race not vanish from the earth. For the sexual drive is only created as an effective motivation; it has, so to speak, the function of causing, in the male part, the sowing of seed, and, in the female part, the seed's reception into the earth. Sexual intercourse serves for both parts as a means of attracting them, in order to 'capture' a child, much as one attracts a bird by spreading seed that it likes

to eat, in order to catch it in one's net. (al-Ghazālī [1352] 1933, 2:22)

According to al-Ghazālī, procreation has four advantages for the Muslim:

> First, striving to beget children in order to preserve the species means fulfilling the will of God the Almighty. Second, one thus fulfils the wish of the most blessed ambassador of God, who wishes to adorn himself with a large number. Third, one receives the grace that, after his death, a pious child prays for him. Fourth, he receives an advocate with God, if his small child dies before him. (al-Ghazālī [1352] 1933, 2:22)

The undeniable importance of children has led to a positive attitude in the assessment of new reproductive techniques in the present. If no pregnancy is possible by natural means and with the help of other therapeutic measures, fertilization outside of the body by means of in vitro techniques is allowed under certain conditions. The most essential of these are: both egg cell and semen should come from legally married partners and the fertilized egg should be implanted into the womb of the wife (Krawietz 1990, 210–21; Diyanet 1995, 101–2; Ebrahim 1993, 85–118; Rispler-Chaim 1993, 19–27).

4. The Sick Child of Muslim Parents

Islamic belief, with its holistic character, prescribes a number of rights and responsibilities in the relationship between parents and children. The child has a claim to freedom from bodily harm and preventive and curative health care is the responsibility of his or her Muslim parents. Because the decisions of Muslim parents on behalf of a sick child are connected with a reward or punishment in the next life, it is not surprising that Muslim parents pay much attention to Islamic values and regulations in making such decisions. Parental decisions about a sick child can lead, in practice, to conflicts with the decisions of medical staff. The matter would be even more complicated if the sick child of Muslim parents lives in a non-Islamic country (Ilkilic 2003a, 39–40; 2003b, 203–15). Some therapies can come into conflict with Islamic food directives (e.g., medicine that contains alcohol and pork products, or heart valves transplantation from pigs) and therefore can be refused by Muslim parents.

The notion of children's autonomy or the ability to give consent or assent, which are already controversial in medical ethics, become more complex through cultural diversity and religious value systems. Even if decisions that can be derived from Islamic articles of faith cannot lead to mortal consequences, such as can arise from the refusal of Jehovah's Witnesses to allow blood transfusions, it is nevertheless possible that the attitudes of Muslim parents

differ from standard therapeutic decisions (Ilkilic 2002, 103–6, 162–3).

IV. The Concept of Illness

Understanding and experiencing an illness as a reality of life is influenced by various factors, including religious convictions. The interpretations of illness that can be traced back to Islamic sources and the relationship that Islamic belief sees among medication, healing, and God also influence the attitude of Muslim patients about medical interventions and will be briefly outlined here.

1. Interpretations of Illness

A. Illness as a Test from God

This life, which ends with death, is viewed by Muslims as a place of testing: "Every human being is bound to taste death; and We test you [all] through the bad and the good [things of life] by way of trial: and unto Us you all must return" (Surah 21:35). Some trials in this life and ideal attitudes toward them are described in the Quran as follows: "And most certainly shall We try you by means of danger, and hunger, and loss of worldly goods, of lives and of [labour's] fruits. But give glad tidings unto those who are patient in adversity" (Surah 2:155). This verse speaks among other things of an illness one experiences oneself (Yazır 1971, 1:548). By becoming ill, the patience of the human being is tested. The story of the Prophet Job in the Quran not only makes this interpretation clear, but also describes the appropriate attitude for a Muslim in a case of illness (Surah 21:81–4; Surah 38:41–3). According to this view, illness is nothing to be hated or despised, but rather a condition that makes trial of ones patience as a natural consequence of belief and thus tests faith itself. The fact that the Prophet Moses underwent a therapy, the Prophet Job cooled himself with the healing water mentioned in the Quran, and the Prophet Mohammed recommended that his companions allow themselves to be treated shows that illness is a test but that this does not mean renouncing therapy.

This interpretation can play an important role not only for the patient himself, but also for his parents, relatives, and friends in dealing with the illness. An example would be a situation in which Muslim parents discover that their unborn child has Down syndrome, a condition for which there is as yet no therapy. The interpretation of their child's illness as a test from God could have concrete consequences for the parents' decision about whether to abort the fetus. The illnesses of frail and elderly parents can be interpreted as a test from God for their children. Caring for one's parents and treating them well belong to the most important obligations of the Muslim (Surah 17:23–4). When parents become ill, their children are tested to see whether they behave according to the precepts of Islam when their parents are in need of special help.

B. Illness as a Gift of Grace and Forgiving Sins

The mercy that God showed to His Prophet Job in his illness and the lightening of religious duties provided for in Islamic law, disproves the view that illness is always divine punishment. Mainstream Islam does not view illness as punishment or wrath of God, although some Muslims embrace this interpretation for themselves. A more common attitude toward illness derives from the belief that, after death, a person's acts are weighed on a (metaphorical) scale on the Last Day, and each person will be rewarded with paradise or punished with hell according to the weight of his deeds (Surah 3:185; Surah 99:7–8). It is possible to influence this calculation in this life. One such possibility, according to the following Hadith, is being ill or a Muslim's patient attitude toward illness: "No fatigue, nor disease, nor sorrow, nor sadness, nor hurt, nor distress befalls a Muslim, even if it were the prick he receives from a thorn, but Allah expiates some of his sins for that" (Buḥārī 1985, 7:371–72). Adverse conditions offer Muslims the opportunity to have their sins forgiven by God (kaffāra). This interpretation of Muslim life has led many mystics to refuse therapy, placing their trust in God (tawakkul) instead. Although this attitude cannot be considered to be unislamic, al-Ghazzālī represents the mainstream of Islamic thought in recommending the acceptance of therapy (al-Ghazzālī 1933, 4:249).

2. Fate (qadar), Trust in God (tawakkul) and the Relationship among Medication, Healing, and God

Qadar means both Divine determination (destiny; predeterminism) and written form at the beginning of creation and their causes and conditions, that is, the powers and abilities which they possess and their spatial and temporal entries into the world of being. According to this definition, qadar is a necessary expression of the divine attribute of omniscience (Watt 1948; al-Ghazzālī 1992, 80–1; Burrell 1993). Trust in God (tawakkul) that one takes the measures necessary for reaching a goal in the awareness that the realization or attainment of this goal takes place with the knowledge of God and with His permission. A Muslim trusts in God during the whole action and considers the means by which he reaches his goal not as the true or first cause, but instead merely as second causes (Reinert 1968). According to the principle of tawakkul, the result of action is not the result of a deterministic complex of relationships that excludes God.

The relationship among the law of nature, causality, and theological terms such as fate (qadar) and trust in God (tawakkul) was an important subject in the history of Islamic thought. In this complex discussion al-Ghazālī's point of view is that there is not necessarily a correlation between cause and effect. In the physical world we experience eating and satiety or taking medicine and being cured in succession. Because of His omnipotence God capable of creating an "effect" without needing a "cause." This is, according to al-Ghazzālī, sunnat Allah (God's act) (Al-Ghazzālī 1958, 237). Trust in God does not exclude other means to achieve some results and therefore Trust in God is not inconsistent with taking medicine.

If one now applies the principles of belief in qadar and tawakkul to the relationship between medication and healing, the following picture emerges. An illness can be caused by biological (bacteria, viruses, etc.), chemical (poisons, etc.), or physical (radiation) means or by means of other substances. All this happens with God's knowledge and permission. He gives these substances their ability to make people sick, and bestows on medical measures their healing powers. The therapeutic measures are not themselves the first cause, but rather the mediators of healing that comes from God. The human being is nevertheless obliged to make use of these means to achieve the healing that comes from God. The following tradition from al-Ghazālī serves to illustrate this complex relationship.

A religious scholar told the following story of the Israelites. When Moses was once sick, the Israelites came to him and having recognized the nature of his illness, said to him: 'If you treat yourself with this and that, you will recover.' But Moses said: 'I will submit to no treatment, in order that God heal me without medication.' But his illness continued for a long time, so that they said to him: 'The treatment for this illness is well-known and tested. We treat ourselves with it and we become well.' But he said: 'I will undergo no treatment.' After his sickness had lasted even longer, God said to him: 'By my power and majesty, I will not heal you until you allow yourself to be treated with the things they have told you of.' So he said to them: 'Treat me with the things you have spoken of.' They treated him, and he became well. But as he harboured fears about this, God said to him: 'Do you intend to invalidate my wisdom by your trust in my power? Who, if not I, put the usefulness for all these things in the drugs?' (Al-Ghazālī [1352] 1933, 4:245)

The Prophet Moses refused the treatment offered him because he knew that God knew about his situation and did not need medication to heal him. But God warns him about this attitude and emphasizes that trust in God is not an adequate justification for refusing causes (in this case medication). Because the healing power of medication is given to it by God, the decision to use medication is nothing other than turning to God (al-Ghazālī [1352] 1933, 4:249).

V. The end of Life, Death and Dying

Death, as an existential experience common to all human beings, affects in Islamic belief both the physical and the spiritual aspect of the person. Belief in the next life, in resurrection after death and the Final Judgment belong to the essential articles of Islamic faith. Death is not the consequence of a sin, but instead a returning home to one's creator, and its time (*ağal*) is determined by Him (Surah 56:60). The Quran portrays death (*maut*) not as the end of the human being, but rather as the door from this life to the next, in which good and bad deeds are rewarded or punished:

> Every human being is bound to taste death: but only on the Day of Resurrection will you be requited in full [for whatever you have done] – whereupon he that shall be drawn away from the fire and brought into paradise will indeed have gained a triumph: for the life of this world is nothing but an enjoyment of self delusion" (Surah 3:185; Surah 62:8).

The process of dying is a transition to the next life and the grave begins a new life in a new state of being. Through death, the relationship of the soul or the spirit (*rūḥ*) to the body is changed and vice versa. The spirit has no authority over the body, and bodily organs are not available to it. The soul leaves the body at death until the Final Judgment or the Day of Resurrection in which they are reunited. After the Angel of Death (*ʿIzrāʾīl*) has separated the soul of the dead person from his body, questions are asked in the grave. After this, the soul waits for the Final Judgment in pleasant or fearful anticipation. This place of waiting was compared in a Saying of the Prophet with a garden of paradise or the pool of hell.

The world and all beings in it will be destroyed at a time determined by God. This time, which was also hidden from the Prophet Mohammed, is called *yaum al-qiyāma*, the Last Day. In the Quran we find impressive descriptions of the Last Day and the Final Judgment (Surah 18:99; Surah 22:1–2; Surah 39:67–73; Surah 99:1–8; and others). After all that exists has been annihilated, all the people who have ever lived, from the beginning of the world, will be re-awakened to life and brought before the judgment seat of God (*Hashr*, i.e., the gathering of the dead). At the Final Judgment, all the deeds of a person will be weighed on the heavenly scales and the decision will be made about whether he is to be rewarded or punished (Gräf 1976, 126–45; Nagel 1978, 130–44; Hagemann 1985, 103–20).

The specific decision that emerges from this process is to be understood as a sign of divine justice. This is expressed in the Quran as follows: "And so, he who shall have done an atom's weight of good, shall behold it; and he who shall have done an atom's weight of evil, shall behold it" (Surah 99:7–8).

1. The Islamic Rituals in the Presence of the Dying and the Dead

The interpretation of death described in the Islamic sources is transmitted by Muslims in everyday life in sayings such as "As we came into the world, so we will leave it. May God make a good ending possible" or "May God give us at the end the Quran (i.e., the recitation of the Quran) and *īmān* (belief)." Here the importance of the recitation of the Quran and of the article of faith *Ašhadu an lā ilāhe illallāh wa ašhadu anna muḥammadan abduhu wa rasuluhu*, that is, "I confess that there is no God but Allah and I confess that Mohammed is Allah's servant and ambassador" is emphasized. The Quran and the article of faith can be recited or spoken by a leader of prayers in the mosque (*imām*), but also by a Muslim who can read Arabic. During such a recitation of the Quran, the thirty-sixth Surah, Surah Yā Sīn, which teaches the dying and the grieving about the true nature of human life, is often selected.

After death, the hands of the dead person are washed and folded on the breast or on the stomach, according to which legal school is followed, the eyes are closed and the chin tied up with a piece of cloth. Then the clothes are taken off and the body wrapped in three or five sheets. As early as possible, either on the same day or on the next, the whole corpse should be washed. For this washing, which is to be done by a person of the same sex as the dead person, the water must be not too hot nor too cold – as though for a living person. After the washing, the corpse is wrapped in a white cloth, the shroud, and laid in a simple coffin. The cloth should also be simple and without a border, just like the white cloth of pilgrims in Mecca. The gentle treatment of the body of the dead person implies that the corpse possesses a certain right to freedom from harm in Islam. The cleaning of the body by washing it indicates symbolic preparation, like that which accompanies daily prayer, for meeting the Creator. One of the most important duties of a Muslim community to its dead is organizing prayer for the dead through an imam. Before burial, the members of the community are asked about their opinion of the dead person, and the imam recommends that they forgive all his faults. The Muslim deceased is laid in the grave on his right side and his face turned toward Mecca, as during the five-fold prayer. It is not recommended that one grieve with laments and cries. One should remember the deceased person with his good deeds (Bilmen 1986, 227–50; Şentürk and Yazıcı 1998, 212–22; al-Qaradawi 1998, 251–2).

2. Consequences for Medical Intervention at the End of Life

Two basic attitudes toward medical intervention at the end of life can be discerned with respect to Islamic religious convictions, eschatology, belief in fate (*qadar*) and trust in God (*tawakkul*) (Surah 54:49; Surah 22:70; Surah 5:23). The first attitude is influenced by the statements in the Quran about the immutability of the moment of death and the positive attitude of the individual to death. If death, according to normal medical criteria, is imminent and dying a bridge to the next life, which, for believers, is a better place to be (Surah 57:20), then it does not seem to be sensible to postpone death at all costs. If the recitation of the Islamic article of faith, the Quran or taking one's leave of one's family or organizing family matters are preferences that require a certain state of consciousness, then the medical measures to prolong life can be interpreted as contradicting the well-being of the patient.

The refusal of measures to prolong life must not, however, be interpreted as an absolutely fatalistic attitude, which is sharply criticized by the majority of Islamic legal scholars. A fatalist decision can be made if a Muslim patient refuses a therapy that has a chance of success that cannot be doubted on the grounds that "My healing lies in the hand of God. It is not decisive whether I accept the therapy or not. If God wants to, he can heal me without this therapy." Al-Ghazālī rejects such an attitude, in general, and explains that this approach is not compatible with Islamic trust in God and the Islamic understanding of fate (al-Ghazālī [1352] 1933, 4:245).

The desire for a long life to do good deeds and achieve forgiveness of sins can also be seen as a concern that is tenable in Islam; it leads, however, to a different attitude about medical intervention at the end of life. It is only seldom that one can speak, in medicine, of the success or uselessness of a therapy with absolute certainty. It is equally difficult to evaluate with certainty whether a therapy might not lead to remission or the prolongation of life, even if with reduced quality of life. If this fact is connected with the statement of the Quran that only God knows the time of death and that God is entirely capable of healing people in apparently hopeless situations, then this can lead to a positive attitude toward medical interventions at the end of life. An intensive therapy with relatively low chances of success can also be agreed to by the patient or the family. From this perspective, another approach to therapies for cancer can be considered. Many cancer therapies can prolong life of differing quality, without being able to cure the disease. Even a reduced quality of life as a result of chemotherapy could, on the basis of the above-mentioned patient preferences, contribute to

his or her well being, and so could be accepted (Ilkilic 2002, 106–10).

Because the human body is understood as a gift that God has entrusted to human beings, euthanasia is not compatible with Islamic religious principles (Surah 4:29; Buḫārī 1985, 7:390). The modern technical possibilities in an intensive care unit, which complicate the debate about euthanasia enormously (Beauchamp and Childress 1994, 219–41), represent a challenge for the Muslim process of decision making (Rispler-Chaim 1993, 94–9). The internal Islamic discussion about decisions at the end of life can be roughly categorized into three main positions. The first of these speaks of a therapeutic obligation at the end of life even in medically hopeless cases. This view rejects a distinction between active and passive euthanasia. The second position denies a therapeutic obligation and instead recommends assent to life-sustaining medical treatment. This position emphasizes that the exactness of medical prognostications cannot be guaranteed, and the possibility of miracles at the end of life, which, according to Islamic belief, cannot be ruled out. The third view declares life-sustaining medical therapy to be neither obligatory nor recommended, but rather entirely optional. This position sees no benefit for the patient in life-prolonging measures in hopeless situations. It does not, however, reject even an intensive therapy. Rather, the wishes of the patient or the family are to be decisive. This last position is finding increasing support in Islamic countries, not least on account of the scarcity of resources (see Ghanem 1989; Umri 1987, 136–44; Kasule 1998; Sachedina 2002).

The religious background sketched here and the possible decisions that can be derived from it illustrate the complexity of the decision-making process of a Muslim patient at the end of life. The use of the above-mentioned theological premises on the part of the Muslim individual on the one hand and the possibility of more than one interpretation of therapies at the end of life within the framework of Islamic belief on the other hand show that this decision-making process has many levels. It must be emphasized that not only the degree of religious commitment, but also the individual interpretation of the religious premises is decisive. It is also clear that other parameters such as education, personal experience, customs, or tradition influence the way in which a Muslim patient will think.

VI. Conclusion

It is obvious that the Islamic view of humanity and the articles of faith influence the understanding and experience of different phases of life in the biography of a Muslim. Even if one can proceed on the basis of a general basic approach to all phases of life, differing opinions about the appropriate and ethically tenable attitudes in these areas of life are to be found in different legal schools. This is an inter-Islamic reality that is to be traced back to the nature and structure of conventional decision making. New medical insights and technical possibilities provide a basis for new ethical arguments and give rise to positions that differ from the classic verdicts of the Islamic scholars of the Middle Ages, as is the case, for example, in the current discussion about the moral status of the embryo and the beginning of life.

NOTES

1. "To judge by parallel passages, ᶜalaq denotes the earliest form of the embryo in the womb." (Bell 1939, 667). In several German translations of the Quran, this word is rendered "embryo." (Cf. Khoury 1981, 475; Paret 1993, 433)

2. All of the English Translation of Quran is by Muhammad Asad, except when otherwise noted.

3. During the life of Prophet Muhammad, his decisions and instructions on the basis of the Quran played a decisive role for the Muslim community to resolve conflicts. After his death new problems arose in the expanding Islamic territory. It was necessary to develop and establish appropriate methods to solve these unfamiliar new problems. Because of this legal schools were founded in the eighth and ninth centuries. Four of them gained acceptance and their influence is known up to today in the Islamic world. These legal schools of Sunnite are called by the name of their founders. Hanafites: Abu Hanifa (d. 767); Turkey, Balkan, Afghanistan, Indian Subcontinent, Central Asia. Malikites: Malik Ibn-Anas (d. 795); Upper Egypt, North and West Africa. Shafiites: Ibn Idris Al-Schafi'i (d. 820); Under Egypt, East Africa, the south of Arabia, Indonesia and South-East-Asia. Hanbalites: Ahmad Ibn Hanbal (d. 855); Arabia. Zaidites is a legal school of Shiite in Yemen.

4. All quotations from works of classical Arabic literature in this chapter are my own, except when otherwise noted.

Part IV

The Discourses of Religion on Medical Ethics

Chapter 9

The Discourses of Hindu Medical Ethics

Katherine K. Young

I. Introduction

Aside from the fact that it has a special relationship with India, which has given it spatial and ethnic roots, Hinduism has been so inclusive that it has resisted self-definition. True, there are key ideas but none that are universal. Even though acceptance of the Vedic scripture as eternal revelation (*śruti*) has been used to distinguish Hinduism from other Indian religions such as Buddhism, Jainism, and Sikhism, there are Hindu traditions that have denied this authority and still others that are oblivious to it as in some tribal and village traditions. As the modern Indian Constitution has put it, people are Hindus in India unless they have "officially" rejected this label. "It is a peculiarly Hindu phenomenon that Hinduism may be defined as the religion of the Hindus and this definition should, however narrowly, escape tautology" (Sharma 1993, 5). The metaphor that best captures the dynamic and rich texture of Hinduism is the kaleidoscope – patterns that constantly change over time and according to context but consist of many recognizable elements. According to Arvind Sharma, "[b]ecause Hinduism lacks a standard definition, and practice tends to take precedence over theory, it is best to elicit the specific 'Hindu' religious life-pattern of the patient by engaging in a dialogue with him or her on this point" (Sharma 2002, 1).

Whereas Western civilization has had to bridge a split between philosophy and religion (created in part because of its dual heritage from Greek philosophy and Hebrew religion), Indian civilization and its offshoots have faced no such problem. Although after the sixth century BCE, specialization of knowledge developed with state formation and urbanization (which led to distinct branches of learning), religion and philosophy were integrated into a "way of life" and telos that included both spiritual and rational orientations. The nature of existence, knowledge, and proper conduct, issues of authority, the valid means of knowledge, concepts of category and causality, grounds for the belief and disbelief in God or revelation, and the problems of language, truth claims, and evil were all explored philosophically within Indian religions and contributed to distinctive subdivisions or sects.

This specialization of knowledge affected the concept of medicine (*bheṣaja*) as well. As with philosophy, its link with religion never disappeared. In the ancient period (1500–600 BCE), descriptions of health included the absence of disease defined as demonic interference or divine punishment of human sins. Therapy was based on divine, magical, or spiritual power. By the classical period (600 BCE–600), when medicine became more empirically and rationally based, religion moved to the background. Medical specialists developed expertise in etiology (*hetu*), symptomatology (*liṅga*), and therapeutics (*auṣadha*), including a vast pharmacopoeia and surgical expertise. In the medieval period (600–1700), religious approaches to medical problems again became strong, probably because several religions competed by offering easy "cures" for medical problems, along with easy means to salvation. The modern period (c. 1700 to the present) has been characterized by a deep identity crisis over indigenous religions and medical systems caused by the confrontation with colonialism. This has resulted in a pluralism of systems.

In general, religion and ethics are viewed as integral. The Hindu word for both religion (especially when qualified by the adjective *sanātana* meaning eternal) and ethics is *dharma* (literally "that which upholds or sustains). It assumes that human action is necessary to maintain both cosmic and social order and includes many things not generally included in modern Western ethics, such as ritual, law, duty, virtue, piety, and even rules, customs, and norms, that characterize the castes (when used in the plural). "It has been repeatedly emphasized that the concept of dharma is so difficult to define because it ignores or transcends differences which are essential or irreducible for Western understanding – differences between fact and norm, cosmos and society, physics and ethics, etc." (Halbfass 1988, 312–313). This fluidity, captured in the concept of the stream of life (*saṃsāra*), makes medicine never completely distinct from religion. As one Indian psychoanalyst has put it "Hindu attitudes toward body, mind, and environment emphasize confluence rather than differentiation, the object has not quite become separate from the subject, and the Western celebration of mastery over nature has never quite become a value" (Desai 1989, 4).

II. PREHISTORY (PRIOR TO 1500 BCE)

The origins of religion and medicine are obscure, but some aspects may have belonged to the Indus Valley Civilization (c. 2700–2000 BCE) located in the northwestern part of the subcontinent. Although this civilization is now known only from archaeological records, its system of urban baths, privies, and drainage and what might have been a great bath in the capital suggest a concern with cleanliness or purity. Purity was a feature of later Hinduism. The caste system was structured in part on the opposition of pure and impure and ritual bathing was both the means of daily purification and a metaphorical crossing of the "ocean" of *saṃsāra* (the cosmos) to the other shore (liberation). Kenneth Zysk suggests that a figure found on seals called the "proto-Śiva," wearing a horned headdress, seated in a yogic posture, and surrounded by animals might have been a shaman healer. Images of trees – possibly sacred because they have a female figure like the tree spirits or *yakṣīs* of subsequent periods – might have

been linked to the later sacred and medicinal significance of their leaves (Zysk [1985] 1996, 3).

III. ANCIENT PERIOD (C. 1500–600 BCE)

The world view of this period known as Vedic Religion has been distinguished from the world view of the classical and post-classical periods called Hinduism. The first explicit references to religion and medicine appear in the *Ṛg-veda* (see Zysk 1991, 13–201 and Zysk 1996 for the Ṛgvedic references in this section). Although *veda* literally means knowledge and connotes eternal scripture, from a historical perspective it is of disputed date (the "family books" early in the period and books I, IX, and X, possibly composed just prior to codification approximately 800 BCE).

The *Ṛg-veda* refers to demons that cause diseases and deities, charms, and incantations (*mantra*s) that cure them. On the principle of sympathetic magic (like attracts like), unseen and therefore internal problems (consumption, fever, worms, constipation, and so forth) are created by unseen causes (such as demons in the body) and seen and therefore external problems (accidents, wounds, insect bites, and skin diseases) by observable agents. Health is the absence of attack by demons from within and other agents from without, disease being the opposite. Rudimentary observation of symptoms and their classification is found.

Several important deities associated with disease and its cure become prominent only in the later strata of the *Ṛg-veda*. The most important is Varuṇa who punishes the sins of human beings with disease – thereby encouraging moral behavior and protecting cosmic order (*ṛta*) – but also saves them from the same with his magical power. Another deity connected to illness and health is Rudra. He has a powerful, cooling, watery medicine for longevity (*Ṛg-veda* I.114.5; 2.33.7); in another hymn he has a thousand medicines (VII.46.3). With these he cures his supplicants (*Ṛg-veda* II.33.4.13). He also causes afflictions with his poisonous arrows (*Ṛg-veda* I.114.8; II.33.11,14; etc.) or his weapons of thunder and lightning connected to *takman* (a poison or demon who causes internal diseases); this creates sores on the skin or wounds. Because of this dual role, Rudra's hand is said to possess valuable medicines as well as pointed weapons. A group of wandering ascetics (*muni*s) are connected to this deity and are experts in his herbal medicines (*Ṛg-veda* X.136).

The twin physician gods, the Aśvins (literally, horsemen), are called upon for rejuvenation therapies (*Ṛg-veda* VII.68, 71; X.39, etc.) and cure for blindness, lameness, and leprosy (*Ṛg-veda* I.112, 116–117, 120; X.39–40) (Basham 1976, 119). They create an artificial bronze limb for a warrior who lost a leg in battle (*Ṛg-veda* I.112,116–118; X.39). According to one myth, they attach the head of the sacrificial horse, which had been lost or stolen, and by this act gain acceptance at the Vedic fire sacrifice. This alludes to the possibility that physicians and their surgical expertise had been outside the Vedic circles (see Chapter 20). It also alludes to the idea that the Vedic religion had once been in danger of being overwhelmed by another religion but had made its resurgence with the latter's integration.

A few deities associated with medicine are at the core of the Vedic religion such as the god Soma (*Ṛg-veda* VI.74), the personification of a plant of disputed identity used in rejuvenation therapies. Sometimes the Vedic gods Indra and Agni are requested to provide longevity and health. The Vedic sacrifice (*yajña*) brings such blessings. The goal of life is longevity, optimistically expressed as living for 100 years (at a time when the life expectancy was probably more like 30). The Veda expanded into four Vedas. One of them, the *Yajur-veda* (XII.92) calls medicine a queen. The fourth Veda, the *Atharva-veda*, was particularly interested in medicine (see Chapter 20 for its relation to the medical Āyurveda texts).

Religion, pharmacopoeia, and surgery are mixed in these most ancient texts. Knowledge of anatomy has been attributed to (1) observation of animal sacrifice as described in the Brāhmaṇas, texts appended to the Vedas that elaborate on the increasingly complicated animal sacrifice or to (2) meditation on decaying corpses as described in the ascetically oriented Upaniṣads, yet later Vedic appendages.

There were several other important developments in the Upaniṣads. One was the law of karma. It was believed that good or bad actions themselves automatically produce good or bad results for the individual. Suffering, in other words, was now the person's *own* responsibility, whether the karma came into manifestation in this life or the next. Two explanations – disease by external (divine) or internal (human) agency – would henceforth have an uneasy coexistence in the history of Hinduism.

IV. CLASSICAL PERIOD (C. 600 BCE–600)

Dramatic changes occurred in the classical period. They can be attributed to internal developments of the Vedic world view, to the gradual merger of several cultural orientations and regional cultures, or both. The classical period was a time characterized by the extension of agriculture and trade and the formation of stable states out of small-scale communities and warring chiefdoms. This had first occurred in the Gangetic plain (but the process was gradually extended throughout the subcontinent). This was also the time when Hindu social structure was formulated as the duties of caste and stage of life (*varṇa-āśrama-dharma*). Religious and cultural innovations in the Gangetic heartland were guided by priestly and intellectual *brāhmaṇas*,

who were fast defining orthodoxy, although not without major competition from other religions such as Buddhism (see Chapter 10) and Jainism (which developed in this period) and not without incorporation of local deities and customs, especially beyond the Gangetic heartland in the central and southern regions of the subcontinent. Key religious concepts now include a supreme deity (variously understood as Nārāyaṇa-Viṣṇu, Śiva, Skanda, or Devī, deities that had been marginal to the Vedic pantheon) or the Absolute (the impersonal Brahman). The soul (*ātman*), whose relation to the divine varies according to theistic or absolutistic orientations, is characterized by eternality (*nitya*) and real being (*sat*). The period witnessed a relegation of the Vedic sacrificial religion to the background with "nonviolent" ascetic movements taking its place. Still, the curative value of sacrifices (*yajña*) and Vedic hymns continued with appeals to gods such as Agni, Indra, Soma, and others to end suffering, especially when people were ill for a long time or their condition was grave.

The growth of specialized knowledge in the classical period affected ethics. This is attested in the category of scripture called *smṛti* (composed from approximately the fifth century BCE), especially the Dharmasūtras (consisting of aphorisms on the various *dharma* topics) and the somewhat later Dharmaśāstras, an expansion of the former consisting of classifications of virtues (and their underlying rules), their rankings – sometimes with rationales, reflections on ethical ambiguities, occasional arguments in casuistic manner, and skillful hermeneutical adjustments to cope with social change, regional variation, and conflicting positions of authors to ensure normative integrity.

More specifically, topics of dharma include the phases, rituals, and duties of the life cycle definitions of caste, ritual purifications, the special nature and duties of men and women, expiations, vows, festivals, and pilgrimages – in fact every aspect of life (at least for those "twice-born" or initiated men of the upper castes who were *brāhmaṇas* or under brahmanical influence). *Smṛti* also includes the Itihāsa or epics such as the *Mahābhārata* and *Rāmāyaṇa*, which place the often dry and theoretical ideas of the previous texts into dramatic narratives to explore the complex ambiguities and perennial problems at the heart of the ethical life. In the *Mahābhārata*, the scope of *dharma* becomes considerably broader. Intention and its underlying psychology as well as remorse for wrong doing are important, perhaps in imitation of the Buddhists. Although names are attached to all these *smṛti* texts, it is likely that most represent compendiums of traditions created over time. The acephalic nature of Hinduism as a whole – the *brāhmaṇa* caste itself has had internal, competing subcastes with their own religio-philosophical systems – contributed to a kaleidoscopic complexity of supposedly normative discourse.

1. The Classical World View

A general Hindu *Weltanschauung* developed, which would characterize the religion through to the modern period. It is based on eternal (*apauruṣeya*) revelation that is "heard" by sages (thus known as *śruti* from the verb "to hear"). This most ancient and authoritative genre of scripture (which included the four Vedas – henceforth a key marker of "Hindu" identity) is complemented by *smṛti*, from the verb "to remember," a large corpus including epics, texts on ethics, and medical texts. Spiritual experience confirms what is learned through revelation. Depending on one's caste or sex, one will turn to *śruti*, the Vedas (for upper caste, "twice-born" men) or *smṛti*, especially the Epics and Purāṇas (for women and low caste *śūdra*s).

Cosmogonical myths speak of creation of the universe from the formless to the formed and its duration through cosmic cycles (*yūga*s) until dissolution and return to the primal substance, a process repeated ad infinitum (*saṃsāra*). The cosmic cycles have their parallel on the individual level, for each sentient being – consisting of soul (*ātman*), life principle (*jīva*), and body (*deha/śarīra*) – undergoes cycles of rebirth on account of primal ignorance or desire. The nature of the new birth (animal, human, or deity) is determined by the law of karma (which literally means action and by extension causality and destiny). This "law" of reaping what one sows is closely connected to medicine because it can offer explanations for the unexpected such as accidents or untimely death and the unexplainable (why some suffer from defects or disease and others enjoy good health), thereby providing meaning to life and suffering. In addition, those situations that could not be treated by ordinary medicine are explained by the bad arrangement of the planets (astrology).

The law of karma is linked to free will, effort, behavior, and health by good diet, exercise, adequate sleep, avoiding psychological stress, sensual and sexual moderation, and so forth. These can mitigate the negative effects of karma from a previous life and can help fulfill basic human desires in this life and the next. Because health is necessary to fulfill the teleological goals of life, activities to ensure it are deemed morally good and therefore dharmic. "Recognizing cause and effect in everyday action promoted ethical and responsible conduct but also provided a way to link actions from different periods. Furthermore, the theory explained the inexplicable and thereby provided an after-the-fact justification for untoward workings of time. In medical theory, karma is understood equivocally. Resigning oneself completely to fate makes the work of a physician meaningless . . . [and] leaves many questions unanswered. Therefore only a few medical conditions and epidemics are seen as a result of fate, and human effort is thought capable of overcoming consequences of disease" (Desai 1989, 102). Unlike ordinary people, who seek ways to relieve suffering, some ascetics actively pursuing liberation court suffering because deprivation is said to expiate sin and create spiritual power.

There are two types of *dharma*: *sāmānya* and *viśeṣa*. *Sāmānya* or common *dharma*, according to the famous rulegiver Manu (who lived sometime between the second century BCE and second century CE), includes nonviolence, truthfulness, nonstealing, purity, and restraining of sense organs (*ahiṃsā-satya-asteya-śauca-indriyāṇigrahaḥ*). This became a standard list to the extent that anything can be called standard in Hinduism. By contrast, *viśeṣa* or particular *dharma* is right action (including rituals) determined by a person's sex, caste, stage of life, occupation, and region. These norms cumulatively (and ideally) create order, stability, and social harmony by bringing the different categories into functional, meaningful, and structured relationships. Dharma is conceptually similar to Sanskrit grammar, which is "a domain of 'normative empiricism,' an exemplary structure of rules and exceptions, complex and infinitely differentiated, yet irreducibly one and unique . . . We may also refer to the use of the word *sādhu*, 'good,' 'correct,' which signifies both the grammatically 'correct' forms of words and persons who are 'good' insofar as their behavior conforms to the norms of *dharma*" (Halbfass 1988, 320). The ethics of "place" was wary of absolutes; rules, and their exceptions referred to context – time, place, and custom.

"Place" is more complicated than initially meets the eye. An individual is an extremely complex mosaic of preordained categories each with mandatory behaviors or norms coded by even more specific virtues with their underlying rules. Moreover, these norms are tempered by individual karmic destinies that contribute to a person's own being, *svabhāva*, which creates a rich palate of behavioral and moral shades and constitutes the public, "worldly" self (*ahaṃkāra*). As such, *viśeṣa* ethics is position relative – not in the postmodern sense that each individual has freedom, by and large, to define a distinctive self and determine the nature of the "good," but in the sense that sensitivity to the context and creative adjustment are constantly necessary to be social, moral, and elegant. This is like the poet who controls the constraints of meters and semantics but plays subtly with them to express insight. The deepening and creative adjustment of norms to the individual's evolving nature so that they are like poetry is the expression of *rasa* (a term that in the medical texts refers to the organic substance created with the digestion of food that circulates through the body to nourish and uphold it but in the drama texts means aesthetics). *Rasa* brings a dimension of vitality and refinement to ethics.

This moral aesthetics, in turn, is related to a deepening of the universal level of ethics and the spiritual dimension of life. Although (theoretically) a major change such as caste can occur only with a new birth, radical change of status can occur in this very life by pursuing a path – the way of action (*karmayoga*), the way of knowledge or (*jñanayoga*), or the way of devotion (*bhaktiyoga*) – to liberation. This stops the chain of causality by reducing the passions that create karma and keep one bound within the cycles of rebirth. To stop the causality, it is necessary either to stop action altogether (which prompted fasting to death in some circles) or to stop the desire for the results, which propels the cause and effect chain (epitomized in the *Bhagavadgītā*'s concept of *naiṣkāmyakarma yoga*, action without desire for the results). P. V. Kane puts it this way: "In the midst of countless rules of outward conduct there is always insistence on the necessity to satisfy the inner [person] ... (*āntara-puruṣa*) ... The reason given for cultivating ... virtues ... is based upon the philosophical doctrine of the one Self being immanent in every individual as said in the word '*tat tvam-asi*' [that art thou]. This is the highest point reached in Indian metaphysics and combines morality and metaphysics" (Kane 1974, 7, vol. 2). The root metaphor for this is to cross the "ocean of *saṃsāra*" to liberation (*mokṣa*) on the other shore. According to one important religio-philosophical system called Advaita, there is a two-level epistemology (provisional truth and ultimate truth) and two distinct orientations: life in the everyday world (*pravṛtti*), including medicine and care of the body, and that which is beyond (*nivṛtti*). In the latter, the soul will be separated from the body and will become eternally free.

2. The Medical Texts

With these features of the classical world view in mind, we will now look at two medical texts – the *Caraka-saṃhitā* and *Suśruta-saṃhitā*[1] that were composed in the early classical period, the time when empirical medicine developed (this probably occurred in the early Vedic schools and Buddhist universities such as Taxilā by approximately 300 BCE and was influenced both by Brahmins and Buddhists) (see Chapter 20). The early strata of the these (represented by the presumed authors Ātreya and Agniveśa) were written from the third century BCE but were probably built on earlier traditions of empirical medicine in the previous century. Both of these texts likely represented compendiums of schools rather than works by individuals (the word *caraka* literally means "wander" and *suśruta* means "well-heard" or "famous"), a point underscored by the fact that there are internal accounts about parts being lost or added. (This process was ongoing. A redaction of the *Caraka* was made by Dṛhabala in the fourth or fifth century, and one of the *Suśruta* was done by one Nāgārjuna, who added the sixth and last part of the text, before the sixth century.)

According to these texts, medical expertise includes observation, description, categorization, and experimentation. The valid means of knowledge for empirical medicine are perception, inference, and reasoning. With

reason, for instance, one can determine causality (*Caraka-saṃhitā Sūtrasthāna* XI.23–25).

Medicine is divided into eight topics: internal medicine, diseases related to eye, ear, nose, mouth, and throat; surgery; toxicology; psychology; pediatrics; rejuvenation therapies; and aphrodisiacs (*Caraka-saṃhitā Sūtrasthāna* XXX.28). Surgery is a topic largely ignored by the *Caraka* even though the first allusion to surgery was in the *Ṛgveda* – it mentions using a reed as a catheter – and some texts of the classical period mention it. *Rāmāyaṇa* II.12.5 refers, for instance, to the transplant of an eyeball and *Rāmāyaṇa* I.48.6–10 mentions (albeit mythically) the transplant of a ram's testes to cure the god Indra's impotence (cited by Basham 1976, 27). The topic of surgery, however, is well developed by the *Suśruta*. The text places it first in the list of the branches of medicine and connects it to the surgical expertise of the Aśvins to establish its antiquity (*Suśruta-saṃhitā Sūtrasthāna* II:4). "There are descriptions of ophthalmic couching (the dislodging of the lens of the eye), perineal lithotomy (cutting for stone in the bladder), the removal of arrows and splinters, suturing, the examination of dead human bodies for the study of anatomy, and much besides ... Many details in his descriptions could only have been written by a practicing surgeon" (Wujastyk 1998, 106).

The verbal root *dhṛ* that gave rise to the term *dharma* also gave rise to the medical term *dhātus* (the substances that hold the body together). The *Caraka-saṃhitā* refers in some passages to the five elements or *bhūtas* (ether, air, fire, water, and earth) as *dhātus* and in other passages to three elements called phlegm (*kapha*), bile (*pitta*), and wind (*vāta*) as *dhātus* (*Caraka-saṃhitā Sūtrasthāna* IX.4; XXVIII.7–8). When these three are disturbed [because of lack of sleep, inappropriate diet, mental stress, and so forth] creating an imbalance, disease of three types (internal, invasive, and mental) develops (*Caraka-saṃhitā Sūtrasthāna* IX.4). The morbid *dhātus* are then called *vāyu*, *pitta*, and *kapha*. Over time, the term fault (*doṣa*) gradually replaced the term *dhātu*. As a result, Āyurveda came to have the curious doctrine that "a person's health depends on the balance of the three 'faults' (*doṣa*)" (Scharfe 1999, 609). The *Suśruta* takes this a step further, saying that the "balance of the faults becomes an ideal to be preserved and the diminished faults must be increased" (Scharfe 1999, 626).

By contrast, although the causes of disease are attributed to wind, bile, and phlegm, they are never identified as faults (*doṣas*) in the Pāli Canon nor is an etiology based on three faults ever found (Sharfe 1999, 612). Because these elements or faults came to be associated with fluids, modern scholars have translated them as humors, on the Greek analogy of disease being caused by the imbalance of humors. Although the term "humor" implies a derivation from the Greek theory of the humors, recent scholarship now holds that this is doubtful (Scharfe 1999, 612; Zysk 1991, 29).

This understanding of balance and imbalance presupposes an analysis of all the physical, psychological, social, ethical, spiritual, and interactive properties (distance, combination, and number) that make each individual unique. Like the general concept of *viśeṣa dharma*, which defines individuality and right *place*, so too the concept of medicine defines individuality and right place according to past karma, diet, season, personal habits, temperament, caste, age, occupation, spiritual level, and even the location of the planets. Properties are organized according to similarities and dissimilarities, especially opposites. Therapy consists of opening up and oiling the body's channels and removing bad substances from them by purgation, bloodletting, enemas, or other depletion therapies. The *doṣas* are then restored to balance by introducing substances (such as leaves, roots, bark, fruits, bark, leaves, roots, or animal parts – here the medical prescription overrides vegetarian norms) of opposite qualities to counter deficiencies or aggravations. They are also restored to balance by diets and by observing the proper use of "hot" and "cold" foods and drugs ("hot" diseases require "cold" foods and drugs, "cold" diseases the opposite). The external ecology and cosmology affects in no small measure the internal ecology of the body, and this has to be carefully regulated.

The concept of imbalance is used to explain epidemics. When a society collectively does wrong, this disturbance of the social order creates an imbalance that in turn causes epidemics. People are encouraged to follow ethical and religious practices to restore the balance. Those unaffected are said to be protected by their store of good karma.

But the *Caraka* also has prescriptions on how to avoid infectious diseases: personal hygiene (bathing before eating, wearing clean clothes, avoiding food provided by certain classes of unclean people or served with unclean utensils); avoiding intercourse with certain people (especially those with sexually transmitted diseases) or in organs other than the vagina; and social hygiene (not sneezing or urinating in certain places). In addition, the *Caraka* mentions hospitals. They should be in a good location, with good water, place for bathing, kitchen, medical supplies, staff, cooks, and attendants to help with baths, massages, the preparation of the herbs, and so forth (*Caraka-saṃhitā Sūtrasthāna* XV.6; see also Kangle (trans.), *Kauṭilya Artha-śāstra* II.4).

The "philosophical" underpinning of the *Caraka* and *Suśruta* is Sāṃkhya. The origins of Sāṃkhya are obscure. Some authors claim that the tradition predates the Vedas (Lusthaus 1998, 462). Kauṭilya mentions it as one of the prevailing schools of his time (c. 300 BCE). It figures in the *Mahābhārata* (some sections dating to the early classical period) (Lausthaus 1998). Given its popularity, it can be supposed that the more philosophically inclined physicians would have looked to it, especially because Sāṃkhya

was initially atheistic and medicine largely materialistic. Along with the primary category of matter (*prakṛti*), it postulated the self (*puruṣa*). Sāṃkhya's classification of the three types of pain or disorder (intrinsic, extrinsic, and divine) might have contributed to the medical definition of disease (endogenous, exogenous, and karmically caused). Similarly, it likely contributed to the relation of therapeutics and moral conduct with its view that the three qualities (*guṇas*) – *sattva*, *rajas*, and *tamas* – simultaneously have physical, psychological, ethical, and spiritual properties. *Sattva* is constituted on the physical level by semen, coolness, and lightness, on the psychological level by calmness, on the ethical level by purity and virtue, and on the spiritual level by devotion and meditation. On the physical level, *rajas* is represented by blood, activity, and heat; on the psychological level by passion; on the ethical level by happiness and sorrow; and on the spiritual level by such characteristics of vitality as emotion, pleasure, and virility. On the physical level, *tamas* is represented by fat, heaviness, and dullness; on the psychological by lethargy and stupidity; on the ethical by evil; and on the spiritual by sloth and idleness. The three *guṇas* in turn are represented by the colors white, red, and black, respectively. In the medical context, *pitta*, *vāta*, and *kapha* are linked to *sattva*, *rajas*, and *tamas*, respectively.

In this perspective, body types are closely connected to psychological ones and these dispositions to types of behavior. Types of behavior in turn are connected to kinds of action and ethical propensities. "This brings us back to action, for the *guṇas* have a feedback mechanism: their manifestations have consequences, and so does action... Actions are consistently seen as substantial; they accumulate on a person's ledger of deposits and debits" (Desai 1989, 96–97). Over time, a life of imbalance will affect destiny negatively, whereas a life of balance positively. The system is not mechanistic or fatalistic, however, for it acknowledges that individual effort (*puruṣakāra*) is necessary to maintain balance or move to a new level of spiritual orientation with a more active pursuit of liberation. Over time, the earlier atheistic Sāṃkhya was subsumed within a larger religious telos that oriented the individual to a Supreme Being or Absolute and liberation from the cycles of reincarnation.

The idea of the faults (*doṣas*) may also be attributed to the influence of Sāṃkhya philosophy; the balance of three "faults" became a necessary feature of good health, in parallel with the three "virtues" (*guṇa*). "[J]ust as the three strands of Sāṃkhya transform themselves into the world through the subtle and gross elements (*tan-mātra*, *bhūta*), the three faults cause illnesses through the bodily elements (*dhātu*)" (Scharfe 1999, 627).

With all of this in mind, we turn to the content of the medical texts. The main subject of the medical texts is Āyurveda, the knowledge of life or longevity (*āyus*), a term that came to mean medicine but is much more broadly conceived. In the *Caraka*, Āyurveda is defined as "that which gives knowledge about life (*āyus*) with special reference to happiness and unhappiness, beneficial and unbeneficial life, long and short life spans, and the material, qualities, and actions that influence the life span" (*Caraka-saṃhitā Sūtrasthāna* XXX:23; translated by Young 1994, 7). Following the classical Hindu consensus of the four goals of human life – religion/ethics (*dharma*), wealth (*artha*), pleasure (*kāma*), and liberation (*mokṣa*) – the *Caraka* calls health the very root of these. It relates the first three (definitive of the mundane telos of life) to happiness (*sukha*). This is defined by the will to live, enthusiasm, the desire for prosperity, moderation in all things, a prudent and healthy lifestyle, strength, and the absence of physical and mental problems based on the premise of the deep reciprocity between body and mind (*Caraka-saṃhitā Sūtrasthāna* XXX:24, etc.). Mind is understood as subtle matter and linked through the impressions (*saṃskāras*) of karma to egoity (*ahaṃkāra*). The length of the lifespan is determined by two components: karma from past lives (*daiva* or fate) and the new karma being created in this life through human effort (*puruṣakāra*).

The *Caraka* gives a religious reason for why disease exists at all: a gradual decline in righteousness through the four cosmic periods (*yugas*) of this cosmic cycle, which is correlated with decline in the goodness (water and fertility) of the earth because of greed and with that a decline in diet and health (*Caraka-saṃhitā Vimānasthānam* III.24). (This is an interesting premodern awareness of the relation of ethics and ecology.) Nevertheless, it was believed that practices of ritual purity had an effect on health. This may well have been true because they served to reduce food poisoning and infection, so common in the subtropical climate.

Prescribing other religious activities to complement empirical medicine, the *Caraka* lists "mantras, talisman, wearing of gems, auspicious offerings, gifts, oblations, observance of scriptural rules, atonement, fasts, chanting of auspicious hymns, obeisance to the gods, going on pilgrimage, etc." (*Caraka-saṃhitā Sūtrasthāna* XI:54). According to the *Suśruta*, the very act of surgery is placed into a ritualistic context: the right astral combination for timing, and offerings to *brāhmaṇas*, physicians, and gods (*Suśruta-saṃhitā Sūtrasthāna* V.4). Sometimes Vedic *mantras* are uttered to protect the patient at the time of surgery (*Suśruta-saṃhitā Sūtrasthāna* V.12). From all of this, we see that empirical medicine (*auṣadha*) was given a very broad definition: it was of three types based on religion, reason, and good behavior/ethics (*Caraka-saṃhitā Sūtrasthāna* XI:54).

The medical texts respect *brāhmaṇas* (the custodians of Vedic learning) no doubt because they were composed by them and prescribe religious rites and duties for the three higher or twice-born (*dvija*) castes. As such, they cater to the social elite. Religion is connected to medicine

in yet another way. Heading the list of the valid means of knowledge is the preeminent authority of the omniscient sages, who transmit the eternal knowledge or revelation to this world (*Caraka-saṃhitā Sūtrasthāna* XI:18–19). A connection to revelation is also made by calling the Āyurveda a supplementary Veda or a limb of the *Atharva-veda* (which contains some medical material). The *Caraka's* interest in religion is apparent in its attempt to refute the skeptics of rebirth, for instance, by presenting arguments based on scripture, perception, inference, and reasoning (*Caraka-saṃhitā Sūtrasthāna* XI.6–12). Like other religiously oriented texts, this one recognizes that liberation is the ultimate telos of life; it is equanimity (*stithaprajñā*) and peace (*śānti*) – realization of the Absolute or a Supreme Being beyond all the oppositions that characterize ordinary life.

V. MEDIEVAL PERIOD (C. 600–1700)

This period witnessed the popularization of devotion to a personal god, temple worship (*bhakti*), and, somewhat later, esoteric combination of this with a sexualized yoga (*tantra*). The religious dimension of medicine (based on magical and spiritual power) came to the foreground once again with these developments best described as a spiritual entrepreneurialism. New genres of *smṛti* texts called Purāṇas, Āgamas, and Tantras presented etiologies of disease based on a fall from paradise, demons, witches, sorcerers, unhappy ancestors, ghosts, karma, and astrology. Medical practitioners included the *bhiṣaj*, *oja*, priest, astrologer, guru, and swāmi. Their claims of authority were based on the powers of asceticism, charisma, possession, spiritual experience, and awareness of hidden realities. God Śiva was the patron of the physicians (*vaidyas*). (In the *Ṛg-veda*, the word *śiva* had been an epithet of the god Rudra whose helpers were ascetic healers or *munis*. By the classical period, the name Rudra was largely replaced by the name Śiva.) Other deities or sages associated with medicine in the medieval texts were Bhairava, Gaṇapati, Viṣṇu, Dhanvantarī, and many goddesses. Therapeutic techniques included faith, confession, objectification of illness and its transference to a disease demon, fasts, amulets, divinized gems, stones, *yantras* (geometric images), *mantras* (special chants by people who have developed their ascetic and ritualistic powers), trances, dances, pilgrimages (especially to the holy city of Vārāṇasī/Banaras), and so forth. One of the forms of medicine that came into textual view in this period was Tamil Siddha. Its practices were based on yoga, alchemy, minerals, poisonous substances, and a hermeneutic of negation and reversal. Its antistructural, secretive, mantric, and yogic orientation reveal its affinity with Tantra.

Religions promote ethical ideals through images of founders and saints. The founder "discovers" the norms. One type of saint has more than the usual amount of altruism but still upholds the norm and thereby idealizes it, the just king or "saintly" Hindu wife being cases in point. When religious norms become too rigid and stifle religious experience or soteriological values, however, they may be dramatically reversed to express primary religious power and transmundane insight. This type of saint is the religious virtuoso. Examples include Hindu *bhakta* saints and *tāntrikas* (and Buddhist *bodhisattvas* and *tāntrikas*). There is an institutionalized or official version of the religious virtuoso consisting of those who pursue recognized paths to liberation (morality is usually a key component of these, at least at the lower stages; it is assumed by many that morality has been internalized at the higher stages and then transcended altogether with liberation).

The Āyurvedic medical traditions and their ethics continued into this period, though some scholars suggest a decline, especially in the field of surgery. Other aspects, such as hospitals, became popular, probably because Hinduism and Buddhism were now in full competition to become the most popular religion for the ordinary person. (See Haldar (1992, 71–72) for Hindu Purānic references to medicine and hospitals and chapter 10 here.) There is inscriptional evidence in the Cōla dynasty (ninth–twelfth centuries) of hospitals and dispensaries attached to larger temples as well as medical schools (Haldar 1992, 81–82).

The corpus of Āyurvedic texts was expanded in this period. It included the *Sūtra of Women's Medicine Declared by the Sage Kaśyapa* (*Kaśyaparsi-proktastrīcikitsā-sūtra*) (c. seventh century) about the diseases of women and children. In addition, the corpus included the *Heart of Medicine* (*Aṣṭāṅgahṛdaya*) by Vāgbhata (c. seventh century), a grand synthesis of Indian medicine, memorized by students over the centuries and translated into Tibetan, Arabic, and other languages. (This work together with the *Caraka-saṃhitā* and *Suśruta-saṃhitā* are called the "three ancients" or the "great triad.") Another text was the *Śārṅgadhara-saṃhitā* (c. fourteenth century) by Śārṅgadhara, a condensed "pocketbook" rendering of the medical tradition, which quickly became popular. Finally, the corpus included Ānandarāya's *Jīvānanda* (seventeenth century), an allegorical drama about the attack of diseases upon King Jīva (life), which are defeated by the joint action of medicine, *bhakti*, and yoga (Wujastyk 1998, 10–16; Basham 1976, 21, 36).

The Muslims who came to India beginning in the tenth century brought with them their own system of medicine, which can be traced back to that of the Roman physician and savant Galen. It was called Yūnānī (*ūnānī*), and it was case-oriented in approach. Based on a hospital system (many were introduced into India under Muslim rule, perhaps with Hindu physicians attending to high caste *brāhmaṇas*), it catered to the urban elite (Dunn 1976, 150). Because it had difficulty locating familiar drugs – it introduced into India mercury and opium – it integrated many local ones. Some Muslim kings such as Muhammad Tughluq and Fīrūz Tughluq were physicians (Basham

1976, 39–40). *The Mine of Medicine of King Sikandar* (*Ma'danu'l shifā'-Sikandarshāhī*) written in 1512 was the most important Indian Muslim medical text. The Muslim savant Albīrūnī complained that Hindu concerns with purity prevented a fruitful exchange between Āyurveda and Yūnānī (Basham (1976, 39 referring to Albīrūnī's *Kitab us-Sardāna*). Nevertheless, this occurred to some degree, the result being called *Tibia*. Many Indian medical texts, for instance, were translated into Arabic (Basham 1976, 39).

VI. MODERN PERIOD (C. 1700–PRESENT)

Colonial powers introduced modern, Western medicine into India. They too built hospitals and medical colleges. The missionaries who offered medical services to attract potential converts played a role in this. Many female Christian converts became nurses (an occupation that had been shunned by Hindu upper caste women because of concerns over purity and the fact that women were often sequestered). When English medicine was first introduced in Calcutta and Bombay, it was combined with Āyurveda (and Yūnānī Tibia), a process that was hastened by the East India Company's use of vernacular languages. Gradually, Indian medical texts were translated into English during a time of Orientalist scholarship and the writing of histories on Indian medicine and science. After the medium of instruction changed to English in 1835 and the conflicting premises of science and Indian religions became apparent, debates occurred between those advocating exclusive positions (either Western or Indian) and those wanting inclusive ones. The latter were based on the idea that the Hindu religio-philosophical schools prefigured, confirmed, or amplified modern science, or that both systems had their merits that should be combined. These debates, arising as they did in the colonial context, reflected the deep crisis over Indian identity, which was premised on religious, medical, and ethical views. Nevertheless, the exchange was by no means a one-way street: for instance, the Indians' expertise in rhinoplasty, for which they had long been famous, was studied by European surgeons (Basham 1976, 27).

Pluralism characterizes the modern Indian medical scene. Scholars describe the continuity of Āyurveda, especially in the villages. There are still traditional schools where students memorize the 730 hymns of the *Atharvaveda* for "white magic" and healing *mantras* under a physician–guru (Knipe 1989, 90). Modern, urban, educated Indians look to "cosmopolitan" (the euphemism for Western-originated) medicine for quick relief, especially with serious diseases, and when this is not forthcoming (as in the case of some chronic and terminal illnesses) to indigenous methods as a last resort (Leslie 1978). Indigenous medicine is also used for "cultural diseases" (ailments such as semen loss) for which there is no "cosmopolitan" equivalent, and indigenous methods are a last resort for mental problems (Obeyesekere 1978, 260; see also Obeyesekere 1976, 213).

Even today, many Hindus view the body (*śarīra*) as consisting of discrete and interchangeable parts, which make it inherently unstable: it disconnects in pain and disease and decays over time, falling apart. "Such a body construction helps explain the fact that body and body-parts, consciousness, hypochondriacal preoccupations, and psychosomatic illnesses are encountered in Indian populations with higher frequencies... The body and its parts thus become the idiom of personal distress" (Desai 1989, 57). Even the soul might splinter or leave the body or other souls might enter it as with possession. On the other hand, a balance and harmony between the body and its constituents is the basis of good health.

Imbalance includes changes in the biological organism itself: birth and death, hunger, and sexual desire as well as aging and the passing of time represented by the goddess Kālī (whose name means time, *kāla*). In addition, imbalance can be caused by contact with the outside world (for instance, the change of seasons). "For Hindus every contact, human or nonhuman, has the potential to alter the balance positively or negatively, with simultaneous and inseparable implications for moral and physical well-being... Any contact between two items in the cosmos therefore has to be appropriate" (Desai 1989, 81). If it is inappropriate, such as contact with impurity, there must be a correction to restore the original equilibrium. "The body ends up being an input-output system. Food, drink, words, deeds, and thoughts are part of an elaborate exchange between the human and the nonhuman" (Desai 1989, 80). Diagnosis is based largely on the observation of symptoms such as loss of appetite, weakness, fever, paralysis, or swelling or symptoms of specific diseases interpreted within the general framework of the person's constitution, age, psychology, diet, and so forth. The physician's observation is complemented by the patient's report on the "history" of the problem (assuming the physician over time finds it to be reliable). Together these are further framed by the concept of the balance of the *dhātus/doṣas* (Desai 1989, 82). In addition to cosmopolitan medicine, there is homeopathy based on Samuel Hahnemann's eighteenth-century cure and naturopathy from a syncretistic tradition.

Anthropologists and historians of religions (Obeyesekere, Knipe, and Kinsley) have documented the complex interface between religion and medicine in modern India. In addition, people resort to folk medicine from special concoctions to possessed communications with spirits, to visits to the shrines of goddesses associated with dangerous epidemics, such as smallpox, to snake-bite specialists, to astrologers. Obeyesekere thinks indigenous medicine will disappear slowly and Western medicine will gradually prevail (1976, 217). This is questionable however. Today, Āyurvedic physicians still outnumber cosmopolitan ones, and are increasing their numbers. The Āyurvedic physicians have been more interested in professionalization than the Yūnānī ones (Dunn 1976, 153).

As for ethics, the emphasis within the broad category of *dharma* is now shifting to justice (see Chapter 44). Whereas traditional ethics had emphasized *viśeṣa-dharma* (with its close links to the stages of life and the caste system), contemporary *dharma* is expanding the universal virtues (*sāmānya*) into legal concepts and human rights (see Chapter 44). All this, along with economic changes from an agrarian-based society to an increasingly urbanized, industrialized, technological, and computerized one, has contributed to dramatic changes. In urban areas, extended families are becoming nuclear ones and greater individual autonomy is developing (see Chapter 44). Even the traditional concepts of authority are being challenged, a process that began with the "Hindu Renaissance" of the nineteenth century: legitimation of change was skillfully introduced by arguing that different criteria are to be used in the present age (*kaliyuga*) or in times of crisis (*āppaddharma*).

In the twentieth century, Mahātma Gandhi contributed to the concept of autonomy by giving primacy to experience and conscience (*anubhava; ātmatuṣṭi*), which had been in fourth place in the traditional schema of authority. Since then, conscience and individual initiative have been steadily gaining ground, at least in the middle class, as old restrictive (and hierarchical) norms move to the background. Yet, the pace of social change is uneven, the rural areas or conservative circles often lagging behind. (For a discussion of the four principles of bioethics (non-maleficence, beneficence, autonomy – including choice, informed consent, privacy, and confidentiality – and justice, and the relationship between physicians and patients, see Chapter 44.)

VII. Conclusion

One of the distinguishing features of Hinduism has been its penchant for both analysis and synthesis. The development of specialized knowledge in the classical period contributed to empirical medicine based on analysis. Despite an emphasis on observation, description, categorization, and experimentation, efforts were made to keep the new approach within a general religious framework and to recognize the fact that body, psychology, and behavior (including ethics) must work together with the environment to maintain harmony, prevent disease, or restore health. This integrative approach also prevented a deep split between philosophy and religion or between religion and ethics. In the medieval period, it led to grand synthetic treatises of the Indian schools of medicine, new syntheses with religion, and attempts to integrate the Islamic systems of medicine. All this was influenced by concerns

with purity and impurity, notions of hierarchy, and ethical reflections based on concepts of virtue that were part
of the path to liberation or at least to a better rebirth.
Synthesis did not mean sameness or relativism.

By the modern period, the synthetic spirit was at work
once again trying to integrate Western medicine. By the
time of Independence, however, there was a growing
concern that Hindu identity was eroding through
such generosity (tolerance being one of the traditional
Hindu virtues). Despite the political debates that this
engendered, medical pluralism and its quasi-integration
with religion (including some archaic notions of demons,
magic, amulets, mantras, and a variety of religious healing
specialists and deities) continued. Hinduism could still
claim that its world view was a "way of life," a holistic
approach to religion, medicine, and medical ethics
(even as critics pointed to the need for a more empirical

approach and more equality to keep pace with changing
values).

NOTE

1. All citations from *Caraka-saṃhitā* are cited by the text
name and *stāna*, not the translators, following the number-
ing system of R. K. Sharma and V. B. Dash (eds. and trans.):
1972, *Agniveśa's Caraka Saṃhitā*, vol. 1 (*Sūtrasthāna*) and vol. 2
(*Nidāna-sthāna, Vimāna-stāna, Śarīrsthāna, Indriya-Sthāna*) (Sanskrit
Text with English translation and Critical Exposition based on
Cakrapāṇi Datta's *Āyurveda Dīpīka* (Chowkhamba Sanskrit Series
Office, Varanasi). All quotations are from these sources unless
otherwise noted. All citations of *Suśruta-saṃhitā* are from K. K.
Bhishagratna (ed. and trans.): 1963, *Sushruta Saṃhitā*, 2 vols.
(Chowkhamba Sanskrit Series Office, Varnasi). I have taken the
liberty of eliminating sexist language in translations, where it is
clear that the reference can be to both men and women.

CHAPTER 10

THE DISCOURSES OF BUDDHIST MEDICAL ETHICS

Katherine K. Young

I. INTRODUCTION

There are three major branches of Buddhism called Theravāda, Mahāyāna, and Vajrayāna. Although they developed sequentially in India, they eventually overlapped and all spread beyond India's borders. Over time, Theravāda became associated primarily with Sri Lanka and Southeast Asia, Mahāyāna with East Asia, and Vajrayāna with Tibet. Buddhism died out in India, the land of its birth circa 1300, although it has been making a comeback in the modern period with its conversion of the Dalits.

Buddhism denies a Supreme Being or Absolute. It also denies revelation. Its concept of enlightenment is based on insight into the very nature of reality framed by the law of karma (the law of reaping what one sows) and cosmic and individual cycles of existence (*saṃsāra*).[1] Its doctrines of no-soul (*anātman*), impermanence (*anitya*), and becoming (*pratītya-samutpāda*) collectively produce a spiritual existentialism, which has as its sacred authority the experience of liberation (*nirvāṇa*). As in Hinduism (see Chapter 9), religion, philosophy, and medicine have been integrated into a "way of life" and telos that include both spiritual and rational orientations.

The place of ethics in Buddhism, however, is hotly debated. There are two prevailing views. One is that the Buddha's teachings and path are provisional, a raft to be eventually left behind. In this view, ethics (rules and virtues) are instrumental, and epistemology has two levels (provisional knowledge and truth). As a result, ethics cannot be made into absolute or universal rules and enlightenment is not characterized by goodness. Robert Florida (1994), for instance, reminds us of the foundations of Buddhist ethics in the concepts of no soul (*anātman*), dependent coarising (*pratītya-samutpāda*), will (*cetanā*), emptiness (*śūnyatā*), compassion (*karuṇā*), wisdom (*prajñā*), skill-in-means (*upāya*), the five precepts (*pañcaśīla*), and so forth. He then interprets the idea of the precepts as useful tools that should not be reified into something absolute but rather seen as a way to mediate between eternalism (dogmatic inflexibility) and nihilism (antinomianism). The number of precepts (whether 5, 8, or 200 plus), he points out, has always depended on one's situation: monastic or lay and if the latter, the number varying depending on the context. The number of precepts in the monastery has also varied depending on whether one is a man or woman. Because the number varies according to context, he implies, we are dealing with a situational ethic.

Others argue that ethics has an instrumental role prior to liberation and afterward an authentic expression because ignorance has been removed. Whereas both of these views make ethics extrinsic to enlightenment, in the view of Damien Keown, Buddhist ethics is intrinsic both to the means and to the goal of enlightenment (Keown 1992, 10–11). More specifically, it is a virtue ethic; virtue constitutes both the means and the goal.

Howsoever the role of ethics is defined in Buddhism, it is encompassed within a more general soteriological orientation, which accounts for why Buddhist ethics is not an autonomous discipline and why it "has shown little initiative in developing and refining the tools of ethical analysis . . . The expectation in Buddhism seems to be that ethical problems will be entirely resolved or 'dissolved' in the pursuit of the religious life" (Keown 1992, 1–2). Even when altruism is to the foreground, as is often the case in Mahāyāna Buddhism, personal salvation does not disappear. It too can be characterized as teleological (Keown 1992, 232).

II. Theravāda Buddhism

The fifth century BCE in India was a time when clan (lineage) confederacies were being absorbed into sixteen monarchies (for example, Kośala and Magadha) in the Gangetic plain, the current center of Vedic civilization. Gautama, the future Buddha, was born into a prominent family belonging to the Śakya clan, which lived in the foothills of the Himālāyas (now Nepal). He then moved down to the eastern Gangetic plain, the "frontier" part of the heartland, which was socially and religiously still fluid. A much later hagiography (Aśvaghoṣa's first-century Buddhacarita) makes him into a prince who faces an existential crisis when he leaves his pampered palace life and sees for the first time a sick person, an old person, a dead person, and an ascetic. This existential rite of passage into realizing the nature of the human condition (disease, aging, and death) and its solution (asceticism) led to the Buddha's decision to leave home and experiment with the extreme lifestyles of several ascetic groups. He is said to have gained enlightenment (whence the epithet buddha or enlightened one) while meditating near the town of Gayā in Magadha. He then went to a place called Sārnāth (near Vārāṇasī), where he began to teach about his experience in terms of four noble truths.

The first declares that all is suffering (because of birth, aging, sickness, death, sorrow, grief, physical pain, despair, that which is unpleasant, absence of the pleasant, and the unfulfillment of desires). The Buddha went on to declare that there is an origin to suffering (desire); there can be an end to suffering (elimination of desire); and the way to this is the middle path (between extreme indulgence and extreme asceticism) consisting of eight steps (right views, resolve, speech, conduct, livelihood, effort, memory and meditation). Together, these constitute the Four Noble Truths and the Eight-fold Path of Buddhism. First under the Buddhist king Aśoka and then under "missionary" monks and nuns (from the third century BCE),

Buddhism spread throughout the subcontinent. It then spread to Sri Lanka, East and Southeast Asia, and Tibet.

Whatever the exact historical details of early Buddhism, some were transmitted by oral traditions for several centuries until the cumulative tradition was written down in Pāli (perhaps the dialect in Magadha), becoming the Pāli Canon. (The earliest extant version of the Canon is mentioned in Sri Lankan texts.) The Pāli Canon, the collection of texts of the Theravāda (Way of the Elders) school, describes the "three jewels": the Buddha, the Dhamma (Skt. Dharma) (his teachings), and the Saṅgha (the monastery).

Despite the existence of a canon, Buddhism rejected the idea of a holy, revealed scripture, instead preferring experience as authoritative. Buddhist logic, which developed as a distinct school in the fifth century, for instance, accepted only the experience of perception and inference from experience (corresponding to empiricism and rationalism) (Sharma 1995, 78), as valid means of knowledge (prāmāṇa). Although all rules, doctrines, and even concepts were based on valid means of knowledge, according to one interpretation promoted by scholars, such as Florida and Pinit Ratanakul, they nevertheless belonged to the lower or conventional level of reality (saṃvṛtti), and so they were provisional in nature, useful aids to help one cross over the ocean of saṃsāra, to the ultimate experience of enlightenment.

According to another interpretation offered by Keown, these rules were more than useful aids, for they were intrinsic both to the path and to the goal. Keown argues against assigning moral rules to lower knowledge, which is merely instrumental and utilitarian: "Contraindications to the utilitarian presumption include the tendency among Buddhists to regard the precepts as moral absolutes . . . and also the ideal of moral perfection as an end in itself as defined in the conduct of the enlightened and in particular the Buddha" (Keown 1992, 17). In other words, ethical action in Buddhism is "soteriologically potent" (Keown 1992, 127) and Buddhism a teleological system. Buddhism, moreover, emphasizes the will (cetanā) including motives and immediate intentions, along with cognitive and affective faculties, which are morally determinative and therefore ethically charged (Keown 1992, 220–1). It recognizes the complexity of causes, these inevitably entangling people's free will and resultant actions with those of others, every action therefore becoming a reaction and interaction. This insight in turn leads to the view that all phenomena are interdependent. The inherent mutuality or coarising of the conditions of causality defines the wheel of rebirth (pratītya-samutpāda; saṃsāra). "In Buddhism virtuous choices are rational choices motivated by a desire for what is good and deriving their validation ultimately from the final good for man (nirvāṇa)" (Keown 1992, 222).

Closely related to these concepts is the law of *karma*. Buddhism explains the effects of actions as a natural outcome of the unmanifest traces of previous actions stored in the subtle body on the analogy of a seed that ripens and eventually produces fruit (hence the common phrase: the fruits of karma).

A number of ethical implications arise from the teaching on the inherent mutuality of all existing things and the law of karma. First is the implication that nothing has its own substantial or independent nature (and so real autonomy is impossible). This is expressed in the concepts of no soul, impermanence, and momentariness. Second, all these make suffering (*duḥkha*) the key characteristic of human life (even pleasures, after all, are fleeting). Third, actions are divided into three types: (1) skillful (*kuśala*) actions (healthy, harmless, beneficial, and therefore good), (2) unskillful (*akuśala*) ones (self-centered, harmful, unbeneficial, and therefore bad), and (3) actions that are neither (and therefore are neutral). According to Keown, actions are therefore inherently good or bad, not good or bad because they bring about good or bad results (Buddhist ethics is not a consequentialist ethic, he argues, although good actions have regard for consequences). Good actions are called *puṇya* (merit) and are related to faith, mindfulness, self-respect, nongreed, nonhate, tranquility, ease, receptivity, competence, and so forth. Bad or harmful ones are called *pāpa* (demerit), the opposite of the fore-mentioned values. The karmic residue of *kuśala* and *akuśala* actions contain power and information (the impressions) that will become manifest at some time. The roots of unskillful actions (in the final analysis based on the misperception of reality or wrong views) lead to unskillful actions and these lead in turn to harm of self, others, and both self and others. This results in suffering, anxiety, frustration, stress, sadness, tension, nervousness, insecurity, and unhappiness. To stop unhealthy or unethical actions, Buddhists must cut out the roots of unskillful actions, which are *lobha* (greed, desire, and passion); *doṣa* (anger and hatred); and *moha* (delusions). There is always the danger that they will cling to the idea of merit and a better rebirth. Once again, not all Buddhists agree with Keown's view; as we have already pointed out, some see ethical actions as merely instrumental to the goal.

The most common requirement to stop unhealthy actions is acceptance of the Three Refuges: the Buddha, the Dharma (his teaching), and the Saṅgha (the monastery). Common to all Buddhists, monastics and lay, but created especially for the lay person, are the five precepts, which include not taking life, not stealing, not committing adultery, not lying, and not consuming intoxicants. The list of five is sometimes extended to ten common prohibitions as a temporary observance on holy days: "not killing, stealing, or fornicating; not lying, slandering, speaking harshly, or chattering frivolously; and

not having covetous thoughts, hostile thoughts, or false views" (Robinson and Johnson [1970] 1977, 98; see also Keown 1992, 31).

These negatively expressed precepts are the foundation for Buddhist ethics. This is indicated by the Sanskrit term *śīla* (Pāli *sīla*) when they are formally taken as vows. *Śīla* means moral precept, morality, ethics and good conduct. Precepts can also be expressed positively as virtues (a common translation of *śīla* is wholesome and good states), which strengthen character, provide good habits that help root out bad ones, and contribute to human happiness and flourishing (similar to Aristotelian ethics according to Keown 1992, 193–227 and Harvey 2000, 50). In Theravāda, one becomes a monastic if one seriously desires to pursue the Path in this lifetime. Because it was necessary to regulate monastic life and the relation of the monastery to the society at large, there are approximately 200 special rules for monks (and even more for nuns) (Tsomo 1996, 21). In the Pāli Canon account, codified at the First Council, and collectively called the *Paṭimokkha*, these rules, classified by the degree of severity of offense, define the standards of conduct and are to be followed punctiliously. Infractions are to be confessed monthly in a communal context, the four most serious ones, such as *intent* to kill, which *causes* death, result in expulsion from the Saṅgha. This places emphasis on both the intention and the consequence: the intention to kill that does not result in a death is not as serious an infraction as one that does (see Chapter 4). Many of the rules had developed out of specific problems that arose in the monastic community, some during the lifetime of the Buddha. These contextually derived rules developed in a manner not unlike casuistry in the West.

In Buddhism ethics is not for its own sake, but is an essential aspect of the path to the final goal of enlightenment (which makes Buddhist ethics teleological). "All the factors of the Eightfold Path, for example, are seen as 'wholesome'" (Harvey 2000, 48–49). Ethics is therefore a necessary but not sufficient condition for enlightenment. "That which is 'wholesome' or 'unwholesome,' then, goes beyond the purely moral/immoral to include states of mind, which may have no direct effect on other people" (Harvey 2000, 48–49). Harvey suggests that Buddhist ethics consists of removing moral defilements by removing their motivations and cultivating counteractive virtues. He calls this ethic a moral objectivism because some actions are categorically wrong (such as harming another sentient being). We all have an innate, natural sympathy for the sufferings of others; when we identify with the suffering of others, this reduces it, leading to happiness. Because there is no substantial, permanent Self, selfish actions do not accord with reality (Harvey 2000, 58–59). Keown makes the same point, arguing that it aligns with the Buddha's empiricism and is based on criteria to assess "rightness and wrongness independently of subjective moral perception or preference" (Keown 1992, 232).

The Theravāda path therefore goes beyond external conduct to interiorization (understood as removal of the impediments to liberation and eventually liberation from the cycles of existence. In the Pāli text *Visuddhi-magga* I:10, Buddhaghosa says that the beginning of the path is characterized by *sīla*, which brings about special qualities such as nonremorse; the middle of the path by concentration, which brings about special qualities of supernormal power, and the end of the path by understanding and equipoise with respect to the desired and the undesired (Ñāṇamoli trans., *Visuddhimagga* 1956, 5). Elsewhere, he says that *sīla* is restraint by following the rules of the monastery and by mindfulness, knowledge, patience, and energy. It is the practice of duties. The consistency of the rules is a support for the profitable states (Ñāṇamoli trans., *Visuddhimagga* 1956, 7–8). Buddhaghosa's *Visuddhimagga* not only speaks of adherence to precepts (*sīla*), it also promotes four sublime virtues (*brahmavihāras*), three of which focus specifically on other people: friendliness (*mettā*), compassion (*karuṇā*; Skt. *karuṇā*), and sympathetic joy (*muditā*). Ultimately, *nibbāna* (Skt. *nirvāṇa*) involves the dissolution of the concept of self and other. Keown argues that morality and wisdom constitute the primary dimensions of perfection with meditation providing the impetus for their full development (Keown 1992, 55); with enlightenment, therefore, there is the spontaneous expression of morality (but, once again, there is the other Buddhist view that sees morality as merely the means to enlightenment, not constitutive of it).

David Little and Sumner Twiss agree on the teleological nature of Buddhist ethics. Because enlightenment is the teleological goal of Buddhism, ethics is ultimately religious, a way to overcome the hindrances that constitute bondage: "Accordingly, the system of action-guides is hierarchic and progressive. Acts appear to be arranged, understood, and evaluated in reference to a pattern of increasing and cumulative efficacy for realizing self-conquest. (It is, of course possible to break through to insight at any stage of the system)" (Little and Twiss 1978, 215).

The individual orientation to enlightenment in Theravāda culminates in the ideal type of person called the *arhat* (Skt. *arhat*), a monastic who achieves salvation in this life. Although later called selfish by the Mahāyānists, the *arhat*s were not so self-centered as often decried. Implicit in the very idea of interdependence (*paticca-samuppāda*; Skt. *pratītya-samutpāda*), after all, is the idea of mutual support, cooperation, and responsibility.

The first Theravāda text that focused on the laity was the *Sigalovāda-sutta*, belonging to the *Dīgha-nikāya* of the Pāli Canon. It describes the importance of good friends and reciprocity among the social classes. In the history of Buddhism, however, lay life has been largely ignored, the specifics of family life being left to the customs of the prevailing culture, for example, the Hindu concept of *viśeṣa-dharma* defined by "place" with its many variables, such as caste (see Chapters 3, 9). (There were some differences, however; the Buddha considered the *kṣatriya*s the highest caste, not the *brāhmaṇa*s, and appealed to the trading or *vaiśya* caste as well.)

In the canon, enlightenment is called the absence of illness, the secularist a patient, and the ignorant a blind man (*Majjhima-nikāya* I.510 cited by Demiéville 1985, 12). The analogy between Buddhism and medicine is sometimes extended to ethics as in the *Milindapañha*: "One who is moral, sire, possessed of moral habit, is like an antidote for destroying the poison of the defilements in beings; he is like a healing balm for allaying the sickness of the defilements in beings" (Horner trans., *Milindapañha* [1963–1964] 1969–1990, 195).

The Pāli Canon describes the need to care for fellow monastics and provide them with medications. Illness is viewed as the normal condition of the body, which always needs medical attention to make life itself possible. The *Mahāvagga* describes, for instance, how wandering monks and nuns have medicines such as cow's urine as antidote for snakebites (*Mahāvagga* 1.30.4.77, 6.14.6; cited by Zysk 1991, 145). The text also describes how the Buddha came upon a sick monk, who had fallen in his own feces and was ignored by other monks. On this occasion, the Buddha instituted the rule: "You, O *bhikkhū*s [Skt. *bhikṣu*], have neither a mother nor a father who could nurse you. If, O *bhikkhū*s, you do not nurse one another, who, then, will nurse you? Whoever, O *bhikkhū*s, would nurse me, he should nurse the sick" (*Mahāvagga* 8.26.3 cited by Zysk 1991, 41). According to the *Mahāvagga*, some monks at Sāvatthi were unable to retain the food they had eaten and gradually became emaciated. The Buddha sanctioned clarified butter, fresh butter, oil, honey, and molasses to be consumed (*Mahāvagga* 6.1.1–5 cited by Zysk 1991, 74–75). When there was no improvement, he said that these substances could be eaten at any time. To make them available, they could be stored up to 7 days. They were not classified as food but rather as medicine. (This circumvented the basic rule that forbade monastics from eating food between noon and sunrise.) These passages could well be early (see Chapter 20). They speak to the need to care for sick monks and nuns and mention some basic medicines for which monastics begged. Sometimes laywomen called on sick nuns and offered medicines for both monks and nuns (an act of piety for which they received merit) (Horner 1930, cited by Zysk 1991, 43 and 146 n. 33).

Some *Vinaya* passages are much more elaborate and suggest that an empirical medicine had already been developed by the time the canon was closed (first century BCE) (see Chapter 20). Medicines were classified into five categories: fats, types of roots, extracts (from trees), leaves, fruits, gums or resins, and salts. Fats, moreover, were enumerated as five types of animal fat (that of bears, fish, alligators, swine, and donkeys) to be mixed with oil (*tela*) and taken as medicines before meals. Because Theravāda monastics were allowed to eat meat, although they were prohibited themselves from killing animals, medicines made from animal products were not an anomaly. (See Zysk 1991, 76–83 for details.) The *Vinaya* gives specific cases of medical problems that were experienced by particular monastics and their treatment. This casuistry follows the general manner by which monastic rules were formulated. For instance, a certain monk suffered from a skin problem (large oozing sores). We are told that when this came to the Buddha's attention, he recommended a treatment consisting of a medicinal powder. There are similar accounts for eye diseases, problems caused by heat that affect the head, so-called wind diseases, problems caused by split skin on the soles of feet, swellings, snakebite, poisonous drinks, digestive and abdominal problems, jaundice, fevers, and rectal fistulae. Treatments include enemas, bloodletting, cauterization, sucking, plasters, tourniquets, scarification, and so forth.

The canon also refers to public health. Dispensaries are to be placed outside the city core to prevent the spread of epidemics. Town planners are to segregate people who worked in unclean occupations, privies are to be constructed with cesspools in the monasteries, urinals are to have lids, and bathrooms are to be kept clean (Haldar 1992, 33–46). People are to avoid contact by not sharing dishes, drinking vessels, beds, and so forth, and feet are to be washed when entering from the outside (Haldar 1992, 54–55 for references).

Over time medicines and treatments expanded and were further classified. The texts, for instance, mention a large pharmacopoeia (*Sutta-vibhaṅga* IV.1.1, *Saṅgiti-suttānta Dīgha-nikāya* III.268, *Sutta-nipāta* IV.288, 291, and *Niddessa* II.523 cited by Zysk 1991, 40 and 146 n. 11). (See also Haldar 1977, 48–49 for mention of ninety-eight diseases in the *Milindapañha* and thirty-four in the *Aṅguttara-nikāya* and *Niddessa* as well as the ingredients of medicines in the *Mahavāgga Khaṇḍaka* 6.) In short, a detailed knowledge of empirical medicine (pharmacopoeia that was precisely classified) and medical problems of particular monastics and their treatment as a kind of casuistry had entered the monastery or had developed there (see Haldar 1992, 32).

With empirical medicine, a new etiology of disease develops. Buddhist texts allude to the beginning of the theory of the three humors (see Chapters 10, 20). The term "humor" implies a relationship with, or even dependence on, Greek humors; such a relationship is doubtful, however, in the current state of scholarship (Scharfe 1999, 612; Zysk 1991, 29). The Buddhist view of the physical world consists of three or four elements (*bhūta* or *dhātu*). Later texts interpreted these as the lubricating and cooling

phlegm (*kalpha*) located mainly in the upper part of the body, the digesting and transformative bile (*pitta*), located mainly in the midregion, and the circulating wind (*vāyu*) of nutrition and wastes, located mainly in the lower part. The concept of the three *doṣas* (faults) was added after the Canon to this (Demiéville 1985, 65; see also 6, 13, 79) (see Chapter 10 for a discussion of the faults).

The Four Noble Truths are described as the four principles of medicine: cause (*hetu*), symptom (*liṅga*), cure (*prasamana*), and nonrecurrence (*apunarbhava*). Because these four principles are found nowhere in classical Āyurvedic texts, Zysk argues that this is a Buddhist innovation (1991, 38). (For a debate over this interpretation, see Demiéville 1985, 13.) Asaṅga (c. fourth century) in the *Yogācārabhūmi-śāstra* defines medical science (*cikitsā*) as a category between internal science (*adhyātma*) and logic (*hetu*); here the four principles are mentioned in strictly medical terms (see also the *Bodhisattvabhūmi* cited by Demiéville 1985, 13). From one perspective, Buddhists view the body as an invalid with nine wounds (the body orifices such as the ears, nostrils, mouth, and so forth), which is why it suffers (*Mahāparinirvāṇa-sūtra* T 375: 30:741c[2], cited by Demiéville 1985, 18). The nine wounds are said to be created by poisoned arrows (greed, hatred, and delusion, which cause suffering). This metaphor comes from a story about how a hunter had been hit with a poisoned arrow. Just as it had to be pulled out immediately to prevent the spread of the poison, so people should look for immediate cures – the Buddha's Four Noble Truths – for the "poison" of existence. (For texts that compare human sufferings to the wounds caused by "poisoned arrows" see Demiéville 1985, 15.) (The concept of "poisoned arrows" might ultimately go back to the Vedic deity Rudra who sends disease with his poisoned arrows, see Chapter 10.) Like Hindus, Buddhists think that one needs a healthy body to pursue the Four Noble Truths and thereby to cross *saṃsāra*. This connected medicine and religion.

Beginning in the Pāli Canon, an extensive analogy is developed between Buddhism and medicine. The Buddha is described as the great physician (see *Sutta-nipāta* III.7.13; *Majjhima-nikāya* I.429; *Sumaṅgala-vilāsini* 67.255; and Horner trans., *Milindapañha* 1963, 169). Nāgasena in the *Milindapañha* makes a number of explicit analogies between Buddhism and medicine when he answers the questions of Milinda (Menander, a Greek in the court of Candragupta Maurya of the fourth century BCE). Just as when patients are cured of their malady by consumption of the five medicines made from roots and need not take them again, so too right understanding of the five controlling faculties (faith, energy, mindfulness, concentration, and wisdom) cures the spiritual malady for ever (Horner trans., *Milindapañha* [1963–1964] 1969–1990, 43).

Buddhism places emphasis on the root causes of the wheel of existence because by eliminating them, one eliminates rebirth forever. Enlightenment is the permanent cure for the affliction of life. Similarly, just as patients are to be blamed if they go to a physician skilled in diagnosis and efficacious medicines but they do not "follow doctor's orders" and do not let themselves be treated, just so people are to be blamed it they go to the Tathāgata (Buddha) who has the ambrosial medicine (that is, enlightenment) which is able to entirely suppress all the sickness of sin, but do not drink it (Horner trans., *Milindapañha* [1963–1964] 1969–1990, 247). In other words, just as a good medical patient must take the medicine prescribed by the physician, so too the spiritual patient must take the spiritual medicine prescribed by the Buddha to eliminate the disease of existence.

This idea is elaborated. The disposition to an evil character is analogous to the consumption of poison. The Four Noble Truths are its antidote and will free people from the cycles of rebirth: "And whosoever, longing for the highest insight (the insight of Arahatship), hear this doctrine of the four truths, they are set quite free from rebirth, they are set quite free from old age, they are set quite free from death, they are set quite free from grief, lamentation, pain, sorrow, and despair" (Horner trans., *Milindapañha* [1963–1964] 1969–1990, 334). In another passage, the Buddha's medicines by which he cures the whole world of gods and men are described as the means of mindfulness, morality, wisdom, and the path which are like an emetic that purges the body from lusts, malice, dullness, doubt, self-righteousness, sloth of the body, inertness of the mind, shamelessness, hardness of heart, and all evil (Horner trans., *Milindapañha* [1963–1964] 1969–1990, 335).

The relationship of religion to medicine is summed up in the question of whether the Pirit ritual (not mentioned in the canon but found in the *Milindapañha*) should be used for the sick. Nāgasena replied that this ritual is not for those whose allotted span of life has come to an end (because medicine is useless in these cases) but only for those who still have a phase of life remaining, who are mature, and who restrain themselves from bad karma. Nāgasena then observes that the ritual can be effective to decrease or categorically reverse diseases just as medicine can be, but will work only for those who have faith and are without sin and bad karma (cited by Kitagawa 1989, 20). In short, this is a Buddhist defense of faith healing, not as a substitute for medicine but as its complement in cases of nonterminal illness.

III. MAHĀYĀNA BUDDHISM

Mahāyāna (the Great Vehicle) Buddhism became popular between 100 BCE and 400. The Mahāsaṅghika sect paved the way by placing emphasis more on the spirit than the letter of the rules; promoting the idea of the illusoriness (*māyā*) or emptiness (*śūnyatā*) of all phenomena;

suggesting that the real Buddha is transmundane (Gautama of the Śakyas being but an apparition); and viewing the *bodhisattva* as the ideal person. All this contributed to a new genre of literature, the Mahāyāna Sūtras, the source of which was attributed to the Buddha's inspiration infused into the minds of later day disciples.

The distinctive approach of Mahāyāna ethics (*śīla*) is embodied in the concept of the *bodhisattva* who vows not to attain final enlightenment until all sentient beings are saved. The *bodhisattva* path includes the six perfections (*pāramitās*). The first is giving (*dāna*) and consists of giving material things and spiritual instruction out of compassion and concern for the welfare of others. All the merit attained from such generosity is transferred to other beings, moreover, to help them solve their daily problems and to progress to enlightenment. The other perfections – morality, patience, courage, meditation, and wisdom – are described in a similar manner. There is "a new emphasis on the function of moral virtue as a dynamic other-regarding quality," rather than as a concern "with personal development and self-control" (Keown 1992, 131). The perfection of the *pāramitās* is doing an act (such as giving) without self-consciousness, pride, or ulterior motives such as reward. In one sense, ethics is no longer instrumental to salvation; giving without thought of liberation and compassion for all are penultimate to liberation. The *bodhisattva* toward the end of the path is beyond the dictates of karma but will be in this prefinal-enlightenment state until *all* sentient creatures achieve salvation. This type of *bodhisattva* is sometimes called a celestial bodhisattva.

Whereas Theravāda has balanced emphasis on intent and consequence in judging infractions of monastic rules, Mahāyāna ostensibly emphasizes consequence at the everyday level: any act seems to be permissible as long as it contributes to the salvation of a sentient being. The quantification of sentient beings to be saved (remember, the *bodhisattva* must vow to save *all* others) brings this focus on results, their maximization, and the efficiency of the process close to the modern idea of utilitarianism. Here too it is the spiritual goal (rather than the pursuit of mundane happiness or pleasure) based on the idea of radical altruism (supererogation) that makes the Mahāyāna idea of ethics distinctive and prevents it from falling into the perspective of utilitarianism.

More specifically, *bodhisattva*s are to practice skill-in-means (*upāya*) to bring every sentient creature to liberation. Out of their compassion they respond to needs of the laity by any method, even if that means reversing ordinary norms. This idea has been interpreted in various ways. According to Arvind Sharma, the concept of skill-in-means allows Mahāyāna Buddhists to "resort to a useful fiction if its moral effects are salutary. Thus to the extent that belief in God, even if it be philosophically a false belief, helps people lead a morally useful life it could be considered justifiable. The criterion has no doubt shifted from one of truth to that of value but it is useful to bear in mind that such a shift is acceptable within Buddhism" (Sharma 1995, 36–37). Others are more cautious in their interpretation of the Mahāyāna concept of *upāya*. Keown attributes the antinomianism of some passages to "a symbolic as opposed to normative statement" (Keown 1992, 159), which is confined to the last four perfections. He argues that although flexibility is introduced by dividing the precepts into serious and minor ones (which need not be observed so carefully), this shift of emphasis should be treated cautiously, for there are other passages to the contrary and there are limits on the *bodhisattvas'* behavior because they must be vigilant in their moral perfection and must act for the welfare of others. Finally, he thinks that although the concept of *upāya* has some structural similarities to modern situational ethics. This interpretation was not accepted by most Buddhists because there remained a sense of objective wrong beyond compassion and skill-in-means. "The texts which adopt this position therefore underline the importance of altruism and supererogation while still reserving a deontological basis for moral validation" (Keown 1992, 191). Harvey observes that the antinomian tradition was central to Indian Tantra, which on the Buddhist side developed into Vajrayāna and therefore cannot be dismissed quite so easily (Harvey 2000, 141–2).

Theoretical discussions on the nature of Buddhist ethics aside, the *bodhisattva* ideal permeated both society and spiritual imagination. There were ordination rites for human, lay *bodhisattvas*, and loose-knit fraternities for them. Some were human teachers. Some such as Avalokiteśvara, Mañjuśri, Mahāstamaprāpta, and Maitreya were (and still are) celestial figures. (According to the Mahāyāna Sūtras, they were present when the Sūtras were given by the Buddha.) By the third century, they had become cult figures who could manifest themselves anywhere and could answer the prayers of people, respond to their confession of sins, and help them attain rebirth in a paradise, especially when their names were chanted. In short, with the idea of the transfer of merit, the law of karma was pushed to the margin and compassionate figures helped the laity to fulfill both mundane and supramundane desires. If celestial *bodhisattvas* now seemed to be too much like Hindu deities, the very concept could be deconstructed by the more philosophically minded by the idea that all concepts are ultimately empty. In some Mahāyāna texts, the Buddha is called a great king of physicians (*Samyuktāgama* T 99:15:105a–b, cited by Demiéville 1985, 9). A text of the Kṣyapiya school (a late branch of the Sarvāstivāda), preserved from the Chinese Ch'in dynasty (350–431 CE), states that "mundane physicians have expertise in the body, children, eyes, and 'poisoned arrows' and the Tathāgata (Buddha) surpasses these because 'he understands how to cut off the cataract . . . of ignorance with the iron of wisdom' and so

forth, thereby going beyond the physical to the three fundamental passions or defilements, which are the person's most serious illness" (Demiéville 1985, 10). The title "king of physicians/medicine" (*vaidarāja*) also became for Mahāyāna Buddhists an epithet of other *buddhas*, especially Bhaṣagyaguru, "'master of medicaments,' whose 'fundamental resolve' (*mūla-praṇidhāna*) was to be healer of the sick" (Demiéville 1985, 14 for T 276:384c; T 159:8:330b and so forth). The title was applied to *bodhisattvas* as well.

Like Theravāda texts, Mahāyāna ones made analogies between the Four Noble Truths of Buddhism and the four principles of medicine: cause (*hetu*), symptom (*liṅga*), cure (*prasamaṇa*), and nonrecurrence (*apunarbhava*). Asvaghoṣa (first century CE) in *Saundarananda* (16:41) says: "Therefore in the first Truth think of suffering as disease, in the second of the faults as the cause of disease, in the third of the destruction of suffering as good health and in the fourth of the path as the medicine" (Demiéville 1985, 9). There is a different version of this idea in the tenth century text the *Sūtra of the Medical Comparison* (T 219, *Bhiṣajupamāna-sūtra* K1446) of the Chinese Canon (cited by Demiéville 1985, 10). According to the *Udānavarga*, religious therapies include recitation of Buddhist texts (for demoniac illnesses) and worship of saints, deities, works of charity, and destruction of the aggregates (*skandhas*) by wisdom (T 211:2:579a–b cited by Demiéville 1985).

One of the problems raised by the view of the body as the locus of suffering was whether *buddhas*, *arhats*, and *bodhisattvas* suffer pain. Because they are enlightened, they are ostensibly beyond it (and yet their suffering, especially in the throes of death, had no doubt been witnessed). This problem had helped split the Saṅgha into proto-Mahāyāna (Mahāsaṅgika) and proto-Theravāda (Sthavīravāda) sects. The Pāli Canon had accounted for the various ailments of Gautama Buddha – backaches, foot wounds, headaches, and finally physical death from bad pork – by saying that these resulted from unspent past karma, which maintained the existence of his body and its ills. Much the same argument was made for *arhats*; with enlightenment they were free of mental but not physical suffering. In Mahāyāna texts, with the development of the doctrine of the *trikāya* (three bodies) of the Buddha, physical suffering is attributed only to the *nirmāṇakāya* (the body of birth, aging, and death), whereas the supreme or essential body (*dharmakāya*) is eternal, pure, and removed from birth, aging, and death. Sometimes even the physical suffering of the *nirmāṇakāya* buddhas and the *bodhisattvas* is said also to be only apparent and is skill-in-means (*upāya*) to lead people to enlightenment (*Vimalakīrtinirdeśa-sūtra* T 475:2 and so forth cited by Demiéville 1985, 25–26).

The *Vimalakīrtinirdeśa-sūtra*, for instance, describes how the wealthy householder Vimalakīrti uses his illness to teach his lay visitors the difference between the ordinary suffering body of human beings born from craving (*tṛṣṇa*) due to ignorance and the Buddha's essential body. *Bodhisattva*s, who love sentient beings as their own sons, and have great compassion, so identify with the latter's illnesses that they too become as if ill. Their illnesses, however, really do not exist (and neither would those of the laity if they could eliminate wrong ideas and passions and understand the real nature of emptiness). It is argued that the supramundane body of the Buddha is necessary to eliminate the criticism of the (Hindu) *brāhmaṇa*s and others, who might point to the Buddha's inability to cure his own body. (These arguments were developed in an extensive commentary on this text by the founder of the Chinese T'ien-t'ai sect, Chih-I.)

The Pāli Canon had described miraculous cures when the Buddha touched the head or wound of a patient. This idea is expanded in Mahāyāna so that *bodhisattva*s give their very body as medicine. Sometimes the body of a *buddha* or *bodhisattva* is compared to a tree of medicine or even to a human sacrifice: "all those who were ill – in seeing him, in smelling him or in touching him, or in consuming his skin, his blood, his flesh, his bone, or his marrow – were healed of all illness" (*Upāsakaśīla-sūtra* T 1488:2:1042a cited by Demiéville 1985, 47; see also *Avataṃsaka* Bdjt 1752c and *Mahāparinirvāṇa-sūtra* T 375:30:804a for images of the tree of medicine.)

Medicine came with Buddhism to China via Central Asia in the first several centuries of the Common Era (see Demiéville 1985, 50ff, for physician monks in China and their miraculous cures). It has been argued that even though the Chinese had their own sophisticated medicine, their deep interest in the topics of healing and longevity and their perception that the Buddhist monks had important, if not superior, theories, techniques, and medicines led to an interest in Buddhism and contributed to its spread (Birnbaum 1989, 34–35). Many Indian texts with medical information, such as the *Suvarṇaprabhāsa-sūtra*, the *Saddharmapuṇḍarīka-sūtra*, and what has been called the Bower Manuscript (discovered in 1890 and dating from the fourth to sixth century CE) were translated into Chinese (see Zysk 1991, 67 for additional texts). Mahāyāna made the professional study of medicine (along with grammar, arts, logic, and spiritual philosophy) a general topic in Indian Buddhist universities, such as Nālandā, according to Chinese pilgrims such as I-Ching and Hsuan Tsang (Haldar 1992, 50ff).

During the medieval period, the care of the ill was accompanied by the building of hospitals. There is only one reference in the Pāli Canon to a sick room (*gilānasālā*) in the monastery (*Suttanipāta* IV.210–13, cited by Zysk 1991, 147 n. 40) and only one in the *Mūlasarvāstivāda* (T 1451:17:283a–b cited by Demi, ville 1985, 54). By the seventh century, the Chinese pilgrim to India Hsuan-tsang reported that there were distribution halls for food and medicine for the poor (called *puṇyaśāla* or *dharmaśāla*) (Demiéville 1985, 57). Kings and rich laity were to protect

people (sometimes the indigent, widows, and orphans are singled out) by supporting hospitals. According to the *Cūlavaṃsa*, some kings had knowledge of medicine themselves (*Cūlavaṃsa* chap. 73, cited by Haldar 1992, 26–27; see also Demi, ville 1985, 36). This is supported by inscriptional evidence in India and Sri Lanka (Haldar 1992, 82–87).

In this period there was considerable competition to Buddhism from Hindu *bhakti* (devotional) movements that popularized the religion with temple worship, concepts of the grace of a personal deity who fulfilled all desires, and access to medicine with the building of hospitals (see Chapter 10). Together with the advance of Islam, this contributed to Buddhism dying out in the land of its birth. In the meantime, however, its Vajrayāna tradition had been transplanted to Tibet.

IV. VAJRAYĀNA BUDDHISM

From approximately 600, yet another development occurred in Indian Buddhism, which would have influence throughout Tibet and the Far East: Buddhist Tantra or Vajrayāna. Like Mahāyāna (which continued to flourish in this period), it too furthered some already existing aspects of Buddhism. Magical spells, present in the Pāli Canon to protect against snakebite and other harms, were elaborated, for instance, into magically efficacious sounds (*mantras*). In addition, visual diagrams for meditation and theophany (*yantras; maṇḍalas*) became popular. Some of these religious practices were correlated in turn with parts of the human body (the microcosm) and the Buddhist cosmology (the macrocosm). Key practices included a way to destroy the passions through the passions (for example, by illicit sexual intercourse, drinking wine, or eating meat) all under the guidance of a preceptor to achieve the Tantric ideal of the *siddha* or accomplished one, a kind of wizard-saint, presumably beyond the categories of monastery and laity, morality and immorality. (Once again, scholars differ on whether the reversal motifs are to be taken literally or symbolically; the former aligning with the instrumental view of ethics, the latter with the view that ethics is intrinsic to both means and goal.)

There seems to have been little influence of Chinese medicine on Indian medicine. There was influence of Chinese medicine, however, on Tibetan medicine (Demiéville 1985, 93–94). According to I-Ching, a Chinese pilgrim to India in the seventh century, Chinese medicine was distinguished for its drugs of longevity, arts of acupuncture, skills of cauterization, and diagnosis by pulse.

The development of medicine in Tibet has been described by Ian Baker (1997). Its introduction there is traced to the seventh-century king, Songtsen Gampo. According to the Tibetan chronicles, he invited Indian, Chinese, and Iranian physicians to his court. Many medical texts, such as the Indian text by *Vāgbhaṇa*, were then translated into Tibetan. This continued under the patronage of King Trisongdetsen (eighth century), who consulted with physicians from many countries. According to tradition, in the eleventh century the *Four Tantras* of the medicine Buddha Bhaiṣajyaguru (consisting of 5,900 verses), which had been hidden in a monastery (a common origin myth for manuscripts) were found. They were subsequently revised by integrating local shamanic healing traditions together with Indian Āyurvedic traditions (pharmacopoeia, and so forth) and Chinese pulse diagnoses and acupuncture. In 1696, a hospital and medical college (Chagpori Medical College) were established in Lhasa. At this time the *Vaidurya Ngonpo (Blue Beryl)*, a commentary on the *Four Tantras* by Sangye Gyamtso, was composed. According to the *Blue Beryl*, therapies include magical plants (such as the fungus *amanita muscaria*) or alchemical ingredients such as mercury. The *Blue Beryl* was illustrated by thousands of paintings. Although these (along with the college) were destroyed in 1959 with the Chinese takeover, replicas (consisting of thousands of illustrations of physiology, health, and disease, the latter consisting of 404 illnesses and 84,000 afflictions, of the human body) have been preserved in the Mentsekhang medical college, which had been established in Lhasa in 1916. The Mentsekhang still operates (albeit under Communist ideology). The Chagpori tradition has been rebuilt in exile (Darjeeling, India), and the Institute of Tibetan Medicine has been founded in Dharmasala (Himachal Pradesh, India), where the exile government is located.

Tibetan physicians apply the Buddhist ideals of wisdom and compassion to the physical, emotional, and spiritual needs of their patients, and to their own spiritual practices. For instance, they visualize themselves in the form of the Medicine Buddha and invoke his presence, saying "As all sentient beings, infinite as space, are encompassed by the compassion of the Master of Remedies, may I too become their guide . . . May I quickly attain the healing powers of the Medicine Buddha, Bhaishajyaguru, and lead all beings into his enlightened realm" (Baker 1997, 32–33). The *bodhisattva* ideal has become the ordinary physician's ideal.

This is taken one step further. As in other Mahāyāna texts, disease is considered important for awakening a person to the workings of the mind and its bad habits that can cause disease. The texts describe practices, such as meditation on the breath, in which one inhales the suffering of all humanity and exhales one's own well-being. Even when in pain, taking on the sufferings of others in this way diminishes one's own suffering (Baker 1997, 69). This passage suggests that now *everyone*, not just the *bodhisattva*s and physicians, can be healers.

Tibetan medicine focuses on spirit possession (a tradition going back to pre-Buddhist shamanism). Although Tibetan Buddhists claim that ultimately demons are but mental projections or empty of real being, they must be taken seriously because they arise through imbalance of the humors, affecting even dreams, and can be cured through various kinds of therapies. Religious therapies, they say, have longer lasting results than merely medical ones. In the Tibetan context, the human body becomes the positive vehicle for enlightenment. Purified and transformed through alchemical processes, it becomes the inner *maṇḍala* of wisdom and compassion.

V. THE MODERN PERIOD

Most Asian countries have been deeply affected by colonialism and have struggled with issues of political independence and identity as a result. This has affected ethics as well. Westerners, both on religious and secular bases, have often claimed that Asian religions have no real ethics, that the religions are other-worldly, that they are materially poor, lacking in scientific and technological developments, and that they have no "social gospel." To reply to this charge, Buddhism in the last half of the twentieth century has developed a movement called Socially Engaged Buddhism, and this has profoundly influenced reflection on ethics (see Chapter 44). In connection with international organizations and Western countries, there have been collaborative projects to improve medical ethics in developing nations (see Chapter 44 for this and for a discussion of Buddhist reflections on the four principles of bioethics – nonmaleficence, beneficence, autonomy, and justice).

VI. CONCLUSION

This chapter has examined the place of ethics within the general Buddhist world view (a soteriological orientation). There are differences within Buddhist ethics based on Buddhism's three major traditions – Theravāda, Mahāyāna, and Vajrayāna – and how they view the relation between religion and medicine. In addition, there are differences in modern scholarship based on whether Buddhist ethics is viewed as limited to the means (and therefore but instrumental) or intrinsic to both the means and the goal.

Theravāda ethics (largely a monastic orientation) as reflected in the Pāli Canon drew on the story of the Buddha's experience of seeing a sick person, an old person, a dead person, and an ascetic, which sparked his spiritual quest and his subsequent teachings about the Four Noble Truths, the wheel of causality/interdependence, the law of karma, the doctrine of soullessness, concepts of skillful and unskillful actions, the moral precepts, and the Eight-fold Path. The focus was on personal quest and individual enlightenment, the *arhat* being the ideal person. Analogies with medicine were common: illness is the normal condition of the body within samsāra, the Buddha is the great physician, Buddhist teachings are the medicine, and enlightenment is the absence of illness. In addition, there was practical information about medicine: monks and nuns had to be cared for within the monastery (this led to an interest in empirical medicine) but this had to be done in a way that monastic rules were not broken.

By contrast, Mahāyāna ethics crystallized around the concept of the *bodhisattva* who vows to save all living creatures and whose path focuses on generosity and compassion – a radical altruism, transfer of merit, and skill-in-means, which has been understood either literally as "anything goes if it helps" or symbolically as the consummate gift. In addition, some Mahāyāna passages focus on results, maximization, and efficiency. In other words, the antinomian passages of Mahāyāna and Vajrayāna are interpreted literally by those scholars who view ethics as but instrumental. This has led to some modern scholars interpreting them within the Western framework of utilitarianism or situational ethics. Others, however, under-stand these passages symbolically because they think that ethics is intrinsic to both the means and the goal and view them still within the broad frame of virtue ethics. Both interpretations include them within a teleology.

NOTE

1. In the literature on Buddhism, Sanskrit terms are often considered standard; they will be used here when discussing Buddhism as a whole. In the context of specific discussion on Theravāda Buddhism or the Pāli Canon, Pāli terms will be used and the Sanskrit equivalent for common ones will be provided at their first occurrence. In all primary source citations in the format "T 156," "T" is to be understood as referring to the Taish catalogue of Chinese Buddhist texts (which include translations of Indian Buddhist texts).

CHAPTER 11

THE DISCOURSES OF CONFUCIAN MEDICAL ETHICS

Ruiping Fan

I. INTRODUCTION: THE CONFUCIAN VIEW OF MEDICINE: THE ART OF *REN*[1] (HUMANITY)

1. The Traditional Chinese Understanding of Health and Disease

The beginning of Chinese medicine is generally attributed to Shen Nong (the Heavenly Husbandman), a legendary emperor who, living circa 2700 BCE, introduced agriculture and had personally tasted the hundred types of plants to discover their medicinal values. He is also supposed to have introduced the technique of acupuncture; however, he does not figure in the story of the cardinal classic of Chinese medicine, *Huang Di Nei Jing* (The Yellow Emperor's Internal Medicine).[2] This work features Huang Di, the Yellow Emperor, who is believed to have lived at the same time as Shen Nong and was, a legendary emperor revered by both Confucians and Daoists (Qian 1987).

The Yellow Emperor's Internal Medicine was most probably compiled during the Eastern Han dynasty (25–220) (Liao 1993, 55–80). It includes the most distinguished texts of ancient Chinese medicine, integrates and theorizes various healing arts, and sets down the foundational principles of Chinese learned medicine and its written traditions. It shares the same Chinese concept of the universe

as philosophy, science, politics, and indeed nearly everything else traditionally Chinese (Ho and Lisowski 1997, 17). First, it can be understood as offering a particular metaphysics of *qi*[3] as the basic elements of the universe. *Qi* is difficult to translate. In this view, the whole universe is ultimately a field of *qi* in which there is not a personal god out there to create, preserve, and regulate the universe and human beings. Instead, it is an incessant process of the transformation and development of *qi* that comprises the myriad things as well as their changes in the world. *Qi* should be understood as both material and spiritual; it is becoming rather than being. "Every part of the human body, especially the nine orifices (ears, eyes, nostrils, mouth, anus, and urethra), the five organs (kidneys, liver, heart, spleen, and lungs), and the twelve joints (elbows, wrists, knees, ankles, shoulders, and hips) are all the crucial conduits open to the *qi* of the universe" (*The Yellow Emperor's Internal Medicine*, Chap. 2). Moreover, the law of the two basic types of *qi*, *yin* and *yang*, governs everything in the universe, including heaven, earth, and human, the so-called three forces (*san-cai*). A harmonious cooperation between *yin* and *yang* in all things of the universe is the requirement of the law. "Huang Di said: 'the law of *yin* and *yang* is the *dao*[4] (way) of the universe, the foundation of all things, the mother of all changes, and the root of life and death." In healing, one must grasp the root of the disharmony, which is always subject to the law of *yin* and *yang*. In addition, the universal *yin* and *yang* transform into the five earthly transformative energies, also known as "five agents" or "five phases" (*wu-xing*), namely, metal, wood, water, fire, and earth. Through these doctrines of *yin-yang* and five phases, Chinese medicine holds a magical unity of nature: the structure of the human organism and the functions assigned to its individual parts reflect a systematic correspondence to the complex mechanisms of various parts of the universe, especially heaven and earth (Unschuld 1985, 51–100).

These views generated the particular Chinese conceptions of health and disease as well as set down the bases of Chinese etiology and therapeutics. Thus, in Chinese medicine, health is understood to be the harmonious state of the bodily *qi* in response to the *dao* of *yin-yang* and five phases. Disease is an imbalanced state of the bodily *qi* due to the violation, obstruction, or frustration of the *dao*. In particular, the Chinese etiology lists seven endogenous (mental) factors (delight, anger, sadness, pleasure, grief, fear, and fright) and six exogenous factors (wind, cold, heat, humidity, dryness, and fire) as the most common causes of diseases. These factors are not disease entities. Rather, they exist as the natural modalities of *qi* in both the cosmos and the human body. Only when any of them becomes excessive or insufficient (thus becoming "evil *qi*") in the human body and thus breaks the balance of the bodily *qi*, can a health problem or disease occur. Accordingly, the goal of Chinese diagnosis is to find the principal imbalance of these factors through a series of medical techniques, especially the four important Chinese diagnostic observations (*si-zhen*): the inspection of the patient's general physical appearance (*wang*); original forms of osphristics and auscultation (*wen*); interrogation (*wen*), and palpation and sphygmology (*qie*). The major principle of treatment is restoring the balance or maintaining the harmony (see Liu 1988).

2. The Confucian Conception of *Ren* (Humanity) and the Shaping of Chinese Medical Ethics

It is controversial regarding how much Confucianism has affected the content of Chinese medical theories (Qiu 1993, Chap. 6). Most scholars seem to believe that the Daoist contribution to original Chinese medicine is more prominent than Confucianism (Ma 1993, Chap. 6); however, it is not controversial that the Confucian teachings of *ren* (humanity) have shaped the basic tone of Chinese medical ethics. Confucius (551–479 BCE) used *ren* to account for the foundation of human rituals, rules of propriety (*li*), and the appropriate structure of society. *Ren* constitutes the basic virtue of human individuals and sets down the fundamental Confucian principle of human society. Etymologically, *ren* is made up of the element "person"

and the number "two," meaning that one cannot become a person by oneself. By extension it also means that the *dao* (way) of the good life consists in forming appropriate human relationships. The primary requirement of *ren* is loving humans (*Analects* 12:12). It is embodied by the particular moral virtues for distinct human relations, such as filial piety (*xiao*[5]) to one's parents, kindness (*ci*) to one's children, loyalty (*zhong*) to one's superiors, and fidelity (*xin*) to one's friends. Confucians hold that one must begin the practice of love of one's family and attempt to extend it gradually to all the people in the world. For Mencius (327–289 BCE, one of the most important Confucian masters, second only to Confucius), the root of *ren* is the human heart that cannot bear the suffering of the other (*Mencius* 2A:6). Every human has such a heart probably because everyone's heart is metaphysically made up of refined *qi*, which naturally holds sympathetic reactions to the *qi* of the other hearts. This might be why Mencius emphasized that to become virtuous, one should be good at nourishing one's vast, flowing *qi* (*Mencius* 2A:2). For Confucians, *qi* is the mutually sympathetic and harmonious metaphysical reality.

After Confucianism became the orthodox ethics of Chinese government in 134 BCE, medicine has been taken to be the art of *ren* (*ren-shu*) (Xue 1999, 46). The phrase "*ren-shu*"[6] first appeared in *Mencius* (1A:7), referring to the kind of behavior that shows an unbearable feeling even to the suffering of the animal. Confucians have naturally seen medicine as "the art of *ren*." Although they have not taken medicine to be as important as politics (see Section III), by defining medicine as the art of *ren* in nature, Confucians have seen it as a cause of loving and caring, rather than a business for profit or repute. Mastering and practicing medical techniques requires great virtues, so that one can undertake a serious social responsibility for helping people prevent diseases, alleviate suffering, rescue lives, and achieve longevity. Indeed, Confucianism takes human life as the most noble and valuable of all things in the universe (*Xiao-Jing*). As Xun Zi (305–235 BCE), another crucial classic Confucian, states:

> Water and fire have *qi* but not life. Plants and trees have life but not perception; birds and animals have perception but not a sense of appropriateness. Human has *qi*, life, and perception, and in addition the sense of appropriateness; therefore he is the noblest of all-under-Heaven. (Xunzi 1990, Chap. 9)

Life, perception, and appropriateness are the further developed states of *qi*, or refined *qi*. This constitutes a Confucian theory of the so-called ladder of souls (Needham [1956] 1980, 21–2). Medicine is inevitably significant in the Confucian view of *ren* because it takes care of human life.

II. THE SICK: FAMILY CARE

1. Moral and Healthy Life

Confucianism holds that moral virtues are the necessary qualities that define a healthy person. By learning and exercising the virtues for self-cultivation, one is simultaneously pursuing and improving one's personal health. Physical well-being, mental peace, and social appropriateness are all closely related to the Confucian positive conception of health. For Confucians, a Daoist hermit is not quite healthy, even if he is physically well, because he stays away from the normal social relations that should not have been avoided for his personal well-being. Accordingly, Confucianism can be understood as a personal health care system, even if it cannot be reduced to a personal health care system (Ni 1999). A person of *ren* is not only morally superior but he also tends to have longevity (*Analects*, 6:21). In Confucianism, there is a unity of morality and medicine.

It is by exercising moral virtues that one can better deal with the etiological factors, especially the mental factors. This is why Confucianism emphasizes self-care and disease prevention. Self-care is self-cultivation for the good way of life. Self-cultivation aims at living a balanced life – a life of going the middle way (*zhong-yung* or *zhong-he*) between extremes. *Zhong* is the state without stirrings of emotions such as joy, anger, or sadness; *he* is the state when these emotions act in their due degree (*The Doctrine of the Mean*, Chap. 1). If one can perfectly maintain the state of *zhong-he*, one's healthy *qi* will be nourished and one will flourish. In particular, Confucius warned:

> There are three things against which a gentlemen (*jun-zi*) is on his guard. In his youth, before his blood *qi* has settled down, he is on his guard against lust. Having reached his prime, when the blood *qi* has finally hardened, he is on his guard against strife. Having reached old age, when the blood *qi* is already decaying, he is on his guard against avarice. (*Analects* 16:7)

The Confucian ideal of *zhong-he* has been at the heart of an important branch of Chinese medicine: *yang-sheng* (life-cultivation). *Yang-sheng* develops a series of complicated techniques to help people promote their health. Its central principle, however, is simple: to have a healthy life, one must moderate one's desires, especially the desires of appetite and sex. Prevention is taken to be more important than treatment for one's health. As a well-known Chinese medical saying goes, "the sagely physician does not treat those who are already sick, but treat those who are not sick yet." The ideal is to have no sickness. The Confucian understanding of health is that one should follow the *dao* and maintain one's health in a well-regulated everyday life. For instance, in the beginning of the *Yellow Emperor's Internal Medicine*, we read:

> Those ancient people who understood the *dao* followed the movement of yin and yang, harmonized methods and limits, controlled their eating and drinking, had regularity in getting up and sleeping, never exhausted themselves unnecessarily. That is why they were able to keep fit both in shape and in vitality, lived up to the natural limit of human life, and died after one hundred years old. People today are different. They use alcohol as regular drink, and exhaust their energy in love-making; they use up their precious vitality, and have no idea of holding up and accumulation. They do not guard their spirit from time to time, and they want immediate pleasure for satisfaction. They live opposite to the principles of life and happiness, and have no regularity in getting up and sleeping. That is why they are declined at the age of fifty. (Chap. 1)

2. The Sick and the Family

Sickness is seen as the failure of a healthy life. Nevertheless, patients are taken as the unfortunate rather than the blameworthy. Confucians understand that there are things outside of human control. Man's fate is eventually determined by the heavenly force. "Life and death have their determined appointments" (*Analects* 12:5). The sick person is taken to be an unfortunate human being, with whom the physician sympathizes and for whom the physician therefore cares. Indeed, patients are often listed in the Confucian literature together with those who are widowed, orphaned, or handicapped as the most unfortunate in society.

The family plays a crucial role in taking care of the sick. From the Confucian view, it is the family, rather than separate individuals, that is the ultimately autonomous unit from the rest of society. This is because the unity of the family is the primordial unity of *yin* and *yang*, representing the foundational model of human existence. A family member's disease is taken to be the issue of the whole family, which must undertake special fiduciary obligations to care for the patient. Generally, the physician discusses the diagnosis, prognosis, treatment, and all other relevant issues of a patient with the family members of the patient, rather than with the patient him/herself. The patient is assumed to be left to rest and relax. The patient is usually more than willing to be represented by the family members regarding his or her health care, and the family has the final authority to accept or refuse the physician's prescription for the patient. This familial pattern of medical decision making is not seen as depriving the patient of a right to make decisions for himself or herself. Rather, the family is appreciated for removing burdens from the sick, including the burden of listening to and discussing the patient's condition and clinical care with the physician. Confucians take it for granted that the family ought to take care of such burdens (Fan 1997). Moreover, when a fatal diagnosis or prognosis is involved, the patient is usually prevented from knowing the truth. Confucians believe it is unsympathetic to the patient if such harsh information is given to him or her directly. They are worried that disclosing such information to the patient would bring about serious psychological burdens on the patient so that it would further harm his or her health and discount the efficacy of treatment. Accordingly, ever since ancient times, Chinese physicians have followed a medical ethical rule: do not disclose a fatal diagnosis or prognosis to the patient; instead, it should be told to the patient's family (Wei and Nie 1994, 105–8). In short, the family is responsible for every member's health care, financially, emotionally, and morally.

III. THE PHYSICIAN: PRACTICING *REN*

1. Political and Medical Life

Far back at the dawn of Chinese history in the second millennium BCE, Chinese society had its "medical men" (*wu*), something like shamans of the North Asian tribal peoples. During the course of the ages, these differentiated into all kinds of specialized professions, not only physicians (*yi*), but also Daoist alchemists, invocators, and liturgiologists for the imperial court, pharmacists, veterinary leeches, mystics, magicians, and technologists of all kinds (*fangshi*) (Needham 2000, 40–41). By Confucius' time, the end of the sixth century BCE, the course of the differentiation of physicians had not yet finished. He designated healers by a term that did not distinguished *wu* from *yi* when he said that, "a man without persistence will never make a good healer (*wu-yi*)" (*Analects* 13:22). The differentiation must have been completed soon after Confucius' time. Bian Que, a very influential physician most probably living approximately 50 years after Confucius (see Liao, Fu, and Zheng 1998, 77), clearly announced that the physician should not treat those who would rather trust shamanism than medicine (Qian 1987).

As discussed in the first section of this chapter, Confucians have seen medicine as "the art of *ren*" (*ren-shu*); however, they have seen politics as "the governing of *ren*" (*ren-zheng*). Although both are the enterprises of *ren* for promoting people's well-being, politics has been taken to be more important due to its broader extent of influence. Specifically, Confucians have not taken medicine to be as important as politics because medicine as the art of *ren* is only able to help a small number of people at a time, whereas politics as the governing of *ren*, if done well, is able to benefit all the people under Heaven. Accordingly, medicine has been termed "the little *dao*" (*xiao-dao*), whereas politics is called "the great *dao*" (*da-dao*). Moreover, classic Confucianism was rationalistic and opposed to any superstitious forms of belief, and this seemed to be beneficial to empirical studies. On the other hand, however, its intense concentration of interest on human social life to the exclusion of nonhuman phenomena negated all investigation of natural things, as opposed to social affairs. This generally explains why most traditional Chinese medical practitioners, especially before the Song Dynasty (960–1279), were not Confucian physicians, but Daoist shamans, quacks, mountebanks, and other types of nontheoretically trained general practitioners. There were only a few famous Confucian physicians before the Song Dynasty (960–1279).

Since Confucianism was set as the orthodoxy ideology of Chinese government in the Eastern Han dynasty (134 BCE), every man had to begin with the Confucian classics to learn the *dao* for a career. At the heart of the Confucian classics is the teaching of self-cultivation (*xiu-sheng*): to learn and practice the virtues. Confucianism holds that self-cultivation must be performed in the way of forming the appropriate human relationships and social institutions: the family, the state, and the all-under-Heaven (*tian-xia*). If individuals are appropriately cultivated, their families can be well regulated; if their families are well regulated, their states can be rightly governed; if their states are rightly governed, the all-under-heaven can be made peaceable. This is why, according to Confucianism, from the king of a state to the mass of people, all must consider the cultivation of the individual as the root of everything (*The Great Learning, the Text*). Accordingly, the process of Confucian self-cultivation is the very process of engaging in politics: regulating the family, governing the state, and making the whole world peaceable. To do this well, one must master and follow the *dao*. Because Confucianism holds that Heaven, Earth, and the myriad things all follow the same *dao*, the *dao* of *yin-yang* and five phases (specifically manifested in heavenly principles, earthly models, and human affairs), the knowledge of the *dao* can certainly be used for the matters of health care and medical purposes. Accordingly, all Confucian scholars can be taken as "Confucian physicians" in the broad sense because they are supposed to have grasped the basic medical principles and are able to guide people regarding health care issues, although they are not actually practicing medicine in taking care of patients. In other words, they are not the Confucian physicians (*ru-yi*) in the narrow sense. Some of them did practice medicine and lived a life of treating patients but they seemed to have a sense of regret for not being able to do politics. For instance, Hua Tuo (second–third century), the best physician in the Eastern Han dynasty, mastered several Confucian classics and had excellent healing skills. Although he was not interested in repute or profit, he also regretted being a physician (Chen (Jin) 1995, Book 29). Up to the

Song Dynasty, the social status of physicians had not been high.

Essential changes occurred in the Song Dynasty (960–1279). The number of the Confucian physicians (*ru-yi*) in the narrow sense tremendously increased. They have made enormous contributions to the both theoretical development and practical improvement of Chinese medicine. Different schools of Chinese medicine were shaped and developed in mutual competition, and the social status of physicians was also substantially elevated. The main factors responsible for these changes are as follows (Liang 1995, 79–102).

First, the rise of Neo-Confucianism in the Song Dynasty stimulated a closer connection between the typical Confucian political career and empirical medical studies. Neo-Confucianism elaborated an elegant Confucian metaphysics based on the concept of *qi*. It unifies *qi, li* (reason), *dao, yin-yang*, five phases, heaven, earth, and the myriad things in a complicated and coherent cosmological system. Everything is made up of *qi*. Wherever there is *qi*, there is *dao*. *Dao* and *qi* are inseparable. *Dao* is one but it has many manifestations in different things. One should investigate things to know the *dao*. This way of thinking constitutes a healthy correction of the classic tendency to exclude the study of empirical things. Together with the Confucian emphasis of *ren*, this thought has enormously benefited the study of disease and health and the pursuit of medical knowledge.

Moreover, the Song government gave special emphasis to healing arts and medical drugs. The first emperor of the dynasty even grasped some healing arts by himself. A few other emperors also paid attention to medical knowledge. Their attitudes toward medicine certainly affected their ministers, general Confucian scholars, as well as the larger society. This in turn determined the way of the Song policy reformulation, which benefited its medical system, education, and practice. Never in the Chinese history was medicine thought to be so important. An important high official, Fan Zhongyan (989–1052), clearly stated, "if one cannot become a good premier, one should become a good physician." His reason is as follows:

> If one can become a good premier and implement the *dao* of a sage king, one will be able to benefit everyone under-the-Heaven, both nobles and ordinary men. However, if one is not able to become a good premier, then nothing is better than becoming a good physician to practice the art of saving humans and benefiting things. Only a good physician, although staying below, is able to offer help to both his superiors and subordinates. To his superiors he can cure the ailments of his parents and emperor, to his subordinates he can rescue them from their maladies, and to himself he can preserve his life and pursue longevity (Wu (Song) 1984, Book 13).

The idea ("if one cannot become a good premier, one should become a good physician") has become the ideological root of many subsequent Confucian physicians.

Furthermore, the Song government reformed the system of medical education. Long before the Song, Chinese had had the system of Civil Service Examinations for selecting officials as well as a National University (*tai-xue*, which had become part of the Directorate of Education (*Quo-zi-jian*) since 490) for training brilliant scholars for government offices. Medical students were educated not in the National University, but in the Imperial Medical Service (*Tai-yi-shu*), an institution primarily for medical care management and the treatment of government officials and their families as well as the members of the imperial court. Their quality as well as the social status were not as high as the students in the National University. The Song government continued medical education inside the Imperial Medical Service; at the same time, however, it set up a new college of medicine in the Directorate of Education. The college attracted Confucian scholars to engage in medicine and improve the quality of physicians. Although this college was not maintained for a long time, it had a profound influence in society and promoted the repute of physicians.

Finally, the Song government reformulated a series of policies and measures for developing medicine, such as editing and publishing traditional medical books, investigating and improving *materia medica*, establishing pharmacies, perfecting the system of the examinations of medical proficiency, and so forth. All these policies and measures proved prosperous for medical studies and stimulated Confucian scholars to turn to the areas of medicine.

2. Practicing *Ren*

The Confucian physicians had two prominent features. First, they made enormous contributions to the theoretical development of Chinese medicine. Unlike most general practitioners who were even illiterate or semi-illiterate, the Confucian physicians were well educated and trained in classical literature. They could not only learn medicine from their teachers, but they could also study it by reading medical books by themselves. They were committed to pursuing the *dao* of health, disease, and medicine, without stopping at the level of simple technical imitation. They were able to edit and republish previous medical books, summarizing their strengths and weaknesses, and develop new theoretical doctrines. This, in turn, brought about different medical schools and promoted their mutual competition and pushed forward the development of Chinese medicine.

Moreover, the Confucian physicians took medicine as an enterprise of *ren*, namely, the art of *ren*. Medicine is their way of making the Confucian life, rather than simply treating diseases as technicians. The meaning of practicing medicine had to be integrated into the ideals of self-cultivation, family regulation, state governing, and world peace. It was by taking care of people's health that they could best exercise the Confucian virtues of filial piety to their parents, loyalty to their emperor, reverence to the old, benevolence to the young, and the extension of love to all-under-Heaven. Throughout history, the Confucian physicians have always stressed that real physicians are performing the art of *ren*, rather than conducting a business for profit. They should never be motivated by monetary considerations to practice the art. Instead, it is the health and well-being of people that constitute the end of the art. As a great Confucian physician Sun Si Miao (541–680) argued, the true physician is characteristic of two features: proficiency in techniques and sincerity in ethics (Gan 1995). They should always treat the patient according to the Confucian virtues, whoever the patient may be.

IV. CONCLUSION: WHAT HAS CONFUCIAN MEDICAL ETHICS TO TEACH US TODAY?

Confucianism is not an organized religion. It does not have churches or priests as other religions do; however, the most interesting issue at this point is how the Confucians' ultimate concern about the way (*dao*) of life is related to medicine. Different religions offer different *daos*. Confucianism holds that the *dao* is *ren* – the harmonious existence of *qi* manifested in the appropriate relations of love among humans. The good life for Confucians is the life of cultivating the virtues for taking care of the family, the state, and the whole world. Medicine is the art of love. It is part of the Confucian cause of *ren*, which requires self-cultivation as a necessary condition for individual dedication. Accordingly, Confucianism does not see the physician as an ordinary person. He should be laden with the Confucian virtues and seeking the Confucian ideal with his special skills.

In the contemporary world, as patients' rights and self-determination have increasingly gained precedence, physicians' virtues have been discounted. It appears that more and more physicians have accepted a contract model of medicine; namely, the physician is obliged to do no more than whatever has been written or is implicit in the law, regulations, rules, or contract that the physician and the patient have directly or indirectly accepted from each other. The model appears to enlarge the patient's autonomy, but it overlooks the physician's virtues. It takes the physician as a businessman providing services for making profits. It deprives medicine of its traditional Confucian link to the chain of *ren* that is substantially larger than medicine itself. Medicine is no longer the art of *ren*. It becomes a business that is not different than any other business in today's overwhelmingly consumer-oriented society. The loss is not limited to the credit of a profound world view based on the concept of *qi*. The loss also includes the deep meaning of medicine itself: there is no longer anything deeper in alleviating pain, curing ailments, preventing diseases, and prolonging life than their apparent effects for desire, satisfaction, and scientific achievements. Confucian medical ethics must see this circumstance as problematic as well as superficial.

Moreover, health care has become ever more individualistic in medical decision making and population based in resource allocation. More and more individuals are taught to see their health care matters as their own matters solely and attempt to make medical decisions by themselves, regardless of the views of their families. They are even encouraged to exclude their families from the process of decision making. After all, they are told, it is their own body, health, and life that are at stake. Confucianism holds that, being a human, one is first and foremost a family member. It is beneficial to oneself for one's family to join in the process of decision making and help one obtain a deliberative medical decision. Family-shared decision making is also embodies one's basic way of existence in the family and through the family, interdependently suffering and flourishing as a unit. Finally, Confucianism is not sympathetic to any egalitarian health care program imposed by the state. Rather, it takes health care primarily as the responsibility and care of the family.

ACKNOWLEDGMENT

The research presented in this chapter is supported by the Governance in Asia Research Center, City University of Hong Kong.

NOTES

1. Confucius (551–479 BCE) used *ren* to account for the fundamental human virtue, the foundation of human rituals, and the appropriate structure of society. Etymologically, *ren* is made up of the element "person" and the number "two," meaning that the basic human virtue consists in forming appropriate human relationships. For Confucius, the nature of such relationships is love (*Analects* 12:12). Because this love is naturally granted in everyone's familial relations, it can be nurtured, developed, and extended to other people outside of one's family. Accordingly, the Confucian principle of *ren* is primarily the requirement of universally applied but gradually extended and differentiated love. It is in meeting the requirement of this love that Confucius found the very meaning of following the rules of propriety in the Chinese traditional rites (*Analects* 3:3). In other words, with the establishment of the moral principle of *ren*, Confucius reinterprets the meaning of traditional Chinese rites in terms of love. For *Mencius* (327–289 BCE), the beginning of *ren* is the human heart that cannot bear the suffering of the other (*Mencius* 2A:6). So everyone must make efforts to cultivate this heart. Finally, *ren*

was further developed by Neo-Confucians in the Song Dynasty (960–1279) as the moral substance of the universe and fundamental principle of morality.

2. *The Yellow Emperor's Internal Medicine* is the cardinal classic of traditional Chinese medicine. The entire work is a dialogue between the legendary Yellow Emperor Huang Di and several of his medical advisors and ministers. Its standard version used today includes eighty-one chapters in twenty-four volumes, covering the most distinguished ancient Chinese medical texts. All fundamental doctrines and theories of Chinese medicine, such as *qi*, *yin-yang*, organs, and channels, have been laid out in the book. Although it contains some heterogeneous pieces that are not completely in accord with each other, it as whole integrates and theorizes about various Chinese healing arts and sets down the foundational principles of Chinese medicine and its written traditions as well as has been followed by all subsequent learned Chinese physicians since its compilation.

It is quite controversial regarding when the volume was compiled. We follow a convincing study (Liao 1993, 55–80) to hold that the current version of the volume, based on some much earlier texts, was reorganized, revised, expanded, and edited by a group of Chinese physicians in the Eastern Han dynasty (25–220).

3. As a fundamental Chinese metaphysical concept, *qi* refers to the basic and ultimate elements of the universe. The theory of *qi* originated in ancient Chinese classics and was further developed by Neo-Confucians in the Song dynasty (960–1279). According to this theory, *qi* is both material and spiritual. It comprises the myriad things as well as their changes in the world, and the world is in an incessant process of transformation and development of *qi*. Essentially, there are two types of *qi*, called "*yin*" and "*yang*." Everything in the universe changes, transforms, and develops in accordance with the combination and cooperation of the *yin-qi* and *yang-qi*.

4. *Dao* is a basic Chinese concept. It literally means "path" or "way." Philosophically it means "the way to truth" or "the ultimate principle." For Daoists, *dao* is also used to indicate the ultimate reality, which, according to Daoists, cannot be clearly described by any human language. For Confucians, the ultimate reality is Heaven (*tian*), whereas *dao*, if anything, are heavenly principles (*tian-dao*). Most Confucian classics (such as *Analects* and *Mencius*) speak of heavenly principles as moral virtues, such as *ren* (humanity) and *yi* (righteousness), whereas some classics

(such as the *Classic of Change*) speak of heavenly principle as *yin-yang* (*qi*). This apparent contradiction is resolved by Neo-Confucians in the Song dynasty (960–1279) through their theory of the unity of principle and *qi*: there is no *qi* without principle and there is no principle without *qi*; principle governs *qi* and *qi* makes manifest principle.

5. *Xiao* is an enormously important virtue in the Confucian tradition. As the love of children for their parents, *xiao* is grounded on the blood-tie relations between parents and children. In fact, Confucius sees *xiao* as the root of *ren* (*Analects* 1:2) and assigns it with a foundational value for the possibility of human morality. If *ren* as love is possible, it is because the intimacy between the child and the parent is naturally available in human life. For Confucians, if one cannot begin love in respectfully treating one's parents, love can begin nowhere. Basically, *xiao* requires children venerate their parents and maximize their parents' interests. An obstacle to understanding *xiao* appropriately arises from a simplistic equation between *xiao* and absolute obedience to one's parents. This is misunderstanding. As the *Classic of Filial Piety* (*Xiao Jing*, a book compiled by Confucius' disciples) clearly states, being truly *xiao* to one's parents, like being a loyal minister at the court, one must actively remonstrate rather than automatically comply with one's parents. The purpose is to ensure the righteousness of the parents' behavior and their good moral reputation.

6. Although the phrase "*ren-shu*" first appeared in *Mencius* (1A:7), referring to the kind of behavior that shows an unbearable feeling even to the suffering of the animal, medicine had gradually been taken as the unique case of *ren-shu* (the art of *ren*). In particular, medicine as the art of *ren* was especially advocated and promoted by the Neo-Confucian physicians in the Song Dynasty (960–1279). They took medicine as a cause of *ren* so important that was second only to politics, the governing of *ren* (*ren-zheng*). They emphasized that although politics, if done well, could benefit people broadly, medicine could also help people significantly. It requires great virtues in learning and practicing medical techniques to help people prevent diseases, alleviate suffering, save lives, and achieve longevity. So medicine, as the art of *ren* in nature, is a cause for love rather than a business for profit for Confucians. This ideal has gained Confucian physicians high repute among Chinese people and encouraged them to practice their art diligently since the Song Dynasty.

CHAPTER 12

THE DISCOURSES OF EARLY CHRISTIAN MEDICAL ETHICS

Darrel W. Amundsen

I. INTRODUCTION

Jewish expectations of a Messiah who would free them from Roman rule and lead them to new heights of temporal power were especially high among Palestinian Jews of the early first century. Popular hopes, focused on various insurrectionists, were consistently disappointed. Very different from these claimants to messiahship was Jesus, who proclaimed a message of repentance and the imminence of the kingdom of God. His teaching and miracles, especially of healing, attracted large crowds and a small group of devoted followers. Jewish leaders, offended by his teachings and threatened by his popularity, which they feared would eventuate in violent suppression by the Romans, accused him of sedition and he was crucified. Belief that he had risen from the dead transformed his timorous and discouraged followers into bold heralds of the gospel of salvation from the penalty of sin, purchased by the death, and resurrection of their Messiah whose kingdom was not of this world. This revolutionary understanding of Old Testament messianic prophecies offended most Jews.

Many, however, became converts and obeyed their risen Lord's command to "make disciples of all nations" (Matthew 28:19; cf. Luke 24:47; Acts 1:8). As the new faith spread quickly through the Mediterranean basin, its adherents saw it as the fulfillment of Judaism, pagans saw it as a Jewish sect, and Jews saw it as a radical departure from Jewish tradition. Eventually the Roman imperial government distinguished it from Judaism and declared it an illicit religion. Christians endured spasmodic persecutions that culminated in the Great Persecution (303–311). Constantine I converted to Christianity and declared it a licit religion in 313. Theodosius I (379–395) proclaimed it the official religion of the state and prohibited the public practice of pagan worship.

Early Christianity is typically divided into two eras: the first century, during which the followers of Jesus composed the New Testament; and the second through the fifth centuries, during which early Church leaders and theologians produced an extensive body of literature that, along with the era in which it was written, is labeled "patristic." Stimulated by various internal controversies and by the teachings of various tangential groups whose beliefs were fundamentally different from the developing orthodoxy of the Church, these Church Fathers articulated and refined Christian beliefs and practices, thus gradually defining a core of doctrine and a hierarchy of authority within the ever-expanding Church. As this orthodoxy of doctrine and ecclesiology evolved, various theological divergences and tangential communities were declared heretical and hence outside what was emerging as the mainstream of Christianity.

To describe the "discourses of early Christian medical ethics," we shall first demonstrate that the New Testament presents a primarily naturalistic understanding of sickness that was not inimical to naturalistic healing and medical practice (without which it would be fatuous to speak of early Christian medical ethics); and second, we shall briefly describe the most fundamental principles of New Testament ethics. We shall begin our discussion of the patristic era by articulating some basic principles that provided the theological and moral framework of the Church Fathers' medical ethics and shall next consider the question, regularly raised in secondary literature, of whether the Church Fathers ever rejected the use of medicine and physicians on theological grounds. Having dealt with these propedeutic but essential matters, we shall finally address various aspects of patristic medical ethics under the rubrics of compassion, philanthropy, and etiquette and the sanctity of life.

II. THE NEW TESTAMENT[1]

1. Sickness, Healing, and Medicine in the New Testament

No one embarks on a study of any aspect of the New Testament without some preconceptions. This is evident when dealing with the nature and causality of disease. When reading the medical literature of ancient cultures, one must avoid viewing descriptions of disease symptoms through the prism of modern western disease typologies and nosologies. This necessity is compounded when reading nonmedical literature of antiquity if this literature assumes that disease has "meaning" in a sense that is totally foreign to the ostensibly value-free scientific medical models of today. The probabilities are high that if one wished to learn about the nature and causality of disease in the New Testament, one would soon be informed that the authors of the New Testament assumed a demonic causality for all, or at least most, illnesses. Klaus Seybold and Ulrich B. Mueller, for example, state categorically that "the dominant view in the New Testament is that demons are the causes of sickness" (Seybold and Mueller 1981, 100). Otto Böcher includes Jewish and New Testament milieus in his pan-demonological interpretation of disease in ancient near eastern cultures (Böcher 1970, 1972a, 1972b). Similar interpretations had earlier conditioned scholarship to such a degree that they appear even in the standard lexicon of New Testament Greek, which has, of course, further perpetuated them. Included in the definition of *daimonion* is "who are said to enter into persons and cause illness, especially of the mental variety ... Hence the healing of a sick person is described as the driving out of demons" (Arndt and Gingrich 1957, 168). Inquirers who read such authors as Seybold, Mueller, Böcher, or any of a plethora of other like-minded scholars, or simply

look up *daimonion* in the most authoritative New Testament Greek lexicon, would be confident that the authors of the New Testament regarded demons as the exclusive, or at least the dominant, cause of sickness. That is, unless they bothered to pursue the passages cited by Arndt and Gingrich to illustrate the supposed disease-causing agency of demons.

Most of the verses that Arndt and Gingrich cite refer generically to the act of casting out demons without indicating any specifics. Several simply involve disparaging a person by accusing him of having a demon. Two describe a demon-possessed man who behaved erratically and violently and another relates Jesus' driving a demon out of a man who could not speak, thus restoring his speech. The rest demonstrate quite the opposite of that for which they are cited by distinguishing unequivocally and categorically between driving out demons and healing the sick. When read, especially in their contexts, none of the verses cited by Arndt and Gingrich, except for such marginal examples as aberrational behavior and muteness, prove to have anything to do with illness or disease as the words are typically used today or, for that matter, as the corresponding Greek words are used in the New Testament.

Leaving the Gospel narratives aside for the moment, one can confidently assert the following about the remainder of the New Testament. The few instances of exorcism in Acts are devoid of illness, and the healing narratives in Acts are devoid of demonic involvement. In the epistles and Revelation, there is not a single instance of demon possession, and all mention of sickness is free from any hint of demonic activity. As for the Gospel narratives, in the vast preponderance of the healings performed by Jesus, not only is there no mention of demonic involvement, but also the symptoms are clearly distinguished from those of demon possession. A woman with a severely bent spine is described as having a "spirit of infirmity" or, as the New International Version too freely renders it, as being "crippled by a spirit" (Luke 13:10–17). There are two cases in which demon possession manifests itself in blindness and/or muteness (Matthew 9:32–33; Luke 11:14; Matthew 12:22). The last two involved exorcism, the first did not. None of them exhibited the erratic, self-destructive, or violent behavior that is typically associated with demon possession. These symptoms are present, however, in the case of a boy who is described as having seizures or convulsions perhaps consistent with epilepsy (Matthew 17:14–20; Mark 9:14–29; Luke 9:37–43 with some intriguing variations). This is the only instance in the New Testament of a demon-possessed person manifesting self-destructive, erratic behavior together with what are, perhaps, symptoms of a disease or physical sickness. The only other examples of the demon-possessed exhibiting the self-destructive or violent behavior typically associated with possession are the Gerasene demoniac(s) (Matthew

8:28–34; Mark 5:1–20; Luke 8:26–39) and a vocally disruptive demoniac (Mark 1:21–28; Luke 4:31–37). As we have seen, there are only three cases in the New Testament in which a physical dysfunction or disability is attributed to a demon and only one in which symptoms that are perhaps consistent with sickness are attributed to demon possession. Significantly, in this case erratic behavior is also present. In both this and in all other episodes of demon possession the erratic behavior *is* the demon possession. When scholars assert that demons are the exclusive, primary, or even a significant cause of sickness in the New Testament, one must wonder whether they are only uncritically repeating what other scholars have said without reading the relevant texts for themselves, are consciously misrepresenting the texts, or are simply unconsciously rearticulating their presuppositions as their conclusions.

Because such a nearly negligible proportion of references to sickness in the New Testament involve demonic causality, what other sources of disease were part of the universe of ideas in the Mediterranean world of the first century? One was malevolent magic, of which there is no suggestion in the New Testament as a cause of the sicknesses encountered there. Another was divine, as distinct from demonic causality. In Jewish culture, this was God, rather than the gods. Few if any Jews would have denied that God could directly or indirectly cause sickness or dysfunction, which were popularly assumed to be punishment for sin. Jesus, however, called into question the direct causal link between individual sickness and personal sin. On one occasion he forgave a paralytic's sins before healing him, although no connection is implied between the forgiveness and healing (Matthew 9:1–8). After healing another paralytic, Jesus urged him to "stop sinning or something worse may happen to you" (John 5:14). When Jesus' disciples encountered a man who had been born blind, they asked, "Who sinned, this man or his parents, that he was born blind?" Jesus replied, "Neither this man nor his parents sinned, but this happened so that the work of God might be displayed in his life" (John 9:1–3). Although Jesus' response does not preclude a direct causal relationship between personal sin and individual sickness, it suggests that he regarded sweeping, judgmental assessments as tenuous.

In several instances, divine purpose and ultimate causality are unequivocally stated. For example, the angel Gabriel struck the senectuous Zechariah with muteness for the duration of his wife's pregnancy because of his disbelief (Luke 1:5–23, 57–66); for Herod Agrippa's pride, "an angel of the Lord stuck him down, and he was eaten by worms and died" (Acts 12:20–23; cf. also Acts 5:1–11; 13:4–12; and in the eschatological realm, Revelation 2:22–23; 9:5, 10; 11:6; 16:2; 18:8; 22:18). In both of these cases, God's purposes are clear, and although he is depicted as the ultimate cause, he employs an angel as the immediate agent. When Jesus' friend Lazarus was ill, Jesus remarked that his sickness was "for God's glory so that God's Son may be glorified through it." Belief in divine sovereignty did not preclude a naturalistic understanding of the immediate causality of Lazarus' illness. The disciples apparently regarded the cause as natural because, when Jesus figuratively alluded to Lazarus "sleeping," their reaction was, "Lord, if he sleeps, he will get better" (John 11:1–15).

We have considered three causes of sickness that were current in New Testament times: (1) demonic, to which a nearly negligible proportion of sicknesses were directly attributed in the New Testament; (2) magical, to which no reference is made in the New Testament; and (3) divine, of which a relatively small number are specified. There is also a fourth. No immediate causality is given and no specific divine purpose is stated or implied for the overwhelming majority of all specified cases of sickness or disability that appear in the New Testament. They all have in common the complete absence of symptoms or attributions that could reasonably suggest any immediate causality other than a natural one. Without doing violence to the texts in question, one cannot infer either demonic or immediate divine causality. What other alternatives were available? Magic would certainly have been mentioned – and attacked – if it had been regarded as the cause of any of these numerous instances of unattributed sickness or dysfunction. That leaves naturalistic causality, which is ignored by so many scholars, perhaps because they are unaware of the history of ancient medicine or because the possibility of a naturalistic paradigm as viable in first-century Jewish Palestine is simply too discordant with their preconceptions of the nature of the culture portrayed in the New Testament.

In the Old Testament, God is the physician of his people, whom he instructs not to have recourse to magic or to pagan healing practices. This did not preclude the use of natural means of healing, which were probably limited to folk remedies. How early a category that can be labeled "physicians" arose in Israel is unknown. At least by the second century BCE, Jewish medical practitioners seem to have become common in Jewish Palestine. The extent to which they had been directly influenced by Greek medical theories, particularly humoral pathology, is still being debated (Newmyer 1996). The interplay between Jewish physicians of the western diaspora and those of Palestine undoubtedly influenced the latter, because Greek medicine, once it was disengaged from the religion of natural philosophy that had provided the context in which it developed, was religiously neutral. Even if Jewish medicine was primarily an independent development parallel to Greek rationalistic medicine, as Stephen Newmyer says, "Talmudic medicine shares with its Hippocratic counterpart a reliance upon rational observation" for it "is firmly grounded in the belief that the nature of disease may be comprehended through rational observation of phenomena" (Newmyer 1996, 2902 and 2903).

It is reasonable to assert that although disease in the New Testament is described phenomenologically and understood theologically, it is not in most cases overtly theologized, that is, only rarely is a divine purpose specified in individual instances of sickness. In those relatively rare occurrences for which a divine purpose is assigned, and certainly in all other cases except those of demon possession, a general appreciation of natural etiology exists (even in the absence of specified immediate causality) that is consonant with perceptions of disease causality that prevailed in the Mediterranean world of the first century. For the writers of the New Testament, a belief in miraculous healing did not require a nonnaturalistic perception of the immediate causality of disease. Rather it was fully compatible with a belief in supernatural intervention in natural processes (Amundsen and Ferngren 1996, 2956; cf. Ferngren 2000).

Stephen Newmyer remarks, "Throughout Jewish medical history in antiquity, disease and health are regarded as religious categories, and the physician is reckoned as the agent of God's will" (Newmyer 1996, 2898). This is well illustrated by Ecclesiasticus or the Wisdom of Jesus ben Sira, written in Jerusalem during the early second century BCE, which contains an encomium of medicine and physicians (Ecclesiasticus 38). Ben Sira believed that physicians were agents of God and that their medicines were divinely bestowed instruments of salutary benevolence to humanity, although he emphasized that when sick one must place one's faith in God, not in physicians (Noorda 1979). Hence, it is not surprising that nowhere in the New Testament is there even an implied condemnation of physicians and medicine. As Owsei Temkin observes, "The Jesus of the Gospels appears to be in no way hostile to secular healing." Regarding the woman with a uterine hemorrhage who had, according to Mark 5:26, "suffered a great deal under the care of many doctors and had spent all she had, yet instead of getting better she grew worse," he perceptively observes, "The remark regarding the doctors' inability to cure the woman with the bloody flux merely shows Jesus' superiority" (Temkin 1991, 104). We should also note that Paul's traveling companion was "our dear friend Luke, the doctor" (Colossians 4:14), traditionally regarded as the author of Acts and the Gospel that bears his name.

The New Testament emphasizes the ultimate sovereignty of God and his love manifested in the ministry and redemptive sacrifice of his Son. It is in this context that sickness must be viewed in the New Testament. The presence of sickness is one symptom of a world that has been dislocated by sin. Sickness is one of many aspects of material (as distinct from moral) evil that resulted from the Fall. Because the Fall was caused not only by human disobedience but also by the Serpent's intrigue and deception,

both moral and material evil are, in that sense, considered the works of Satan. Hence Jesus referred to a woman with a severely bent spine as one "whom Satan has kept bound for eighteen long years" (Luke 13:16). In Acts, Peter reminded the centurion Cornelius that Jesus "went around doing good and healing all who were under the power of the devil" (Acts 10:38).

2. New Testament Ethics

Early Christians regarded the Old Testament as divinely inspired and authoritative. Its God was their God. His final revelation was manifested through his Word Incarnate, Jesus Christ, and through his word inscripturated, the New Testament. God's redemptive mercy is fundamental to both Old Testament and New Testament ethics, the former in terms of promise and the latter in terms of fulfillment. Jesus' ministry is pervaded by his consciousness of his messianic mission, including his perfect fulfillment of the moral requirements of the Law.

In one sense, Jesus deepened the requirements of the Law. He gave to the Law a radical interpretation, a return to its basic intention, by demanding not a reformation of behavior but a transformation of character. He showed the necessity of this by probing into the mind and motive behind behavior, for it is inner character that manifests itself in outward conduct (Luke 6:45). Holiness of conduct involves obedience to the divine commandments (John 14:15). Even as new creations in Christ, Christians do not immediately and intuitively know his commandments, much less every aspect of his moral will. Hence the authors of the New Testament were zealous to ensure that Christians grow in their understanding and in the practical application of their increasing moral discernment.

Jesus deepened the requirements of the Law by internalizing its requirements – what could be more convicting than his teaching that purity of heart requires a sensitivity to one's own sinfulness that equates hatred with murder and lust with adultery (Matthew 5:21–22, 27–28)? – and by unequivocally identifying and condemning specific sins. Yet in another sense he simplified the Law. He summarized the moral essence of the Torah in two commandments: "'Love the Lord your God with all your heart and with all your soul and with all your mind.' This is the first and greatest commandment. And the second is like it: 'Love your neighbor as yourself.' All the Law and the Prophets hang on these two commandments" (Matthew 22:37–40, quoting Deuteronomy 6:5 and Leviticus 19:18). He reformulated the second as the Golden Rule: "Do to others as you would have them do to you" (Luke 6:31), for tradition had added to the command to love your neighbor, "and hate your enemy." Hence Jesus said, "But I tell you: Love your enemies and pray for those who persecute you" (Matthew 5:43–44). This revolutionary application of love – *agape* – permeates New Testament ethics. Although the New Testament nowhere teaches that *agape* as a motivation determines the content of God's moral will, *agape* is the first fruit of the Spirit (Galatians 5:22), the preeminent expression of faith (Galatians 5:6), "the fulfillment of the Law" (Romans 13:10), indeed, it is to be the motivation and the manner of all that Christians are to do (1 Corinthians 16:14). The Gospels portray Jesus as the ultimate example to follow, and the remainder of the New Testament is replete with encouragements to imitate him. In that sense, the distinctive genius of New Testament ethics is, indeed, the imitation of Christ.

When a Jewish scribe, discussing the command to love one's neighbor as oneself, asked Jesus, "Who is my neighbor?" Jesus responded by telling a parable about a Jew who while traveling was assaulted by a band of robbers who left him beside the road badly injured. After a priest and a Levite had both hurried by, ignoring him, a Samaritan (an ethnic and religious enemy of the Jews) "took pity on him. He went to him and bandaged his wounds, pouring on oil and wine. Then he put the man on his own donkey, took him to an inn and took care of him. The next day he took out two silver coins and gave them to the innkeeper. 'Look after him,' he said, 'and when I return, I will reimburse you for any extra expense you may have.'" Jesus then asked the scribe, "Which of these three do you think was a neighbor to the man who fell into the hands of robbers?" After he replied, "The one who had mercy on him," Jesus said, "Go and do likewise" (Luke 10:29–37). The lesson of the parable of the Good Samaritan provides a model of practical Christian *agape* to be extended to men and women whose inherent value to God is so great that his incarnate Son not only made the ultimate sacrifice to redeem them but also, during his ministry, entered into their suffering and alleviated it through healing their diseases.

Because of the strong philanthropic motivation inherent in the Christian concept of *agape*, concern for others was shown not only in a desire for the salvation of lost sinners, but in providing help for those in physical need. Hence, James writes, "Religion that God our Father accepts as pure and faultless is this: to look after orphans and widows in their distress and to keep oneself from being polluted by the world" (James 1:27). In several passages in the Gospels, Jesus is recorded as having set forth the principles of personal charity incumbent on all his followers. "For I was hungry and you gave me something to eat, I was thirsty and you gave me something to drink, I needed clothes and you clothed me, I was sick and you looked after me, I was in prison and you came to visit me. . . . whatever you did for one of the least of these brothers of mine, you did for me" (Matthew 25:35–40). The verb here translated "looked after" was sometimes used in classical Greek to describe a physician's visiting a patient.

These, then, are the themes that provide the foundation for discussions of medical ethics in a variety of Christian contexts.

III. PATRISTIC MEDICAL ETHICS[2]

1. Introductory Considerations

The Church Fathers wrote from theological perspectives that are not always consistent with each other, but were part of a culture much broader and more diverse than that of the authors of the New Testament. Their lives extended over a range of four centuries, during which there were enormous changes in the Mediterranean world. They gave particularly great attention to defining and articulating principles of Christian morality more broadly, specifically, and elaborately than had the authors of the New Testament. This manifested itself in a more rigorist stance on various moral issues than that taken in the New Testament, the introduction of gradations of sins, and the development of a penitential system under the authority of an increasingly complex and authoritarian ecclesiastical hierarchy. All Church Fathers were consciously or unconsciously affected, at least to some extent, by Greek philosophy, especially Stoicism and Platonism. Although some developed philosophically informed ethical systems, none isolated for systematic scrutiny any group of issues that have typically come to be placed under the rubric of medical ethics. Moreover, there is no evidence that any Christian physician living during the patristic era wrote on medical ethics or etiquette.

The Church Fathers discussed, sometimes directly but often tangentially, various issues of medical ethics. Before considering these, it is important to be aware of some basic principles that provided the theological and moral framework of their medical ethics. (For a more thorough discussion of these issues, see Amundsen 1996, especially Chaps. 1, 4, and 5).[3]

- Because this world is the good work of God in his goodness, matter is not inherently evil, as the Incarnation itself clearly attests. On this principle the Church Fathers stood unwaveringly. Some Christian ascetics indeed exaggerated the Pauline flesh/spirit dichotomy and sometimes a very thin line existed in practice between the mortification of the flesh and a dualistic excoriation of matter in general and the flesh in particular as inherently evil. One may reasonably assert, however, that any ostensibly Christian writer who unequivocally classified all created matter as inherently and intrinsically evil was *eo ipso* not Christian. To insist that such radical dualism as that of the Gnostics, Manichees, and some Docetists belongs within the broad range of early Christian beliefs that in the aggregate can be regarded as normative is to make of early

Christianity something so amorphous as to be infinitely malleable.

- That "God created man in his own image, in the image of God he created him; male and female he created them" (Genesis 1:27) is fundamental to patristic theology. Irrespective of disagreements among the Church Fathers about the interpretative nuances of the exact nature of the *imago Dei* (image of God) before and after the Fall, it imparted to human life an inherent value.

- Patristic theology viewed physical health as a good, but not an absolute good, much less the supreme good. Physical health could even be an obstacle to the supreme good, which was spiritual health. The Church Fathers emphasized that because the soul is infinitely more valuable than the body, care for the latter was not to conflict with care for the former. They saw health as a blessing from God, but as it was only a relative good, it could be an evil if given a higher priority than it deserved.

- The Church Fathers held the firm conviction that Christians should rejoice in sickness as well as in health. Sickness could be an impetus to spiritual and moral self-examination and could correct or restrain one from sin, refine, admonish, increase patience, reduce pride, cause one to be less self-reliant and more dependent upon God, and make one more mindful of eternity and one's own mortality.

- Sin lurked in the background of all conditions of suffering. Without sin there would be no suffering because the Fall of Adam and Eve was the ultimate explanation for the miseries of the present, including sickness. Sin, in this sense, was generic in the human race. Sickness could – indeed, should – stimulate self-examination because God could thus use sickness, even if it was not caused by a specific sin, as a means of spiritual purification. The Church Fathers, however, bluntly identified a direct link between sin and sicknesses that they believed were caused by carnality or overindulgence. When they otherwise identified personal sin as the cause of sickness, it was typically in the context of pastoral exhortations intended to comfort and correct rather than to foster guilt.

- The Church Fathers identified four disease causalities, namely divine, natural, demonic, and magical. These were not mutually exclusive, for example, magic and demonic activity were closely associated. Although the Church Fathers appear to have been hesitant to attribute disease directly to God, the more they stressed his sovereignty, the more they viewed him as either sending or permitting illness through secondary, immediate means. Our understanding of the patristic understanding of disease causality remains somewhat muddled, especially regarding the ostensible role of demons, although a recent study argues convincingly that direct attribution of sickness (other than mental) to demons was quite rare (Ferngren 2000). What was thought to cause disease in any given case greatly affected the choice of means of healing: spiritual/miraculous (e.g., prayer, the sacraments, exorcism, and, beginning in late antiquity, the cult of saints and relics); or natural/medical (e.g., drugs, herbs, dietetics, and surgery).

- God was not regarded as the source of all healing. Much healing came through spiritually pernicious sources such as the pagan healing cults and demonically empowered magic. All Church Fathers took this as a given. Satan and his demons (and early Christians regarded the multitude of pagan deities as demons) were able to heal. No Church Father dismissed the pagan healing cults as frauds or denied that demons could cure especially those sicknesses or dysfunctions that they had caused. Asclepius was a demon to be taken very seriously indeed. Furthermore, the Church Fathers never denied the efficacy of magic. Although they regarded some practitioners of magic as charlatans and tricksters, they never denied the demonically based power of magic because they knew that many pagans employed magic efficaciously for a variety of purposes, including the healing of disease.

- All Church Fathers believed that God had provided sustenance for humanity through the proper use of nature, for example, vegetables and animals for food, various means of shelter, and herbal and mineral medicinal remedies.

- There are significant limitations on the occasions and extent to which Christians should use the services of physicians and medicines. All Church Fathers who commented on medicine and physicians placed this caveat on Christians' recourse to them: One must not rely *exclusively* on them but must rely on God as the source of the skill of the physician and of the efficacy of the medicine, for God could choose to heal through them, to heal without them, or to withhold healing. God, not the physician, was the only worthy object of one's faith. Although the Church Fathers firmly held that death was not to be sought, they encouraged Christians not to fear physical death, because it would simply usher them into the ineffable delights of heaven. Hence, numerous Church Fathers marveled at Christians who were afraid of death. They were especially appalled at those who, when afflicted with seemingly hopeless illness, clung so desperately to life that they would place their faith in any physician who would promise them a glimmer of hope of sustaining their lives. They viewed such conduct as tantamount to blasphemy, or at least as a sad contradiction of Christian values.

- The Church Fathers were convinced that the art of medicine could be used for egregious and sinful ends (e.g., abortion).

Bearing these ten principles in mind, we shall first consider the current state of the debate about whether the potential for tension between Christianity and medicine ever led to a rejection of medicine. We shall then address aspects of patristic medical ethics under the rubrics of compassion, philanthropy, and etiquette; and the sanctity of life.

2. A Patristic Rejection of Medicine?

Did concerns about the propriety of the use of medicine by Christians ever cause any Church Fathers to condemn medical practice? Various scholars have contended that some Church Fathers were categorically opposed to Christians' using medicine or consulting physicians (e.g., Harnack 1892; Frings 1959; and Schadewaldt 1965). Most patristic sources that had been thus interpreted have lately been shown not to have been hostile to medicine per se (e.g., by Temkin 1991, 119–25; Amundsen 1996, 158–74). It is now reasonable to assert that no Christian document from the patristic period entirely condemns, *on theological grounds*, Christians' use of physicians and medicine (Amundsen 1996, 7–11, 26 nn. 7, 9). Some Church Fathers, however, asserted that only those who lacked spirituality sufficient for them to be able to rely exclusively on divine healing should use medicine (e.g., Origen [c.184–c.253], *Contra Celsum* 8.60). Others practiced an asceticism that so glorified suffering and disease that they would not avail themselves of help from any source, although they did not deny the propriety of medicine for other Christians and even would administer medicines to the ill as an act of Christian compassion (see Harvey 1985).

Even if no Church Fathers unequivocally rejected medicine, the existence of passages thus construed, along with various caveats regarding Christians' use of medicine, demonstrates an undergirding tension. Hence, some scholars (e.g., Harnack 1892; Frings 1959; Schadewaldt 1965; Nutton 1985a, 1985b) have propounded two possibly complementary theories to account for the general uneasiness about Christians' using medicine expressed by some Church Fathers and the supposedly unequivocal condemnation of medicine by others. First, an early, conservative hostility against medicine was gradually ameliorated by a Hellenistic, liberalizing influence. Second, Christianity's supposed emphasis on, and ostensible promise of, miraculous physical healing was a constant, major obstacle to compatibility. Both views betray a misunderstanding of the nature of the inherent and hence enduring tensions and compatibilities between Christianity and medicine (Amundsen 1996, Chaps. 1 and 5), whereas the second compounds the error by exaggerating the importance of miraculous healing in the propagation of the gospel and in the Christian community especially during the second and third centuries (Ferngren 1992). Furthermore, it is interesting to note

that, after the New Testament, it is not until the fourth century that reports of miraculous healings are regularly encountered in Christian literature. With the rise of the cult of saints and relics later that century, they become commonplace. If the assumptions of certain scholars are correct, we have the peculiar puzzle that the tensions between Christianity and medicine were diminishing in intensity at the very time during which the frequency of miraculous healings was dramatically increasing, that is, at a time when competitiveness between the two healing alternatives should have been exacerbated.

At this stage, it is reasonable to affirm that all patristic sources who said anything about medicine shared the conviction that the use of physicians and medicine was not *essentially* and *intrinsically* inappropriate for Christians.

3. Compassion, Philanthropy, and Etiquette

In early Christian literature, Jesus was often referred to as the "Great Physician" and sometimes as being himself both the physician and the medication (Pease 1914; Arbesmann 1954; Schipperges 1965; Temkin 1991, 144–45). Early Christians had adapted a tradition from classical literature that employed, in simile or metaphor, the idea of physicians as dedicated, unselfish, and compassionate preservers or restorers of health who were always committed to the good of their patients. The Church Fathers occasionally referred to the art of medicine metonymously as the "Hippocratic art" and sometimes used the name Hippocrates to represent an ethical ideal for the medical practitioner. Christ himself was, "as it were, a spiritual Hippocrates" (Pease 1914, 75).

The "Hippocratic ideal" of decorum and etiquette was very appealing to early Christians. Jerome (c. 345–c. 419) wrote to a priest that it:

> is part of your duty to visit the sick, to be acquainted with people's households, with matrons, and with their children, and to be entrusted with the secrets of the great. Let it therefore be your duty to keep your tongue chaste as well as your eyes. Never discuss a woman's looks, nor let one house know what is going on in another. Hippocrates, before he will instruct his pupils, makes them take an oath and compels them to swear obedience to him. That oath exacts from them silence, and prescribes for them their language, gait, dress, and manners. How much greater an obligation is laid on us who have been entrusted with the healing of souls! (*Epistle* 52.15; see Temkin 1991, 182)

There is a passage in a letter falsely attributed to Clement of Alexandria (c. 150–c. 220) that contains the injunction, "we are to visit the sick . . . without guile or covetousness or noise or talkativeness or pride or any behavior alien to piety . . . [I]nstead of using elegant phrases, neatly arranged and ordered... act frankly like men who have received the gift of healing from God, to God's glory" (*De virginitate* 1, 112). This advice could have been written by or for physicians. It was, however, addressed to Christian exorcists. Its every detail, except references to piety and to God, also appears in classical treatises on medical decorum and etiquette. Possibly this anonymous author was consciously adopting principles of medical etiquette. In any event, the guidelines for conduct in both instances seem to be little more than practical etiquette for clergy as well as for physicians.

There was one feature of the "Hippocratic ideal," however, that the Church Fathers regarded as much more significant than principles of decorum and etiquette, and that was compassion or philanthropy (Amundsen and Ferngren 1982). Origen (c. 184–c. 253) writes that he followed "the method of a philanthropic physician who seeks the sick so that he may bring relief to them and strengthen them" (*Contra Celsum* 3.74). In demonstrating the superiority of Christianity to pagan philosophy, he says that "Plato and the other wise men of Greece, with their fine sayings, are like the physicians who confine their attention to the better classes and despise the common man while the disciples of Jesus carefully study to make provision for the great mass of men" (*Contra Celsum* 7.60). It was in caring for common people, especially for the destitute and the poor, that Christian physicians could display, in the most practical manner, the compassion that Jesus had stated as essential for his followers. Augustine (354–430) regarded his friend, the physician Gennadius, as "a man of devout mind, kind and generous heart, and untiring compassion, as shown by his care of the poor" (*Epistle* 159). He frequently mentioned physicians who, motivated by charity, asked no remuneration for their services, but undertook the most desperate cases among the poor with no thought of receiving any recompense (e.g., *Sermon* 175.8–9).

According to Augustine, physicians should always have their patients' cure at heart (*Sermon* 9.10), for the practice of medicine would be cruelty if physicians were only concerned about engaging in their art (*In Psalm.* 125.14). Gregory of Nyssa (c. 335–394) began a letter to the physician Eustathius with the statement that "philanthropy is the way of life for all of you who practice the medical art" (although almost certainly written by Gregory of Nyssa, this letter is usually printed as *Epistle* 189 of his elder brother, Basil of Caesarea). Although compassion or philanthropy may have been regarded as a desirable quality by some pagan physicians, Christianity had made it an ethical obligation for Christian physicians (Temkin 1991, 220, 252–53). For some it was the chief motivation for practicing medicine.

Because it was an obligation incumbent upon all Christians to extend care to the needy, especially to the sick, Christians responded with remarkable courage during various outbreaks of plague in their efforts to care for the ill,

Christian and pagan alike. One particular group, of whom we have only scant knowledge, were known as the *parabalani* ("reckless ones") because of the risks they faced by caring for plague victims (Philipsborn 1950). Their zeal in the face of such imminent danger was motivated in part by the belief that death thus incurred ranked with martyrdom (Eusebius [c. 265–c. 339], *Ecclesiastical History* 7.22.8). By late antiquity the care of the sick had become a highly organized activity supervised by local bishops (Ferngren 1988). Institutions at which medical care was given to the indigent and the poor were first established in the fourth century and became quite common, especially in the eastern Mediterranean (Miller 1985; Temkin 1991, 162–70, 253; van Minnen 1995). The most famous of these was the *nosokomeia* or *ptocheion* of Basil, who was the bishop of Caesarea from 370 to 379. These institutions, as well as orphanages and homes for the care of the elderly and destitute, first arose after the legalization of Christianity, were distinctly Christian, and were a practical manifestation of Christian charity.

4. The Sanctity of Life

A principle of sanctity of human life predicated on the concept of the *imago Dei*, the belief that every human being was formed in the image of God, was thoroughly developed during the patristic era (Ferngren 1987). By virtue of sharing the *imago Dei*, all human life was of value and therefore was owed compassion and care. Although contraception, abortion, and infanticide are not directly condemned in the New Testament, they were unequivocally denounced in the earliest patristic literature. These condemnations were not initially grounded in a developed concept of the *imago Dei* as the basis of inherent human value. Rather they arose in the context of passionate denunciations of the most offensive sins to which Christians felt pagans were especially prone, for example, gladiatorial shows, other displays of extreme cruelty, and sexual immorality of an extravagantly imaginative variety. The history of contraception and abortion in early Christianity is rife with interpretive difficulties that are examined in Chapter 7.

The Church Fathers condemned active or passive infanticide, including child exposure, of any newborn, whether healthy, sickly, defective, or even grossly deformed, as the murder of one made in the image of God (Amundsen 1996, Chap. 3). Although not discussed by the Church Fathers, active euthanasia had to have been regarded as murder, given the early Christian community's attitude toward suicide (discussed in detail in Chapter 8). Passive euthanasia, if it resulted from failing to extend care to one whose life could be saved, could hardly have been approved. Passive euthanasia, if the alternative was assisting a desperate Christian to cling life, could hardly have been discouraged. Nowhere in the patristic literature is there any indication that Christian physicians should feel any sense of obligation to attempt to prolong life per se.

IV. CONCLUSION

Christianity inherited from Judaism its ethical monotheism, which centered on the sovereign Creator who revealed his moral will through the Law and the Prophets. Early Christians believed that the messianic promises of the Hebrew Scriptures were fulfilled in and by Jesus Christ, who deepened, internalized, and simplified the moral Law, and exemplified in his messianic mission its essence, which was *agape*, the defining feature of New Testament ethics. The practical manifestation of *agape* remained the focus of patristic ethics, especially in the treatment of the most vulnerable members of society, whether pagan or Christian.

Christianity also inherited from Judaism a practical appreciation of the sovereignty of God over his creation, by which he had provided licit means of human sustenance. Just as Jews, prior to and contemporary with early Christians, tended to view disease as most commonly, although not exclusively, attributable to natural causes, so also did the authors of the New Testament and the Church Fathers. Jews and early Christians alike both recognized the moral and religious legitimacy of the use of medicine and physicians. Both alike also recognized the potential of medicine for good or evil, and the most subtle danger here was for the ill to place their faith in medicines and physicians rather than in the sovereign Source of all good.

Early Christians borrowed from the Hippocratic tradition those of its features that were consistent with Christian values (see Chapters 23 and 24). At some time during the patristic era, Christian physicians adopted an "Oath of Hippocrates insofar as a Christian may swear it," of which several manuscripts are extant (Jones 1924). The Christian oath states the prohibition of abortion unambiguously and precisely, compared with the enigmatic language of the pagan version. The forswearing of active euthanasia is retained: "Neither will I give poison to anybody though asked to do so, nor will I suggest such a plan." Where the pagan Oath reads, "Into whatsoever houses I enter, I shall do so to help the sick, keeping myself free from all intentional wrong-doing and harm," the Christian Oath reads, "Into whatsoever houses I enter, I will do so to help the sick keeping myself free from all wrong-doing, both intentional and unintentional, tending to death or to injury." The addition of the promise to keep oneself free from even unintentional harm, although not inconsistent with pagan

medical ethics, is even more harmonious with early Christian ethics of respect for life that not only condemned infanticide and suicide (including active euthanasia), but also manifested itself in the practical care of the destitute and the ill.

In early Christian literature a reasonably clear if not exhaustive picture emerges of ideal physicians who were "Hippocratic" in their decorum and motivated by Christian philanthropy, and who so cherished the sanctity of human life that they would neither perform abortions nor assist in suicide, yet regarded desperate attempts to forestall death as inconsistent with ultimate Christian values. Nevertheless, such a description tells us nothing directly about the practical ethics of early Christian physicians except insofar as individual physicians may have agreed with and attempted to conform to such an ideal.

The ideal physician had been posited in classical antiquity, and that ideal included compassion as a desirable characteristic. *Agape* – Christian love, which was the basis of philanthropy – was so central a tenet of Christian theology that it was applied to the physician as not merely a desirable but an essential characteristic. An obligation to care, not an obligation to cure, was a categorical imperative to extend compassion in both word and deed to the poor, the widow, the orphan, and the sick. Henry Sigerist did not exaggerate when he wrote that Christianity introduced "the most revolutionary and decisive change in the attitude of society toward the sick. Christianity came into the world ... as the joyful Gospel of the Redeemer and of Redemption ... It became the duty of the Christian to attend to the sick and the poor of the community ... The social position of the sick man thus became fundamentally different from what it had been before. He assumed a preferential position which has been his ever since" (Sigerist 1943, 69–70).

NOTES

1. All Scripture quotations are taken from the *Holy Bible*, New International Version, copyright 1973, 1978, 1984 by the International Bible Society.

2. For references to available texts and English translations of the works of Church Fathers cited or quoted, consult Quasten (1950–1986) or Ferguson (1990).

3. Two categories of secondary literature not cited in the text are included in the bibliography. (1) Surveys of early Christian medical history: Amundsen and Ferngren ([1986], 1998); Ferngren and Amundsen (1996); and d'Irsay (1927). (2) Specialized studies of individual Church Fathers: Keenan (1941) and (1944); Leven (1987); and Müller (1967).

CHAPTER 13

THE DISCOURSES OF ORTHODOX CHRISTIAN MEDICAL ETHICS

H. Tristram Engelhardt, Jr.

I. INTRODUCTION: BEFORE AND BEYOND THE SCHOLASTIC–ENLIGHTENMENT PROJECT

There is a continuity between the commitments of the Scholasticism that emerged in the thirteenth century and the Enlightenment project of providing a discursive rational account of proper moral probity. Although the Enlightenment attempted to give an account of morality undirected by revelation and ecclesiastical authority, thus involving a substantive break with previous moral and political assumptions, the Enlightenment as well as Scholasticism share a substantive commitment to reason's abilities to provide a universal account of morality. Bioethics as it took shape in the 1970s reflected a late-Enlightenment attempt to provide a secular surrogate for the religious moral authorities that had once guided the West (Engelhardt 2002). Secular and Western Christian bioethics have drawn on philosophical assumptions regarding the capacities of discursive reflection. They both have a penchant for identifying moral truths with the deliverances of systematic moral reflections. In contrast, Orthodox Christianity lives in an understanding of morality unaltered by Scholasticism, the Renaissance, the Protestant Reformation, and the Enlightenment.

Orthodox Christianity understands the moral life to be a whole, a way of life within which one can enter into union with God. Orthodox theology, morality, and bioethics identify this way of curing the soul of self-love such that distinctions among dogmatic theology, moral theology, and liturgical theology threaten to distort and disorient the lived appreciation of theology as a practice transcending the confines of the academy. Most significantly, the Orthodox recognize the truth to be personal, namely, the Trinity, and morality to be a kind of therapeutic regimen for purifying the person so that illumination by God's grace can take place. For Orthodox Christianity, theology is praying well so as to experience the indwelling of the Holy Spirit.

The reader therefore must be warned: Orthodox Christianity does not offer a medical ethics in the same way in which secular and Roman Catholic thought offers systematic reflections based on settled moral judgments elaborated philosophically toward the goal of developing ever clearer insights into the nature of morality (see Chapters 12 and 14). Instead, Orthodox Christian morality and medical ethics are modes of reorienting persons away from themselves toward God and their fellow man. Because theology par excellence is directed to purification of the heart and illumination by God's grace, all theological progress is personal. At best, the academic endeavors of Orthodox scholars offer clarifications regarding the use of terms and the development of languages suitable for communication of reflections concerning the unbroken experience by the Church of a timeless truth: the Trinity. As a consequence, Orthodox medical ethics has more of a homiletic than a scholarly character. It is an invitation into a way of living. The academic endeavors of scholars do afford commentaries on the experience and teachings of the Church Fathers over the centuries; however, this scholarly analysis and commentary are always secondary in authority and importance to theology as an experience of God. Because of the nondevelopmental character of the Orthodox Christian experience of God's presence, the age of the Fathers has not ended for Orthodoxy, as it did for the West around the eighth century. Strictly speaking, the age of the Fathers is coterminous with the unbroken presence of the Holy Spirit.

A number of points distinguish the Orthodox Christian approach to medical ethics.

- Orthodox morality and medical ethics first and foremost form a seamless integral part of a way of life.
- Because Orthodox Christianity aims at a relationship with a fully transcendent God with Whom there is no analogy of being, rational principles, casuistic analyses, and other discursive rational devices that might introduce a false juridicism and Scholasticism are rendered into therapeutic guides.
- Because Orthodox Christian morality and bioethics are spiritual-therapeutic rather than academic, they are understood as tools for aiming rightly at the holy, at the Truth Who is God.
- Unlike Western Christianity, which came to look for traces of God in nature, Orthodox Christianity approaches nature as an icon, as a window through which to look to God.
- As a consequence, Orthodox Christianity is hierological in relativizing the right and the good in terms of an overriding pursuit of the holy.
- Orthodox Christian epistemology is at root noetic or mystical; it understands that the only way beyond a finite horizon of experience and texts is through coming into a transforming and informing relation with God.

The result is not only that Orthodox Christianity rejects the discursive rational commitments of Scholasticism and the Enlightenment, it also breaks through the fragmentation marking the moral pluralism that defines post-modernism. It reaches beyond the confines of particular narratives and texts, which are set within the horizon of the finite and the immanent. Thus, for example, the Scriptures are neither revelation nor a set of writings relevantly to be reassessed through such academic means of analyses as historical, text-critical, and higher-critical methods. Instead, the Scriptures are records of revelation whose meaning can only be correctly experienced within the grace of the Church that is the body of Christ, so that

their meaning is acquired on the model of Christ's unlocking the Scriptures on the way to Emmaus (Luke 24:13–35). Within the privileged ascetic and liturgically directed epistemological standpoint of the Church, the writings she has accepted, affirmed, and interpreted become, like an icon, a window by which one looks through the text to God.

II. THE PAST IN THE PRESENT TENSE

Neither "medical ethics" nor "bioethics" is a univocal term. Each has a meaning set within a cluster of background commitments and assumptions framing a particular understanding of appropriate action, moral probity, and morality. These assumptions are often unnoticed, in that they comport with the background presuppositions that structure the contemporary, dominant, secular culture. Against this background, it is difficult to imagine a radically different medical ethics set within disparate moral commitments. Orthodox Christianity through its morality, medical ethics, and theology provide a stark example of such differences. It is not just that Orthodox morality and medical ethics possess a content different from that of the secular culture, as well as most religious communities, in addition, these perspectives diverge in terms of what a morality should be about. For example, the morality is therapeutic in intent rather than juridical.

As an introduction to the depth of these differences, one might consider the Orthodox Christian historiography of Christian morality and medical ethics. Orthodox Christians hold that Christian medical ethics is nondevelopmental in the sense of affirming the same moral commitments and insights that directed the Church of the first thousand years: It understands that all that is essential for the appropriate moral life has been available since the time of the Apostles. This difference is in part grounded in the Orthodox Christian recognition that truth is not merely a what as a set of discursive propositions, but a radically transcendent Who (i.e., the Trinity), with Whom because Pentecost right-worshipping Christians have had the possibility of a full relationship.

This nondevelopmental recognition of the full presence of truth in the Orthodox Church is expressed by the Fathers of the Seventh Ecumenical Council (Nicea II, 787):

> To make our confession short, we keep unchanged all the ecclesiastical traditions handed down to us, whether in writing or verbally.... Thus we follow Paul, who spoke in Christ, and the whole divine Apostolic company and the holy Fathers, holding fast the traditions which we have received.... For we follow the most ancient legislation of the Catholic Church. We keep the laws of the Fathers. We anathematize those who add anything to or take

anything away from the Catholic Church. (Schaff and Wace 1994, 550–51)

Orthodox Christianity understands its morality and medical ethics to have been in its substance delivered to the Apostles once and for all. In this, Orthodox Christianity contrasts with both Roman Catholicism and most Protestant faiths in rejecting a notion of moral dogmatic progress. In particular, Orthodox Christianity does not regard moral theology as a cardinal cultural endeavor through which the academy makes advances in moral insight and understanding. Instead, Orthodox Christianity acknowledges its moral truth as set within a liturgical Now, a moral experience that has existed and been sustained in its fullness since the age of the Apostles. As a consequence, Orthodox Christianity regards its moral theological past as if it were present. It is for this reason that Orthodox Christians seemingly turn indiscriminately for guidance to any of the Fathers in any century. This epistemological standpoint within which the past is experienced as presented in a "now" is captured in the practice of the Orthodox Church of explaining the past as present. For example, the Vespers of the Sunday of the Holy Fathers of the First Six Ecumenical Councils declares: "Those God-mantled Fathers have proclaimed today in concert . . ." (Nassar 1979, 558). Despite the circumstance that these councils occurred from the fourth to the seventh centuries, liturgically they are encountered as if they were present within the experience of God.

The Orthodox Church does not deny terminological development in the narrow sense that distinctions, terminologies, and analyses of theological experience take shape within a history. Yet, because Orthodox theology is primarily not an academic discipline but an immediate experience of God, these analytic, conceptual, and academic developments are not acknowledged as theological developments per se. Rather, they are temporally and historically located responses to heretics and expositions of answers to particular questions and puzzles. In this context, the contributions of the Fathers from the third to the eighth centuries can be understood as playing a role distantly analogous to the age of the Fathers for the West: they are a rich resource of theological reflection and Scriptural exposition that records the commitments and life of the Church of the first part of the first millennium. For Orthodox Christians, however, the age of the Fathers has not ended, for the same Spirit Who inspired the Gospels inspires the holy Fathers of the twenty-first century. In this sense, one should understand the statement of Bartholomew I, the Ecumenical Patriarch of Constantinople:

> The manner in which we [the Orthodox and the West] exist has become ontologically different . . . the Orthodox Christian does not live in a place of theoretical and conceptual conversations, but rather

in a place of an essential and empirical lifestyle and reality as confirmed by grace in the heart [Heb 13:9]. This grace cannot be put in doubt either by logic or science or other type of argument . . . However, the change of man's essence, theosis by grace, is a fact that is tangible for all the Orthodox faithful. Grace is not only obtained through the transformed relics of the saints, which is totally inexplicable without acceptance of the divine. Grace also radiates from living Saints who are truly in the likeness of the Lord. [Luke 8:46] (Patriarch Bartholomew, 21 October 1997)

The age of the Fathers has not ended, for all of theology is always fully available to all who, embedded within right worship, experience God.

In approaching new technological developments, such as cloning, the use of embryonic stem cells, and germ line genetic engineering, Orthodox Christians will not seek new moral insights but to express in a new context the enduring moral consciousness of the Church. The goal will not be the articulation of new medical-ethical or bioethical principles, but the capturing of a permanent possibility for epistemic insight grounded in the consequences of the Incarnation. The goal will be to provide an expression of an abiding truth guided in part by the writings of the Fathers and crucially sustained by the presence of the Holy Spirit.

III. MEDICAL ETHICAL NORMS

The norms for the use of medicine and the biomedical sciences are set within the constraints that Orthodox Christians understand are integral to aiming one's life at holiness, at union with God. Because Orthodox Christianity has from the Apostles and Fathers had a concrete moral vision bearing on the full range of human concerns from marriage, sexuality, and reproduction to suffering, dying, and death, contemporary moral issues from abortion and cloning to the use of scarce medical resources and euthanasia are approached within an already well-established framework. In addition, given the focus of that holiness that leads to saintliness, concerns to avoid suffering and postpone death are radically relativized by a viewpoint that looks beyond the horizon of the immanent and finite to final judgment and beyond.

IV. BEYOND IMMANENT UNDERSTANDINGS OF GOOD AND EVIL: MORALITY TRANSFORMED BY HOLINESS AND DIVINE MERCY

It is not just that Orthodox Christianity has an understanding of history at odds with that of the West; its account of morality is fundamentally different as well. Four points of difference must be underscored. First, all immanent (i.e., this-worldly) considerations of good and evil are recast in terms of a transcendent horizon of concern. Because of its hierological focus, Orthodox Christian medical ethics cannot be reduced to moral concerns, in the sense of immanent interests in the good, the right, and the virtuous. The holy transcends, relocates, and relativizes the ethical. Living a good life is never sufficient for salvation and, because of the possibility of final repentance, living a good life is not strictly necessary either. The radical mercy of God always transcends and sets aside the strict requirements of justice. Because of its overriding interest in coming into union with God through repentance and illumination through God's grace, Orthodox Christian medical–ethical reflection locates good, professional conduct in terms of a good spiritual life. Orthodox Christian medical ethics is inarticulable, except in terms of the pursuit of holiness.

Second, this character of Orthodox Christian medical–moral historiography is rooted in the noetic or mystical character of its epistemology. Theological knowledge is grounded in the experience of God, not primarily in analysis, reflection, and discursive reasoning. Given this moral–theological epistemology, Orthodox Christian moral theologians par excellence are such because they are holy, not because they are necessarily learned in an academic sense. As Evagrios the Solitary (345–399) stresses, "if you are a theologian, you will pray truly. And if you pray truly, you are a theologian" (Evagrios 1988, 1:62). This sets Orthodox Christian moral theology and its medical ethics apart from that which took shape in Western Europe under the influence of Augustine of Hippo (354–430), and especially during the Western Scholasticism of the thirteenth through the sixteenth centuries, which led to a discursively grounded, philosophical account of morality. The noetic character of Orthodox theology affirms an iconic view of created reality as a window to the uncreated, so that God and His moral requirements are held to be recognizable through nature (Foltz 2001). This appreciation of the invisible through the visible marginalizes discursive attempts to deduce moral requirements from nature. In particular, an independent Orthodox moral philosophy is not available (a point emphasized by St. John Chrysostom and the Fifth Council of Constantinople [1341, 1347, 1351], among many others) to revise theological moral commitments. Finally, Orthodox Christianity recognizes that those who fail to live a holy life will fail as well to appreciate fully the requirements of morality. The good is appreciated rightly only from the perspective of the holy.

Third, Orthodox Christian spiritual concerns have a spiritually therapeutic character. Because sin is understood as falling short of the mark of aiming flawlessly at holiness (the Greek term used in the New Testament for sin, *hamartia*, means falling short of the mark or target), and

because sins can be involuntary in the sense of involving unwittingly turning from wholehearted love of God and neighbor, the focus is on righting a person's spiritual direction. It would be an error to read Orthodox canons bearing on medicine in moralistic or juridical terms. Because the ultimate focus is on union with God, which depends not on merit from good works but on purification through repentance, ascetic struggle, and grace, periods of excommunication and penance must be interpreted not as punishments, but as spiritual therapy, allowing one to accept transformation through God's mercy. It is in this light that the Orthodox notion of economia as a departure from the strict requirements of a canon (i.e., acrivia) should not be understood as a dispensation but as a redirection of spiritual energies so as better to realize the therapeutic goal of the canon. This spiritually therapeutic character of Orthodox Christianity nests medical ethical concerns in a framework alien to much of Western ethics.

Finally, Orthodox Christian reflections on ethics point to an integral way of life with a profoundly holistic character. Orthodox Christianity implicitly recognizes a danger in compartmentalizing moral concerns under rubrics such as medical, legal, and business ethics. Even categories such as moral, dogmatic, and liturgical theology are one-sided abstractions unless they are embedded in a theological way of life, a prayerful experience of God. It is therefore an error to approach Orthodox Christianity's various canons, directions, and prohibitions regarding medicine apart from what it would mean to be successful as a Christian, that is, to become a saint. Orthodox reflections have not produced a set of guiding moral rules and principles that can be appreciated in isolation from an Orthodox way of life.

As a result of these four points of difference, an understanding of Orthodox Christian medical ethics requires entrance into a mindset or way of thinking that places moral concerns in a framework abandoned by Western Christianity more than a millennium ago. It is a view untouched by the Renaissance, the Enlightenment, or the modernist movements of the nineteenth and twentieth centuries, which transformed many Protestant and Roman Catholic appreciations of medical moral issues. Orthodox Christian reflections on the appropriate use of medicine, as well as on abortion, suicide, and truth telling, were well articulated by the end of the fourth century and have not experienced any substantial change. After the ninth century, there is little to be found that would further inform an Orthodox Christian medical ethicist of the twenty-first century. Orthodox Christian history of medical ethics is twice over oxymoronic. Historical moral development is set aside within a now embedded in the kingdom of heaven experienced in worship, while mercy nullifies the requirements of justice, and medical ethical concerns with the right, the good, and the virtuous are recast within a spiritually therapeutic pursuit of the holy.

V. MEDICAL ETHICS AND THE MIND OF THE FATHERS

The peace brought by the age after St. Constantine the Great (d. 337) allowed the opportunity for a comprehensive record of the mind of the Church on a range of issues, including medicine. As St. Basil the Great (329–379) stresses, "Each of the arts is God's gift to us, remedying the deficiencies of nature . . . the medical art was given to us to relieve the sick, in some degree at least" (Basil 1962, 330–1). This endorsement of medicine creates a presumption that medicine will be engaged to restore health and preserve life. Good health aids in the discharge of one's duties to others. Although suffering can lead to spiritual growth, it is not an end in itself. Medicine is endorsed because of its ability to relieve morbidity: "with mandrake doctors give us sleep; with opium they lull violent pain" (Basil 1994, 8:78). This positive attitude toward the amelioration of suffering is affirmed in a petition that is part of "The Litany of Supplication" in Vespers, Matins, and Liturgy: "A Christian ending to our life, painless, blameless, peaceful, and a good defense before the fearful judgment seat of Christ, let us ask" (Antiochian Orthodox Christian Archdiocese 1989, 28). While affirming the use of analgesics, the Fathers rejected suicide, although they recognized that suicide can be the nonculpable result of mental illness (Peter 1983, 746). The Church, which had always tended to the poor and the sick, began in the fourth century to establish hospitals, which until the fall of Constantinople (1453) provided a level of care beyond that available in the West. The understanding of general surgery, orthopedics, obstetrics-gynecology, otorhinolaryngology, as well as epidemiology, was comparable to much that appeared in the West only in the nineteenth century (Constantelos 1991, 118).

Although medicine and hospital care were endorsed and supported, there was a recognition that the use of medicine can become an all-consuming passion, distorting and misdirecting the spiritual life. St. Basil warns that we should avoid "whatever requires an undue amount of thought or trouble or involves a large expenditure of effort and causes our whole life to revolve, as it were, around solicitude for the flesh . . . " (Basil 1962, 331). Trying to save life at all costs is recognized as having too high a spiritual cost. This recognition of how medicine can play a disproportionate role in the lives of individuals lies at the root of the sixteenth-century Roman Catholic distinction between ordinary and extraordinary care (see Chapter 14). Through this distinction, Roman Catholic moral theology sought to determine the circumstances under which the natural duty to preserve one's life is defeated by the burdens of treatment or a low likelihood of successfully securing health. In contrast, the Orthodox Christian concern is explicitly and forthrightly with the spiritual life, with determining when the use of medicine will dis-

tract from the pursuit of salvation. In addition, there is a recognition that reliance on medicine should not supplant or marginalize reliance on God. "To place the hope of one's health in the hands of the doctor is the act of an irrational animal" (Basil 1962, 333). The promises of medicine are relativized by the ultimate goal of salvation. Orthodox Christian medical ethics thus did not take on the secular idiom facilitated by the natural-law arguments in the West beginning in the thirteenth century.

It is in light of what will deflect from salvation that patristic understandings of abortion must be appreciated. First, all sexual activity and reproduction are placed within the marriage of a man and a woman. Second, as early as the late first-century or late second-century *Didache* (II.2), there are lists of proscriptions, including "thou shalt not commit adultery; thou shalt not commit sodomy; thou shalt not commit fornication; . . . thou shalt not procure abortion, nor commit infanticide" (Lake 1965, 1:311, 313). A similar list is found in the Epistle of Barnabas (XIX.3–6) from the same period. Abortion is proscribed because it involves taking the life of what should become a human person. Independently of whether the fetus is yet a person, Orthodox Christianity treats any individual as

> a murderer who kills an imperfect and unformed embryo, because this though not yet then a complete being was nevertheless destined to be perfected in the future, according to indispensable sequence of the laws of nature. (Basil 1983, 789)

Canons against abortion abound, as early as a council held in Ankara in 315 (Council in Ancyra 1983, 501), followed by canons from the Fathers (Basil 1983, Canon 2, 789; John the Faster 1983, Canon 21, 944) and the Quinisext Council or Council in Trullo (691–692), which produced the canons for the Fifth and Sixth Ecumenical Councils (Quinisext Council 1983, Canon 91, 395).

Because of a recognition of the spiritual harm even in involuntary homicide, miscarriage through no fault of the mother is penanced and treated with absolution, as the rituals of the Orthodox Church attest.

> According to Your great mercy, be merciful to Your servant, N., who is in sin, having been involved in the loss of a life, whether voluntary or involuntary, for she has miscarried that which was conceived in her. Forgive her transgressions, both voluntary and involuntary, and protect her from every snare of the Devil. Cleanse her stain and heal her infirmities. And grant to her, O Lover of Mankind, health and strength of soul and body. . . . Forgive this, Your servant, N., who is in sin, having been involved in the loss of a life, whether voluntary or involuntary, for she has miscarried that which was conceived in her. And, according to Your great mercy as the Good God Who loves mankind, be merciful and forgive all

those who are here present and who have touched her. (Monk of St. Tikhon's Monastery 1987, 6–7)

This is not to deny that more harm is associated with a willful and intentional abortion. Nevertheless, there is an appreciation of the experience of guilt frequently associated with a miscarriage and the need to set it all aside through the power and forgiveness of grace.

This recognition of the spiritual harms suffered in a world broken by sin is made possible by the insight predominant in the Church of the first millennium that one can be spiritually injured by a proximate causal involvement in the death of another person. Homicide even in a just war incurs excommunication (i.e., requires ascetic spiritual therapy and absolution) (Basil 1983, Canon 13, 801–2). Orthodox Christianity eschewed developing an analogue to the Roman Catholic doctrine of double effect regarding homicide. This doctrine holds that when an action has two effects, one good and the other evil, as long as the act itself is not evil and the good effect does not flow from the bad effect, one can without culpability act intending the good effect, while only foreseeing the bad effect, as long as there is a proportionate reason (i.e., one will bring about more benefit than harm). The Roman Catholic doctrine allowed Roman Catholicism to permit as guiltless indirect abortions undertaken to save the life of the mother (e.g., removing a cancerous pregnant uterus, foreseeing, but not intending, the abortion). In contrast, for Orthodox Christianity all abortions are recognized as instances of homicide, although some (e.g., those that are direct, willful, and without threat to the mother's health and life) are more evil than others. It is important to notice that a casuistry has not developed to guide Orthodox Christian confessors in determining whether and when strictly to apply the standard penances associated with abortion, or instead, by economia, to require less or more. These decisions are to be made in each case guided by the Holy Spirit. For this reason among others Orthodox Christian morality coincides with the morality of the ancient Christian church and is regarded by Roman Catholics as underdeveloped.

Orthodox medical–ethical norms regarding truth telling are untouched by Augustine of Hippo's (354–430) condemnation of deceit through the intentional telling of a falsehood. Because of the spiritually therapeutic character of Orthodox Christian moral interest, there is no absolute requirement of truth telling on the part of physicians. Indeed, the obligation of physicians to lie when this is necessary for the well-being of patients is taken as paradigmatic of a similar obligation on the part of persons generally. Clement of Alexandria (155–220) holds that one should generally tell the truth, yet he recognizes that one must at times "medicinally, as a physician for the sake of the sick . . . deceive or tell an untruth" (Clement 1994, 2:538). Although one may be obliged to lie, nevertheless,

one should attempt spiritually to compensate for the spiritual harm caused by lying, as Abba Dorotheos of Gaza (506/508–580) stresses.

> But if a man did such a thing [as lying], in extreme necessity, let him not be without anxiety but let him repent and sorrow before God and consider it, as I said, a time of trial and not let it become a habit but done once and for all. . . . Just as an antidote for snake poison or a powerful purge is beneficial when taken in time and in case of need, it does harm if taken habitually, without necessity (Dorotheos 1977, 161).

This acknowledgement that in a world broken by sin one may be obliged to become involved in sin (i.e., to engage in an activity considered by itself to fall short of the mark) to pursue salvation requires approaching moral issues within the overriding concern to cure from self-love so as to turn in full love to God and one's neighbor. The result is a nonbinary (i.e., not black or white, not sinless or sinful) account of the human predicament.

Because of the focus on the pursuit of salvation, it has been taken for granted that an Orthodox Christian physician should not be religiously neutral in the care of patients. Holy physicians are celebrated who, such as St. Panteleimon (d. 304), took advantage of their physician–patient relationships to convert their patients. Although one is obliged to avoid all coercion (canon CXIX of Carthage, 419), it is far from improper to use a patient's recognition of human vulnerability as an opportunity to open the way to repentance and conversion. The professional life of the physician is located within the religious life of the physician. There has been no discounting of the religious commitments of the physician in favor of an independent secular moral vision of professional conduct, indeed, to the contrary. Contemporary Orthodox Christian medical ethics is one with the ethos of fourth-century Christianity, which holds itself to be the authentic expression of the ethos of the Apostles.

VI. Contemporary Medical Ethics Framed within the Context of the First Millennium

As with many other religions, rapid biomedical advances have produced questions requiring pastoral guidance. Orthodox priests, bishops, and churches have responded by placing contemporary biomedical issues within the mind and framework of the Apostles and the Fathers. Seemingly new challenges have been addressed with the conviction that Christ and the behavior He requires is the same yesterday, today, and tomorrow (Heb. 13:8). These responses have for the most part occurred beginning in the twentieth century, primarily since the 1990s.

Although the canons of the ancient Church make no explicit reference to contraception, in addressing artificial contraception Orthodox Christianity has regarded it and family planning as on a par (i.e., when the contraception does not involve abortion). They both have been understood as temptations for husbands and wives to fail in their duties generously to bring children into the world. The focus is thus more centrally on the obligations of husbands and wives, given the nature of marriage, to trust unselfishly in God, rather than in a disengaged biological account of natural versus unnatural acts. Differences in approaches to the propriety of contraception can then be understood as differences in judgments regarding how to act selflessly as Christian parents. As elsewhere, the attempt is to place decisions within the mind of the Fathers rather than to create new understandings through discursive moral–philosophical reflection.

A similar approach can be seen as available for questions such as transsexual surgery. From the early Church, there is a condemnation of castration done out of a rejection of one's sexual identity. As Canon VIII of the First-and-Second Council held in Constantinople in 861 states, affirming a canon from Nicea I in 325:

> Wherefore the holy Council has been led to decree that if any bishop, or presbyter, or deacon, be proved guilty for castrating anyone, either with his own hand or by giving orders to anyone else to do so, he shall be subjected to the penalty of deposition from office; but if the offender is a layman, he shall be excommunicated; unless it should so happen that owing to the incidence of some affliction he should be forced to operate upon the sufferer by removing his testicles. For precisely as the first Canon of the Council held in Nicaea does not punish those who have been operated upon for a disease, for having the disease, so neither do we condemn priests who order diseased men to be castrated, nor do we blame laymen either, when they perform the operation with their own hands. For we consider this to be a treatment of the disease, but not a malicious design against the creature or an insult to creation. (First-and-Second Council 1983, 465)

There is an acceptance of therapeutically appropriate castrations, along with a rejection of those that are undertaken to reject the embodiment given to an individual by God. One is constrained to accept the embodied sexuality that is one's lot.

Similarly, the evil of cloning can be placed within the recognition of the interconnection of husband and wife in reproduction. St. John Chrysostom (354–407) addressed this issue in his commentary on Ephesians: "Nor did He enable woman to bear children without man; if this were the case she would be self-sufficient" (Chrysostom 1986, 44). This understanding is generalized to men as well as to women, thus forbidding solitary reproduction such as cloning. The focus is on placing human sexuality and reproduction fully within the union of husband and wife, a union whose status is endorsed by both the New and Old Testaments. So, too, the use of donor gametes in artificial insemination or in vitro fertilization can be recognized on analogy with adultery, although such insemination may lack the full harm of adulterous carnal intercourse. In considering each medical–moral issue, it is placed within the framework of the Church of the first millennium.

VII. Conclusion

Because of the recognition that moral knowledge is only fully disclosed through relationship with God, contemporary Orthodox Christian analyses of medical–moral issues will often proceed to examine those issues by placing them within the prayers and Liturgy of the Church, which are recognized as providing normative guidance (Guroian 1996). The context for analysis remains that of worship, Scripture, the Fathers, and Holy Tradition, not an independent, academic tradition of discursive theological moral investigation. In this mode, a number of studies have emerged (Harakas 1990; Breck 1998; Engelhardt 2000). These Orthodox Christian moral theological reflections are not recognized as gaining their authority from their place within an independent academic discipline of moral theology, but through directing Christians back to the authentic experience of the Christian life. Such "new" reflections on medical ethics have the character of being connected with and embedded in the mind of the early Church. Contemporary reflections and those of the Fathers are united in the liturgical now of Orthodox Christian prayer, which is the source of all its theology. Because the history of Orthodox Christian medical ethics is that of a struggle against error and heresy to maintain its authentic understandings ever the same, ever in the mind of the Fathers, there is not simply a backward-looking character to its history, but one marked by a rupture of the horizon of ordinary temporality. Orthodox Christian reflections on medical ethics are one element of the Church's attempt to set aside the alienating character of time, which appears to isolate the past from the present, which seems to separate us from the living Fathers of the first centuries. By recognizing that this gulf is bridged in each Liturgy, Orthodox Christianity affirms its radically different account of the history of moral theology and medical ethics.

CHAPTER 14

THE DISCOURSES OF ROMAN CATHOLIC MEDICAL ETHICS

Darrel W. Amundsen

I. INTRODUCTION

Pope Pius XII's (b. 1876; r. 1939–1958)[1] address in 1944 to the Italian Medical-biological Union of St. Luke, an exclusively Roman Catholic audience, is a concise summary of many aspects of Roman Catholic medical ethics as they had evolved up his time, which he supported philosophically by arguments from natural law, explicated theologically from Scripture and Tradition, and elaborated with deep pastoral concern (Papal Teachings 1960, 51–65). He introduced his allocution with an anecdote: "Your presence, beloved sons, brings to mind a scene enacted in Paris in December, 1804. In the Grand Hall of the Louvre, when numerous delegations crowded to render homage to the Vicar of Christ and to receive his blessing, five young doctors . . . were introduced to the Sovereign Pontiff, Pius VII. The Pope could not disguise a reaction of surprise: 'Oh!' he said laughingly, '*Medicus pius, res miranda!*'"

This exclamation of a pope 140 years earlier – "A pious physician – what an amazing thing!" – echoed an adage from the Middle Ages, "*Ubi tres medici, ibi duo athei*" ("Where there are three physicians there are two atheists"). The warnings of the lure of scientific naturalism as a danger to which physicians are especially susceptible have been reiterated throughout the history of the Church. Furthermore, that medicine may be employed as much to evil as to good ends had been a concern of the Church Fathers (see Chapter 12) and has been a focal point of Roman Catholic medical ethics. As the horizons of modern medicine have been broadening nearly exponentially during the last century, so also have the concerns of the hierarchy of the Church and of moral theologians to address the moral dimensions of scientific research and medical practice. There is something very distinct about the discourses of Roman Catholic medical ethics. For instance, the discourses of Protestantism can in fact only be the discourses of Protestants, since Protestantism exists as an idea rather than as an institution, as a core of common beliefs at least formally shared by numerous denominations and independent congregations. In a sense that Protestants cannot claim, there is a Roman Catholicism that is primarily identified with its magisterium, its institutional structure, its promulgated canon law, and, in the realm of ethics, its long and rich history of moral theology.

This chapter will focus on the major sources of moral definition and authority within Roman Catholicism, in two sections that overlap some chronologically. The first section extends from the early Middle Ages to the First Council of the Vatican, which convened in 1869. During most of this lengthy period, canon law and moral theology were the major sources of Roman Catholic medical ethics. The second section focuses primarily on the role of the magisterium as a source of moral definition. Because the importance of the magisterium as the primary source of moral definition and authority, especially since Vatican I, can hardly be overemphasized, some preliminary observations are in order here.

The semantic, conceptual, and institutional history of the ecclesiastical Latin term *magisterium* is complex. The word itself is from the Latin *magister*, which in antiquity and the Middle Ages applied to the person in charge of any of a wide range of areas and functions. Magisterium meant the office or dignity of a *magister*. In the history of the Church, magisterium has usually described the position of authority to exercise the function of teaching. In the thirteenth century, St. Thomas Aquinas (1224–1274) spoke of two kinds of *magisteria: magisterium cathedrae magistralis*, that is, the magisterium of theologians, and *magisterium cathedrae pastoralis*, that is, the magisterium of bishops. The major conceptual and functional difference between the two was that the latter, the magisterium of bishops, involved the authority of those having specific ecclesiastical jurisdiction.[2] Since Vatican I (although it had become increasingly common earlier in the nineteenth century), the word *magisterium* has typically referred to what St. Thomas called the *magisterium cathedrae pastoralis*, the magisterium of bishops, that is, the teaching function of the hierarchy and, by extension, the hierarchy itself as the bearer of this authority. Rarely, since Vatican I, has the term been used in any other way, except in disputes among theologians regarding the propriety of this limited and generally exclusive usage. Because the hierarchy of the Church has as its temporal head the pope, and as most pronouncements emanating from the magisterium are issued directly by the pope or by agencies directly reportable to him,[3] the hierarchical magisterium has, for all practical purposes, become the papal magisterium.

Since Vatican I, at which the dogma of papal infallibility was promulgated, the magisterium has become the most vigorous party, both proactively and reactively, within the Catholic communion in defining and refining the Church's position on all issues of medical ethics. In the process, the magisterium has created an atmosphere of both moral certainty and uncertainty in which the most intellectually stimulating and creative moral theologians, many of whom are on the cutting edge of bioethics, find themselves in a constrained and sometimes precarious position.

At the outset, the reader should note that the issues of medical ethics that have been and remain most in dispute within the Church involve the beginning and end of the life cycle, especially contraception, abortion, euthanasia, and, more recently, reproductive technologies and research in prenatal human life. Because the history of these issues within the Church is as old as the Church herself, on occasion they inevitably arise in the present chapter. This chapter provides a history of the context in which those issues and other aspects of the broad realm of the ethics of health and healing have developed in Catholic tradition.

II. Canon Law and Moral Theology

1. The Middle Ages

Canon law is the juridical–legislative articulation of the life of the Church at any point in her history. Before the early thirteenth century, however, there was no officially promulgated collection of canons having the force of law. Canon law consisted of private compilations of canons of councils, papal rescripts, and episcopal statutes, often inconsistent with each other. The first great effort to bring order out of this chaos was Gratian's monumental *Decretum* (c. 1140; Friedberg 1879). Its original title, *Concordia Discordantium Canonum (A Harmony of Discordant Canons)* graphically portrays his purpose. The method he employed was to state a specific problem, introduce authorities on both sides of the question, and then propose a solution that would bring the conflicting positions into harmony or show the greater acceptability of one position.

The promulgation of official collections of canon law first occurred in the early thirteenth century, by far the most important being the *Decretales* (Friedberg 1879), promulgated in 1234 by Pope Gregory IX (b. 1170?; r. 1227–1241), which rendered all previous collections, whether of an official or unofficial nature, obsolete (except for the *Decretum*, which the official collections did not supplant but rather supplemented), and is part of what became known as the *Corpus Iuris Canonici* (Corpus of Canon Law).[4] This was the classical period of canon law during which canonists, that is, commentators on canon law such as decretists (commentators on the *Decretum*) and decretalists (commentators on the *Decretales*), produced exhaustive analyses of canons in an effort to establish legal principles and to show how they could be applied to real and hypothetical situations.

The influence of canon law on the development of Roman Catholic medical ethics has been profound, especially in three respects. First, owing to the influence of the penitential manuals (to be described later), early medieval canon law developed a dominantly punitive character, essentially more negative than positive. Such has also been the defining characteristic of Catholic medical ethics for most of its history. Second, the first systematic efforts to determine the moral responsibilities of physicians and surgeons were in response to specific decrees of canon law. Third, these efforts were made by canonists and by moral theologians, who often cited or quoted the works of canonists. Our major source of knowledge of Roman Catholic medical ethics prior to Vatican I is moral theology.

If one is to understand the fundamental role that moral theology has played in the development of Roman

Catholic medical ethics, one must be aware of the circumstances that gave rise to the discipline itself. Although moral theology had always been present in the Church as the articulation of principles of Christian morality, its roots as a discipline go back to the penitential manuals of the early Middle Ages, which were essentially lists of sins for which appropriate penances were assigned. These primitive and theologically unsophisticated manuals had no official standing, and some were formally condemned for their severity. They set the negative and legalistic tone that has been the defining characteristic of moral theology until nearly the present: "a preoccupation with sin; a concentration on the individual; and an obsession with law"; indeed a relinquishing of "almost all consideration of the good in man to other branches of theology" (Mahoney 1987, 27, 29).

Composed from the sixth through the early eleventh century to assist the clergy in their interrogation of penitents (McNeill and Gamer 1938), the penitential manuals must have exercised considerable influence on popular moral understanding. Sexual sins more than any other aroused the attention of the authors of these handbooks. They were especially interested in sexual acts in which there was little or no possibility of conception and in abortion. Concern with superstitious practices was a strong contender for second place after sexual sins in these handbooks. Abortion, when induced by the use of potions or pessaries, was typically classified as pagan magic. Pagan methods of healing or preserving health are commonly encountered among the sins specified in this literature. No vocations or professions were singled out for special scrutiny. This was soon to change.

A theological and philosophical renaissance in the twelfth century created a scholarly milieu that fostered formal analyses of moral behavior, which were then enormously stimulated by a decree of the Fourth Lateran Council in 1215. Canon 21, *Omnis Utriusque Sexus*, required annual confession and reception of the Eucharist at least at Easter of all Catholics who had reached the age of discernment. "Otherwise they shall be barred from entering a church during their lifetime and they shall be denied a Christian burial at death" (Tanner 1990, 1:245). This canon, which was thoroughly publicized, then incorporated into the *Decretales* (5.38.12), and strictly enforced, evoked a positive and practical response from moral theologians.

Much of the energy of the emerging field of moral theology was directed to creating systematic treatments of the sacrament of penance and convenient manuals to aid priests in interrogating penitents. This literature was written by those who "were considered experts, with special knowledge about penitents, confessors, and confessing" (Tentler 1977, xiv) for priests who typically did not have at their disposal the great commentaries and specialized writings of the major scholastic theologians or canonists.

Through these treatises the complexities of legal and moral prescriptions could filter down in an easily understandable form to those who needed immediate answers. They were reference works designed to give answers, not theological or philosophical inquiries designed to rouse debate. They were intended to simplify doctrine for practical application and were organized so that the confessor could locate answers easily.

Confessional examination was to penetrate into every area of life. Nothing was outside its purview: birth, marriage, sex, the rearing of children – indeed, every aspect of private, domestic, social, and economic life. Under the latter fell the special areas of sin to which various occupations were regarded as susceptible. It was not until the early fourteenth century, however, that the list of occupations singled out for special attention became stabilized in the confessional literature and regularly included medicine and surgery.

These treatises differ from one another significantly in length, form, and emphases. Some are short and refer the reader to no authorities for the opinions given, although they may include a plethora of sins with little or no comment. Others are longer, even very long, but only rarely cite any sources other than the *Decretum*, the *Decretales*, and numerous decretists and decretalists to give weight to their opinions. The variety of sins and the order in which they are treated also differ from treatise to treatise.

Three canons in the *Decretales*, which they frequently cite, deal specifically with aspects of medical practice. *Ad Aures* (1.14.7; between 1187 and 1191) and *Tua Nos* (5.12.19; 1212), both of which were papal responses to specific queries, are complementary. Applying the principle that one must refrain from usurping offices alien to him, *Tua Nos* addresses the death of a patient after surgery, attributable to her failure to follow the physician's instructions, and exonerates the latter because he was both competent and diligent. *Ad Aures* involves a physician who wished to enter the priesthood. He was troubled that perhaps some of his patients had died owing to his treatments, although he had diligently followed the traditions of his art. He was instructed to search his conscience to determine whether he was responsible for any harm having come to his patients. The concern here was with error of commission and provided decretalists and the authors of confessional literature with a fitting balance to the issues raised by *Tua nos*. (For a translation and more detailed discussion of these two canons, see Amundsen 1996, 235–36, 254–58.)

Cum Infirmitas (5.38.13; canon 22 of Lateran IV [1215]) contains two provisions.

we by this present decree order and strictly command physicians of the body, when they are called to the sick, to warn and persuade them first of all to call in physicians of the soul . . . This among other things has occasioned this decree, namely that some people on their sickbed, when they are advised by physicians to arrange for the health of their souls, fall into despair and so the more readily incur the danger of death. If any physician transgresses this our constitution, after it has been published by the local prelates, he shall be barred from entering a church until he has made suitable satisfaction for a transgression of this kind... since the soul is much more precious than the body, we forbid any physician, under pain of anathema, to prescribe anything for the bodily health of a sick person that may endanger his soul. (Tanner 1990, 1:245–46)

The summary that follows combines the most salient features of the sections that deal with the sins of physicians in nine treatises of varying length (a study of which is in Amundsen 1996, 248–88). The earliest was written approximately 1317 by Astesanus de Asti (died c. 1330), the latest roughly 1538 by Bartholomaeus Fumus (died 1555). The lengthiest and most thorough is the *Summa Theologica* (or *Summa Moralis*) of St. Antoninus of Florence (1389–1459), which was completed in 1477. When the authors address the sins of physicians, their citations typically are of sources that articulate legal or moral principles that they then apply to the conduct of physicians. Their moral reasoning was founded on principles of natural law inherited from their predecessors, especially as articulated in the thirteenth century by St. Thomas Aquinas in his *Summa Theologiae* (Thomas Aquinas 1964).

Physicians sin by practicing without adequate training or skill, by not following the traditions of the art, and by being negligent. They must never administer medicines about whose effects they are in doubt or test the efficacy of dangerous substances and thus expose patients to the peril of death or grave injury. Nevertheless, they must ensure that they not be so cautious that they fail to give the appropriate medicines. It is especially egregious for them to seek to increase their fees by aggravating or prolonging illnesses.

Physicians should accept only a "reasonable" fee, as determined by the quality of care, their labor and diligence, local customs, and the patient's means. They must treat the poor gratis if the patient would die without treatment. Even in apparently hopeless cases, physicians sin if they do not do all they can to cure their patients or if they entirely withdraw before death comes naturally. Some moral theologians maintain that physicians must treat gratis rich misers who are unwilling to employ their services, and even provide medicines without charge; otherwise they are killing them indirectly.

Discussions of the requirement that physicians "warn and persuade" their patients to summon a priest vary in length, detail, and sensitivity to the problems that this admonition posed. Several laconically insist that

physicians sin if they do not require all patients without exception to summon a confessor before treating them. Others maintain that the requirement applies only to cases of extremely dangerous or mortal illnesses, because the patient's life would be endangered if physicians had to delay treatment until the patient had been shriven. Some remark that if physicians require patients who suffer from chronic but not threatening ailments (e.g., gout) to call a confessor before treatment, their advice and the canon itself would fall into derision. Some insist that physicians are obliged to withdraw from a case if the patient refuses to call a confessor. Others assert that if physicians are required to abandon stubborn patients, this canon could be seen as violating the principle of charity. There was uniformity neither of practice nor of interpretation of this piece of canonical legislation at the end of the Middle Ages.

Some authorities excuse physicians from informing patients of imminent death because predicting a fatal outcome may remove all hope of recovery and hasten death. Most insist that unless physicians are certain that their terminally ill patients have set both their spiritual and temporal affairs in order, they must inform them of their condition. Otherwise harm may occur not only to patients' estates but to their souls as well.

The second requirement of *Cum Infirmitas* is for physicians to refrain from advising sinful means for the recovery of health. Several of the moral theologians simply quote that stipulation without elaboration. Others condemn specific matters such as advising fornication, masturbation, incantations, consumption of intoxicating beverages, breaking the Church's fasts, and eating meat on forbidden days. Although all include thorough discussions of abortion elsewhere in their treatises, only two of the nine sources surveyed include it in their discussions of the sins of physicians and surgeons. None of the nine address what today is known as active euthanasia or assisted suicide, although all deal with suicide under other rubrics.

Some address intraprofessional conduct, rigorously condemning mutual envy and slander of colleagues, and scrutinize their relations with apothecaries. Physicians must ensure that they recommend to their patients only honest and competent apothecaries; otherwise they should compound their own drugs. Some also address the moral and legal aspects of the ordination of physicians and surgeons as well as the practice of medicine and surgery by clerics. As though at a loss as to where to discuss whether patients are obligated to obey their physicians, several include this topic in their sections on the sins of physicians, and one expatiates on the sin of employing Jewish physicians.

It should be noted that none of the confessional treatises had any legal or official standing. They were simply *vade mecums* for priests in their role as confessors. There is ample evidence that some penitents in the late Middle Ages engaged in "confessor shopping" to locate the most lenient priest. If a diligent priest consulted several sources in difficult cases, he was not bound by the authority of one over another on points wherein these differed.

2. From the Council of Trent (1545) to Vatican I (1869)

Medieval Catholicism ended with the Council of Trent, which met intermittently from 1545 to 1563. Trent responded to the Protestant Reformation in two distinct ways. First, it sought to correct the abuses and corruption within the Church that had contributed to Protestant separation. Second, by vigorously reaffirming those aspects of its dogmas of justification, revelation, and the sacraments with which the Reformers unequivocally disagreed, it made their return to the Church impossible unless they denied their most distinctive convictions about these issues. The Council of Trent reiterated the Fourth Lateran Council's requirement of annual confession. The evolution of moral theology, particularly with a view to its practical utility in the confessional, was stimulated by a reform instituted by the Council of Trent that called for the establishment of standards for a consistent and disciplined seminary education of the clergy. The burgeoning discipline of moral theology flowered during the next century, creating "for the first time in Western culture, a systematic taxonomy of human behavior" (Jonsen and Toulmin 1988, 142). Its methodology was that of casuistry (which is case-based moral reasoning, that is, the resolution of moral questions through the application of general ethical principles to particular cases of conscience or conduct).

Albert Jonsen and Stephen Toulmin mark the beginning of the century of "high casuistry" with the publication in 1556 of the Spanish edition of what was later published in Latin as the *Enchiridion sive Manuale Confessariorum et Poenitentium* of Martin Aspilcueta, who is better known as Navarrus (1493–1586). His major contribution to moral theology was the way he structured his *Enchiridion*. Earlier confessional manuals typically were arranged alphabetically by topic. Navarrus, however, arranged his cases according to the order of the Decalogue, (i.e., the "Ten Commandments"). This focus occupies roughly the second and third quarters of the work. Toward the end of the book, in a lengthy chapter, *De Peccatis Diversorum Statuum* (Concerning the Sins of People in Various Roles) is *De Peccatis Medici et Chirurgi* (Concerning the Sins of Physicians and Surgeons). In this section (for a summary of which see Amundsen 1978a, 942–45), Navarrus does not deal with topics not already addressed by moral theologians before the Council of Trent, although he made one statement that may be interpreted as a condemnation of what is now called physician-assisted suicide. The logical rather than merely alphabetical sequence of topics in the

Enchiridion "was of great importance to the maturation of casuistry" (Jonsen and Toulmin 1988, 152–53).

A. Probabilism and the "Crisis of Moral Theology"

A far greater stimulus to casuistic fertility than Navarrus' precedent-setting arrangement was made in 1577 by the moral theologian Bartholomew Medina (1490–1546) who, in his commentary on St. Thomas' *Summa Theologiae*, wrote, "It seems to me that, if an opinion is probable, it is licit to follow it, even though the opposite opinion is more probable" (Jonsen and Toulmin 1988, 164). It is essential to pause at this point to forestall some misunderstandings.

First, "probable" in moral parlance means "plausible," "possibly true," "arguable," or "provable," that is, "something for which there is a good argument, or two or more good arguments, irrespective of the merits of any alternative." In other words, for the probabilist, "any action was morally justified for which a good case could be made" (Mahoney 1987, 136–37; Jonsen and Toulmin 1988, 166).

Second, the complexity of cases of conscience with which the typical priest had to deal necessitated interpreting law and moral principles in light of the circumstance of specific situations. Jonsen and Toulmin remarked that

> Medina envisaged a person deliberating about the advice he should give to another, or about a judgment he should render about another's action . . . Suppose, for example, that the confessor believed a certain law to be binding under particular circumstances. The penitent states in response that he, perhaps with the approval of another confessor, believes in good faith and with good reasons that the law does not oblige under the given circumstances. Is the confessor morally bound to judge the penitent by his own opinion, which in his view is more sound? Or may he accept the less sound, though still reasonable, opinion of the penitent or other confessor? In the cultural context of confessional practice, this problem is not outlandish, and Medina's thesis is quite comprehensible. (Jonsen and Toulmin 1988, 167)

Third, as Medina adds, "Of course it is not probable, merely because it has proponents who state apparent reasons, but because wise men propose it and confirm it by excellent arguments" (Jonsen and Toulmin 1988, 164). In this sentence, Medina distinguished between two bases for probability: extrinsic probability, which arises from the prestige and authority of the theologians whom one could cite in favor of a position, and intrinsic probability, which arises from the force of the argument itself.

Jonsen and Toulmin succinctly state that the "thesis of probabilism simply asserts that a person who is deliberating about whether or not he is obliged by some moral, civil, or ecclesiastical law may take advantage of any reasonable doubt whether or not the law obliges him" (Jonsen and Toulmin 1988, 166). They assure us that "The 'probable opinions' of the classical casuists... were not recommended actions, let alone obligatory ones. They were actions that the casuist judged to be morally permissible in certain special circumstances" (Jonsen and Toulmin 1988, 245–46).

Probabilism, as John Mahoney observes, "spread rapidly through the Catholic Universities and the Church, and acted as an immense stimulant to the development of moral case-studies..." (Mahoney 1987, 138). However, it was not unopposed. Some moral theologians supported probabiliorism, which teaches the obligation of adopting the stronger, that is, the intrinsically more probable, argument in any moral deliberation. Others were even more cautious and maintained that, if law (whether revealed, natural, canon, or civil) addressed any important moral question, even if its applicability to the specific situation was doubtful, it was safer (*tutius*) to follow the law although good and reasonable arguments could be made against it. This is known as *tutiorism*.

Although extreme tutiorism fosters rigorism, probabilism in its extremes spawns laxism. It was especially the latter that led to what Mahoney labels the "crisis of moral theology." He remarks that the controversies did not arise simply from laxist opinions.

> The implicit invitation to find good arguments to justify the most bizarre of moral opinions as "probable," or even to create a doubt where previously there was none, was a challenge which did not go unaccepted. Were the subject-matter not so serious one would be tempted to compare the products of some of the probabilist theologians... with the fertile imagination and ingenuity of intelligent ten-year-olds. It was not without reason that one moralist became known as the lamb of God because he took away so many of the sins of the world,[5] and another was given the doubtful title of "prince of laxists." (Mahoney 1987, 138)

Jonsen and Toulmin set the end of the era of "high casuistry" at 1656, the year in which Pascal published his *Provincial Letters*, a scathingly hilarious attack on probabilism. Pascal was an ardent supporter of Jansenism, a movement that desired to encourage moral rigor in personal conduct. Mahoney remarked, "The purring irony of Pascal was but the most elegant expression of the vehement Jansenist reaction to laxism and to its principal exponents," who were the Jesuits (Mahoney 1987, 139). In a sense, Pascal was caricaturing probabilistic casuistry; however, as Jonsen and Toulmin acknowledge, he "rightly recognized the inherent tendency of probabilism to slide toward moral skepticism, where every opinion is as good as any other, and into moral laxism, where all law falls before

liberty. In Letters V and VI he set up these consequences as the target of his attack. Yet he missed the main point. His own words reveal this: 'I am not satisfied with probability. I want certainty.'" (Jonsen and Toulmin 1988, 171).

The certainty for which Pascal yearned was that which the extremes of tutiorism provide, a rigorism every bit as unacceptable to the Holy See as the most laxist extremes of probabilism. In attacking the casuistry employed by probabilists, Pascal focused on an easy and vulnerable target. "Casuistry, as an exercise in practical reasoning, involved a tissue of distinctions, qualifications, and exceptions; and when the resolution of a moral problem was torn away from this fabric of reasoning, it could easily be made to look ridiculous" (Jonsen and Toulmin 1988, 241).

Some probabilist propositions condemned in the mid-seventeenth century demonstrate the extremes of laxist casuistry. For example, one who eats a considerable quantity of food on a day of fasting by eating small amounts frequently, does not break the fast. If a son kills his father while drunk, it is licit for him to rejoice over the parricide because of great riches inherited by him. Because it seems probable that every fetus, while it is still in the womb, lacks a rational soul (*anima rationalis*) and receives one only at birth, it follows that in no abortion is homicide committed. One is not bound under pain of mortal sin to restore what one has stolen in small amounts, however large the total theft may be. Because fornication by its nature involves no malice and is evil only because it is forbidden, the contrary seems entirely dissonant with reason. Because intercourse with a married woman with her husband's consent is not adultery, it is sufficient during confession to say that one has committed fornication (Denzinger and Schönmetzer 1973, #1129, #1165, #1185, #1188, #1198, #1200). It is important to be aware that when popes Alexander VII (b. 1599; r. 1655–1667) and Innocent XI (b. 1611; r. 1676–1689) condemned these and many other laxist propositions in 1665, 1666, and 1679, they were condemning neither the fundamental principles and methodology of probabilism nor even the intellectual sloth of some probabilists, who avoided the cerebral challenge of deciding cases by arguing intrinsic merits but based their positions exclusively on extrinsic probability, whether by marshaling the support of as many moral theologians as they could muster or by relying on the prestige of even a single source. By contrast, when in 1690 Pope Alexander VIII (b. 1610; r. 1689–1691) condemned various rigorist propositions, he was also attacking rigorist doctrines and, indeed, the entire Jansenist movement.

B. Alphonsus Liguori: The Patron Saint of Confessors and Moral Theologians

The debates among probabilists, probabiliorists, and tutiorists continued, typically without interference by the

Holy See. The resolute actions of the papacy rendered some moral theologians skittish, or at least more cautious, and casuistry "lost much of its analytic vigor and boldness of attack" and "began to show signs of senescence" (Jonsen and Toulmin 1988, 269). Moral theology, however, was yet to produce its greatest luminary. Called by Mahoney, "the most prestigious of all moral theologians" (Mahoney 1987, 26) and by Jonsen and Toulmin, "the greatest of moral theologians" (Jonsen and Toulmin 1988, 156), Alphonsus Liguori (1696–1787) devoted most of his life to resolving the desiccating conflict among moral theologians. During his nearly 91 years, he devoted a third of his voluminous writings to moral theology. His magnum opus, *Theologia Moralis*, evolved from its first edition in 1748 to its ninth in 1785. Rejecting both rigorism and laxism, he sought to develop a system distinct from both probabilism and probabiliorism, to which he gave the name equiprobabilism, which acknowledges "on the one hand that in principle a doubtful law does not oblige and one may follow a probable opinion, but, on the other, that a law is really doubtful only when the opinions for and against are evenly balanced" (Mahoney 1987, 143). In other words, equiprobabilism "permits choice of any solidly probable opinion in matters of doubt, but it rejects the thesis with which Medina initiated the debate – namely, the acceptability of a less probable opinion in face of a more probable one" (Jonsen and Toulmin 1988, 175).

As the literature of moral theology had evolved since Navarrus' time, the typical structure was first an introduction to questions of general moral theology, then a discussion of the theological virtues, followed by an analysis of each commandment of the Decalogue, a scrutiny of the obligations of various states of life, a treatment of the sacraments, and an examination of bases for ecclesiastical censures. Many issues now subsumed under medical ethics arise in the section on the Decalogue. Abortion, suicide (including euthanasia), and mutilation (including castration and sterilization) are analyzed under the fifth commandment ("You shall not kill") and contraception under the sixth ("You shall not commit adultery") and ninth commandments ("You shall not covet your neighbor's wife") and under the sacrament of marriage.

Liguori deals with the duties and sins of physicians in book four of his *Theologia Moralis* (4.291) and in section 57 of his *Praxis Confessarii* (a separate treatise on confession included in volume four of Gaudés edition of the *Theologia Moralis*). Combining these two sections, which differ in only minor ways, we see that physicians sin if they practice without having sufficient knowledge or skill, fail to devote themselves to more study when encountering more difficult cases, or attempt to treat a serious disease without sufficient expertise. They sin if, when they recognize that a patient is in danger, they do not make themselves available because it is inconvenient, if they are negligent, forbid other physicians to be consulted, or obtain drugs

from an incompetent or negligent apothecary because he is a friend. Physicians must perform their duties, as much as possible, with minimal danger and damage to patients. Hence, they must ordinarily follow the established and safe precepts of physicians, using medicines about which they are confident and avoiding doubtful treatments. They sin if they rashly administer medicines that are conveniently available when they have not yet thoroughly examined the nature of the disease or if they use untested medicines (*medicamenta inexplorata*) to experiment (*explorandi gratia*) while they have medicines available that are probably useful. If there is no medicine known to be effective, they must use a more, rather than a less, probable and safe medicine.

Physicians sin if they apply dangerous treatments to a patient of whose life they have not yet despaired. If, however, there is no hope for a patient's recovery and they have available a medicine that may either help or harm, they may, indeed they must (*debent*) apply it. Here Liguori refers the reader to section 46 of his *Tractatus de Conscientia*, which is book one of the *Theologia Moralis*. There he considers at greater length whether a physician who despairs of the health of a patient may apply to him remedies about whose potentially helpful or harmful effects he is in doubt. It is, he maintains, certain and commonly accepted, first, that if it is probable that the remedy would be beneficial, then the physician is permitted, rather he is obligated (*tenetur*), to apply it, when he does not have a more certain medicine. It is certain, secondly, that it is not permitted to apply to the ill, even if despaired of, a remedy about which the physician is ignorant whether it is salutary or harmful, to experiment upon the patient. He asserts that the reason is because it is not permitted to make an experiment that may put the patient in danger of death or hasten his death. It is certain, thirdly, that if it is doubtful that the remedy will be profitable and certain that it will not be harmful, generally (*omnino*) it should be applied to the patient.

He then returns to the question of whether a physician who despairs of the health of a patient may apply to him remedies about whose potentially helpful or harmful effects he is in doubt. There are, he says, two responses. First, the negative, because (as said previously) it is never permitted to expose the patient to the danger or the hastening of death. The second response, however, "which is sufficiently probable and perhaps more probable," affirms that it is permitted, because, when the patient is despaired of, it is more conformable to the patient's prudence and will (especially if he himself expressly consents in this) to apply to him a doubtful remedy than to omit it when there is certainty of death. He concludes, "Furthermore, even if a physician may not propose a treatment that is against his own judgment, nevertheless if that treatment is approved by other medical authorities and the patient consents, he may licitly apply it."

Returning now to Liguori's two sections on the duties and sins of physicians, we see that they sin if they contemptuously ignore and fail to treat gratuitously paupers who are in grave necessity; if without necessity they give license to anyone to break the Church's fasts or to eat meat when forbidden; or if they advise anything contrary to God's honor, such as, incantations, superstitious practices, and sexual immorality. He then refers the reader to the pertinent sections of his *Theologia Moralis*. In his section on physicians' duties and sins in the *Theologia Moralis*, he unaccountably omits any mention of the requirement that physicians advise their patients to summon a priest for confession. That this is a topic dear to his heart is evidenced by his devoting to that issue more than 80 percent of the section in his *Praxis Confessarii* on the confessional interrogation of physicians in which he also refers the reader to two sections of his *Theologia Moralis* (3.182 and especially 6.664) where he wrestles with the spiritual principles and practical problems of this requirement.

In 1566, Pope Pius V (b. 1504; r. 1566–72) had renewed *Cum Infirmitas* in his *Supra Gregem* (the Latin text of which is quoted by Liguori in *Theologia Moralis* 6.664). This was a papal decree issued *motu proprio*, which means that, at his own initiative as Supreme Pontiff, and not in response to a request for a ruling or clarification, he addressed an issue that he regarded as sufficiently important to warrant his legislative intervention directed to the Church at large. *Supra Gregem* mandated that physicians must discontinue treatment after the third day unless the patient produced a document signed by a confessor certifying that he had duly confessed; all candidates for degrees in medicine or surgery must take an oath to obey this requirement; and physicians who violated this rule were to be declared infamous, denied the privilege of practicing, and ejected from their university or medical and surgical associations. Over the next two centuries, the extent of enforcement of this requirement appears to have varied considerably from region to region, and moral theologians were still as divided in their interpretations as they had been over *Cum Infirmitas*.

Liguori's most thorough examination of the matter is in his discussion of the sacraments in the sixth book of his *Theologia Moralis* (6.664). After summarizing the substance of *Cum Infirmitas* and *Supra Gregem*, he asks, "To what kind of sickness do these decrees apply?" There are, he says, three *sententiae* (opinions). The first is that they apply only to a dangerous sickness or at least to any about which there is doubt whether it is dangerous. The supporters of this *sententia* assert that this is how the requirement has typically been received by physicians. The second is that it applies to every sickness, even those not mortal, because in a dangerous sickness natural law would dictate forewarning; accordingly, "since *Cum Infirmitas* established a new precept, the text must not be understood to apply only to a mortal illness." The third *sententia*, which he asserts is more

commonly held by numerous authorities, is twofold. First, the requirement is not to be understood to apply only to dangerous illnesses. *Cum Infirmitas* was promulgated so that patients would not interpret their physician's advice to call a confessor as an indication that their condition is mortal and thus despair of recovery and more easily incur the danger of death. Second, it is certainly not to be understood to apply to any mild sickness, "which would be ridiculous," but to serious illnesses even if not dangerous, because both decrees refer to the ill lying in bed. Hence, the requirement does not apply to conditions such as gout but only to those that would require one to take to bed.

Before endorsing any of these *sententiae*, Liguori notes four different ways in which various authorities understand that physicians adequately fulfill the requirement. First, it is sufficient if they advise patients through others. Second, the testimony of a trustworthy intermediary is sufficient without a written statement from a confessor. Third, physicians are not obligated if they are certain that a specific patient is in a good state spiritually. Fourth, if patients are obstinately unwilling to confess and would be in danger of death if not treated, then physicians are not obligated to abandon them because these decrees are not contrary to charity, because charity befriends even the obstinate as much as possible.

Returning now to the three different *sententiae*, Liguori unequivocally gives his support to the third. Then he exclaims, "Oh that the aforesaid decrees would be observed, would that so many patients would avoid damnation who, because of the indifference (*osctantia*) of physicians, by putting off confession die either unconfessed or having confessed poorly!" His pastoral concern is expressed even more passionately in his *Praxis Confessarii* (57):

> Oh how terrible it is to see so many of the ill (and especially those who are of proven character) brought to the extremity of death... when they are, as it were, lifeless, when they can hardly speak, barely hear, scarcely grasp the state of their own conscience and the pain of their sins! And this is entirely the fault of those physicians who, lest they displease patients or their relatives, do not make them certain about their danger, but rather go on deluding them right up to the point that they themselves despair entirely of their patients' lives. (Liguori [1785] 1905–1912, *Praxis Confessarii* 57)

He concludes his section on the interrogation of physicians in the *Praxis Confessarii* by admonishing the confessor to question physicians with fervor about this matter. "I say 'with fervor,' for the spiritual health not only of the physician but also of all patients who are under his care depends on this matter" (Liguori [1785] 1905–1912, *Praxis Confessarii* 57). His lengthy examination of this issue in book six of his *Theologia Moralis* ends with his acknowledging that many authorities maintain the decrees of Lateran IV and Pius V are not binding in those regions in which they have not been accepted by custom or have been abrogated, as in Spain, or, as Liguori is well aware, in his own Kingdom of Naples where they are observed only in dangerous illnesses.

Alphonsus Liguori died in 1787. After his writings had been thoroughly examined by the Holy See, they were declared to contain nothing meriting censure. He was beatified in 1816. Controversies between rigorists and Liguori's disciples arose. In 1831, Cardinal de Rohan-Chabot, addressed to the Sacred Penitentiary two questions regarding Liguori's authority. First, may a professor follow his opinions with a clear conscience? The response was affirmative. Second, should a confessor be censured who follows Liguori's reasoning simply because the Holy See had found nothing in his writings to merit censure but does not examine the bases for his opinions? The response was negative (Palazzini 1962, 61–62). In 1839, Liguori was canonized as St. Alphonsus and was declared Doctor of the Church in 1871. In 1950, Pius XII declared Alphonsus the patron saint of confessors and of moral theologians.

C. Roman Catholic Medical Ethics on the Eve of Vatican I

We have devoted much space to moral theologians' discussions of the duties and sins of physicians. We should now note four matters. First, the primary concern of these authors is the spiritual health of Catholic physicians who come as penitents to a confessor. In other words, the context is the physician in the confessional. Second, the practice of medicine and surgery potentially involves great danger to patients; hence competence and diligence are the physician's first obligation, and refraining from rashly experimenting on patients is a close second. Third, the incompetent or negligent practitioner sins mortally by practicing at all and may likely cause physical harm. If the physical harm is death and the patient is unshriven, the spiritual harm to the patient may be incalculable. Fourth, physicians are obligated to be concerned with the spiritual health of their patients, for the fundamental principle in all relevant aspects of Catholic thought is that the health of the soul is of inestimably greater value than that of the body. Hence two obligations are incumbent upon physicians. One is that they recommend nothing to their patients that is spiritually harmful, ranging from masturbation (thought by many physicians, before humoral theory fell into desuetude, sometimes to be necessary for restoring the health of the sexually inactive) to violating the Church's dietary rules. The second is to ensure that their patients summon a confessor, a requirement that was unequivocally articulated in canon law. This was first done by Lateran IV, an ecumenical or general council, presided over by Pope Innocent III in 1215. Then, in 1566, Pius V

issued *Supra Gregem*, which set requirements that are even more precise and unambiguous than those of *Cum Infirmitas*. Yet a moral theologian as cautious and conscientious as St. Alphonsus felt justified in supporting an application of both decrees that was considerably more flexible than their wording and probably than the intentions of their promulgators. Such was still the freedom of moral theologians on a moral issue that a general council had addressed and on which a pope had taken the initiative to legislate directly as Supreme Pontiff, even after the unequivocal papal condemnations of positions enunciated by various moral theologians in the seventeenth century. This freedom, as we shall see, will be considerably circumscribed by the ambiguous implications of the dogma of papal infallibility. Yet, at least two principles of moral reasoning that theologians followed then are still used in resolving moral dilemmas. Writing in 1988, Jonsen and Toulmin asserted that "Nowadays . . . it is permissible for a Catholic moral theologian to follow either equiprobabilism or probabilism in the resolution of cases of conscience" (Jonsen and Toulmin 1988, 175).

Can one properly speak of the beginning of a field clearly identifiable as Roman Catholic medical ethics before the twentieth century? It is reasonable to suggest that works on medical ethics written by Catholic physicians represent Catholic medical ethics. For example, some treatises have survived from the early Middle Ages that are part of a genre at least as old as the Hippocratic Corpus of ancient Greece. These early medieval treatises display a blending of Hippocratic medical etiquette with Christian morality (MacKinney 1952), as do the ethical treatises of several physicians and surgeons of the late Middle Ages (Welborn 1939; Garcia-Ballester 1993; Jonsen 2000, Chap. 2). This tradition of Christian medical ethics was sustained beyond the Reformation by both Catholic and Protestant physicians, and when Catholic physicians wrote about medical ethics they were thoroughly informed by the distinctly Catholic emphases of moral theology. In the seventeenth century, Paolo Zacchia wrote *Quaestiones Medico-Legales* and Michiel Boudewyns *Ventilabrum Medico-Theologicum* (Kelly D 1979, 55–59). Both were very influential for the genre of "pastoral medicine." Some works in this genre were designed specifically for the moral instruction of medical students and physicians,[6] others primarily for rural priests whose impoverished parishioners often sought medical help from them. The latter typically consisted of two parts, one a medical guide, the other a moral guide. A notable representative of this already venerable genre is Carl Capellmann (1841–1898), a German physician whose work, published in Germany in 1877, was translated into English in 1879. His heavy reliance on, and citations of, such great moral theologians as St. Alphonsus, did not preclude his writing this disclaimer: "In whatever is written in this work, it has been my intention to be in complete accord with the doctrines of the Holy Roman Catholic Church. Should anything have been inadvertently advanced ever so little at variance with them, I recall and disavow it, by anticipation, unconditionally" (Capellmann 1879, v; see Kelly D 1979, 70–74). Although his disclaimer was appropriate earlier, written as it was while the impact of Vatican I was still reverberating throughout Catholicism, it is rather prophetic of developments that we shall consider next.

III. THE ERA OF THE HIERARCHICAL MAGISTERIUM

1. From Vatican I to Vatican II

A. Guarding the Faith and Protecting the Faithful

When describing papal condemnations of extreme laxist and rigorist positions in the seventeenth century, Charles Curran parenthetically remarked, "this was the most significant intervention up to that time by the papal office in the area of moral theology and began a trend that has continued until contemporary times" (Curran 1985, 222). This trend was much broader than condemnations of specific opinions of individual moral theologians. It was as broad as necessary for condemning all aspects of secular and theological thought inimical to Catholic dogma and contrary to principles of natural law. Its purpose was twofold. One was to address those outside the Church, both schismatics and secularists, the former varying considerably in the extent of their departure from truth, the latter already beyond the pale except for those whose consciences were not yet irreparably cauterized. The second and more vital purpose was to warn the faithful against imbibing from the poisoned wells of modernism (the "synthesis of all heresies," as Pope Pius X [b. 1835; r. 1903–1914] called it) and contemporary secular thought.[7]

John Boyle has shown that "The exercise of the papal teaching authority became more frequent and more insistent from the time of the inaugural encyclical Mirari Vos Arbitramur" (Boyle 1979, 380), an encyclical issued in 1832 by Pope Gregory XVI (b. 1765; r. 1831–46), which strongly denounced liberalism and religious indifferentism. In 1864, his successor, Pius IX (b. 1792; r. 1846–78) published the *Syllabus of Errors* that denounced various trends in philosophy and culture. He condemned eighty "theses" ranging from pantheism, which identifies God with the universe, and naturalism, which totally excludes him from it, to various liberties then becoming fashionable, such as unrestricted liberty of speech and of the press and equal status for all religions.

Pius IX's successor, Leo XIII (b. 1810; r. 1878–1903), authoritatively supported the doctrine of natural law as "a particularly apt instrument in the development of the Church's social and political teaching in a world which

might listen to reason even if it would not heed the revealed word of God" (Mahoney 1987, 81). In *Humanum Genus* (1884), he condemned naturalism and those who set nature and human reason above the supernatural order, because the natural order and natural law are part of the divine order and the products of supernatural design. In *Libertas Praestantissimum* (1888) he stated that the natural law "is written and engraved in the mind of every man, and this is nothing but our reason, commanding us to do right and forbidding sin ... the law of nature is the same thing as the eternal law, implanted in rational creatures, and inclining them to their right action and end; and can be nothing else but the eternal reason of God ... " (Leo XIII 1888, #8).

Subsequent popes attacked various secular movements and theological modernism generally. Pius XII (b. 1876; r. 1939–1958) entered the fray in his first encyclical, *Summi Pontificatus*, issued in 1939, in which he declared that "it is certain that the radical and ultimate cause of the evils which We deplore in modern society is the disregard, so common nowadays, and the forgetfulness of the natural law itself" (Pius XII 1939, #28). Eleven years later, in *Humani Generis* he condemned several liberal or modernistic positions taken by some Catholic theologians and concisely restated those traditional Catholic doctrines that he felt were being ignored, questioned, or threatened. Early in the encyclical he emphasized that "human reason by its own natural force and light can arrive at a true and certain knowledge of the one personal God, Who by His providence watches over and governs the world, and also the natural law, which the Creator has written in our hearts." Right reason will also lead one to basic theological and moral understanding. But there are many obstacles to right reason "making efficient and fruitful use of its natural ability," for "the human intellect ... is hampered both by the activity of the senses and the imagination, and by evil passions arising from original sin. Hence men easily persuade themselves in such matters that what they do not wish to believe is false or at least doubtful." Near the end of the encyclical, he warned, "new opinions endanger the two philosophical sciences which by their very nature are closely connected with the doctrine of faith, that is, theodicy and ethics" (Pius XII 1950, #2, 34).

B. Papal Infallibility and Papal Teaching Authority from Vatican I to Vatican II

Regardless of the reaction of non-Catholics to such papal pronouncements, the seriousness with which Catholics had to harken to the Supreme Pontiff, although always great, had increased since Vatican I. Presided over by Pope Pius IX, Vatican I met from 1869 to 1870 and is best remembered for its formulation of the doctrine of papal infallibility. In its Dogmatic Constitution *Pastor Aeternus*, the council declared "as a divinely revealed dogma that when the Roman pontiff speaks *ex cathedra*, that is, when, in . . . virtue of his supreme apostolic authority, he defines a doctrine concerning faith or morals to be held by the whole church, he possesses that infallibility which the divine Redeemer willed his church to enjoy in defining doctrine concerning faith or morals." Such papal definitions "are of themselves, and not by the consent of the church, irreformable" (Tanner 1990, 2:816).

Mahoney observes, "In the making of moral theology no single event has been more dramatic, and yet in several respects more puzzling, than the solemn definition in 1870 by the First Vatican Council of the infallibility of the Roman Pontiff in his moral teaching" (Mahoney 1987, 144). Although no pope has ever explicitly exercised his prerogative of infallibility to define any doctrine about morals, none has done anything to discourage what various scholars have referred to as "creeping infallibility," an "aura of infallibility," and "infallibility by association" in ostensibly noninfallible papal pronouncements. Indeed, some popes, especially Pius XII, did much to encourage this tendency.

Vatican I had marked an acceleration of the centralization of authority in the Church, which has been most evident in the activity of the magisterium, which "became so identified with official papal formulations that other sources of moral knowledge were neglected" (McCormick 1984, 47). The section of Vatican I's *Pastor Aeternus* that sets forth the dogma of papal infallibility opens with the statement that "the apostolic primacy which the Roman pontiff possesses . . . includes also the supreme power of teaching" as "the constant custom of the church demonstrates" and as the ecumenical councils "have declared" (Tanner 1990, 2:815). Earlier in the council, the Dogmatic Constitution *De Fide Catholica* declared, "Everybody knows that those heresies, condemned by the fathers of Trent, which rejected the divine magisterium of the church and allowed religious questions to be a matter for the judgment of each individual, have gradually collapsed into a multiplicity of sects, either at variance or in agreement with one another; and by this means a good many people have had all faith in Christ destroyed" (Tanner 1990, 2:804–5). It was this rejection of the "divine magisterium" that had led to numerous ills, including the denigration of Scripture as myth, the rise of rationalism, naturalism, pantheism, materialism, and atheism, "and the consequence is that they strive to destroy rational nature itself, to deny any criterion of what is right and just, and to overthrow the very foundations of human society" (Tanner 1990, 2:804–5). *De Fide Catholica* then pronounces on a variety of doctrines that had been thus undermined, including the moral function of natural law (Tanner 1990, 2:808–9). A little earlier in this Dogmatic Constitution it was declared that "by divine and Catholic faith all those things are to be believed which are contained in the word of God as found in scripture and tradition, and which are proposed by the church

as matters to be believed as divinely revealed, whether by her solemn judgment or in her ordinary and universal magisterium" (Tanner 1990, 2:807).

In 1896, Leo XIII wrote, in his encyclical *Satis Cognitum*, "Christ instituted in the Church a *living, authoritative and permanent Magisterium*," which "must be believed by every one as true. If it could in any way be false, an evident contradiction follows; for then God Himself would be the author of error in man" (Leo XIII 1896, #9; emphasis in original). His referring to the magisterium as "living, authoritative, and permanent" both magnified the importance of the magisterium and increased the ambiguities about its nature. The major distinction is between the "extraordinary" or "solemn" magisterium and the "ordinary" or "universal" magisterium. An assumption of many, but not all, Catholic theologians after Vatican I has been that the former may be used for infallible definitions, while the latter is authoritative but noninfallible.

Following Vatican I's promulgation of the dogma of papal infallibility, "theologians were a bit overawed by the documents of the ordinary noninfallible magisterium. They tended to be almost exegetical in their approach to these teachings, and it was close to unthinkable (and certainly very risky) to question the formulation of such documents" (McCormick 1984, 63). Contributing to this was that, as the papal exercise of the magisterium became more autonomous and absolute, an unprecedented division of the Church into the "teaching" Church, or the hierarchy, and the "learning" Church developed. In 1914, Benedict XV (b. 1854; r. 1914–1922) essentially limited the areas of discussion by theologians to those in which the Apostolic See had not delivered its own judgment (Benedict XV 1914, #22–23), a decision reinforced in 1950 by Pius XII in his encyclical *Humani Generis*. It should be noted that encyclicals are not legislative texts but pastoral letters typically dealing with doctrinal, disciplinary, or moral issues, in the exercise of a pope's ordinary magisterium. In this encyclical Pius XII declared that, because in writing encyclical letters popes do not exercise the supreme power of their magisterium, it must not be thought what is expounded in them does not of itself demand consent. "For these matters are taught with the ordinary Magisterium, of which it is true to say: 'He who heareth you, heareth me' [Luke 10:16]." If popes, "in their official documents purposely pass judgment on a matter up to that time under dispute, it is obvious that the matter, according to the mind and will of the same Pontiffs, cannot be any longer considered a question open to discussion among theologians." Theologians must explain "how the doctrine of the living Magisterium is to be found either explicitly or implicitly in the Scriptures and in Tradition. . . . This deposit of faith our Divine Redeemer has given for authentic interpretation not to each of the faithful, not even to theologians, but only to the Magisterium of the Church" (Pius XII 1950, #20 and #21). In an allocution delivered in

1956, Pius XII denounced what he referred to as the "evident error" of thinking that theologians could be *"magistri Magisterii,"* that is, "teachers of the Magisterium" (Sullivan 1983, 217). In the mind of this pope, theologians *qua* theologians were clearly part not of the "teaching" Church but of the "learning" Church.

"This approach of Pius XII," Mahoney comments, "did much to explain the almost innumerable interventions and initiatives with which he reacted to contemporary events in the daily exercise of his *magisterium"* (Mahoney 1987, 161). Yves Congar notes that *Humani Generis* brought earlier "developments to a high point in two ways: (1) The ordinary magisterium of the pope demands a total obedience. . . . (2) The (or one) role of theologians is to justify the pronouncements of the magisterium" (Congar 1982a, 325). Referring to the same encyclical, McCormick later remarks that the pre–Vatican II "notion of a highly centralized and authoritarian teaching office led to the conclusion that *Roma locuta, causa finita* ('Rome has spoken, the matter is closed')" (McCormick 1984, 69).

C. Pius XII's Pronouncements on Medical Ethics (1939–1958)

With gradually increasing frequency since Vatican I, Rome had spoken on numerous aspects of medical ethics. An unprecedented cascade of pronouncements on moral issues in medicine emanated from the magisterium of Pius XII, mostly in the form of allocutions to medical audiences. These addresses were made to two types of assemblies. Some were to distinctly Catholic organizations or groups. More were to secular organizations, especially international medical congresses. The only discernible difference in content and tone between his allocutions to Catholic and secular organizations, is that when addressing the former, he reminded his auditors that, as Christians, they could understand even more clearly than their non-Christian colleagues the truth of his moral arguments, typically based on natural law, because they had the benefit of Scripture, Tradition, the teachings of the Church, and, indeed, at that very moment, the words they were hearing from the lips of the Supreme Pontiff, who consistently used the first person plural when referring to himself. Furthermore, when addressing Catholic audiences, he appealed to them as Christians not only to obey divine and natural law but to show compassion and charity beyond that which is traditionally recognized as desirable in all physicians. Although his addresses to secular organizations contain some principles that he identified as distinctly Christian, the basis for his moral pronouncements, which he declared with unequivocal certitude, is the natural moral law that is common to all humanity.

Seldom did he fail to emphasize to medical audiences their lofty calling. Medicine and surgery are providential arts; doctors are a gift of God whom he appointed to minister to the needs of suffering humanity as collaborators with him "in the defence and development of His creatures." To such a role in human societies many responsibilities are attached. The first duty is competence, which is essential especially because the doctor is not dealing with inert matter but with a man like himself who "merits the greatest care, because he is the image of God, of an incarnate, suffering God." The physician "must often give advice, make decisions, formulate principles that affect the spirit of man and his eternal destiny." Hence "the physician, as also all his activity, is constantly in the orbit of the moral order, subject to the authority of its laws . . . For his every word and action he is responsible before God and his own conscience." With regularity Pius warned that physicians must keep in mind "man's place and function in the universal order of being" or they can be "easily entangled in more or less materialist prejudices" and follow "the destructive tendencies of utilitarianism, hedonism, and absolute autonomy from the moral law" (*Papal Teachings* 1960, 52–53, 58, 66, 69, 187, 327).

Physicians' "greatest dignity and nobility," even "that almost sacred character" of their persons and activities, derive from moral norms that "far surpass the prescriptions of the code of honor of the profession." Hence they must "safeguard this tradition, which an all-devouring materialism threatens to engulf" and "be on guard against the fascination of science" and against the "deification of nature itself and of material forces," because that would essentially be "denying their Author." He insisted that a materialistic ideology and a materialistic culture are not true simply because their scientific results are. The criteria of truth lie elsewhere. It is in the divinely created order of being – the absolute value of the spiritual and the relative value of the material, the infinite worth of the soul and the finite worth of the body – in this economy of goods and in absolute moral principles inseparable from their transcendental truth reflected in the very nature of nature itself that Pius XII viewed the benefits and dangers of the astounding progress of medical science that had occurred during the preceding century. "Christian thought and life," he stressed, "do not attribute an absolute value to the progress of science." Such an attitude, however, "is regarded as natural by materialistic thought and by the concept of life which materialism inspires. For them it serves as a religion or as a substitute for religion." The Christian appreciates and uses new scientific discoveries but "rejects every materialistic apotheosis of science and culture. He knows that science and culture occupy a place on the scale of objective values but that, while they are not the lowest, neither are they the highest" (*Papal Teachings* 1960, 116–17, 327–28, 361–62, 365).

Pius consistently maintained that the

Inviolable laws of natural and Christian morality must be observed everywhere. It is not from emotive

considerations nor from a materialist, natural philanthropy that the essential principles of medical
ethics derive, but from these laws: the dignity of
the human body, the pre-eminence of the soul over
the body, the brotherhood of all men, the sovereign
dominion of God over life and destiny.

In short, "the basic principles of medical ethics are a part
of the Divine Law." Hence, in 1954, in an address to
the Eighth Congress of the World Medical Association,
he proposed three fundamental principles for medical
ethics. First, "Medical ethics should be based upon being
and nature," that is, should proceed from corresponding ontological principles, conforming "to the essence of
human nature, and to its law and immanent relations,"
because "a purely positivistic code of medical ethics is self-
repudiating." Second, "Medical ethics should conform to
reason and finality, and should be based upon positive values." When facing ethical questions that they must answer
according to the dictates of conscience, physicians must
ask, "'What does this norm of action entail? How can it be
justified?' (That is to say, what ultimate goal does it pursue
and set for itself?) 'What is its independent value, its value
to man, and its value to society?' In other words: 'With
what is it concerned?' 'Why? For what purpose? What is
its worth?'" Third, "Medical ethics should be rooted in the
transcendental." Anything that man has established, he
can discard. "This is contrary, however, to the constancy
of human nature, of its intended purpose and ultimate
objectives, and the absolute and imprescriptible character
of its moral demands," which "make their presence felt in
the depths of the individual conscience on an entirely different basis . . . The absolute character of the moral order,
a phenomenon to which men have always been able to
attest, compels Us to acknowledge that medical ethics is,
in the final analysis, rooted in the transcendental, and subject to higher authority" (*Papal Teachings* 1960, 117, 283,
317–19).

The demands of natural ethics are the demands of the
moral law, or natural law, the common heritage of all
humanity, readily discernible through reason rightly used.
Most fundamental is that, in the divinely designed structure of reality, the eternal is of inestimably greater significance and value than the temporal, the spiritual than
the material, and the soul than the body. In the inevitable
tension that arises between these pairs, the former must
never be impaired for the benefit of the latter; for in each
set, the former is in the realm of absolute, the latter of relative, good. Right reason can lead to no other conclusion.
It follows then that physicians must resist their patients'
desires for what is detrimental to their souls. Hence, he
emphasized to an audience of Catholic physicians that
they "will often be solicited for advice, and decisions, and
principles which, though they affect directly the care of
the body with its members and organs, will nevertheless

concern too the soul and its faculties, and man's supernatural destiny. . . . " To them falls the "delicate task" of
"dissipating prejudices and unreasonable and disastrous
apprehensions," to prepare the way for the priest, "who
can open the door to divine life, a life which knows no
end" (*Papal Teachings* 1960, 53, 66, 69, 132, 276).[8]

In 1952, Pius accepted an invitation from the First
International Congress of Histopathology of the Nervous System to address the moral limits of medical
experimentation.[9] He did so under three rubrics: "the
interests of medical science;" "the individual interests of
the patient under treatment;" and "the common interests
of the community" (*Papal Teachings* 1960, 196).

In regard to the interest of medical science, he asserted
that new knowledge and a more profound comprehension of truth possess a value quite independent of their
usefulness and are in harmony with the moral order. That
does not mean that every research method or endeavor
becomes lawful and morally admissible by virtue of its
increasing our knowledge because science is not the highest value to which all other values must be subjected.
Science

must be inserted in the order of values. Here, well-
defined frontiers present themselves, which even
medical science cannot transgress without violating
higher moral rules. The relationship of confidence
between doctor and patient, the right of the patient
to life, physical and spiritual, in its psychic or moral
integrity – here, amongst others, are values which
rule scientific interests. (*Papal Teachings* 1960, 197)

Second, the medical interests of the patient do not *ipso
facto* establish the moral legitimacy of a medical act. The
question must be asked whether the intervention that the
doctor has in mind conforms to the moral law. The consent of the patient is necessary, because the "doctor has
only that power over the patient which the latter gives
him, be it explicitly, or implicitly and tacitly. The patient,
for his part, cannot confer rights that he does not possess.
The decisive point, in this problem, is the moral legitimacy
of the right which the patient has at his own disposal." The
patient "is not absolute master of himself, of his body, or
of his soul. He cannot, therefore, freely dispose of himself
as he pleases" but "is bound by the immanent purposes
fixed by nature," that is, within the limits of "natural finality." (This is a theme that appears in several of his allocutions to medical audiences [e.g., *Papal Teachings* 1960, 54,
67, 198–99, 316] and is consistently used in condemning contraception, abortion, and euthanasia.) To limit the
destruction or mutilation of individual parts to what is
necessary for the good of the whole organism, Pius XII
invoked the principle of totality, which he later defined
as that "which declares that the part exists for the whole,
and that, consequently, the good of the part remains subordinated to the good of the whole: that the whole is that

which determines the part and can dispose of it in its own interest." By the same principle, a patient does not have the right to submit "his physical and psychic integrity" to experiments or research that "entail, either immediately or subsequently, acts of destruction, or of mutilation and wounds, or grave dangers" (*Papal Teachings* 1960, 198–99, 206).

The laws of morality demand that the individual must observe the hierarchy of the scale of values and the hierarchy of individual goods within an identical order of values. One cannot allow operations that remove serious defects but cause permanent destruction of, or considerable damage to, the human personality, thus degrading one to the level of an automaton. The moral law does not support this. Therefore, it is counter to the medical interests of the patient. He maintained that, "fixed by the judgment of right reason" and "traced by the demands of the moral law . . . the boundaries are the same for the doctor as for the patient," because the doctor "disposes of rights, and those rights alone, which are granted by the patient, and because the patient cannot give more than he possesses himself." As for children, the feeble-minded, and the insane, their legal representatives "do not posses[s] over the body and the life of their subordinates any other rights than they themselves would have, if they were capable of it" (*Papal Teachings* 1960, 199–201).

Third, in regard to the common good, Pius XII posed the question of whether the medical interests of the community are limited by any moral boundaries. Many, he said, argue that the good of the individual must be sacrificed for that of the community. Furthermore, they assert, such individual sacrifice, especially for scientific research, ultimately benefits the individual." After citing the horrendous Nazi atrocities as especially heinous examples of where such reasoning may lead, he maintained that if the interests of the individual are subordinated to common interests of medicine, one transgresses the most basic demands of the natural law. Man does not exist for the use of society, but the community, "as ordained by nature and by God," exists for man. The community, however, does not possess as a whole a unity that subsists in itself as does each physical organism. Hence, the principle of totality does not apply to the community as it does to the individual. For the "principle of totality itself affirms nothing except this: where the relationship of the whole to part is verified, and in the exact degree to which it is verified, the part is subordinated to the whole, which latter can in its own interest dispose of the part. Too frequently, alas, in resorting to the principle of totality, these considerations are left aside" (*Papal Teachings* 1960, 202–7).

He acknowledged that the moral law does not require "the total exclusion of all danger and of every risk" before new methods may be tried, for that would "paralyze all scientific research, and would very often turn to the detriment of the patient." Furthermore, in doubtful cases, when usual treatment has failed, a new and insufficiently tested method that, although very dangerous, offers "appreciable chances of success," may be lawfully employed if the patient consents. He further stated, "this method of action cannot be established as a line of treatment for normal cases" (*Papal Teachings* 1960, 207).

The removal of a healthy organ to arrest the evil effects on another organ raised moral issues that Pius addressed in 1953. He emphasized that the healthy organ either directly or indirectly must cause a serious menace for the whole body. In either case, if no other alternative is available, such a procedure is "permissible." He declared that there are three conditions that

> govern the moral licitness of a surgical operation which causes anatomic or functional mutilation: first that the continued presence or functioning of a particular organ within the whole organism is causing serious damage or constitutes a menace to it; next, this damage must be remediable or at least can be measurably lessened by the mutilation in question, and the operation's efficacy in this regard should be well assured; finally, one must be reasonably certain that the negative effect, that is, the mutilation and its consequences, will be compensated for by the positive effect: elimination of danger to the whole organism, easing of pain, and so forth.

He thereupon asserted, "Our conclusion is based on the right which man has received from the Creator over his body. This right is founded on the principle of totality, in virtue of which every particular organ is subordinated to the body as a whole, and, in case of conflict, must cede to the good of the whole. As a result, man, who has received the use of the whole organism, has the right to sacrifice a particular organ if its continued presence or functioning causes notable harm to the whole, a harm which cannot otherwise be avoided." He then condemned as an erroneous application of the principle of totality the removal or tying of healthy fallopian tubes to prevent conception, even if pregnancy could be dangerous or life-threatening to the woman (*Papal Teachings* 1960, 277–79).

On the related subject of organ transplantation, in an allocution to a Symposium on Corneal Transplants in 1956, Pius XII "endorsed, with some cautions about respect for the cadaver, organ removal for transplant" (Jonsen 1998, 224 n. 13). Then, the next year, in an allocution to an International Congress of Anesthesiologists, he addressed the moral issues involved in resuscitation, ordinary and extraordinary means of sustaining life, removal of artificial respiration, and the definition of death (Pius XII 1957b) (see also Chapter 7).

It has been estimated that during the first 15 years of his pontificate Pius XII gave nearly 1,000 public speeches and radio addresses (Ford and Kelly 1982, 1). Many of these were on issues ranging from labor relations and international peace to family morality and medical ethics. Needless to say, he had considerable assistance in composing these messages. In fact, his numerous addresses on medical ethics were authored in close consultation with, and sometimes primarily by, the Jesuit moral theologians of the Gregorian University, particularly Father Franz Huth (Jonsen 1998, 36). Nevertheless, although many of these addresses did not come entirely, or even primarily, from Pius' pen, they were on subjects in which he was deeply interested, they expressed his positions on these issues, were orally delivered by him, were disseminated in print in numerous languages as his words, and thus emanated from his magisterium. As Curran observes, "Obviously, the interest and concern of Pius XII sparked the growth and development of the discipline of medical ethics" (Curran 1995, 2326).

D. Medical Ethics, Moral Theologians, and the Magisterium between Vatican I (1870) and Vatican II (1962)

Throughout the history of the Church, the concern has been addressed that medicine is a mixed blessing because its misuse poses a potential threat to both physical and spiritual health, that is, to the temporal life of the body and the eternal destiny of the soul. Physicians' sins and their moral responsibilities, as we have seen in Section II, had been scrutinized for centuries by moral theologians who also typically discussed under separate rubrics a variety of issues that are now within the purview of medical ethics. All active moral theologians felt constrained to address issues that their predecessors could not have foreseen, as they sought to keep pace with an expanding vista of medical-ethical issues and to analyze old issues afresh in light of medical advances. Scholarly journals were created that were devoted to Roman Catholic discourse on medicine and medical ethics, for example, the *Linacre Quarterly* in 1932, *Cahiers Laënnec* in 1934, the *Catholic Medical Quarterly* in 1947, and *Arzt und Christ* in 1955. As early as the last decade of the nineteenth century, some theologians had begun to write articles and books specifically on medical ethics. Those especially worthy of mention, before Vatican II, are Charles Coppens (1897), Alphonsus Bonnar (1939), Charles McFadden (1949), Edwin Healy (1956), Thomas O'Donnell (1956), and, preeminently, Gerald Kelly (1958).[10]

These moral theologians employed the already well-established modality that some scholars refer to as physicalism, which, in Albert Jonsen's words, "refers to the interpretation of natural law doctrine in terms of the apparent physical structure and purpose of human functions. For example, the ethics of sexuality is derived from the 'natural orientation' of the sexual act to effect reproduction" (Jonsen 1998, 36). Physicalism regularly availed itself of the principle of double effect in resolving difficult issues. Double effect, also called the indirect voluntary, is thus defined by Gerald Kelly:

> The principle of double effect, as the name itself implies, supposes that an action produces two effects. One of these effects is something good which may be legitimately intended; the other is an evil which may not be intended.... An action is permitted, in accordance with the principle, if these conditions are fulfilled: 1) the action considered by itself and independently of its effects must not be morally evil; 2) the evil effect must not be the means of producing the good effect; 3) the evil effect is sincerely not intended but merely tolerated; 4) there must be a proportionate reason for performing the action in spite of its evil consequences. (Kelly G. 1958, 12–13)

Mahoney summarizes the principle as that by which moral theology "has systematically incorporated consequences into its considerations in a balancing of the foreseen good and bad effects of behaviour as one essential factor in evaluating the morality of that behaviour" (Mahoney 1987, 316). Physicalism, according to David Kelly, was the dominant modality of the emerging field of Roman Catholic medical ethics for the first four decades of the twentieth century, during which the magisterium addressed a comparatively small number of issues of medical ethics (Kelly D. 1979, 230).[11] Whenever the magisterium did pronounce on any issue, however, moral theologians typically deferred to that authority.

David Kelly sees a shift from a dominant modality of physicalism to what he calls ecclesiastical positivism beginning with the pontificate of Pius XII (Kelly D. 1979, 230).[12] Again, in Jonsen's words, "Ecclesiastical positivism means that moral theologians sought the final justification of all moral teaching in the *magisterium*, the teaching authority of the Church, constituted by the bishops under the supreme authority of the Pope. When the *magisterium* pronounced on an issue, such as abortion or contraception, the final word had been said and the theologians respectfully concluded their debates" (Jonsen 1998, 36). It should be noted, however, that when the magisterium addressed moral issues, especially those of medical ethics, if arguments or reasoning were presented to justify or at least explain the position set forth, they employed primarily a physicalist modality based on natural law bolstered, when applicable, by the long-established principle of double effect.

So how, especially after Pius XII's encyclical *Humani Generis* (discussed previously in Section III.1.A and B), did moral theologians deal with issues that had been addressed by popes who left their infallibility veiled? The comments in an article on mutilation written in 1956 by Gerald Kelly, a Jesuit who devoted much of his scholarship to medical ethics, are instructive: "The principal approach to any theological treatise should be the teaching of the magisterium, especially of the Holy See itself, when such teaching is available." After listing the pertinent documents, he writes:

> My enumeration includes encyclicals, allocutions, a radio message, and decrees of the Holy Office – all of which are usually understood to be media of the authentic, but not infallible, teaching of the Holy See. By this I do not mean that these media either cannot or do not contain infallible moral teaching. Certainly a pope may, if he wishes, use such media for *ex cathedra* pronouncements, as well as for clear expressions of the ordinary and universal teaching of the Church. Whether the popes have actually used these media for infallible moral teaching may be open to question. (Kelly G. 1956, 322)

He then refers to a paragraph condemning contraception in Pius XI's encyclical *Casti Connubii*[13] that "fulfils all the conditions laid down by the Vatican Council for an *ex cathedra* pronouncement. Moreover, even though a theologian should be loath to admit this, he can hardly doubt that this paragraph . . . makes it clear that the moral teaching . . . is an expression of the constant and universal teaching of the Church on a matter of natural and divine positive law – a teaching which is binding on the consciences of all the faithful and which admits of no possibility of change." Shortly thereafter he asseverates, "It suffices to recall here that, even when not infallible, the authentic teaching of the Holy See is of great importance. It requires both internal and external acceptance, not only on the part of the faithful but also on the part of theologians; it can be of such a decisive character that it ends actual theological controversy and precludes potential controversy" (Kelly G. 1956, 322–24). Kelly then navigated deftly through the shoals and reefs of papal pronouncements on the issue of mutilation, in which the principle of totality (described previously in Section III.1.C) played an essential role.

It is perhaps noteworthy that there is no article specifically entitled "Medical Ethics" in either the *Catholic Encyclopedia* (1911) or in the *New Catholic Encyclopedia* (1967). In the former one finds "Medicine and Canon Law" and in the latter "Physicians, Moral Obligations of," although there are, of course, articles on both medical ethical topics, such as abortion and contraception. "Medical Ethics" as a discrete entry at last appears in the 1974 supplement volume to the *New Catholic Encyclopedia*. This short article ends with some perceptive observations:

> A structural analysis of systematic works on Catholic medical ethics . . . clearly reveals the indebtedness of the field to the classic treatises on

moral theology. Most medical-ethical issues can, in fact, be traced to a precise location within the general moral-theology textbooks . . . Perhaps because of this rootage in the tradition of moral theology, Catholic medical ethics is not primarily a professional code for members of the medical profession. It is, rather, a more general ethic whose norms are relevant to the intentions and actions of physicians and patients alike. (Walters 1974, 291)

2. Vatican II and Beyond

When Pius XII died in 1958, little could anyone have known that an era had ended. With the Reformation, the Roman Catholic Church had become "one Christian sect competing among many, which nevertheless continued to maintain its traditional universalist claims as the one true church . . . Competitiveness bred exclusivity. It led inevitably to the development of a kind of siege mentality and just as inevitably to an increasing centralization of decision making with the pope and his curia" (O'Connell [1986] 1998, 108, 113). This centralization of authority achieved its most complete realization in the decrees of Vatican I, and ushered in an era that Mahoney described as one of ostensible "tranquillity," "an imposed serenity," "an apparent placidity and calm, as the unnatural sequel to the blanket and indiscriminate condemnation and suspicion of anything savouring of – in the revealing term – modernism." This, he maintains, was "a quite uncharacteristic period of the Church's history," "really abnormal." Writing two decades after Vatican II, he surmised that "for many in the Church this must be a disquieting conclusion, and one which appears to have scant regard either for the authority of the Church's hierarchical *magisterium* or for the destructive effects of dissent within the Christian body." For, as we shall see, this placidity and serenity was "rudely shattered in the ferment following" Vatican II (Mahoney 1987, 296, 326) by reactions to a papal pronouncement on a particular issue of medical ethics that profoundly affected most Catholics.

A. Vatican II, 1962–1965

In 1958, when he was elected pope 1 month shy of his seventy-seventh birthday, John XXIII (b. 1881; r. 1958–1963) was expected by many to be merely a transitional pontiff. Although his pontificate lasted fewer than 5 years, he initiated a new era in Roman Catholicism by convening the Second Vatican Council for spiritual renewal and *aggiornamento* (updating, modernizing) the role of the Church in the modern world. In his opening address to Vatican II in 1962, he said, "The greatest concern of the Ecumenical Council is this: that the sacred deposit of

Christian doctrine should be guarded and taught more efficaciously" (Abbott 1966, 713). A little later in this opening discourse, he remarked, "Our duty is not only to guard this precious treasure ... but to dedicate ourselves ... to that work which our era demands of us, pursuing thus the path which the Church has followed for twenty centuries." He then set the tone for the Council and for the Church: "The substance of the ancient doctrine of the deposit of faith is one thing, and the way in which it is presented is another. And it is the latter that must be taken into great consideration with patience if necessary, everything being measured in the forms and proportions of a magisterium which is predominantly pastoral in character." The Church must still confront errors, but not as she had in the past. "Frequently she has condemned them with the greatest severity. Nowadays, however, the Spouse of Christ prefers to make use of the medicine of mercy rather than that of severity. She considers that she meets the needs of the present day by demonstrating the validity of her teaching rather than by condemnations" (Abbott 1966, 715–716).

It has been and is supposed by many, both within and outside the Catholic Church, that Vatican II had, in fact, altered "the very model of the Church from pyramidal to concentric" (McCormick 1984, 2), while engaging in a "shift of weight from the metaphor of the 'body of Christ' to the term 'people of God'" (Gustafson 1978, 127). In the words of Leon Cardinal Suénens, "Seen from the starting point of baptism rather than that of the hierarchy, [it] rested on its base, the People of God, rather than on its summit, the hierarchy" (McCormick 1984, 66).

The Council frequently spoke of the "pilgrim Church," that is a Church in exile from its heavenly home, a maturing and learning Church, always, in accord with the old axiom Ecclesia semper reformanda est, in need of reform. In its decree on ecumenism, Unitatis Redintegratio, the Council said, "Every renewal (renovatio) of the Church essentially consists in an increase of fidelity to her own calling" (#6; Abbott 1966, 350). This is a delicate matter – always in need of reform and renewal, yet always remaining faithful to its calling, always, as emphasized repeatedly, faithfully guarding the "deposit of faith." A pilgrim Church, as Curran observes, "does not pretend to have all the answers" (Curran 1985, 143). The Council recognized this, addressing it twice in its "Pastoral Constitution on the Church in the Modern World" (Gaudium et Spes). "The Church guards the heritage of God's Word and draws from it religious and moral principles, without always having at hand the solution to particular problems" (#33; Abbott 1966, 232). Mahoney suggested, "If one had to single out any conciliar sentence as summing up the general temper of the Council's thinking, notwithstanding its firm teaching on numerous moral topics ... it would be difficult to overlook [this] statement" (Mahoney 1987,

303). A few paragraphs later in Gaudium et Spes, the Council states:

> Laymen should also know that it is generally the function of their well-formed Christian conscience to see that the divine law is inscribed in the life of the earthly city. From priests they may look for spiritual light and nourishment. Let the layman not imagine that his pastors are always such experts, that to every problem which arises, however complicated, they can readily give him a concrete solution, or even that such is their mission. (#43, Abbott 1966, 244)

Curran commented that before Vatican II, "Catholics pictured the Church as a perfect society having all the answers, and as the one bulwark of security in a changing world" (Curran 1985, 142). So, as McCormick remarked after quoting the second passage from Gaudium et Spes given previously (#43), "This is downright revolutionary when compared with the preconciliar notion of the function of official teachers. It is a final farewell to the one-sided dependency on the hierarchy in the formation of conscience" (McCormick 1984, 67). Hence it is not surprising that many within the Church were optimistic that this new spirit would lead to fundamental changes in the Church's assessment of some moral issues, an openness to reevaluation and the employment of approaches to moral analysis less rigid than those of natural-law physicalism, which had typified not only the manuals of moral theology but also the moral pronouncements of the magisterium.

Vatican II emphasized that in the training of priests "Special attention needs to be given to the development of moral theology. Its scientific exposition should be more thoroughly nourished by scriptural teaching. It should show the nobility of the Christian vocation of the faithful, and their obligation to bring forth fruit in charity for the life of the world" (Optatam Totius #16, Abbott 1966, 452). This is the Council's endorsement of an effort already being made by some moral theologians to change the orientation of their discipline from its predominantly negative sin-oriented emphasis to a more positive virtue-oriented approach. The mandate that moral theology be "more thoroughly nourished by scriptural teaching" is one of many examples of the Church's new emphasis on biblical study as already cautiously initiated by Pius XII's encyclical Divino Afflante Spiritu (Pius XII 1943). Vatican II's stipulation that "easy access to sacred Scripture should be provided for all the Christian faithful" in reliable translations from the original languages (Dei Verbum #22, Abbott 1966, 125–26) reflects a significant change from previous policy. It is inseparable from two major emphases of Vatican II: the elevated status and role of the laity as the people of God and a much greater stress on Scripture in all branches of theology. Of course, "The task of authentically interpreting the word of God . . . has been entrusted exclusively to the living teaching office of the Church [i.e., the magisterium], whose authority is exercised in the name of Jesus Christ" (*Dei Verbum* #10, Abbott 1966, 117–18).

In the writings of some moral theologians since Vatican II, there is a nearly palpable tension between two positions taken by the Council. One consists of statements, some of which have been quoted previously, that raised the hope, indeed the expectation, of a less rigid stance on the resolution of vexing moral problems by the magisterium. The other is the Council's intermittent reminders of the magisterium's ultimate authority in all matters of faith and morals as well as the duty of all Catholics to give it "close attention" (*Gaudium et Spes* #43; Abbott 1966, 244). In its "Dogmatic Constitution on the Church" (*Lumen Gentium*), the Council, "following in the footsteps" of Vatican I, unequivocally reaffirmed the dogmas of papal supremacy and infallibility. The college of bishops exercises supreme teaching authority when united with the pope, for example, in an ecumenical council, but "has no authority unless it is simultaneously conceived of in terms of its head, the Roman Pontiff." Although individual bishops do not "enjoy the prerogative of infallibility, they can nevertheless proclaim Christ's doctrine infallibly" (*Lumen Gentium* #18, #22, #25; Abbott 1966, 38, 43, 48–49).

Four sentences in *Lumen Gentium* #25 are of particular significance:

> In matters of faith and morals, the bishops speak in the name of Christ and the faithful are to accept their teaching and adhere to it with a religious assent of soul. This religious submission of will and of mind must be shown in a special way to the authentic teaching authority of the Roman Pontiff, even when he is not speaking *ex cathedra*. That is, it must be shown in such a way that his supreme magisterium is acknowledged with reverence, the judgments made by him are sincerely adhered to, according to his manifest mind and will. His mind and will in the matter may be known chiefly either from the character of the documents, from his frequent repetition of the same doctrine, or from his manner of speaking. (Abbott 1966, 48)

There is here a remarkable perpetuation of the earlier ambiguities of the nature of the magisterium and the responsibilities of "religious submission of will and of mind" to it "even when [the pope] is not speaking *ex cathedra*." Along with *Lumen Gentium* #25, the statement in *Dei Verbum* that "sacred tradition, sacred Scripture, and the teaching authority of the Church, in accord with God's most wise design, are so linked and joined together that one cannot stand without the others" (#10; Abbott 1966, 118) vigorously reinforces the teaching of Vatican I that

helped to foster such confusion about the precise authority of moral pronouncements of popes in the noninfallible but authentic (i.e., authoritative) exercise of their ordinary magisterium.

B. The Immediate Aftermath of Vatican II and the Impact of Humanae Vitae

The frustrations of some moral theologians are well illustrated by two statements made in proximity by McCormick in 1984. Having described Pope Pius XII's determination expressed especially in *Humani Generis* (1950) to end further discussion by theologians of any previously disputed question once a pope had intervened in the exercise of his ordinary magisterium, McCormick said, "This was the attitude of the time and it led to the conclusion that obedience was the appropriate response to authoritative teaching. Vatican II profoundly undermined this attitude." Three pages later, referring to the paragraph from *Lumen Gentium* #25, quoted above, he exclaimed, "It is this paragraph that is used as a club against those (bishops, theologians, and laity) who dissent from or even modify past official formulations of the Church" (McCormick 1984, 69, 72). It could be argued that what the Council gave with one hand it took back with the other.

Curran observed that the "encouraging reforms of Vatican II seemingly provided an impetus for the possibilities of massive reform and renewal . . . Disillusionment quickly followed . . . The whole process of reform and growth is much more complicated and difficult to attain than many had realized in the warm afterglow of Vatican II" (Curran 1985, 48). For that warm afterglow was dampened, some would say extinguished, when, only 3 years after the close of Vatican II the Church experienced an event that Marvin O'Connell described as "the most severe crisis of authority within the church since the Reformation" (O'Connell 1986, 141). This was Paul VI's (b. 1897; r. 1963–1978) issuing in 1968 his long-anticipated encyclical, *Humanae Vitae*, on the use of the contraceptive anovulant pill, previously condemned by Pius XII.

In 1963 John XXIII had appointed a commission to study over-population.[14] Its charge was soon changed to deal specifically with "new questions regarding conjugal life" and with "the regulation of births" (Paul VI 1968, #4). In 1964 John's successor, Paul VI, promised that the findings of the commission would soon be given. In the meantime, the position on contraception traditionally taken by the magisterium was still binding. The Council, which was still in session, was instructed not to deal with the issue, except to reiterate that it was not permissible for Catholics to take contraceptive measures that were condemned by the magisterium (*Gaudium et Spes* #51; Abbott 1966, 256). In 1966, Paul VI announced that the commission had delivered its recommendations. He would be studying the matter and give his conclusions in due time. In the meantime, of course, the traditional teaching of the magisterium was still binding. Two years later, he issued his encyclical.

In *Humanae Vitae* he stated that the "conclusions at which the commission arrived could not ... be considered by us as definitive." There were two reasons. First, "within the commission itself, no full concordance of judgments concerning the moral norms to be proposed had been reached." Even more crucially, "certain criteria of solutions had emerged which departed from the moral teaching on marriage proposed with constant firmness by the teaching authority of the Church" (Paul VI 1968, #6). He was, he wrote, compelled to uphold the Church's traditional rejection of artificial contraception. His argument was based, first, on that tradition itself and, second, on principles of natural law, here essentially a biological understanding of natural law and its place in the "hierarchy of values" (Paul VI 1968, #4, #8, #10). Along the way he asserted that only a misuse of the principles of totality and of double effect could justify artificial contraception, including sterilization and abortion (Paul VI 1968, #3, #14, #17). Proper application of these principles, however, would justify "the use of those therapeutic means truly necessary to cure diseases of the organism, even if an impediment to procreation, which may be foreseen, should result therefore, provided such impediment is not, for whatever motive, directly willed" (Paul VI 1968, #15).

He urged the clergy – especially "those who teach moral theology" – "to expound the Church's teaching on marriage without ambiguity," emphasizing that "it is of the utmost importance, for peace of consciences and for the unity of the Christian people, that in the field of morals as well as in that of dogma, all should attend to the magisterium of the Church, and all should speak the same language" (Paul VI 1968, #28).

In an allocution 6 days after issuing this encyclical, he "disclosed his own tortured feelings in the course of its preparation and in the making of his final decision," a "candid baring of the soul" that was "a remarkable event" (Mahoney 1987, 268, 270 n. 32). In the encyclical, he had expressed his hope that his decision would be received in a spirit of Christian docility with loyal internal and external obedience to the magisterium. Such hope was "to be sadly disappointed in the completely unprecedented and violent reactions which it aroused, both outside and within the Roman Catholic Church" (Mahoney 1987, 271).

In the immediate wake of its publication, one of the most highly respected and influential moral theologians, Bernard Häring, who had been a consultor to the theological subcommission of the papal commission, wrote a provocative article entitled "The Encyclical Crisis." It opens with the observation, "No papal teaching document has ever caused such an earthquake in the Church as the encyclical *Humanae Vitae*. Reactions around the world – in the Italian and American press, for example – are just as sharp as they were at the time of the *Syllabus of Errors* of Pius IX, perhaps even sharper" (Häring 1968, 588). Häring wrote, in the heat of his extreme disappointment, that the pope had followed the advice of a highly conservative and traditionalist minority of the commission whose influence helped produce an encyclical that "is regarded as a great victory by those groups who opposed the Council [i.e., Vatican II] from beginning to end" (Häring 1968, 588). Häring saw the major issue as one not of contraception but of authority within the Church. He gave numerous examples of positions that had been articulated in noninfallible but authoritative pronouncements of the magisterium but were later reversed, often owing to the pressures of cultural changes. Häring urged his fellow Catholics, who believe that the pope is the rightful successor of Peter, to "keep in mind the warning of the Lord against an earthly conception of the Messiah: 'Away with you, Satan; you are a stumbling-block to me. You think as men think, not as God thinks' (Mt. 16:23)." Hence, in regard to *Humanae Vitae*, he obliquely advised the pope, "the question, when all is said and done, is really, 'When you have come to yourself, you must lend strength to your brothers' (Lk. 22:31)."[15] For all Catholics, "what is needed is an enlightened understanding of the spiritual office" of the pope "against the most bitter opposition of that curial group which at the moment is triumphant" (Häring 1968, 589).

A little later he remarks, "I do not know whether Pope Paul himself was personally aware that he was making a test-case for non-collegial exercise of his teaching authority. However, I have very strong reasons for believing that his curial advisors had precisely such a test case in mind" (Häring 1968, 591). This collegiality is that of the pope's relations with the college of bishops. Incidentally, the majority of the bishops on the papal commission had advocated the position that the pope rejected. So "it is clear that an outmoded understanding of curial power is the real issue, and, in conjunction with it, the issue of non-collegial exercise of the teaching office, and the inadequately explored issues of how the pope teaches ... what is most important at this time is that the authority of the Church not be destroyed" (Häring 1968, 589, 594).

Viewed from one perspective, Vatican II, in its perceived emphasis on the concentric rather than pyramidal nature of the pilgrim Church, promoted the conclusion that the Council marks at least the beginning of the decentralization of authority within the Church. Yet, as Jonsen and Toulmin astutely observed, *Humanae Vitae* was the "culmination of [previous] centralization of authority in the moral sphere" (Jonsen and Toulmin 1988, 271), and it deepens the confusion about the exact nature of the authority that noninfallible papal pronouncements carry. On the day of the release of *Humanae Vitae*, the pope's representative, Monsignor Lambruschini, held a press conference in which he said that, although the encyclical was not an infallible statement, its authenticity (i.e., authority) was reinforced by its continuity with previous pronouncements by the magisterium. The encyclical, he maintained, did not leave open any questions about the regulation of births. Although "assent of theological faith" is due only to infallible definitions, "loyal and full assent, interior and not only exterior" is owed to an "authentic pronouncement of the *magisterium*, in proportion to the level of the authority from which it emanates . . . and to its object, which is most weighty." The authentic (i.e., authoritative) pronouncement of *Humanae Vitae* "prevents the forming of a probable opinion, that is to say an opinion acting on the moral plane in contrast with the pronouncement itself" (Mahoney 1987, 271).

In other words, although not an infallible definition, *Humanae Vitae* must, for all practical purposes, be treated as if it were. No one may anyone appeal to probabilism, the basic principle of which is that a doubtful law does not oblige, because the authority of the encyclical clearly is binding. Furthermore, the implication is that no contrary position could have extrinsic probability in the face of such a papal pronouncement. Mahoney suggested that "probabilism was dealt an official blow from which it is unlikely to recover its former legalistic vigour, if only because the category of 'approved authors' was considerably diminished and tended rather to be replaced by an unofficial category of suspect authors" (Mahoney 1987, 301). Furthermore, no moral argument could have intrinsic force sufficient to override the bases for the pope's decision, namely, the continuity of magisterial pronouncements and the application of principles of natural law upon which both the previous and present pronouncements of the magisterium were founded. So, it would appear *Roma locuta, causa finita* still prevailed.

In his press conference, Lambruschini said that in the encyclical "purposely no mention was made of scriptural arguments, but the entire reasoning was based on natural law" (Curran 1985, 121). Arguments based on natural-law theory appeal to human reason rightly applied. As many Catholic critics of the encyclical protested, however, the people of God were essentially being asked to discard reason, if the papal reasoning did not appear reasonable, and substitute for it the docility of faith in the logical inscrutability of the magisterium as guided by the Holy Spirit. Mahoney observed that many readers of the encyclical were "baffled," finding its teaching "incomprehensible." The encyclical was a "catalyst" that "did most to bring about the crisis of identity within the Church which had been imminent since the closing of the Council." Many Catholics "took a half step back . . . and began perhaps for the first time to take a somewhat more detailed view . . . than they had hitherto as the entire Church was being forced to examine itself and to follow through the practical and theological implications of events" (Mahoney 1987, 281, 284, 300–1).

It is not surprising that this led to a crisis of conscience for many married Catholics who, probably after much soul searching, ignored the stipulations of *Humanae Vitae* while continuing to participate in the sacraments and to consider themselves faithful Catholics. It was the beginning of what is sometimes disparagingly called "cafeteria Catholicism." For those moral theologians who disagreed not only with the pope's conclusions but also, and perhaps more importantly, with the methodology that had brought him to such conclusions, the crisis of conscience was amplified by the question of how they were to respond to this papal pronouncement in their teaching and public discourse, whether written or oral.

C. Moral Theologians and Medical Ethics from Vatican II (1965) to Veritatis Splendor (1993)

Various factors affecting the discourses of Roman Catholic medical ethics converged during the 1960s. First, some moral theologians, encouraged by the Second Vatican Council's introduction of fresh ideas into moral theology calling for a more biblical and pastoral perspective in moral reasoning, felt free to approach both old and new moral questions by exploring and employing modalities other than, and indeed in conflict with, the natural-law physicalism that had become the grid through which the hierarchical magisterium and most moral theologians saw all, or nearly all, issues of medical ethics. As Richard McCormick, who was emerging as one of the leading Roman Catholic moral theologians to address medical ethics, remarked a decade and a half after Vatican II, this had led to "a new willingness to reexamine some traditional formulations that were authoritatively proposed to the Catholic community" (McCormick 1988, x). Second, the ecumenical emphases of Vatican II were promoting an unprecedented dialogue of Catholic moral theologians with their Protestant and Jewish counterparts and with secular philosophers. Third, the ethical questions arising from advances in medical knowledge and technology were contributing to the emergence of the field of bioethics, which Warren Reich has defined "as the systematic study of the moral dimensions – including moral vision, decisions, conduct, and policies – of the life sciences and health care, employing a variety of ethical methodologies in an interdisciplinary setting" (Reich 1995b, xxi). That this emerging field attracted the attention of some of the best minds in Roman Catholic moral theology is not surprising (see also Chapter 7). But there was a further stimulus. As Jonsen comments, the "debate over the nature of ecclesiastical authority" aroused by *Humanae Vitae* had "an indirect effect on bioethics" by driving several Catholic moral theologians into this new field (Jonsen 1998, 301, cf. 37–38).

The debate that ensued over the nature of ecclesiastical authority focused on two concerns. The first was the question of whether noninfallible papal pronouncements on moral issues bound the consciences of the faithful and essentially closed discussion of these specific moral issues by theologians. The second involved the rejection of the physicalist natural-law methodology employed by the hierarchical magisterium in reaching the conclusions on moral issues enunciated in various forms, especially through encyclicals. We shall first consider the second of these two areas of debate.

1. The Rejection of Physicalism and the Exploration of Different Modalities of Ethical Analysis. Four years before Paul VI issued *Humanae Vitae*, Louis Dupré said of physicalism, "Such a way of reasoning about nature contains, I feel, two basic flaws. It confuses man's biological structure with his human nature. And it takes human nature as a static, unchangeable thing, rather than as a principle of development. Man's biological life and its intrinsic laws are but one aspect of human existence" (Dupré 1964, 43–44). Many moral theologians who agreed with Dupré's assessment were soon employing a modality of moral reasoning inherently in conflict with physicalism, and that is personalism.

Writing in 1979, David Kelly exclaimed that personalism "defies exact definition or even adequate description" (Kelly D. 1979, 417). Most importantly, it is a reaction against physicalism's "basing morality only on the finality and purpose of distinct physical faculties . . . according to which the moral aspect of the human act is identified with the physical aspect of the act" (Curran 1995, 2329), that is, considering "merely the physical criteria of the act-in-itself or of the biological faculty . . . under analysis," thus "limiting criteria for ethical analysis to physical cause-and-effect relationships" and making "these criteria . . . determinative in moral judgment" (Kelly D. 1979, 421). By contrast, personalism attempts to see "the total good of the person as the overriding ethical criterion" (Reich 1974, 183); hence, in medical ethics, the "emphasis is placed on the entire personal complexus of the act in its human dimensions, circumstances, and consequences," that is, in the total "spectrum of human experience, which includes, but is not limited to and often does not emphasize, either Scriptural or magisterial ethical judgments" (Kelly D. 1979, 419).

Because of its amorphous nature, it is difficult to describe exactly what this wholistic personalism is without having to describe what it has become in the hands of a variety of moral theologians. One word alone, however encapsulates what it is not: physicalism. Physicalism is sometimes called "natural-law physicalism," just as prevailing natural-law theory is sometimes called "physicalist

natural law." That these two expressions are used interchangeably says something significant about the degree of dependence of physicalism upon what had become the "traditional" Roman Catholic understanding of natural law and about the extent to which Roman Catholic natural-law theory had become physicalist in the manner of its application to many moral issues.

Natural-law theory, as it had developed in Roman Catholicism especially during the late-nineteenth and the early twentieth centuries, deduced, with ever greater degrees of specificity, from primary principles of natural law (e.g., do good and avoid evil), which are universally obligatory, secondary principles that are then pronounced as equally obligatory in both principle and application. In medical ethics this was spectacularly manifest in the writings of moral theologians of the mid-twentieth century such as Edwin Healy who, in 1956, asserted about a wide range of issues from contraception to euthanasia:

> It matters not whether one be Roman Catholic, a Protestant, a Jew, a pagan, or a person who has no religious affiliations whatever, he is nevertheless obliged to become acquainted with and to observe the teachings of the law of nature. In the present volume all the obligations which are mentioned flow from the natural law, unless the contrary is evident from the context. (Healy 1956, 7)

Those Roman Catholic moral theologians who rejected physicalism also rejected physicalist natural-law theory. In doing so, most did not reject natural-law theory per se but typically they honed and employed theories of natural law that were less rigid and narrow, "a more historically conscious approach" that "gives more emphasis to growth, development, and change, and likewise emphasizes the individual, the particular, and the contingent," that is, "a more inductive methodology . . . more tentative about its conclusions than the former deductive method" (Curran 1995, 2329).

There emerged a spectrum of interpretations of natural law by Catholic moralists, ranging from those who continued ardently to support the physicalist modality and its most controversial presentation, *Humanae Vitae* (e.g., McFadden 1976; O'Donnell 1976), to those who, without rejecting natural law entirely, modified it to such an extent that by denying, at least in principle, the existence of any negative moral absolutes (i.e., that any acts can be defined *eo ipso* and without exception as intrinsically evil), they appeared to deny that any truly definitive moral determination can be made regarding concrete norms of the natural moral law (e.g., Maguire 1974).

It has become nearly impossible to put most moral theologians since Vatican II into tidy compartments based on their interpretation and application of natural-law theory. By approximately two decades after Vatican II, however, there had developed what may be regarded as a "center of gravity," so to speak, which Francis Sullivan called simply "the more common view" of contemporary moral theologians. He asserted:

> It is now generally agreed that the process by which we arrive at the knowledge of the concrete norms of the natural law is through shared reflection on human experience; it is rather an inductive process than a deductive one. Christians seek the answers to concrete moral problems in the light of the Gospel, but these answers are not conclusions that follow with metaphysical certitude from revealed premises. (Sullivan 1983, 150)

Furthermore, he regarded as the commonly held view of moral theologians that "human nature itself is not a static, closed reality, but a dynamic, evolving one . . . the immediate norm of natural morality is man himself in his concrete nature. But this concrete nature of man in all its dimensions (biological, social, etc.) is itself precisely subject to a most far-reaching process of change. While some universal moral norms may be said to flow from the metaphysical nature of man, the particular norms are based on human nature as it exists in history, as subject to change" (Sullivan 1983, 152). Whether the majority of Catholic moralists held these precise views is subject to dispute; however that the majority of those who were most actively engaged in the discourses of medical ethics and bioethics held these views or some close variation of them seems indisputable (e.g., Richard McCormick, Bernard Häring, Joseph Fuchs, and Charles Curran, in their profuse writings, both on principles of moral theology generally and on medical ethics and bioethics specifically).

Closely linked to natural law, especially to natural-law physicalism, is the principle of double effect (briefly described previously in Section III.1.D). Double effect justifies any act that produces a legitimately intended good effect, although an unavoidable but unintended evil effect also results, *but only if four conditions are met*: "1) the action considered by itself and independently of its effects must not be morally evil; 2) the evil effect must not be the means of producing the good effect; 3) the evil effect is sincerely not intended but merely tolerated; 4) there must be a proportionate reason for performing the action in spite of its evil consequences" (Kelly G. 1958, 12–13).

David Kelly noted that, in the application of physicalist criteria to issues of medical ethics, the conditions of the principle of double effect that were most directly involved were the first two, because "the act-in-itself (first condition) and the cause-and-effect chain (second condition) were physically specified" (Kelly D. 1979, 424). The range of attitudes of Catholic moralists to the principle of double effect ran from a strict natural-law physicalist interpretation and application of the principle to the complete rejection of it. The beliefs of most moral theologians, however, lay somewhere between these two extremes. Their "more

complex and analytical criticisms of physicalism," Kelly asseverated, "are attempts to reformulate the principle of double effect in a non-physicalist way.[16] The human act is defined as more than a mere physical act-in-itself, and the cause-and-effect chain is not accepted as a central moral determinant. The emphasis is thus placed on the third and fourth conditions of the principle. The agent must not have evil as the intended end of the action; there must be a due proportion or commensurate reason for placing an act which will unavoidably have some ontic or premoral evil effects" (Kelly D. 1979, 425). This change allowed more latitude in the application of the principle of double effect.

Various names were given to this principle by its early proponents, such as, "commensurate reason" (Knauer 1967), but the use of such expressions as "due proportion" and "proportionate reason" as the defining characteristic of its method of moral analysis gave rise to its most common appellations, the "principle of proportionality" or "proportionalism." There has been much disagreement about how this new principle should be expressed, whether the concept of intrinsically evil acts ought or even could be retained, and whether, and if so how, it differed from utilitarianism or consequentialism.

Richard McCormick was arguably the most influential refiner and expander of the principle of double effect in applying to topics of medical ethics and bioethics what he regarded as its central and most functional component, that is, "proportionate reason." To him, as he wrote in 1973, this meant three things: "(a) a value at stake at least equal to that sacrificed, (b) no other way of salvaging it here and now, and (c) its protection here and now will not undermine it in the long run" (McCormick 1973, 69). Twenty years later, when proportionalism was under severe attack by the magisterium, he wrote that, in spite of

> differences that individual theologians bring to their analyses . . . common to all so-called proportionalists is the insistence that causing certain disvalues (nonmoral, premoral evils) in our conduct does not by that very fact make the action morally wrong, as certain traditional formulations supposed. The action becomes morally wrong when, all things considered, there is not a proportionate reason in the act justifying the disvalue. Thus, just as not every killing is murder, not every falsehood is a lie, so not every artificial intervention preventing or promoting conception in marriage is necessarily an unchaste act. (McCormick 1993)

Proportionalism, in its various forms, was readily applied to a host of sexual and medical topics, ranging from contraception (including sterilization) and abortion to end-of-life issues, justifying in particular circumstances even acts traditionally condemned under all circumstances as intrinsically evil. It is not surprising that the answers to numerous situations of moral perplexity by "proportionalists" were often at considerable variance with the positions enunciated by the hierarchical magisterium.

2. The Rejection of Ecclesiastical Positivism: Dissent from Noninfallible Teachings of the Hierarchical Magisterium.

The new approaches by "revisionist" theologians that have in common the rejection of physicalist methodology employed by the magisterium were themselves a form of dissent from the prevailing ecclesiastical positivism when the publicly articulated conclusions they reached were in direct opposition to the teaching of the hierarchical magisterium. Writing in 1979, David Kelly exclaimed, "What is clear is that Roman Catholic medical ethical methodology has freed itself from the kinds of physicalist restrictions which offered it clear and universally applicable norms and criteria for the solution of nearly all of its medical ethical questions" (Kelly D. 1979, 428), and a few pages later, he reiterated his enthusiasm:

> The critique of ecclesiastical positivism in medical ethics, together with that of physicalism, has freed Catholic medical ethics from its former restrictive methodology. Individual consciences and differences of situation are better recognized. The human aspects of the moral dilemma can achieve their proper place in ethical analysis and judgment. (Kelly D. 1979, 435–36)

Between these two passages, Kelly lamented, "the personalist approach might have been adopted and defended by magisterial authority in a way similar to that in which physicalism was adopted and defended. Official ecclesiastical decrees might have switched their language from the one to the other, and prescribed authoritatively the 'newer' kind of approach typified by appeal to proportionate reason" (Kelly D. 1979, 429). There were, he acknowledged, various reasons why this had not occurred. He surmised that more important than any other was probably "the fact that personalist medical moralists arrive at conclusions which are at variance with previous official pronouncements." This was particularly the case regarding contraception, abortion, and even, although rarely, active euthanasia. Hence, "to change from physicalism and physicalist conclusions would be to admit previous error and thus weaken the case for magisterial inerrancy in moral matters" (Kelly D. 1979, 430).

Yet, as David Kelly knew very well, the papal magisterium had never pronounced *ex cathedra* and infallibly on any moral issue. It is commonly held that no pope will ever venture to do so, because infallible definitions are, by their very nature, irreformable. Furthermore, many revisionist moral theologians' methodologies, by their very nature, appear to disallow as conceptually impossible any *truly infallible*, therefore irreformable and absolute, moral definition of particular norms and concrete acts (see, e.g., Sullivan 1983, 149–50).

Some moral theologians, whose methodology could lead to conflict with the hierarchy, especially with the pope, simply deferred to magisterial authority. For instance, Louis Dupré, whose negative critique of physicalism was quoted previously, wrote a revisionist appraisal of contraception while the issue was being considered by the commission appointed by John XXIII and continued by Paul VI. Early in his study he said, "whatever the magisterium's final word on the question will be, it will also be mine" (Dupré 1964, 6). Thus, although still rejecting physicalism, he hewed to ecclesiastical positivism. Most revisionists, however, did not follow his example. In response to *Humanae Vitae*, an unprecedented surge of open dissent occurred as numerous theologians respectfully, and some not so respectfully, disagreed with, or openly repudiated, both the methodology employed by, and the conclusion reached in, that encyclical.

Disciplinary action was taken against some revisionist moral theologians, the focus of whose dissent was on issues about which the hierarchical magisterium had taken an inflexible stand. Father Charles Curran is a well-known example. As a young professor of moral theology at the Catholic University of America in Washington DC, Curran was in the vanguard of vocal dissent against *Humanae Vitae*. He wrote prolifically on many topics of moral theology, especially on those issues of sexual and medical ethics on which the hierarchical magisterium had made its most specific and inflexibly condemnatory judgments. His closely reasoned and concisely articulated dissent from magisterial pronouncements eventually led to an extensive investigation of his writings by Joseph Cardinal Ratzinger in his capacity as Prefect of the Congregation for the Doctrine of the Faith, a post to which he had been appointed by Pope John Paul II (b. 1920; r. 1978–2005) in 1981. In 1986, with the approval of the pope, the Congregation for the Doctrine of the Faith advised the chancellor of the Catholic University that Curran "was no longer . . . considered suitable [or] eligible to exercise the function of a Professor of Catholic Theology." He was removed from his tenured position at the Catholic University although "neither stripped of his priesthood nor forbidden to function as a priest. Nor was he forbidden to publish, make public appearances, or teach in a non-Catholic institution" (Weigel 1999, 524).[17]

This was at a time when John Paul II had become determined to address not merely dissent by Catholic moral theologians but the fundamental principles of moral theology. The result, after years of preparation, was the publication in 1993 of the encyclical *Veritatis Splendor*, a watershed in the history of Roman Catholic moral theology.

D. The Magisterium and Moral Theology at the End of the Second Millennium

1. John Paul II's *Veritatis Splendor* (1993). In 1987 John Paul issued his Apostolic Letter *Spiritus Domini* announcing his decision to write an encyclical in which he would "treat more fully and more deeply the issues regarding the very foundations of moral theology" (John Paul II 1987b, #3). Six years later, he published his promised encyclical, *Veritatis Splendor*, to set forth clearly "*certain aspects of doctrine which are of crucial importance in facing what is certainly a genuine crisis*," limiting the encyclical's scope to "dealing with *certain fundamental questions regarding the Church's moral teaching*" and "issues being debated by ethicists and moral theologians." He applied "the principles of a moral teaching based upon Sacred Scripture and the living Apostolic Tradition" to the problems being discussed, while shedding light on "the presuppositions and consequences of the dissent which that teaching has met" (John Paul II 1993, #5, emphasis in original). This crisis is "no longer a matter of limited and occasional dissent, but of an overall and systematic calling into question of traditional moral doctrine, on the basis of certain anthropological and ethical presuppositions." This manifests itself in four ways. First, some moral theologians reject the traditional doctrine of the natural law and its "universality" and "permanent validity;" second, they regard "certain of the Church's moral teachings" as "simply unacceptable;" third, they consider the magisterium "capable of intervening in matters of morality only in order to 'exhort consciences' and to 'propose values,' in the light of which each individual will independently make his or her decisions and life choices;" and, furthermore, they have a tendency to separate faith and morality and regard the former alone as the basis for "membership in the Church and her internal unity" (John Paul II 1993, #4).

Early in this lengthy encyclical he reminds his readers that always, but especially during the last two centuries, popes, either individually or in collaboration with the College of Bishops, "have developed and proposed a moral teaching regarding the *many different spheres of human life*." In the face of the moral crisis that is now troubling the Church and the world, the magisterium "senses more urgently the duty to offer its own discernment and teaching" on the very questions that are being debated by moral theologians today and about new tendencies and theories that have developed in moral theology. The magisterium, of course, does not intend to impose any particular theological, much less philosophical, system. But it "has the duty to state that some trends of theological thinking and certain philosophical affirmations are incompatible with

revealed truth." Hence, he will "state *the principles necessary for discerning what is contrary to 'sound doctrine'*" and while doing so draw attention to "those elements of the Church's moral teaching which today appear particularly exposed to error, ambiguity or neglect" (John Paul II 1993, #4, #27, #29, #30, emphasis in original).

Certain moral theologians deny the existence in divine revelation of "a specific and determined moral content, universally valid and permanent," thus limiting Scripture to "proposing an exhortation . . . which the autonomous reason alone would then have the task of completing with normative directives which are truly 'objective,' that is, adapted to the concrete historical situation." "No one," John Paul asserts, "can fail to see that such an interpretation of the autonomy of human reason involves positions incompatible with Catholic teaching." Hence "the fundamental notions of human freedom and of the moral law, as well as their profound and intimate relationship" must be clarified "in the light of the word of God and the living Tradition of the Church" (John Paul II 1993, #36–37).

After a lengthy description of the teaching of the Church about the natural moral law and its relation to revelation (John Paul II 1993, #38–45), he says that although "*Debates about nature and freedom* have always marked the history of moral reflection;" currently nature and freedom are being set in opposition, "as if a dialectic, if not an absolute conflict," between them "were characteristic of the structure of human history." Hence, some moralists, "conceive of freedom as somehow in opposition to or in conflict with material and biological nature, over which it must progressively assert itself." After elaborating on various aspects of these moralists' theories, he states, "In this context, *objections of physicalism and naturalism* have been levelled against the traditional conception of *the natural law*, which is accused of presenting as moral laws what are in themselves mere biological laws," of attributing a permanent and unchanging character to certain kinds of human behavior, and of attempting on this basis "to formulate universally valid moral norms." According to some theologians, "this kind of 'biologistic or naturalistic argumentation'" is even present in certain teachings of the magisterium, especially in those dealing with sexual and conjugal ethics. "It was, they maintain, on the basis of a naturalistic understanding of the sexual act that contraception, direct sterilization . . . and artificial insemination were condemned as morally unacceptable." These moral theologians maintain that on such issues the teaching of the magisterium "fails to take into adequate consideration both man's character as a rational and free being and the cultural conditioning of all moral norms. In their view, man, as a rational being, not only can but actually *must freely determine the meaning* of his behaviour." Typical human behavior and natural inclinations "would established at the most – so they say – a general orientation towards correct behaviour, but they cannot determine the moral assessment of individual human acts, so complex from the viewpoint of situations" (John Paul II 1993, #46–47, emphasis in original).

John Paul declared that such teaching is inherently in conflict with the Church's traditional teaching, which, he asserted, is not physicalist in its understanding of the place of biological functions in the unity of both soul and body (which constitutes the person), and consistently proclaimed the immutability of the natural law and the existence of objective norms of morality that are valid for all people everywhere, past, present, and future, because there is in all people a human nature that transcends every culture and all time (John Paul II 1993, #48–53).

Arguably, the key teaching of *Veritatis Splendor* is the section entitled "The Moral Acts" (#71–83), where John Paul considered the criteria necessary for assessing correctly man's freely chosen acts. He acknowledged that "the moral life has an essential *'teleological' character*, since it consists in the deliberate ordering of human acts to God, the supreme good and ultimate end (*telos*) of man" but, according to "certain *ethical theories*, called *'teleological,'* . . . concrete behaviour would be right or wrong according as whether or not it is capable of producing a better state of affairs for all concerned. Right conduct would be the one capable of 'maximizing' goods and 'minimizing' evils" (John Paul II 1993, #74, emphasis in original).

Two types of so-called teleologies can be distinguished from each other: "consequentialism," which "claims to draw the criteria of the rightness of a given way of acting solely from the calculation of foreseeable consequences deriving from a given choice," and "proportionalism," which "by weighing the various values and goods being sought, focuses rather on the proportion acknowledged between the good and bad effects of that choice, with a view to the 'greater good' or 'lesser evil' actually possible in a particular situation." Such theories "maintain that it is never possible to formulate an absolute prohibition of particular kinds of behaviour which would be in conflict, in every circumstance and in every culture, with those values," and insist that it is not possible to determine whether any act that has been traditionally defined by the Church as intrinsically evil is actually evil unless one first considers the pre-moral (also called nonmoral, physical, or ontic) good and evil states of affairs an act is likely to cause in the concrete situation. Hence, in the alternatives available in concrete situations, the foreseen proportions of premoral goods to evils at times can justify exceptions to precepts traditionally regarded as absolute. According to such theories, "Even when grave matter is concerned, these precepts should be considered as operative norms which are always relative and open to exceptions. In this view, deliberate consent to certain kinds of behaviour declared illicit by traditional moral theology would not imply an objective moral evil." He rejected these theories,

because they "are not faithful to the Church's teaching, when they believe they can justify, as morally good, deliberate choices of kinds of behaviour contrary to the commandments of the divine and natural law" (John Paul II 1993, #75–76).

Although it is necessary to take into account both the intention and the consequences of human actions, the *"morality of the human act depends primarily and fundamentally on the 'object' rationally chosen by the deliberate will."* A good intention is not sufficient in itself. A correct choice of acts is also necessary because the human act depends on whether its object "is *capable or not of being ordered* to God, to the One who 'alone is good'" Because Christian ethics "is directed to promoting the true good of the person," it "recognizes that it is really pursued only when the essential elements of human nature are respected. The human act, good according to its object, is also *capable of being ordered* to its ultimate end. That same act then attains its ultimate and decisive perfection when the will *actually does order* it to God" (John Paul II 1993, #77–78, emphasis in original).

John Paul focused specifically on the fundamental principle of intrinsic evil: *"One must therefore reject the thesis,* characteristic of teleological and proportionalist theories, *which holds that it is impossible to qualify as morally evil according to its species – its 'object' – the deliberate choice of certain kinds of behaviour or specific acts, apart from a consideration of the intention for which the choice is made or the totality of the foreseeable consequences of that act for all persons concerned."* The object of the human act, "which establishes whether it is *capable of being ordered to the good and to the ultimate end, which is God,"* is the "primary and decisive element for moral judgment." This capability is grasped by reason. It is in the very being of man, "considered in his integral truth, and therefore in his natural inclinations, his motivations and his finalities, which always have a spiritual dimension as well. It is precisely these which are the contents of the natural law" (John Paul II 1993, #79, emphasis in original).

He then stated categorically that reason attests that some objects of human acts "are by their nature 'incapable of being ordered' to God, because they radically contradict the good of the person made in his image. These are the acts which, in the Church's moral tradition, have been termed 'intrinsically evil' (*intrinsece malum*): they are such *always and per se*, in other words, on account of their very object, and quite apart from the ulterior intentions of the one acting and the circumstances" (John Paul II 1993, #80, emphasis in original). He quotes from the Second Vatican Council's *Gaudium et Spes* #27, among several examples of such acts, "any kind of homicide, genocide, abortion, euthanasia and voluntary suicide; whatever violates the integrity of the human person, such as mutilation," which "are a negation of the honour due to the Creator." He illustrates the moral reasoning employed by the Church "with regard to intrinsically evil acts, and in reference to contraceptive practices whereby the conjugal act is intentionally rendered infertile," by quoting from Paul VI's *Humanae Vitae*:

> Though it is true that sometimes it is lawful to tolerate a lesser moral evil in order to avoid a greater evil or in order to promote a greater good, it is never lawful, even for the gravest reasons, to do evil that good may come of it (cf. Rom. 3:8) – in other words, to intend directly something which of its very nature contradicts the moral order, and which must therefore be judged unworthy of man, even though the intention is to protect or promote the welfare of an individual, of a family or of society in general. (John Paul II 1993, #80, the indented quotation being from *Humanae Vitae* #14)

Although a good intention or particular circumstances can diminish the evil of an intrinsically evil act, they cannot remove it, for they "remain 'irremediably' evil acts; per se and in themselves they are not capable of being ordered to God and to the good of the person," and can never be transformed by circumstances or intentions into acts subjectively good or defensible as a choice. Hence, "the opinion must be rejected as erroneous which maintains that it is impossible to qualify as morally evil according to its species the deliberate choice of certain kinds of behaviour or specific acts, without taking into account the intention for which the choice was made or the totality of the foreseeable consequences of that act for all persons concerned. Without the *rational determination of the morality of human acting* as stated above, it would be impossible to affirm the existence of an 'objective moral order'" (John Paul II 1993, #81–82, emphasis in original).

With greater urgency than on previous occasions, John Paul II commands moral theologians, although "recognizing the possible limitations of the arguments employed by the Magisterium . . . to develop a deeper understanding of the reasons underlying its teachings and to expound the validity and obligatory nature of the precepts it proposes, demonstrating their connection with one another and their relation with man's ultimate end." They are to give "the example of a loyal assent, both internal and external, to the Magisterium's teaching in the areas of both dogma and morality," which "is of the utmost importance, not only for the Church's life and mission, but also for human society and culture" (John Paul II 1993, #110–111).

He reminded moral theologians that the Church is not a representative democracy in which "exchanges and conflicts of opinion may constitute normal expressions of public life." Moral teaching "cannot depend simply upon respect for a process: indeed, it is in no way established by following the rules and deliberative procedures typical of a democracy." There is a line that moral theologians must not cross in expressing their disagreement with the magisterium. "*Dissent*, in the form of carefully orchestrated protests and polemics carried on in the media, *is opposed to ecclesial communion and to a correct understanding of the hierarchical constitution of the People of God*. Opposition to the teaching of the Church's Pastors cannot be seen as a legitimate expression either of Christian freedom or of the diversity of the Spirit's gifts" (John Paul II 1993, #113, emphasis in original). The sternness and intensity of this reproof of dissenting moral theologians by a pope speaking expressly "with the authority of the Successor of Peter" vividly demonstrate the gravity and urgency he felt in issuing this encyclical.

John Paul had addressed *Veritatis Splendor* to his fellow bishops. Near the end of the encyclical he stated that he and they have been entrusted by Christ to make moral teaching an object of their *munus propheticum* (prophetic office) and of their *munus sacerdotale* (priestly office). "Especially today, Christian moral teaching must be one of the chief areas in which we exercise our pastoral vigilance, in carrying out our *munus regale*" (regal office). He then acknowledged, "This is the first time, in fact, that the Magisterium of the Church has set forth in detail the fundamental elements of this teaching, and presented the principles for the pastoral discernment necessary in practical and cultural situations which are complex and even crucial." He was convinced that this unprecedented intervention in moral theology was necessary because "each of us knows how important is the teaching which represents the central theme of this Encyclical and which is today being restated with the authority of the Successor of Peter. Each of us can see the seriousness of what is involved, not only for individuals but also for the whole of society, with the *reaffirmation of the universality and immutability of the moral commandments*, particularly those which prohibit always and without exception *intrinsically evil acts*" (John Paul II 1993, #114–115, emphasis in original).

He reminded his fellow bishops that he and they had the duty "to see to it that this moral teaching is faithfully handed down and to have recourse to appropriate measures to ensure that the faithful are guarded from every doctrine and theory contrary to it." There is only a limited role for theologians: "In carrying out this task we are all assisted by theologians; even so, theological opinions constitute neither the rule nor the norm of our teaching." This responsibility and authority belong to bishops, who "have the grave obligation to be *personally* vigilant that the 'sound doctrine' (1 Tim. 1:10) of faith and morals is taught in our Dioceses." A particular instance regards Catholic institutions. "Whether these are agencies for the pastoral care of the family or for social work, or institutions dedicated to teaching or health care, Bishops . . . are never relieved of their own personal obligations. It falls to them, in communion with the Holy See, both to grant the title 'Catholic' to Church-related schools, universities, healthcare facilities and counselling services, and, in cases of a serious failure to live up to that title, to take it away" (John Paul II 1993, #116).

It is not surprising that there were immediate reactions from various quarters, especially from moral theologians.

2. The Reception of *Veritatis Splendor* by Moral Theologians.

Veritatis Splendor was signed on August 6, 1993, but not released until October 5, 1993. Because moral theology was its topic and specific moral systems its target, the responses of moral theologians were swift. A few, who were themselves critical of the methods of moral reasoning criticized in the encyclical, spoke in praise of the criticisms made by the pope. A larger number, who saw themselves – although the pope had named no names – and their methodologies repudiated by the pope, maintained that either he misunderstood their teaching or had been ill-served by those who, in assisting him in the composition of the encyclical, misrepresented and caricatured their teaching.

Perhaps the earliest published reaction of a moral theologian was that of Germain Grisez, the first in a series of eleven brief essays printed in *The Tablet* from October 16, 1993, to January 15, 1994. Grisez praised the encyclical, predicted that "dissenting theologians undoubtedly will respond that the Pope has misinterpreted them, missed them altogether, and/or found no new or convincing arguments against their views." Regardless, because the papal argument is the product of revelation, they have only three choices: "to admit that they have been mistaken, to admit that they do not believe God's word, or to claim that the Pope is grossly misinterpreting the Bible" (Grisez 1993).

In the next week's issue, Bernard Häring (whose strongly negative reaction to *Humanae Vitae* is described in Section III.2.B) opened his essay entitled, "A Distrust That Wounds," by saying that after reading the encyclical carefully, "I felt greatly discouraged. Several hours later I suffered long-lasting seizures of the brain," but in due course had "a new feeling of confidence, without blinding my eyes and heart to the pain and brain convulsions that are likely to ensue in the immediate future." Although *Veritatis Splendor* "contains many beautiful things," Häring lamented that "almost all real splendour is lost when it becomes evident that the whole document is directed above all towards one goal: to endorse total assent and submission to all utterances of the Pope, and above all on one crucial point: that the use of any artificial means for regulating birth is intrinsically evil and sinful, without exception, even in circumstances where contraception would be a lesser evil." He exclaimed that he and his fellow moral theologians "should let the Pope know that we are wounded by the many signs of his rooted distrust, and discouraged by the manifold structures of distrust which he has allowed to be established. We need him to soften toward us, the whole Church needs it" (Häring 1993).

In its October 22 issue, *Commonweal* published a "symposium" of short reactions to the encyclical by several moral theologians and Christian ethicists (Cunningham et al.

1993). Although several of the eight contributors found some positive observations to make about the encyclical, and two were quite supportive, most were highly critical. Both Lawrence Cunningham and Joseph Komonchak drew comparisons with Pius XII's *Humani Generis* (on which see Section III.1.A. & B), hoped that the suppression of eminent theologians that *Humani Generis* precipitated would not occur now, but took some solace from the fact that the very teachings for which those theologians had been disciplined had ultimately triumphed at Vatican II. Charles Curran maintained that the encyclical's "defensive nature . . . comes through especially in its inadequate, caricatured, and even erroneous interpretations of the positions taken by many contemporary Catholic moral theologians," none of whom "embraces relativism, subjectivism, positivism, and individualism." His essay concluded on a discouraged note: "the pope has no appreciation for a loyal opposition that disagrees on some specific issues but finds itself in basic and fundamental agreement with the core of the Catholic moral tradition. The practical consequences of this document will only come to light in the future, but my forecast for the immediate future is quite bleak" (Cunningham et al. 1993, 14).

Richard McCormick contributed the third essay on *Veritatis Splendor* to *The Tablet*. Published simultaneously there and in *America* on October 30, his paper agreed with the encyclical's "ringing rejection of the false dichotomies identified by John Paul II between autonomy and theonomy, freedom and law, conscience and truth, etc. These extreme positions dead-end in relativism, subjectivism and individualism, and all of us repudiate such pathologies." McCormick then turned to the substance of his disagreement with the encyclical. "That brings us to one of the tendencies that concerns the Pope: proportionalism." After quoting some statements made in *Veritatis Splendor* about proportionalism, he stated, "In brief, the encyclical repeatedly states of proportionalism that it attempts to justify morally wrong actions by a good intention. This, I regret to say, is a misrepresentation." The pope, according to McCormick, has plain and simply missed the point of proportionalism. "When contemporary theologians say that certain disvalues in our actions can be justified by a proportionate reason, they are not saying that morally wrong actions (*ex objecto*) can be justified by the end. They are saying that an action cannot be judged morally wrong simply by looking at the material happening, or at its object in a very narrow and restricted sense. This is precisely what the tradition has done in certain categories (e.g., contraception, sterilization). It does this in no other area."

McCormick saw in the encyclical "an unstated agenda item. It is this: I am convinced that the Holy Father will reject *a priori* any analytic adjustments in moral theology that do not support the moral wrongfulness of every contraceptive act. Proportionalism certainly does not give such support." As to the effect of this encyclical letter,

"On the public, zero. It is too technical and abstract to address anyone but specialists." Although what about bishops; they are enjoined to taken certain measures to rein in dissent? McCormick thought it unlikely that any theologians would be fired for teaching what the encyclical wrongly accuses them of doing. "They cannot be punished for uncommitted crimes. In this respect *Veritatis Splendor* differs from Pius XII's *Humani Generis*," He predicts that *Veritatis Splendor* will "eventually enjoy a historical status similar to that of *Humani Generis*" (McCormick 1993).

Whether McCormick's prediction will prove correct is still too early to say. Two matters, however, are certain. The debate between theologians about the validity of John Paul's representation of proportionalism and, regardless of that, about its legitimacy as a modality of moral reasoning for Catholics, soon after these few examples given above were published, became very vitriolic (cp., e.g., McCormick 1994 and Neuhaus 1995). Furthermore, various forms of proportionalism and nonphysicalist natural-law modalities continue to be employed by many Catholic moral theologians in their discourses on topics of medical ethics and bioethics.

E. "A Culture of Life" in the Midst of "A Culture of Death": John Paul II's Evangelium Vitae (1995)

In 1991, John Paul II wrote a letter to all Catholic bishops, in which he drew their attention to what he called a "striking analogy" between the oppression of the fundamental rights of the working classes, which had been addressed by Leo XIII 100 years earlier in his encyclical *Rerum Novarum*, and the current oppression of another category of persons' fundamental rights – the right to life itself. He had written this letter to ask the bishops to cooperate with him in developing an encyclical that would fulfill a request made earlier that year by an Extraordinary Consistory of Cardinals "to reaffirm with the authority of the Successor of Peter the value of human life and its inviolability, in the light of present circumstances and attacks threatening it today." In the "Introduction" to the encyclical *Evangelium Vitae*, issued 4 years later, he refers to this letter to all bishops and asserts, "If at the end of the last century, the Church could not be silent about the injustices of those times, still less can she be silent today, when the social injustices of the past . . . are being compounded in many regions of the world by still more grievous forms of injustice and oppression, even if these are being presented as elements of progress in view of a new world order" (John Paul II 1995a, 1995b, #5).

Evangelium Vitae, the most comprehensive manifesto of the Church's doctrine of the dignity and value of the human person ever made by the hierarchical magisterium, condemns unequivocally the current "culture of death" as a "conspiracy against life" that creates "structures of sin" to undermine the life of the most vulnerable. Such a culture "betrays a completely individualistic concept of freedom," which becomes the "freedom of 'the strong' against the weak who have no choice but to submit." This culture of death grows increasingly stronger because scientific and technological progress provide "new forms of attacks on the dignity of the human being." The culture of death, by its very nature, justifies "certain crimes against life in the name of rights of individual freedom." Hence, with impunity and the approval of the state, people freely commit these crimes assisted by subsidized health-care systems. That "choices once unanimously considered criminal and rejected by the common moral sense are gradually becoming socially acceptable" is "both a disturbing symptom and a significant cause of grave moral decline"(John Paul II 1995a, 1995b, #4, 12, 19, 24).

So how, John Paul rhetorically asked, did such a precipitous moral decline occur? The answer is quite obvious. When secularism dominates a social and cultural climate, not only is the sense of God lost but "there is also a tendency to lose the sense of man." Then the meaning of everything becomes profoundly distorted. This in turn "leads to a practical materialism which breeds individualism, utilitarianism and hedonism." What is then called "quality of life" is little more than "economic efficiency, inordinate consumerism, physical beauty and pleasure," which neglect "the more profound dimensions – interpersonal, spiritual and religious – of existence." In such an ethos, the body "is simply a complex of organs, functions and energies to be used according to the sole criteria of pleasure and efficiency" (John Paul II 1995a, 1995b, #21–23).

With regularity the pope reminded his readers that it is due to the denial or rejection of one's fundamental relationship to God that law and ethics, having no foundation, become nothing more than personal autonomy and majority totalitarianism resting on the shifting sands of relativism. Sadly, this has subtly corrupted some Catholics, who, while continuing to "take an active part in the life of the Church, end up by separating their Christian faith from its ethical requirements concerning life, and thus fall into moral subjectivism and certain objectionable ways of acting." Of course in secular society, where either God is denied or people live as though he did not exist, thus ignoring his commandments, "the dignity of the human person and the inviolability of human life" are rejected or compromised (John Paul II 1995a, 1995b, #95–96).

In the current milieu of godless secularism and materialism, man can no longer "see himself as 'mysteriously different' from other earthly creatures." Life itself has become "a mere 'thing,' which man claims as his exclusive property, completely subject to his control and manipulation." Man, of course, is the master neither of life nor death; his role is not that of lordship but of stewardship because "life is entrusted to man as a treasure which must not be squandered." Such knowledge is innate in all people because "in the depths of his conscience, man is always reminded of the inviolability of life – his own life and that of others – as something which does not belong to him, because it is the property and gift of God" (John Paul II 1995a, 1995b, #22, #40, #46, #52).

Scripture clearly teaches, the Church's tradition has constantly upheld, and the magisterium has consistently proposed the moral truth of the absolute inviolability of innocent human life. The magisterium, which "has spoken out with increasing frequency in defence of the sacredness and inviolability of human life," now, more than ever before, must interpret and apply even more precisely the eternal and natural law to the current moral crisis. Hence John Paul II declared, "by the authority which Christ conferred upon Peter and his Successors, and in communion with the Bishops of the Catholic Church, I confirm that the direct and voluntary killing of an innocent human being is always gravely immoral. This doctrine, based upon that unwritten law which man, in the light of reason, finds in his own heart, is reaffirmed by Sacred Scripture, transmitted by the Tradition of the Church and taught by the ordinary and universal Magisterium" (John Paul II 1995a, 1995b, #28, #57).

Natural-law theory is a fundamental principle to which John Paul makes reference nearly from the beginning to the end of *Evangelium Vitae*. The Gospel of life "has a profound and persuasive echo in the heart of every person – believer and non-believer alike," who can "come to recognize in the natural law written in the heart the sacred value of human life from its very beginning until its end, and can affirm the right of every human being to have this primary good respected to the highest degree." Conscience, however, darkened by "widespread conditioning . . . is finding it increasingly difficult to distinguish between good and evil in what concerns the basic value of human life." Yet conscience is not entirely dead even among the most ardent proponents of the culture of death, "as is evident in the tendency to disguise certain crimes against life in its early or final stages by using innocuous medical terms which distract attention from the fact that what is involved is the right to life of an actual human person." So there is every reason for confidence that "all the conditioning and efforts to enforce silence fail to stifle the voice of the Lord echoing in the conscience of every individual." One can be "certain that moral truth cannot fail to make its presence deeply felt in every conscience" because "the value at stake is one which every human being can grasp by the light of reason" (John Paul II 1995a, 1995b, #2, #4, #11, #24, #90, #101).

The culture of death has at its disposal inordinately more powerful resources and means than does the culture of life. Yet "we know that we can rely on the help of God, for whom nothing is impossible." There is much for us to do. Fortunately, the past provides encouragement

for the future. "It is this deep love for every man and woman which has given rise down the centuries to an outstanding history of charity, a history which has brought into being in the Church and society many forms of service to life which evoke admiration from all unbiased observers. Every Christian community, with a renewed sense of responsibility, must continue to write this history through various kinds of pastoral and social activity" (John Paul II 1995a, 1995b, #87, #100).

"Under grave obligation of conscience," Christians and all people of good will must refuse to cooperate in practices that, although legally permitted, "are contrary to God's law." In the realm of social activity, there is a veritable litany of possibilities for constructive involvement especially by voters and legislators who must do all they can to reverse the legalization of criminal acts against human life. The pope mentions numerous acts that Christians can do and programs in which they can engage to promote respect for life and to help those who are most vulnerable. Finally, "There is an everyday heroism, made up of gestures of sharing, big or small, which build up an authentic culture of life. A particularly praiseworthy example of such gestures is the donation of organs, performed in an ethically acceptable manner, with a view to offering a chance of health and even of life itself to the sick who sometimes have no other hope" (John Paul II 1995a, 1995b, #74, #86).

The responsibilities of health care providers loom large. "To refuse to take part in committing an injustice is not only a moral duty; it is also a basic human right. Were this not so, the human person would be forced to perform an action intrinsically incompatible with human dignity." This essential right "should be acknowledged and protected by civil law. In this sense, the opportunity to refuse to take part in the phases of consultation, preparation and execution of these acts against life should be guaranteed to physicians, health-care personnel, and directors of hospitals, clinics and convalescent facilities." And in the midst of this culture of death, hospitals, clinics, and convalescent homes "staffed by Religious or in any way connected with the Church" must not "merely be institutions where care is provided for the sick or the dying. Above all they should be places where suffering, pain and death are acknowledged and understood in their human and specifically Christian meaning" (John Paul II 1995a, 1995b, #73, #88).

Early in the encyclical the pope lamented that "even certain sectors of the medical profession, which by its calling is directed to the defence and care of human life, are increasingly willing to carry out these acts against the person. In this way the very nature of the medical profession is distorted and contradicted, and the dignity of those who practise it is degraded." Much later he says that, although health-care professionals are called "to be guardians and servants of human life," today, when "science and the practice of medicine risk losing sight of their inherent ethical dimensions, health-care professionals can be strongly tempted at times to become manipulators of life, or even agents of death." Hence both their temptations and responsibility today are greatly increased. Their responsibility's "deepest inspiration and strongest support lie in the intrinsic and undeniable ethical dimension of the health-care profession, something already recognized by the ancient and still relevant Hippocratic Oath, which requires every doctor to commit himself to absolute respect for human life and its sacredness." The pope then reminded them that they "must always reject experimentation, research or applications which disregard the inviolable dignity of the human being, and thus cease to be at the service of people and become instead means which, under the guise of helping people, actually harm them" (John Paul II 1995a, 1995b, #4, #89).

These are familiar themes. Although far from comprising a summary of the manifold issues of Catholic medical ethics, they were the issues most pertinent to the crisis of morality that, in the pope's opinion, most threatened the dignity, value, and inviolability of the human person as the second millennium was nearing its end. These threats were most conspicuously and perniciously implemented against the unborn and the terminally ill. Yet the design of this encyclical was so much greater than merely to condemn abortion and euthanasia, which it does do at length and with much specificity.[18] It was rather to reassert the most fundamental theology of life, without which Catholic ethics of health and healing would have no stable foundation. The foundational principles of *Evangelium Vitae* are fundamentally Christian and their mode of articulation distinctly Catholic.

F. "A Complete and Systematic Exposition of Christian Moral Teaching" at the End of the Second Millennium: The New Catechism of the Catholic Church

On the recommendation of an Extraordinary Synod of Bishops, in 1986, John Paul II appointed a commission of cardinals and bishops, chaired by Cardinal Ratzinger, Prefect of the Congregation for the Doctrine of the Faith, to prepare a catechism in extensive consultation with the entire Episcopate. This would be the first new comprehensive compendium of doctrine of faith and morals issued by the Holy See since the *Roman Catechism* of 1566. Just as the *Roman Catechism* had been composed to disseminate the decrees of the Council of Trent, so also was the proposed new catechism to do for Vatican II.

When the pope issued the Apostolic Constitution *Fidei Depositum* in 1992 promulgating the *Catechism of the Catholic Church*, he characterized it as "a statement of the Church's faith and of Catholic doctrine, attested to or illumined by Sacred Scripture, the Apostolic Tradition, and the Church's Magisterium. I declare it to be . . . a sure norm for teaching the faith." He says that the *Catechism* is given to the faithful "that it may be a sure and authentic reference text for teaching Catholic doctrine and particularly for preparing local catechisms" (John Paul II 1992, #IV). The English-language edition, published in 1994, had sold two and a half million copies by 1998. After extensive review by an Interdicasterial Commission, the pope promulgated the "Latin Typical Edition"[19] of the *Catechism* in 1997 by the Apostolic Letter *Laetamur Magnopere* in which he describes it as "a full, complete exposition of Catholic doctrine, enabling everyone to know what the Church professes, celebrates, lives, and prays in her daily life" and as a "new, authoritative exposition of the one and perennial apostolic faith" (John Paul II 1997). An English translation of this revised edition was published in 2000.

Between the publication of the *Catechism* in 1992 and the "Latin Typical Edition" in 1997, that is, while an Interdicasterial Commission was engaged in extensive review of its contents, John Paul II issued what are arguably the two most significant encyclicals of his pontificate, certainly the most important for the subject matter of this chapter, *Veritatis Splendor* in 1993 and *Evangelium Vitae* in 1995. Yet, so congruous were the contents of these two encyclicals with the teachings of the hierarchical magisterium as they had developed by the late twentieth century, that the Interdicasterial Commission did not deem it necessary to draw from either encyclical to bolster the authoritative nature of the treatment in the revised edition of the *Catechism* of the issues to which these two encyclicals are devoted. Hence neither is included in the section of the "Index of Citations" labeled "Pontifical Documents."[20]

It should be noted that the *Catechism* unequivocally proclaims papal supremacy and infallibility and the authority of the magisterium on which Christ had bestowed "the charism of infallibility in matters of faith and morals" and whose task it is "to preserve God's people from deviations and defections and to guarantee them the objective possibility of professing the true faith without error" (*Catechism* 2000, #890). In the exercise of the ordinary magisterium, the pope or the bishops in union with him may, "without arriving at an infallible definition and without pronouncing in a 'definitive manner,'" propose "a teaching that leads to better understanding of Revelation in matters of faith and morals. To this ordinary teaching the faithful 'are to adhere . . . with religious assent' [*Lumen Gentium* #25] which, though distinct from the assent of faith, is nonetheless an extension of it" (*Catechism* 2000, #892). They are to "receive with docility the teaching and directives that their pastors give them." Indeed, they "have the *duty* of observing the constitutions and decrees conveyed by the legitimate authority of the Church." Never should "personal conscience and reason . . . be set in opposition to the moral law or the Magisterium of the Church" (*Catechism* 2000, #87, #2037, #2039, emphasis in original).

In the *Catechism*, the moral law and the magisterium are closely connected. We have seen that in *Veritatis Splendor*, published a year after the promulgation of the *Catechism*, John Paul II condemned, among other "fundamental errors," the denial that any acts are "intrinsically evil" and the rejection of the traditional doctrine of natural law in its universality and permanent validity.

In regard to the first, under the rubric "The Morality of Human Acts," it is unambiguously specified that the three sources of the morality of human acts are the object, the intention, and the circumstances. In regard to the first, "The object chosen morally specifies the act of the will, insofar as reason recognizes and judges it to be or not to be in conformity with the true good. Objective norms of morality express the rational order of good and evil, attested to by consciences" (*Catechism* 2000, #1751). An evil action cannot be justified by a good intention: "A good intention . . . does not make behavior that is intrinsically disordered . . . good or just. The end does not justify the means" (*Catechism* 2000, #1753). This is clarified in the summary section by the statement, "There are concrete acts that it is always wrong to choose, because their choice entails a disorder of the will, i.e., a moral evil. One may not do evil so that good may result from it" (*Catechism* 2000, #1761). The circumstances, including the consequences, of a moral act come in a distant third to the object and the intention. Though they increase or diminish "the moral goodness or evil of human acts" and can also "diminish or increase the agent's responsibility," of themselves they "cannot change the moral quality of acts themselves; they can make neither good nor right an action that is in itself evil" (*Catechism* 2000, #1754). The implications of such declarations for proportionalism are starkly obvious.

In regard to the second, under the rubric "The Natural Moral Law," the "traditional" doctrine of natural law is unequivocally reaffirmed, supported by quotations ranging from the pagan Roman statesman and philosopher Cicero to Pius XII and Vatican II. The doctrine is thus summarized at the end of the article on the moral law: "The natural law is a participation in God's wisdom and goodness by man formed in the image of his Creator. It expresses the dignity of the human person and forms the basis of his fundamental rights and duties. The natural law is immutable, permanent throughout history. The rules that express it remain substantially valid. It is a necessary foundation for the erection of moral rules and civil law" (*Catechism* 2000, #1978–1979).

References to natural law are made crucially throughout the *Catechism*. For example, in discussing civil society, the principle is expressed that "no one can command or establish what is contrary to the dignity of persons and the natural law." Citizens are "obliged in conscience not to follow the directives of civil authorities when they are contrary to the demands of the moral order" (*Catechism* 2000, #2235, #2242). Although a "diversity of political regimes

is morally acceptable," those "whose nature is contrary to the natural law, to the public order, and to the fundamental rights of persons cannot achieve the common good of the nations on which they have been imposed." Authority is exercised legitimately only when it seeks the common good and employs morally licit means to attain it. The common good, first, presupposes respect for the person as such. Hence "public authorities are bound to respect the fundamental and inalienable rights of the human person." Second, "the common good requires the social well-being and development of the group itself," including health and the right to establish a family (*Catechism* 2000, #1901, #1903, #1907–1908). The political community "has a duty to honor the family, to assist it, and to ensure" availability of various opportunities and services, including the right to medical care and assistance for the aged, "in keeping with the country's institutions" (*Catechism* 2000, #2211; cf. #2288).

Social justice can be obtained only "in respecting the transcendent dignity of man" and "the rights that flow from his dignity as a creature. These rights are prior to society and must be recognized by it. They are the basis of the moral legitimacy of every authority." Moreover, it is the "Church's role to remind men of good will of these rights and to distinguish them from unwarranted or false claims" (*Catechism* 2000, #1929–1930). The *Catechism* supports this assertion by a quotation from section 747.2 of the *Code of Canon Law* (a thorough revision of the *Codex Iuris Canonici* of 1917, for which see n. 3), promulgated by John Paul II in 1983: "To the Church belongs the right always and everywhere to announce moral principles, including those pertaining to the social order, and to make judgments on any human affairs to the extent that they are required by the fundamental rights of the human person or the salvation of souls" (*Catechism* 2000, #2032). Basic to this right is that the "authority of the Magisterium extends . . . to the specific precepts of the natural law, because their observance, demanded by the Creator, is necessary for salvation. In recalling the prescriptions of the natural law, the Magisterium . . . exercises an essential part of its prophetic office of proclaiming to men what they truly are and reminding them of what they should be before God" (*Catechism* 2000, #2032, #2036).

Within the Church the magisterium is ordinarily exercised in teaching moral principles and precepts through catechesis and preaching. In this fashion the magisterium, with the help of theologians and spiritual authors, generation after generation, has handed on the "deposit" of Christian moral teaching, which is "composed of a characteristic body of rules, commandments, and virtues . . . Alongside the Creed and the Our Father, the basis for this catechesis has traditionally been the Decalogue which sets out the principles of moral life valid for all men" (*Catechism* 2000, #2033). The Decalogue is "valid for all men" because it contains "a privileged expression of the natural law." The

Ten Commandments are "accessible to reason alone," are "fundamentally immutable," and "oblige always and everywhere," since they "are engraved by God in the human heart" (*Catechism* 2000, #2070–2072). Hence the centrality of the Decalogue exists both for moral discourse and for catechesis. As in the old manuals of moral theology, so also in the *Catechism*, most issues of medical ethics arise in the exegesis of the fifth and sixth commandments.

The explication of the fifth commandment ("You shall not kill.") begins with a quotation from a document composed by the Congregation for the Doctrine of the Faith, *Donum Vitae* ("Instructions on Respect for Human Life"), which John Paul II had approved and ordered published in 1987: "Human life is sacred because from its beginning it involves the creative action of God and it remains for ever in a special relationship with the Creator, who is its sole end. God alone is the Lord of life from its beginning until its end: no one can under any circumstance claim for himself the right directly to destroy an innocent human being" (*Catechism* 2000, #2258). The deliberate murder of an innocent person is vigorously condemned and the legitimacy of insisting on respect for one's own right to life is staunchly defended. Because the fifth commandment forbids direct and intentional killing as "gravely sinful," infanticide is specifically condemned, and it is specified that "concern for eugenics or public health cannot justify any murder, even if commanded by public authority." Furthermore, the *Catechism* "forbids doing anything with the intention of indirectly bringing about a person's death." Although unintentional killing is not morally imputable, "one is not exonerated from grave offense if, without proportionate reasons, he has acted in a way that brings about someone's death, even without the intention to do so" (*Catechism* #2000, #2261, #2264, #2268–2269).

At this point (#2270–2283) abortion, euthanasia, and suicide are discussed. In the section on abortion, we read that respect for the life of the embryo demands that "as a person" it "must be defended in its integrity, cared for, and healed, as far as possible, like any other human being." This is immediately followed by a series of quotations from *Donum Vitae*. Here prenatal diagnosis is declared morally licit "if it respects the life and integrity of the embryo and the human fetus and is directed toward its safeguarding or healing as an individual . . . It is gravely opposed to the moral law when this is done with the thought of possibly inducing an abortion, depending upon the results: a diagnosis must not be the equivalent of a death sentence." The next quotation declares licit "procedures carried out on the human embryo which respect the life and integrity of the embryo and do not involve disproportionate risks for it, but are directed toward its healing, the improvement of its condition of health, or its individual survival." The subsequent quotation pronounces immoral the production of human embryos "intended for exploitation as disposable biological material." The last quotation from *Donum*

Vitae asserts that "attempts to influence chromosomic or genetic inheritance," which are "not therapeutic but are aimed at producing human beings selected according to sex or other predetermined qualities . . . are contrary to the personal dignity of the human being and his integrity and identity." To this last sentence the *Catechism* adds the concluding clause, "which are unique and unrepeatable" (*Catechism* 2000, #2274–2275).

Following directly upon this is a short section dealing with euthanasia. It opens with the insistence that "Those whose lives are diminished or weakened deserve special respect." Regardless of motives and means, direct euthanasia, which "consists in putting an end to the lives of handicapped, sick, or dying persons," is "morally unacceptable." Hence, whether by act or omission, causing "death in order to eliminate suffering constitutes a murder gravely contrary to the dignity of the human person and to the respect due to the living God, his Creator." Burdensome, dangerous, or extraordinary medical procedures, as well as those that are "disproportionate to the expected outcome," may be legitimately discontinued, since this is simply "the refusal of 'over-zealous' treatment." In such cases, one is simply accepting his inability to impede death and does not intend to cause death. If the patient is competent and able, the decision should be his, otherwise it resides with those legally entitled to act for him. Ordinary care owed to the patient, even if death is imminent, must be continued. Administering painkillers to alleviate the suffering of the dying, even if this hastens their demise, "can be morally in conformity with human dignity if death is not willed as either an end or a means, but only foreseen and tolerated as inevitable" Finally, palliative care is "a special form of disinterested charity. As such it should be encouraged." (*Catechism* 2000, #2276–2279).

Later in its explication of the fifth commandment, the *Catechism* gives a fundamental caveat that has appeared with regularity in Christian literature over the centuries: "If morality requires respect for the life of the body, it does not make it an absolute value. It rejects a neo-pagan notion that tends to promote the cult of the body, to sacrifice everything for its sake, to idolize physical perfection and success at sports. By its selective preference of the strong over the weak, such a conception can lead to the perversion of human relationships." Furthermore, the "virtue of temperance disposes us to avoid every kind of excess: the abuse of food, alcohol, tobacco, or medicine." The use of drugs, except on strictly therapeutic grounds, not only "inflicts very grave damage on human health and life" but also is a "grave offense" (*Catechism* 2000, #2289–2291).

Attention is next addressed to science and technology. Although these "are precious resources . . . for the benefit of all," nevertheless, by themselves "they cannot disclose the meaning of existence and of human progress" but must "find in the person and in his moral values both evidence of their purpose and awareness of their limits." Claiming "moral neutrality in scientific research and its applications" is an "illusion." Neither "simple technical efficiency," "the usefulness accruing to some at the expense of others," nor, "even worse, . . . prevailing ideologies" can provide guiding principles for science and technology, which "by their very nature require unconditional respect for fundamental moral criteria." Rather, "in conformity with the plan and the will of God," they must be "at the service of the human person, of his inalienable rights, of his true and integral good" (*Catechism* 2000, #2292–2294; cf. #159 on faith and science). Then appears a paragraph on research or experimentation on human subjects, which warrants quoting in its entirety:

> Research or experimentation on the human being cannot legitimate acts that are in themselves contrary to the dignity of persons and to the moral law. The subjects' potential consent does not justify such acts. Experimentation on human beings is not morally legitimate if it exposes the subject's life or physical and psychological integrity to disproportionate or avoidable risks. Experimentation on human beings does not conform to the dignity of the person if it takes place without the informed consent of the subject or those who legitimately speak for him. (*Catechism* 2000, #2295)

Organ transplants "are in conformity with the moral law if the physical and psychological dangers and risks to the donor are proportionate to the good that is sought for the recipient." Organ donation after death is declared "legitimate," a "noble and meritorious act," and "is to be encouraged." It is, however, "not morally acceptable if the donor or his proxy has not given explicit consent. Moreover, it is not morally admissible directly to bring about the disabling mutilation or death of a human being, even in order to delay the death of other persons" (*Catechism* 2000, #2296). Still dealing with the Fifth Commandment, under the heading "Respect for bodily integrity," it is specified that "Except when performed for strictly therapeutic medical reasons, directly intended amputations, mutilations, and sterilizations performed on innocent persons are against the moral law" (*Catechism* 2000, #2297).

The much-disputed requirement of the late medieval and Tridentine Church that physicians ensure that their patients summon a confessor had, by the time of Pius XII, as we have seen above (Section III.1.C), diminished to appeals to Catholic physicians to encourage their terminally-ill Catholic patients to call for a priest. Now it is relatives of the dying who "must see to it that the sick receive at the proper time the sacraments that prepare them to meet the living God" (*Catechism* 2000, #2299). This change should not be construed as a diminution of the Church's concern with the major issue here, for the *Catechism* makes clear that the moment of death is the single most crucial moment of life for one's eternal destiny.

In the discussion of the sixth commandment ("You shall not commit adultery."), the major issue of medical interest is contraception. Some points warrant mention here. "Fecundity is a gift, an end of marriage. . . . A child does not come from outside as something added on to the mutual love of the spouses." Although "research aimed at reducing human sterility is to be encouraged, on condition that it is placed 'at the service of the human person, of his inalienable rights, and his true and integral good according to the design and will of God'"(quoting *Donum Vitae*), procedures that "entail the dissociation of husband and wife, but the intrusion of a person other than the couple (donation of sperm or ovum, surrogate uterus), are gravely immoral. These techniques (heterologous artificial insemination and fertilization) infringe the child's right to be born of a father and mother known to him and bound to each other by marriage." Procedures that involve "only the married couple (homologous artificial insemination and fertilization) are perhaps less reprehensible, yet remain morally unacceptable" because they "dissociate the sexual act from the procreative act." Several sentences are then quoted from *Donum Vitae*, the last being, "Only respect for the link between the meanings of the conjugal act and respect for the unity of the human being make possible procreation in conformity with the dignity of the person" (*Catechism* 2000, #2366, #2375–2377).

Under the eighth commandment ("You shall not bear false witness against your neighbor.") the obligation is placed on those in several vocations, including medicine, to keep "professional secrets" or "confidential information given under the seal of secrecy . . . save in exceptional cases where keeping the secret is bound to cause very grave harm to the one who confided it, to the one who received it or to a third party, and where the very grave harm can be avoided only by divulging the truth" (*Catechism* 2000, #2491). In the exegesis of the eighth commandment, no mention is made of truth telling specifically in the physician–patient relationship. However, the Catholic physician could find guidance in the principle enunciated only three paragraphs earlier: "The right to the communication of the truth is not unconditional. Everyone must conform his life to the Gospel precept of fraternal love. This requires us in concrete situations to judge whether or not it is appropriate to reveal the truth to someone who asks for it" (*Catechism* 2000, #2488). The failure to address this specific moral issue as it manifests itself in the arena of medical care is not surprising because the *Catechism* is not even a code of ethics for Catholics, in general, much less a code of professional ethics for physicians in particular.

Some matters of importance to Catholic medical ethics during earlier eras may no longer appear to be relevant to medical practice. For example, as we have seen above (Sections II.1 & 2), during the early Middle Ages, the authors of the penitential manuals were deeply concerned about the ill turning to pagan, magical healing practices, and moral theologians of the late Middle Ages and the early Tridentine era included incantations among examples of sinful means for the recovery of health that physicians were forbidden to advise. At the close of the second millennium, this injunction appears in the *Catechism* in the explication of the first commandment ("You shall have no other gods before me."): "All practices of magic or sorcery, by which one attempts to tame occult powers, so as to place them at one's service and have a supernatural power over others – even if this were for the sake of restoring their health – are gravely contrary to the virtue of religion ... Recourse to so-called traditional cures does not justify either the invocation of evil powers or the exploitation of another's credulity" (*Catechism* 2000, #2117). This is hardly what one would encounter in codes of medical ethics today. Yet, these issues are of importance not only in many Third World countries where Christianity and indigenous religions exist side-by-side but even in Western cultures where "New Age" and occult beliefs and practices are thriving. The principles undergirding these warnings and the concern that the welfare of the soul not be harmed by expedient measures for the good of the body are as germane to Catholic ethics of health and healing as the positions taken by the Church on the most complex and sophisticated issues of contemporary bioethics.

IV. CONCLUSION

The manner in which the *Catechism* was conceived and developed reveals its significance. In 1985, the Synod of Bishops had expressed to John Paul II their desire that "a catechism or compendium of all Catholic doctrine regarding both faith and morals be composed." In 1986, he entrusted the task of preparing a draft to a commission of twelve cardinals and bishops headed by Cardinal Ratzinger. Over the next 5 years, the catechism went through nine subsequent drafts. Suggestions along the way were solicited from "numerous theologians, exegetes and catechists, and, above all, [from] the Bishops of the whole world, in order to produce a better text." Hence, the pope could say, "this *Catechism* is the result of the collaboration of the whole Episcopate of the Catholic Church" and "thus reflects the collegial nature of the Episcopate" (John Paul II 1992, #1–2). A year after its promulgation and publication in 1992, John Paul II declared in *Veritatis Splendor* that the *Catechism* "contains a complete and systematic exposition of Christian moral teaching" and "presents the moral life of believers in its fundamental elements" (John Paul II 1993, #5). He had already appointed a commission that for 5 years reviewed suggestions for changes that came in "from around the world and from various parts of the ecclesial community" to enable certain truths of the faith "to be formulated in a way more suited to the requirements of contemporary catechetical instruction."

Such revisions were approved by the pope and incorporated into the "official" Latin typical edition (John Paul II 1997), on which all subsequent translations, including the English translation of 2000, are based. As the twentieth century was nearing its end, the *Catechism* was available in forty-four languages (Weigel 1999, 663).

As the first catechism promulgated by the Supreme Pontiff in more than 400 years, in its pages are enunciated moral principles and precepts for all spheres of life, including issues of medical ethics as they were defined by the hierarchical magisterium at the end of the second millennium. What is included in the *Catechism* is *ipso facto* of vital importance for the Church's self-definition at this crucial time in her history. That certainly holds true for issues of medical ethics.

The *Catechism* was, for the most part, received with enthusiasm. As George Weigel observed, it "quickly established itself throughout the world as a popular instrument by which Catholics could tell their children and neighbors (and, when necessary, remind their clergy, their religious educators, and, in some instances, their bishops) just what the Catholic Church believed and taught" (Weigel 1999, 664). In the minds of some Catholics, red flags go up immediately upon reading that last clause, for who can say that the *Catechism* does, in fact, say what the Catholic Church believes and teaches? The fact may impress some Catholics that John Paul II, in his Apostolic Letter promulgating the "official" Latin version of the *Catechism*, called it "a full, complete exposition of Catholic doctrine, enabling everyone to know what the Church professes, celebrates, lives, and prays in her daily life" as well as a "new, authoritative exposition of the one and perennial apostolic faith" (John Paul II 1997). Yet, many Catholics, including theologians of diverse specialties clergy, and laity, disagree with various articulations of doctrine made in the *Catechism*, especially in its third part, "Life in Christ" (#1691–2557), which is devoted to moral teaching.

On the tenth anniversary of the publication of the *Catechism*, Cardinal Ratzinger, as Prefect of the Congregation for the Doctrine of the Faith, gave an address on the "Current Doctrinal Relevance of the *Catechism of the Catholic Church*." Early in this address he remarked that "in some segments of the Catholic intellectual world of the West" the *Catechism* "met skepticism, indeed, rejection." Such critics declared that its content was "static, dogmatic" and that it "failed to take into account the theological developments of the last century," just as at the inception of the project to produce this new *Catechism* it had been opposed by a "group of theologians and specialists in catechesis ... in their understandable intellectual desire to be able to experiment as much as possible." To them, the "certainty of faith appeared as the opposite of the freedom and openness of continuing reflection." As Ratzinger maintained, however, "the faith is not primarily the matter for intellectual experimentation, it is rather the solid foundation ... on which we can live and die." The *Catechism*, he said, had "responded to a universal expectation felt everywhere in the Church," because after Vatican II a "vision of the whole was lacking" and "it seemed to be problematical to know what was still valid and what was not." Hence overall there was, in his opinion, "great gratitude for the *Catechism*" (Ratzinger 2002).

In drafting the *Catechism*, its third part, "Life in Christ," was, according to Ratzinger, "the most difficult section." He gave two reasons for this. The first was due to "the differences that are debated about the structural principles of Christian morality." The second was because of "the difficult problems in the realm of political, social ethics, and bioethics, that are in a continuous process of evolution thanks to constant new facts, as also is the case in the realm of anthropology, while here the debate on marriage and the family, and on the ethics of sexuality, is in full swing." Then, after stating categorically that the *Catechism* "does not claim to present the only possible form of moral theology or even the best systematic form of moral theology – this was not its mandate," Ratzinger described the theological and philosophical principles that guided the drafters of this section of the *Catechism*, focusing on the role of reason in the section of his address titled "Dialogue and Covenant" and on natural law under the rubric "Christology and Natural Law" (Ratzinger 2002).

In the latter section he asserted that, in *Gaudium et Spes*, the Second Vatican Council had sought to distance moral teaching from "the purely natural-law centred mentality and emphasized Christology," although "in its individual themes," it "made ample use of rational argumentation and did not intend to be bound to a moral teaching based purely on revelation – precisely for the reason that it presented a dialogue with the non-Christian modern world about all the common essential values." According to Ratzinger, after Vatican II an "authentically Biblical moral teaching should have developed." Hence, his frustration that, "If the fundamental outlines of the Council can be designated as a return to a moral teaching interpreted in an essentially biblical, Christocentric manner, nevertheless in the post-conciliar period a radical reversal soon took place." He concluded a short description of this "radical reversal" in moral theology by calling it "a morality of calculation which took ultimately as its only criteria the probable effects of an action and in this regard, the principle of the calculation of goods was extended to the whole of moral action." This was the context in which *Veritatis Splendor* had "offered fundamental clarifications" on the specific character of "Christian moral teaching and on the right relation between faith and reason in the elaboration of ethical norms" (Ratzinger 2002).

Earlier in this chapter (Section II.2.A) we discussed a "crisis of moral theology" that had begun in the seventeenth century. Since Vatican II, or at least since the publication of *Humanae Vitae* in 1968, there has been a new "cri-

sis of moral theology." Some comparisons are warranted. In the seventeenth century, the crisis involved papal interventions in the moral reasoning of tutiorism, which in its extremes fostered moral rigorism, and probabilism, which in its extremes spawned moral laxism. Both extremes were condemned by Alexander VII, Innocent XI, and Alexander VIII. The rigorist positions that were condemned were held by Jansenists, members of a movement that encouraged moral rigor in personal conduct. The papal condemnation of various rigorist moral propositions, although not a repudiation of tutiorism per se, was part of an attack against a range of rigorist doctrines and, indeed, against the entire Jansenist movement. By contrast, the laxist positions that were condemned had been advanced by some probabilists who remained in the mainstream of Catholic moral theology. The papal condemnation of these laxist positions was a repudiation of neither the fundamental principles nor the methodology of probabilism.

In 1985, Charles Curran observed that "this was the most significant intervention up to that time by the papal office in the area of moral theology and began a trend that has continued until contemporary times" (Curran 1985, 222). This trend has, indeed, intensified in the late twentieth century. In *Veritatis Splendor*, John Paul II rejected various forms of teleology, most significantly the proportionalism that he attributed to unnamed revisionist Catholic moral theologians. He said that there is no justification for claiming that these theories are grounded in the "Catholic moral tradition," although that tradition had witnessed "the development of a casuistry which tried to assess the best ways to achieve the good in certain concrete situations." This casuistry, he maintained, had involved "only cases in which the law was uncertain, and thus the absolute validity of negative moral precepts, which oblige without exception, was not called into question." He repudiated certain modern teleologies because, in his judgment, those theories "are not faithful to the Church's teaching, when they believe they can justify, as morally good, deliberate choices of kinds of behaviour contrary to the commandments of the divine and natural law" (John Paul II 1993, #76). In *Veritatis Splendor*, he went well beyond the condemnation of specific laxist extremes of probabilism by popes in the seventeenth century, which, as already noted, was a condemnation of neither the fundamental principles nor the methodology of probabilism. Yet his rejection of proportionalism stopped far short of the condemnation of the moral reasoning of the extreme tutiorism of the Jansenists that was but a part of the censure of that entire movement.

The effects of the magisterium's interventions in moral theology in the seventeenth century rendered some moral theologians skittish, or at least more cautious, and casuistry "lost much of its analytic vigor and boldness of attack" and "began to show signs of senescence" (Jonsen and Toulmin 1988, 269). Will the recent interventions of the magisterium have similar effects on moral theologians? There is, at this stage, little evidence to suggest that they will. Where the current "crisis of moral theology" will lead no one, of course, can predict with absolute perspicacity. That there are many revisionist moral theologians who continue to engage in vigorous moral analysis employing a variety of methodologies shows that moral theology, especially as applied by Catholic moralists to issues of medical ethics and bioethics, remains dynamic. Creative Roman Catholic moral theology is not even silent, much less dead.

At the end of the second millennium, the hierarchical magisterium has left no doubt about its sense of ultimate responsibility for, and authority in, moral teaching. In *Evangelium Vitae*, John Paul II emphasized how essential he felt it was to ensure that "in theological faculties, seminaries and Catholic institutions sound doctrine is taught, explained and more fully investigated." Hence he urged that all theologians, pastors, teachers, and all those responsible for catechesis and the formation of consciences be "aware of their specific role" and that they "never be so grievously irresponsible as to betray the truth and their own mission by proposing personal ideas contrary to the Gospel of life as faithfully presented and interpreted by the Magisterium" (John Paul II 1995a, 1995b #82). Consequently, "*Roma locuta, causa finita*" still prevails, although on various issues of medical ethics dissent thrives. This occurs tacitly in the practices of many Roman Catholics, ranging from the conceptual separation of faith from morals, which is strongly condemned by the magisterium, to the disregard or rejection of the magisterium's teaching on a variety of moral issues, also strongly condemned by the magisterium. Dissent is most conspicuous in the discourses of some Catholic theologians and intellectuals who continue to argue that the pertinaciously tacit refusal of the magisterium to exercise its charism of infallibility in the doctrine of morals leaves many moral issues, the preponderance of which are in the realm of medical ethics and bioethics, open to disagreement, discussion, and debate. Such discussion and debate are not confined to those who dissent from "authentic" (i.e., "authoritative") noninfallible teachings of the magisterium, but often exists between them and those Catholics who vigorously support both the intrinsic validity and the extrinsic authority of such magisterial pronouncements.

Writing in 1984, Richard McCormick observed, "At present there is a deep conflict of attitudes in the Church about authority, particularly teaching authority. Not only does this divide Catholics, but it turns nearly every serious moral problem into an authority problem" (McCormick 1984, 61). This most certainly has not lessened since he made that observation. The lines are rather clearly drawn, especially between some revisionist moral theologians, who probably appear to the magisterium to be

dangerously laxist, and the magisterium, which these same moral theologians regard as dogmatically rigorist. In his generally favorable reaction to John Paul II's 1995 encyclical *Evangelium Vitae*, McCormick said that framing the concerns about the range of moral issues addressed in that encyclical "in terms of a face-off between a culture of death and a culture of life can nourish the impression that all the matters touched on in the encyclical are either-or, back and white. This, of course, is not so. Complexity, doubt, ambiguity and uncertainty still surround some of the issues raised by [*Evangelium Vitae*]. We must have the honesty and courage to say this and to insist that [*Evangelium Vitae*] has not coopted theology's agenda and eliminated its critical function" (McCormick 1995).

Undoubtedly many within the Church support the commitment of revisionist moral theologians who, at risk to their standing within the Church and to their academic appointments in Catholic institutions, continue courageously to wrestle as Catholic moralists with issues of moral perplexity. Others revere an authoritative ecclesiastical hierarchy that will continue to make moral pronouncements that are either/or, black and white. For among the approximately one billion Roman Catholics worldwide, there are many who today echo the longing of Pascal's conscience: "I am not satisfied with probability. I want certainty."

NOTES

1. For all popes referred to in the text, the dates given are their year of birth (b.) and their regnal years as pope (r.). The dates of their death and of the end of their papacy are the same.

2. For references to Aquinas' various discussions of this topic, see Congar 1982b, 303 and Sullivan 1983, 24–25.

3. For example, sometimes this magisterial function is performed by the Congregation for the Doctrine of the Faith (originally the Sacred Congregation of the Universal Inquisition until 1908 when its appellation was changed to the Sacred Congregation of the Holy Office, the title that it retained until given its current name in 1965), one of the bureaus of the Roman Curia charged with protecting all matters of doctrine pertaining to faith and morals. Furthermore, national councils of bishops of various countries, especially since Vatican II (1965), issue documents that carry considerable weight as products of the hierarchical, although not papal, magisterium.

4. The *Corpus Iuris Canonici*, as supplemented by a plethora of new laws, remained the official collection of canon law until it was superceded by the *Codex Iuris Canonici (Code of Canon Law)* in 1917.

5. The reference is to the statement made by John the Baptist when he first saw Jesus and exclaimed, "Behold, the Lamb of God, who takes way the sin of the world!" (John 1:29).

6. A notable and late representative of this branch of the genre of pastoral medicine is Albert Niedermeyer. The Vienna School of *Pastoralmedizin* is very important historically, continuing well into the twentieth century. Even today there is one professor of Pastoral Medicine in Austria.

7. It should be noted that modernism is not to be equated with modernity in all its aspects, but rather with those features of modernity inimical to traditional orthodox Christianity, for example, theological liberalism, rationalism, naturalism, and materialism.

8. In regard to the conundrum of truth telling in medical practice, Pius XII maintained that although a physician must never give an answer that is positively untrue, sometimes he "cannot crudely tell the whole truth, especially when he knows that the patient has not the strength to stand such a revelation." He "has most certainly the duty of speaking out clearly, a duty before which every other medical or humanitarian consideration must give way. It is not lawful to lull the sick person or his relations into a false sense of security when there is the risk of compromising the eternal salvation of the former, or his fulfillment of his duties in justice and charity." Such conduct cannot be justified on the grounds that "the physician always says what, in his opinion, will best contribute to the patient's well-being, and that it is the fault of his hearers if they take his words too literally" (*Papal Teachings* 1960, 62–63).

9. This allocution is also available at www.papalencyclicals.net under the title "The Moral Limits of Medical Research and Treatment."

10. For a thorough analysis of the contributions of these moral theologians to the development of Roman Catholic medical ethics, see D. Kelly, especially 110–17, 149–53, 161–68, 170–80, 200–4, 216–19, 279–91, 321–24, 345–71, 382–86.

11. Chapter 4 of D. Kelly's book, titled "Early Works (1897–1940): The Development of Physicalism," is a full and astute historical and methodological analysis of physicalism (Kelly D. 1979, 244–310).

12. Chapter 5 of D. Kelly's book, titled "Later Works (1940–1960): The Shift towards Ecclesiastical Positivism," is a full and astute historical and methodological analysis of ecclesiastical positivism (Kelly D. 1979, 311–98).

13. Issued in 1930, *Casti Connubii* (literally "Of Chaste Marriage," but known in English by the title "On Christian Marriage") condemned as a "base stain" on marriage and as a perversion of the natural order any means of contraception other than abstinence or "periodic continence." It also condemned divorce, eugenics, and the destruction or mutilation of any part of one's body "except when no other provision can be made for the good of the whole body."

14. Not only was the idea of such a commission unusual, perhaps unprecedented, but also even more remarkable was the inclusion of laypersons, both men and women. The history of the activities of this commission is fascinating (see Kaiser 1985).

15. Both quotations from the Gospels were statements made by Jesus to Peter. The first was when Peter protested against Jesus' revelation to his disciples that he must go to Jerusalem, suffer and die, and rise from the dead on the third day. The second occurred in the context of Peter's confident declaration that he would never deny his Lord, and Jesus' assertion that before the rooster crowed Peter would in fact three times deny that he even knew him.

16. Some examples of such moralists that David Kelly cites are Knauer (1967), Van der Poel (1968), and Curran (1975, 173–209, 1977).

17. Curran reports that, when summoned to the Vatican in 1986, he "asked Cardinal Ratzinger, 'Is theological dissent from noninfallible church teaching ever permitted, and, if so, under what conditions is it permitted?' He refused to answer" (Curran 2005, 18). For Curran's full account of the whole affair, see Curran (1986).

18. There is nothing taught on those and related issues in *Evangelium Vitae* that is not concisely, although much more briefly, articulated in the new *Catechism of the Catholic Church*, discussed in Section III.2.F, later.

19. That is, the "official" Latin edition from which all subsequent translations were to be made.

20. In spite of not being included in the "Index of Citations," *Evangelium Vitae* is, in fact, quoted on at least one occasion in the revised *Catechism*: In the treatment of the Fifth Commandment, during a consideration of capital punishment, the *Catechism* states that "the cases in which the execution of the offender is an absolute necessity 'are very rare, if not practically non-existent'" (*Catechism* 2000, #2267, quoting *Evangelium Vitae* #58).

Furthermore, it should be noted that John Paul stated in *Veritatis Splendor* that he had postponed issuing that encyclical, "so long awaited," in part because it "seemed fitting for it to be preceded by the *Catechism of the Catholic Church*, which contains a complete and systematic exposition of Christian moral teaching. The *Catechism* presents the moral life of believers in its fundamental elements" (John Paul II 1993, #5). *Veritatis Splendor* explains in detail, after the fact, as it were, the very principles of moral reasoning employed in the *Catechism* and, in turn, cites the *Catechism* as authoritative.

Chapter 15

The Discourses of Protestant Medical Ethics

Gary B. Ferngren

I. Introduction: The Protestant Outlook on Health and Medicine

In general, Protestants, like most Christians, have regarded the body as a relative, not an absolute, good. Health is not a virtue (as it was for the Greeks), but a blessing bestowed by God. Both Martin Luther (1483–1546) and John Calvin (1509–1564) echoed a widely held Christian view in arguing that, like every other human condition, good health can be used either for God's glory or for selfish purposes. They also introduced what were to become distinctively Protestant convictions. On the one hand, the Reformers explicitly rejected monastic practices that sought to mortify the body to strengthen the will. The ascetic ideal has for the most part been foreign to Protestant thinking. On the other hand, Protestantism has often encouraged abstinence and moderation in the care of the body. This encouragement has varied from tradition to tradition, receiving its greatest emphasis in Calvinism and pietism. Calvin advised Christians to avoid a preoccupation with health that might encourage too strong an attachment to this world. At the same time Protestants urged care for the body because it was both God's workmanship and the temple of the Holy Spirit. Hence the early Methodists, under the influence of Francis Asbury (1745–1816), discouraged (as did the Quakers) the use of addictive substances, such as tobacco and alcohol, as incompatible with biblical standards of both health and holiness.

Basic to Protestant understandings of health-related matters has been the belief, which Protestants have shared with most orthodox Christians, that sickness and suffering are a permanent element of the human condition (Kocher 1950, 6–7). Christians lived in a fallen world that was corrupted by the effects of original sin, of which disease and bodily suffering were a part. No Protestant Reformer or orthodox theologian within the Protestant tradition could anticipate a future in this life in which disease would be fully eliminated. In the present world sin has always existed and with it the curse of physical suffering. Only in the final resurrection would the body be redeemed and death, the final enemy, conquered. In the meantime, medicine offered some relief in alleviating suffering, as well as progress in overcoming it.

If disease and pain were evils, however, Protestants believed that they were used by God incidentally to produce beneficial spiritual effects: to purify from sin, to soften hearts, to sensitize to spiritual concerns, and to create sympathy for others who experienced suffering. Calvinists in particular took a providential view of life that found a place in God's plan for illness and affliction. Believing firmly in God's sovereignty over human affairs, they looked for the hand of God in the everyday occurrences of their lives. The potential benefits of affliction led those striving to be godly to develop a keen eye for suffering. They were ever watchful for afflictions in themselves and others. Thus Cotton Mather's (1663–1728) *Magnalia Christi Americana* (1702) devoted a major section to biographies of New England's founders, many of which detail suffering as contributing to their Christian character. In spite of almost universal popular opinion to the contrary, Protestant theologians have not considered most disease and physical suffering to be God's retributive punishment for personal sin. Because Christ had already borne the punishment for sin by his death on the cross, disease was a sign not of God's displeasure toward the sufferer, but of a chastisement that was intended to encourage greater spirituality and dependence on him. The ethical problem here was that even if one's purpose was honorable in seeking out the benefits of affliction, it was possible to be consumed by the affairs of the body to the neglect of spiritual concerns. It was a problem greater than one's merely becoming preoccupied with health. Some Protestant diarists in England and early America display concern that the very severity of their condition might lead sufferers to focus on the immediacy of their pain and lose sight of God in their suffering. Religious melancholy presented a variation of the dilemma. How can one distinguish between the darkness that is born of a necessary humility (perhaps that which precedes an awakened spirit) and the depression that grows through obsessive regard for corporeal feeling? This was a concern of Cotton Mather's in both his *The Angel of Bethesda* (1972) (the first medical book written in America, although not published until the twentieth century) and his personal diary. The devout might search for God in the sufferings of the mind or body but lose him there as well.

Protestantism has been characterized by a somewhat different emphasis in its approach to the Christian life than has traditional Catholicism (Harbison 1964, 152–56). In place of the monastic ideal of an ascetic or reclusive life, it has encouraged Christians to combine attention to personal holiness with active service in the world. Central to the Reformer's view of the spiritual life was the idea of vocation. Catholic theology had divided the world into spiritual and temporal estates, in which those who desired to serve God fully sought a vocation as priest, or within the contemplative life as a monk or nun, while secular professions (the active life) were regarded as distinctly second best. Luther and Calvin abolished for Protestants the medieval distinction between sacred and secular callings, seeing both as possibilities for all Christians. All professions had the potential to be spiritually fulfilling. A physician who sought to glorify God through medicine could play as important a role in society as a priest. Hence, Protestantism encouraged the participation of Christians in every aspect of society with the confidence that they could provide a redemptive force in a sinful world. Their confidence was rooted not in aspirations of transforming the world by human effort, but in a firm belief that ordinary human activity, no matter how humble, could serve as an outworking of redeeming grace. That belief gave to Protestants a distinct preference for the active life over the contemplative life.

II. THE NATURE OF MORAL OBLIGATION IN PROTESTANTISM

Protestantism differed from both the Roman Catholic and Orthodox churches in regarding Scripture as the supreme rule of faith and life. The Protestant Reformers taught that the church's authority rested on Scripture alone (*sola scriptura*) rather than on the tradition of the church. Scripture was given primacy over all human and ecclesiastical traditions and indeed over the church itself, a view that was summarized in the Reformation statement *ecclesia reformata, ergo semper reformanda* ("The church reformed, therefore always in need of reform"). Scripture was the medium through which special revelation had occurred and it constituted the very word of God. Differences of emphasis existed between the various branches of the Reformation, but all agreed that the Roman Catholic Church had over time erected a vast theological and hierarchical superstructure that had obscured the primitive teachings of the early apostles as embodied in the New Testament. Scripture was the touchstone by which all matters of theology, morals, and ecclesiastical practice should be judged. But Protestantism has never been a monolithic tradition. There was in Protestantism no definitive formulation of dogma similar to the *magisterium* (teaching authority) of the Roman Catholic Church. The very existence of several historical strains (Lutheran, Reformed, Anglican, and Anabaptist) guaranteed diversity within the movement. Even within each of the respective traditions there existed a degree of individual opinion that made it difficult to arrive at an authoritative position on many controverted issues of moral theology (Gustafson 1978, 3–6).

Protestantism has tended to reject the formulation of a detailed system of ethics and to roll ethics back into systematic theology. Protestant medical ethics arose more directly from religious considerations of health and disease, as well as from biblical themes such as providence, justification, law and grace, covenant, and the place of suffering in the Christian experience. Hence, Protestantism never produced a tradition of casuistry similar to that of the Roman Catholic Church. There existed among early Anglicans and Puritans, however, manuals on "cases of conscience," of which Richard Baxter's (1615–1691) is a representative example (Gustafson 1978, 3). In addressing the duties of physicians (part IV, chap. V), Baxter, a Puritan minister who also practiced medicine, urges physicians to make "the honouring and pleasing God, and the public good, and the saving of men's lives" their intention rather than their own honor or profit. He advises them to help the poor, to seek the counsel of abler physicians in difficult cases, to rely on God for direction and success, to avoid atheism (a danger to which physicians were widely believed to be prone), and to use opportunities to speak to their patients (especially to dying patients) of their souls.

The development of a tradition of Protestant casuistry was hindered by elements inherent in the nature of Protestantism. Beginning with Luther many Protestants retained a strong antipathy toward anything that resembled the constraints of legalism, while they largely ignored the rich tradition of natural law that had played such an important role in Catholic moral theology (Verhey 1995, 4:2117–18, 2123–24). Their rejection of private confession and penance further weakened the development of casuistic ethics. Perhaps their negative reaction to the highly developed tradition of casuistry within Catholicism was enough to weaken the attempt to create one among Protestants. Instead Protestants stressed commandment and conscience (or norm and context) as the twin pillars on which ethics should be based: the application of general biblical principles (e.g., those of the Decalogue) to particular situations (Gustafson 1978, 132; Harbison 1964, 145). The individual alone before God was a basic Protestant theme. The cultivation of the private conscience, which sought to apply the text of Scripture to concrete ethical situations, became its characteristic emphasis. This approach was ideally suited to the Baconian tradition of English (and later American) Protestantism. Francis Bacon (1561–1626) believed that induction was the most fruitful method of acquiring scientific knowledge. Eschewing the deductive method and all-embracing explanatory systems, he urged the patient building of knowledge on secure empirical foundations. Scottish Common Sense philosophy, which was rooted in Baconianism, found ready acceptance among Anglo-Saxon Protestants, who applied the inductive method both to the interpretation of Scripture and to the construction of theological and ethical systems on the basis of biblical texts, while avoiding excessive speculation.

Distinctive too of Protestant approaches to moral questions was the importance of lay men and women. In the Roman Catholic and Orthodox communions, the clergy have always played the central role in defining doctrine and morals. By contrast the tradition of the priesthood of the believer (coupled with the Protestant understanding of vocation) implicitly elevated the laity and gave it a role to play in theological and ethical discourse that was largely denied to it in the Catholic tradition. Hence, Protestantism has produced a long line of distinguished lay theologians who have addressed ethical issues in science and medicine. In medicine Protestant physicians and philosophers as well as theologians – laymen as well as clergy – have influenced the formulation of medical ethics. Without a magisterium or any central ecclesiastical structure, however, consensus has been lacking on many issues and authority has been diffuse.

III. Medicine

The spirit of early Protestantism had a formative influence on the scientific revolution, particularly in England. A distrust of human tradition and ecclesiastical authority in theological matters was carried over into the sciences, where experiment and the search for natural causes seemed to be a logical extension of the theological ideas of the Reformation. The Protestant Reformers had a deep respect for medicine as they did for the sciences in general. Luther and Calvin accepted medicine (the correlative of a naturalistic understanding of disease) as a beneficial gift of God for the healing of disease and an expression of common grace (Numbers and Amundsen [1986] 1998, 176–83; 208–09). Luther believed that a "higher medicine, namely, faith and prayer," sometimes transcended ordinary medicine, but one looks in vain in Luther or the other Reformers for evidence of tension between faith and medicine. Protestant ideas of altruism and the spiritual utility of the secular professions, together with the value Protestants placed on a learned ministry, combined to give the physician a respected status. It is no coincidence that Edinburgh, situated in strongly Presbyterian Scotland, produced what by the eighteenth century had become one of the finest medical faculties in Europe.

Although pre–nineteenth-century medical literature contains little discussion of what we should term medical ethics, it alludes to the ideals of the profession of medicine in a manner that is tinged with religious and moral values (Jonsen 2000, 57–62). The physician was expected to be an educated gentleman and to observe the precepts of Christian behavior. Character was essential in allowing him to fulfill the professional responsibilities that accompanied a high calling. A physician enjoyed opportunities to give counsel in spiritual matters and to admonish patients of the need for repentance or moral improvement. The analogy between healing bodies and healing souls was one that went back to the Greeks. Society expected Christian doctors to do both. Medicine was a humane art that was especially open to opportunities for beneficence on the part of those who viewed it as a calling in the service of God. Although this ideal was by no means limited to Protestants, the personal response of the physician was of primary importance, given the Protestant aversion to casuistry in moral theology and the lack of an infallible church to give guidance. For generations of Protestant physicians a sense of Christian duty took the place of an external code of ethics (Jonsen 2000, 64–67).

From the sixteenth through the eighteenth centuries, many Protestant clergymen practiced medicine on the side (Watson 1991). Clergymen/physicians flourished especially in rural parishes and small towns, where trained physicians were rare and clergymen had the leisure and learning to read medical books. In colonial New England, ministers who were engaged in medical practice were so common that Cotton Mather of Boston (himself a minister who practiced medicine) referred to the blend of the care of soul and body as the "angelical conjunction." Mather was the center of controversy when, during an epidemic of smallpox in 1721, he supported the physician Zabdiel Boylston in inoculating for the disease. Conservative physicians (joined by the local press) opposed the controversial practice as medically unsafe and a blatant disregard of divine providence. Several members of the clergy supported Mather, who argued that similar objections could be applied to any medical intervention (Numbers and Amundsen [1986] 1998, 212–13). More than a century later, purely religious criticism of the use of chloroform as an anesthetic by James Young Simpson (1811–1870), who introduced it in Edinburgh in 1847, was virtually nonexistent. Many clergymen supported it, with the chief opposition coming from physicians, who adduced medical, ethical, and safety objections (Duffy 1964; Russell 1998).

There are few examples in early Protestantism of disputed questions that anticipate modern medical-ethical concerns and they fall properly under the rubric of moral theology. One was the matter of suicide (Ferngren 1989). Augustine's (354–430) view (1.17–27) that suicide was a violation of the sixth commandment and a sin that precluded repentance was almost universally accepted by Roman Catholic moral theologians in early modern Europe. Although most Protestants took over the Augustinian formulation, some contended that suicides suffering from melancholy or insanity might ultimately experience God's forgiveness. John Sym (1581? –1637) (1637) and John Donne (1572–1631) (written in 1607 or 1608 for private circulation) argued for the latter position (Ferngren 1989, 164; 168–71). Donne asserted that suicide was not the "irremissible" sin that Christian teaching made it out to be and his work provoked much debate. His position was challenged by several authors, but others (chiefly Anglicans and Puritans) maintained that God might indeed forgive suicide in exceptional cases and that one could not judge the state of the heart. The question was never resolved among Protestants of that era but the debate that followed it assumed what was to become a familiar pattern. Certain questions did not permit easy solution because the biblical evidence was not clear. In such cases, Protestants either drew inferences from biblical principles or from passing references in Scripture; however, Protestants were willing to remain silent where Scripture did. This meant that they were more inclined than Catholics to admit exceptions and to entrust doubtful cases to the judgment and mercy of God. That approach, the almost inevitable outcome of the Protestant method of dealing with controverted issues in moral theology, was to remain a common one in issues of medical ethics to the

end of the twentieth century, as suggested, for example, by the divergent attitudes to suicide taken by ethicists Dietrich Bonhoeffer (1906–1945) and Stanley Hauerwas (1986).

IV. NINETEENTH-CENTURY DEVELOPMENTS

The nineteenth century saw a number of new movements within Protestantism, several of which reflected the impact of the evangelical revivals of the late eighteenth century. Largely through Methodist influence, faith healing[1] came to prominence in mid-century American Protestantism. Traditional Protestants held that miracles had ceased with the close of the apostolic age at the end of the first century. They acknowledged that God sometimes healed in answer to prayer and apart from medical means; however, they considered supernatural healing to be an occasional and special manifestation of God's providence and they distinguished it from faith healing. In the mid-nineteenth century several leading evangelicals in America (e.g., A. B. Simpson [1844–1919] and A. J. Gordon [1836–1895]) maintained that God continued to heal miraculously in every generation. This novel view was vigorously attacked by traditional Protestants of all denominations, most prominently by the redoubtable Princeton theologian B. B. Warfield (1851–1921), who asserted that the Bible does not teach that the sick can expect God to heal miraculously. Hope for healing in answer to prayer was not the same as the expectation that God would heal apart from medicine by the exercise of faith alone (Numbers and Amundsen [1986] 1998, 491–95).

Health and healing were topics of widespread interest in American Protestantism in the nineteenth century. Sanitary reform, for example, was endorsed by religiously motivated sanitarians, who saw the relationship between filth and disease as a moral issue (Rosenberg and Rosenberg 1968). Traditional Protestantism, with its requirement of an educated clergy and its high regard for medicine, tended to support medical orthodoxy, whereas several innovative (and only marginally Protestant) American sects that had their roots in apocalyptic movements aligned themselves with sectarian medicine. Seventh-day Adventism, founded by Ellen G. White (1827–1915), incorporated health reform into its belief system, which included vegetarianism, hydropathy, and abstinence from tobacco and alcohol (Numbers and Amundsen [1986] 1998, 447–67). Jehovah's Witnesses, initially founded as the Zion Watch Tower Bible and Tract Society, did not focus on health-related issues, as did the Adventists, but the editor of their denominational magazine, Clayton J. Woodworth, often attacked the medical profession, as well as aspirin and vaccination. Witnesses later attracted attention for their refusal to accept blood transfusions, which the Society officially condemned in 1945 as incompatible with the teaching of biblical passages such as

Gen. 9:4, Lev. 17:13–14, and Acts 15:29 (Numbers and Amundsen [1986] 1998, 468–85). Christian Scientists rejected medical healing altogether in favor of spiritual healing, holding to a belief that disease and death were merely illusions (Numbers and Amundsen [1986] 1998, 421–46).

Another feature of nineteenth-century Protestantism that was to have long-term significance for medical ethics was the influence of two radical developments that struck at the very roots of supernatural religion, namely, biblical criticism and Darwinism. Both operated on naturalistic assumptions that were mutually supportive. Some Protestants (particularly evangelicals and fundamentalists) rejected them as incompatible with supernatural Christianity. Others (many mainstream Protestants and theological liberals) incorporated them into their thinking and attempted to redefine Christianity by retaining only those elements that could be accommodated to the new "scientific" thinking. For theological liberals religious experience rather than special revelation became the basis for defining faith and ethics. They regarded biblical morality as culturally conditioned and no longer necessarily normative for modern man. From the late nineteenth century, Protestantism would be characterized by a moral pluralism, with a range of Protestant positions that reflected divergent ethical perspectives, some only tangentially related to biblical norms.

The latter decades of the nineteenth century and the early decades of the twentieth saw the secularization of society in every sphere. The growing professionalization of medicine resulted in the exclusion from the medical profession of those without formal medical training, including many clergymen, who had previously been influential. With the dominance of positivistic science medicine became more a science and less an art. As medical faculties demanded of their students a rigorous training in science and devoted their attention increasingly to research, medicine became a secular profession that insisted on autonomy and gradually distanced itself from Christian ideas of compassion and calling. The new model for understanding nature was assumed to be a naturalistic evolutionary one. While medical ethics continued to be largely professional ethics, the traditional Christian framework in Protestant (especially Anglo-Saxon) countries diminished in influence with every succeeding generation.

V. The Twentieth Century

Within mainstream Protestantism theological liberalism entered the twentieth century as a growing and increasingly dominant force. No longer primarily seeking the eternal salvation of human souls, it sought to build the kingdom of God on earth through social and political structures. Major Protestant denominations began to promote a progressive social agenda and to issue official statements on leading questions of the day. One of the most notable was the eugenics movement, which sought to improve the human race by eliminating mental illness, retardation, and criminal behavior through such means as compulsory sterilization and restrictions on marriage (Larson 1995). In the early decades of the century, the movement attracted broad support in Europe and North America from well-known Protestant liberals, and progressive ministers lobbied for legislation to require eugenic sterilization. Roman Catholics and conservative Protestants actively opposed the movement, however, and it declined after World War II in part due to the revelation of Nazi eugenic practices.

In Britain and America, the influence of Methodism on the evangelical revivals of the eighteenth and nineteenth centuries led to the growth of a temperance movement that culminated in 1919 in the passage of the Eighteenth Amendment to the United States Constitution, which prohibited the "manufacture, sale or transportation" of alcoholic beverages. Prohibition was justified on the grounds that excessive or unrestrained consumption of alcohol produced personal and social evils such as domestic violence and crimes against women, public drunkenness, and numerous health-related problems. Although the temperance movement declined dramatically after repeal of the Eighteenth Amendment in 1933, large sections of evangelical Protestantism continued to encourage total abstinence from alcohol, smoking, and addictive drugs. The issues, however, were usually those of personal holiness and the deleterious spiritual effects of drugs rather than simply the promotion of good health.

Whereas Roman Catholics could claim a long tradition of dealing with medical ethics, the first major attempt to treat the subject systematically by a Protestant was Joseph Fletcher's (1905–1991) (1954), based on his Lowell Lectures delivered at Harvard in 1949. Fletcher, a theologically liberal Episcopalian, broke new ground in basing medical ethics (including issues such as the use of contraceptives, artificial insemination, sterilization, and euthanasia) on the patient's right to decide what should be done rather than on specific biblical or Christian principles. The way in which technology allowed for expanding choice in these areas had initially drawn Fletcher's interest. Fletcher was later to attract attention for his formulation of "situation ethics." Rejecting absolutist ethics, he maintained that nothing was wrong in itself and that the agent's intention should be based only on love. Very different from Fletcher's approach was Methodist Paul Ramsey's (1913–1988) (1970). It too was focused on the concept of patients' rights, but Ramsey's more conservative theological stance placed both physicians and patients within a context of covenant fidelity (Verhey and Lammers 1993, 7–29). Fletcher and Ramsey affirmed that the patient was a free and autonomous moral agent, an assumption that was to become basic to the discussion of medical ethics by Protestant – as indeed by nearly all – medical ethicists in the last third of the twentieth century. Both were concerned with the role of God's self-giving love, Fletcher arguing that it is enacted through the will without moral rules and Ramsey that it is "inprincipled," or enshrined in rules that are based on divine revelation and require obedience.

Concern for patients' rights reflected the spirit of the age, which sought greater individual freedom in every sphere of life, and fit nicely into the culture of American individualism. It stressed personal freedom and choice, but differed from the Enlightenment concept of human autonomy in being constrained by the rule of love and one's accountability to God. Paternalistic attitudes of physician to patient came to be regarded not merely as anachronistic but as an affront to the patient's freedom to be informed, to choose which procedure was best, and to control one's destiny. Justifying the proliferation of patients' rights required a good deal of legerdemain on the part of Protestants, because the biblical tradition emphasized the sovereignty of God, absolute norms within a moral framework (such as that of the Decalogue), limitations on human freedom (in such matters as ending one's life), and the sanctifying value of suffering.[2] Hence, ethicists such as William F. May preferred to speak from a perspective of covenantal responsibilities rather than from one of patients' rights (Verhey and Lammers 1993, 106–26; May 1983). Issues in medical ethics increasingly split Protestants along the fault line of the liberal–conservative divide, with liberals like Fletcher arguing from a utilitarian or personalist perspective that veered toward relativism, and conservatives like Ramsey and May arguing from a more traditionally biblical and deontological view based on covenant partnership.

The differing Protestant approaches were especially apparent in divisive issues such as abortion and euthanasia. Attitudes about both reflected distinctively Protestant perspectives on questions of moral theology (Lammers and Verhey 1998, 600–11). Although neither was specifically condemned in Scripture, both seemed contrary to several scriptural passages (e.g., Jer. 1:5; Ps. 139:15–16; Lk. 1:41 on abortion) and had been almost universally condemned by Christian theologians since the second century. Conservative Protestants believed that abortion was incompatible with the doctrine of the "image of God,"[3,4] according to which God had created the human race in his likeness (Ferngren 1987). Yet, as in the matter of suicide, so in abortion, the issue was not so clearly defined as it was in Catholic moral theology. Some Protestants argued that extenuating circumstances (such as danger to the life of the mother) might justify abortion on the ground that an actual life is of greater value than a potential one. Others believed that additional, if exceptional, instances (for example, rape) might justify abortion. Hence there existed within the Protestant tradition historically some willingness to recognize exceptions to the general prohibition of

abortion (Numbers and Amundsen [1986] 1998, 504–5). Nevertheless, Protestantism was characterized by a strong pronatal position. With the sexual revolution of the 1960s and the rapid growth of secular attitudes, the demand grew in Western countries for more liberal abortion laws. The controversy became sharper in the United States following the U.S. Supreme Court's legalization of abortion in its decision in *Roe v. Wade* (1973).

In the 1980s, the issue of euthanasia came to the forefront initially over the ability of physicians to extend life artificially through support systems. In the 1990s, the debate was broadened to include the legalization of physician-assisted suicide (Larson and Amundsen 1998). Liberal Protestants argued for the freedom of the autonomous individual to end his or her life. The "right to die" was, they asserted, a personal decision like any other and should not be restricted by law or professional constraints. Evangelicals were opposed to active, but not necessarily to passive, euthanasia. Most recognized that the development of life-support systems had permanently altered the process of dying and that there were instances in which nothing useful was gained by extending the life of a merely vegetative patient. Evangelicals' firm belief in an afterlife provided support for their position (Numbers and Amundsen [1986] 1998, 505–7).

Active euthanasia and physician-assisted suicide seemed different. Evangelicals and other conservative Protestants argued that God is sovereign, the author of life and death, and that physicians usurp God's prerogative when they assist a patient in ending his or her own life (Lammers and Verhey 1998, 655–62, 671–78). By the end of the twentieth century the liberalization of laws in the Netherlands and the United States (in Oregon) suggested that the right to an assisted death would become yet another freedom guaranteed by law to patients. In a society that sought to maximize individual rights, it seemed to be merely the logical extension of already existing rights. Attempts to remove legal and social impediments to physician-assisted suicide drew a good deal of opposition from conservative Protestants of many denominations (as well as many non-Protestant Christians), a fact that testified to the continuing strength of traditional Christian opposition to suicide and euthanasia.

If abortion and euthanasia provided the most highly visible focal points of tensions among Protestants regarding medical-ethical concerns, it was human sexuality that proved to be the most divisive. The traditional Protestant pattern for sexual behavior included well-defined hierarchical gender roles within marriage and abhorrence of those practices that were regarded as directly contrary to God's intended sexual standards (e.g., fornication, adultery, homosexuality, and lesbianism). In the Protestant pattern of companionate marriage, matrimony was a school for character that provided a safe and natural outlet for sex, encouraged the conception of children within a nurturing relationship, and promoted mutual support. Well into the twentieth century, most Protestants considered artificial contraception to be immoral, an attitude that doubtless owed something to Victorian attitudes toward sex as well as to the secular and humanist origins of the family-planning movement. The immorality of artificial contraception was defended partly by appeal to Scripture (Gen. 38:8–10 was often cited) and partly by the argument that it was inconsistent with a belief in divine providence (a view that had earlier been urged against inoculation) and encouraged promiscuity. The Church of England became, in 1930, the first Protestant communion officially to accept the morality of birth control, and other Protestant bodies and theologians quickly followed suit. Acceptance, which was widespread by mid-century, was made easier for Protestants than for Roman Catholics by the conviction that intercourse exists for conjugal pleasure as well as for procreation. (Roman Catholic teaching by contrast stressed an intrinsic connection between the unitive and procreative purposes of sexual expression in marriage.) In the last third of the century, owing to a neo-Malthusian concern for overpopulation and its effects on the standard of living throughout the world, theological liberals came to argue that couples and nations had a responsibility to limit their populations to preserve scarce resources. Conservatives, on the other hand, emphasized the personal moral issues inherent in the use of contraceptives.

During the same period new technologies raised a number of ethical issues (e.g., medical experimentation on human subjects, artificial insemination, in vitro fertilization, organ transplantation, cloning, stem cell research), forcing ethicists of all points of view to define their positions. The response among Protestants has, not surprisingly, lacked a general consensus (Campbell C. 2000). On the one hand, with their longstanding adherence to the Baconian belief that scientific knowledge leads to human progress, Protestants have been inclined to welcome the application of technology to medicine. On the other hand, Protestants are a diverse people, divided into many denominational (and nondenominational) communions, and reluctant to accept any single interpretation of highly complex issues.

On a number of medical–ethical issues there has been no single Protestant position. One cannot look to official pronouncements of denominations for authoritative statements, because they frequently represent the views of a small group of theological or ethical professionals who are not necessarily representative of the larger denomination. The very fact that Protestant denominations issue position statements has seemed to some laymen to be contrary to the tradition of Protestant voluntarism, and indeed an attempt to impose a particular point of view that inhibits the exercise of private conscience (Gustafson 1978, 126–37). No single person or group within Protestantism can be said to speak for the church. Protestant emphasis on subjection to the word of God in Scripture has led to what Paul Tillich called the "Protestant principle:" the refusal to absolutize the relative, whether it is found in human traditions or in ecclesiastical institutions. Although Protestants have remained divided over the validity of Enlightenment-based biblical criticism (which enjoyed widespread acceptance within mainstream Protestant circles during the twentieth century but was generally rejected by evangelicals and other theological conservatives), they were reluctant to disregard biblical injunctions, especially on moral issues. As a group, Protestants have tended not to be as concerned with complex issues raised by modern medical technology, which appeared to be well understood only by specialists, as they have been about matters of personal morality, which have impacted them more directly. On moral issues laymen have been hesitant to abandon traditional interpretations of Scripture.

On one issue, however, that of genetic engineering, widespread (although by no means unanimous) agreement initially existed across the theological spectrum. Several Protestant writers on biotechnology suggested caution in genetic experimentation, exhorting researchers to avoid usurping God's role. Some American Protestant denominations issued pronouncements that approved of genetic research but warned against genetic engineering. Protestants of all persuasions opposed the patenting of genetic material; however, differences existed. Conservatives opposed the use of prenatal genetic screening on the ground that it encouraged abortion. A deeper issue for conservatives, like Gilbert Meilaender, who gained prominence because of his writing and testimony for the National Bioethics Advisory Commission on cloning and stem cell research, was the concern that transgenic animal research and human cloning might alter the genetic makeup of humans and lessen their distinctiveness as a unique species created in God's image that was set apart from animals. The issue here was bound up with the definition of the image of God: Is it in part determined by genetic makeup or is it defined in terms of such factors as rationality or a spiritual and moral sense? On the other hand, theologians like Ronald Cole-Turner (1993) and Ted Peters (1997) argued that humans are "created co-creators" with God through biotechnology and that genetic engineering offers the potential for a partnership with him in an ongoing work of shaping and directing creation, which remains open to human exploration and manipulation.

The debates over biotechnology reveal a clash of Baconian optimism with the recognition that there exists a potential for harm arising out of original sin and human pride. Both are traditional Protestant leitmotifs. They also invoke the Protestant theme (although it is by no means exclusively Protestant) of man's stewardship over nature that involves the care of creation that God has entrusted to the human race, with a special concern for other creatures. Keith Thomas (Thomas 1971) found in this tradition of stewardship for the environment, which extends from the Puritans to John Wesley, the intellectual origins of later campaigns against cruelty to animals.

VI. CONCLUSION

The "Protestant empire" that dominated Anglo-Saxon values in the nineteenth century has eroded over time and no longer retains its unchallenged influence in the formulation of widely accepted societal values. For much of the twentieth century religion has been pushed to the margins of society by the secularizing elites in the academy and the professions. Divorced from public life, it has become increasingly confined to the private sphere as the structures of society have undergone rapid secularization. In fact, the pervasive *fin-de-siècle* cultural motifs of pluralism and diversity implicitly forbade the expression of religious values in public discourse. Many medical ethicists have tended as a result to adopt utilitarian or consequentialist approaches.

The contributions of Protestant medical ethicists such as Paul Ramsey, Stanley Hauerwas (Verhey and Lammers 1993, 57–77; Hauerwas 1986), James M. Gustafson (Verhey and Lammers 1993, 30–56), James F. Childress (Verhey and Lammers 1993, 127–56), and William F. May, among others, have continued to exercise wide influence, and feminist and liberation perspectives (like those of ethicist Karen Lebacqz [Lebacqz 1983]) have complemented more conventional Protestant views. Leading Protestant theologians such as Helmut Thielicke (1908–1985) (Lammers and Verhey 1998, 184–92; 785–95) and Karl Barth (1886–1968) (Lammers and Verhey 1998, 7–12; 154–57) have addressed the theological issues that underlie medical ethics, such as the basis for assigning value to human life. Moreover, although they are seldom given public expression, Protestant ideas of providence, vocation, stewardship, sanctity of life, covenant, *agape*, and compassion have played important roles in decision making at both the personal and institutional levels by physicians, nurses, and other health care professionals involved in the alleviation of human suffering. The distinctively Protestant understanding of the individual and his or her conscience alone before God, together with its insistence that a Christian's calling must be lived out in the world, have served as powerful motivating factors in the medical professions. As long as the religious values that undergird them retain their influence, they are likely to continue to do so.

ACKNOWLEDGMENT

The author gratefully acknowledges the support of a Special Fellowship in the Medical Humanities at Ben Gurion University (Israel) during the summer of 2000, when much of this article was written.

NOTES

1. *Faith healing* is a term that has been used for the practice of seeking physical or emotional healing by reliance on God or on some other supernatural force to heal directly and even miraculously those who ask. Faith healing has been espoused by some religious believers in every generation and in nearly every religious tradition. It has often involved an intermediary, whether an individual healer, a shrine, or a pilgrimage. In its most common form, it relies on prayer. In the Graeco-Roman world, it was widely practiced and especially associated with particular gods of healing such as Asclepius (Aesculapius) and Serapis, to whose temples pilgrims flocked for healing. Some Christians past and present have appealed for support of faith healing to Jesus' miracles of healing and to his commands to his disciples to heal (e.g., in Mark 16:15). Widely practiced among Christian communions is a rite of healing that employs anointing with oil (described in James 5:13–15). Many Christians have assigned a limited role to faith healing, viewing it as complementary to conventional medical treatment but not replacing it. A much smaller number have maintained that the use of medicine reflects a lack of faith in God and that Christians should resort to faith healing rather than to medicine. According to Roman Catholic theology, miracles (including those of healing) continue to take place in every generation, especially at shrines like Lourdes and Fatima. Most Protestant churches have not historically emphasized miraculous healing, but have generally believed that God does intervene to heal in answer to prayer, but occasionally and according to his sovereign will. Faith healing plays a prominent part in the Pentecostal tradition, however, which teaches that divine healing has been promised to believers of every age. Within several religious traditions in the late twentieth century, including New Age spirituality, the belief has arisen that faith itself (rather than supernatural power) is the active agent in healing. M. T. Kelsey (1976) traces healing movements in Christianity to the present. B. B. Warfield (1918) provides a critical survey of various Christian healing movements throughout history. Donald W. Dayton (1982) examines the theological roots of the Pentecostal movement's attitudes to health and healing. David Harrell, Jr. (1975) traces the history of Pentecostal and related healing ministries.

2. Different religious and philosophical traditions account for suffering in a variety of ways. A popular view in virtually all societies, which reflects an inherent human desire for poetic justice, is that much disease and physical suffering can be explained as retributive punishment for personal sin. Stoicism regarded illness or suffering as neither good nor bad but belonging the category of "things indifferent" (*adiaphora*). One's goal in life was to remain unmoved by external circumstances, including both good and bad fortune, and to cultivate personal virtue, which was the only important thing. Hinduism and Christian Science deny the existence of evil, believing it to be merely an illusion. The Jewish view of suffering can be seen to develop over time in the Hebrew Scriptures (Old Testament). The writer of the Book of Job views suffering as neither God's discipline nor the penalty for personal sin but rather the means by which Job is drawn closer

to Yahweh and recognizes his own unworthiness (Job 42:1–6). Christians of nearly every variety have held that sickness and suffering can be spiritually beneficial in the lives of religious believers. They view sickness as the result of the entrance of sin into the world, which originated with the Fall of man in the Garden of Eden. As a result all persons can expect to experience some illness, suffering, and sorrow, as well as the inevitability of death. Traditional Christian theologians have usually emphasized that there is no necessary correlation between godliness and health: The evidence is abundant that many virtuous individuals suffer affliction and pain, whereas those who lack moral integrity often enjoy good health and prosperity. Rather, they have viewed suffering as the discipline of God, a mark of his love and concern for a believer's spiritual well-being, not of his anger. Suffering directs a believer's thoughts to God; it softens hearts, humbles them, and prepares them for death by purifying them. The Roman Catholic tradition additionally sees suffering, if accompanied by a penitential attitude, as supplementing the redemptive work of Christ by atoning for sin. J. S. Feinberg (1979) and John Hick (1966) examine the theological explanations that have been given for evil and suffering. C. S. Lewis (1948) provides a theodicy from a Christian point of view. Jeremy Taylor's classic work (1651) deals with the Christian's response to suffering.

3. This phrase refers to the Judeo-Christian belief that man was created in the image of God, which has provided the basis of Western ideas of the sanctity of human life. The Jewish and Christian doctrine of man's creation in the image of God has its origins in the creation narrative of Genesis, 1:26–27: "Then God said, 'Let us make man in our image, after our likeness; and let them have dominion over the fish of the sea, and over the birds of the air, and over the cattle, and over all the earth, and over every creeping thing that creeps upon the earth.' So God created man in his own image, in the image of God he created him; male and female he created them" (RSV). According to this belief man was created last; as the highest of Yahweh's (God's)

works he stands at the summit of the created order. There is wide disagreement, however, over precisely what the "image" denotes. It is unlikely that a physical resemblance is indicated because the Hebrews believed that Yahweh has no physical form and they were forbidden to make any pictorial representation of him. It is more likely that man's dignity lies in his role as Yahweh's representative on earth. He is endowed with rationality, self-consciousness, and volition. He is a spiritual being able to enjoy communion with Yahweh and is morally responsible for his own actions. The Genesis narrative implies that the divine image is passed to successive generations by means of procreation because Adam is said to have transmitted it to his son Seth (Gen. 5:3). In Hebrew thought, life is regarded as sacred and the destruction of the human body is an affront to God (Gen. 9:6). Hence child exposure, infanticide, and emasculation are prohibited by the Torah. The view that human life possesses intrinsic value by virtue of its divine endowment stood in contrast to classical Greco-Roman thought, which understood personhood to be bestowed rather than inherent. It required membership in a family, kinship organization, or state, which granted it. In the New Testament the theme of the *imago Dei* undergoes further development.

4. The image of God, although obscured and blurred by sin, is restored through the Incarnation, in which God became man in Jesus Christ. The belief that every human life has absolute intrinsic value led to the Christian condemnation of abortion, infanticide, and suicide, which pagan ethics generally tolerated. It also saved Christianity from being taken captive by dualistic ascetic movements that denigrated the body for the sake of the soul. It continues to provide the basis for sanctity-of-life positions in medical ethics. S. Belkin (1960) has described the concept in Judaism and G. B. Ferngren the theological origins of the idea (1987). J. M. Rist describes the very different philosophical basis for human value in Greco-Roman ethics (1982). H. Thielicke considers its relevance for the modern understanding of human value (1966).

CHAPTER 16

THE DISCOURSES OF JEWISH MEDICAL ETHICS

Noam J. Zohar

I. INTRODUCTION

"Jewish Medical Ethics" was established as a recognized subspecialty by Immanuel Jakobovits (1921–1999), the late Chief Rabbi of the United Kingdom, in *Jewish Medical Ethics*, (1959). In developing this field Jakobovits and others have drawn from sources going back as far as 3,000 years and particularly on the *halakhah*, the Jewish tradition of normative discourse. Anyone interested in this subject needs to appreciate the nature of biblical law and rabbinic *halakhah*, and to gain some familiarity with those classical teachings that have particular relevance to medical issues. Because the field is so vast, what follows is intended as a set of illustrative examples rather than as a comprehensive survey.

II. BIBLICAL FOUNDATIONS

Within the twenty-four books canonized in the Hebrew Bible, the laws are found primarily in the "Five Books of Moses" (the Pentateuch). Revered by Jews as the document of God's revelation, these constitute *Torah* in its narrow sense, as distinguished from *Torah* in the broad sense of instruction, which encompasses all valid teachings in Judaism down to the present. These laws are not presented as arbitrary divine commands; rather, the text emphasizes their sense and purpose, embedded in a narrative of God's relationship, first with humankind in general and then with the Israelite people in particular.

The Bible opens with the story of the Creation, whose apex is the creation of humans in God's image. This theme is elaborated in the wake of the Flood story, when God addresses Noah and his sons and emphasizes the sharp distinction in value and protection between human and animal life:

> Every creature that lives shall be yours to eat; as with the green grasses, I give you all these. You must not, however, eat flesh with its life-blood in it. But for your own life-blood I will require a reckoning: I will require it of every beast; of man, too, will I require a reckoning for human life, of every man for that of his fellow man!
>
> Whoever sheds the blood of man, By man shall his blood be shed;
> For in His image Did God make man.
>
> Be fertile, then, and increase; abound on the earth and increase on it.[1] (Genesis 9:3–7)

The same theme finds legal expression in the concluding section of the law protecting an inadvertent killer from the victim's relatives (Numbers 35:29–34). The qualitative gap between the value of human life – male or female, child or adult – and of all other things is a central feature distinguishing biblical law from other ancient near Eastern codes (Greenberg 1960).

Despite this divine grounding of the value of human life, there is scant evidence in the Bible for positions currently associated with a "sanctity-of-life" ideal. With regard to fetal life, the law in Exodus (21:22–23) reads:

> When men fight, and one of them pushes a pregnant woman and a miscarriage results, but no other damage ensues, the one responsible shall be fined according as the woman's husband may exact from him, the payment to be based on reckoning. But if other damage ensues, the penalty shall be life for life.[2]

Virtually all Hebrew commentators understand this "other damage" as referring to death of the woman herself, which transforms the case into a homicide. For fetal life, by contrast, only monetary redress is stipulated.

For biblical references to suicide, we must look to the narrative sections of the so-called earlier prophets. Several instances of suicide are recounted, all committed by protagonists defeated in battles or uprisings, most notable among them is Israel's first king, Saul (see 1 Samuel 31:1–6).[3] The biblical text does not, however, reveal any explicit judgment of these acts of suicide. Regarding the distinct (although arguably related) issue of martyrdom, the biblical view is clearly *not* that life should be valued above all else (see Daniel Chap. 3).

Physicians and their practice are rarely mentioned in the Bible. Natural ailments were commonly regarded as divine chastisement, or at least the biblical text would have its audience regard them as such. Just after the exodus from Egypt, for example, God promises the Israelites: "If you will heed the LORD your God diligently, doing what is upright in His sight, giving ear to His commandments and keeping all His laws, then I will not bring upon you any of the diseases that I brought upon the Egyptians, for I the LORD am your healer." (Exodus 15:26). This notion seems to provide the background for the accusation recorded against King Asa: "In the thirty-ninth year of his reign, Asa suffered from an acute foot ailment; but ill as he was, he still did not turn to the LORD but to physicians" (2 Chronicles 16:12). Traditional explanations of Asa's fault have emphasized either the very fact that he turned to the physicians, or rather his failure to turn also (or first) to God. In any case, the foundational legal code of Exodus 21–23 orders that an assailant "must pay for his [victim's] idleness and his cure" (Exodus 21:19).

III. RABBINIC DISCOURSE

The classical period of Rabbinic Judaism extends from the last centuries of the Second Commonwealth through the redaction of the Babylonian Talmud, circa 500. The authoritative foundation of Rabbinic teachings is the bible, or the "written *Torah*," but its definitive medium is the "oral *Torah*," the cumulative tradition of interpretation and discussion. The basic document of this tradition is the Mishnah, redacted circa 200, which constitutes the core of the twenty-volume Talmud, whose pages include legal debates and analyses, biblical homilies, legends, lore, and much else. Other important sources are the collections of *midrash* – the rabbinic mode of (sometimes radical re-) interpretation.

Rabbinic discourse offers detailed normative amplification of the principle that humans are created in God's image. Thus the *midrash* derives a prohibition on suicide from the biblical verse (Genesis 9:5, cited previously), "But for your own life-blood I will require a reckoning," although the word "but" is construed as warranting two exceptions: martyrdom, and a case "like [that of] king Saul" (*Genesis Rabbah*, section 34). The statement regarding Saul illustrates how the workings of the "oral *Torah*" may accord normative import to narrative portions of the Bible. In a similar manner, Rabbinic narratives in turn became sources for subsequent *halakhic* teachings. The talmudic story of the martyrdom of Rabbi Hanina ben Teradion, for example, is the source for the dictum "It is better that [my soul] be taken by Him who has bestowed it – a person should not harm himself!" Rabbi Hanina's final assent to the hastening of his own death indicates alternative possibilities.[4]

> Rabbinic teachings regarding the supreme value of human life take the form of according very high priority to the duty of "life-saving," paradigmatically over against the severe prohibitions involved in observing the Sabbath. This is classically derived from the biblical verse in which God enjoins the Israelites to "keep My laws and My rules, by the pursuit of which man shall live" (Leviticus 18:5) – to which the *midrash* adds pointedly, "but not die." The limits of "life-saving" were defined in the context of persecution and martyrdom: Regarding all transgressions prohibited by the Torah, if a person is told: "Transgress so as not to die!"–he should transgress so as not to die; except for idolatry, incest,[5] and bloodshed.[6] (Babylonian Talmud *Sanhedrin* 74a; translation from Walzer et al. 2003, Chap. 11)

The same limits apply also to endeavors to save a life through healing, such as by medications produced from an *asherah* – a tree that is the object or location of idolatrous worship (Babylonian Talmud *Pesahim* 25a). Because numerous practices of their times might be tinged with idolatrous elements, it was necessary for the Rabbis to distinguish legitimate medicine from illegitimate magic grounded in idolatrous culture, called "the ways of the Emmorites;" they thus adopted the rule that "Anything that has a medical effect is not included in [the prohibition] of 'the ways of the Emmorites'" (Babylonian Talmud *Shabbat* 67a).

The limits of "life saving" apply equally, of course, to bloodshed: It is forbidden to kill one person to save another. This firm protection of human life extends even to a partly born infant, who may not be killed to save the mother. By striking contrast, a fetus prior to birth is not conceived as a person with a right to life:

> If a woman is in difficult labor, the fetus should be cut up within her and removed limb by limb, since her life takes precedence over his life. Once most of him has emerged, he may not be touched, for one person may not be destroyed for the sake of another. (Mishnah *Ohalot* 7:6)[7]

Other Rabbinic sources also reflect a relatively low regard for fetal life, even late in pregnancy (see Babylonian Talmud *Arakhin* 7a). On the other hand, the obligation of emergency life saving (even involving desecration of the Sabbath) was extended to rescuing a fetus, and according to one source, destroying a fetus is included under the rubric of "homicide."[8] Because the Talmud is a compendium of many voices and traditions, this lack of a univocal message is not surprising and is in fact characteristic of the source materials for medieval rulings and for contemporary Jewish medical ethics.

Even without positing any fetal "right to life," the Talmud is definitely pronatalist. Procreation is an explicit religious obligation (*mitzvah*), grounded in the belief that humans are created in God's image, as explained by Rabbi Elazar ben Azariah: "Anyone who does not engage in procreation, is considered as though he had diminished the [divine] image" (Tosefta *Yevamot* 8:7). The divine image inheres even in the human body in death and is thus the basis for the obligation to "respect the dead," requiring prompt burial and disallowing disfigurement of a human cadaver (see *Mishnah Sanhedrin* 6:5 and *Tosefta Sanhedrin* 9:7). Despite this, as Jakobovits rightly states, "it is noteworthy that no voice of protest was raised against . . . practices [of dissections for scientific purposes] or their descriptions in the Talmud . . . Judaism, then, became heir to a distinctively tolerant attitude to dissection" (Jakobovits 1975, 135–36).

This conclusion is generated, in part, through looking at a broad array of talmudic sources (e.g., "descriptions of practices"). Indeed, it is worth remembering the great variety in the kind of materials collected in the Talmud, by no means limited to normative statements or even to narratives of exemplary persons and deeds. In addition, the Talmud is a repository of folk sayings and lore – including medical lore – as well as fables and parables, practical advice and much else. There are numerous warnings against acts deemed "dangerous," a category of prudence conceived as distinct from – and in a sense requiring greater diligence than – the evaluative category of the

"forbidden" (see Babylonian Talmud *Hullin* 9b). The basic outlook of these sources is in line with that of medieval and modern preventive medicine.

I have mentioned here, of course, only a small sample of the talmudic texts relating to issues in medical ethics. It is also worth noting that the talmudic teaching most explicitly relevant to health care ethics does not focus upon medicine or physicians but rather upon a duty incumbent upon every member of the community, namely the *mitzvah* of "visiting the sick." God himself, the Rabbis taught, had set an example in this, when He visited Abraham who was convalescing from his circumcision.[9]

IV. POST-TALMUDIC JUDAISM: CODES, RESPONSA, AND LEARNED PHYSICIANS

During the centuries following the redaction of the *Talmud*, Jewish communities throughout the diaspora would write for guidance in difficult *halakhic* questions to the heirs of the talmudic masters, the *geonim*, heads of the Babylonian academies. Around the turn of the millennium, Judaism saw a shift away from a single cultural center, and rulings in moral/legal/ritual matters of *halakhah* came to rest in the hands of local courts or individual scholars, masters in the art of *talmudic* interpretation. Enquiries were sent to regional eminent scholars, and their answers were collected and preserved in books of responsa. This period also saw great works of codification, from Isaac Alfasi's "Abridgement of the Talmud" (eleventh century, North Africa) and Maimonides' *Mishneh Torah*[10] (twelfth century, Spain and Egypt), through Jacob ben Asher's *Arba'ah Turim* (fourteenth century, Spain) to Joseph Caro's *Shulhan Arukh* (sixteenth century, Land of Israel) with the glosses by his contemporary Moses Isserles (Poland).[11]

In Spain, Jewish scholars encountered Muslim philosophy and science in general, and medical learning in particular. Because many of the prescribed remedies were not readily explicable in terms of natural science, the question arose whether they might come under the prohibition of "the ways of the Emmorites." Maimonides, the great twelfth-century codifier and philosopher, had defined idolatry as a grand illusion, and generally prohibited recourse to any irrational remedy. In thirteenth century Montpelier, a protracted debate arose over the use of "a shape of a lion, without a tongue, engraved upon a plaque of silver or gold . . . For it is recorded [in the name] of the ancients in medical texts that this is effective in [treating] an ailment in the loins, provided that it is made at a particular time" (Maimonides 1964, 543) Successive enquiries were addressed to Shlomo Adret of Barcelona, the leading rabbinic authority in thirteenth-century Spain, asking whether this might come under the talmudic permission of "anything that has a medical effect." Adret allowed the practice, reporting that his renowned teacher Nahmanides had himself administered it and pointing out that "the [workings of] charms are unknown to us, and should not be assessed according to the established laws [literally: "well-known ways"] of nature." In a lengthy discourse, he raised logical and talmudic objections to Maimonides's restrictive position.[12]

Although medieval rabbis sought to distinguish medicine from illicit superstitions, many of them were also concerned about drawing a line between relying on effective medicine – grounded in human wisdom – and reliance on God's healing. The Talmud, relying on a verse in Exodus (21:19) had expressly stated that "permission has been granted to the physician to heal." Yet several commentators restricted the scope of this permission, positing against it a religious ideal of responding to illness by repentance and prayer. Notably, Nahmanides (in his renowned *Commentary on the Pentateuch* (1963–1964), Leviticus. 26:11), adopting the more exclusivist reading of the biblical accusation against King Asa, exclaims: "what share is there for physicians in the house of those who do God's will?!" Still, he explains, a physician may treat the many who cannot, or will not, adhere to this purist ideal. In his *Torat ha-Adam*, by virtue of which he has been called "the most comprehensive codifier of medical-ethical matters during the Middle Ages,"[13] Nahmanides (1963–1964, Vol. 2: 41) offers another explanation for the "permission to heal:" It was proclaimed to overcome not a divine prerogative, but physicians' hesitation to incur the risks of causing harm. Maimonides, by contrast, ridiculed the notion that employing human wisdom to effect healing through natural means somehow detracts from religious faith, asking rhetorically: "If a person is hungry and seeks bread to eat – whereby he is undoubtedly healed from that great pain – should we say that he has failed to trust in God?!"[14] (For comparable debates in the Christian and Islamic contexts, see Chapters 8, 12, 14, and 17.)

In addition to Spain, an important hub of Jewish learning was the Rhine valley and northern France, where Rashi (eleventh century) composed his classical commentary on the *Talmud*. Of special importance to practices surrounding life and death is the book *Sefer Hasidim*, attributed to Judah He-hasid, leader of a twelfth century pietistic movement. The book is compiled of several hundred disparate sections; several of them contain instructions on how to treat a dying person. Four centuries later, Joshua Bo'az (Italy, sixteenth century) struggled with the seeming inconsistencies in these instructions, from which he sought guidance concerning a practice of his contemporaries: "When a person is dying [*gosses*], and the soul is unable to depart, they remove the bedding from under him. For it is said that the bedding contains feathers of a certain bird which cause the soul not to depart. Several times, I protested vehemently, seeking to bring an end to this evil practice, but was unsuccessful. My teachers, however, disagreed with my position; and Rabbi Nathan of Hungary, of blessed memory, wrote permitting

this." Finally, Bo'az concluded that the proper rule is non-interference; and that removing an impediment is not the same as actually hastening death. Throughout, neither Bo'az nor his sources in *Sefer Hasidim* rely on any scriptural or talmudic source; their arguments are presented simply as earnest reasoning. Their point of departure crucially is, however, the talmudic teaching on the preciousness of every moment of life, emphatically including the last moments of a dying person.[15]

From the high Middle Ages and through the Renaissance, it was not uncommon for Jewish physicians to be also rabbinic scholars. The example and the writings of such individuals form an important part of the heritage of modern Jewish medical ethics. Maimonides was a renowned physician, and incorporated into his *Mishneh Torah* instructions on maintaining one's health, defined as a religious obligation of "preserving life." In a similar vein (following Aristotle), he conceived the prescriptions of the *Torah* as aimed to inculcate a healthy character or as cures for the "illnesses of the soul" that consist in the various vices.

The writings of several Jewish physicians include a critique of their colleagues' focus on fees and wealth. Indeed, Jewish law disallows charging a fee for life saving, and physicians were supposed to be paid only for their "time and trouble" but not for their expertise.[16] This was only meant, however, to exclude payments of a fee-for-service character: physicians were handsomely rewarded by way of retainers by families or entire communities, and often by grants of tax-exempt status by princes and kings. Noted Renaissance figures include Amatus Lusitanus and Jacob Zahalon.[17] In Lusitanus's testimony or "oath" (1559; reproduced in Friedenwald 1944), he emphasizes that he always treated patients with the same dedication, whether or not they could pay.

V. The Modern Period

With the advent of modern medicine, *halakhic* scholars faced challenges entailed by new practices and discoveries. An illustrative example from the second half of the eighteenth century is the response by Prague's rabbi – Yehezkel Landa – to a query sent from London, where the local rabbis had been unable to reach a consensus. In the wake of a failed lithotomy, the surgeons proposed an autopsy:

> in order to see directly the source of this affliction, so as to gain from it knowledge regarding the surgeons' future conduct, should such a case occur [again]; so that they would know how to conduct themselves with respect to the cutting necessary for healing, and not cut excessively, so as to minimize the dangers of cutting. Is it forbidden because it involves disfigurement and disrespect

of this deceased person, or is it permitted because it might bring about saving of life in the future, through becoming thoroughly proficient in this art?[18]

Rabbi Yehezkel Landa refused to permit the autopsy. He explicitly rejects the suggestion that the potential for future healing (which he defines as a "slight chance") be accorded the status of "life-saving," which would have mandated overriding whatever prohibition pertains to "disfiguring the deceased." Interestingly, this ruling prohibiting autopsy was challenged in the twentieth century by Israel's chief Sephardi rabbi, Ben-Zion Hay Uziel, who pointed to the proven record of modern medicine, which had facilitated the saving of many lives by knowledge attained through post-mortem examinations.[19]

Responses to medical innovations were by no means always negative. In the early eighteenth century, another rabbi in central Europe, Jacob Reischer, was often consulted by Jewish "expert physicians" on normative professional matters. In one case, he boldly permitted a speculative medical procedure for a patient who was otherwise deemed incurable and close to death, despite an admitted risk that the procedure might cause immediate death. It is important to note that, although the patient may have wanted to take this risk, the discussion does not refer to his consent but rather to the value of hoped-for cure over the value of the short span of life that might be lost.[20]

In general, modern Jewish bioethics has tended to proceed in the spirit of Maimonides, endorsing the enhancement of the capacity to heal. At the same time, an important strand of discourse on "halakhah and medicine" has emphasized various halakhic ritual norms that must constrain medical practice and health care delivery, at least when there is no definite issue of "life saving" at stake. Thus, we find resistance to placing Jewish patients in institutions where the ritual dietary laws cannot be observed, numerous concerns over observing the Sabbath by both patients and staff in hospitals, insistence on details of ritual circumcision although accepting (some) medical innovations. Other issues in contemporary Jewish bioethics have a more clearly ethical dimension, often related to the valuation of humans as created in God's image, for example, resistance to the dissection of human cadavers, rejection of patients' self-determination with respect to choosing death, or firm opposition to any sacrifice of one individual to rescue another.

VI. Issues of Methodology in Contemporary Jewish Medical Ethics

In the wake of nineteenth-century emancipation, rabbinic courts no longer retained the authority that they had enjoyed in the medieval Jewish communities (although in the state of Israel the Chief Rabbinate has an official advisory function, and an effective consultative role, in important bioethical matters; there is some impact of Jewish law on the state's democratically based jurisprudence[21]). Nevertheless, people committed to the halakhah have continued to turn to rabbinic leaders, and significant portions of the writings in modern Jewish bioethics are produced in the traditional form of responsa. In addition, during the second half of the twentieth century, an increasing number of scholarly essays of either rabbinic or academic character (and sometimes a mixture of both) have appeared in various forums. The Schlesinger Institute in Jerusalem has published a journal, Assia – Jewish Medical Ethics (in Hebrew, starting 1970; in English, starting 1988) and a six-volume Encyclopedia of Jewish Medical Ethics (Steinberg 1988, English three-volume edition, 2003). English-language compendiums have been produced notably by Rosner (1972, [1986] 1991; Rosner and Tendler 1980).

In the more traditional – or Orthodox – of these publications, the instructions provided are often justified purely by reference to authoritative texts and precedents, although some authors may combine this with appeals to a broader-based moral reasoning. In recent years, there has arisen some second-order discussion regarding the method and nature of Jewish bioethics. Insofar as halakhic discourse is perceived as grounded exclusively in the authority of Torah as revealed and accepted by the Jewish community in the Sinai covenant, it cannot address those not bound by that covenant – whether non-Jews or secular Jews.[22] Some important authors – notably Bleich – readily concede this insular view, defining their work in terms of Jewish law rather than of a Jewish voice in ethics.

Others have asserted, however, the rational nature of the Torah's commandments (or at least of many of them). One strand of such assertions has posited the prudential purpose of many halakhic norms, especially as pertains to maintaining physical and mental health. This view – well rooted in medieval treatises on "the reasons for the commandments" – is represented in the Introduction to Jakobovits' book (1959) written by his father-in-law, E. Munk, who refers to a modern precursor, Goslar's (1930) edited collection of essays on "Hygiene and Judaism." Jakobovits himself, in his foundational book (1959) and in subsequent writings, similarly rejected the insular view of halakhic norms, but tended to emphasize their value content more than any prudential advantages. Indeed, he was moved to engage in this project during his term as Chief Rabbi of Ireland, where he witnessed the Roman Catholic influence upon legislation and policy through "texts written in the vernacular" and couched in terms of natural law and universal reason. The subtitle of Jakobovits's book defines it as a "comparative and historical study," and each chapter seeks to locate Judaic teachings within the context of other traditions, both religious and secular.

Other traditionally committed authors have sought more explicitly and analytically to engage a Judaic voice within philosophical bioethics, and to draw insights for Jewish bioethics from biblical narratives and from rabbinic non-*halakhic* sources.[23] More broadly, the field has also been enriched by contributions of some authors not committed to *halakhah*, yet grounded in traditional Judaic sources or theological positions.[24]

NOTES

1. Biblical citations are from *Tanakh, The Holy Scriptures* (Philadelphia, Jerusalem: Jewish Publication Society 1985). All translations in this chapter are by the author unless otherwise indicated.

2. The word translated here as "other damage" has been translated alternatively as "mischief" (KJV) or "harm" (RSV). In ancient Jewish Hellenic circles, this passage was read differently, ascribing greater value to fetal life; for a critical discussion, see Freund (1990, 241–50).

3. For a general discussion, see Goldstein (1989).

4. Babylonian Talmud, *ʿAvoda Zarah* 18a. For a discussion and analysis, see Zohar (1997, 50–58).

5. The Hebrew term [*giluy ʿarayot*] extends to adultery as well.

6. Similarly, the Rabbinic debate on whether an individual may be sacrificed to save the many is set in the context of a Jewish community under threat of an external army (see Daube 1965).

7. Literally, "one soul (*nefesh*) may not be set aside for the sake of another," Rashi explains that the fetus "is not a soul."

8. The source is in BT *Sanhedrin* 57b. For an extended discussion, see Jakobovits (1975, 182–91).

9. See Genesis Rabbah section 8.

10. An almost complete English translation, titled *The Code of Maimonides*, has been published by Yale University Press starting in 1949.

11. For a detailed survey see Elon (1994, 1138–1366).

12. The description of the practice at issue is preserved in Adret's Responsa 1:167; the issue is revisited in greater length in responsum 1:413, a letter to Abba Mari of Lunel, published also by Dimitrowsky (1990, 281–310). For a succinct survey of the various sources and opinions, see Jakobovits (1975, 33–36). Regarding the amulet itself, see Kottek (1967).

13. The appellation is from Kottek (1996, 172), who explores several teachings from that tractate.

14. Maimonides, Commentary on the Mishnah, Pesahim 4:6. This is my own translation, relying on the Kappah edition (1963–68) and verified by Dr. Zvi Zohar. For an analysis of the arguments and views of both Nahmanides and Maimonides, see Zohar 1997, 34–66.

15. The talmudic foundations are compiled in Alfasi on tractate *Mo'ed Katan* 16b. Bo'az's analysis is contained in his glosses *Shiltei Ha-gibborim*, printed in the margins of the same page (section 4). For the original Rabbinic source, see *The Minor Tractates, Semahoth* pp. 326–27.

16. For some examples see Garcia-Ballester (1996), 29–31. Regarding Jewish law on this matter, see Shulhan Arukh YD 336.

17. See Feingold (1996).

18. Responsa *Noda Bihuda* II, YD 210. This responsum is actually a critical rejoinder to the author's relative, to whom the initial query had been directed and who had written back permitting the autopsy.

19. Responsa *Mishpetey Uziel* YD 28.

20. Responsa *Shevut Ya'acov* 3:75.

21. See, for example, Elon (1969).

22. See Brody (1983), and compare Green (1985) and Novak (1985).

23. For example, see Sinclair (1989); Zohar (1997); Dorff (1998); Newman (1998); Freedman (1999); and Zoloth-Dorfman (1999).

24. See Davis (1991); and Zemer (1998).

CHAPTER 17

THE DISCOURSES OF ISLAMIC MEDICAL ETHICS

Ilhan Ilkilic

I. INTRODUCTION

The close connection between faith, society, and the responsibility of the individual provided a basis on which faith and morality could remain an indivisible unity. The structure and moral implications of the articles of faith, basic responsibilities, and normative values in Islam exclude a clear division between the religious and private spheres (Antes 1982, 40; Ess 1980, 70–71). Like all other areas of experience, illness is also one of the parts of life on which the Islamic faith takes a particular perspective and for which it provides corresponding norms of behavior.

For Muslims, the Quran and the traditions of the Prophet Muhammad (Sunna) are the main sources of what is morally good and normative. The Quran, the sacred scripture of Islam, contains the verbatim word of God that was revealed to the Prophet Muhammad in Arabic between 610 and 632. The Prophet Muhammad (570–632) applied the general instructions of the Quran in his behavior and manners and gave Muslims directions in issues that were not regulated in detail in the Quran. Because the Islamic textual sources, which date from the seventh to ninth centuries, are also the basis for ethical practice in the area of medicine, this chapter will concern

itself initially with the concepts of health, disease, and illness presented in these sources and the moral obligations for practitioners and patients that can be derived from them (see also Chapter 25). The meaning and justification of medical skill and a number of medical–ethical principles will also be discussed.

II. ILLNESS AND HEALING IN THE SOURCES OF ISLAM

1. Illness and Healing in the Quran

The word "disease" (*marad*) is used in the Quran in two main senses, literal and metaphorical. In its first use, *marad* refers to disease as an actual bodily disorder or malfunction. This indicates that disease, understood as pain, structural anomaly, or dysfunction or failure of the body or the soul, is a hindrance on the road of life and is assessed by the Quran accordingly. This sense is concerned with physical suffering and the exemptions from religious obligations that arise from it: from fasting (Surah 2:184; Surah 2:185), pilgrimage (Surah 2:196), ritual washings (Surah 4:43; Surah 5:6), prayer (Surah 73:20), and from a number of social obligations (Surah 24:61). Other verses relevant to the topic of health and illness address hygienic regulations, nutrition, sexual intercourse, and behavior toward the dead and the sick.

Whereas the second, metaphorical sense of "illness" as disbelief or hypocrisy is connected with Divine admonition and damnation, the first sense is always associated with the comfort and mercy of God, a link that is often emphasized in those verses that deal with exemptions from prayer in the case of illness: "God wills that you shall have ease, and does not will you to suffer hardship" (Surah 2:185). The sick person does not need to feel inferior to his fellow human beings or guilty toward God if he does not fulfill his religious and social obligations (Surah 9:91; Surah 24:61; Surah 48:17; Surah 4:102).

In the verse, "When I sicken, then He healeth me" (Surah 26:80), emphasis is placed on God as the first cause of all medical healing. God provides human beings with this healing in different forms (medicines, fruits, animal products, etc.). "[And lo!] there issues from within these [bees] a fluid of many hues, wherein there is healing [*šifā*] for man" (Surah 16:68–69).

The second, and most common, use of *maraḍ* is not literal, but metaphorical. It is used to characterize hypocrisy (Surah [chap.] 2:10; Surah 5:52; Surah 8:49; Surah 24:50; Surah 33:12; Surah 47:29), disbelief (Surah 9:125; Surah 33:60, 74:31), doubts about the existence of God (Surah 22:53), and lack of piety (Surah 33:32). When the Quran uses *maraḍ* in a metaphorical sense, it often signals this by the expression "In their hearts is a disease" (*fī qulūbihim maraḍ*). Al-Ghazzālī (d. 1111), one of the most influential scholars of Islamic intellectual history, has commented on the meaning of the word *qalb* (heart).

> When we speak of the heart, therefore, you should know that we mean by this the real essence of the person, that part which is sometimes called "the spirit" and sometimes called "the soul," not, however, that piece of flesh which is located in the left side of your breast. [. . .] The knowledge of its essence and its characteristics is the key to the knowledge of God." (al-Ghazālī 1998, 37)

In commentaries on the Quran, there is a broad consensus that the expression "In their hearts is a disease" describes a loss of equilibrium in the soul, that is, a falling away from belief in the oneness of God, doubts about the existence of God, and hypocrisy (Yazir 1971, 1: 227–231). Like *maraḍ*, the word *šifā*, which in Arabic means "healing, recovery, medicine, therapy," is also used in the Quran primarily in a metaphorical sense (Surah 9:17; Surah 10:57; Surah 17:82). The Quran is often described as a source of healing for the previously mentioned illnesses in a metaphorical sense: "Say unto them (O Muhammad): For those who believe, it [the Quran] is a guidance and a healing"[1] (Surah 41:44).

2. Illness and Healing in the Traditions of the Prophet Muhammad (Sunna)

The metaphorical meaning of the notions of illness and healing are also to be found in the sayings of the Prophet (the Hadiths), which will not be discussed in detail here. The Prophet's recommendations of medical therapies or the mention of specific medicines for particular illnesses emphasize the values of bodily well-being and imply that it is necessary to maintain one's health. In connection with other Hadiths, which concentrate on hygienic issues, the care of the body, or occasional medical advice, a strong concern with preventative measures can be discerned in the medical Hadiths.

In one tradition, the Prophet Muhammad says: "God has sent down a medicine for every illness. Therefore, treat them, but not with anything which has been forbidden"[2] (Abū Dāwūd 1994; K. aṭ-Ṭibb 1994, bāb 11, no. 3874, 3:388). This Hadith and similar passages articulate first of all – like the Quran (Surah 28:80) – the idea that God is the first cause, not only of disease and illness, but also of healing. After this description of illness, the clear opinion of the Prophet about medical therapy is expressed: "Have yourselves treated." He thus obliges sick Muslims to take appropriate therapeutic measures to receive the healing that God has created. At the end of this Hadith, we find a restriction on medical treatment: the prohibition "Do not allow yourselves to be treated with anything forbidden" requires that a medication or a therapeutic method be legitimate within Islam. If a substance is prohibited by the Quran and the Prophet, it should not be used in the course of medical treatment. One is to think here primarily of substances explicitly mentioned in the Quran and the Sunna such as pork, alcohol, and so forth. These prohibitions allow exceptions in emergency situations and in the case of illnesses that can be treated in no other way, according to the principle of Islamic law, "The emergency makes the forbidden allowed" (*al-ḍarūrāt tubīḥ al-maḥzūrāt*) (Zaidān 1976, 100).

It is clear in the Islamic sources that the human body is not to be viewed simply as a possession, but rather as a gift entrusted to human beings by God. This is why suicide is not compatible with Islamic principles. "Do not kill yourselves" (Surah 4:29). The following Hadith prohibits even the wish to die in the case of sickness: "None of you should wish for death because of a calamity befalling him; but if he has to wish for death, he should say: 'O Allah! Keep me alive as long as life is better for me, and let me die if death is better for me.'" (Buḫārī 1985, 7:390). Some Hadiths draw attention to the obligations of the relatives of the sick to visit them, the rules of conduct connected with this, and "encouragement." "Feed the hungry, visit the sick, and have the captives set free" (Buḫārī 1985, 7:375). "When you visit a sick person, so comfort him by wishing him recovery and a long life. This will satisfy him" (Tirmiḏī, *K. aṭ-Ṭibb*, 1994, bāb 30, no. 2088, 4:23).

3. Prophetic Medicine and its Moral Implications for Muslims

Prophetic medicine (*ṭibb an-nabī* or *aṭ-ṭibb an-nabawī*) comprises the recommendations or practices of the Prophet Muhammad for the alleviation of particular forms of suffering, preventive measures with respect to particular illnesses, or matters of hygiene. Hadiths on medicine and the sick appear first in the eighth and ninth centuries in the classical Hadith collections as single chapters. Later, separate books were compiled on the medicine of the Prophet, and these contain more Hadiths than the earlier single chapters. The oldest *Ṭibb an-Nabī* work known to us was compiled by ʿAlī ar-Riḍā (d. 818) and was written as a report to the Abbasid Caliph al-Maʾmūn (813–33) who, because of his great interest in medicine, natural science, and philosophy had many works in other languages translated into Arabic. Other authors of works on the medicine of the Prophet include ʿAbdalmalik Ibn Ḥabīb b. Sulaimān as-Sulami (d. 852), Aḥmad b. Muḥammad Ibn as-Sunnī ad-Dinawarī (d. 974), Abū Nuʿaim Aḥmad b. ʿAbdallāh b. Aḥmad al-Isfahani (d. 1038), Ibn Qayyim al-Ǧauzīya (d. 1350), and Ǧalaladdīn as-Suyūti (d. 1505) (see also the comprehensive lists of these books in Elgood 1962, 40–45; Recep 1969, 4–13; Ullmann 1970, 185–9).

The Hadiths in these works can be divided into two groups. The first group contains those Hadiths that are concerned with preventive measures and therapies for particular illnesses. In these Hadiths, the therapeutic effects of antimony, dates, henna, honey, garlic, pumpkin, milk, olive oil, and so forth are emphasized (Rasslan 1934, 35–39; Elgood 1962, 66–119). Into the second group fall recommendations and advice on personal cleanliness, the washing of food, keeping one's clothes clean, dental hygiene, and the circumcision of male children; this group is more concerned about hygiene in general than the first.

It has already been mentioned that the decisions, recommendations, and omissions of the Prophet Muhammad have binding character for the ethical practice of a Muslim. In this context, it seems reasonable to ask what normative content and moral implications the historical texts can have for contemporary Muslims. A classic and still ongoing debate in Islamic intellectual history (Canan 1988, 11:252–3; Kırbaşoğlu 1993, 70–83; Rahman 1987, 32–58) concerns the question of whether the therapeutic recommendations of the Prophet with respect to specific illnesses are to be considered binding today. Some scholars hold that these Hadiths remain binding to a certain extent and assign them intrinsic value. Their main argument appeals to verses in the Quran that declare the decisions and recommendations of the Prophet to be binding norms for the conduct of Muslims. "Nor doth he [Muhammad] speak of (his own) desire. It is naught save an inspiration that is inspired" (Surah 53:3–4; see also Surah 4:80; Surah 4:13; Surah 4:14). These and similar verses emphasize the truthfulness of the Prophet Muhammad and the relationship of his speech to God. Because the Prophet cannot lie in what he says and is not without divine inspiration, his statements about medical matters should be considered absolutely valid. Today there exist variations of this position, ranging from the thesis that it is the task of the modern natural sciences to examine and prove the scientific worth of the Hadiths to use them for the benefit of humankind, to the view of those who see the implementation of the Hadiths as a kind of liturgical practice.

Ibn Qayyim al-Ǧauzīya (d. 1350) is considered to be one of the most important representatives of this position. At the beginning of his work *at-Ṭibb an-Nabawī* he mentions his intention to discover the wisdom of the medicine of the Prophet, which has been hidden even from famous physicians (Ibn Qayyim al-Ǧauzīya 1994, 5). He classifies the illnesses and identifies the basic principles of the medicine and methods of the Prophet in different therapies. It is to be noted that he interprets the therapeutic methods of the Hadiths on the basis of the medical science of his day. In the course of his discussions, he cites Galen, Rhazes, and Avicenna. Although he also mentions therapies that are not to be found in Galenic medicine, such as the recitation of the verses of the Quran, no hostile attitude toward Galenic therapies can be discerned. In addition, he places considerable emphasis on the advice of physicians, on visits to doctors, and on the choice of an experienced doctor in the case of illness (Ibn Qayyim al-Ǧauzīya 1994, 96).

Other scholars question the binding character of the medicine of the Prophet, offering two levels of argumentation. On one level, it is argued that the aim of the Prophetic mission is not the communication of specific scientific information. Rather, the task of the Prophet is to proclaim the message of God to humankind and to point out the principles of faith that can be derived from it and their practical implications. In this context, the famous historian Ibn Khaldûn (d. 1406) wrote in his important work Muqaddima that "Muhammad was sent to teach us the religious law. He was not sent to teach us medicine or any other ordinary matter" (Ibn Khaldûn 1967, 3:150). In support of this position, a Hadith is often cited in which the Prophet advises the inhabitants of the city of Medina against the traditional method of pollinating dates. As a result of this, scarcely any dates were harvested, at which point the Prophet took back his advice with the following words: "I am only human; if I instruct you to do something in a religious matter, then you should do it; but if I only express my opinion [with respect to worldly things], I am only human [and can make mistakes]" (Muslim, without year, K. al-Faḍāʾil, bāb 37, no. 2362, 4/1:95).

The second level of argumentation adduced by scholars favoring this position turns on the fact that the majority of Hadiths that recommend specific therapies agree with the popular medicine of their day (Ibn Khaldûn 1967, 150). They should therefore be read as the transmission of therapeutic methods and medical practices that were known at the time and had proved themselves by experience. It is not impossible that some exchange of knowledge took place between the Prophet Muhammad and his friend, the physician Harīt bin Kalada (Ibn Abī Usayba 1884, 109; Bürgel 1991, 172; Rahman 1987, 41), who had been trained in Gondhēshāpūr (Sayılı 1965, 2:1119–20). The intent of these Hadiths was to convey current medical information and, as that information was updated, it stands to reason that the implications of the Hadiths should be updated accordingly.

III. Conception of Medicine

The concept of medicine in the Islamic Middle Ages was influenced by the theory of the humors. This notion, known also to the Ancient Greeks and Indians (Chapters 9, 10), was applied in the treatment of illnesses. According to this theory, nutrients taken up into the body and transformed into liquid were changed in the metabolic process into four cardinal fluids: blood (*dam*), phlegm (*balǧam*), yellow bile (*al-mirra as-safra*) and black bile (*al-mirra as-saudā*) (Ullmann 1970, 97). A harmonious mixture of these fluids is what makes a person healthy. A disturbance, however, is understood to be disease, the cause of an illness. The character of the disease corresponds to the quality of the fluids and their relationships to each other. In the course of time, a person takes on a particular temperament by virtue of his humoral predisposition and his environment, such as, for example, a sanguine, phlegmatic, choleric, or melancholic temperament. This also plays a role in the symptomology of disease, the emergence of an illness. If a person is melancholic, he can easily be afflicted with the illness of melancholy manifesting itself in such symptoms as spontaneous crying or taking to one's bed during the day (Ullmann 1970, 97). An important point is that neither the cardinal fluids nor their qualities are the first cause of life. They are merely the means by which the evidence of life appears (Nasr 1976, 160).

The human being who, according to the Quran, was created in the best of all possible forms and with the best instructions from God (Surah 95:4) is God's representative on earth (Surah 2:30; Surah 6:165; Surah 10:14; Surah 27:62). Medicine is granted a special place because of its service to humankind. Only if he is healthy can a person fulfill his obligations and the purpose of his creation (Surah 51:56). Because of this important contribution to human life, many scholars, among them Al-Ghazzālī, described the study and practice of medicine as *fard kifāyah* (a common duty), that is, as a major obligation to God; if some

people fulfill it, they thereby relieve others of having to do so.

> Sciences whose knowledge is deemed *fard kifāyah* comprise every science which is indispensable for the welfare of this world such as: medicine which is necessary for the life of the body, arithmetic for daily transactions and the division of legacies an inheritances, as well as other besides. These are the sciences whose absence would reduce a community to narrow circumstances. But should one who can practise them rise in that community, it would suffice and the obligation to acquire their knowledge would cease to be binding upon the rest of the community.[3] (al-Ghazzālī 1962, 37)

Although there is no doubt of the value of the study of medicine, the method of acquiring this important skill was already a matter of controversy. In the famous debate between ʿAlī ibn Ridwan (d. 1061 or 1068) and Ibn Butlān (d. 1066) in the years 1049–1050, the question was whether the training of a physician should be based on the study of great scholars or on the instruction of a master (Ibn Butlān 1984, 32–33; ʿAlī ibn Ridwan [1409] 1982, 7)."Science is twofold, the science of bodies (medicine) and the science of religions," also points to the high status of medicine among the other sciences. This classification is often quoted as a saying of the Prophet (Sāʾid ibn al-Hasan 1968b, 5b), but can be traced back to Shafii (d. 820), the founder of a legal school, who is viewed as the father of Muslim jurisprudence (Bürgel 1991, 181). The saying that "there are two classes of men who are indispensable, philosophers for religion and physicians for bodies" (Elgood 1962, 124; Canan 1991, 11:253), (the source of which is not clear) emphasizes the importance of these two professions. Both professions are indispensable for a successful life and are hierarchically ordered by Shafii. According to him, medicine takes second place after the science of religion (Canan 1991, 11:253). Al-Ruhāwī, however, a doctor and expert in the Hippocratic and Galenic texts (Ibn Abī Usayba [1882–1884] 1972, 254), maintained a different position in the ninth century in his work *Adab at-Tabīb*. In al-Ruhāwī's conception, health represents the highest good for the human being (al-Ruhāwī 1967a, 70b). He also emphasizes the importance of health for realizing human potential and fulfilling religious duties such as fasting and prayer (al-Ruhāwī 1967a, 79a–79b). For this reason, al-Ruhāwī assigns medical skill an even higher status in the service of humankind than the religious disciplines and philosophy in that it becomes the noblest of all arts (*ašrafu as-sināʾa*) (al-Ruhāwī [1347] 1985, 154). For: "The philosopher can only improve the soul, but the virtuous physician can improve both body and soul" (al-Ruhāwī 1967a, 79b).

Medical skills gain their legitimacy not only by virtue of their service to humankind, but also by means of their contribution to political power or the stability of a state.

Like every person, a ruler needs a healthy body and mind if he is to fulfill his duties of government. He is therefore dependent, like every one else, on good physicians. The Abbasid Caliph Harun ar-Rašid (786–809), said the following about his physician Djibril ibn Bakhtishū, who belonged to the famous family of physicians Bakhtishū from Djundishapur (Browne 1921, 18–24): "The well-being of my body and my constitution depends on him, and the well-being of the Muslims depends on me, therefore the well-being of the Muslims depends on his well-being and maintenance" (Bürgel 1967b, 11). Given the basic importance of medicine, no town can do without a doctor. For this reason, a good physician is a reason often cited in many classical works for settling in a particular town. ʿAlī ibn Sahl Rabban aṭ-Ṭabari writes: "It is also said that no one should live in a country in which the following four things are not to be found: a righteous king, running water, a capable and knowledgeable physician, and medicines" (Rabban aṭ-Ṭabari 1928, 560 and 576; similarly Ṣāʾid ibn al-Ḥasan: Ṣāʾid 1968b, 7a).

In the current discussion, the following passages from the classical Islamic sources are used to legitimate medicine and as a basis for arguing for moral obligations in medical practice (Nanji 1988, 257–75; Rahman 1987, 29–40; Ebrahim 1993, 38–43; Serour 1994, 75–91; Hathout 1992; Hathout and Lustig 1993):

When I sicken, then He healeth me. (Surah 26:80)

If anyone slays a human being – unless it be [in punishment] for murder or for spreading corruption on earth – it shall be as though he had slain all mankind; whereas, if anyone saves a life, it shall be as though he had saved the lives of all mankind. (Surah 5:32)

And spend [freely] in God's cause, and let not your own hands throw you into destruction; and preserve in doing good: behold, God loves the doers of good. (Surah 2:195)

There cometh forth from their [bee] bellies a drink diverse of hues, wherein is healing [šifāʾ] for mankind. (Surah 16:68–69)

God has sent down a medicine for every illness. Therefore, treat them, but not with anything which has been forbidden. (Abū Dāwūd 1994, K. aṭ-Ṭibb, bāb 11, no. 3874, 3:388)

The best among men is he who has a long life and does good deeds." (Tirmidī, without year, K. az-Zuhd, bāb 21, no. 2336, 4:147)

With reference to these verses and Hadith, many contemporary Muslim scholars and intellectuals have a positive attitude toward modern medicine and actual scientific research. They think that the new methods of diagnosis and therapy serve humankind as pure means to achieve a cure whose agent is God. The art of medicine contributes to saving life and to preserving the well-being of humankind and therefore deserves a great respect. Similar arguments are to be found also for medical research. According to the Quran, all natural phenomena and in general the cosmic harmony are signs of God (āyāt Allah; vestigia Dei). "What we call scientific research now is called, in juridical terminology, the 'uncovering of God's tradition in His creation' by discovering the laws of nature" (Hathout 1992, 65).

In this connection, scientific research in the field of natural sciences as well as medicine is an attempt to understand the divine creation. Abdus Salam, Pakistani Nobel Prize winner for physics said: "Science is important because of the underlying understanding it provides of the world around us and of Allah's design" (Salam 1981, 98). Egyptian physician Hassan Hathout considers scientific research of nature as an Islamic duty: it is similar to prayer. A restriction of this research would be preventing an understanding of the creation of God (Hathout 1992, 70). There is, however, another attitude toward these problems. The new medical developments and techniques, especially in genetic engineering, give an impulse to voices that are critical of the first position. Munawar Ahmad Anas, Pakistani biologist and Muslim scholar emphasizes in his publications the ideological character of modern biology and denounces the "biological despotism" (Anees 1989, 11). He points out the difference between the biological image of man and the Islamic one and calls for a critical analysis of contemporary and future developments in this field. "The Islamic view of human nature does not consider biology as an inevitability. This single most important distinction between reductive, deterministic, exploitative biology and the universal worldview of Islam is crucial in the total elimination of sexism, racism and socioeconomic inequities. We must confront the biological ideology with the Islamic worldview . . . Muslim individuals must not remain prisoners to their biology that is defined only through Western technology" (Anees 1989, 15). A similar attitude is that of Osman Bakar, Professor for Islamic science in Malaysia. He underlines the holistic character of Islamic sciences and of the Islamic concept of medicine. In the Islamic world view, the value of man cannot reduce itself to bodily perfection and physical health. An application of techniques that would be based on the ignorance of this central point could not be justified from an Islamic image of man (Bakar 1999, 173–99).

IV. THE MORAL OBLIGATIONS OF PRACTITIONERS

The terms birr (reverence, piety, uprightness; see Surah 2:177 and 189), iḥsān (the showing of kindness, the doing of good works; see Surah 2:83; Surah 4:36; Surah 6:151; Surah 17:23; Surah 46:15; among others), *maʾrūf* (the good, the approved, friendliness, charity; see Surah 3:104, 110, 114; Surah 9:71; Surah 7:157; amongst others) and others appear in the Quran in a broad range of contexts and meanings. Among these, the performance of good works was given particular emphasis, so that it became a basic concept in the Islamic understanding of morality. "Persevere in doing good: behold, God loves the doers of good" (Surah 2:195).

The semantic and theological explication of these terms shows how closely linked they are to belief. In this way, doing good becomes the natural habitus of a Muslim on the basis of the close relationship between the notions of *imān* (belief) and *islām* (Izutsu 1980, 66). In the following verse, belief in the oneness of God, a central point in Islamic doctrine, is juxtaposed with the obligation to take care of one's parents, one's relatives, and the needy, a complex with reference to everyday morality:

> And worship God [alone] and do not ascribe divinity, in any way, to aught beside Him. And do good unto your parents, and near of kin, and unto orphans, and the needy, and the neighbour from among your own people, and the neighbour who is a stranger, and the friend by your side, and the wayfarer, and those whom you rightfully possess. (Surah 4:36 and similarly Surah 17:23–24)

The strong emphasis placed on a gentle and helpful attitude toward one's parents and relatives and toward the needy must be brought to bear on patients as suffering and needy people. The establishment of hospitals (*Bīmāristān*), unknown in classical antiquity, takes place very early in Islamic history. The construction of the first hospital goes back to the Umayyad Caliph al-Walīd I in Egypt (705–715). Here leprosy patients, the blind, and others were cared for and treated (Dunlop and Şehsuvaroğlu 1960, 1:1222–26). Later, hospitals were established in major cities such as Baghdad, Cairo, and Damascus by the Abbasid Caliphs al-Manṣūr (754–775) and Hārūn al-Rašīd (786–809) and other caliphs and statesmen. These hospitals rapidly became the places where physicians and nurses were trained, and this made the towns where they were established important centers of medical science (Hamarneh 1997, 158–254). They were often financed from state funds or by foundations (*waqf*) set up specifically for the purpose (Surty 1996, 56; Yediyıldız 1993, 13:153–72).

The period between the eighth and tenth centuries saw the translation of many works – primarily from Greek, but also from other languages – into Arabic. The translation movement was especially supported and encouraged under the Abbasid Caliph al-Maʾmūn (813–833). Alongside the classical sources of Islam, the translated medical works of Hippocrates, Galen, and other texts of classical antiquity have had a major influence on the emergence of a medical code of ethics (Plessner 1974, 423–460; Klein-Franke 1982, 68–84).

In the ninth century, Isḥāq b. ʿAlī al-Ruhāwī (Ibn Abī Uṣayba 1884, 254) argued in his work *Adab aṭ-Ṭabīb* ("The Ethos of the Doctor"; Bürgel 1966, 337–60, 1967a, 90–102) that two things are necessary for the medical practice of the physician, and that ethics is appropriate to the profession and scientific competence. Following Aristotle (Nic. Eth. III, 5, 1112 b13), he compared the qualities required in a ruler and a physician with respect to their obligations. Because the physician is a ruler of the body and the soul, which are more valuable than any possessions, he bears more responsibility than the ruler of a state (al-Ruhāwī 1985, 8). Al-Ruhāwī requires from a doctor moderation (*iʾtidāl*) in all areas of life (Bürgel 1967a, 90–102). Above all else, wisdom should be preferred to wealth.

> The physician must not be vengeful, envious, hasty, sad, vexed, or greedy; on the contrary [he must be] forbearing with regard to faults, indulgent with people, steady, erudite, soft, humble, quick to do good, content, thankful, and with great praise as being far from sin, virtuous, and clean inside and outside. (al-Ruhāwī 1967a, 60a)

> The justice of the physician and its beginning is that it is necessary to be good, training and taking care of oneself by cultivating good morals and actions, with sympathy, mercy, gentleness, chastity, courage, and generosity; by being just, keeping a secret, and other things such as these. These are the virtues of the soul and its proper cultivation. One must also work to acquire the skill [of medicine], studying its books and their content so as to practise it and to bestow it [i.e. its benefits] on all people without distinguishing between friend or foe, in agreement or disagreement.[4] (al-Ruhāwī 1967a, 111b)

According to al-Ruhāwī, good medical training and the study of old, popular personalities is not adequate to become an exemplary physician. He required other actions and characteristics that are no longer discussed in the context of medical ethics and instead viewed as private matters. Al-Ruhāwī gave normative guidelines on such topics as the selection of one's circle of friends, the extent of piety, dealing with money, and emotional reactions to particular events.

ʿAlī b. Sahl Rabban aṭ-Ṭabarī (d. 855) declared in his work *Firdaus al-ḥikma fīʾt-ṭibb* ("Paradise of Wisdom"), dedicated to the Abbasid Caliph al-Mutawakkil (847–861), that the maintenance of health and treatment of illness are the main goal of medicine (Rabban aṭ-Ṭabarī 1928, 558).

To practice medicine, Rabban aṭ-Ṭabarī required the following characteristics from a physician:

> In them [sc. the physicians], five qualities are united
> which are united in no others. The first of these is
> the continuous care of that from which they hope to
> provide well-being for everyone, second, their bat-
> tle with illness and with suffering which is hidden
> from their view, third, respect for kings and the com-
> mon people who have great need of their services,
> fourth, the agreement of all people with respect to
> their skill, fifth, the name for them, which is bor-
> rowed from the name of God. (Rabban aṭ-Ṭabarī
> 1928, 4)

The way in which medical care is to be applied is also
mentioned. "He [sc. the physician] should be gentler to a
sick person than to his own family, and supply his need
more quickly than his own" (Rabban aṭ-Ṭabarī 1928, 4).

Ṣāʾid ibn al-Ḥasan (d. 1072) made similar demands on
doctors to those of al-Ruhāwī and Rabban aṭ-Ṭabarī in his
work *Kitāb at-Tašwīq aṭ-Ṭibbī* (Book of the Empowerment
of Medicine) and discusses the qualities of a physician "on
whom one can depend and to whom one can entrust the
care of patients." Intellectually, a doctor should "possess
much understanding, an acute mind, and a good imagination" (Ṣāʾid 1968, 11b). In terms of his character, he
should not be curious about the affairs of other people,
"neither greedy for gain, nor jealous of possessions" (Ṣāʾid
1968, 11b), not garrulous, lazy, self-satisfied, or proud. In
the area of medical knowledge, he ought to be familiar
with the classical works and gather experience by visiting
hospitals; he should also study auxiliary sciences such as
mathematics. He should keep secrets and be moderate in
his humor and relaxation. A physician should pursue the
lifestyle assigned to him in Islam: "He should refrain from
becoming addicted to the pleasures of wine, and should
not be obsessed with leading an indecent and dissolute
life" (Ṣāʾid 1968, 12a). Even the extent to which a doctor
should ask questions and the way he speaks are important
to Ṣāʾid ibn al-Ḥasan: "He should have compassion and
speak gently" (Ṣāʾid 1968, 11b). "He should ask the necessary questions politely and ask nothing which he does
not need to ask. He should maintain health and treat the
sick with thoughtfulness and friendliness" (Ṣāʾid 1968b,
17b). If he does this, God promises to help him.

In the aforementioned works, classical authorities such
as Hippocrates and Galen play a special role in the presentation not only of medical science but also of medical ethics. Despite numerous common positions on topics in medical ethics, such as the problem of abortion,
euthanasia, the doctor's duty to maintain confidentiality, it does not seem appropriate to describe the medical
ethics of the Islamic Middle Ages as a copy of the Hippocratic ethics. There are significantly different emphases
in Islamic medicine. It is more concerned with preventive

medicine. The Greek ideal of the beautiful body is notably
absent. Moreover, the equal treatment of friends and
enemies, the rich and the poor, citizens and slaves, for
example, was not the common way of behaving within
the structure of ancient Greek society. Recommendations
such as "he [sc. the doctor] should be merciful towards
the weak and the poor by treating them before he treats
the rich" (Ṣāʾid 1968b, 12a–12b) or "he should be gentler to a sick person than to his own family, and supply his
need more quickly than his own" (Rabban aṭ-Ṭabarī 1928,
4) assume an altruistic attitude shaped by basic Islamic
norms. Another important point of difference with Hippocratic medical ethics is the attitude of the physician
toward chronic illnesses. Whereas the Hippocratic dicta
urged physicians to refrain from treating those "overmas-
tered" by their diseases, Islamic medical ethics prohibits
any refusal on the part of the doctor to treat chronic illnesses. Even if the physician cannot heal the illness, he
should alleviate the suffering caused by it (Taschkandi
1968, 25).

Another distinctive characteristic of Islamic medicine
is the way in which God is declared to bear final responsibility for the physician in the case of immoral actions.
Belief in God, in his Prophet, and in the Holy Scriptures
is viewed as an indispensable foundation for medical practice. Any moral failure on the part of a doctor, therefore,
is to be traced back to a lack of faith or piety. "When
Hippocrates says that the physician should be good by
nature, this requirement is to be fulfilled in Islam through
his commitment to religion" (Taschkandi 1968, 14). With
respect to the problem of abortion, al-Ruhāwī quotes the
Hippocratic Oath and at the same time declares the performance of an abortion to be a moral failure on the part
of the doctor, a disbelief or a lack of the fear of God: "If
you understand, O friend, you have the advice of the great
Hippocrates. He said that you must not mind the impa-
tience of a woman whom you see distressed and afflicted
due to her gestation, and not pity her or give her a remedy to make her foetus fall. *Whoever does so has no fear of God*"
(al-Ruhāwī 1967a, 60a–60b; emphasis added).

V. THE MORAL OBLIGATIONS OF PATIENTS

From the fundamental Islamic texts discussed so far, we can
discern two basic preferences for the patient, with corresponding implications for behavior. First, the Islamic catalogue of commandments and prohibitions, the keeping
of which is viewed as the natural implication of Islamic
belief, and second, the maintenance of one's own bodily health as a claim of God on one's life. The religious
conviction that declares health to be a gift entrusted to
humankind implies at the same time a human responsibility for its maintenance or restoration. An understanding
of faith that asserts that a person is not the real owner
of his body, but rather only its owner in this life, obliges

him or her to handle it appropriately. It is therefore an Islamic duty to observe appropriate hygienic measures or to submit to the medical measures necessary to maintain or restore health (Ilkilic and Veit 2004). This is because Muslims will be held accountable in the next life for the way in which they treated their bodies, which will have consequences in terms of reward or punishment.

In the classic works, special obligations are also formulated for patients. Al-Ruhāwī recommended that a patient who wants to follow the instructions of his doctor should first inquire about his doctor's scientific competence and moral character to protect himself from later negative consequences (al-Ruhāwī 1967a, 73a). If the patient meets an excellent doctor, he should obey him with body and soul. Al-Ruhāwī is convinced that effective medical practice depends on mutual trust between the doctor and the patient. Trust in the doctor will mean that the patient will follows the physician's instructions. The patient should respect his doctor, treat him in a friendly way, be helpful to him in the course of his treatment, follow his instructions, and avoid negative thoughts about his illness. No reasonable person should hide anything from his doctor, so that he makes no unnecessary mistakes (al-Ruhāwī 1967a, 70b–74a). Al-Ruhāwī noted that, like the physician, the patient too, when healthy, strives for virtue and does not allow himself to be controlled by his desires. Whoever refrains from anger and animosity and practices patience and strives to develop a good character will also bear the time of illness well. The situation for someone who is disciplined as a healthy person is similar. He will find it easier to cope with dietary restrictions than an undisciplined person (al-Ruhāwī 1967a, 77b). Ṣāʾid ibn al-Ḥasan warned the patient about false doctors and charlatans, and advised him to follow the instructions of physicians and to refrain from satisfying desires that have a negative influence on the healing process (Ṣāʾid 1968, 40b). Rabban aṭ-Ṭabarī made a knowledgeable,

compassionate, skillful doctor who looks successful a condition of healing. In addition, he advised the patient to obey his doctor's dietary instructions and to bear his treatment patiently (Rabban aṭ-Ṭabarī 1928, 560).

VI. CONCLUSION

According to Islamic world view health as well as illness belong to life with their specific meanings. As the two most basic sources of Islam, the Quran and the tradition of the Prophet Muhammad have not only shaped the Muslim understanding of illness, but also influenced the corresponding moral values for doctors, patients, and society since the seventh century. The body is a gift from God and the Muslim is responsible for his health. It is an Islamic obligation to submit in case of illness to the necessary medical treatments. To do religious and social duties, a healthy body and soul is needed, and for health the medical art. Therefore, the study and practice of the medical art is an Islamic duty. Through this service to humankind medicine is given the status of "the noblest of all arts." On account of this positive approach to medicine as well as natural sciences they were taken over and integrated from other cultures. Through this taking over, ethical principles were also adopted but on the condition that these did not interfere with the Islamic image of humankind.

NOTES

1. Translation by M. Pickhall.
2. All quotations from works of classical Arabic literature in this chapter are my own, except when otherwise noted.
3. I have made some changes in the English translation of al-Ghazālī.
4. I have made some changes in the English translation of al-Ruhāwī.

Part V

The Discourses of Philosophy on Medical Ethics

CHAPTER 18

THE DISCOURSES OF PHILOSOPHICAL MEDICAL ETHICS

Robert B. Baker and Laurence B. McCullough

I. INTRODUCTION

There is a comforting certitude about this chapter's title. It indicates the intersection of two fields, philosophy and medical ethics, suggesting to readers that they will find within it an account of philosophical discourses on medical ethics in various cultures over the course of time. This veneer of titular certitude is misleading. Undoubtedly, most healing traditions embrace some notion that healers have some special responsibilities; however, these notions of responsibility did not assume the form that we now call "medical ethics" until the nineteenth century, when the expression medical ethics, and its counterparts (e.g., déontologie médicale (medical deontology)) were coined (see Chapters 1, 32, 36). Moreover, for most of human history, it was not philosophy but religion and civil society/law that served as the dominant discourses of social authority. The Hippocratic Oath, for example, opens with an invocation of the gods, not with an appeal to philosophical concepts. Even Thomas Percival (1740–1804), who coined the expression medical ethics in his eponymous work, *Medical Ethics* (Percival 1803), originally titled it "Medical Jurisprudence," in an attempt to draw on the social authority of *law*, which was far more authoritative than philosophy or ethics. Complicating matters

further, even in those eras when philosophy commanded social authority, few physicians seem to have read much philosophy. Moreover, had these few sought moral guidance from philosophers, they would have found few relevant texts. For a while, a number of philosophers had been trained as physicians – Aristotle (384–322 BCE), William James (1842–1910), John Locke (1632–1704), and Bernard Mandeville (1670–1733) – they were typically silent about medicine and the conduct of its practitioners.

It might appear, therefore, that, until relatively recently, philosophers had little social authority, had little to say about medicine or its ethics, and that, even if they had said something, physicians would have been disinclined to pay attention to it. This, indeed, is the conclusion reached by Daniel Fox, one of the few historians to examine the influence of philosophy on medical morality. Consequently, Fox suggests there is a "curious *disconnection* of medical ethics from contemporary ideas about individual and social behavior" (Fox 1979, 81; see also Veatch 1995b, 2005). In this chapter, we offer an alternative to Fox's disconnection hypothesis, providing an account of the influence of philosophy on medical morality that explains the "disconnection" phenomenon while establishing a deeper sense of connectivity.

II. A METHOD OF ANALYZING PHILOSOPHICAL INFLUENCE

Given Fox's astute and entirely accurate observation that physicians seldom pay attention to philosophical ethics, one has to wonder whether philosophy ever exerted an influence on medicine or medical ethics. To answer these questions we draw on the work of two theorists: philosopher Hans-Georg Gadamer (1900–2002) and historian of science, I. Bernard Cohen (1914–2003). Gadamer emphasizes the notion that philosophy exerts its influence on medicine across a temporally "long horizon." Thus, concepts and bits of ideas or theory fragments found in the writings of long-dead philosophers, such as Cicero (103–143) and Plato (427?–347 BCE), can influence medicine long after their original culture context has vanished and the author's intent has been forgotten (Gadamer 1996). Moreover, to turn to a model used by I. Bernard Cohen to analyze the stages by which an innovative idea is transformed into conventional wisdom (Cohen 1985), such influence is typically exerted through a four-stage process. In the initial stage, an innovator – a physician or medical scientist – toys with adopting a philosophical concept or theory fragments to address topics in medical practice or research. In stage two, innovators appropriate philosophical concepts or theory fragments into their own thought and writings, recontextualizing them for medicine and giving them a sense specific to medicine or medical ethics. Stage three involves the dissemination of the medically recontextualized philosophical concepts or theory fragments to a wider medical audience, who receives it, *not* as philosophy but as medical ethics. Finally, stage four, medically recontextualized philosophical concepts or theory fragments become the received view, or the conventional wisdom in a given medical community. After their acceptance as medical, the philosophical origins of these concepts and theory fragments will have been forgotten – giving rise to the phenomena underlying Fox's disconnection hypothesis. There is one interesting exception to this pattern: medically recontextualized concepts or theory fragments may be reconnected with their philosophical origins if they prove controversial. Proponents of the controversial concept or discourse then typically appeal to the social and intellectual authority of the original philosophical source in an effort to valorize and legitimate the contested concept or theory fragments.

Linguistic data can provide a means of documenting this process. Linguistically speaking, conceptual innovation typically requires new terminology (e.g., medical ethics), or a new way of applying, reading, or interpreting older terms or usages (e.g., sympathy, professional). It is sometimes possible to find evidence of an innovator toying with a new usage (stage one). More typically, one finds linguistic evidence of stage two: an innovator

repeatedly using a new usage or adopting an old usage in new ways, so that it becomes integral to the language of this one person, to the innovator's idiolect (i.e., one person's way of using language). For a new concept or usage to spread from the speech or writings of some physician or scientist influenced or inspired by philosophy to the medical community generally, it has to leap from that person's idiolect to a dialect used by some subgroup within the medical community (stage three), and then become part of medical/scientific discourse more generally (stage four) – perhaps even becoming a standard usage in the wider language.

Consider, as an illustrative example, a case of influence acknowledged by skeptics: the influence of philosophy, through bioethics, on professional medical ethics in the last three decades of the twentieth century. Fox and other skeptical commentators (e.g., Veatch 2005) acknowledge that bioethics – the interdisciplinary field created by philosophers jointly with clinicians, lawyers, policy makers, scientists, social scientists, and theologians in the middle of the twentieth century – draws many of its core concepts, such as, "autonomy," from philosophy. The appropriation of Kantian concepts to the practical ethical issue of protecting the human subjects of scientific research began (stages one and two) in such influential works as theologian Paul Ramsey's *Patient as Person* (Ramsey 1970). Kantian usages became widely disseminated (stage three) in the 1980s through the Belmont Report (The National Commission for the Protection of Human Subject of Biomedical and Behavioral Research 1979) and the *Principles of Biomedical Ethics* (Beauchamp and Childress 1979). These publications became the source from which they were disseminated and became integral (stage four) to the everyday discourse of bioethicists, clinicians, and researchers. By the mid-1990s, the American Medical Association (AMA) could use the term "autonomy" in documents addressed to working medical practitioners without further explanation. Thus, the AMA wrote in its Code of Ethics: "The principle of patient *autonomy* requires that physicians should respect the decision to forego life-sustaining treatment [of a patient] who possesses decision-making capacity" (American Medical Association [1994] 1999, emphasis added; for a similar empirically based approach to analyzing conceptual influence, see Evans 2002).

By tracking the path of terminology, we can thus trace the influence of conceptions across disciplines.[1] One can also use this technique to track the dissemination of a concept over time. "Euthanasia," for example, was a neologism introduced into English by the philosopher Francis Bacon (1561–1626). Writing in 1623 Bacon envisioned a medicine whose efficacy depended on an alliance with experimental science. Believing that this new medicine could transform the nature of dying, he sought to develop a concept that would medicalize the *ars moriendi* (the art of dying) to include a pain-free death. He denominated this new and, to his mind, better, medicalized way of dying with a neologism drawn from Greek terms, "eu" for good, or well, and "thanatos," for death – "euthanasia," dying well, a good death (Bacon [1623] 1868, 1875). By tracking the dissemination of the term euthanasia from Bacon's idiolect, to the dialect of eighteenth-century physicians, then into nineteenth- and twentieth-century public discourse, one can trace the influence, and transformation of the concept of *euthanasia* from philosophy, to medicine, to public discourse (see Chapter 7).

There are some limitations to this method. Consider the term "deontology," which was coined by the English utilitarian philosopher, Jeremy Bentham (1748–1832) to encapsulate the concept of a "science of duty" (Mautner 1999, 132). A few years after Bentham's death, a French physician, Maxmilien Isidore Amand Simon, appropriated the term as the title for a volume expounding upon the duties of physicians, *Déontologie Médicale* (Simon 1845; see Chapter 32). Simon's terminology was soon applied to French codes of medical conduct generally and soon meant something akin to the English medical ethics. French medical historians began to apply it to any code of medical conduct, including the Hippocratic Oath. English-language historians of medicine, apparently unaware of the Benthamite origins of deontology, later appropriated the expression, as an *alternative* to medical ethics – because they viewed the latter as improperly insinuating philosophical influence on physicians' conceptions of medical conduct. Ironically, a term invented by a philosopher had been appropriated by historians to deny the influence of philosophical ideas. One moral of this odd twist of linguistic fate – and one limitation of this method of tracking influence – is that because terms acquire new meanings over time, the transmission of terminology may not accurately represent the dissemination of a concept. To apply this method properly, one needs not only to document the transmission of terminology, but also the arguments and interpretive frameworks in which a term is contextualized.

A discourse-centered focus can also lead one to overlook forms of influence that are nonlinguistic. Bentham can once again serve as an exemplar. As many tourists to London are well aware, a wax image molded around Bentham's bones resides in the antechamber library of University College London. This attraction is visited by thousands annually in London, and by even more curiosity seekers *internationally* (a word coined by Bentham, by the way) via the Web (Bentham 2004). Yet, few who stop to gaze at Bentham's auto-icon are aware that his bones were preserved after he *voluntarily* had his body publicly dissected in a medical school. By the terms of his will, Bentham – acting on the very utilitarian theory to which he had been dedicated in life – directed his heirs to have a public dissection of his body performed

in front of medical students. Bentham's objective was to challenge the social taboos against dissection that then constrained the training of physicians and surgeons. The publicity-garnering public dissection of Bentham's body in June of 1832 set the stage for a parliamentary debate, paving the way for the passage of the Anatomy Act later that year. The Act, the earliest law permitting the consensual donation of human bodies or their parts, legalized the practice of consensual donation of bodies to medical schools (Marmoy 1958). The Bentham model of consent-based *body* donation would later serve twentieth-century bioethicists, clinicians, and policy makers as the model for cadaveric *organ* donation, setting the stage for modern transplantation practices (Baker and Hargreaves 2001).

Bentham's dramatic gesture clearly influenced British law and medical ethics around the globe, and, ultimately, medical practice. Yet, because Bentham influenced by *example*, rather than through language, our method would be insensitive to his influence, and would not have tracked it. There are thus clear limitations to the sensitivity of our method. It can both overestimate and underestimate the nature and strength of philosophical influence. Nonetheless, it is generally accurate, and, most of the elements of the four-stage model tend to be in place even in cases, like this one, in which our method is insufficiently sensitive. Thus, although Bentham's influence was asserted through a gesture, rather than linguistically, as our model suggests, his ideas were nonetheless introduced to medicine by such medical intermediaries as Sir Edwin Chadwick (1800–1890), and Southwood Smith (1788–1861), author of the famous tract *Use of the Dead to the Living* (Smith 1827) and, going back to the auto-icon, the dissector of Bentham's body (Baker and Hargreaves 2001).

Our method also leads us to approach the history of philosophical influence on medical ethics in a nontraditional manner. One perfectly reasonable approach to the history of philosophical medical ethics focuses on works in which canonical philosophers addressed ethical issues related to medicine, such as suicide and euthanasia. The virtue of this approach is that it provides a sense of the evolution of philosophical ideas relevant to medicine over the course of time. As Fox, Veatch, and other critics have pointed out, however, this approach provides no linkage between philosophical ideas and the actual thought and practices of physicians and other practitioners. Philosophy thus appears disconnected from medical thought and practice. The principal virtue of our approach is that it makes evident actual connections among philosophy, medical ethics, and medical practice.

These limitations and virtues of our methodology noted, we now turn to three case studies that document, in detail, the influence of philosophy on classical medical ethics, that is, medical ethics before the bioethics revolution. Each of these cases involves one or more philosophers, as well as a medical figure(s) who appropriates and "recontextualizes" philosophical arguments, concepts, or discourses, disseminating them into medicine. We apologize for using the awkward neologism, "recontextualizer." We use it to indicate that when physicians appropriate concepts and discourses from philosophy, they often do more than simply "apply," "translate," or "specify" a philosophical argument, concept, or discourse for medicine or science, transferring it, meaning intact, from philosophy to medicine, science, or medical ethics. Instead, they typically transform the appropriated argument, concept, or discourse, giving it meanings and uses beyond those envisioned by its philosophical originators.

All the selected cases involve canonical philosophers – Francis Bacon (1561–1626), Cicero (106–43 BCE), Hume (1711–1776), Locke (1632–1704), Plato (428/427–348/347 BCE), and Nietzsche (1844–1900) – and avoid less well-known figures and anyone whose influence might be construed as religious (Thomas Aquinas (1225 or 1227–1274)) or scientific (Descartes (1596–1650)). We have thus taken care to avoid problematic cases like that of Kong Qiu (551–479 BCE) or the Master Kong (Kong-fu zi or Kongzi), an important figure, ritually worshiped in temples, whose writings on "the way of the gentleman," along with those of his disciples, influenced medical practitioners in Imperial and modern China. Sixteenth-century Jesuit missionaries renamed the Master Kong, "Confucius," characterizing "the way of the gentleman" as "philosophy." Both designations are problematic. Because we are trying to analyze paradigm cases of incontrovertibly "philosophical" influence, we did not analyze the impact of Confucian thought on Chinese medical ethics – although insofar as Confucianism is considered philosophy, it had an undeniably profound impact on the ethics of practitioners of Chinese medicine (see Chapters 5, 11, 21, 43; Song Guo-bin 1933).

In the first of the three cases analyzed, the ideal of the sympathetic physician, the recontextualization proved noncontroversial and so the philosophical origin of the concept in question was forgotten. The concept came to be thought of as ahistoric and universal, lacking a moment of invention or introduction. In the second case – the notion of medical practitioners as professionals committed to professional ethics, specifically medical ethics – the concepts are taken to be uncontroversial and were again treated as ahistoric by medical practitioners and the public. Scholars challenging these concepts, however, recognized that the concept has a history and often discuss and critique the physician appropriator, Thomas Percival (1740–1804). Our third case involves the euthanasia of vulnerable populations proposed by lawyer Karl Binding (1841–1920) and, more importantly for our purposes, psychiatrist Alfred Hoche (1865–1943) – a proposal often seen as laying the foundation for the Holocaust, the genocide of Jews by the Nazis during World War II (see Chapters 34, 54). This proposal was controversial

from the moment of its inception, and scholars and intellectuals thus tend to be aware of its philosophical origins – although only one of the philosophers, whose ideas Binding and Hoche cited to valorize their proposal, tends to be noticed, Friedrich Wilhelm Nietzsche; the other, perhaps more culpable philosopher, Plato, tended to receive little attention, escaping opprobrium.

III. CASE ONE: THE SYMPATHETIC PHYSICIAN: JOHN GREGORY AND THE PHILOSOPHIES OF FRANCIS BACON AND DAVID HUME

The image of the ideal physician as sympathetic and caring, someone who skillfully, scientifically, and humanely attends to the needs of a trusting patient, may seem universal and ahistoric (Spiro 1993), but it is largely the invention of one physician, John Gregory (1724–1773), who presented it and published and lectured on it while he was Professor of Medicine in the University of Edinburgh, a position that he held from 1766 until his death 7 years later, at the age of only 49 (Gregory [1770] 1998a, [1772b] 1998b; McCullough 1998a; see also Chapter 30). Gregory drew self-consciously on Francis Bacon's philosophy of medicine and David Hume's moral philosophy to write the first modern, English-language monographic on medical ethics, (Gregory [1772b] 1998b) at the center of which is the concept of the sympathetic physician (Haakonssen 1997; McCullough 1998a; see also Chapter 30).

The development and dissemination of John Gregory's concept of the sympathetic physician follows the four-stage pattern in the transmission of concepts from philosophy to medical ethics detailed previously. In general, Gregory's appropriation of philosophical ideas takes a variety of different forms. In some cases, for example, Bacon's definition of medicine, Gregory simply applies concepts he finds in Bacon's philosophical writings. To a greater extent, however, Gregory adapts and extends the concepts that he takes from philosophers, recontextualizing them to create new concepts. Thus, Gregory drew on philosophical concepts he found in Francis Bacon's philosophy of medicine and in David Hume's moral physiology and moral philosophy to develop a concept of a physician in which the intellectual capacity of openness to conviction and its intellectual virtue, diffidence, is combined with the moral virtues of the capacity of sympathy, tenderness, and steadiness (McCullough 1998a). The result was the ideal of the sympathetic physician – a physician who is both open to conviction (i.e., being convinced by scientific evidence) and to the suffering of the sick. This ideal is not to be found in Bacon and Hume; it is rather a recontextualization of their ideas, a redefinition of the virtues of diffidence, tenderness, and steadiness to suit the context of clinical practice and research. Ultimately, as we shall see, his reconceptualization required Gregory to explicitly defend the "feminine" as a paramount virtue in medical ethics.

In the third stage, Gregory's medical ethics is disseminated both in the United States, by his Edinburgh students, especially Benjamin Rush (1746–1813), and, in Britain, by another Edinburgh student (although one who never studied under Gregory) Thomas Percival (1740–1804). As Edinburgh-educated and -influenced physicians spread Gregory's ideas they became profoundly influential in the nineteenth century in both Britain and the United States (see Chapter 36). A series of nineteenth-century translations seem responsible for spreading Gregory's ideas to French, German, Italian, and Spanish language and culture (see Chapter 33). Finally (fourth Stage), as the concept of the sympathetic physician becomes a durable moral norm in both medical ethics (Spiro 1993) and popular culture, the role played by Gregory and his philosophical sources, Bacon and Hume, becomes lost from public and scholarly memory.

1. The Scottish Enlightenment Context of Gregory's Medical Ethics

Gregory was a self-conscious participant in and significant contributor to the Scottish Enlightenment of the eighteenth century. Although it is common to use the expression, "the Enlightenment," as if it names a single, homogeneous intellectual, scientific, social, and political movement that emerged in Europe and the Americas in the seventeenth and eighteenth centuries, this usage is misleading. There was no single "Enlightenment." There were several related national movements with both shared and distinctive characteristics (Porter and Teich 1981). The shared characteristics included the desire to find a peaceful alternative to war, a commitment to the reform and improvement of major social institutions – including agriculture, the arts, domestic life, law, education, government, medicine, and science – and a rejection of appeal to traditional authorities to establish the truth or falsity of various claims and beliefs, whether in science, medicine, or morality.

On the European continent, the main appeal was to reason and its dictates. In sharp contrast, the Scottish Enlightenment thinkers, deeply influenced by Bacon, took their instruction in science and medicine from experience, that is, the carefully accumulated, tested, and analyzed results of natural and contrived experiments. Baconian Enlightenment thinkers cultivated a disciplined skepticism and did not embrace the quest for certainty that characterized both the German and French Enlightenments. The goal of science and moral reasoning was to develop reliable beliefs and judgments, which we can act on with confidence; the goal was not to establish self-evident truths, the denial of which would involve a contradiction or violate some other precept of pure reason.

Scottish Enlightenment figures such as Gregory held firmly to the view that instinct provided a more reliable guide to morality than reason, which they regarded as the weaker of these two basic capacities of human beings (Gregory 1765). Reason was thought of as mere calculation, matching means to ends, but not as establishing the intellectual or moral authority of ends. The other basic human capacity, instinct, provided this foundation.

Scottish Enlightenment thinkers also understood themselves to be secular thinkers, in a very particular sense. Following the Baconian method of investigating nature, including human nature, they took the view that no appeal to transcendent reality or to moral principles derived from sacred texts and traditions was required to develop reliable beliefs and judgments about the world, about human nature, and about morality and government. At the same time, reflecting the weariness with religious wars and persecution – which continued well into the eighteenth century in Scotland – Scottish Enlightenment thinkers took the view that secular ways of thinking were not necessarily hostile to religious beliefs and practices. Gregory thus devotes a considerable portion of his lectures on medical ethics to an argument to show that becoming a physician, which requires one to adopt Baconian, skeptical, experienced-based clinical science and practice, does not require a physician to become an atheist.

2. Gregory and Bacon

Gregory was familiar with Bacon's writings from his student days onward (McCullough 1998a). Sometimes he appropriates ideas from Bacon whole, incorporating them directly into his own medical ethics. Consider the definition of medicine with which Gregory opens his *Lectures on the Duties and Qualifications of a Physician* (Gregory [1772b] 1998b). Gregory defines medicine as "the art of preserving health, prolonging life, and of curing diseases" (Gregory [1772b] 1998b, 2). An earlier version of this statement is found in a manuscript titled, "Proposall for a Medicall Society," in which Gregory lists "Four Capitall Enquiries:" "1. The Preservation of Health. 2. The Retardation of Oldage. 3. The Cure of Diseases. 4. The improvement of our Nature" (Gregory 1743, 6 AUL 2206/45). Gregory takes the first three "Enquires" from Bacon's account of the "three offices" of medicine: "the first whereof is the Preservation of Health, the second the Cure of Diseases, and third the prolongation of Life" (Bacon 1875, 383). These capacities reappear, with only their order changed, in Gregory's mature work in which, to reiterate, medicine is defined as "the art of preserving health, prolonging life, and of curing diseases" (Gregory [1772b] 1998b, 2).

Another example of a case in which Gregory seems to have absorbed a concept directly from Bacon is that of *"outward Euthanasia,* the easy dying of the body" (Bacon 1875, 387). Gregory embraced this ideal in his definition of medicine, holding that medicine should develop the capacity of "making death easy" (Gregory [1772b] 1998b, 109), and that it is the duty of physicians to continue to care for the dying, "to alleviate pain, and to smooth the avenues of death" (Gregory [1772b] 1998b, 35–36). One means of doing so in Gregory's day was by the generous administration of laudanum, a liquid form of opium. This powerful analgesic, first compounded by Paracelsus in the sixteenth century, provided hope to the gravely ill for a painless dying process. In large enough doses, laudanum could provide a painless death. In this case, Gregory does not employ Bacon's terminology "outward euthanasia," but it is clear that he has absorbed and accepted the concept.

Sometimes, however, Gregory extends and recontextualizes Baconian ideas in directions not explored by Bacon, enriching a concept's scope and meaning. Bacon, for example, called for scientific investigators to be open to evidence from any source, provided it was based on experience. Gregory too requires that physicians be "open to conviction," that is, open to being convinced by reliable evidence from any quarter about what the patient's problem is and what remedies might help to address it. Intriguingly, for Gregory, any quarter includes *patients and their families*. Gregory thus extends the Baconian concept of openness so that, as a matter of intellectual integrity and with a view toward improving medical care, physicians were obligated to be open to patients' views about the management of their conditions, diseases, and injuries.

> Sometimes a patient himself, sometimes one of his friends, will propose to the physician a remedy, which, they believe, may do him service. Their proposal may be a good one; it may even suggest to the ablest physician, what, perhaps, till then, might not have occurred to him. It is undoubtedly, therefore, his duty to adopt it. Yet there are some of the faculty, who, from a pretended regard to the dignity of the profession, but in reality from mean and selfish views, refuse to apply any remedy proposed in this manner, without regard to its merit. But this behaviour can never be vindicated. Every man has a right to speak where his life or his health is concerned, and every man may suggest what he thinks may tend to save the life of his friend. It becomes them to interpose with politeness, and a deference to the judgment of the physician; it becomes him to hear what they have to say with attention, and to examine it with candour; If he really approves, he should frankly own it, and act accordingly; if he disapproves, he should declare his disapprobation in such a manner, as shews it proceeds from conviction, and not from pique or obstinacy. If a patient is determined to try an improper or dangerous medicine, a physician should refuse

his sanction, but he has no right to complain of his advice not being followed. (Gregory [1772b] 1998b, 32–34)

Gregory thus expands Bacon's concept of openness so that it becomes morally important; the capacity of being open to conviction is thus transformed into an intellectual virtue with powerful moral implications, a virtue that Gregory denominates as "diffidence." Gregory argued that the virtue of diffidence should be well developed in the professional character of the physician, so that the physician is open to the ideas and judgments of patients. Being open to them in the right way, that is, following Baconian method to assess patients' views and judgments, focuses the intellectual attention and regard of the physician on the patient. Baconian intellectual openness, recontextualized as diffidence, thus becomes an essential intellectual virtue of physicians in the proper care of patients.

3. Gregory and Hume

Just as Gregory converted the Baconian intellectual virtue of intellectual openness to conviction into the intellectual virtue of diffidence, recontextualizing it as a clinical virtue that incorporates both openness to evidence and input from patients and families, he converts the Humean virtues of moral openness to the pain and distress of others into the clinical virtues of tenderness and steadiness. These new virtues – diffidence, tenderness, and steadiness – in turn, are integrated into the concept of the sympathetic physician. Moreover, to complete the analogy, just as diffidence grounds scientific and clinical competence, the virtues of sympathy guide the use of competence primarily to benefit the patient. "Sympathy" or "humanity" – terms that Gregory uses interchangeably – does so by opening the physician, and requiring the physician to be routinely responsive, to the pain, distress, and suffering of patients.

> I come now to mention the moral qualities peculiarly required in the character of a physician. The chief of these is humanity; that sensibility of heart which makes us feel for the distresses of our fellow-creatures, and which, of consequence, incites us in the most powerful manner to relieve them. Sympathy produces an anxious attention to a thousand little circumstances that may tend to relieve the patient; an attention which money can never purchase: hence the inexpressible comfort of having a friend for a physician. Sympathy naturally engages the affection and confidence of a patient, which, in many cases, is of the utmost consequence to his recovery. (Gregory [1772b] 1998b, 19–20)

Gregory draws on Hume for this account (McCullough 1998a). Hume's principle of sympathy was developed in the context of Hume's Baconian account of morality, expounded in his *Treatise of Human Nature* ([1739] 2000).

In the *Treatise*, Hume describes sympathy as a real, causal, constituent element of human nature by which we "enter into the sentiments" of others (Hume [1739] 2000, 234). In the 1750s, Gregory closely studied and debated the *Treatise* with other members of an intellectual society that he helped to found, the Aberdeen Philosophical Society – sometimes known, not always in admiration, as the "Wise Club" (Ulman 1990). The records of the Wise Club make it clear that Gregory accepted Hume's account of sympathy as a real, constitutive, causal principle of human nature (McCullough 1998a). In 1759, for example, Gregory writes that there is a

> distinguishing principle of mankind . . . that unites them into societies & attaches them to one another by sympathy and affection . . . This principle is the source of the most heartfelt pleasure, which we ever taste. It does not appear to have any natural connexion with the understanding. (Gregory 1759, 7)

In the deliberations of the Society, Gregory considers and rejects the view advanced by his cousin, Thomas Reid, that sympathy is inadequate to motivate and regulate moral behavior by itself, that external sanctions are required to supplement sympathy (McCullough 1998).

Hume understood sympathy to be a function or expression of instinct, not reason. This view was altogether in keeping with a basic tenet of the Scottish Enlightenment that, of the two constitutive principles of human nature – instinct and reason – the former, instinct, is the stronger, inasmuch as it is the source of the ends or goals worthy of human pursuit. Morals concern action and volition; "reason alone can never produce any action, or give rise to volition . . . " (Hume [1739] 2001, 266). Hume's conception of sympathy is more complex than one might expect. It involves what Hume calls the "double relation" of impressions and ideas, which he considers to be a basic feature of human moral physiology.

Explicating this concept requires a brief review of Hume's epistemology. For Hume, impressions involved the world physically pressing against – literally impressing – the five senses of the body. Impressions thus involve an immediate unmediated experience of the world. Ideas, in contrast, are something we abstract from repeated patterns of impressions, as a matter of instinctual habit. Ideas are thus concepts under which impressions are routinely sorted and classified. When joined together into coherent groups, ideas provide our knowledge of the world.

Observing another in distress or pain routinely involves a sequence of impressions and ideas: one has the *impression* of that person being in distress or pain; one forms the *idea* of that person being in distress or pain (the first relation of impressions to ideas); one then forms the *idea* of oneself being in the same sort of distress or pain; and this routinely leads to the formation of the impression of oneself being in like distress or pain. One literally *feels* for another's pain, by

feeling distress or pain. (This is the second relation of ideas to impressions: Hence, the "double relation" of impressions and ideas form a natural, instinctual, physiological sequence.) For Hume, this double relation of impressions and ideas describes the causal sequence that underlies the phenomenon of sympathy, that is, our feelings for others in discomfort or pain.

Hume uses a vivid clinical situation to illustrate the double relation of impressions and ideas underlying the principle of sympathy.

> When I see the *effects* of passion in the voice and gesture of any person, my mind immediately passes from these effects to their causes, and forms such a lively idea of the passion, as is presently converted into the passion itself. In like manner, when I perceive the *causes* of any emotion, my mind is convey'd to the effects, and is actuated with a like emotion. Were I present at any of the more terrible operations of surgery [namely, amputations], 'tis certain, that even before it begun, the preparation of the instruments, the laying of the bandages in order, the heating of the irons, with all the signs of anxiety and concern in the patient and assistants, wou'd have a great effect upon my mind, and excite the strongest sentiments of pity and terror. No passion of another discovers itself immediately to the mind. We are only sensible of its causes or effects. From *these* we infer the passion: And consequently *these* give rise to our sympathy. (Hume [1739] 2000, 368)

Hume makes it clear that sympathy is not only present-oriented but also future-oriented.

> 'Tis certain, that sympathy is not always limited to the present moment, but that we often feel by communication the pains and pleasures of others, which are not in being, and which we only anticipate by the force of imagination. For supposing I saw a person perfectly unknown to me, who, while asleep in the fields, was in danger of being trod under foot by horses, I shou'd immediately run to his assistance; and in this I shou'd be actuated by the same principle of sympathy, which makes me concern'd for the present sorrows of a stranger. The bare mention of this is sufficient. Sympathy being nothing but a lively idea converted into an impression, 'tis evident, that, in considering the future possible or probable condition of any person, we may enter into it with so vivid a conception as to make it our own concern; and by that means be sensible of pains and pleasures, which neither belong to ourselves, nor at the present instant have any real existence. (Hume [1739] 2000, 248)

Humean sympathy is naturally at home in medical contexts and in his *Lectures* Gregory makes it the foundation of his medical ethics. As we noted previously, he believes that sympathy opens the physician to the pain, distress, and suffering of the sick and turns the attention and regard of the physician to their relief. Patients, in turn, respond to sympathy with "affection and confidence" or trust. In applying Hume's principle of sympathy in medical contexts, however, Gregory is forced to recontextualize it. One problem he faced was that medicine was an all male occupation, and he was calling upon manly physicians to assume "feminine" virtues (i.e., virtues distinctive to women) (Tong 1993). In the social discourses of eighteenth-century Scotland, being open to the pain, distress, and suffering of others was something that women were understood to be better at than men. To apply Humean ethics was thus to introduce a feminine discourse of the virtues of sympathy, including "tenderness" and "steadiness."

Gregory took as exemplars of Humean sympathy, tenderness, and steadiness his wife and the "women of learning and virtue" whom he met when he lived in London in the 1750s at the gatherings of Elizabeth Montagu's (1720–1800) Bluestocking Circle of artists and writers (McCullough 1998a). These women of learning and virtue displayed two central virtues of sympathy. The first was tenderness, the openness of the heart to the pain, distress, and suffering of others, such that relief of the other's plight becomes one's primary concern and motivation – even if considerable self-sacrifice is involved. The second was steadiness, the need to discipline the sympathetic response so that it was not too diminished, hard-heartedness, or too strong, hypochondria.

> Sudden emergencies occur in practice, and diseases often take unexpected turns, which are apt to flutter the spirits of a man of lively parts and of a warm temper. Accidents of this kind may affect his judgment in such a manner as to unfit him for discerning what is proper to be done, or, if he do perceive it, may, nevertheless, render him irresolute. Yet such occasions call for the quickest discernment and the steadiest and most resolute conduct; and the more, as the sick so readily take the alarm, when they discover any diffidence in their physician. The weaknesses too and bad behaviour of patients, and a number of little difficulties and contradictions which every physician must encounter in his practice, are apt to ruffle his temper, and consequently to cloud his judgment, and make him forget propriety and decency of behaviour. Hence appears the advantage of a physician's possessing presence of mind, composure, steadiness, and an appearance of resolution, even in cases where, in his own judgment, he is fully sensible of the difficulty. (Gregory [1772b] 1998b, 18–19)

Gregory may have appropriated the idea of sympathy from Hume, but in looking to women as exemplars of virtue in a universe of entirely male physicians, Gregory went beyond Hume. Many men who championed the Scottish Enlightenment – women played a very small role – were put off by this idea of feminine virtues as exemplars for men to follow. Gregory was sometimes ridiculed for his feminine conception of virtue, for example, when he presented his ideas at one of the famous intellectual societies of Edinburgh, the Poker Club (McCullough 1998a). Gregory was undeterred. He mounts an explicit defense of his feminine views in his *Lectures*, in a passage that is unlike any penned by Hume.

> If the physician possesses gentleness of manners, and a compassionate heart, and what Shakespeare so emphatically calls "the milk of human kindness," the patient feels his approach like that of a guardian angel ministering to his relief: while every visit of a physician who is unfeeling, and rough in his manners, makes his heart sink within him, as at the presence of one, who comes to pronounce his doom. Men of the most compassionate tempers, by being daily conversant with scenes of distress, acquire in process of time that composure and firmness of mind so necessary in the practice of physick. They can feel whatever is amiable in pity, without suffering it to enervate or unman them. Such physicians as are callous to sentiments of humanity, treat this sympathy with ridicule, and represent it either as hypocrisy, or as the indication of a feeble mind. That sympathy is often affected, I am afraid is true. But this affectation may be easily seen through. Real sympathy is never ostentatious; on the contrary, it rather strives to conceal itself. But, what most effectually detects this hypocrisy, is a physician's different manner of behaving to people in high and people in low life; to those who reward him handsomely, and those who have not the means to do it. A generous and elevated mind is even more shy in expressing sympathy with those of high rank, than with those in humbler life; being jealous of the unworthy construction so usually annexed to it. – The insinuation that a compassionate and feeling heart is commonly accompanied with a weak understanding and a feeble mind, is malignant and false. Experience demonstrates, that a gentle and humane temper, so far from being inconsistent with vigour of mind, is its usual attendant; and that rough and blustering manners generally accompany a weak understanding and a mean soul, and are indeed frequently affected by men void of magnanimity and personal courage, ['in order' added in errata] to conceal their natural defects. (Gregory [1772b] 1998b, 19–21)

Adopting feminine virtues would not "unman" physicians, leaving them with "feeble minds," but just the opposite, as Gregory shows on the basis of "experience," that is, evidence. Physicians who do not adopt the feminine virtues, however, will become like Lady Macbeth, who prayed to be "unsexed" – turned into a hard-hearted, ruthless man – because her husband was "too full of the milk of human kindness," that is, living by feminine virtues. Lady Macbeth destroyed herself and her husband. Physicians who destroy themselves by being gruff and unfeeling, by being "insensible" men, also destroy their patients.

This was a radically new conception of the physician and was appreciated as such in Gregory's day. It drew upon and unites Baconian intellectual virtues to Humean moral virtues, bringing together intellectual and emotional openness, to create a new model of the virtuous physician as diffident and sympathetic, tender but steady, each virtue complementing and balancing the other. Realized in the daily life of a physician these virtues – although drawn from Bacon and Hume – represent an entirely new ideal of the physician as fiduciary of the patient: someone open, sympathetic, committed to competence, to excellence in patient care and medical research, who will develop and use that competence primarily for the benefit of patients, making self-interest secondary.

4. Dissemination of Gregory's Baconian/ Humean Concepts

As we noted earlier, Gregory's account of the virtues of sympathy was taken up immediately by two of his successors in the English-language medical morality literature: Benjamin Rush (1745–1813) and Thomas Percival. Both had studied at Edinburgh. Rush, who had attended Gregory's lectures while still a student, brought Gregory's concept of the sympathetic physician to the newly independent former British colonies in North America (see Chapter 31). As a homage, he even appropriated as the title for his own lectures a modified form of the title of Gregory's: *Observations on the Duties of a Physician, and the Methods of Improving Medicine. Accommodated to the Present State of Society and Manners in the United States* (Rush 1805). In a lecture titled, "On the Vices and Virtues of Physicians," first delivered in 1801, Rush employs Gregorian terminology to examine the vices of physicians. Among the vices listed is "inhumanity," which Rush also characterized as "insensibility to human suffering" (Rush 1811, 124, compare Gregory [1772b] 1998b, 9). Not surprisingly, the chief virtue of physicians is said to be "humanity," which Rush valorizes as "a conspicuous virtue of physicians among all ages and countries" (Rush 1811, 129). Rush adds the following: "No sooner do they enter upon the duties of their profession, than they are called upon to exhibit their humanity by sympathy, with pain and distress in persons of all ranks" (Rush 1811, 130). This is Gregory's (Humean)

language, and Rush goes on at some length to emphasize the physician's humanity-based obligations to care for the sick poor without recompense.

The second major disseminator of Gregory's concept of the sympathetic physician was Percival, who left Edinburgh just before Gregory arrived in 1765. Percival expressly acknowledges "the excellent lectures of Dr. Gregory" as one of the sources he drew upon in writing his seminal *Medical Ethics* (Percival 1803, 6). The book opens with the following line:

> Hospital physicians and surgeons should study, also, in their deportment, so to unite *tenderness* with *steadiness*, and *condescension* with *authority*, as to inspire the minds of their patients with gratitude, respect, and confidence. (Percival 1803b, 9)

Although Percival does not explain the basis of these virtues, his physician readers would recognize their source in Gregory's medical ethics. Because *Medical Ethics* was extraordinarily influential, by incorporating Gregorian discourse into the opening lines of the book, Percival helped to disseminate widely the concept of the sympathetic physician.

Many American physicians were educated in Edinburgh, or by physicians who had studied there, and so turned to Gregory directly for guidance on moral matters (Gregory's works were immediately brought to America (McCullough 1998a) and an American edition of Gregory's lectures was published in 1817 (Gregory [1772a] 1817)). Evidence of Gregory's influence on American thought is found in two important American codes of medical ethics drafted in the 1820s and 1830s. The innovative and influential *System of Medical Ethics* adopted in 1823 by Medical Society of the State of New York explicitly cites Gregory and his student Rush, as sources of inspiration. Article I of the *System* appeals to Gregorian virtues that "A physician cannot successfully pass through his career without ... conscience, honor and humanity." Lest there be any doubt about the source of these ideals, a footnote directly references Gregory's *Lectures*. Throughout, the New York *System* appeals to Gregory, not only to justify ideals of conscience, honor, and humanity, but also the (Baconian) idea of openness to conviction. Thus, Gregory's claim that "an obstinate adherence to an unsuccessful method of treating a disease is self-conceit ... a species of pride to which the lives of thousands have been sacrificed" is expressly cited (as "Gregory, Lect. I *On the Duties*, page 28," Medical Society of the State of New York, 1823, 11) to justify the physician's obligation to accept treatment proposals favored by a majority of his colleagues.

A later *System of Medical Ethics* published by the Medico-Chirurgical Society of Baltimore in 1832 – which, as we shall see later, was very important to the evolution of nineteenth-century American codes of medical ethics – also cites Gregory's *Lectures On the Duties and Qualifications of a Physician* as influential. Following the precedent of the New York *System*, the first sentence of the code invokes the Gregorian concepts of virtue, integrity, and humanity, as attributes essential to the character of a physician. Later passages mention the key quality of sympathy. These 1823 and 1832 codes laid the foundation for the American Medical Association's code of ethics, which, as mentioned earlier, evoked Gregorian concepts parsed in Percivalean language in its first article: "Physicians should study ... in their deportment, so to unite tenderness with firmness, and condescension with authority, as to inspire the minds of their patients with gratitude, respect and confidence" (American Medical Association [1848] 1999, Chap. I, Art. I, Sec. 1; see Chapter 37).

Gregory's medical ethics was translated into French, German, Italian, and Spanish (McCullough 1998a; Chapter 29). Because the history of Gregory's influence through these translations has yet to be written, we do not yet understand the extent to which Gregory's (Baconian–Humean) ideals influenced the distinctively virtue-based medical humanism found in southern European medical ethics/bioethics (see Chapter 40) and Latin American medical ethics/bioethics (see Chapter 42). What is evident, however, is that in Italy, Spain, and in much of Latin America, the virtues of the physician play a much more prominent role in medical ethics than they do in medical ethics in Britain and the United States. It is quite possible that the forms of medical ethics/bioethics taken to be distinctive of southern Europe and Latin America may have an unacknowledged source in the Scottish Enlightenment medical ethics of Gregory, and in the British philosophers who inspired him, Bacon and Hume.

We are now very far removed from Gregory's self-conscious reliance on Hume and Bacon. As the concept of the sympathetic physician became the received view (More 1994), its philosophical origins in Gregory's appropriations and reconceptualizations of Bacon and Hume were forgotten and the concept of the sympathetic physician became an artifact of popular culture. The hero of *Arrowsmith* (Lewis [1925] 1976), struggling with the moral demands of an exemplary model of the good physician, is the conceptual heir of Gregory's medical ethics. So, too, are generation after generation of television doctors in the United States – from Drs. Kildare and Marcus Welby of old through Dr. Hawkeye Pierce of "M*A*S*H" to Drs. Ross and Green of "ER." These popularizations are seen as admirable figures precisely to the extent that they fulfill our Gregorian expectations about the character and behavior of the sympathetic physician. Indeed, so powerful is this image that, when circumstances are right (getting his arm amputated by a helicopter rotor), even the gruff and hard-hearted surgeon, Dr. Romano (also of "ER") turns out to have a heart of gold, precisely as required by the model of the sympathetic physician. Of course, in American popular culture the origins of this still-compelling model in eighteenth-century Scottish Enlightenment medical ethics – and its philosophical roots – have long since been lost from consciousness.

IV. CASE TWO: THOMAS PERCIVAL AND THE INVENTION OF THE MODERN CONCEPT OF A PROFESSION

It might seem odd to suggest that someone invented the modern concept of a profession and of professional ethics. Many commentators write as if the modern conception of a profession – the notion of a self-regulating occupation of educated individuals committed to ethical standards who dedicate themselves to serving the interests others – is a universal idea, so self-evident, that it had no particular moment of invention. Others date the origins of the concept of a profession to the Hippocratic Oath, arguing that because *profeteri* is Latin for "oath," our modern concept of a profession derives back to an oath taken by ancient Greek physicians (Pellegrino 1979, 223–25; Pellegrino and Thomasma 1981, 209–12). The origins of the modern concept of a "profession," however, are more circuitous. The concept has a history and a moment of invention, but this history and moment have nothing to do with the Hippocratic Oath, or with any other aspect of ancient Greek medicine. These do, however, have something to do with the fact that "profess" derives from the Latin verb for swearing an oath. "Originally," as historian of professionalism Samuel Haber has observed, one's "profession" was any form of "work that afforded a livelihood. The word goes back to the practice of Roman tax gatherers requiring inhabitants to declare [i.e., to profess] their occupations.... all occupations were professions then, as they still are in French usage" (Haber 1991, x). To reiterate, originally the term, profession, simply meant one's occupation – the occupation one declared to the tax collector under oath. The term lacked any moral connotations and it was not associated with collective self-regulation or with service to others.

The earliest known English characterization of medicine as a "profession" dates from 1541, when a commentator on Galen referred to the "The parties of the art of Medycyne" as "the medicynall profession." This usage suggests that because there were several medical occupations – apothecaries, physicians, and surgeons – it was convenient for anyone discussing them collectively to refer to them in terms of a collective noun phrase as "the medicynall profession" (see Edelstein 1967, 337–40; Nutton, 1993, 1995, 520).

Early English-language translations of Latin versions of the Hippocratic Oath also undercut the notion that the English concept of profession, or of the medical professions, derives from the Hippocratic Oath. The first Latin edition of the Hippocratic Corpus, including the Oath, was published in 1525; several sixteenth-century

English-language translations of the Oath were published subsequently. Translations by the cleric, Thomas Newton, (1586), and by the surgeon, John Read (1588), both use the term profession, but only in the occupational sense.[2] Neither characterizes the Hippocratic Oath itself as the "Hippocratic profession." Had they done so, they would have mistranslated the Latin because, again, at that time medicynall profession simply meant medical occupation. The modern morally freighted concept of *profession* as a self-regulating occupation dedicated to competently serving others had yet to be invented.

Signs of a drift away from the purely occupational sense of profession began to surface in mid-eighteenth-century dictionaries, such as Doctor Samuel Johnson's 1755 *Dictionary of the English Language* (Johnson [1755] 1979). The preponderance of examples Johnson cites to illustrate uses of the term, profession, are from the "liberal professions," that is, those occupations that, like law and medicine, presume literacy and formal, advanced education. This concept, "liberal profession," has clear normative implications, but the normative element derives from the term liberal. How do we know this? Because eighteenth- and nineteenth-century practitioners castigated each other for acting "illiberally" in the flyting literature (hostile exchanges of letters or pamphlets); which is to say that, because they saw education as demarcating status, they condemned each other for acting in the manner of the uneducated, that is, "illiberally." Until well into the nineteenth century, however, medical practitioners did not condemn one another for being "unprofessional," or for acting "unprofessionally." It was thus "liberal" that carried normative force in the expression, liberal profession, the term, profession, simply meant occupation.

The condemnatory use of "unprofessional" did not arise until well after the publication of Thomas Percival's *Medical Ethics: Or a Code of Institutes and Precepts, Adapted to the Professional Conduct of Physicians and Surgeons* (Percival 1803), the book that first introduced a morally freighted concept of profession and the interrelated concepts of professional ethics and medical ethics to the world. Percival's neologism, "professional ethics," expressly infuses normative content into the concept of profession. He coined the expression to reflect his new conception of professionals as members of a self-regulating learned occupation, dedicated to the service of society and to the care of others. To put the point more accurately, Percival's new concept of a profession that was inherently ethical, compounded three somewhat different notions into a new conception, laying the groundwork for centuries of uncertainty about what it is to be a professional. The three conceptions that Percival compounded were a conception of the professional as someone playing a role governed by its own internal morality of service to others, the idea of the professional as bound by a social compact in which social privileges are conferred on a learned occupation in exchange for

social obligations to serve society, and the notion of the professional as a member of a fraternal society, bound by its own self-imposed rules.

1. The Development of Percival's Medical Ethics

What makes Percival's compound conception of profession interesting for our present purposes is that, in forming it, he incorporates Gregory's (philosophically influenced) concept of the physician as sympathetic fiduciary into conceptions drawn from the works of three philosophers: Cicero, Francis Bacon, and – via the conduit of the writings of the Reverend Thomas Gisborne (1758–1846) – John Locke (1632–1704). Before discussing Percival's appropriation of ideas from these three philosophers, however, it is helpful to consider the context in which *Medical Ethics* was composed and from which the modern concept of a profession emerged: the long decade from 1792 to 1803. In this decade "fevers" like cholera and typhus were common in the factories and mills of Manchester, where Percival worked. It was a decade of intense industrialization, of worker agitation, of political ferment that included anti-slavery campaigns. It was also a decade of antirevolutionary repression, launched as the British responded to the revolution in France.

Percival and fellow Unitarians were a politically active, affluent, and influential social and intellectual elite in Manchester and other northern English cities, who were nonetheless a persecuted religious minority deprived of basic civil rights. Called "Dissenters" because they would not sign the Church of England's thirty-nine Articles of Faith, they were officially prohibited by parliamentary acts – like the Act of Uniformity of 1662 and the Five Mile Act of 1665 – from teaching in "public" schools, from holding public office, from serving on juries, from attending Cambridge or Oxford, from belonging to the royal colleges (of physicians, of surgeons) – even from legally performing publicly recognized rites, such as marriage or burial. Unofficially, they were subject to mob violence. In 1791, the year before Percival began to work on the first rules for the code that became *Medical Jurisprudence* and *Medical Ethics*, Anglican clergy incited a mob to burn the Birmingham chapel, home, and scientific laboratory of one of Percival's teachers, a fellow Unitarian, the chemist Joseph Priestly (1703–1804; see Haakonssen 1997, 94–100).

Dissenting intellectuals such as Percival and Priestly championed Enlightened religion, science, and social reform – the abolition of slavery, public health reform, labor reform – as a middle road between Tory religious, socio-economic and political conservatism, and radicalism, atheism/materialism, and anarchy/mob rule. Voluntary hospitals, like the Manchester Infirmary (a large hospital complex, at least for that period, that provided free health care to more than 1,000 inpatients and more than 5,000 outpatients annually), were an ideal expression of the middle road Dissenters sought. The Infirmary responded to the concerns of workers, who often saw factories and mills as a source of "fevers," even as it combined Christian charity with the prudent isolation of the ill, in ways that appealed to factory and mill owners.

Circa 1792 a planned expansion of the hospital was threatened by vicious flyting and pamphlet wars between rival teams of "man-midwives" (physicians who practiced obstetrics). Although nominally focusing on such issues as the ethics of Caesarean deliveries, the dispute was fueled by considerations of "turf" and religion – one group of obstetricians was Anglican, the other Dissenter. The Trustees called upon Percival, who had a great deal of experience chairing committees, to head a committee charged with drafting rules for the expanded hospital that would prevent intrapractitioner squabbling. The rules were drafted in 1792. A more dramatic version of the origins of *Medical Ethics* has the committee formed because patients were lying unattended at the gates of the fever hospital as the staff squabbled within; it is unclear what evidence supports this version (see Chapter 36; Pickstone and Butler 1984; Pickstone 1993).

Percival had served on many committees and had had the satisfaction of seeing his recommendations implemented at the institutional and national level, (e.g., in the Health and Morals of Apprentices Act of 1803, (Pickstone 1993, 167)), but his committee work seldom inspired literary ambitions. The report of 1792 was different. It served as the core for the first chapter of a four-chapter code of ethics that Percival circulated in a small edition in 1794 under the title, *Medical Jurisprudence: Or a Code of Institutes and Precepts, Adapted to the Professional Conduct of Physicians and Surgeons* (Percival 1794). Because Percival's papers were destroyed in the German bombing of Manchester during World War II, and because the only Percival correspondence available is the selected "literary letters" that Percival's son chose to publish in *The Works* (Percival 1807), one can only speculate about why Percival published *Medical Jurisprudence* (1794); or why he published a revised version as *Medical Ethics* (1803b) – or why he created the concepts of *professional ethics* and *medical ethics* for the revised edition.

We do know, however, that in 1793 Percival was corresponding with a younger admirer and fellow antislavery reformer, the Reverend Thomas Gisborne. The correspondence was about a chapter that Gisborne was drafting on the duties of physicians for his forthcoming work, *An Enquiry into the Duties of Men in the Higher and Middle Classes of Society in Great Britain Resulting from their Respective Stations, Professions and Employment* (Gisborne 1794a). Because Percival had just written a draft code of ethics in 1792, reading drafts of Gisborne's chapter on the duties of medical practitioners may have inspired Percival to produce his own work on the subject – a work that he could dedicate

to his eldest son, James, who was then entering medical school. What is certain is that the two corresponded, that each read the others drafts, and that each influenced the other's writings (Gisborne 1794, 383; Percival 1803, 157–59).

We also know that after James's death in 1793, and after a small 1794 printing of the short text that circulated under the title *Medical Jurisprudence* received mixed reviews – including a hostile reaction to its title – Percival dropped the project. The project was reinstituted in 1803 when Percival's younger son, Edward, became a medical student. The volume is dedicated to Edward, just as Percival had intended to dedicate it to James, a decade earlier. Appended to the volume, as a memorial, is a sermon by a deceased middle son, Thomas. Also appended, in the form of notes, are a miscellany of replies to critics and comments and fragments on variety of subjects, such as dueling. Taken together with Percival's prefatory remark that "experience[ing] the pressure of advancing years" he had come to "regard [*Medical Ethics*] as the conclusion . . . of [his] professional labours . . . [as well] as a paternal legacy" (Percival 1803, ix, x), it is reasonable to read *Medical Ethics* as something of a memorial to Percival himself. It was also a defense of Enlightenment idealism and of the Dissenters' middle road of science and social reform, which, in the early 1800s, were facing political repression. More, pragmatically, reissuing the book might assuage a resurgence of flyting and pamphlet wars that were again threatening to destabilize Percival's beloved Manchester Infirmary (Pickstone 1993, 171).

Medical Ethics was thus a volume produced under duress. Percival wanted to defend his conception of a code of medical conduct from critics, he wanted to memorialize his life, his work, his dead sons, the retreating ideals of the Enlightenment and the Dissenter's middle road of science and sympathy – and he had to do this as he was going blind, which, as spelling changes suggest, probably forced him to dictate sections of the book. (Compare the older spelling of chirurgical in the 1803 Preface, p. 6, for example, with Percival's consistent preference for the more modern spelling, surgical in 1794.) In this context, Percival abandoned his controversial title, *Medical Jurisprudence*, retitling his code, *Medical Ethics*.

Percival implies that he chose the title, *Medical Ethics*, to align his efforts with Gisborne's, which Percival characterizes as "the most complete system, extant, of PRACTICAL ETHICS" (Percival 1803, 5). Gisborne, however, never used the expression, "practical ethics," in his published work; he employs, instead, the somewhat similar expression, "applied moral philosophy." Perhaps Gisborne had used the term in his personal correspondence with Percival, or perhaps the near-blind Percival misremembered Gisborne's terminology and substituted a usage popular in eighteenth-century Scottish moral philosophy (Beauchamp 2007). Whatever the case, Percival's twin neologisms, "medical ethics" and "professional ethics," are constructed in a way that echoes the expression, "practical ethics," that Percival attributes to Gisborne.

Thus, pressured to defend his code against various criticisms, Percival coined these neologisms and – more to the point of this chapter – attempted to valorize them by drawing on philosophical authorities: Cicero, Gisborne, and Francis Bacon. Because Gisborne's applied moral philosophy involved "applying" the social contract theory of John Locke, the justification that Percival offers of his conception of a profession, of professional ethics, and of medical ethics was to be found not only in Cicero or Bacon, but also, via Gisborne, in the work of John Locke.

In the discussion that follows, we will use textual analysis to paint a detailed portrait of Percival's appropriation of concepts and quotations from philosophers to defend, to valorize, and to justify his code. We will also track his decade-long recontextualization of philosophical concepts to create the new conceptions of profession, professional ethics, and medical ethics. Finally, we will show how, as Percival's conceptual innovation became commonplace, its Percivalean and philosophical origins become obscured and forgotten, so that they came to be perceived as ahistoric and universal, and thus without a moment of invention.

2. Percival's Recontextualization of Cicero: Offices, Duties, and Roles

Before turning to Cicero, the first philosopher Percival cites in defending his work, it is important to reemphasize that, as is clear from the subtitle to Gisborne's *Enquiry*, "*Duties of Men in the Higher and Middle Classes of Society in Great Britain Resulting from their Respective Stations, Professions and Employment*," Gisborne is using "profession" in the occupational sense, that is as a form of "employment" – although nonetheless asserting that, like stations and other employments, there are duties required, not of all men, but of men in the higher and middle classes of society, as they pursue their professions/occupations. These moral duties derive from these men's privileged status in society, *not* from the nature of their occupations/professions. In *Medical Ethics* and its earlier incarnation, *Medical Jurisprudence*, however, Percival claims that it is the very nature of medical practitioners' occupations that creates their moral obligations, or, at least, their obligations to their patients. To defend this view Percival turned to Cicero.

Both the 1794 and 1803 editions of Percival's code open with precisely the same words. In the first sentence of the first section/chapter in *Medical Jurisprudence/Ethics*, Percival states that "HOSPITAL PHYSICIANS and SURGEONS should minister to the sick, with due impressions of the importance of their *office*; reflecting that the ease, the health, and the lives of those committed to their charge depend on their skill, attention, and fidelity" (Percival 1794, Sec. I, Art. I; 1803b, Chap. I, Art. I, emphasis

added). The pivotal term in this passage is *office*. The term is drawn from the philosophy of Marcus Tullius Cicero ("Tully," as his eighteenth-century English admirers called him). The physician/surgeon–patient relationship had been discussed by Gregory and by Gisborne, as Percival acknowledged (Percival 1803, 5, 6). As we discussed previously, however, Gregory found the moral basis of this relationship in moral sense, specifically, sympathy (Gregory [1770] 1998a, 102–4); Gisborne believed that its moral basis lay in a tacit social compact between patient and physician (Gisborne 1794, 396).

Neither account suited Percival in 1794. He was a student of the realist philosopher John Taylor (1694–1761), who believed that morality had to be grounded in something more substantial than "mechanical instincts," such as sympathy; for although such instincts may assist morality, Taylor considered them "but crutches" for the proper principles of morality (Taylor 1759, 43). Percival was thus initially unwilling to ground the morality of the physician–patient relationship in what Taylor saw as mere sentiments, or in some unstated tacit social compact. Instead, he invoked the Ciceronean notion of medicine as a duty-generating "office."

Apparently the allusion to Cicero on "offices" was lost on some of Percival's 1794 critics; so, Percival prefaced the 1803 *Medical Ethics*, with a quotation, in Latin, from Cicero's *De Officiis*, (On Office/Duty). An English rendering of the passage is:

> For no phase of life, whether public or private, whether in business or in the home, whether one is working on what concerns oneself alone or dealing with another, can be without its moral duty [*officio*]; on the discharge of such duties depends all that is morally right, and on their neglect all that is morally wrong in life. (Cicero 1923, II:7)

Percival was probably attracted to this quotation from *De Officiis* because, as historian Ludwig Edelstein (1902–1965) has observed, *De Officiis* contains an implicit "program of professional ethics."[3] According to Cicero, occupations suitable for gentlemen – judge, lawyer, and teacher – invoke special *roles* that carry with them role-specific duties or offices of *service to others*. This commitment to service allows a true gentleman to accept the demeaning fact that compensation is associated with these occupations; they are thus social "roles" that true gentlemen can properly play without lowering their gentlemanly status.

Cicero invented the concept of a social "role." He introduced the concept by asking readers to consider the case of a judge passing judgment on a friend.

> An upright man will never for a friend's sake do anything in violation of his country's interests ... *for he lays aside the role of a friend when he assumes that of judge.* (Cicero 1923, III:311, emphasis added)

Edelstein translates the italicized line as, "for he lays down the role (or mask) of the friend when putting on that of the judge" (Edelstein 1967, 342).[4] Thus, for Cicero, gentlemen, in appropriately gentlemanly occupations/professions, step into roles the way actors in classical theater don masks. Each of these roles carries with it an attendant set of duties. It was thus the duties/offices of any gentleman playing the role of "HOSPITAL PHYSICIAN and SURGEON" that Percival signaled himself as describing when he used the word office in the first sentence of *Medical Jurisprudence*. The quotation from Cicero that prefaces the later work, *Medical Ethics*, was designed to assist those insufficiently erudite to catch this reference.

By 1803, however, Percival was doing more than simply appropriating the concept of *office/duty* from Cicero. In *Medical Ethics* – but not in its precursor of 9 years earlier, *Medical Jurisprudence* – he renames these offices/duties, christening them "professional ethics." In the dedication to his son Edward that prefaces *Medical Ethics* – the point at which Percival introduces the neologism professional ethics to the world – Percival characterizes the content of professional (medical) ethics as the extensive moral duties and relations in which a medical professional "stands to his patients, to his brethren, and to the public." He then informs Edward that these obligations do *not* derive from being a gentleman, but rather "The study of professional Ethics [and] the observance of the duties which they enjoin will... form you to that propriety and dignity of conduct, which are essential to the character of a GENTLEMAN" (Percival 1803b, viii–ix). Professional ethics is thus a subject that can be studied independently of one's understanding of gentlemanliness and, if one understands professional ethics and acts on its precepts, one will assume the essential characteristics of a gentleman.

The newly christened concept of professional ethics thus recontextualizes Cicero's conception of a role-generated duty/office by inverting the relationship between gentlemanliness and being a professional. For Cicero, and for Gisborne, one's status as a *gentleman* created one's role-related responsibilities in various "Stations, Professions and Employments," to use Gisborne's turn of phrase. For them, being a "gentleman" brought ethical standards into the roles one played – brought ethics into employments, occupations or professions suitable to gentlemen. Percival was claiming the opposite: that acting as a "professional," according to the standards of professional ethics, would make one a proper gentleman. He thus transformed the concept of a profession, from an "occupation that a gentleman could take up without demeaning himself" to one, which, in the words of historian Samuel Haber, "more wondrously, [were] occupations that might make someone a gentleman simply by his taking it up" (Haber 1991, xi).

Thus, the first conception of professional medical ethics – defined as practitioners' moral relations and duties to their patients, their peers, and the public – delineated by Percival in 1803 was a recontextualized Ciceronian role ethic in which a practitioner's moral duties were *not* derived from his gentlemanly status, that is, they were not a function of practicing medicine "like a gentleman," but were implicit in the very nature of the practitioner's office, role, or "profession." *Medical Ethics*, the first work to declare itself a work of professional ethics, was thus an attempt to formalize, or make explicit, duties toward patients, peers, and the public implicit in the role of being a medical professional.

3. Percival's Appropriation of Gisborne/Locke's Social Compact

It took a decade for Percival to reconceptualize Cicero's concept of office into professional ethics. In the course of that same decade his interpretation and acceptance of Gisborne's Lockean notion of a "social compact" evolved as well. Gisborne had developed the notion in his first book, *The Principles of Moral Philosophy Investigated and Briefly Applied To the Constitution of Civil Society* (Gisborne 1789). *The Principles* not only applied John Locke's social contract theory to "the constitution of civil society," it defended the Lockean social compact against a major critic, William Paley (1743–1805). Paley held that members of society were bonded to each other, not by a social compact, but through their shared history as a civil society, that is, by tradition (Paley [1795] 1985). Gisborne rejected this traditionalist account, arguing that the moral warp and woof of society was a web of reciprocal obligations – the idea encapsulated in the metaphor of the "social compact." Those who accepted the protection of society's laws – in particular, those who enjoyed the privilege of its higher stations, professions, and employments – had *tacitly* contracted to accept a set of duties to society. Gisborne's second book, *An Enquiry into the Duties of Men in the Higher and Middle Classes of Society in Great Britain Resulting from Their Respective Stations, Professions and Employment* (Gisborne 1794a, 1795) was a social contractarian rendition of a traditional genre, "the gentleman's manual," designed to detail the specific reciprocal duties incumbent upon men who were ministers, barristers, physicians, and so forth, by virtue of their tacit social compact with society. A later companion work, *An Enquiry into the Duties of the Female Sex* (Gisborne 1794b), specifies the duties of women.

Despite the effusive praise that Percival heaps on Gisborne's *Enquiry* in the preface to *Medical Ethics* – "a work that reflects the highest honour the abilities and philanthropy of its author; and which may be justly regarded as the most complete system, extant, of Practical Ethics" (Percival 1803b, 5) – Percival was initially cool to the concept of a tacit compact. In *Medical Jurisprudence*, Percival alludes to the idea of a tacit compact (specifically to Gisborne 1794, 383) precisely once: in the opening passage of Section Four. There, Percival invokes the notion of reciprocity to counter a claim by a famous figure, Sir William Blackstone (1723–1780), that was directly antithetical to the notion of medical jurisprudence in general, and to the subject of Section Four, "Of the Knowledge of Law Requisite for Physicians and Surgeons." Blackstone had proclaimed the study of law is "less essential to [physicians] than to any other class of men" (Percival 1794, Sec. 4, Art. I). Percival replied that because society gave legal privileges to physicians, they were obligated to study the law. This point noted, Percival does not again mention or allude to Gisborne's tacit compact in 1794. He relies instead on an unexplicated Ciceronian concept of office.

By 1803, under pressure to clarify and defend the notions attributed to office in *Medical Jurisprudence*, Percival warmed to the concept of a tacit compact. In addition to citing reciprocity to counter Blackstone's claim that medical practitioners need little knowledge of the law in Chapter Four – now retitled, "Of *Professional Duties* which require a Knowledge of Law" (emphasis added) – Percival expressly posits tacit compacts between professionals and those who pay their fees (Percival 1803b, 177), among members of a profession, and between professions and society. In an intriguing passage he further appeals to the contractarian idea of reciprocity to generate a new concept – one that must have appeared self-contradictory at the time – the notion that the *private* practice of medicine is really a "*public* trust." This concept is introduced as part of new material added to Section II of *Medical Jurisprudence* to create Chapter II of *Medical Ethics* "Of Professional Conduct in Private, or General Practice." Here, Percival poignantly reflects on his declining mental and physical powers.

> The commencement of that period of senescence, when it becomes incumbent on a physician to decline *the offices* of his profession, it is not easy to ascertain ... But in the ordinary course of nature, the bodily and mental vigour must be expected to decay progressively ... As age advances, therefore, a physician should, from time to time, scrutinize impartially, the state of his faculties; that he may determine ... the precise degree in which he is qualified to execute the active and multifarious offices of his profession. And whenever he becomes conscious [of failing abilities] ... he should at once resolve, though others perceive not the changes which have taken place, to sacrifice every consideration of fame or fortune, and to retire from the engagements of business. To the surgeon under similar circumstances, this rule of conduct is still more necessary ... Let both the physician and surgeon

never forget, that *their professions are public trusts, properly rendered lucrative whilst they fulfil them; but which they are bound, by honour and probity, to relinquish, as soon as they find themselves unequal to their adequate and faithful execution.* (Percival 1803b, Chap. II, Art. XXXII; emphasis added[5])

The Ciceronean concept of the offices of [ones] profession is here tied to the Gisbornean/Lockean notion of reciprocal obligation – the notion underlying the metaphor of the tacit social compact – to argue that professionals' prerogatives obligate them to relinquish their privileges, however lucrative they may be, when they can no longer fulfill "the multifarious *offices*" of their professions. The social compact thus regulates the internal morality of professional offices/duties, converting professional conduct in *private* medical practice into a *public* trust that medical professionals are "bound by honour and probity" to respect. This new notion – that professions are public trusts – expands the domain of professional ethics beyond the confines of public institutions, like hospitals, into the sphere of private practice. It also transforms deeply personal decisions – when to retire – from the private sphere to the public domain, creating, in the process, the modern notion of professionals as publicly accountable for their private actions.

4. Bacon and the Concept of Professions as Tacit Compacts among Professionals

Percival defined professional medical ethics as the moral duties and relations in which medical professionals stand to their patients, to their brethren, and to the public. In both 1794 and 1803, he justified the obligations of medical professionals toward their patients by appealing to a Ciceronian conception of role-specific duties or offices; in 1803, he justified a liberal profession's obligations to the public by appealing to the Gisbornean/Lockean concept of a tacit social compact. How did he justify medical professionals' third set of moral duties, their duties to each other? What justifies peer enforcement of the "moral rules of conduct" in "*private* practice?" Specifically, what justifies the pivotal peer arbitration rules that lie at the core of *Medical Jurisprudence/Ethics*: the obligation to submit disputes over "professional conduct" to peer arbitration by fellow professionals, privately, without seeking public vindication of their personal honor by flyting or publishing hostile pamphlets? What justifies rules like the following?

> [When] controversy, and ... contention ... occur, and can not be immediately terminated, they should be referred to the arbitration of a sufficient number of physicians or surgeons ... or to the orders of both collectively ... But neither the subject, nor the adjudication, should be communicated to the public; as

they may be personally injurious to the individuals concerned, and can hardly fail to hurt the general credit of the faculty. (Percival 1794, Sec. II, Art. XX; 1803b, Chap. II, Art. XXIV)

Hospital trustees had institutional authority to regulate practitioner conduct with respect to institutional matters (as is evident from the rules Percival's committee drafted for the Manchester Infirmary (Percival 1803, 144–47)). Yet, in the passage cited above, Percival vests moral authority for adjudication of disputes in private practice *in the clinicians themselves*, not in the trustees. There was some precedent for clinician arbitration of disputes in the *Statutis Moralibus* (Moral Statutes) of the Royal College of Physicians, but the authority to arbitrate was deeded to the College by the crown. Nonetheless, as Percival remarks, "whatever merit or authority [the *Statutis Moralibus*] possess, [they] are not sufficiently comprehensive for the existing sphere of medical or chirurgical duty" (Percival 1803, 6). The idea of peer self-regulation in private practice generally exceeded traditional authority and it is likely that critics of Percival's 1794 manuscript would have pointed this out to him.

In 1803, Percival offered a justification for peer adjudication of disputes. He invokes Gisborne's "tacit compact," valorizing the notion by turning to an authority far better known than Gisborne. He invokes the patron philosopher of all medical reformers, Francis Bacon, citing the following passage from Bacon's *Elements of the Common Lawes of England* (Bacon [1630] 1969).

> *I hold every man a debtor to his profession; from which as men of course do seek to receive countenance and profit, so ought they of duty to endeavor themselves, by way of amend, to be a helpful ornament thereunto.* This is performed, in some degree, by the honest and liberal practice of a profession, when men shall carry a respect not to descend into any course that is corrupt and unworthy thereof; and preserve themselves free from the abuses wherewith the same profession is noted to be infected. (Bacon [1630] 1969, cited at Percival 1803b, 3, emphasis added)

In the text of Chapter II, however, Percival recontextualizes Bacon's notion that "every man [is] a debtor to his profession" in terms of Gisborne's Lockean "tacit compact."

> The *Esprit de Corps* is a principle of action founded in human nature, and when duly regulated, is both rational and laudable. *Every man who enters into a fraternity engages, by tacit compact, not only to submit to the laws, but to promote the honour and the interests of the association, so far as they are consistent with morality, and the general good of mankind.* A physician, therefore, should cautiously guard against whatever may injure the general respectability of his profession; and should

avoid all contumelious representations of the faculty at large; all general charges against their selfishness or improbity; and the indulgence of an affected or jocular skepticism, concerning the efficacy and utility of the healing art. (Percival 1803b, Chap. II, Art. XXIII, emphasis added; no comparable section in Percival 1794)

This article was inserted in front of the contentious claim that "[When] controversy, and . . . contention . . . occur, and can not be immediately terminated, they should be referred to the arbitration of a sufficient number of physicians or surgeons, . . . or to the orders of both collectively" (Percival 1803, Chap. II, Art. XXIV; a reiteration of Percival 1794, Sec. II, Art. XX). Thus, having valorized the idea that individuals were debtors to their professions by citing Bacon, Percival borrows Gisborne's Lockean concept of the tacit compact to justify professional self-regulation – "submission to the laws of one's profession" – and, more controversially, at least at that time, peer adjudication of intrapractitioner disputes between private practitioners. Because of their collective interest in their profession, because all professionals are debtors to their profession, professionals must obey "the laws of their profession" and submit to arbitration of their disputes by fellow professionals, so that their disputes can be resolved without damaging "the general respectability of the profession."

The notion of professions as *self*-regulating occupations was thus conceived out of the pressing need to *justify* a set of rules requiring peer arbitration of flyting and other conflicts, that is, self-regulation. Note the order of invention: the rules came first, in 1792 and 1794; their philosophical *justification* in terms of a Bacon/Gisborne/Locke debt/tacit compact came later, in 1803. This pattern is quite different from Percival's turn to philosophy in the two earlier instances examined (and from Gregory's appropriate of concepts from Bacon and Hume). The applied ethics model evident in Percival's introduction of the Ciceronean "office" in the first sentence of *Medical Jurisprudence* is easy to appreciate. He borrowed a concept from a philosopher, and later, under pressure, identified the philosophical origins of the concept. Percival thus seems to be *applying* a concept drawn from Cicero (much as Gregory applied Bacon's concepts of "outward euthanasia," and "openness to conviction"). The first cases provide clear instances of "applied ethics," that is, applying a philosophical concept in a new context. As we noted previously, however, the rules of professional adjudication of 1792 and 1794 precede the debtor/compact philosophical justification offered in 1803. This is thus *not* a case of applied ethics, or of recontextualization, but of something different. It might be called "justificatory" – turning to philosophical to validate, valorize, or justify some precept that one has already accepted.

Once evoked, however, the justificatory concept of the tacit fraternal compact does more than justify the right of professionals to adjudicate disputes between peers. It also empowers them to set the laws of the profession, widening the mandate of professional self-regulation far beyond the original adjudicatory function stipulated in the rules being justified. A new and broader conception of the prerogatives of the profession was thus conceived out of the need to justify a preexisting rule. Although justificatory appeals to philosophy are ad hoc – decidedly after the fact – they thus have the power to change "the fact" by providing new frameworks for interpreting and justifying the facts, so to speak. As we shall see, the historical importance of this passage would lie in the compact metaphor's justificatory role in legitimating professional self-regulation: specifically, the warrant it gave to medical organizations to regulate the conduct of their members.

To summarize, in the decade between 1794 and 1803, critical pressure forced Percival to search for justificatory language, metaphors, and arguments from philosophers. As he did so, he transformed the concept of a profession from that of a liberal occupation to an occupation bound by an internal Ciceronian role morality of office to serve others, bound by internal laws that its members have tacitly compacted to obey, and bound to serve society by a tacit compact that converts their private practices into a public trust. Applying, borrowing, and recontextualizing arguments, concepts, discourses, and metaphors from philosophers, found first- and second-hand (through Gisborne), to justify his rules of professional conduct, Percival transformed the older notion of medicine as a liberal profession into the modern concept of a profession, inventing the concepts of professional ethics and medical ethics in the process. The combination of practical need, pragmatic innovation, visionary ideals, and justificatory demands led him to rummage through the thoughts of philosophers to produce, under pressure, something entirely new and previously unimaginable.

5. The Assimilation of "Professional" and "Professional Ethics" into Medical Discourse

In previous sections we detailed the evolution of Percival's neologisms – professional ethics and medical ethics – showing how they came to encompass the modern notion of a profession as a self-regulating, educated occupation and a public trust, bound by its own internal morality and dedicated to serving others. As we have seen, to develop each of these elements Percival drew on the ideas and authority of philosophers – Cicero, Locke (indirectly through Gisborne), and Bacon (reparsed using Gisborne's discourse) – openly acknowledging his sources and intellectual debts. In terms of our version of Cohen's schemata, this is a second-stage appropriation, a recontextualization and valorizing/justifying use of philosophical concepts.

The third stage of the process involves the dissemination and absorption of Percival's new concepts of profession and professional ethics into medical discourse, and the subsequent fourth stage of shedding of their philosophical origins, until, finally, the concepts become so conventional that they appear ahistoric, atemporal, and all memory of their philosophical origins has been lost.

The dissemination of Percival's concepts was convoluted. Until well into the twentieth century the British tended to treat medicine as a liberal, gentlemanly occupation, and their discourse and organizational patterns reflected this (see Chapter 36). It was the Americans who experimented with Percival's new concepts. In the early years of the nineteenth-century American municipal, county, and state medical societies hewed to the British model of gentlemen's associations, governed by a sense of gentlemanly honor – adding bits and pieces of new ideas borrowed from Gregory and from Gregory's American disciple, Benjamin Rush. They turned to Percival's *Medical Ethics* only for practical guidance, eschewing his conceptual innovations – medical ethics, professionalism, and professional ethics.

In 1808, for example, when the Massachusetts legislature deeded licensing authority to the Association of Boston Physicians, the association borrowed extensively from *Medical Ethics* to draft a formal code of conduct. It called its code a "Medical Police," echoing a traditional expression "hospital police" that Percival used (Percival 1803, 7). Drawing, often verbatim, from Chapter II of *Medical Ethics*, the resulting "police" regulated members' conduct in "Consultations," "Interferences," "Differences of Physicians," "Discouragement of Quackery," "Fees," "Exemptions from Charges," "Vicarious Offices," and "Seniority." The "Medical Police" contained no sections regulating practitioner–patient relations or addressing practitioners' obligations to the public. A section justifying the self-regulatory authority of the society to police itself reproduces the "tacit compact" passage from *Medical Ethics* almost verbatim – with one significant difference, "association" was substituted for "profession."

CONDUCT FOR THE SUPPORT OF THE MEDICAL CHARACTER

The *esprit du corps* is a principle of action, founded in human nature, and, when duly regulated, is both rational and laudable. Every man, who enters into a fraternity, engages, by a tacit compact, not only to submit to the laws, but to promote the honour and interest of the *association*, so far as they are consistent with morality and the general good of mankind. A physician, therefore, should cautiously guard against whatever may injure the general respectability of the profession, and should avoid all contumelious representations of the faculty at large, all general charges against their selfishness or improbity, or the indulgence of an affected or jocular scepticism, concerning the efficacy and utility of the healing art. (Association of Boston Physicians [1808] 1995, 44, emphasis on "association" added[6])

Notice that although Percival's notion of a (Lockean) tacit compact is invoked to legitimate the authority of a specific medical *association* over its members, it is not invoked to justify the authority of a *profession* over its members. The substitution of the term association for profession is significant. *Medical Ethics* was a professional ethics, providing moral guidance for everyone in the medical profession. In contrast, the Boston "Medical Police" is a set of rules that apply only to members of a particular association, not an ethics applicable to the profession as a whole – a professional ethics – that happens to be endorsed by a particular association. As one might expect, therefore, although the term profession is used twelve times in the Boston Medical Police, it is always used in the occupational sense. The first occurrence, for example, states that "Medicine is a liberal profession; the practitioners are, or ought to be men of education" (Association of Boston Physicians [1808] 1995, 42). Physicians, moreover, are characteristically referred to as gentlemen (a term used six times) or designated as "regular practitioners;" they are warned, moreover, not to make "a mere trade of a learned profession" or to "evince a meanness of disposition, unbecoming the character of a physician or a gentleman" (Association of Boston Physicians [1808] 1995, 42–43). These expressions are indicative of a conception of medicine as a liberal occupation suitable for gentlemen. It was thus appropriate for the Association of Boston Physicians to refer to their code as a medical police – a set of rules for the gentlemen who were members of a particular association. In 1817, the Connecticut Medical Society adopted virtually the same code, renamed a "System of Medical Police." This gentlemen's association model of medical police was dominant among American medical associations until almost mid-century.

The first medical societies to experiment with alternative conceptions of self-regulation – to try out the thought of themselves as "professional" societies – were the Medical Society of the State of New York and the Medico-Chirurgical Society of Baltimore. Significantly both self-regulatory codes abandoned the title 'medical police,' favoring instead a more properly Percivalean title, "A System of Medical Ethics." The New Yorkers were the first to break new conceptual ground. In 1821 the medical society charged a two-person committee – John H. Steele (d. 1838) of Saratoga and James R. Manley (1782?–1851) of New York City – with "collect[ing] and form[ing] a system of Medical Ethicks, to govern the profession in their intercourse with each other, and particularly in cases of consultation" (Medical Society of the State of New York, 1823); that is, the Society charged them with pro-

ducing a code governing intra-practitioner relations on Boston/Connecticut model. Steele, apparently considered this mandate confining and the two-man committee found itself at an impasse. So another New York City physician, Felix Pascalis (1762?–1833), was appointed to the committee.

Like Manley, Pascalis was an editor of the *Medical Repository* (1821), the first American medical journal (Kahn and Kahn 1997). In this capacity Manley and Pascalis had often appealed to Percival's *Medical Ethics* to deal with issues of professional integrity. About the time the committee was formed, for example, they published an editorial in which they cited *Medical Ethics* (Chap. I, Art. XII) to condemn a team of upstate physicians for proclaiming a cure for rabies in the popular press, without first submitting their cure to what we would today call "peer review" by fellow physicians.

Manley and Pascalis's familiarity with *Medical Ethics* may explain why the three-man committee decided that a medical police governing practitioner–practitioner conduct dealt with "but a small part of the moral duties of physicians and surgeons." The society, they claimed, needed a code that would "embrace all the maxims and precepts of Medical Ethics and Police which have been sanctioned by reputable authority, in relation to the personal character of the profession; to their practical acts, and to the information frequently required of them by magistrates and courts of justice." (Manley, Pascalis, and Steele 1823, 3). The Medical Society of the State of New York adopted the proposed system of medical ethics without dissent. It had five "Divisions:" "Personal Character of Physicians," "Quackery," "Consultations," "Specifications of Medical Police in Practice," and "Forensic Medical Policy."

The New York "System of Medical Ethics" was thus conceived to be more than a "medical police," because it included of discussions of the personal character of practitioners, practitioner–patient relations, and medical jurisprudence – now renamed "forensic medicine." Moreover, unlike codes of medical police, this system of ethics laid claim to being, not merely a code of conduct for a particular medical association, but a system of ethics for the *profession* of medicine, interpreted for members of New York medical societies. As is evident from the section titles, in the outline, *A System of Medical Ethics* parallels Percival's *Medical Ethics*; however, the nonforensic additions tend to be more strongly influenced by the writings of Gregory (who is cited seven times; Percival is cited only twice). Moreover, the expression, professional ethics, does not appear in *A System*; whereas the term, profession, appears eighteen times, and it is used in ways consistent with the occupational sense: professional avocations, learned professions, privileges of his profession, importance of the medical profession, professions of Medicine and Surgery, members of the same profession, professional acts, professional reputations, professional qualifications, trade or profession, and professional fees (Manley, Pascalis, and Steele 1823, 6, 8, 9, 14, 17, 18, 19).

Only in Sections XX and XXI of Division IV, "Specifications of Medical Police in Practice," do the authors appeal to such notions as the "highest [moral] aim of the profession" as a whole (Manley, Pascalis, and Steele 1823, 18); they also discuss individual practitioners' obligations to "contribute as far as is in their power, to the honor, improvement, and utility of their professions." That passage continues:

> According to this precept [i.e., that medical professionals have an obligation to contribute to the honor, improvement, and utility of their professions] physicians and surgeons have something more to do, than to procure their livelihood. As they are indebted to the labors, talents and experience of their predecessors in the healing art for all that constitutes its admirable body of doctrine; so present and future generations look to them for some improvement, because much can yet be done to extend its usefulness. This obligation is unbecomingly violated by many physicians who pretend to eminence. (Manley, Pascalis, and Steele 1823, 19)

These passages invoke Percival's Baconian conception of individual practitioners as debtors to their profession, intimating reciprocal obligations between members and their profession. In passages like these, the New Yorkers seem to be entertaining something akin to Percival's concept of a profession. Despite these intimations, however, the robust Percivalean sense of profession is, for the most part, only immanent in New York's *A System of Ethics*.

Nine years later, in 1832, the Committee on Ethics of the Medico-Chirurgical Society of Baltimore embraced a more robustly Percivalean concept of a profession and professional medical ethics. Heading the five-member committee was Eli Geddings (1799–1878), Chair of Anatomy and Physiology at the University of Maryland and, like Pascalis and Steele, editor of a medical journal (the *Baltimore Medical and Surgical Journal and Review*, 1831–1837). Serving with Geddings were surgeons such as Henry Willis Baxley (1803–1876), and physicians such as John Fonerden (1804–1869). The committee prepared *A System of Medical Ethics* making "free use . . . of Percival's Ethics, the abridgement of the same by the κ. λ. [Kappa Lambda] Society of Philadelphia, Gregory's Lectures . . . the Code of Ethics [of] the New York Sate Medical Society, that of the Connecticut Medical Society, Rush's . . . Lectures . . . and Ryan's Medical Jurisprudence" (Medico-Chirurgical Society of Baltimore 1832, 5).

A System opens with a statement of the demands for "virtue, integrity, benevolence and humanity" made on the physician by "the very nature of his profession," that is, it sets forth the idea of an internal morality of the medicine, created by the "nature" of the "profession." Having noted the moral demands made on physicians and remarked on the confidence society places in them, it makes a reciprocity claim: "For all these acts then, how great are the obligations of the community to *the medical profession*, and how well earned the high and unlimited respect and confidence which it has at all times secured whenever its duties have been exercised with honor, integrity and humanity" (Medico-Chirurgical Society of Baltimore 1832, 5–6, emphasis added). In this interesting gambit the Baltimore society both demands reciprocity from society, and reassures medical professionals that "historically" whenever they have acted with integrity, honor, and humanity, society has reciprocated appropriately.

These demands for reciprocity between profession and society are concretized in Section V of the System, which stipulates the "Duties of Patients towards their Physician."

> *The members of the medical profession*, upon whom are enjoined the performance of so many important and arduous duties towards the community, and who are required to make so many sacrifices of comfort, ease, and health, for the welfare of those who employ them, certainly have a right to require and expect, that their patients should entertain a due sense of *the reciprocal duties which they owe their medical attendants*. These have been very clearly detailed by the celebrated Rush. (Medico-Chirurgical Society of Baltimore 1832, 19, emphasis added)

There follows a list of duties that patients have toward their physicians. These deal with: the type of physician to be selected; the duty to consult a physician, to communicate "faithfully and unreservedly to their physician, the history and cause of their disease," and to obey the "prescriptions of [one's] physicians;" the duty *not* to seek a second opinion, until after first consulting with one's own physician; and the duty to send for physicians in the morning, to credit one's physician for cures, and to "remunerate him properly" (Medico-Chirurgical Society of Baltimore 1832. 19–23).

In passages like those quoted above, the Baltimore society tends to use the expression "medical profession" in ways that reflect Percival's conception of a profession as bound by social compact to serve society, but with a different emphasis: they draw on this conception to stress the patient and community's reciprocal obligations to the profession. In keeping with the general theme of reciprocity, the notion of fraternity in Percival's tacit social compact passages seems gratuitous. It was thus replaced by the notion that members are indebted to their profession on grounds of reciprocity.

> XI. Every individual, on entering *the profession*, as he becomes thereby entitled to all of its privileges and immunities, incurs an obligation to exert his best abilities, to maintain its dignity and honor, to

exalt its standing, and extend the bounds of its use-fulness. He should therefore observe strictly, such laws as are instituted for the government of its members: – should avoid all contumelious and sarcastic remarks relative to the faculty, as a body, and while, by unwearied diligence he resorts to every honorable means of enriching the science. (Medico-Chirurgical Society of Baltimore 1832, Sec. I, Art. XI, p. 11)

Article XI, quoted above, marks the point at which the notion of profession clearly supplants the idea of fraternity in American codes of medical ethics. The tacit compact metaphor for reciprocity has been replaced by a direct appeal to reciprocity and so expressions such as fraternity and tacit compact are now superfluous. In consequence, they are deleted.

The transition is supported by a host of passages drawn from, or strongly influenced by, Percival (e.g., Medico-Chirurgical Society of Baltimore 1832, e.g., Sec. I. Art. VI–XI; Sec. II Arts. I, I, Sec. III, Art. I, X, Sec. IV Art. I, III, VIII; "office" is in Sec. I. Art. VII), although always with an emphasis on medicine as a profession. In summary, although the Baltimore *System of Medical Ethics* is something of a pastiche, it nonetheless envisions medicine as a self-regulating profession, whose members are bound, in reciprocity, to obey the stipulations of their profession's ethics. It is the first code to integrate the idea of the tacit compact into the concept of profession, and thus the first to incorporate a robust Percivalean concept of professionalism into its text.

In developing and strengthening this Percivalean conception of the medical profession, the authors of Baltimore *System* acknowledge their debt to the extracts from Percival's *Medical Ethics* published by the Kappa Lambda society of Philadelphia (Anonymous 1823). The extracts comprised Chapter I, Article I of *Medical Ethics* (i.e., the article explaining the *offices* of physicians and surgeons), plus thirty-one of the thirty-two articles of Chapter II (including the *tacit compact* passage). These were edited for an American audience, eliminating parochially British usages and concerns. All three Percivalean conceptions of professional ethics were incorporated in this edition: professional ethics as a Ciceronian role ethics predicated on duties of office to one's patient (Anonymous 1823, Art. 1), as a liberal occupation whose members are bound by a tacit fraternal compact to obey the laws of their profession (Anonymous 1823, Art. 23), and as a public trust (Anonymous 1823, Art. 32). Percival's dedication and preface, however, were not reprinted, neither were any references to the philosophical origins of Percival's ideas.

The Philadelphia edition of the Kappa Lambda extracts from Percival's *Medical Ethics* is important not only because it was widely circulated and because of its influence on the Baltimore *System of Ethics*, but because the editors of the

publication John Bell (1796–1872) and Isaac Hays (1796–1879) headed the committee that, in 1846–1847, drafted the Code of Ethics that the AMA adopted on a unanimous vote at its founding meeting in 1847. This code is the primary vehicle through which the Percivalean conception of professional medical ethics and of medicine as a profession – as interpreted and enhanced in the Baltimore *System of Ethics* – was disseminated throughout the United States.

Unfortunately, a penumbra of vagueness surrounds the actual circumstances under which the AMA Code of Ethics was drafted. Hays had proposed founding the AMA, he also proposed drafting a code of ethics for the new organization, and he actually organized the founding meeting of the AMA – always acting through the agency of others. As a Sephardic Jew, Hays had experienced intolerance and was uncertain of his reception in public fora. When he edited journals, or acted as a committee chair, he preferred eminently Christian voices to speak on his behalf (see Chapter 36; Baker 1999, 23–25). So when Bell, the nominal head of the committee, presented the code to the founding convention, he read aloud "some explanatory remarks" *on behalf of* "Doctor Hays," who chose not to address the convention directly.

On examining a great number of codes of ethics adopted by different societies in the United States, it was found that they were all based on that by Dr. Percival, and that the phrases of this writer were preserved, to a considerable extent, in all of them. Believing that language that had been so often examined and adopted, must possess the greatest of merits for a document such as the present ... having no ambition for the honours of authorship, the Committee which prepared this code have followed a similar course ... A few of the sections are in the words of the late Dr. Rush, and one or two sentences are from other writers. But in all cases, wherever it was thought that the language could be made more explicit by changing a word, or even a part of a sentence, this has been unhesitatingly done; and thus there are but few sections which have not undergone some modification; while, for the language of many, and for the arrangement of the whole, the Committee must be held exclusively responsible. (Hays [1847] 1999, 315)

Note that Bell is reading a report drafted by Hays explaining the work of the committee. The fact that Hays was the authority on the committees work suggests that he may actually led the committee's work, with Bell serving a figurehead. This suspicion tends to be confirmed by Bell's speech introducing the Code of Ethics to the Conference, which, although filled with lofty sentiments, seems more in tune with the Baltimore *System* than with the code presented to the AMA by the committee.

The code drafted by Committee draws many of its articles directly from the *Extracts from the Medical Ethics of Dr. Percival* that Bell and Hays had edited for Kappa Lambda almost a quarter of a century earlier. It was also strongly influenced by the Baltimore *System of Ethics*. It differed from its precursors, however, because it was framed as an explicit social compact among patients, physicians, and the public. Just as the United States constitution was a formal social compact between the government and its people, formally stating the rights and responsibilities of each, so too the 1847 AMA Code of Ethics set out to be a social compact, specifying the rights and reciprocal obligations of physicians, patients, and the profession to each other. The titles of the code's chapters reflect this framework of reciprocal obligations: the "Duties of Physicians to their Patients and . . . the [reciprocal] Obligations of Patients to Their Physicians;" "Duties of the Profession to the Public and [reciprocal] Obligations of the Public to the Profession."

The use of the term "profession" in the titles of the AMA Code's last two chapters is indicative of a profession that has duties and to which duties are owed. The term profession is used fprty-one times in the AMA code of ethics; medicine is characterized as a "liberal profession" only once. More often physicians (a term that, after the 1820s embraced surgeons as well as physicians, in American usage) are referred to as professional men, having undergone a professional education, making professional visits, in professional attendance, offering professional services, and – most importantly – as having professional obligations. As to the source of these professional obligations, the AMA Code (echoing Percival, Chap. I Art. I) still grounds physicians' duties to patients in their office, but it modernizes the concept of office by referring to it as a "mission." As in Percival, this mission is regulated by a series of social contracts; however, following the precedent set by Baltimore code, the metaphor of the social contract is rendered otiose by explicit statements of reciprocal obligations. The AMA code thus reproduces, verbatim, the Baltimore rendition of Percival's tacit compact as the first article in the chapter titled "Of the Duties of Physicians to Each Other and to the Profession at Large." Thus, following the Baltimore *System*, the expressions tacit compact and fraternity have disappeared – replaced by the (modern) concept of a profession and professionalism.

Art. I. *Duties for the support of professional character*

1. Every individual, on entering *the profession*, as he becomes thereby entitled to all its privileges and immunities, incurs an obligation to exert his best abilities to maintain its dignity and honor, to exalt its standing, and to extend the bounds of its usefulness. He should therefore observe strictly, such laws as are instituted for, the government of its members;

should avoid all contumelious and sarcastic remarks relative to the faculty, as a body; and while, by unwearied diligence, he resorts to every honorable means of enriching the science, he should entertain a due respect for his seniors, who have, by their labors, brought it to the elevated condition in which he finds it. (American Medical Association [1847] 1999, 327–28)[7]

Completing the contractarian conception of professions is "Chapter III: Of the Duties of the Profession to the Public, and of the Obligations of the Public to the Profession." Article I of this chapter lays out the duties of the profession to the public, which include: "giving counsel to the public in relation to matters especially appertaining to their profession, as on subjects of medical police, public hygiene, and legal medicine;" and the most demanding of all obligations – an obligation well beyond that in any previous statement of medical ethics – "when pestilence prevails, it is [the physician's] duty to face the danger, and to continue their labors for the alleviation of the suffering, even at the jeopardy of their own lives" (AMA [1847] 1999, Chap. III, Art. I, Sec. 1, 333). Chapter III also states a professional duty to "recognize [poverty] as presenting valid claims for gratuitous services . . . to individuals in indigent circumstances, such professional services should always be cheerfully and freely accorded" (AMA [1847] 1999, Chap. III, Art. I, Sec. 3, 334). In reciprocity, the profession seems to demand relatively little: "The benefits accruing to the public directly and indirectly from the active and unwearied beneficence of the profession, are so numerous and important, that physicians are justly entitled to the utmost consideration and respect from the community." In respecting the profession, however, "the public ought likewise to entertain a just appreciation of medical qualifications; – to make a proper discrimination between true science and the assumption of ignorance and empiricism, to afford every encouragement and facility for the acquisition of medical education," that is, the public ought to discriminate between the regular profession and its irregular competitors (AMA [1847] 1999, Chap III. Art. II, Sec. 1, 334).

After its founding in 1847, the AMA disseminated its Code of Ethics widely. It became the subject of editorials in the medical and popular press, it became integral to the medical school curriculum; and it was translated into French, German, Japanese, and other languages. Wherever it was printed, read, or discussed, the code carried with it the modern concept of a profession. In 1855, the AMA's Code of Ethics became binding on all member organizations, which is to say every regular medical society and medical school, every asylum, dispensary, and hospital in the United States. In response, the code was again widely reprinted. Discussion in the *Transactions of the American Medical Association*, soon moved from the code's content to code enforcement and, in consequence, such expressions as "unprofessional conduct" began to appear.

In the 1880s, there was an anti-code-of-ethics revolt initiated by "no code" and "new code" factions of the Medical Society of the State of New York (see Chapter 36). New coders wanted to redefine the fiduciary and public service components of professionalism in terms of an ethics of competence (in which to be professional is simply to be technically competent in a learned self-regulating occupation), while "no coders" wanted to return to the gentleman's association conception of medical organizations, and to a purely occupational, pre-Percivalean, conception of medicine as a profession. In combination, these factions managed to seize control of the AMA, and to replace its code of ethics with "Principles of Medical Ethics" (American Medical Association [1903] 1999, 335–45). They also abolished the AMA's mechanisms of ethics enforcement; however, they could not change the meaning of professionalism (although later specialty societies formed outside of the AMA adopted the competence model of professionalism). The 1903 *Principles* still embraced the fiduciary "mission/office" of the physician to the patient (Chap. I, Sec. 1), of the individual practitioner to the profession (Chap. II, Secs. 1, 2), and of the profession to the public (Chap. III, Sec. 2) – including the obligation to "labor for the alleviation of suffering people, even at the risk of their own lives" (American Medical Association [1903], Chap. III, Sec. 2, 344). The *Principles* were revised and strengthened in 1912, and 1957, and are still enforced today (American Medical Association [1912] 1999, 346–54; [1957] 1995 355–57). In 1908, the American Bar Association published its "Canons of Professional Ethics," definitively disseminating the concept of professionalism and professional ethics to another "profession."[8]

By the early twentieth century, a robust version of the Percivalean concept of a profession and professional medical ethics had become commonplace throughout the United States and the world. Although the AMA sometimes acknowledges its debt to Percival's code, virtually no one credits him with inventing the modern concept of a profession, or of professional ethics, much less acknowledges his application, recontextualization, and justificatory use of concepts and metaphors drawn from the philosophers Cicero, Bacon, and (via Gisborne) Locke, in inventing the concept of professional ethics. More commonly, as noted earlier, these concepts are either (incorrectly) presumed to trace back to the Hippocratic Oath, or assumed to be universal, ahistoric and thus lacking a moment of original conception or invention. As predicted on our model, once a philosophically inspired concept becomes commonplace, it will be presumed ahistoric and its invention and philosophical origins will be consigned to the dustbin of history.

V. CASE THREE: PLATO AND NIETZSCHE: "BALLASTEXISTENZ," "PARASITES," AND "USELESS EATERS"

There is an important exception to our claim that when an originally philosophical argument, concept, model, or discourse becomes commonplace, or part of the conventional wisdom, its philosophical origins will be forgotten. Insofar as an originally philosophical concept remains controversial, its philosophical origins will tend to be remembered. One notion whose philosophical origins linger in the social memory was promulgated around the Western world in the early twentieth century: the notion that people with disability, especially mental disability, are "parasites on society" whose lives are "meaningless to themselves and others," and that doctors consequently have a "professional and social duty to kill them."

In tracing the origins of the concepts of "the sick person as a parasite on society," as "useless eater," as mere "ballast existents" – and the notion that doctors have a duty to abandon or to kill such parasites, useless eaters and *Ballastexistenzen* – we follow the same procedures as we did earlier. We locate a second-stage appropriation of philosophical arguments, concepts, discourses, or metaphors by a medical professional or professionals, and we then track them through their third-stage dissemination and fourth-stage acceptance as conventional wisdom. In contrast to the cases analyzed previously – the sympathetic physician, the physician as a professional bound by professional ethics – readers are unlikely to find it congenial to entertain the concept of a physician as an executioner of the disabled. They are also likely to find repellent any association between this distasteful idea and such cultural icons as Plato and Nietzsche. It is not our role as historians, however, to present the history of the impact of philosophical discourse on medical ethics only insofar as that history is edifying; our role is to present it even when – perhaps especially when – it is not. To speculate: had World War II a different ending, it is possible that readers of this volume might have regarded the notion that physicians considered themselves to have professional obligations to rid society of "social parasites" to be an admirable advance in "medical ethics."

In point of fact, this conception of the physician's role had many distinguished proponents in the first half of the twentieth century. In the 1930s, for example, Franco-American Nobel Laureate Alexis Carrell (1873–1944) of the Rockefeller Institute for Medical Research, a committed eugenicist, proposed that the mentally ill should "humanely and economically be disposed of in small euthanasia institutions supplied with the proper gases" (Carrel [1936] 1988, 180). As it happens, however, Carrell's ideas carried little influence in the cultural-linguistic sphere that experimented with "euthanizing" children and others with mental disability and illness. It was in Germany in the 1930s that physicians would implement a "eugenic euthanasia" program that closely resembled that envisioned by Carrell. Here is an eyewitness account:

> The director of the Eglfinger-Haar asylum, Herman Pfannmüller, an admirer of Hoche [whom he had, met personally (Burleigh 1994, 103)] gave tours of the eugenic-euthanasia program to young physicians.
>
> SINCE I had studied psychology in 1934/1935 as part of my professional training... I took part in a conducted tour... The asylum director... Pfannmüller, led us into a children's ward... [He] explained... "As a National Socialist, these creatures... naturally only represent to me a burden upon the healthy body of our nation. We don't kill (he may have used a more circumlocutory expression...) with poison, injections, etc., since that would only give the foreign press and certain gentlemen in Switzerland new hate propaganda material. No: as you see, our method is simpler and even more natural." With these words, and assisted by a nurse... he pulled one of the children out of the bed. As he displayed the child around like a dead hare, he pointed out, with a knowing look and a cynical grin, "This one will last another two or three days." The image of this fat, grinning man, with the whimpering skeleton in his fleshy hand is still clear before my eyes... A lady who also took part in our tour asked, with an outrage she had difficulty suppressing, whether a quick death aided by injections would not be more merciful. Pfannmüller sang the praises of his method as being more practical in terms of the foreign press. (Lehners, quoted in Burleigh 1994, 45–46)

Where did German physicians get the notion that *"these creatures ... naturally only represent to me a burden upon the healthy body of our nation?"* Where did they get the notion that it was their *duty* to devise "methods" to dispose of such *"creatures?"* Where did they get the notion of referring to children with disabilities as "creatures" rather than *patients?* They did not get these ideas from Carrell; he did not use this language. The immediate source of their ideas is indicated in the passage above, where it is noted that the asylum director, psychiatrist Hermann Pfannmüller, was an "admirer of Hoche." The reference is to psychiatrist Alfred Hoche (1865–1943), who, in 1920, published a small tract, in conjunction with another tract by a lawyer, Karl Binding (1841–1920), under the title, *Die Freigabe der Vernichtung lebensunwerten Lebens* – in an English translation, *The Release and Destruction of Life Devoid of Value* (Binding and Hoche [1920] 1975). The tract consisted of parallel

essays, one by Binding and one by Hoche, urging legal reform to permit the possibility of voluntary euthanasia. Both also argued for the "eugenic euthanasia" of the incurably mentally disabled or mentally ill – a subject Hoche discussed in his lectures to his medical students.

The consensus of historians who have examined the intellectual background of the physicians involved in the German "euthanasia" program is that this small tract, in particular the section by Hoche – and Hoche's lectures on the subject and his debates with other psychiatrists about his proposals – provided the intellectual catalyst that paved the way for German physicians' support for the Nation Socialist (Nazi) eugenic euthanasia program (see Chapters 34, 54). All the key medical actors in the program, from its codirectors, Karl Brandt (1904–1948), Hitler's personal physician, and Viktor Brack (1904–1948), to the pediatricians who selected infants for eugenic euthanasia, Werner Catel (1894–1981) and Ernst Wentzler (1891–1973) (inventor of an incubator for premature babies), appealed to Hoche's arguments and language to justify their actions. Many claim to have accepted this position *before* joining the "euthanasia" initiative (Burleigh 1994, 100, 273–74). Some, such as Werner Heyde (1902–1964), had attended Hoche's lectures on psychiatry (Lifton 1986, 117). One physician even reported that a discussion of Hoche's ideas was used as a tool to *recruit* him into the program (Lifton 1986, 104). Even in retrospect, he justified his actions by using Hoche's terminology, remarking that certain people were "empty shells" who lived a life devoid of meaning, unworthy of life – *lebensunwertes Leben* – in defending his actions (Lifton 1986, 107).

Neither Binding nor Hoche were National Socialists. Binding was a respected law professor, a legal positivist specializing in constitutional and criminal law. He wrote his section of the tract in the penultimate year of his life, dying decades before the rise of the Nazis. Judging from his writings, he would not have been a sympathizer. Hoche was a psychiatrist; his wife was Jewish; he was forced into early retirement by the Nazis; after retirement he opposed "National Socialist eugenic laws, pointing out that they would have precluded the birth of... Goethe, Schopenhauer, and Beethoven; and he opposed the euthanasia program ... even though much of its rationale derived from his own writings" (Burleigh 1994, 14).

Binding and Hoche wrote *Die Freigabe der Vernichtung lebensunwerten Lebens* in the immediate aftermath of World War I, during the early years of the Weimar Republic (1919–1933) when the intelligentsia felt free to explore areas that had once been unthinkable and felt it imperative to do so. Living through the last year of his own life, Binding was primarily worried about assisted dying for terminally ill patients, that is, administration of lethal doses of drugs. Hoche's exploration of the legal and moral status of the "mental incurables" also reflected personal experience. "Millions of people had died in the recent war, and hard choices about resources had been made ... one ... involved the mass starvation of mental patients" (Burleigh 1994, 15). It was against this background that they – Binding writing "at the end of [his] life," Hoche traumatized by the starvation of mental patients – posed the question "should the destruction of life be permissible for certain classes of people?"

Their two parallel tracts are reminiscent of a legal brief. Together they consist of 251 numbered paragraphs – 199 by Binding dealing with legal questions; 52 by Hoche addressing medical issues – laying out a case that moves from allowing the death of terminal patients, to consensual assistance of their death (Binding's concern), to killing mentally incompetents who are incapable of consenting and who are, moreover, burdensome to society (Hoche's concern). Binding's argument opens with a defense of suicide and moves to support the assistance in dying of the terminally ill, or "euthanasia." The argument emphasizes consent. It then turns to a class of individuals incapable of consenting (Par. 169–70), arguing that someone incurably mentally ill has no "will for life or for death." Observing that such persons have "given no definite consent to euthanasia," Binding notes that nonetheless "their lives are completely useless, but they don't consider it unbearable. They are a very heavy burden both for their relatives and for society. Their death causes no vacuum ... that these exist is a misuse of manpower for unworthy purposes" (Par. 169). Binding then argues that whoever actually takes care of these "idiots" (i.e., the mentally retarded) – parents, managers of institutions – has the right to consent to euthanasia on their behalf (Par. 171). "All euthanasia which breaks the will to live" however, is "excluded," that is, impermissible (Par. 177).

Binding's claim – that people with mental disability or severe mental illness lack a will to live – is one of those academic abstractions that cannot survive even the most superficial acquaintance with real people in these categories. With few exceptions (e.g., untreated major depression), whatever the nature of their disease or disability, people have a robust sense of self-preservation and a thirst for life. In any event, it was not Binding's liberal consent-based analysis – with its focus on euthanasia for terminal patients, like himself – that would influence the physicians who would carry out the Nazi euthanasia program. Physicians tend to be most influenced by the writings and lectures of fellow physicians. Those who became involved in the eugenic euthanasia program were no exception. It was Hoche's arguments that the physicians involved in the Nazi euthanasia program often cited. It was Hoche's concepts and phraseology that they parroted.

Hoche's section of the tract opens with a critique of traditional medical ethics including the Hippocratic Oath (Par. 203). It next turns to a critique of Christian ethics,

(Par. 229–30) touching briefly on the question of allowing and assisting the death of the terminally ill. Hoche then turns to his main concern, "life devoid of value." He replaces Binding's claim that the mentally disabled lack a will to live – unlikely to be persuasive to any psychiatrist – with the claims that the mentally disabled cannot assert a right to life, and, because they live meaningless lives, "worthless" to themselves and to society, they do not deserve to live.

226. The question of whether we should spend all of this money on ballast type persons of no value was not important in previous years because the state had sufficient money. Now conditions are different ...

227. Opposed to our task is the modern effort to keep alive all sorts of weaklings and to care for all those who are perhaps not mentally retarded but are still large burdens ...

228. The granting of death with dignity to life devoid of value to affect the release of the burden will for a long time be met with resistance for mostly sentimental reasons ...

229. In order to attain the necessary results, we must investigate ... the possibility and conditions for euthanasia.

233. One of these days ... we will come to the conclusion that the elimination of the mentally dead is no crime, nor an immoral act, and no unfeeling cruelty, but a permissible and necessary act.

234. What are the qualities and effects of mental death? ... *the character of a parasite* ... *on modern society*: the absence of any productivity; a condition of helplessness; and the necessity of caring for the mentally dead by a third person.

233. The most important [characteristic] of the mentally dead person is the lack of the possibility of ... knowing himself, the absence of self-consciousness. The intellectual level of the mentally dead person is that of a very low animal and the feelings are also most elementary and similar to those of animal life.

235. The mentally dead person [cannot] know himself, [lacks] self-consciousness ...

236. Thus the mentally dead person is not able to subjectively demand life just as he is unable to carry out other intellectual processes. [This] means that eliminating mentally dead persons is not to be equated with other types of killing ...

238. Because the condition of the mentally dead person prevents him from making a demand for life, if you take away his life you are not invading any of his rights.

239. [One] cannot argue from the stand point of pity. People ... project their life into the lives of

other people. [However] where there is no suffering, there can be no reason for pity.

245. Selection [should] be limited to lives definitely worthless for the person himself and for society and [should be done] with such certainty that all mistakes and errors are excluded.

250. The [era] in which we are now living . . . support of every existence – no matter how worthless – has become the highest moral norm. A new time will come when we no longer . . . carry out this demand, which has its origins in an exaggerated ideal of humanity. The present morality places too much value on mere continued existence and asks to high a sacrifice. (Binding and Hoche [1920] 1975, 38–40)

Hoche had borrowed a line from Plato to serve as the title of his book and he medicalized a line from Nietzsche in characterizing people with mental disability as "parasite[s] on . . . modern society" (Hoche [1920] 1975, Par. 234, 37). As Hoche no doubt intended, his contemporaries immediately recognized these references and read him as addressing questions "first raised by Plato, how to deal with 'sick person[s] who [are] a parasite on society'" (Aschheim 1992, 4–5, 163; Kirchner 1927; Procter 1988, 179).

What prompted the reference to Plato was the title of the book, *lebensunwerten Lebens*. The line is from an argument in Plato's most famous work, the *Republic* (Plato 1945, 95–100; *Republic* III, 405–10). "If a man had a sickly constitution and intemperate habits, *his life was worth nothing to himself or anyone else*; medicine was not meant for such people and they should not be treated, though they be richer than Midas" (*Republic* III 408, Plato 1945 98, emphasis added). In the *Republic*, Plato had offered what is, perhaps, the first philosophical analysis of medicine in the Western tradition. He conceptualizes medicine as an art designed to remedy weaknesses, defects, and imperfections of the human body, noting that the "human body . . . has weaknesses and defects, and its condition is not all it might be." Thus, "the art of medicine . . . was designed to help the body and provide for its interests." In practicing this art, Plato goes on to observe that "the physician . . . studies only the patient's interest, not his own . . . The business of the physician . . . is not to make money for himself, but to exercise his power over the patient's body. . . . All that he says and does will be said and done with a view to what is good and proper for the subject for whom he practices his art" (Plato 1945, 22–24).

Plato thus offers a profoundly paternalistic conception of the physician as someone exercising *power* over patients' bodies in the name of the patient's bodily interests. On this account, the patient's own choices, wishes, and desires – even the patient's prerogatives as a consumer and patron – appear irrelevant to the duties demanded of the physician

in practicing his art. Later in the *Republic* (Book III 405–10) Plato appeals to his paternalistic conception of the physician's art to critique of contemporary medical practice. Drawing on the literary conventions of the period, he parses the critique as an anecdote about the gymnastic trainer, Herodicus, who is criticized in name of the god, Asclepius, the god held to have given the healing arts to his human "sons," that is, to physicians.

> Until the time of Herodicus, the sons of Asclepius had no use for the modern coddling treatment of disease. But Herodicus, who . . . lost his health, combined training and doctoring in such a way as to become a plague to himself first and foremost and to many others after him . . . by lingering out his death. He had a mortal disease, and he spent all his life at its beck and call, with no hope of a cure and no time for anything but doctoring himself. Every departure from a fixed regimen was a torment; and his skill only allowed him to reach old age in a prolonged death struggle . . . [Herodicus] never understood that Asclepius did not reveal these valetudinarian arts to his descendants . . . because he realized that in every well-ordered community each man has his appointed task which he must perform; no one has leisure to spend all his life in being ill and doctoring himself . . . [A man] either regains his health and lives to go about his proper business, or, if his body is not equal to the strain, gets rid of all his troubles by dying. (*Republic* III, 405–6; Plato 1945, 95–96)

Herodicus' "lingering death" is thus offered as a "horror story:" prolonging a life, whose sole purpose was to prolong itself – a paradigm case of a life unworthy of life. Having established the paradigm of a life unworthy of life – in German, *lebensunwertes Leben* – Plato pushes the argument further, arguing that it is *unethical* for physicians to prolong such lives.

> Where the body was diseased through and through, [a physician] is not to try, by nicely calculated evacuations and doses, to prolong a miserable existence and let his patient beget children who were likely to be as sickly as himself. Treatment . . . would be wasted on a man who could not live in his ordinary round of duties and was consequently useless to himself and society. (*Republic* III 407, Plato 1945, 97)

Plato then continues, using language that Hoche would later echo: "If a man had a sickly constitution and intemperate habits, *his life was worth nothing to himself or anyone else; medicine was not meant for such people and they should not be treated, though they be richer than Midas*" (*Republic* III 408, Plato 1945, 98, emphasis added). Finally, Plato concludes, physicians are not only to judge whether people have lived lives that make them worthy of the medical art, but also to use their medical knowledge to *kill* those who are unfit. "The physically unfit [physicians] will leave to die and *they will actually put to death those who are incurably corrupt in mind*... That will be the best thing for them as well as for the community" (*Republic* III 410, Plato 1945, 100, emphasis added).

Plato's conception of the physician as obligated to abandon the physically unfit to die and to "put to death" those with mental disability or illness was inconsistent with the Hippocratic ethics of physicians in his own day (see Chapters 23, 24), and with later Judeo-Christian–Islamic morality (see Chapters 12–17). it was not inconsistent, however, with Greco-Roman morality generally. Infanticide by exposure, that is, leaving an unwanted infant, especially one with a birth defect, "exposed" in the open to die was a common Greco-Roman practice, dating from ancient times. Hence, the story of Oedipus, whose name in Greek means "clubfoot," is about a child with a birth defect who was left exposed to die – but who nonetheless lived to inadvertently avenge himself upon the very parents who abandoned him to death (see Langer 1974; Lecky, 1905, II:19–37; Westermark 1912, I:383–417). The practice was condoned not only by Plato (*Republic* V, Plato 1945, 460–61) but also by his student, Aristotle (*Politics*, Book VII, 1335b, 20). Turning to the other end of the life cycle, Stoic philosophers such as the Roman Seneca (c. 3 BCE-65) lauded suicide as an honorable way to escape from debilitating illness (Seneca 1962, *Epistle LXX*, 14–18).

In their original historical context, therefore, Plato's proposals were not shocking. Hoche, however, was employing the Platonic concept of "*lebensunwertes Leben*" – a life unworthy of life – to valorize a conception of the physician as duty bound to "euthanize" those with mental disability in the context of Western Judeo-Christian culture, in liberal, democratic Weimar Germany. German medicine not only claimed Hippocratic ancestry, it saw itself in the tradition of Christhoph Wilhelm Hufeland (1762–1836), who held that the "fundamental law" governing all of a physician's moral relations was "saving life, restoring health, and relieving the sufferings of humanity... as far as possible" (Hufeland [1836] 1844, 2). He expressly rejected the Platonic notion that physicians should judge the value or meaningfulness of someone's life.

> A physician is bound in duty to do nothing but what tends to save life; whether existence be fortunate or unfortunate, whether life be valuable or not, is not for the physician to decide. If he once permits such considerations to influence his actions, the consequences cannot be estimated, and he becomes the most dangerous person of the community. For if he once trespass his line of duty and thinks himself entitled to decide on the necessity of an individual's life,

he may by gradual progressions apply the measure to other cases. (Hufeland [1836] 1844, 7)

Hoche was challenging the deepest traditions of German medicine and German morality. He thus opens his tract with a critique of both medical ethics and Christian morality. To valorize his departure from conventional morality and medical ethics, he not only borrowed the Platonic concept of *lebensunwertes Leben*, he borrowed a turn of phrase from a cultural icon more recent than Plato and better known than Hufeland – Friedrich Wilhelm Nietzsche. In one of his last books written in 1888, *Götzen-Dämmerung, oder wie man mit dem Hammer philosophiert* (*The Twilight of the Idols: Or, How to Philosophise with the Hammer*) Nietzsche has a short section, "A moral for doctors" in which he offers his own version of Platonic medical ethics. The section opens with a line that Hoche would borrow: "the sick man is a parasite of society."

> *A moral for doctors.* – The sick man is a parasite of society. In certain cases it is indecent to go on living. To continue to vegetate in a cowardly dependence on doctors and special treatments, once the meaning of life, the right to life, has been lost, ought to be regarded with the greatest of contempt by society. The doctors, for their part, should be agents for imparting this contempt, – they should no longer prepare prescriptions, but should every day administer a fresh dose of *disgust* to their patients. A new responsibility should be created, that of the doctor – the responsibility of ruthlessly suppressing and eliminating *degenerate* life, in all cases in which the highest interests of life itself, of ascending life, demand such a course – for instance in favor of the right of procreation, in favour of the right of being born, in favour of the right to live. One should die proudly when it is no longer possible to live proudly. (Nietzsche [1888] 1964, 16:88)[9]

Hoche had borrowed the expression "the sick man is a parasite of society" from Nietzsche, but Nietzsche's himself – a student of classical philology who often comments on Plato – borrows many of the ideas in this passage from Plato. Like Plato, Nietzsche's concern is the lingering Herodician death. He transforms Plato's admonition that "treatment would be wasted on a man who... was useless to himself and society" into "The sick man is a parasite of society" who has no right to live – noting that once the "meaning of life" is lost, so too is "the right to life." Like Plato, therefore, Nietzsche believes that medicine should abandon moral neutrality by refusing to treat those whose life is meaningless, "ruthlessly suppressing and eliminating *degenerate* life, in all cases in which the highest interests of life itself demand such a course." Physicians thus had the "responsibility of ruthlessly suppressing and eliminating *degenerate* life."

Hoche took Nietzsche at his word – as the title of his tract with Binding proclaims – and argued that the law and morality should both be liberalized to accommodate killing those whose lives were unworthy of life. Hoche, however, gave these words a biological twist, "there is no doubt that in trying to preserve life without dignity by all means, exaggeration has occurred... We doctors know that in the interest of the whole human organism, single, less valuable members have to be abandoned and pushed out" (Binding and Hoche [1920] 1975, 37). Hoche refers to these less valuable members of society as *Ballastexistenzen*, "ballast existences," who have *"the character of a parasite . . . on modern society; the absence of productivity; a condition of complete helplessness; and the necessity of caring for the mentally dead person by a third person"* (Binding and Hoche [1920] 1975, 37, emphasis added). This section of the tract concludes that "one of these days... we will come to the conclusion that the elimination of the mentally dead is no crime, nor an immoral act, and no unfeeling cruelty, but a permissible and necessary act" (Binding and Hoche [1920] 1975, 37).

Hoche's tract was well received by some in the medical community. Distinguished Tübingen psychiatrist Robert Gaup, inventor of the concept of *Kriegsneurosen*, or "shell shock," applauded the proposals, remarking that he had often wondered why he was obligated to provide for mental patients during World War I, when people "of full value" were starving to death (Burleigh 1994, 20). Binding and Hoche's proposals were debated – and ultimately rejected – at meetings of professional medical and psychiatric societies in 1921 and 1922 (Burleigh 1994, 24). In 1925, Ewald Meltzer, director of the Katharinenhof Asylum at Grosshennersdorf, Saxony, published a detailed response to Binding and Hoche, *Das Problem der Abküzung 'lebensunwerten' Leben* ((The Problem of the Curtailment of Life 'Unworthy' of Life) (Meltzer 1925)). Yet, even though the debates of the 1920s culminated in the formal rejection of Binding and Hoche's proposals at various meetings of medical and psychiatric associations, the very process of debating and rebutting their proposals disseminated such concepts as "ballast existence" and *"lebensunwertes Leben,"* facilitating their third-stage dissemination beyond Hoche's idiolect into the vocabulary of German medicine and psychiatry.

One of the physicians who adopted Hoche's vocabulary was Dr. Gerhard Wagner, leader of the National Socialist (Nazi) Physicians' league. In an address to the Nazi Party Congress held in Nuremberg in 1935, Wagner decried the "burden and unexcelled injustice" that the cost of care for the mentally ill "placed on normal, healthy members of the population." In addition to deploying arguments popularized by Hoche, Wagner turned to Nietzschean language by denouncing *Gleichheitslehre* (theory of equality), the doctrine of equality that placed "the value of the sick, the dying, and the unfit on par with the healthy and

the strong" (Proctor 1988, 181). Wagner's critique of *Gleichheitslehre* echoed a passage from Nietzsche.

> The biblical prohibition "thou shalt not kill" is a piece of naiveté compared with the seriousness of the prohibition of life to descendants: "thou shalt not procreate!" – Life itself recognizes no solidarity, no "equal rights," between the healthy and the degenerate parts of an organism: one must excise the latter – or the whole will perish. – Sympathy for decadents, equal rights for the ill-constituted – that would be the profoundest immorality, that would be anti-nature itself as morality. (Aschheim 1992, 389; see also 141–42, 391–93)[10]

It was at this congress that Hitler told Wagner that "if war should break out, he (Hitler) would authorize a national program of euthanasia" for those unworthy of life (Proctor 1988, 181; Burleigh 1994, 97).

Hitler kept his promise. On August 18, 1939, 14 days before the invasion of Poland, the Committee for the Scientific Treatment of Severe, Genetically Determined Illness ordered local governments to have doctors and midwives register all children with hereditary illness. Using this registry, three physicians, all professors, selected which children were to be killed in twenty-two institutions designated for dispatching with those classified as *"lebensunwertes Leben"* – a concept recontextualized by the psychiatrist, Hoche, from the works of Plato and Nietzsche.

VI. CONCLUSION

This chapter opened with the historian Daniel Fox's astute observation of "the curious disconnection" between medical ethics and philosophy. By applying Gadamer's concept of the "long horizon" of philosophical influence – which allows one to analyze the impact of Platonic discourse on a physician, such as Hoche, many centuries later – and by adopting I. Bernard Cohen's four-stage analysis of the dissemination of innovative ideas in science, we were able to show, in three case studies, how concepts, such as the sympathetic physician, professional ethics, and *lebensunwertes Leben*, trace their origins to such philosophers as Bacon, Cicero, Hume, Locke, Nietzsche, and Plato.

Our method has focused on arguments, concepts, and discourses. The evidence used is both textual and linguistic. A skeptic – perhaps some externalist or internalist historian of medicine or science – might raise questions about whether the philosophically influenced concepts and discourses that we have traced to practitioner's usages *really* had any impact on medical thought and practice. Perhaps doctors talked a bit differently, perhaps they used some concepts originated by philosophers, but does that really mean that philosophy was really influential? Did philosophical arguments, concepts, and discourses "really" make a difference in the history of medicine, or even in the history of medical ethics?

We lack a theoretical model that offers a rigorous way of addressing these questions; however, some thought experiments are suggestive. Imagine a world in which the Enlightenments did not include the Scottish Enlightenment. In this world there would be no Hume, no Adam Smith (1723–1790), no Francis Hutcheson (1649–1746), and no "Wise Club" or Edinburgh philosophical societies that nurtured the development of Gregory's medical ethics. None of these philosophers could have influenced Gregory. In such a world, the prevalent ideals of secular morality would probably have been based on reason: Ciceronian duty, Kantian principles, or utilitarian calculations. Secular moral discourse would thus have been dominated by ideals of rationality alone, untempered by the ideals of moral sentiment such as sympathy and the virtue of tenderness. In such a world, would Gregory still have suggested the concept of the sympathetic physician? Would anyone? Or would we have come to expect our physicians to be as technically proficient, dedicated, objective, and *dispassionate* as our accountants, our bankers, our judges, and our scientists?

Although it might seem as if the concept of the sympathetic physician ought to be universal, in fact this ideal came into existence as an artifact of the Scottish Enlightenment. It became prominent *only* where Gregory or those he influenced (such as Percival and various American codifiers) were influential. In Britain, Italy, France, Germany, North America, and Spain, the concept of the sympathetic physician became prevalent *only after* Gregory's work was disseminated; it does not appear anywhere until after contact with physicians trained in traditions in which Gregory's ideas were influential. Had Hume and his contemporaries never challenged the role of reason in morality, it seems doubtful that anyone – including Gregory – would have thought to promote the idea of the sympathetic physician. In consequence, had there never been a Scottish Enlightenment, our conception of the ideal physician, and the actual practice of contemporary medicine might have been quite different from what it became.

What of the concepts of medical ethics, professional medical ethics, and the modern concept of a profession? Had Percival died in 1795 – before he turned to Bacon and Locke (via Gisborne) to invent his new concepts of medical ethics and professional ethics – would we have had the concept of medical ethics, the modern concept of a profession, or of professional ethics? As of 1794, Percival had only published *Medical Jurisprudence*, a title that evokes the authority of law, not morality, not ethics. Always a syncretic thinker, Percival innovated by compounding ideas drawn from others. In 1794, he had drawn on ideas from Cicero and Gregory to create the concept of medical jurisprudence, but he had yet to cobble together the modern concept of a profession or of professional ethics.

Had he died at that point, or had he not sought such new concepts as profession, professional ethics, and medical ethics – drawing on arguments, concepts, and discourse that he found in Bacon, Gisborne, and Locke – would we today have the modern concept of medicine as a profession bound by professional medical ethics?

The dissemination of these concepts tracks the influence, first of Percival, and then of the AMA's 1847 Percivalean Code of Ethics. In Britain, Canada, France, Germany, and Japan the modern concepts of a profession and professional medical ethics are post-Percivalean/1847 AMA code, and are strongly influenced by them. Percival invented these concepts in a unique situation. Nearly blind, anticipating his death, under pressure to complete his last missive to the world, he rummaged through the arguments and discourses of philosophers in a perhaps desperate attempt to shore up his ideals – inventing the modern concepts of a profession, professional ethics, and medical ethics in the process. Is it likely that any of these concepts would have been invented by anyone else, or that Percival himself could have, or would have, invented them without recourse to a store of philosophical ideas?

Arguments, concepts, and discourses, although intangible, are just as much inventions as tangible artifacts. Just as the artifacts and technologies available to a culture – from abacuses, to wheels, windmills, and writing – are a function of their heritage, their receptivity to new ideas, and their capacity for innovation, so too are the discourses, with their conceptual and theoretical frameworks, available to them. Just as Gregory and Percival drew on a philosophical heritage to create the concepts they deeded first to British medicine, and then to the world, so too German physicians drew on their philosophical heritage to create the arguments, concepts and discourses that they deeded to the world. Would German medicine have produced concepts like "ballast existence," *lebensunwertes Leben*, or denounced "*Gleichheitslehre*" – the concept that all sick people are to be treated equally – had Nietzsche and Plato never written?

As we remarked earlier, until Hoche, German medicine embraced profoundly prolife ideals of medical ethics. It is as unlikely that German medicine would have turned to different ideals without some medical appropriation of a distinctly different conception of morality – a conception that, in fact, was supplied by philosophical heritage of Plato and Nietzsche. Had Plato and Nietzsche never written, or had their concept of medicine never been appropriated and recontextualized by some medical intermediary, it is as unlikely that German medicine would have accepted such concepts as *lebensunwertes Leben* as it is that we would have a concept of the sympathetic physician without the heritage of Hume and the Scottish Enlightenment. Sadly, there would probably still have been an anti-Jewish genocide, a Holocaust, but it is less likely that physicians would have played such a central role and it is even less likely that the Holocaust would have been initiated in hospitals, by physicians implementing a pediatric eugenic euthanasia program on children with mental disabilities.

The three cases discussed here are merely illustrative of philosophy's influence on conceptions of medical morality – for better, and for worse. A complete history of the influence of philosophy on medical ethics has yet to be written. Yet, as these studies and some of our other observations suggest, if one scratches the surface of the history of medical ethics, or of contemporary bioethics, it is evident that philosophical arguments, concepts, conceptual frameworks, and discourses have exerted a profound and enduring influence on the history of medical thought and practice.

NOTES

1. One can use the same techniques to track the prevalence of concepts within a discipline. For an excellent and detailed study of the displacement of theological concepts by philosophically based bioethical concepts in scientific and popular discussions of genetics, see Evans (2002).

2. Thomas Newton's translation (1586) includes the line "mine Arte and profession." John Read (1588) "And in my profession, I will shew myselfe pure, chaste, and holy." See Sanford Larkey, "The Hippocratic Oath in Elizabethan England," (Burns 1977a, 218–36).

3. Miller notes that *De Officiis* publication in 1465 marks it as the first classical work to have been printed on a printing press.

4. In Greco-Roman theater actors wore different masks as they assumed different characters. The word "role" designates both the role they played and the mask that they wore in playing this role.

5. There is no comparable section in Percival's *Medical Jurisprudence* (1794).

6. The passage reproduces, verbatim, Percival 1803, Chap. II, Art. XXIII, except that "association" has been substituted for "profession."

7. This passage reiterates Medico-Chirurgical Society of Baltimore 1832, Sec. I Art. XI, p. 11; derived from Anonymous 1823, Article 23 – Kappa Lambda – reproduced by the Association of Boston Physicians [1808] 1995, with "association" replacing "profession"; derived from Percival 1803, Chap. II, Art. XXIII – no comparable passage in Percival 1794.

8. In an effort to preserve Nietzsche's reputation many recent translations bowdlerize this text to obscure its meaning.

9. In an important conceptual analysis of the concept of "professional ethics," Michael Davis argues that either the 1908 ABA Canons, or the 1912 AMA Principles were the first to properly qualify as codes of "professional ethics" (Davis 2003).

10. This work was edited by Nietzsche's pro-Nazi sister and published in 1901 and 1906; however similar passages abound, in *The Geneaology of Morals* (Nietzsche [1887] 1964, 120–25), and *Zarathustra* (Nietzsche [1883/1885] 1964, 183–86).

Part VI

The Discourses of Practitioners on Medical Ethics

Chapter 19

The Discourses of Practitioners in Africa

Angela Amondi Wasunna

I. Introduction

This chapter examines the roles and practices of traditional African healers prior to the introduction of the "modern" scientific world view into the conception and practice of medicine in Africa. To this end, this chapter distinguishes the roles of traditional medical healers in Africa, who mainly dealt with biological causation, from those of diviners, whose work was largely based on metaphysical aspects. This section of the chapter also explores the manner in which traditional healers[1] entered the "profession" and examines the ethical framework within which these healers carried out their work. In addition, this chapter examines the wider role and social standing of the traditional healer in the community. It must be noted that whereas this chapter is essentially a historical account, traditional healers remain active in almost all parts of Africa. This chapter will also discuss the introduction of "modern medicine" in postcolonial Africa and will investigate the immediate conflict between concepts of Western medicine and traditional healing. Of particular concern will be the tension that exists between modern, Western-educated doctors and their traditional counterparts. This chapter considers the question of whether there has been any integration of modern science into the conception and practice of medicine. In conclusion, this essay will briefly examine the doctor–patient and healer–patient relationship in Africa.

II. The African World View

One cannot talk about a uniform "African World View." Africa is a continent made up of more than forty-three countries. As a result of its sheer size, it plays host to thousands of distinct social groups, most with their own cultures and languages. There are, however, some similar traits among groups that have common origins and also among groups that have lived alongside each other for centuries. Much of Africa today can be described as Anglophone (English-speaking), Francophone (French-speaking), or Lusophone (Portuguese-speaking) with these descriptions based on each country's colonial legacy.

Africans created hundreds of distinct religions, most of which have survived and remained important, despite centuries of Islamic and Christian influence on the continent. African religions evolved around traditional concepts such as ethnic identity, language, and culture. Like Islam, African religions formed a way of life for the community. There were established rules that governed all aspects of life, such as farming, hunting, love and courtship, marriage and death, and even life after death.

Many African religions addressed the question of what it meant to be human and they sought to discover the correlation between the physical and spiritual world, between evil and suffering, and between their actions in the present life and their fate in the afterlife. As a result, there were ethical norms that were upheld and expressed through sacred oral traditions and passed down through generations in the form of dance, art, rituals and during the all-important, rites of passage. The values of various societies framed the ethics and morals of African religions. Thus, in some societies, acts such as stealing, killing, assault, incest, and witchcraft were considered moral or religious transgressions and were not left unpunished by the community.

All African religions emphasize belief in a Supreme Being. Belief in this Being as the creator and preserver is fundamental to African societies and is expressed through prayer, invocation, sacrifice, offering, song, and dance. The African God is genderless and is considered a just, powerful, and compassionate entity. Africans also believe in lesser beings created by this powerful Supreme Being. Many African traditions revolved around the roles of these lesser beings, which were believed to control various elements that affected the everyday lives of members of society such as rivers, the ocean, forests, fertility, community governance, fishing, and rainfall. As expressed by Mbiti

> God is the originator and sustainer of man; the spirits explain the destiny of man; Man is the center of the ontology; Animals, plants, natural phenomena and objects constitute the environment in which man lives, provide a means of existence, and if need be, establishes a mystical relationship with them. (Mbiti 1969, 167–68)

Among the Yoruba of Nigeria, lesser spirits were known as the *orishas*, and they were believed to number 401 in all. They each had distinct characters, special powers, and there were specific rituals assigned to them. For example, there was *Chango*, god of thunder, *Oshun*, goddess of rivers and feminine beauty, and *Ifa*, god of divination. Among societies in East, Central, and Southern Africa, these lesser beings were believed to have once lived as human beings.

There were also prophets in traditional communities who were ordained by the Supreme Being to interpret His spiritual messages to the common folk. Another important category in the African cosmology were ancestral spirits. In a few cases, this category was restricted to spirits of people who had been caring and compassionate in life. After death, these spirits continued to help the living by appearing to their descendants in dreams and visions and providing them with vital advice and warnings.

Among certain communities in East and Central Africa, the ancestral spirits were not necessarily benevolent. They often caused physical affliction to punish individuals for neglecting their ritual responsibilities or obligations toward the extended family. It must be understood that African religions recognized that powers that circulated in the universe originated from the Supreme Being. It is these life forces, interacting with the physical world, but residing in the spiritual realm, that were believed to govern the people's destiny. As a result, they were to be feared and, at the same time, respected.

III. THE ROLE OF AFRICAN TRADITIONAL RELIGION AND PHILOSOPHY IN THE PRACTICE OF MEDICINE

The role of African traditional healers has been the subject of great misunderstanding. Until the 1970s, most studies concerned with traditional medicine in Africa linked it with beliefs, religion, and rituals that included the view that all healers were "witch doctors" and practiced magic. Witchcraft was often understood in the context of African traditional medical practitioners as the use of mystical powers to harm others in society (Mbiti 1969, 198). According to this interpretation, witchcraft, sorcery the evil eye (or whatever terminology it was given) was fundamentally *evil* (Sindiga, Nyaigotti-Chacha, and Kanunah 1995, 17).

Despite increased knowledge and interest in Africa, indigenous medical traditions have often been cast in a negative light and are viewed by many as the incarnation of a shameful legacy of paganism, barbarism, and black magic. The activities of traditional medical practitioners were often held up as "examples of irrationality and malpractice, a mixture of superstition, deliberate deception, and ignorance . . . " (MacLean 1971, 13). There was also "good magic" that represented the manipulation of mystical power by a traditional healer in the treatment process, for the good of the society (Mbiti 1969, 198). Thus, some traditional healers served to neutralize the harmful powers of the sorcerers or witches.

Health in African communities is generally viewed as a fundamentally ethical question pointing to the relationships in the family and in the community, and between people and nature. Concepts of illness, disease, diagnosis, treatment, and life and death always had a *cultural dimension* in all societies, including African societies. Most African societies believe in the dualism of body and soul. Most human suffering, illness, accidents, childlessness, suffering, misfortune, and war can be attributed to evil forces (sorcery) or ancestral spirits or punishment, as a result of breaking of taboos. These beliefs mark an important difference between traditional African and modern medicine.

> Disease is not merely something resulting from malfunctioning in this or that organ or a lesion therein . . . but essentially of a rupture of life's harmony to be imputed either to a material cause instinct with some "intangible force" or directly to

that intangible force itself. It is ... necessary in traditional medical practice to confront the symptomology and etiology of diseases not only in the
material but also in the immaterial world. (Ampofu
and Johnson-Romauld, 1987, 40)

In African traditional societies, therefore, disease and
misfortune were regarded as having socio-religious foundations. As a result, treatment sought to address not just
the physical symptoms manifested in the body, but also
the root causes of the disease to prevent its recurrence
(Mbiti 1969, 198–9). The previously described spiritual
role of the healer was not the only facet of his work
because diseases of metaphysical or social origin were not
the only ones known in the indigenous African medical
system. Because modern medicine recognizes only biological causation, Westerners tended to dismiss the metaphysical aspects of African medicine (Waite 1993, 12).

Africans have diverse disease etiologies that include
natural diseases as well as supernatural infirmities. Thus,
traditional practice includes specializations such as
herbalists, surgeons, birth attendants, and bone specialists, among others. Thus, in most African traditional societies, there were two kinds of practitioners – those who
diagnosed or acted as mediums for territorial or tutelary
spirits (shamans) and those who provided medicines and
did not divine (empirics) (Waite 1993, 15). There were,
of course, overlaps in both in the sense that the diviners
could provide medicine and some medicine men had to
address spiritual causes.

IV. Training of Traditional Healers and Ethics of the Profession

The medical profession in African societies was held in
high regard. Medicine men were considered among the
most important people in the community. According to
Leakey,

> The profession was one that could not be entered
> into lightheartedly; moreover, one at which it was
> by no means easy to be successful. In fact quite a
> number of those who were initiated into the pro-
> fession failed to make a success of it and ceased to
> practice. (Leakey 1977, 1121)

Each and every village in Africa had a medicine man who
was usually quite accessible to individuals in the society.
Healing was not restricted to men and many traditional
societies had medicine women, such as the *Isangoma* of
the Ngunni-speaking society of South Africa. (The term,
"medicine man," used in this chapter is thus a collective
term that refers to both female and male indigenous healers unless specified otherwise.) Medicine men were first
and foremost concerned with sickness, disease, and misfortune. They had to find out the cause of the disease,

apply the right treatment, and supply a means of preventing the misfortune from occurring again. Traditional healers were also consulted on issues such as increasing agricultural productivity, aiding in fertility, detecting sorcery,
removing curses, and controlling spirits in the cosmos.

In many African traditions, medical knowledge was limited to certain families or clans. Medical skills passed down
orally through these narratives were heavily laden with
ethical and moral themes. Folk medical knowledge was
passed down in a highly secretive manner, although, in
some cases, knowledge was acquired by outsiders through
apprenticeship to a practicing family member. Ademuwagun tries to explain this secrecy and disconnect between
traditional practitioners and their modern medicine counterparts.

> Most African healing systems have not been for-
> malized in print, so that their principles could be
> open to outside scrutiny. Part of the ethics of many
> African healing is secrecy; this protects the society
> against the indiscriminate use of such medicines by
> certain individuals. Such secrecy also reflects the
> fact that the knowledge of indigenous medicines
> can be an index of one's power and influence in
> society. Just as Western practitioners of medicine
> guard their professions through tedious methods of
> registration and induction, so does the African tra-
> ditional medical class obtain the same protection
> through secrecy. Unfortunately the success of that
> secrecy has resulted in a serious blow to the credi-
> bility of the entire system. Many people, including
> many urbanized Western-educated Africans, deny
> the efficacy – not to mention the existence – of
> indigenous African medicine about which they have
> often heard but which they have little formal knowl-
> edge. (Ademuwagun et al. 1979, vii)

Studies have demonstrated, however, that traditional healers shared professional knowledge when respect for their
integrity and a genuine desire to learn from them were
communicated (Good 1987, xiii). For example, in a study
done among 100 Yoruba healers in Nigeria, there proved
to be no difficulty whatsoever in obtaining very detailed
accounts of herbal remedies for a number of specific complaints (MacLean 1971, 83).

As stated earlier, in the African context, traditional
healers had various specializations or professional areas
of practice. For example, there were herbalists, diviners,
seers, spiritualists, traditional surgeons, and birth attendants. Furthermore, a healer could have one or more
areas of specialization based upon his or her knowledge,
skills, and years of careful empirical observations (Mbiti,
1969, 167–68). First, among the Abaluhyia of Kenya, for
example, there were the herbalists or *omulesi* who provided drugs that treated mystical diseases as well as ordinary diseases of a serious nature. Second, there were the

divination experts or *omulakusi*. Third, there were surgeons or *omulumiki*. There were also experts who treated fractures and dislocations and removed broken or aching teeth. Finally, there were traditional birth attendants or midwives (Sindiga, Nyaigotti-Chacha, and Kanunah 1995, 127–28). Traditional healers acquired knowledge in matters pertaining to the medicinal value, quality, and use of different herbs, leaves, roots, fruits, barks, grasses, minerals, dead insects, bones, feathers, powders, smoke from different objects, shells, eggs, and other objects.

Even though in some societies, by virtue of his special powers, the traditional healer could arrive at a diagnosis and prescribe treatment without questioning or examining the patient, a typical diagnosis was preceded by a lengthy procedure during which the traditional practitioner would first observe every detail about the patient's movements and ability to perform tasks. Thereafter, the medicine man would perform aptitude tests by asking detailed case history questions, both of the patient and his or her close relations. Next, the healer would enter into a state of divination, usually a trance, where he would become possessed by the "power" and it was in this state that the healer would diagnose and forecast the probable cause of the disease as well as prescribe the appropriate therapy. Finally, he would perform a clinical examination to confirm his diagnosis. This would include physical inspection of the affected areas and other organs such as the tongue, eyes, and examination of blood, urine, and discharges. Treatment procedures usually included herbal remedies to treat the physical dimensions of the disease, purgatives to induce vomiting to "cleanse" the system and animal fat or ointment for a variety of skin diseases and wounds. In addition, a concoction of herbs was used to massage the body to provide relief for constipation, fatigue, and swollen muscles; herbal steaming was used for a variety of fevers, cutaneous incisions for chronic headaches and surgical operations for boils and other such conditions. Africans had effective remedies against intestinal parasites, vomiting, skin ulcers, catarrh, convulsions, tumors, venereal diseases, bronchitis, conjunctivitis, urethral stricture, and many other illnesses (Finch 1990, 139–40).

Traditional African healers thus engaged in sophisticated and complex treatment and surgical regimes. For example, in East Africa traditional bonesetters reduced fractures and dislocations by manual manipulation and traction. Masai surgeons were known to successfully treat pleurisy and pneumonitis by creating a partial collapse of the lung by drilling holes into the chest of the sufferer. Other healers performed autopsies on patients who had died of unknown causes. These were usually done to detect possible witchcraft intervention, but they also contributed to knowledge of the anatomy. Most impressive, however, is the documented eyewitness account by a missionary doctor named Felkin, of a Caesarean section performed by a Banyoro traditional surgeon in Uganda in 1879.

> The patient was a health-looking primipara (first pregnancy) of about twenty years of age and she lay on an inclined bed, the head of which rested against the side of the hut. She was half-intoxicated with banana wine, was quite naked and was tied down to the bed by bands of bark cloth over the thorax and thighs. Her ankles were held by a man ... while another man stood in her right steadying her abdomen ... the surgeon was standing on her left side holding the knife aloft and muttering an incantation. He then washed his hands and the patient's abdomen first with banana wine, then water. The surgeon made a quick cut upwards from just above the pubis to just below the umbilicus severing the whole abdominal wall and uterus so that amniotic fluid escaped. Some bleeding points in the abdominal wall were touched with red-hot irons. The surgeon completed the uterine incision, the assistant helping by holding up the sides of the abdominal wall with his hand and hooking two fingers into the uterus. The child was removed, the cord cut and the child handed to an assistant. (Finch 1990, 135)

This example illustrated that the Ugandan surgeon understood the concepts of anesthesia and antisepsis and he also demonstrated advanced surgical techniques. There are several examples that clearly show that traditional doctors practiced not just divine intervention, but also employed treatment based on sound knowledge of methods proven through generations.

V. TRAINING

Among the Kikuyu of Kenya, even though a person was born into a family of traditional healers, he had to undergo training and thereafter, "graduate" in an elaborate initiation ceremony. (In some societies, the diviner was distinguished from the herbal healer by his initiation. The diviner had to be called by the ancestors, for example through a dream, to practice divination and family tradition were merely contributing factors. A medicine man could, in contrast, simply practice after his apprenticeship.) An experienced traditional healer who then became the mentor of the newly admitted healer led the initiation ceremony. Admission into the practice among the Kikuyu, in contrast to many other communities on Africa, was symbolized by possession of divining gourds and magical powers, which were considered necessary for his new vocation (Leakey 1977, 1121).

Among the Azande of Congo the training of a traditional healer was formal, lengthy, and expensive. Potential medicine men were groomed at an early age into the profession. Once they expressly made their wishes to become healers known, they were given certain medicinal herbs, which were believed to strengthen their souls and give them the powers of prophecy. Thereafter, they would spend the better part of their childhood and teenage years as apprentices, working closely and learning from their assigned teachers (Evans-Pritchard, 1937, 2–10).

Even though the idea of a formal oath like the Hippocratic Oath was unknown in much of Africa, traditional medical systems had long-established rules and traditions, some of which were similar to those of the Hippocratic Oath. The discussion below will illuminate some of the similarities found between African informal rules of conduct and the principles found in the Hippocratic Oath, as well as points of departure. One of the most important was confidentiality. Just as the Hippocratic Oath rather ambiguously demands that the doctor keep his patient's information in confidence, African traditional healers were also bound by this confidentiality rule. When it came to matters of public health, however, their responsibilities extended from their individual patients to the larger community. In other words, their obligations were no longer directed solely toward their individual patients. Instead, they became responsible for the health and welfare of the community at large. Thus, if a particular medicine man had several patients who were dying suddenly or had unexplainable illnesses that progressed rapidly, he was under an ethical obligation to report this matter to the authorities who were usually made up of kings or chiefs, diviners, and seers for further action. The traditional healer was also expected to advise the authorities on how to find the root cause of the problem and thereafter, how to rid the community of the epidemic.

These informal ethical rules guided both the healers and their apprentices in their work and were greatly honored amongst practitioners. The secrecy surrounding the practice of medicine in Africa coupled with the manner in which knowledge was passed to a privileged few exhibited the characteristics of a profession. The practitioners (apprentices) were trained in a defined manner and upon qualification, they were bound by established rules of practice.

Among the Kikuyu of Kenya, traditional healers were enjoined to keep the confidentiality of the health and social problems of their clients. A traditional healer who divulged any confidential information was severely reprimanded by colleagues and in some instances, was irreparably cursed by them (Leakey 1977, 1121). This requirement instilled confidence in the patients that their relationship to their healer would be a fiduciary one with trust and respect as the basis. It was also not appropriate for patients to discuss their ailments and treatment, except among their closest kin.

Kikuyu healers were also under an ethical obligation to admit their inability to offer therapy to hopeless cases

and such cases were left in God's hands. Similarly, a general practitioner was obliged to make referrals of cases he could not handle to appropriate specialists within the profession. Having said this, traditional healers, by virtue of their special skills and favored status in society, were quite paternalistic. There were a few healers who encouraged dialogue and interactive treatment with their patients, but for the most part, healers used their own ability and judgment to treat the patient. This is yet another parallel to the Hippocratic Oath whose central ethic leans toward paternalism.

As mentioned earlier, a notable characteristic of the traditional healer's profession was the institutionalized secrecy surrounding medical matters. Practitioners were not expected to describe their methods are they were considered trade secrets.

Payment for medical services varied from community to community, however, common determinants of fee level included severity of the illness, type of the disease, the time required to treat the patient and patient's income. In rural areas, traditional healers' fees were paid in kind in the form of goats, cows, chicken, and foodstuff such as maize and beans. In more urban areas, payment was usually made in the form of cash. As stated previously, professional fees were usually negotiable depending on various circumstances.

In some communities in West Africa, when a medicine man was preparing medicine for a wealthy client, he often entered into a blood oath with the client. This oath entailed the mutual drawing of blood and it represented an important and respected oral covenant, which symbolized trust.

Among other communities, the medicine man was expected to taste the medicine prescribed to patients in front of them to assure them that there was no poison. The traditional healer's relationship with the patient in these communities, though sacred, was one of both trust and distrust. This must be viewed in light of the fact that medicine men did not always prescribe curative medicine and sometimes were asked to prepare poisons, particularly when an "evil person" was found to be responsible for his patient's illness; however, not all traditional healers were allowed to practice sorcery in this manner. Among the Mbiri of Gabon, for example, traditional healers were bound only by one ethical principle, "do no harm" – another parallel to the Hippocratic tradition.

Indigenous medicine men who were asked to prescribe poisons for known enemies were also bound by an ethical rule that guided the dispensing of such poisons. Before dispensing them, the herbalist had to satisfy himself that the person requesting this service had a genuine grievance, which justified the prescribed measure. Because poisoning another member of the society was such a dangerous and risky venture, the herbalist investigated the matter fully before prescribing the poison to clear himself of any guilt and wrongdoing that might later come to haunt him once the poison was successfully administered.

In conclusion, although there were no formal associations for diviners and traditional herbalists in many African societies, they were kept in frequent contact with each other through meetings, which they arranged amongst each other, usually to give sacrifices to God. Among the Zulu of South Africa, an affluent diviner would once in a while host other fellow diviners, including neighboring medicine men, ex-apprentices, and present students. These sorts of meetings afforded opportunities for different forms of communication. For example, newly qualified healers would be welcomed in a spirit of fraternity or sisterhood; news would be exchanged about occurrences in the various communities represented; discussion would be held about problems posed by the occurrence of particular diseases or diseases that were unfamiliar, and innovations in dealing with specific problems and other issues of communal interest would be shared. These meetings also served to maintain and emphasize Zulu cosmology above all, in that any diviner who was believed to be getting out of line with the basic principles was disciplined and made to conform (Ngubane 1981).

VI. THE TRADITIONAL HEALER'S ROLE IN THE SOCIETY

Most traditional healers underwent long periods of training and apprenticeship to acquire knowledge of medicinal herbs and other specialized medical skills. They also learned to diagnose illnesses of both physical and divine origin and manifestation. As described by Ampofu

> A traditional healer is a person who is recognized by the community in which he lives as competent to provide health care by using vegetables, animal and mineral substances and certain other methods based on the social cultural and religious background as well as on the knowledge, attitudes, and beliefs that are prevalent in the community regarding physical, mental and social well-being and the causation of disease and disability. (Ampofu and Johnson-Romauld, 1978, 38)

This definition delineates the importance of the healer in the community and the great responsibility the title, "healer," bore. According to Mbiti (1969,171), traditional practitioners symbolized the hopes of the society, hopes of good health, protection and security from evil forces, and prosperity and good fortune, and they carried out ritual cleansing when harm or impurities had been contracted. Healers thus had to be upright, moral, responsible, and trustworthy individuals to be able to inspire trust among the citizenry and charge affordable fees (Mbiti 1969, 167). In many communities, such as the Kikuyu of Kenya, the medicine man was a most respected person

within the community (Sindiga, Nyaigotti-Chacha and Kanunah 1995, 134).

Because the traditional medical system was part of a unified whole, interconnected with virtually every other aspect of social life and with ideas and practices that reflected a system of cosmological and earthly order, the traditional healer had other roles. For example, among the Kamba of Kenya, the healer, *mundue mue*, was called upon to interpret and mediate the powerful influence of meanings derived from the interplay of the individual with his family and his culture and the environment (Kiev 1964, iv).

Traditional healers also conducted sacrificial ceremonies, particularly in association with prayers for rain. Rainmaking was an activity that was controlled by diviners and mediums and was of medical interest because inadequate rainfall usually led to hunger and disease. Historically, African savanna societies have depended on rain-fed agricultural production. Because rain was so vital, the cycle of production revolved around it. The High God or aggrieved spirits of the village, chiefdom, or kingdom were believed to be responsible when rainfall was inadequate or untimely, or when some other natural disaster occurred that led to hunger and disease. Rainmaking was thus an important part of the traditional health care system and was a major illness prevention program in which the entire community participated (Waite 1993,17).

The traditional healer was also responsible for the wellness of the community especially in times of plagues and epidemics. When an epidemic broke out, traditional healers were called upon to "chase away" the disease and they became in charge of all the community operations to prevent the spreading of disease among the people. The healers thus coordinated public health programs within their communities in conjunction with the authorities in times of epidemics or environmental disasters that threatened the health of the community.

Benoit (1966) identifies five criteria for the prestige enjoyed by the traditional healer in African societies. The healer was a source of admiration. He or she was also an object of deference; and object of imitation; a source of suggestion and finally the center of attraction. Benoit points out that the high prestige has a contagious facet; those who associate with people of high prestige. This participation was an important motivation to consult a doctor, for people living in a magico-religious atmosphere. Unlike Western societies where the prestige of doctors is partly due to their long academic study, in traditional societies, practitioners gained their prestige from their healing powers and charismata. The financial status of the traditional healer also contributed to his/her status in the community. Traditional healers were in a relatively privileged material position in comparison to other members of the community and all these factors contributed to create an attitude of authority and respect attributed to the healer.

This privileged status translated into the doctor–patient relationship. In most cases, the patient recognized the authority of the doctor and subordinated himself to the "orders" of the healer. It has been argued that the grounds of this subordination lay either in taking the dependent role of the patient or in the fear of negative sanctions from the healer (Kaupen-Haas 1969). In any event, the traditional healer–patient relationship remained largely paternalistic in nature. Whereas traditional healers (both men and women) were integrated into society, because of their great magical powers, they were greatly revered by ordinary members of the community.

The fact that health is inextricably linked with both the supernatural and the biological is central to understanding the role of traditional healers and diviners in the African tradition. Illness, disease, diagnosis, and death assumed cultural dimensions in the various communities in Africa. Thus, African traditional healers had their own strict ethical framework. Colonialists and missionaries who tried to do away with traditional medical infrastructure shunned these ethical principles. Despite a variety of external influences, the traditional healer has survived and to date, maintains a strong presence in most African communities. They are still in constant demand partly due to the fact that modern health care facilities are not easily available or accessible to the average African.

VII. The Introduction of Modern Medicine in Post-colonial Africa

Each country in Africa has its own historical and colonial legacy. For example, Britain colonized among others Zambia, Kenya, Malawi, and Zimbabwe. Germany established rule over Tanzania before World War I and Portugal controlled Mozambique. It is thus impossible to determine a common point in time that Western or modern science was introduced and integrated into African societies. Some African countries have been exposed to modern medicine for more than 100 years whereas others have less than 50 years' experience with Western science (Ndinya-Achola 1995, 1460).

Colonialism in the various African countries did not just expose Africans to Western cultures as embodied in socio-economic institutions such as education, health, and legal infrastructure; it also forcibly subjected Africans to these alien institutions. In so doing, the colonial powers delegitimized and invalidated the existing traditional cultures and this led to the suppression and stripping away of rich resources in the development of traditional beliefs and practices (Owoahene-Acheampong 1998, 137). In the late nineteenth century, European and African worlds were different from each other and acted in a parallel manner in terms of technology, belief and value systems, and culture. The British, Belgians, and Germans came with a new mode of production based on industrial capitalism that

left little space for African community-based concepts of property and modes of production.

Colonial officers and missionaries introduced Western medicine into Africa to displace the traditional regimes and in so doing, despised these African infrastructures as being heathen and the practice of traditional medicine was nothing more than quackery. Europeans in Africa scorned ancestral spirit veneration calling it idolatry, which served to lessen its value among aspiring new elites. Given the religious bases of traditional medicine and culture, most missionaries in colonial Africa adopted a hostile attitude toward them. Thus modern medicine and science were introduced to displace traditional healing systems and to eliminate them as political and medical authorities and advisors to the political leadership (Owoahene-Acheampong 1998, 137).

In Botswana, a conflict arose in this context. It is argued that Tswana medicine was crushed by the missionaries not primarily because the traditional medicine was fundamentally at odds with the "more enlightened" systems of health care of the West, but because as a system it competed as a major ideological, moral, and political force, capable of inducing collective rejection of the missionary and his ways (du Toit and Abdalla 1985, 190–229). To replace these ideas, the missionaries and colonialists ridiculed, disparaged, and rejected the indigenous healers and their practices. Owoahene-Acheampong documents instances in which Orthodox Church missionaries exerted pressure on traditional rulers to persecute practitioners of traditional medicine and outlaw their practices. In Ethiopia, for example, the emperors, under pressure from the Ethiopian Orthodox Church leaders, decreed to punish or punish by the excision of lips and noses, people who chewed or sniffed tobacco because tobacco was considered sacrilegious as it was often used by the traditional healers and their followers. Western medicine was thus introduced to oust traditional medicine all together (Owoahene-Acheampong 1998, 138).

In Kenya, the colonial health department advised European settlers to invest in the health of native laborers because of the possibility of an outbreak of communicable diseases among the locals, which in turn might affect the settlers adversely. Thus, the primary concern was maintaining the health of the settlers. The colonial government went ahead to allocate a relatively small budget toward health services for Africans compared with what was allocated toward the settlers' health care services. Public medical services were limited to urban centers and to those areas considered to have adequately accepted colonial rule. The relationship between medical and education services was quite strategic on the part of the colonial government. These services were used as common rewards for subservience.

Despite being suppressed and condemned during the colonial era, African traditional medicine continued to thrive alongside the modern medical system. After the attainment of independence, countries such as Ghana, Tanzania, and Kenya sought to promote the feeling of "African-ness" by trying to indigenize many of the relics of colonialism. African governments sought to overhaul their education systems and churches, many of which were modeled after those in their respective colonial countries.

The medical sector felt these changes more slowly than did other sectors because the colonial systems had achieved their goal of indoctrinating the ruling (usually educated) elite in the view that Western medicine was superior to their traditional methods of healing. President Kwame Nkrumah of Ghana, for example, directed that traditional healers come together and form an association with a view to improving their practices and restoring their dignity and status in the society. In Tanzania, beginning in the mid-1970s, the government instituted a policy of sponsoring research on medicinal plants (Sindiga, Nyaigotti-Chacha, and Kanunah 1998, 31–32).

Similarly, in Kenya, the government gave official recognition to traditional medicine in 1979. The statement read in part:

> Traditional medicine and health care are an important part of the life of the people in the rural areas. However, more information is needed and will be collected during this plan period with regard to both its substantive aspect and potential link with government institutions . . . further, considerations will be given to the manpower aspects of the traditional sector, for instance, the extent to which certain cadres of selected traditional sector practitioners such as midwives, might be encouraged to serve in Government health institutions in the rural areas. (Republic of Kenya 1979, 136)

This recognition, however, was granted partly due to the governments' inability to set up health care facilities throughout the country, particularly in the rural areas. Despite the issuing of this policy objective, little has been done in terms of recognizing traditional medicine, in terms of support for its technical development through research and development, and finally there has been little support for the development of registration and certification procedures for practitioners (Sindiga, Nyaigotti-Chacha, and Kanunah 1998, 31). The situation in Ghana is similar. For millions of Ghanaians, both rural and urban dwellers, traditional practitioners are the major sources of medical care. Despite this fact, no steps have been taken toward developing indigenous medicine. As noted by Anyinam,

> No formal training programme has been instituted to upgrade, improve upon, and develop healers' medical skills on any appreciable scale. No

budgetary allocations have been made for the promotion and development of ethno-medicine since independence. (Anyinam 1987, 130)

This is true of many African countries. There have been few or no efforts to integrate traditional medical practice with modern medical treatment. Traditional medicine in this context refers to both lay therapies and services provided by traditional healers – harmful forms of traditional medicine are not included.

Traditional health care is still perceived as inferior to the modern health care. The systems run parallel to each other and there is little coordination between the two. The problem is that in most African countries, modern health facilities are not spread out evenly or equitably. Urban areas enjoy relatively well-equipped Western-model medical facilities, whereas rural areas, which have the majority of the population, do not have access to such facilities and people have to travel long distances to reach the nearest hospital or modern health facility. In Kenya, for example, countrywide ratios of modern health centers to population vary from 1:200,000 to 1:50,000 (Bennet and Maneno, 1986). The ratio of Western medically trained doctors to the population is also inadequate. As a result, traditional medicine plays a major role in rural Africa.

Traditional medicine suffers many setbacks in post-colonial Africa. First, it lacks the scientific research support needed to gain more recognition. This problem also prevents further development of the various techniques and herbal substances used to treat disease. Second, traditional practitioners need training in basic disease prevention and management skills so that they are able to operate within clearly defined organizational frameworks – which is not the case in most African countries. Third, traditional healing does not qualify to be classified as a profession because there no examinable, uniform standard quality of care exists. Furthermore, the efficacy and safety of the majority of treatments have yet to be tested. As a result of these problems, especially the lack of nationally coordinated regulation, there has been a proliferation of poorly trained practitioners, which goes to reinforce the negative attitudes toward traditional healers. Furthermore, there is no systematic protection of ownership of orally transmitted information, which is a vital form of intellectual property in traditional medicine (Sindiga, Nyaigotti-Chacha, and Kanunah 1998, 33–34). Thus, traditional healers have no incentive to share their knowledge and information with their modern counterparts. In fact, it is worth noting that because of the centuries of political, social, and cultural disruption, a tremendous amount of oral medical knowledge has been lost. Clearly, the state of traditional medicine today does not reflect the best of what the traditional healers knew.

Even though there does not seem to be any cooperative relationship between traditional practitioners and modern, Western-trained doctors, patients often utilize both systems. These interactions have been classified into four broad categories (Sindiga, Nyaigotti-Chacha, and Kanunah 1998, 33–34). The first form is known as *sequential zigzag*, which refers to patients who begin using either of the medical systems and thereafter move on to the other and thereafter return to the form initially used. The second form of interaction is known as *supplementary* and this relationship exists where only one of the two systems is used for the management or prevention of a condition. A third form of interaction is referred to as *competition*, in which a patient decides to pursue either form of therapy depending on the importance of various factors. This interaction can shift to the sequential zigzag. The fourth form is the *complementary* relationship, in which chronic illnesses are thought to involve psychosocial and spiritual factors; thus a patient may consult both traditional healers for divine intervention as well as Western-trained doctors for physical diagnosis and treatment.

To conclude, there has not been much in terms of a transition of the practice of medicine from traditional healers to modern science. Folk medicine has been left to develop on its own and only recently have countries begun giving it the recognition it deserves. One exception however, is with regard to traditional birth attendants or midwives. This category of traditional healers has more easily integrated into the modern-day health care delivery system. "Mainstream" physicians accept these traditional midwives because they do not pose any serious competition to them in terms of their professional status, their power, and their resources. Western-trained medicine is developed and formally taught at the university level and the curriculum is still very Western in design and content. Physicians who are trained under this system do little to integrate the knowledge and skills of traditional healers. It has been argued that the demise of colonialism did not end the imperialist pattern of thinking in which such physicians are educated. Having examined the ethical framework within which traditional healers conduct their work, it is necessary to investigate the ethical framework, if any, within which modern African doctors perform their services.

VIII. THE WESTERN-TRAINED DOCTOR IN AFRICA

Western medical practice was introduced in many parts of Africa during the colonial period in ways incongruent with traditional healing concepts and practices. In the beginning, clinics and hospitals were set up by the colonial governments to cater to the needs of the European settlers, to the exclusion of black Africans. Later, missionaries established health centers to serve their workers (public service) and also to lure converts away from traditional healing systems. In many parts of Africa, such centers were sporadically located and short on trained staff, and many local people did not have easy access to them.

Upon attaining independence, the new African ruling elites set to providing modern health care services to the people and, in so doing, built more clinics and set up medical training centers. Medical schools were also established at the university level in African countries. These schools' curricula are largely modeled after those of the colonial powers with the most dominant being France and Great Britain. Examples of such schools are the University of Ghana Medical School, Makerere University in Uganda, University of Nairobi Medical School in Kenya, and University of Yaounde Medical School in Cameroon. (Some of these universities however, are now trying to identify relevant and valuable health practices within their own societies and they are seeking ways to harness this knowledge in the context of the modern services they render).

University-trained doctors do not devote much time trying to develop ethical codes or guidelines that are culturally sensitive; instead, they adopt the general medical and professional ethics of the former colonial powers. The Hippocratic Oath remains the main source of ethical principles. The most important of which are privacy and confidentiality, principles that are shared by many traditional healers. A patient who consults a doctor enters into a contractual relationship with the doctor and the doctor then owes the patient a duty of care. There is an implied agreement that the doctor will diagnose the patient's complaint and treat the person in the normal manner according to generally acceptable medical principles. Patients discuss intimate and personal details about themselves with doctors and have a right to expect that their discussions will remain in confidence. In Kenya, doctor–patient confidentiality may be breached in five instances:

- Where a court of law orders doctors to make a disclosure;
- An Act of Parliament requires them to make a disclosure. The best example being the Public Health Act which activates police powers and can make reporting a formidable epidemic a legal requirement;
- If the patient consents to the disclosure being made;
- Where it is necessary for a doctor to defend himself/herself in a disciplinary hearing before the Medical Practitioners and Dentists Board; or
- Where there is a moral or legal obligation on the doctor to make a person or agency that has a reciprocal moral or legal obligation to receive the information.

Most African medical schools curricula do not include ethics as a substantive course. Rather, it is taught in a peripheral manner with usually just one lecture devoted to it. Anglophone African countries such as Kenya and Zimbabwe have medical councils or boards, which are charged with the responsibility of issuing practicing licenses to medical practitioners. The Kenyan Medical

Practitioners and Dentists Board, for example, has the power to withdraw licenses from professionals who undertake unethical practices. Such licensing bodies do not really take on bioethical issues. Instead, they are limited to issues relating to professional secrecy, advertising, professional negligence, fees, and qualifications to practice. This is slowly changing, however, in part because the human immunodeficiency virus/acquired immunodeficiency syndrome (HIV/AIDS) epidemic, which currently affects most of sub-Saharan Africa, has brought with it difficult ethical questions, and this is forcing medical practitioners to consider ways of dealing with these novel ethical problems.

HIV/AIDS, by its very nature, is a clear portrayal of the relationship among medicine, public health law, ethics, and human rights. In providing health care services, doctors have to take into consideration the other dimensions or challenges brought on by the HIV epidemic. The complex dynamics within any society or culture that lead to transmission of HIV and to discrimination and stigmatization, also give rise to difficult questions about rights, responsibilities, and the mechanisms for achieving social and behavioral change for reducing the impact of the epidemic. As a result, doctors can no longer remain confined in the tight framework of their professional duties if they are to be effective in fighting the epidemic. Principles such as strict doctor–patient confidentiality are being challenged in the face of HIV/AIDS. In Kenya, for example, rules of disclosure are being revised to allow doctors to disclose the status of HIV-positive patients to the patient's spouse(s) or known sexual partners.

The imposition of Western standards onto the African experience has created problems, some of which are reflected in the doctor–patient relationship. For example, Western-trained doctors emphasize secondary or tertiary care as opposed to primary care. This means that modern treatment is more curative than preventive and thus requires individual care of the patient by the doctor. Yet, the ratio of Western-trained doctors to the population ranges from 1:3,000 in cities such as Accra (Ghana), Nairobi (Kenya) and Dakar (Senegal) to 1:200,000 in rural areas such as Northern Nigeria, Mali, Burkina Faso, Niger, and Chad, rendering intimate care impractical, if not impossible. These ratios also allow doctors in African countries to assume paternalistic attitudes toward their patients. Furthermore, it is argued that many countries in Africa need stronger public and primary health care structures, rather than the expensive sophisticated, urban-based hospitals, which cater mainly to the African elite.

Postcolonial European ethical codes and texts are often inapplicable in the African context. They are typically directed at nurses and physicians, yet western medical services are usually delivered by paramedical personnel in health care centers in many parts of both rural and urban

Africa, because of the shortage of trained doctors. These medical officers are trained in medical training colleges and upon completion of their studies, take on duties traditionally performed by medical doctors. Many of them actually run clinics, dispense drugs, and counsel patients but because they are not physicians, they are not subject to any professional ethical code or recognized ethical principles. They do not fall under the professional councils or boards governing the practice of medicine. They also do not fall under the classification of traditional doctors, who are themselves subject to strict ethical codes as seen in the previous section. There is thus a clear need for revision of the present ethical codes and guidelines governing the practice of modern medicine in African countries. The revised codes ought take into consideration cultural specificities, which are not apparent in the "colonial codes" currently in place. There is also a need to consider the various personnel delivering medical services and to determine their ethical responsibilities.

IX. CONCLUSION

Africa has yet to experience any meaningful integration of traditional medical systems with modern medical systems as introduced by Western colonial countries. Although the systems run parallel to each other, traditional healing methods are still viewed with suspicion by Western-trained doctors (including African doctors). Most African countries still follow the ethical codes inherited as colonial legacies. Yet, these codes do not apply to the African experience and are in urgent need of reform, as briefly outlined previously. African countries also need to face up to the reality that traditional medical systems still serve the majority of the population in some way and thus need support to develop, improve, and ensure their integration into national health care delivery system.

NOTE

1. The traditional healer, sometimes known as a "Medicine Man" is an important part of African health care and culture. Healers are first and foremost concerned with sickness, disease, and misfortune in the community. They are mandated to find out the cause of a disease (both physical and spiritual causes), apply the right treatment, and create a means of preventing the misfortune from occurring again. In the African context, traditional healers have various specializations or professional areas of practice. For example, there are herbalists, diviners, seers, spiritualists, traditional surgeons, and birth attendants. Furthermore, a healer can have one or more areas of specialization based upon his or her knowledge, skills, and years of careful empirical observations (Mbiti 1969). Traditional healers are also consulted on wider societal issues such as increasing agricultural productivity, aiding in fertility, detecting sorcery, removing curses, and controlling spirits in the cosmos. They are well-connected to

their communities and are greatly respected. Traditional healers often provide the only available and/or affordable method of health care delivery in much of Africa and in some places traditional healers outnumber doctors by 100 to 1. Traditional healers, therefore, play a crucial role in administering health care to the majority of Africans; however their role is still not concretely defined and there is much disparity between western-trained or allopathic doctors and indigenous practitioners. Many from the sector and outside it feel that traditional healers should take up their rightful place within an integrated medical community.

CHAPTER 20

THE DISCOURSES OF PRACTITIONERS IN INDIA

Katherine K. Young

I. INTRODUCTION

Early civilizations were characterized by a growth in specialized knowledge. Natural, supernatural, and social realms were gradually differentiated – but not totally separated (that had to await modern times). This in turn allowed for empiricism (the development of science, including medicine). The corollary of the development of specialized knowledge was the development of professional classes. In India we have records for these developments after the second round of urbanization, which occurred from approximately 800 BCE. In the texts of the classical period (600 BCE–600), we find glimpses of new professional self-consciousness, discourses about the superiority of empirical medicine and its elite practitioners (as distinguished from quacks), and concerns about the public image of the profession (as technically competent, nonexploitative, and model citizen). We find some attempts to ensure group control of the new physicians beginning with their apprenticeship and the taking of oaths (Hinduism) or indirect regulation by the general observance of monastic rules including the required monthly confessions (Buddhism). The discourses of practitioners also describe model nurses and model patients, and who should have access to medicine.

Despite the development of empirical medicine, the discourses of physicians show the model physician to be a spiritual man. The Hindu view of this was directed to the married householder, either the *brāhmaṇa* physician who received gifts (and thus his livelihood) for his skills or other physicians who were paid for their expertise. The early Buddhist view was less explicit (in that those practicing medicine within the monasteries were more caregivers in lieu of a family than professional physicians proper). In Mahāyāna, the ideal religious figure (the *bodhisattva*) worked outside the monastery, often as a physician, thus collapsing the distinction between the monastic and lay realms (see Chapters 9, 10).

In the discourses of practitioners, we find a concern with social and religious differences. In Hinduism, these have included differences defined by hierarchy and purity/impurity, whereas in Buddhism they have included monastic and lay orientations or sectarian ones, such as Theravāda, Mahāyāna, and Vajrayāna. Because Hinduism and Buddhism competed over many centuries, they tried to make the appeal of their religion greater by providing access to medicine. Although one might think that the universal access to medicine promoted by the Mahāyāna Buddhists would ensure its long-term success, this in fact was not the case, in part because (*bhakti*) Hinduism itself developed a rhetoric of universalism and in part because Buddhism never escaped its monastic orientation to appeal sufficiently to the needs of the laity. Then too Hinduism integrated many of the magical aspects of religion into empiricism, thereby broadening its folk appeal during the medieval period. After the arrival of Islam in India, this also served to keep Islamic medicine at bay. But with colonialism and the establishment of Western medicine, the discourses of practitioners reflect a deep conflict of values at the heart of medical practice – a conflict that has played out in independent India with the call for a return to a pure Hindu medicine as an expression of Indian nationalism. Today there is beginning to be a new voice in the discourses of practitioners – that of the patient. This has been inspired by international connections and new therapeutic programs (especially for alcoholism and drugs) and by contact with nongovernment organizations (NGOs) with their international connections. In addition, traditional medicines and their underlying principles of holism and balance are spreading to the West. Their new prestige is contributing to a rise in their status at home (even as their new context is transforming them through integration with New Age spirituality abroad).

II. THE DEVELOPMENT OF A PROFESSIONAL CLASS

In the later books (composed approximately 800 BCE) of the *Ṛg-veda*, the physician (*bhiùaj*) is identified cynically as a one who wants people to have broken bones so he can fix them and obtain wealth (*Ṛg-veda* IX.112.1). This passage lists professionals such as the carpenter (*takṣan*), healer (*bhiṣaj*), and priest (*brāhmaṇa*). Healers are like carpenters in the sense that they fix things but like priests in the sense that they have esoteric knowledge (Zysk 1991, 21). In addition, the physician is described as a *brāhmaṇa* and a *vipra* who has knowledge of herbal remedies for which he is given a horse, cow, or garment (*Ṛg-veda* X.97.4 and 6). Because *vipra* means shaking, this may refer to a healer who goes into possession as a way to communicate with a deity and find out the nature of the problem or cure. Possession was not a type of brahmanical religious experience, however, and so this reference might indicate assimilation of a non-Vedic healing tradition (see Chapter 9).

One text of the late Vedic period (c. 800–600 BCE), the *Taittirīya-saṃhitā*, alludes to the extra-Vedic status of physicians through an elaborate version of the myth of the divine physician twins, the Aśvins. It says that according to the gods, "'these two physicians, who roam with humans, [are] very impure.' Therefore, medicine is not to be practiced by a Brāhman, for he, who is a physician [*bhiṣaj*], [is] impure, unfit for the sacrifice" (Zysk 1991, 22). The passage goes on to describe how the twins are purified with the chanting of a sacred verse and then comments: "[The

gods] deposited the healing [powers] of those two in three places: a third in fire [Agni], a third in the waters, [and] a third in the Brāhman caste. Therefore, having placed the water vessel to one side [and] having sat down to the right of a Brāhman, one should practice medicine. To be sure, as much medicine as he practices by this means, his work is accomplished" (Zysk 1991, 22). This suggests that the physicians have been accepted into Vedic religion through mantric purification and the performance of the (Soma) sacrifice; it also implies that *brāhmaṇa*s are themselves becoming physicians.

From these references, we see that the status of physicians was already a concern for the *brāhmaṇa*s. On the one hand, they wanted the herbal knowledge and skills of healers but on the other they were worried that integration of this knowledge (or the healers themselves) into their own elite (*brāhmaṇa/ārya*) society would lower their status. Even when the healers were ritually initiated into the brahmanical tradition, their status remained a matter of some concern. *Baudhāyana Dharmasūtra* II.1.2 (600–300 BCE), for instance, compares the *brāhmaṇa* physician to an actor or dance teacher who has very low status. The practice of medicine was a sin that could be expiated only by a 2-year exile as an outcaste. This ambiguity of status would continue over the centuries.

Early medicine was also connected to the ascetics. This is corroborated by Strabo (64 BCE–21), drawing from accounts by Megasthenes (the Greek ambassador of Seleukos Nikator to the Indian court of Chandragupta Maurya c. 300 BCE). Strabo divides philosophers into the Brachmanes and the Garmanes (*brāhmaṇa*s and *śramaṇa*s). The first group includes the forest hermits, who wear bark, live on leaves and fruits, associate with kings, determine the causes of things, and petition the deities. [This description approximates that of the Atharva-vedins (see later) who were the *brāhmaṇa* priests (*purohit*s) of kings, performing rituals to determine auspicious timings for battles, and so forth. They were considered to have low brahmanical status by other *brāhmaṇa*s.] The second group consists of physicians who beg for alms, cure diseases by diets, ointments, and so forth, and provide fertility rituals. They practice yoga such as remaining in one position for a long period, and have a philosophical bent. Strabo says the first type is most honored (Strabo XV.60 cited by Zysk 1991, 28). Strabo also refers to Pramnae (another corruption of *śramaṇa*) who are divided into the naked types (the Jains or their precursors?), the mountain types clad in deerskins who offer cures from their bags of roots and herbs as well as by their spells and amulets, and the city types clad in linen. Basham (1976, 24–25) identifies the mountain types with the hill-tribes. All this suggests that religious medicine was associated with various groups, including some ascetic ones. These groups influenced both the brahmanical and Buddhist traditions.

Out of, or in interaction with, archaic healing specialists including wandering herbalists and shamans, some with ascetic orientations, emerged several elite groups practicing a more empirical medicine. Resorting to observation, classification, and experimentation, they developed new explanations, medicines, and therapies. It is difficult to know where empirical medicine first developed. We do know that empirical medicine was "codified" in the Vinaya or monastic rules of the Theravāda Pāli Canon. Key passages describe the Buddha's appeal to monastics to care for each other (because they were now without family), permission to obtain and store certain kinds of foods to be used for medicines, and classifications of types of medicine in use (see chapter 10). This suggests that empirical medicine was well known to the Buddhist monasteries by the first century BCE, when the Pāli Canon was finalized, and perhaps as early as the fourth century BCE, assuming that the Vinaya belongs to the oldest strata. Empirical medicine was also well known to the authors of the (Hindu) Caraka-saṃhitā and Suśruta-saṃhitā.[1] The early strata of the these (represented by the presumed authors âtreya and Agniveśa) were written from the third century BCE but were probably built on earlier traditions of empirical medicine in the previous century. Both of these texts likely represented compendiums of schools rather than works by individuals (the word caraka literally means "wander" and suśruta means "well-heard" or "famous"), a point underscored by the fact that there are internal accounts about parts being lost or added. (This process was ongoing. A redaction of the Caraka was made by Dçóhabala in the fourth or fifth century CE, and one of the Suśruta was done by one Nāgārjuna, who added the sixth and last part of the text, before the sixth century).

Whatever its exact origins, empirical medicine was further developed in the universities. Taxilā was a famous university from the third century BCE frequented by both Buddhists and Hindus alike (Zysk 1991, 55). It was famous for medicine among its many subjects. The Buddhist Jātaka texts testify to its cosmopolitan nature that attracted students from all castes (except the outcastes, caṇālas). Many brāhmaṇas attended and studied nontraditional subjects (Mookerji [1947] 1989, 482). In this context, it should be recalled that âtreya, the presumed author of the Caraka, may have been at Taxilā at the same time as the famous physician Jīvika, who catered to the Buddhist monasteries (according to Zysk and Basham). This suggests that Buddhist and Hindu empirical medicine developed in an interactive way in India from about the fourth century BCE on. One Buddhist text, for instance, refers to brāhmaṇas as physicians (Ekottarāgama T 125:33:731a–b cited by Demi‚ville 1985, 31, 84). The existence of common terms in the âyurvedic texts and the Pāli Canon – Sanskrit vaidya, bhiṣaj, cikitsaka; and Pāli vejja, bhisaka, and tikicchaka for physician, medicine, and medicine/therapy respectively – speaks to this common source and subsequent interaction.

According to Paul Demi‚ville: "Nothing in India warrants a distinction between a 'monastic medicine' and the medical tradition proper such as historians of medicine make in the Christian West" (Demiéville 1985, 92–93).

There are no references in the texts to case studies of particular patients. On the surface, this is not a casuistic literature. Yet, according to Basham (1976, 26–27), cases were probably the topic of colloquia (saṃbhāṣā), which for the Caraka were a way to increase the physician's knowledge and demonstrate his debating skills (Caraka-saṃhitā Vimānasthāna VIII.27): "A physician should make statements with due regard to the principles of debates. He should not make statements out of context or contrary to scriptural prescriptions or without due examination of irrelevant, confused or too sketchy statements. Whatever he states should be based on arguments" (Caraka-saṃhitā Vimānasthāna VIII.67).

III. DISCOURSES ON ETHICS: HINDUISM

Hindu medical ethics emerges into view in the Caraka-saṃhitā and the Suśruta-saṃhitā. They describe not only the nature of empirical medicine, concepts of disease and health (imbalance and balance of the dhātus), and so forth (see Chapter 9), they also set the standards for the practice of medicine, which included model behavior and ethics. The new interest in ethics was closely related to the need to distinguish empirical physicians from quacks by their expertise, decorum, ethics, and spiritual values.

1. On the Proper Behavior of a Real Physician

Physicians must have knowledge, a critical approach, understanding of other branches of knowledge, good memory, promptness, and perseverance to cure diseases. Any of the following – knowledge, intellect, practical experience, continued practice, success in treatment, and dependence on an experienced preceptor – justifies use of the word "vaidya" and the presence of all these qualities justifies the term "excellent physician who comforts all living beings" (Caraka-saṃhitā Sūtrasthāna IX.21–23). The Suśruta says much the same: he must have studied with a preceptor and gained experience by constant practice (Suśruta-saṃhitā Sūtrasthāna IV.6). References to preceptor mean that empirical medicine is learned within an elite, group context. More specifically, it belongs to a sampradāya (a tradition with established teachings transmitted from teacher to disciple).

The development of empirical medicine intensified the debate over definitions of expertise and quackery. There are said to be three types of physicians: pseudo-physicians who establish their credentials simply by exhibiting a box of drugs and medical books; feigned physicians whose reputation is based on their connection to people with wealth, fame, and knowledge, and finally, real physicians

(*Caraka-saṃhitā Sūtrasthāna* XI.5–53). We are then told that "[I]t is better to die than to be treated by a physician ignorant of the science of medicine. Because, like a blind person moving with the help of his hands or like a boat being driven by the wind, a quack physician applies the course of treatment with apprehension because of his ignorance" (*Caraka-saṃhitā Sūtrasthāna* IX.15–16).

Unlike real physicians, quacks dress like physicians, quickly gather around a sick person, use flattery with the friends of the patient, claim they will take only minimum remuneration, blame all setbacks on the patient, disappear when there is a death, quote formulas that are not relevant to demonstrate knowledge, and avoid questions. Moreover, "nobody would know anything about their preceptor, disciple, classmate or even their opponents" (*Caraka-saṃhitā Sūtrasthāna* XXIX.8–9).

In short, formal, brahmanical style education, association with reputable teachers within the context of a *sampradāya*, or university (such as Taxila), and moral character distinguish real physicians from quacks. Institutionalized contexts establish credentials not only through the acquisition of expertise about empirical medicine but also by providing accountability to the teacher and the group. These in turn provide some control over this new branch of specialized knowledge not unlike the control exercised by guilds in the Greco-Roman world. Other texts refer to governmental regulation of the practice of medicine. *Yājñavalkya-dharmasāstra* (c. 100 BCE–300) states that quacks (*kuvaidyas*) must be punished by the king but not qualified physicians when a patient dies (Basham 1976). Because of the king's surveillance of the medical system, students were warned not to anger the king by treating his enemies. The *Suśruta* also notes that fake physicians can be killed by the king (*Suśruta-saṃhitā Sūtrasthāna* III.18). In addition, the text observes that the lives of physicians are at risk in their relationship to the king (they are often the ones to supervise the kitchens to prevent poisoning, and if poison were found, they could be blamed) (*Suśruta-saṃhitā Sūtrasthāna* XXXIV.2–4). Consequently, physicians are encouraged to gather their own herbs to ensure their purity and should be prudent, reverential, and loyal to the king as if he were a deity (*Suśruta-saṃhitā Sūtrasthāna* XXXIV.6).

The practice of medicine is closely related to the concept of good behavior (*sattva*) in the sense of withdrawing the mind from that which is harmful (*Caraka-saṃhitā Sūtrasthāna* XI.54). This is an intriguing definition. It links *ahiṃsā* (nonkilling, noninjury) to both medicine (a basic principle being to do no harm) and religion. *Ahiṃsā* is said to promote longevity more than anything else (*Caraka-saṃhitā Sūtrasthāna* XXX.15). A basic principle of moral and yogic development is to withdraw the mind from harmful things. Medicines made from animals were allowed for therapeutic reasons, an exception to the general rule of non-violence. Caraka "was not so much

a skilled technician as he was a moralist, preacher, and philosopher ... It does not follow that Susruta was not a philosopher, though he was inclined more to skill than to philosophy" (Yano 1976–1977, 339). In parts of the medical texts, ethical ideas from the Dharmasāstras are intertwined with medical ones.

The *Caraka's* prescriptions refer to good relationships with others of model character. In line with the brahmanical tone of this text, codes of right conduct include respect to superiors (a term that signifies *brāhmaṇa*s) and cows (a symbol of Hinduism and *ahiṃsā* by the classical period). The *Caraka* strings together a list of virtues to characterize the ideal physician:

> Those who are the well-wishers of all creatures, who do not aspire for the wealth of others, who are truthful, peace loving, who examine things before acting upon them, who are vigilant, who enjoy the three important desires of life viz., virtue, wealth and pleasure without the one affecting the other, who respect superiors, who are endowed with the knowledge of arts, sciences and tranquility, who serve the elders, who have full control over passion, anger, envy, pride and prestige, who are constantly given to various types of charity, meditation, acquisition of knowledge and quite [sic] life (solitude), who have full knowledge of the spiritual power, and are devoted to it, who make efforts both for the existing as well as the next life and are endowed with memory and intelligence, lead a useful life. (*Caraka-saṃhitā Sūtrasthāna* XXX.24)

This ad hoc list suggests that a physician should lead a balanced, full life that includes experiences of all its basic goods such as wealth, knowledge, and pleasure. These should be pursued with moderation, restrained by ethics, and placed within a larger context of respect and tolerance for all beings, which is the corollary of personal spiritual development: "If one sees oneself as spread in the entire universe and the entire universe spread in oneself, one is in possession of other-worldly and worldly vision. One's peace based on knowledge is not destroyed. Indeed, when one sees all beings everywhere in all situations, there is oneness (*samyoga*) with the Absolute (*Brahman*). One does not produce virtuous (and sinful) acts (i.e., one is beyond the duality of good and evil)" (*Caraka-saṃhitā Śarīrasthāna* V.20–21). This passage views liberation as nondualism (*advaita*). Good and evil belong to the ordinary realm. Nondualism is beyond all oppositions (*dvandva*s). It is assumed, however, that good (the *sāttvika guṇa*) has been perfected on the path to liberation (see Chapter 9) and is spontaneously expressed after liberation in this life. In Hinduism, actions are classified as having three types of qualities (*guṇa*s): *tāmasika* (unfree and so the agent is not responsible); *rājasika* (only partially free because of attachments and repulsions yet the agent can be held responsible because of the possibility of removing them), and *sāttvika* (fully free because all desires have been removed, and so the agent is fully responsible) (Dastidar 1987, 102). Although some yogic orientations have advocated not acting (*akarma*) because actions are said to bind one in the wheel of existence, others understand true non-action to reside in the performance of action done without desire (*naiṣkāmya-karmayoga*). This is the goal of the *sāttvika* person and results in liberation. Another passage remarks on the nature of a physician. Here too medical expertise and ethics are intertwined. He should have "excellence in medical knowledge, an extensive practical experience, dexterity and purity – these are the four qualities of a physician" (*Caraka-saṃhitā Sūtrasthāna* IX.6).

The importance of medical ethics is underscored in the oaths (called *vrata* or vow) that the student makes to the teacher and the teacher to the student in the ritual of initiation into the study of medicine, which is done in front of the sacred fire.

Medical students were initiated into the profession by a teacher in front of the sacred fire. As students, they were to be celibate, nonviolent, vegetarian, speak the truth, be without envy, and be totally dedicated to their teacher (guru), serving him and obeying him. (This is the general brahmanical model of initiation into studentship (brahmacarya.) At this time the student made the following oath according to the *Caraka*.

> If thou desirest success, wealth and fame as a physician and heaven after death, thou shalt pray for the welfare of all creatures beginning with the cows and Brahmanas. Day and night, however thou mayest be engaged, thou shalt endeavour for the relief of patients with all thy heart and soul. Thou shalt not desert or injure thy patient for the sake of thy life or thy living. Thou shalt not commit adultery even in thought. Even so, thou shalt not covert others' possessions. Thou shalt be modest in thy attire and appearance. Thou shouldst not be a drunkard or a sinful man nor shouldst thou associate with the abettors of crimes. Thou shouldst speak words that are gentle, pure, and righteous, pleasing, worthy, true, wholesome, and moderate. (Spicer 1995b, 2633)

The *Suśruta* says that all castes can be initiated into the study of medicine, but a *brāhmaṇa* can initiate only the three higher castes and *śūdras* must be initiated without Vedic *mantra*s (*Suśruta-saṃhitā Sūtrasthāna* II.4). In the initiation, the teacher tells the student: "Thou shalt renounce lust, anger, greed, ignorance, vanity, egotistic feelings, envy, harshness, niggardliness, falsehood, idleness, nay all acts that soil the good name of a man. In proper season thou shalt pair thy nails and clip thy hair and put on the sacred cloth, dyed brownish yellow, live the life of a truthful, self-controlled anchorite and be obedient and respectful towards thy preceptor" (*Suśruta-saṃhitā Sūtrasthāna*

II.4–5). In other words, the student is to lead an ethical and ascetic life (his ochre cloth, in fact, assimilates him to the *śramaṇa* or ascetic groups). As a student-ascetic, he learns humility and dependency by having to beg for his daily food. The teacher oversees the student's development of moral character along with his academic study. The guru goes on to say that the student must follow his commands with integrity but also that he, the teacher, must treat the student justly and not take advantage of his obedience. The student then takes up the precise memorization of the medical texts (*Suśruta-saṃhitā Sūtrasthāna* III.19). Whereas the student wears ochre cloth, the physician dresses in white (*Suśruta-saṃhitā Sūtrasthāna* X.2). This aligns with Strabo's description of city physicians wearing white.

Because medical education includes oaths and cultivation of virtues under the watchful eye of preceptors, and the law of karma acts as an internal constraint against wrong doing, the potentially negative effects of paternalism are mitigated and benevolence encouraged (at least according to the normative texts, the physician is to treat his patients as his own sons and protect them when they mistrust their own parents) (*Suśruta-saṃhitā Sūtrasthāna* XXV.23).

The ethics of the physician extends to his helpers. "Knowledge of nursing, dexterity, affection and purity – these are the four qualities of an attendant" (*Caraka-saṃhitā Sūtrasthāna* IX.8). Elsewhere it is said that medical attendants are to be "endowed with good conduct, cleanliness, character, devotion, dexterity and sympathy and who are conversant with the art of nursing and good in administering therapies . . . People well-versed with vocal and instrumental music, panegyrics, recitation of verses, ancient lores, short stories, Itihāsa (the *Mahābhārata*, etc.), *purāṇa* (mythology), those who can grasp the inner desires, who are obedient, and who have knowledge of the time and place" (*Caraka-saṃhitā Sūtrasthāna* XV.7). Here too ethics is closely intertwined with ideal behavior that consists of expertise in empirical medicine and knowledge of religious texts, but also, interestingly, the ability to entertain.

In addition, the discourses of practitioners make comments on patients. Good patients are to have honesty, fearlessness, memory, and obedience to the physician (*Caraka-saṃhitā Sūtrasthāna* IX.9), all of which help him to know the facts of the particular case, make his diagnosis, and customize the treatment. (On the qualities of a physician, nurse, and patient see also *Suśruta-saṃhitā Sūtrasthāna* XXXIV.9–12.)

After such a strong description of the virtuous character of physicians and helpers, the next passage is surprising. "The doctor should be sympathetic and kind to all patients, should be concerned with those who are likely to be cured and should feel detached [from] . . . those who are towards death. These are the four disciplines for a physician" (*Caraka-saṃhitā Sūtrasthāna* IX.26). Of course, it could be argued that this detachment in the face of a patient's death is not from lack of concern but from the physician's own psychological need to let go at the appropriate moment. Detachment in Hinduism is a yogic ideal, and therefore has positive connotations. This reference to detachment might also be related to the fact that physicians should not treat those who are incurable or dying (see Chapter 44). No doubt this was designed to secure the status of the fledgling profession. The passage suggests that access to medicine is a reward for good behavior – those who are bad should be punished by not being given treatment. It also suggests that care of the poor, feeble, and those without servants (who provide help for both the physician and the patient) is optional. In addition, the Indian medical oath discourages a physician's services to enemies of his ruler and unattended women. A physician is to have compassion for all and must help others if possible; however, he is under *no obligation or duty* to do so. This no doubt served to limit the concept of universalism. This takes us to the topic of access to medicine.

2. On Access to Medicine

There is some debate over access to medicine. The *Caraka* states that everyone is to have medical knowledge, albeit for different reasons: *brāhmaṇa*s to help all creatures, *kṣatriya*s to protect their subjects, *vaiśya*s for earning an income, and everyone for attaining *dharma*, *artha*, and *kāma* and for protecting others (*Caraka-saṃhitā Sūtrasthāna* XXX.29). Thus, this medical system ostensibly provides for basic knowledge of what is necessary for health and prevention of disease, possibly even universal access. Underlying this universalism, however, is a two-tiered system. (1) As just mentioned, some patients such as the incurable have no access to medicine because they can be abandoned. According to the *Suśruta*, professional hunters, habitual sinners and others were also not to be treated (*Suśruta-saṃhitā Sūtrasthānam* I.2.5). (2) Others receive care for free. According to the *Suśruta*, physicians are to treat *brāhmaṇa*s, elders, preceptors, friends, the indigent, the honest, ascetics, the poor, and orphans for free (*Suśruta-saṃhitā Sūtrasthānam* I.2.5). Charity to the needy in general is encouraged by the texts. The model of kingship includes the support of *dharma* by being just and generous. Kauṭilya's *Artha-śāstra* (II.1.4) says, for instance, that the king should give lands to physicians among others. (3) Others pay (see Basham 1976, 29–31 for references to public clinics and physicians advertising their expertise, and their high fees.) (4) And still others pay according to their capacity. The *Caraka* points out that poor patients when faced with an emergency will have to forego expensive, rare drugs and take only those things they can obtain according to their capacity (*Caraka-saṃhitā Sūtrasthāna* XV.19–20).

Dunn argues that access to medical care was limited to upper caste, urban men; the higher the status, the better the treatment (1976, 149). Kings and their courts, moreover, had their own physician, second in professional status only to their priest (*purohita*). The two would accompany kings on all travels and onto the battlefield to treat the wounded. *Artha-śāstra* (X.3.47) says "Physicians, with surgical instruments, apparatus, medicines, oils and bandages . . . shall be stationed in the rear . . ." (see also Kangle, trans. *The Kauṭilīya Arthasāstra* [1969] 1988, 441; *Rāmāyaṇa* II.77.14). *Suśruta-saṃhitā Sūtrasthāna* (XXXIV.6) says that a physician should live in a camp near the king and treat the warriors.

3. On Status

(Hindu) brahmanical discourses of practitioners continue to be concerned about status. It is striking that *śūdra*s, the lowest of the four castes (a category that might also include foreigners or Buddhists) attended universities such as Taxilā. According to the *Suśruta*, *śūdra* students were to be taught without proper initiation (*upanayana*: this initiated education in the Vedas and was permitted only for the three higher castes, which made them "twice-born"), but in a method otherwise akin to Vedic pedagogy – memorization by the student, and explanation by the teacher (*Suśruta-saṃhitā* II.4; see also Basham 1976, 25). (Over time, when surgery lost status among *brāhmaṇa* physicians for reasons of impurity, it is likely that some expertise was preserved by *śūdra*s. As a result, surgery became the expertise mainly of the low status "barber-surgeons." Even *ambaṣṭha*s, once of high status (see later) who had migrated to South India and then Bengal eventually fell into this category (Wujastyk 1998, 106–107).)

An idea of the concern over status can be gleaned from the Dharmaśāstras, the brahmanical, "normative" texts. Manu (c. 200 BCE–200), who was trying to preserve brahmanical orthodoxy (based in part on concepts of purity) in an age of foreign invasions as well as heterodox religious challenges, viewed the very presence of physicians (*vaidya*s) as defiling food (*Manu* III.152). *Viṣṇu-purāṇa*, a later text, says that the penance for one who accepts food from a physician is to consume only milk for 7 days (Basham 1976, 36).

Some Dharmaśāstra passages suggest that *brāhmaṇa*s who become physicians lose status. Manu mentions a caste called *ambaṣṭha* descended from *brāhmaṇa* fathers and *vaiśya* mothers, who were healers (*Manu* X.8, 47). Attributing deviance to caste mixture, the sin of miscegenation, was a way of voicing opprobrium and explaining a lowering of status in brahmanical eyes. This indicates that the physician's role (which had always been somewhat ambiguous despite its integration into some brahmanical circles such as the Atharva-vedins) was associated with impurity (caused by touching the body, especially its fluids, which made surgery anathema in the eyes of the orthodox) (see Chapter 9). The physician's role, moreover, was associated with low caste, hill people with their bags of herbs and amulets, who were perceived as wandering quacks.

But there are several deeper reasons for this idea of loss of status. One was that some *brāhmaṇas* were leaving their priestly role (which was supported by the gifts of ritual clients) for the lucrative one of medicine (for which they were paid handsomely). With this new role, they might have abandoned their Vedic learning, that too at a time when the Vedic tradition was under enormous threat, even though they might have justified this choice by arguing that they were allowed to resort to other professions in times of hardship, the ethics of *āpaddharma*. At the same time, *brāhmaṇas* needed physicians and desired, for reasons of purity, to be treated by those of similar status. This contributed to the ambiguity. (The *ambaṣṭha* in later centuries was called a "clean" or twice-born caste, somewhat below other *brāhmaṇas*. Parāsara, states, for instance, that the function of the *ambaṣṭha* is to treat *brāhmaṇas* only (Dutt 1965, 71 cited by Basham 1976, 37).)

The case of the Atharva-vedins is particularly intriguing when the topic is status. The *Atharva-veda* (the fourth *Veda*) refers to religious material, much of which is archaic and extra-Vedic material, such as *mantras*, charms, amulets, and medicinal plants, whose propitious use is regulated by astronomical timings. This text also refers to *munis* or forest hermits who had been associated with the god Rudra of the *Ṛg-veda* (see Chapter 9), and it refers to healers who wander about to gather medicines and make their expertise available. This might have given rise to the term *cāraṇavaidya* (wandering physician) and be an example of the wandering ascetics mentioned by Strabo. It is curious that a *mantra* in this text "praises the virtues and power of amulets as equal to thousands of medicines used by thousands of physicians (*Atharva-veda* II.9.5 cited by Haldar 1977, 12). This points to the existence of empirical medicine, which had created a competitive environment, perhaps causing the author of the text to say that nonetheless the priest (*atharvan*) is "the best of all good physicians." If the Atharva-vedins, who viewed themselves as custodians of religious medicine, felt that empirical medicine was attracting their clients, they may have decided to upgrade their skills by appropriating empirical medicine.

The *Caraka* and *Suśruta* were connected explicitly to the *Atharva-veda*. "Of the four – *Ṛk, Yajus, Sāman* and *Atharvan-veda*s, physicians owe their loyalty to the *Atharva-veda* because this deals with the treatment of diseases by taking recourse to gift, propitiatory rites, worship, auspicious observances, oblations, observance of spiritual rules, atonement, fast, incantations etc. They are prescribed for the sake of longevity" (*Caraka-saṃhitā Sūtrasthāna* XXX.21). It is likely that the Atharva-vedins decided to integrate empirical medicine. This might have been done in one (now lost) school of the *Atharva-veda* called *Cāraṇa* (a word related to *Caraka*), about the same time that the *Atharva-veda* tradition was attempting to gain status as the fourth Veda, which necessitated presenting itself as more in line with brahmanical customs. The curious mix found in the *Caraka* – traditional brahmanical styles of Vedic learning and ritual along with *mantras*, amulets, and so forth as well as empirical medicine – speaks to this appropriation. The fact that the *brāhmaṇas* already involved in the study of medicine had lost status in the eyes of the orthodox might have encouraged them to regroup under the banner of an *Atharva-veda/Āyurveda* combined tradition now claiming equal if not superior status to other brahmanical groups. The fact that the (Buddhist) Jātaka tales refer only to the teaching of the three Vedas suggests that this *Atharva-veda* maneuver was after the major development of empirical medicine. It probably developed as the Atharva-vedins competed with the Mahāyāna Buddhists in the Deccan about the beginning of the Common Era and was then integrated into the *Caraka* with a new redaction of the text.

The *Suśruta* makes an intriguing comment in this regard. A king is to have both a priest and a physician, for together they protect the king: "The god Brahmā disclosed to the world the *Atharva Veda* together with the eight allied branches of Vedic literature and the science of medicine. And since a priest (*brāhmaṇa*) is well-versed in the aforesaid branches of study, a physician should act subserviently and occupy a subordinate position to the priest" (*Suśruta-saṃhitā Sūtrasthāna* XXXIV.5). In short, Atharva-vedins have integrated empirical medicine but make sure physicians have less status than the priests.

4. On Purity and Impurity

In the final analysis, medical practice in the Hindu tradition was affected not only by social hierarchy but also by related concerns over purity. Purity (*śauca*) was a key concept in traditional Hinduism (see Chapter 9): It referred to ethnic, physical, ritual, and ethical purity. By contrast, impurity was defined by belonging to the wrong ethnic group, not being eligible to perform rituals, by biological processes such as birth and death, or by contact with impure substances – excreta, the food of others, and the touch of low-caste people. This, in turn, created a special problem for physicians and nurses who had to minister to the sick, especially when touch was involved as in surgery or diagnosis by palpation. When explaining the technique of systematically touching the body, the *Caraka* says that it is to be done with the right hand *or by someone else* (*Caraka-saṃhitā Sūtrasthāna* V.3–4). "Taboos against touching and ideas of ritual impurity almost completely outlawed palpation as a method of observation, and intuition and inference were enlarged to proportions greater than what we may expect from materialists" (Desai 1989, 85). Although temporary impurity could be removed by a ritual bath, impurity that was related to constant contact with impure substances created a permanent untouchability. "The important point to note here is that, because of such notions, the Hindu has a greater aversion in general to contact with blood, urine, dead bodies, fecal matter, and the like than the average Westerner" (Sharma 2002, 3).

5. Modern Discourses

With colonialism, tension developed between Western empirical medicine and traditional Hindu (Āyurveda) medicine (see Chapters 9 and 10). By the time of independence in 1947, the proponents of exclusive (âyurveda) and inclusive (Western, àyurveda, Yunāni, and any other) positions were embroiled in many political disputes and a struggle for governmental support. Shiv Sharma, a well-educated, wealthy *brāhmaṇa* advocated a "pure" (*śuddha*) âyurveda, lobbied to reduce the influence of Western medicine in âyurvedic colleges, and was extremely influential as Chairman of the Ministry of Health's Central Council for Research on Indigenous Medicine in defining national policies through the 1970s. "In 1972 the state boards of indigenous medicine had registered 257,000 practitioners, of whom approximately 93,000 had at least 4 years of formal training. There were ninety-five cosmopolitan [Western] medical colleges, compared to ninety-nine âyurvedic colleges, fifteen Yunāni colleges, and one college of Siddha medicine. Many of the indigenous medical schools were small and ill equipped, but twenty-six of them were affiliated with universities and ten offered postgraduate training. Two research institutes for indigenous medicine awarded between thirty-five and forty-five Ph.D. and D.A.M. (Doctor of Ayurvedic Medicine) degrees annually. Also, in 1972 the state and central governments supported entirely or in part 185 hospitals and 9,750 dispensaries for indigenous medicine. The Indian government allocated 160 million rupees for indigenous medical institutions in the fourth 5-year plan, but in contrast to cosmopolitan medicine, in which 75 percent of the physicians were in government service, more than one-half of the registered physicians of indigenous medicine were fee-for-service private practitioners" (Leslie 1978, 238). Most indigenous practitioners worked at it part time.

The indigenous and Western systems were not formally integrated (contrary to China). In the end, it was the integrationists such as C. Dwarkanath in the Ministry of Health (1959–1967), supported by the World Health Organization's concept of primary health care, who dominated the âyurvedic institutions. Dwarkanath, for instance, incorporated vitamins, bacteriology, antibiotics, diagnostic technology, chemotherapy, analgesic drugs, and so forth into âyurveda (see Leslie 1984, 30 for a list of syncretistic textbooks). He was critical of the shortcomings of contemporary âyurveda, its haphazard diagnostic procedures, its elimination of seven of the eight traditional branches of medicine (only internal medicine remaining), and its rote memorization of ancient texts with little comprehension. Others have noted the inadequacy of traditional physiology, a combination of poor knowledge of anatomy on account of taboos on dissection and the esoteric mystical physiology of *haṭha* yoga consisting of *cakra*s or centers of energy. The nineteenth-century religious reformer Dayānanda Sarasvatī who wanted to restore rationality to Hinduism, for instance, actually examined a corpse floating on a river to locate the *cakra*s but found they did not exist (Basham 1976, 29). Only in 1835 did a Hindu physician dissect a corpse. Still others have questioned the traditional idea that consciousness resides in the heart.

Those who shared Dwarkanath's views blamed the decline of indigenous medicine first on Muslim and then on colonial rule, for these had made Hinduism and her branches of knowledge retreat into dogmatism. The status of physicians had varied considerably within the tradition itself, and this is confirmed by modern anthropological studies, which reveal considerable caste movement, both downward and upward. In Kerala, for instance, one subdivision of the Nambūdiri *brāhmaṇa*s is the *vaidiyan*, who is looked down on by other Nambūdiris; Madhya Pradesh has *brāhmaṇa* "baids"; and Tamilnadu has physicians in outcaste (*paraiyan*), low barber caste (curiously with the former *brāhmaṇa* designation of *ambaṣṭha*), and high caste rankings. Fractures may be set by potters, drugs may be sold by other low castes, and teeth pulled by barbers. In Bengal, however, prior to the eighteenth century, physicians who had once belonged to the pure *śūdra* caste today claim *brāhmaṇa* status (Basham 1976, 38).

Leslie sees the indigenous perspective as part of the larger Hindu world view and its systems of classification. "The language of humoralism is used to describe musical forms, drama, dance, cuisine, and the qualities of soils, water resources, and kinds of fertilizers that farmers bring together in agriculture. It is the language of ritual, and helps define caste and status relationships . . . More is at stake in the interpretation of illness than just a medical system" (Leslie 1984, 38–39). He concludes that accounts of people's suffering reflect the fact that medicine is always a moral enterprise, not an analytical one as the âyurvedic texts suggest: "the concepts resist this treatment because they are an iconic dramaturgy for enacting, reconciling, and undoing conflicts" (Leslie 1984, 35). In other words, âyurvedic physicians operate more as psychologists in conjunction with astrologers, diviners, and palm-readers for family problems than as physicians of the physical body. (Some have argued that these medical systems do not separate mind and body or soul and body; they are

superior to Western medicine because they are an integrated or "holistic" approach, see Chapter 44.)

IV. DISCOURSES ON ETHICS: BUDDHISM

Analogies between secular medicine and the spiritual message of Buddhism became a standard feature of early Buddhism (see Chapter 10), but there was comparatively little discussion of medical ethics except for one important
topic: access and wealth.

The availability of medicine and care of other monastics was a practical issue. Monastics had to remain healthy
if they were to pursue liberation. Because they had no family, members of the monastery had to care for each other.
Gradually, Buddhist monastic medicine was extended to
certain categories of laity (fathers, mothers, and their
domestics; domestics and paid laity in the service of the
monastery; potential candidates for the monastery who
already resided there; and other relatives). The second
rock inscription of the Buddhist king Aśoka (c. 269–232
BCE) states, for instance, that medicine is to be given to
both humans and animals, and herbs, roots, and fruits for
this purpose are to be planted where none exist.

A particular problem with patrons (amounting to
medicine as repayment for donations) was circumvented
by insisting that the request be made impersonally
or indirectly via another monastic (*Samantapāsādikā* T
1462:11:753a–c,[2] cited by Demiéville 1985, 39). Contributing to the change of offering medical knowledge to
the laity was the tradition of visiting sick lay people to
recite Buddhist scriptures. There is even a case in which a
layperson was nursed back to health within the monastery
itself (*Dharmaguptaka-vinaya* T 1435:43:877a–877b cited
by Demiéville 1985, 40).

Extending the practice of medicine to the laity led to
collecting fees (Zysk 1991, 27), which began to threaten
the spiritual orientation of the monks and the reputation of the monastery in the eyes of the laity. Criticisms
were directed particularly to nuns such as the one called
Chanda's Mother who took medications, treatments such
as surgery, and midwifery to royal courts and the laity
for which she was paid. According to the accounts, when
Mahāprajāpati reported this to the Buddha, he forbade it,
saying it was a transgression except for verbal counsel; he
went on to define medicine as roots, leaves, fruits, magical
incantations, and astrological predictions (*Mahāsaṅghika-
vinaya* T 1425:38: 531a–531b cited by Demiéville 1985,
36). The monastic rules of other schools also criticized nuns for neglecting their religious duties because
they spend their time preparing remedies and practicing
medicine, earning them the criticism that "They are like
physicians or physicians' disciples" (*Mahīsāsaka-vinaya* T
1421:14:94c–95c cited by Demiéville 1985, 37–38). All
this led to restrictions on the practice of medicine within
many monasteries. For example, some texts allowed for

administering sedatives and other medicines to monastics
as long as this was kept secret from the laity. Eventually even verbal counsel on medicine was disallowed. To
stop the mercenary practice of medicine by stopping the
practice of medicine within the monastery itself, the new
rules were attributed to the Buddha himself to make them
absolutely authoritative, thus creating one of the many
anachronisms in the Pāli Canon.

It is striking that despite the prohibitions of the monastic regulations (Vinaya) against the practice of medicine,
they were ignored in some monasteries. It is likely that
these monasteries belonged to those groups that were
developing new views that would become Mahāyāna,
which was oriented to the laity and intent on popularization. The development of Mahāyāna doctrine contributed
to these changes that came to feature the provision of
medicine as core to Buddhism.

In Mahāyāna, the ideal of the *bodhisattva*, who vowed
not to attain final enlightenment until all living creatures were saved, introduced extreme altruism, an ethic
of supererogation, into Buddhism. The ideal of removing the "poisoned arrows" (greed, hatred, and delusion,
which cause suffering) involves the perfection of giving and compassion (including the transfer of merit to
others) (see Chapter 10). Now the Mahāyāna *bodhisattva*-
physician travels about the countryside, going wherever
he finds pain and wounds to heal, ending suffering and
restoring well-being by removing "poisoned arrows" and
applying wonderful medications. The *bodhisattva* is compared to the fully perfected Buddha called the great king
of physicians. Here the Buddha is described in typically
Mahāyāna terms. Seeing the suffering of all sentient beings
that have been struck by the "poisoned arrows," he gives
them a medicament in the form of the ambrosial doctrine
of the Mahāyāna *sūtras*, and reveals himself to them as the
Buddha to heal them (*Mahāparinirvāṇa-sūtra* T 375:5:631
cited by Demiéville 1985, 15).

The extension of the practice of medicine to the laity
was a practical way to perfect altruism. Because *bodhisattvas*
could be lay persons (including kings), they were encouraged to be physicians, building hospitals, and offering
medical help to the poor – all without payment (see Chapter 10). The ultra-generosity of the *bodhisattva* is embodied
in the story of King Sivi who wanted to give his eyes to a
blind *brāhmaṇa* as an act of compassion and requested the
physician Sivaka to remove them. The doctor avoided
using a surgical instrument (presumably because it was
too violent) and instead removed them by stroking the
eyes with medicinal powder until they fell out of their
sockets and could be cut off. They were then put into the
sockets of the *brāhmaṇa* (This story prefigures the medical
practice of transplantation.) (*Sivi Jātaka* no. 499 recounted
by Zysk 1991, 90).

Mahāyāna monastic rules stipulate that *bodhisattvas*
must care for *anyone* who is ill and failure to do so

anywhere under any circumstances amounts to a misdeed (*Bodhisattvabhūmi*: referred to in the chapter on Ethics in Candragomin, *Twenty Verses on the Bodhisattva Vow* (*Bodhisattvasaṃvara-viṃśaka*) 17d, *Brahmajāla-sūtra* T 1484:2:1005c cited by Demiéville 1985, 43). (Such injunctions were necessary because bodhisattvas at the beginning of the path to enlightenment were not yet virtually perfected unlike the "celestial bodhisattvas" in the final stages of the path, who were.) The *Upasakasīla-sūtra* describes how a poor *bodhisattva* who has nothing, will provide *mantras* and medicine; will obtain from the wealthy money, infusions, and medicinal herbs to give to the needy; will give diagnoses, treatment (medications and diets), and care for the sick with great devotion and without distaste for impurity; and will travel everywhere to tend to them, watching for relapses and waiting until health has been completely restored before moving on. The text says that he demands no recognition as recompense and should he be offered gifts, he will offer them to the poor. Finally, the text says that a rich sage who aspires to awakening will study medicine, build hospitals, and provide for all the needs of patients. Such a one will be known as a pure donor (*Upāsakasīla-sūtra* T 1488:5 cited by Demiéville 1985, 45–46)

The image of the Buddhist physician as free from purity restraints no doubt is a backhanded criticism of *brāhmaṇa* physicians who were concerned about purity and therefore willing to treat only certain kinds of patients (compared with the Mahāyāna ones who were truly universal). As indicated in this passage, Mahāyānists were careful not to appear mercenary, which was a problem when medicine was first practiced in the monasteries, according to the Pāli Canon. Whatever gifts they received for their medical practice, they were to give to the poor. They also were to ignore any praise for their services to prevent another common problem: arrogance. Because *bodhisattvas* could appear in the form of a lay person (including a king and a physician), they were sometimes instructed in the role they should play in bringing medicine to the people. One text says that wealthy *bodhisattvas* should construct free clinics (Demiéville 1985, 58).

Finally, the Buddhist texts make a few comments on the proper behavior of a patient. Some of the descriptions of the patient intertwine moral and other characteristics. Being a bad patient consists, for instance, in not following the physicians' commands (by being lazy, ignorant), not controlling emotions even when in pain, and not speaking the truth or being abusive to the nurse (Demiéville 1985, 34–35). *Mahāvagga* says that the patient "does what is beneficial; he knows moderation in what is beneficial; he takes his medicine; he makes clear the affliction, as it arises, to the nurse and wishes him well, . . . and he endures the arising of bodily sensations that are painful, acute, sharp, severe, disagreeable, unpleasant, and destructive" (Zysk 1991, 41).

There are no discourses by Buddhist practitioners in India in the modern period because Buddhism died out there by and large by 1300, and its modern revival (called neo-Buddhism) has been largely confined to a group of Dalit converts.

V. CONCLUSION

Classical Hindu medical texts tell us a great deal about how physicians were becoming self-conscious about their expertise and status in society. Status was an important topic given the hierarchical nature of Hindu society and *brāhmaṇas* were faced with several dilemmas. First was how to absorb non- *brāhmaṇa* healers into brahmanical ranks in order to gain and domesticate their expertise (especially of herbs and other concoctions), an issue that created the problem of impurity. Second, and related, was how to distinguish themselves from others without the same level of expertise (the "quacks," who may simply have been those who had inherited the traditions of the archaic healers). Because such expertise was not always easy to determine (the sick often got worse, after all, and some died), it was important to take only those cases for which the physician could make a difference – ideally a cure, at least an improvement – so that the particular physician and the profession as a whole would be respected and utilized (there was always great competition among healers). It was also important for the new physicians to develop visible signs of expertise: special dress and comportment and empirical as well as religious textual knowledge that signified elite status and inspired confidence.

As a result, much of the practitioners' (physicians') discourse on medical ethics was embedded in the prescriptions on how a real physician should behave. In this context various virtues (benevolence, peace, respect of authority, promptness, perseverance, moderation, prudence, and so forth) and vices (passion, anger, envy, pride) were discussed. These virtues were transmitted from teacher to disciples and were formalized in oaths (such as that of the *Caraka*). One particularly tricky topic was the pursuit of wealth because greed was not befitting the decorum of true physicians, and yet they were dependent on payment (or "gifts") because this was their means of livelihood.

Among Buddhists, the issue of proper behavior arose first in the monastery. Monastic behavior in general was regulated by precepts and monthly confession of infractions (see Chapter 10), so the practice of medicine – which was necessary to care for those who lived within the monastery and had no family – had to be in line with these more general rules). As the practice of medicine extended gradually from the monastery to the laity, the problem of motivation (especially, the pursuit of wealth) had to be addressed. There were two responses. The Theravāda tradition decided to limit its practice to the monastery. As a result, not much is said in the Pāli Canon about the ethics of the Buddhist physicians (perhaps because of the contro-versy reflected in the Pāli Canon over whether Buddhist monks should extend medical care to the laity and the fact that they never became professional physicians as such). By contrast, the Mahāyāna (and then the Vajrayāna) tried to ensure that medicine was an *altruistic* gift to the laity as embodied in the concept of the *bodhisattva*. Thus, if the cultivation of virtues, the uttering of oaths, and general pressure from the leaders of the Hindu *sampradāya* were used to encourage conformity to a medical ethics in Hin-duism, monastic regulations and the cultivation of virtues (especially compassion and altruism) were used for such purpose in Buddhism. The bottom line was that a king could set limits for both Hindus and Buddhists and enforce them through the power of the state (which strong kings did). In addition, the discourses of both Hindu and Bud-dhist physicians discussed the proper behavior of other health professionals such as nurses as well as the proper behavior of patients themselves (cooperation being nec-essary for help).

The next important discourses of practitioners occur in the modern period. Because Buddhism had died out in the land of its birth, these Indian discourses are mainly Hindu.

They reflect a debate over the comparative merits of West-ern and Hindu (especially âyurvedic) medicine, which, at another level, was a debate over the nature of Hindu (and Indian) identity in the postcolonial period (see also Chap-ter 44).

Notes

1. All citations from *Caraka-saṃhitā* are cited by the text name and *stāna*, not the translators, following the number-ing system of R. K. Sharma and V. B. Dash (eds. and trans.): 1972, *Agnivesa's Caraka Saṃhitā*, vol. 1 (*Sūtrasthāna*) and vol. 2 (*Nidāna-sthāna, Vimāna-stāna, Sarīrsthāna, Indriya-Sthāna*) (Sanskrit Text with English translation and Critical Exposition based on Cakrapāṇi Datta's *âyurveda Dīpīka*, (Chowkhamba Sanskrit Series Office, Varanasi). All quotations are from these sources unless otherwise noted. All citations of *Suśruta-saṃhitā* are from K. K. Bhishagratna (ed. and trans.): 1963, *The Sushruta Saṃhitā*, 2 vols. (Chowkhamba Sanskrit Series Office, Varnasi). I have taken the liberty of eliminating sexist language in translations, where it is clear that the reference can be to both men and women.

2. All primary source citations in the format "T 156," "T" is to be understood as referring to the Taishō catalogue of Chinese Buddhist texts.

CHAPTER 21

THE DISCOURSES OF PRACTITIONERS IN CHINA

Jing-Bao Nie

I. INTRODUCTION

In China, medical ethics, or deliberation on moral issues in medicine, dates back to what the German philosopher, Karl Jaspers, called the "Axial Age" (800–200 BCE). This period produced the earliest Chinese works on disease and healing, from which paradigmatic classics of traditional Chinese medicine such as *Huangdi Neijing* (*The Yellow Emperor's Classic of Medicine*) (1995) – still a must read for today's traditional-style practitioners – were compiled in the later centuries. In the Axial Age, the fundamental orientations and basic vocabulary of Chinese cultural life were established by the teachings of such masters as Confucius, Lao Zi, Mo Zi, Yang Zhu, Mencius, Zhuang Zi, Zou Yan, Xun Zi, and Han Fei Zi. The medical and nonmedical literature of this period included fragmented discussions on the topics that are defined today as medical ethics: the moral character of physicians; the nature of life and illness; the management of dying and death; and the nature of medicine as an art and science. From the intellectual and spiritual innovations of the Axial Age (and earlier), China has developed its healing systems, moral traditions, and medical moralities.

This chapter provides an overview of the moral discourses of medical practitioners in China from the Axial Age to the end of twentieth century, with emphasis given

to the great diversity – a basic but somehow ignored feature – of culture and medical morality in China. Within this context major themes and salient characteristics of moral discourse of the group of what can be called "orthodox practitioners" in traditional China (i.e., to the end of the nineteenth century) will be explored. The moral discourses of practitioners in twentieth-century China will be briefly considered, with attention to both traditional Chinese and Western medico-moral values in contemporary context.

II. DIVERSITY OF CULTURE AND MEDICAL MORALITY IN CHINA

A certain mythology dominates discussions of culture and medical ethics in China, that of a single Chinese culture and medical morality. China, especially traditional China, is depicted as basically static, homogeneous, unified, and monolithic. This myth assumes a distinctively "Chinese" way of doing and seeing things. Some modern scholars have claimed to have discovered a uniquely Chinese mentality or world view that supposedly pervades virtually every aspect of Chinese socio-cultural life. Accordingly, there is thought to exist a united and single Chinese medical morality. Medical ethics in China has usually been simplified to what the dominant ideologies, official documents, well-known doctors, and major medical works have said about the subject. As a result, the great diversity of Chinese culture and medical ethics has been minimized (Nie 1999b, 2000). Taking seriously the various kinds of internal plurality within China constitutes the first step and the core of an adequate cross-cultural dialogue with Chinese people. It is practically urgent for today's China to take this great plurality seriously and find an effective way to address the fundamental diversity in Chinese society (Nie 2004b).

The myth of Chinese uniformity is belied by such basic facts as the wide geographical conditions, obvious language differences, tremendous historical metamorphosis, enormous economic variation, ethnic diversity, a variety of social customs and cultural norms, the great local complexity, and the richness of living experiences of numberless socio-cultural minority groups and the silent majority. It is common sense to see China as pluralistic. Care must therefore be taken with any statement about the overarching characteristics of Chinese culture and Chinese medical ethics. We should always try to be as clear and specific as possible about what we are talking about when we talk about China: which China, which Chinese culture, which Chinese medical morality, which historical period, which region, which groups, and which social milieu. When generalizing about China, we must acknowledge the sense and degree to which the generalization is valid and we must always be aware of socio-cultural diversity.

It is difficult, if not impossible, to define the fundamental terms, "China," and "Chinese." China as a political and cultural entity has never been a homogeneous whole. Historically speaking, it is a mistake to view China as always unified and united. China consisted of several separate states in the Axial period, when the paradigmatic Chinese spiritual and intellectual creations originated. It did not become a united country until the establishment of the Qin Dynasty in 221 BCE. Since the Qin Dynasty, China has been united and separated again and again, a phenomenon that has been generalized as a rule of history in the popular culture. The first sentence of the classical historical novel *Sanguo Yanyi* (The Romance of the Three Kingdoms), which appeared in the fourteenth century and which is still widely read today, states: "States cleave asunder and coalesce in turns. This is the general historical trend of the world [China]." Unfortunately, for many people the history of China is like the unexplored Middle Ages in the West before the twentieth century's detailed and systematic medieval studies. As the French historian Jacques Gernet (1996, 21) said of the monolithic view of the European Middle Ages, "the repeated accusations of stagnation, periodical return to a previous condition, and permanence of the same social structure and the same political ideology are so many value judgements on a history that is still unknown."

Morality in traditional China had never been singular. Although traditional China is usually viewed as a Confucian society, Confucianism was just one of its major ideologies and moral systems. Indigenous Daoism and imported but gradually sinolized Buddhism, as more institutionalized religions, have exerted an extremely strong and enduring influence on Chinese socio-cultural and moral life. The conventional term, "Three Teachings," indicates the importance, coexistence, competition, complementarity, and sometime integration of these three major Chinese ways of thinking and living. All Three Teachings had provided medical practitioners with different but not necessarily incommensurable values and ethical frameworks on moral issues in health care. Often, Daoist and Buddhist understandings of birth, life, illness, suffering, healing, dying, and death differ significantly from those of Confucian views.

In traditional China, healing systems were also diverse. The German historian of medicine, Paul Unschuld (1985), has identified seven medical systems of ideas that either originated in China or were adapted from foreign cultures – oracular therapy, demonic medicine, religious healing, pragmatic drug therapy, Buddhist medicine, the medicine of systematic correspondence and, ultimately, modern Western medicine.

> The history of these seven major conceptual systems is not characterized by simply linear succession, in which practitioners exchange each old system for a new one. Instead, the evidence reveals a diversity of concepts extending for more than two thousand years. New ideas were developed or introduced from outside and adopted by authors of medical texts, while at the same time older views continued to have their practitioners and clients. (Unschuld 1985, 5–6)

Thus, to describe Chinese medicine as unified and coherent seriously distorts the historical reality of medicine in China. Traditional Chinese medicine, as we are familiar with it today, the so-called medicine of systematic correspondence, is merely one of several systems of therapy. These healing systems were not always exclusive. Borrowing such elements as drugs, methods of treatment, and medical concepts and even theories from other systems was commonplace. Followers of these different healing systems competed for clients, resources, and legitimacy and, as part of this process, borrowed popular elements from other systems. For example, the more rational medicine of systematic correspondence incorporated *zhoujin* or *zhuyou* (magic healing).

Historical evidence indicates that different groups of healers with different moral world views and medical paradigms emerged and often coexisted in various periods. For instance, the *Jinpingmei* (*The Golden Lotus*) a realistic novel of the sixteenth century, vividly describes the ordinary life as well as the activities of a variety of healers in late imperial China. The largest group are male literate healers recognizable as practitioners of classical Chinese medicine. Among this group are physicians of general medicine, specialists in children's or women's disorders, and medical officials. Male religious specialists include the foreign monk, the Daoist priest, and the "Immortal," who mainly practiced divination. Other male healers include the "Starmasters," specialists in "lesion poison" and pious distribution of medicine. Female medical practitioners include midwives as well as "Old Women" and nuns who performed healing activities (see Cullen 1993, 108–10). For pragmatic reasons, some practitioners operated in two or three or more paradigms and employed therapies from more than one medical system. Wu the Immortal in the *Jinpingmei* not only told fortunes and practiced divination but also treated the sick with empirical measures such as herbs. Nevertheless, as Unschuld has observed,

> Well beyond the end of the Confucian era, traditional physicians remained a non-homogeneous group which included practitioners of the most diverse training and skills . . . *The* Chinese physician as a definable entity did not exist . . . Up to this [twentieth] century these have included shamans, Buddhist priests, Taoist hermits, Confucian scholars, itinerant physicians, established physicians, "laymen" with medical knowledge (gained from experiences or obtained through family tradition), midwives, and many others. (Unschuld 1979, 112–13, 118; emphasis original)

These people all were "Chinese physicians" when they practiced medicine.

Culture and medical morality in twentieth-century China manifests pluralism in various and obvious ways (Nie 2000). Certainly, the moral discourses of medical practitioners in the Republic of China, the People's Republic of China, and Hong Kong cannot be regarded as homogeneous. In contemporary mainland China, three legitimate medical systems – traditional Chinese medicine, modern Western biomedicine, and combined Chinese and Western medicine – coexist and compete with each other. In addition, many other forms of healing – from folk medicine to religious methods of healing and witchcraft – that are officially prohibited as "superstitious" are often practiced publicly or secretly. Chinese culture today is a mix of many diverse values and beliefs – ancient and modern, Western and Eastern. In today's China, one can easily find in the ways people actually live, and even in official publications, the coexistence of sinolized Western Marxism and communism, traditional Confucianism, Daoism, and Buddhism, and Christianity and Islam. The result is a polyglot of concepts, such as socialism, collectivism, filial piety, and ideals of individual happiness, self-fulfillment, and self-perfection.

In summary, there is simply no such thing as *the* single Chinese morality and culture, no such thing as *the* unified Chinese healing system, no such thing as *the* homogeneous Chinese medical practitioner, no such thing as *the* Chinese medical ethics, and no such thing as *the* singular moral discourse of Chinese medical practitioners. With regard to the diversity of morality, healing systems and healers, an overview of the moral discourses of medical practitioners in China should address the characteristics, dissimilarities, similarities and commonalities of the moral discourses of different groups of healers who believed in specific moral systems or religions and practiced specific types of therapy. The next two sections of this chapter will focus on traditional China and Confucian physicians and then twentieth-century China and socialist or communist health care providers. Lack of systematic and detailed exploration in contemporary scholarship precludes a presentation of other Chinese medico-moral discourses, such as the moral discourses of itinerant healers, sorcerer-healers, and practitioners from various ethnic minorities. There may be many shared values among these different discourses partly because eclecticism was commonplace. It is misleading to assume that the moral discourse of orthodox Confucian practitioners or socialist health care providers represents *the* Chinese discourse and even *the* only legitimate Chinese discourse of medical ethics.

III. MORAL DISCOURSES OF ORTHODOX PRACTITIONERS IN TRADITIONAL CHINA

The group of medical practitioners whose moral discourses will be considered in this section can be characterized as "orthodox practitioners." Most of them were male, well educated, and shared a common medical paradigm, the medicine of systematic correspondence, which flourished in traditional China. Their moral and political values were fundamentally and mainly Confucian, although some of them may also have believed in Daoism and Buddhism. As a result, these practitioners not only enjoyed relatively high social status in their day, their ethical perspectives have been the main, if not exclusive, focus of contemporary scholarship on medical ethics in traditional China.

1. Medicine as *Dadao* (the Great *Dao*) and *Renshu* (the Art of Humaneness) Compared with Medicine as *Xiaodao* (the Little *Dao*) and Jiyi (Craftsmanship)

For orthodox practitioners the *Huangdi Neijing* (The Yellow Emperor's Class of Medicine, usually abbreviated as *Neijing*) is "the unshakable originator" of the medical system that they practiced. *Neijing*, with most compiled during the first to second centuries, consists of two parts – *Suwen* and *Lingshu* – and 162 chapters. The role of *Neijing* in the history of China has been probably even more significant than that of the Hippocratic Corpus in the history of Western medicine. The *Neijing* defines medicine as "the Dao (way) of excellence and the business of great saints" (*Suwen*, Chap. 8). It calls medicine "the ultimate virtue" and acupuncture "the superb craftsmanship" (*Suwen*, Chap. 11). One thus should be very careful in selecting future physicians, for they must possess the requisite character and clinical skills. One must "pass on [medical knowledge and skills] to those who are truly appropriate and should not teach medicine to those who are not appropriate" (*Lingshu*, Chap. 73).

Healers in traditional Chinese society, even orthodox practitioners, never enjoyed the social and economic position that physicians occupy in the contemporary West, or even in today's China. This was mainly due to Confucianism, in which healing was treated as just a type of *ji* (technique or craftsmanship) or *shu* (art). The Confucian tradition usually looked down on forms of craftsmanship, that is working with one's hands, and many Confucians were ashamed to learn or to practice medicine for this reason. In the household essay, "Discourse on Teachers," Han Yu (768–824), a celebrated literary figure of the Tang Dynasty, stated: "Sorcerers, doctors, musicians and various craftsmen are held in contempt by gentlemen." In the twelfth century, the prominent master of Neo-Confucianism, Zhu Xi, classified medicine as *xiaodao* (petty teaching, small way, little Dao), together with agriculture, horticulture, divination, and other specialized works. Zhu considered it extremely deplorable that Sun Simiao (c. 581–c. 681), one of the greatest physicians in Chinese history, in spite of being an extremely talented person, was relegated to the lower social category of artisan or technician in the official history because of his occupation. It was not uncommon that court physicians were persecuted and killed for treating the illness of emperors and high officials and their family members ineffectively (see Ma 1986, 8–9).

In traditional China, the social status of medicine as an occupation or profession was as low as that of other technical skills, certainly much lower than *rushu* (the art of Confucianism) – civil service and Confucian scholarship. In his essay, "On the Confucian Physician," the twelfth-century physician, Xu Chunfu, emphasized the dissimilarities between Confucianism and medicine, when he stated: "Comparing to the art of Confucianism, the art of medicine is definitely secondary" (in Chen[1] [1723] 1962, 50). The thirteenth-century physician Zhang Gao was frequently laughed at by people because he engaged in such technical skills as medicine. Before devoting himself to medicine, the scholar–physician Li Shizhen (1518–1593), one of the greatest figures in the history of medicine in China, attempted to become a civil official and did not give up until he had failed the official examination three times.

Understandably, many orthodox practitioners disagreed with this view. For Lai Fuyang (fl. 1596?), whether medicine is mere craftsmanship or not depends on how it was practiced. He wrote:

> If medical practice is based on deception, it is to be considered low. If medicine is practice on the principle of veracity (*cheng*), it is not to be considered low. If a person's knowledge of medicine is applied only to his own body, this is petty (*xiao*). If the application [of a person's medical knowledge] is extended over all mankind, this is not petty. (in Unschuld 1979, 41)

In the seventeenth century, the great Ming Dynasty physician, Zhang Jiebin, wrote an essay, "Record [of an Instruction] that Medicine is Not a Petty Teaching." For Zhang, medicine demands considerable conscientiousness from the individual because its concern focuses on life. "Medicine is certainly difficult! Medicine is certainly sublime! It represents the earliest tradition of genuine supernatural and exemplary people, and the first duty of a people" (Unschuld 1979, 83).

Partly to enhance the moral and social status of medicine in a Confucian society, orthodox practitioners promoted the idea *yi nai renshu* (medicine as the art of humaneness). *Ren* is a core concept in Confucianism and has been translated variously as "humaneness," "benevolence," "perfect virtue," "goodness," "human-heartedness," "love," "altruism," or "humanity." The strategy was to connect medicine to Confucian moral ideals and principles, thus elevating it to the art of humaneness: "Confucianism and medicine are inseparably, complementary of each other, and medicine is an essential part of Confucianism" (Qiu 1988b, 283). According to Huangfu Mi (214–282), a literate man who compiled the famous text, *Zhenjiu Jiayi Jing* (Systematic Classic of Acupuncture and Moxibustion), "If a person is not good at medicine, he cannot help his emperor and parents when they are suffering from disease even though this person has a heart of loyalty and filial piety (*zhongxiao*) and the nature of humaneness and compassion (*renci*)" (Chen [1723] 1962, 107). The connection to Confucianism was further advanced by claiming that because medicine undertakes to save lives as a duty, it is kindred to the way of Confucianism. In China there was a widely known saying, originated by the eleventh-century statesman, Fan Zhongyan, "Whoever has no chance to work as a good prime minister, may work as a good physician." This saying suggests that both civil service and medicine, although the former is superior to the latter, serve the same Confucian moral ideals and that a good physician might even be comparable to a good prime minister.

Medicine as the art of humaneness requires the physician not only to master Confucian teachings but also to follow Confucian morals in medical practice. It was stressed that before and during learning and practicing medicine one must study Confucian texts diligently. In the section entitled "Regulations of Practicing Medicine," the Ming Dynasty (1368–1644) physician, Li Yan, wrote that because "medicine comes from Confucianism," a practitioner "should get up early in the morning to study one or two Confucian books every day. In this way he can purify the source of his thoughts" (in Chen [1723] 1962, 55). The most important ethical requirement of "medicine as the art of humaneness" is that practitioners must practice medicine from a humane heart and in accordance with Confucian moral principles and ideals. Another Ming-Dynasty physician, Gong Tingxian, in his famous "Ten Maxims for Physicians," explains:

> In the first place physicians must adopt a disposition of humaneness [*renxin*, a heart of humanity]. This is a necessary maxim. They should make special efforts to assist people at every walk of life so that their good deeds have far-reaching influence. Secondly they must master the Confucian teachings. As the precious treasures to the world, Confucian physicians should understand all the [Confucian] principles and consult all the [Confucian] works. (in Chen [1723] 1962, 56)

2. Ideal of *Dayi* (the Great Physician) and Morals of *Liangyi* (the Good Practitioner)

The morals and virtues of the good physician constitute the most salient theme in traditional Chinese medical ethics. In orthodox medical literature, *yongyi* (common physicians) were often described critically and in a derogatory tone. In contrast, there were *dayi* (Great Physicians), *ruyi* (Confucian physicians), *mingyi* (enlightened physicians), *deyi* (virtuous physicians), and *liangyi* (good physicians). According to Xu Chunfu in the twelfth century, "Learners of medicine differ greatly in their degree of excellence in mastering the art of medicine. They thus have different names" (in Chen [1723] 1962, 49). Xu distinguished the five types of practitioners: (1) *mingyi* (enlightened physicians), "those who practice medicine excellently;" (2) *liangyi* (good physicians), "those who are good at medicine;" (3) *guoyi* (state or court physicians), "those who bring a long life to the emperor and protect the ministers from diseases;" (4) *yongyi* (common physicians), "whose who perform their work in an unskilled manner and to whom the principles of medicine remain hidden;" and (5) *wuyi* (sorcerer physicians), "those who beat the drum and perform dances, who recite prayers and prepare sacrifices to [ward off] sufferings and diseases. They are merely followers of witchcraft and have no knowledge

of medicine" (in Chen [1723] 1962, 49; Unschuld 1979, 40–41). "Common physicians," as perceived by orthodox Confucian practitioners, were neither morally virtuous nor technically competent. Some practiced medicine just to make a living, with no noble moral ideals.

In traditional China the first work that explicitly and systematically deals with medical ethics was written by Sun Simiao, a physician whose works combined thoughts and ethics derived from Confucianism, Daoism, and Buddhism. The first chapter of the *Qianjin Yaofang* (Prescriptions Worth a Thousand Gold), titled "Dayi Jingcheng" (On the Consummate Skill and Absolute Sincerity of Great Physicians), is probably the most influential and important treatise on medical ethics in traditional China, enjoying a status similar to that of the Hippocratic Oath in the West. Sun has been called "the king of medicine" in the history of China not only because his medical works agglomerate the medical achievements before the seventh century but also because his ethical precepts on learning and practicing medicine have become paradigmatic. For Sun, medicine is an extremely difficult art so that it is truly dangerous "to grasp the most subtle details with the crudest and most superficial thought." The basic doctrines of Sun's ethics, as the title of his treatise on medical ethics indicates, are that a physician must be simultaneously *jing* (competent in medicine, mastering the consummate skill) and *cheng* (honest, virtuous in character, having absolute sincerity). For the first time in Chinese history, Sun put forward the ideal of *dayi* (the Great Physician) and articulated the ethical principles and manners of a Great Physician. More significantly, Sun himself was seen as an example of the ideal physician, because he not only expressed high moral standards of medicine but also met these standard in his medical practice.

Sun stipulated moral requirements for practicing medicine and made concrete suggestions about what the manners of physicians should be. For Sun, the purpose of medical practice is to help, not to gain material goods and fame. His principles of morality and manners include: to treat every patient on equal ground; to help wholeheartedly; to love life – both human and animal – and not to kill or injure any living creature; not to reject or despise a patient who suffers from an abominable disease like skin ulcers; not to enjoy oneself in a patient's house; not to be talkative; not to exalt one's own virtue; and not to belittle other physicians. Virtuous conduct will be rewarded by humans and spirits. In his second major medical work, published when he was about 100 years old, Sun listed ten types of good conduct in medical practice, including assisting those in need and difficulties, respecting demons and celestial beings, not killing or injuring anyone, developing a compassionate attitude, not envying the rich or despising the poor, preserving a temperate disposition, not drinking wine or eating meat or pungent food, not indulging in music or women, and keeping one's disposition and character well-balanced (in Chen [1723] 1962, 16–17; Unschuld 1979, 33–34).

After Sun Simiao, many writers expounded further on the subject. Zhang Gao (c. 1149–c. 1227), a Confucian physician heavily influenced by Buddhism, expressed his ethical views on good medical practice and good physicians in the section, "Retribution for Medical Services," of his *Yishuo* (Teachings on Medicine). Using the common device of telling stories to promote morality, Zhang related twelve detailed anecdotes. In these stories, he discussed some central themes of traditional Chinese medical ethics. Selfless practice will bring rewards in this world and beyond, whereas bad or greedy practice will result in punishment and death. Conscientious practice requires a physician not to have sex with patients or their family members. The physician should not use fraudulent methods. The practitioner should refuse to sell abortifacients for the sake of the aborted fetus (child). In the sixteenth century, Zhu Huiming devoted special sections to ethical discussion, including "Physician Should Preserve Humaneness," "Good Conduct Brings Rewards," and "A Warning to Determine the Prospect for a Good or Bad Cure Early Enough." In the seventeenth century, Gong Tingxian, a prolific medical writer who from time to time was employed in the imperial office for medicine, offered "Ten Maxims for Physicians" and "Ten Maxims for Patients." In the same century, Chen Shigong put forward the "Five Admonitions to Physicians" and "Ten Maxims for Physicians" in his classic work *Waike Zhengzong* (*Orthodox Manual of Surgery*).

It must be emphasized that no one can be certain about the actual influence of these maxims and admonitions on medical practice. In reality, as the realistic novel, *Jinpingmei*, illustrates, most physicians were "common," rather than truly "good" or "enlightened" or "great." These ethical rules were offered in the form of moral advice and suggestions, and so were not professional codes in the modern Western sense or duties as stated in the Hippocratic Oath (see Chapter 23). Although the *Neijing* does mention that the physician should participate in rituals and take a blood oath before learning and practicing acupuncture (*Lingshu*, chapters 9 and 48), the rite and the content of the oath are not recorded and the practice of taking a blood oath was not continued after antiquity.

3. Opposition to Witchcraft Medicine

One of the most significant changes in the history of medicine in China involved the transition from a magic and religious world view to a more empirical and rationalistic way of thinking about health, illness, and healing. One of the results of this historical transition was the decline of *wu* (witchcraft) and the rise of *yi* (medicine) and *shi* (scholar). The British historian of Chinese science

and civilization Joseph Needham (1970, 265) once stated: "The whole history of the social position of doctors in China might be summarised as the passage from the *wu*, a sort of technological servitor, to the *shih* [*shi*], a particular kind of scholar, clad in the full dignity of the Confucian intellectual, and not readily converted into anyone's instrument." Physicians (*yi*) belonged to the category *shi* in the broad traditional sense of the term. The word *"yi"* in classical Chinese means both medicine as an art and occupation or profession independent from witchcraft and a specialized group of people skilled in healing. Many historians of medicine in China and contemporary textbooks on the subject influenced by Marxism or historical materialism depict a similar historical picture (see Zhen 1997). Although this picture has simplified the historical reality and the victory has never been complete, the view that medicine in China is a history of the transition from *wu* to *yi* or of the victory of *yi* over *wu* captures an element of truth about the social metamorphosis of healers and medicine in traditional China.

In general, orthodox practitioners disapproved of and despised *wu* (the magic or witchcraft medicine) and its practitioners. For instance, like Hippocratic medicine, the *Neijing* clearly opposes religious or spiritual healing. It teaches that "You cannot talk about the ultimate virtue [the art of medicine] with those who believe in ghosts and spirits. You cannot talk about the superb craftsmanship with those who hate the needle and stones [acupuncture]" (*Suwen*, Chap. 11).

4. Admonitions for Patients

An interesting and significant element in the ethical writings of orthodox practitioners is their admonitions for patients. As early the Axial Age, the famous and influential theory, "Six Incurable Conditions," was advanced by Bian Que, who was viewed as the symbol of the good physician and the father of medicine in China. According to Bian Que, there are six conditions in which a patient's disease is not curable or unsuitable for treatment, including, when patients are arrogant and do not listen to reason (the first); treasure wealth more than life (the second); when they are not able to take care of their own activities of daily living (the third); when they are too weak to take any medicine (the fifth); and when they believe in *wu* (witchcraft or the sorcerer physician) not in *yi* (medicine or the physician) (the sixth) (in Chen [1723] 1962, 78). In the essay, "Warning Words for Patients," the seventeenth-century Confucian physician Gong Xin listed a number of bad behaviors of patients. They include not spending money on health care; being unwilling to summon a physician quickly but waiting for diseases to cure themselves; not consulting recognized experts; praying to spirits and demons; and believing that their fate is sealed, thus delaying effective, especially curative treatment. Gong sighed: "Such foolishness can only be deplored. Patients who conduct themselves in this manner should change" (in Chen [1723] 1962, 435; Unschuld 1979, 70). In addition to "Ten Maxims for Physicians," the seventeenth-century physician Gong Tingxian offered "Ten Maxims for Patients." The last of ten is that patients "should not spare expense. What sense is there in economizing here! May I ask you, what is more precious, life or wealth?" The first of ten is that patients "should choose enlightened physicians and thereby receive help in their ailment. They have to be careful, because life and death follow each other closely" (in Chen [1723] 1962, 57; Unschuld 1979, 72–73).

5. The Physician as General: A Metaphor for the Patient–Physician Relationship

What should the role of the physician be? There are many ancient Chinese metaphors or images about the patient–physician relationship and the role of physician in medical decision making. Among them is a metaphor "the physician as general" (Nie 1996). In this metaphor the patient does not relate to the physician as a soldier relates to a general, but as a king to a general. The patient is the sovereign and the physician is the general chosen to marshal medical forces against disease. The fifth-century physician Zhe Cheng remarked, "Using medicine is like employing troops and choosing the physician is like appointing a general . . . Knowing the general's talents and intelligence, [the patient] gives him the army . . . This is the Dao of choosing a physician" (in Chen [1723] 1962, 14).

Obviously, this metaphor does not necessarily lead to the paternalistic or authoritarian view of the physician that is dominant in medical practice in present-day China. In classical Chinese thought on military ethics, wisdom, sincerity, humaneness, courage, and strictness constitute the five cardinal virtues of the general. The Chinese metaphor of the physician as general suggests that the good, enlightened healer – like the good general – must know the limitations of the art, remain alert to constant changes, cultivate virtue, and fight humanely. In this metaphor, the patient is responsible for his or her health and for employing lifelong strategies to protect it. When ill, however, the patient should seek medical intervention to battle disease and oversee the physician's tactics, just as a king oversees a general's battle plan. Being a general – like being a physician – is not easy; it requires great wisdom. As the good general sometimes needs to act independently of the opinions of the king, a good king – like the good patient – sometimes accepts the knowledge and wisdom of the general, acknowledging his experience in battle. It should be evident that the metaphor of the general contrasts with Western images of the healer as parent, technician, teacher, fighter, or ship captain (Nie 1996).

6. Truth Telling

Cheng (honesty, sincerity) is an important virtue in Confucianism, especially Neo-Confucianism. In his "Regulations on Practicing Medicine," Li Yan stipulated, "If being asked to use one word to summarize [how to practice medicine], my answer would be 'not-deceiving'" (in Chen [1723] 1962, 56). Among various kinds of deceit is that the physician does "not tell the patients about their disease honestly after taking the pulse" (Chen [1723] 1962, 56). Li further stated, "If deceiving, one's conscience will be closed up and the way of medicine be lost. If not deceiving, one's conscience will be growing every day and the way of medicine be developing. [What happens] between deceiving and not-deceiving is beyond what humans can give" (Chen [1723] 1962, 56).

Regarding revealing the diagnosis of terminal illness to patients, contrary to the mainstream practice in China today, the recorded great Chinese physicians in ancient times preferred to tell truth to the patient directly and honestly (see Chapter 5).

7. Human Body Parts as Medicine and Animal Drugs

Although many Westerners see acupuncture as the representative therapy in traditional Chinese medicine, using materia medica was the most common method of treatment in Chinese history and remains so today. Although Chinese materia medica is traditionally called *"bencao"* (literally, roots and grass, or plants), for centuries physicians have been using many "animal drugs" – drugs directly coming and derived from the body parts of various animals. There are even some "human drugs" – parts, excreta, and appendages of the human body. In the *Bencao Gangmu* (The Great Pharmacopoeias) – a monumental work compiled in the sixteenth-century and still a standard reference for traditional-style Chinese medical practitioners – Li Shizhen (c. 1518–1593) categorized nearly 1,700 medical substances. Among them were more than 400 animal drugs and approximately 35 human drugs. He has fifteen groups of material medica: water, fire, earth, metal and stone, grass, cereal vegetable, fruit, tree, clothes and utensils, insect, creatures with scales (reptiles and fish), creatures with shells, bird, quadrupeds, and finally, "human drugs" (Li [1592] 1988).

Among the human drugs have been recorded in Chinese materia medica are hair, pubic hair, finger-nails, placenta, urine, bone, flesh, blood, menstrual blood, seminal fluid, and the penis. In the last volume (Volume 52) of *Bencao Gangmu*, Li Shizhen not only systematically summarized these human drugs but also explicitly and critically discussed ethical issues involved in using these drugs from the Confucian moral perspectives like *ren* (humanity), *yi* (righteousness), *li* (ritual), and *li* (reason, principle). For Li, although the use of some human drugs such as hair, fingernails, urine, and urinary sediments may well be ethically justifiable, the use of some others such as blood, flesh, and bone "contradicts *ren*," and "harms *yi*," making them ethically unacceptable. Yet, neither Li nor any other physician or scholar in China has established a systematic Confucian analysis of the ethics of using human drugs. Nevertheless, Li's comments on human drugs provide a window into the moral attitudes of the orthodox practitioner toward the human body, healing, illness and disease, nature and the supernatural, and the ethical or unethical materia medica (Li [1592] 1988, 52; Nie 1999b).

Among the commonly used animal drugs in Chinese medicine are tiger bone, ox gallstone, dried secretion from the musk gland of the musk deer, pilose, deerhorn, antler gelatin, deglued antler powder, antelope horn, water buffalo horn, rhinoceros horn, bear gall, donkeyhide gelatin, and various snakes. Like most physicians and ordinary people in China, Li Shizhen rarely raised ethical questions about animal drugs, partly because Confucianism advocates that animals, as inferior to human beings, should serve humans and deserve little esteem. Because of the influence of Buddhism, however, Sun Simiao clearly opposed the use of animal drugs. He did not include the use of any living creature – insects and animals – as acceptable, whereas the use of some dead insects was acceptable. He even considered it a "great wisdom" not to use hens' eggs especially when their content has been hatched out. Sun believed that "Humans and animals are equal when love of life is concerned" and that "Whoever destroys life in order to save life places life at an even greater distance" (in Chen [1723] 1962, 17; Unschuld 1979, 31).

8. Toward a Better Understanding of Medical Ethics in Imperial China

The explicit discussions of famous physicians about the moral character of practitioners and the physician–patient relationship constitute the main focus of contemporary scholarship on medical ethics in traditional China (Unschuld 1979; Zhou 1983; He 1988). Yet, medical ethics is much broader than statements of the necessary virtues and moral characters of physicians. As the ethical discussion of ancient Chinese physicians on human and animal drugs indicates, the literature of traditional Chinese medicine, so enormous that it has been described "as vast as the open sea," has touched and sometimes explicitly explored other moral issues in medicine. As another example, numerous works in gynecology and obstetrics and case histories embody rich information on how orthodox practitioners viewed and dealt with birth, fetal life, abortion, infanticide, reproduction, gender, motherhood, sexuality, the body, longevity, dying and death, and so on (Bray 1997; Furth 1999; see also Chapter 5). Thus, our

knowledge about the moral discourses of orthodox practitioners, although much more comprehensive than for other group of healers, is still quite limited. More detailed analysis and systematic exploration wait to be done.

IV. MORAL DISCOURSES OF PRACTITIONERS IN TWENTIETH-CENTURY CHINA

Historically speaking, twentieth-century China characterizes itself as the age of *geming* (revolution). A great number of revolutions happened in almost every area of social and cultural life, including government, the economy, education, language, science and technology, and medicine and health care. Those famous phrases used by Marx and Engels more than one and half centuries ago to describe what distinguish the modern ("bourgeois") epoch from all earlier ones in the West can be borrowed to describe the features of twentieth-century China vividly: "uninterrupted disturbance of all social conditions, everlasting uncertainty and agitation." "All fixed, fixed, fast-frozen relations, with their train of ancient and venerable prejudices and opinions, are swept away, all new-formed ones become antiquated before they can ossify. All that is solid melts into air, all that is holy is profaned" (Tucker 1972, 476). This was a century with genuine progress, development, and even liberation. This was also a century with wars (both antiforeign invasion and civil), turmoil, collective violence and destruction – almost always accomplished in the name of the country, people, great cause, progress, revolution, and liberation. As the brilliant contemporary Confucian, Tu Wei-Ming (1997, 149), has pointed out, China since the mid-nineteenth century has been "one of the most violent countries in human history." China has witnessed massive suffering in the past 150 years, which "makes it blatantly clear that a defining characteristic of modern Chinese history is the destruction of lives, property, institutions, and values" (Tu Wei-Ming, 1997, 149). Constant revolutionizing of Chinese medical morality and medical ethics in the twentieth century was both a consequence and a contributing element of this constant revolutionizing of Chinese society.

Accompanying the decline of traditional institutions and values was the widespread and profound influence of the West. Since the seventeenth century, gradual acceptance and distribution of Western technology, science, and values have injected many different ideas, perspectives, and ways of thinking and living into China. By the end of nineteenth century, numerous Western-style hospitals had already been established throughout China. In the twentieth century modern Western biomedicine has been so well established in China that it has become the major medical system, whereas traditional Chinese medicine plays an active but minor role. Formal medical education replaced the traditional father–son or master–disciple model, even for traditional Chinese medicine.

Professional organizations of medicine, such as the Chinese Nursing Association (1909) and the Chinese Medical Association (1915) were established. The ethical code of the American Medical Association was also translated into Chinese in 1912. Song Guobin's *Professional Ethics of Medicine*, the first monograph on medical ethics in modern China, appeared in 1933. As a Western-trained physician, Song attempted to integrate norms of Western medical ethics, such as confidentiality, into Chinese medical practice. Yet, his discussions of the ethics of the medical profession remained grounded in such key Confucian moral concepts as humaneness and righteousness (Song 1933).

The most significant theme in the far from harmonious symphony of twentieth-century China is probably the introduction of Marxism via the Soviet style of socialism, and the later emergence, development, and reform of Communism. This unprecedented social experiment and utopian dream, building a brand new China as a socialist society without exploitation and suppression, provides the context for the appearance and growth of socialist medical morality. In 1941 Mao Zedong (1893–1976) summarized the new medical ethics: "To rescue the dying and heal the wounded and to practice revolutionary humanitarianism." This slogan gradually became the fundamental principle of socialist medical morality. Since the 1940s, the most prominent example of this socialist medical ethics was not a native Chinese, but a foreigner, a Westerner, that is, Dr. Norman Bethune, a Canadian surgeon who joined Chinese communists' guerrilla war against Japanese invaders, wounded himself while operating on a soldier and died from infection. Bethune has since become a household name in China, symbolizing not only the virtuous physician but also the socialist new person.

Professional codes of ethics and official regulations did not appear until the 1980s. In 1981, when China had just started its policies of reform and openness, the Ministry of Health promulgated *People's Republic of China's Rules and Medical Moral Principles of Hospital Personnel* (Qiu 1999, 194–96). Its first two requirements are that one should "love the motherland, love the Communist Party, and love socialism; maintain Marxism-Leninism and the Thought of Mao Zedong" and that one should "study the politics [official ideology] hard and spare no effort in studying medicine hard so as to be both read and expert." At the same time, the *Principles* require that, because the physician–patient relationship in a socialist society is a relationship between comrades, the physician should "respect the patient's dignity, will and rights." A kind of informed consent was also mentioned:

Whenever examining, treating and doing research over the patient, the physician should explain clearly to the patient, obtain consent from the patient or the patient's family members and vol-

untariness. The physician should not impose any decision on the patient. (in Qiu 1999, 195)

To dying patients, medical professionals are required "to make one-hundred-percent effort to save lives even though the hope is only one percent." In the *Principles* no traditional ethical concept such as *ren* (humaneness, humanity) or *yi* (righteousness, justice) was mentioned except the ancient saying that "Whoever has no chance to work as a good prime minister, may work as a good physician."

Among the theoretical and practical issues facing contemporary Chinese medical ethics is how to treat the Western bioethics, an issue parallel to that of how to treat indigenous Chinese moral traditions (see Nie 2001b, 2002b, 2004e). How should we Chinese today, in a fundamentally changed socio-cultural environment, treat traditional Chinese medico-moral values? Do traditional medico-moral values have any worth for today's medicine in and even outside China? Do they have a future? Is a modern transformation of traditional Chinese medical morality desirable and possible? If yes, how? These are not so much theoretical questions as practical problems for medical ethics in contemporary China.

V. Conclusion

In Chinese history, two radically different attitudes towards history and traditions have appeared, traditionalist and antitraditionalist. Like Confucians, orthodox medical practitioners valued the heritage of the past so greatly that they tended to be conservative and traditionalist. Confucius saw himself as "a transmitter and not an originator, a believer in and lover of ancient traditions," although he actually created many new things in transmitting ancient literature, ideas, and institutions. A lifetime goal of Confucius was to revive and perpetuate the culture of the older Zhou Dynasty (eleventh to eighth centuries BCE). Orthodox traditional Chinese practitioners thought of the past, as described in the first book of the *Huangdi Neijing*, as a golden age. Many ancient doctors thus believed that the best medical knowledge and wisdom came from the antique Sages.

Yet, China is not a society that refuses to change. One of the serious problems in twentieth-century Chinese society and culture is that there were too many dramatic changes. In the striking contrast to Confucianism and the conventional philosophy of history in ancient medicine, "totalistic iconoclasm" or "radical antitraditionalism" – profoundly iconoclastic attitudes toward Chinese cultural heritage and a total rejection of China's past – have characterized twentieth-century Chinese intellectual history (Lin 1979). This radical antitraditionism, together with political and other cultural factors, led to the depreciation and actual destruction of traditional values and institutions. This destruction reached its peak in so-called "the Great Proletarian Cultural Revolution" of the 1960s and 1970s. The damage caused by the Cultural Revolution to Chinese society and its cultural heritage often reminds people of the notorious "Burning of the Books and Killing of the Intellectuals" ordered by Qin Shihuang (the First Emperor) in 213 BCE. But the destructive scope and magnitude of the twentieth-century "Burning of the Books and Killing of the Intellectuals" went far beyond those of twenty-two centuries ago. It is not surprising that traditional Chinese medico-moral values have little significance in explicit medical ethics in contemporary Mainland China.

Once again, in the past few decades, medical ethics in China has been changing dramatically. Besides socialism, other socio-cultural factors are reshaping the moral discourses of health care providers, including nationalism, scientism, the market economy, globalization, developments of advanced medical including reproductive technologies, the revival of various religions and cults, a sort of patients' rights movement, the aging of society, and the growing gap between the poor and the rich and between different geographic areas of the country. The most serious challenge for medicine in contemporary China is rural health care (an important subject for medical ethics but rarely studied). Partly due to the fall of the well-known "Barefoot Doctor Movement" and the collapse of the county-town-village three-tie health care system, rural residents in China – the great majority of Chinese people and about one seventh of the world population – now have no insured access to primary care and no basic social welfare.

The rapid increase in health care costs and changing disease patterns, such as the AIDS epidemic, extraordinary high suicide rate among rural women, and the breakout of new "plague" SARS (Sever Acute Respiratory Syndrome) in 2003, all these pose serious ethical challenges to medical practitioners, health care institutions, and the whole society: including the importance of prevention, the role of government and media, the boundaries between individual rights and social good, rights and duties of both patients and medical professionals. Since the 1990s, medical disputes and doctor-patient conflicts became more and more common; the cases in which medical professionals were physically attacked, injured and even killed by unhappy patients or their relatives have been increasing rapidly. Aimed to protect patients' rights, *The Statute of Handling Medical Accidents* issued by the State Council and into effect since September 1, 2002, endorses that patients can directly appeal to judicial authorities whenever they think a medical accident – from a breach of administrative regulations to negligence, from poor medical treatment to malpractice – has occurred. It is hard to tell how this controversial law will be interpreted in practice and whether in long run it will help restore patient-professional trust or deteriorate the in-crisis relationship. Like the moral discourses of practitioners in twentieth century and China in general, the Chinese moral discourses of practitioners in twenty-first century are bond to be full of uncertainties and unpredictability.

ACKNOWLEDGMENTS

I am grateful to Professor Paul Unschuld, Dr. Ole Döring, and Professor Qingshan Yan for their helpful comments and suggestions.

NOTE

1. The last part of the *Fuji Tutu Joshing You Quantum* (first published in 1723) has compiled general discussions on medicine appeared in medical and non-medical works as well as biographies of more than twelve hundred physicians from ancient time up to the seventeenth century. The collected primary materials constitute one of the most useful resources on medical ethics, especially moral discourse of orthodox practitioners, in traditional China.

CHAPTER 22

THE DISCOURSES OF PRACTITIONERS IN JAPAN

Rihito Kimura and Shizu Sakai

I. INTRODUCTION

Contemporary Japanese medicine is comparable to medicine in Europe and the United States; however, Japanese medicine has a vastly different history. Japanese medical ethics developed in the framework of a unique discourse integrating concepts of nature, the human body, and medical practice. The understanding and practice of medicine in Japan has been strongly influenced by the acceptance of medical knowledge from countries such as China, Korea, Spain, Portugal, Netherlands, Germany, Britain, France, and United States. Nonetheless, elements of traditional Japanese medicine remain. The road to modern Japanese medical practice and ethical behavior was paved with different layers of medicine and culture over the past 2,000 years (Fujikawa [1904] 1941; Sakai 1986; Kimura 2004).

II. HEALING GODS IN THE ANCIENT FOLK MEDICINE

As in other parts of the world, Japanese mythological stories described the activities of healing gods. The *Kojiki* (712), *Records of Ancient Matters*, one of the oldest books of Japanese mythology and history, tells of the formation of Japan from its beginning until the reign of Emperor Suiko

(592–628). This text states, "As everything was made by the spirit of the *kami* (god or deity), the intention of gods are the causes of all good and bad things." Therefore, it was quite natural for the ancient Japanese to believe that diseases and wounds were due to some magical power of these invisible gods. This belief led to religious rituals being performed to heal the malignant physical and spiritual situations of illness (Sakai 2002, 57–70). Gods in these mythological stories of *Kojiki*, "*Records of Ancient Matters*," and *Nihonshoki* "*The Chronicle of Japan*" (720) assumed human forms and their approach to nature, animals, and humans could be understood in the context of the ancient Japanese animistic belief (Sakai 2002, 26–36).

The most famous healing story in the *Kojiki* involves a rabbit, *Inaba no Shiro Usagi* (White Rabbit of Inaba), which was suffering after sharks attacked and ripped off its fur. First, an evil god plays a trick on the rabbit, suggesting that washing with salt water will heal the skin (Soda 1989, 91–93). Then a compassionate and merciful god named *Ohkuni-nushi-no-mikoto* (The Ruler-God of Great Country) teaches the rabbit that it must first cleanse the wound in pure water and then treat it with the pollen from *Gama* (cattail). This stopped the bleeding, healed the blisters, and returned the fur to the rabbit. This story explains the medicinal value of cattail (Soda 1989 5–7; Sakai 2002, 30). *Ohkuni-nushi-no-mikoto* (The Ruler-God of Great Country) and another god, *Sukuna-hikona-no-mikoto* (The Little Male God), are regarded as the medical gods in Japanese traditional folk medicine because they possess special healing powers. They taught several methods for treating wounds and burns, including bathing in a hot spa. Many healing stories express these gods' mercy and wisdom to the sick.

It is interesting that *Sukuna-hikona-no-mikoto* appears suddenly as a small figure coming from somewhere overseas and then disappears suddenly back to same place. According to some interpretations, this mythological story symbolizes the arrival of Chinese civilization and medical knowledge in Japan (Sakai 2002, 19–26).

III. THE CONCEPT OF DISEASE IN SHINTO RELIGION

Shinto is the traditional indigenous Japanese religion and can be literally translated as "The Way of Gods" and began to develop in Japan during the Nara period (710–793). It integrates elements of traditional folk religion and customs into the social life of the rice-farming system in ancient Japan. Traditional, folk medicine balances the positive and the negative, as illustrated in the story such as *Bungo-no-Kuni Fudoki* (*The Topography of the Province of Bungo*), which relates the behavior of *Susanooh-no-mikoto*, a male god of wildness who controls both wild and mild spirits. The wild and violent spirit causes epidemic diseases to punish bad people and corrupt governments. The mild and compassionate spirit heals and saves good persons from diseases. These stories thus illustrate a concept of disease in which "The good deed will be hailed and bring protection while the bad deed will be punished." This moral model of disease has remained part of Japanese thinking for more than 1,000 years and persists despite the acceptance of a modern medical system and physiological concepts of disease (Fujikawa [1904] 1941, 5–8). Another popular story illustrates a magical concept of disease and the power of amulets as prophylaxis. This story involves two brothers, one rich and the other poor, and the hospitality given by the poor brother to a god in charge of the earth, *Susanooh-no-mikoto*, who disguised himself as a human traveler. This god had first called at the home of the rich brother, seeking shelter, but was rejected. The poor brother took the traveler in. As an expression of gratitude for the poor man's hospitality, the god offers a specially designed wreath of thatch plant for the future use to protect against epidemic disease. An amulet against disease and evil in the name of this poor man, *Somin*, is sold in some Shinto shrines even today. In June of the lunar calendar shrines also remember the story by giving out small wreaths or by having followers pass through a large thatch plant wreath for health and fortune in the coming the year (Sakai 1993, 39–41).

A famous seventh-century poet, Yamanoue-no-Okura, addressed his suffering from rheumatism in a poem that appeared in *Man-yo-shu* (Collected Waka Poems). He reflected on his disease, possibly articular rheumatism, and suffering by writing, "I have not done any wrong and respect both Buddha and God. I pray god for the cure but my heavy disease is getting worse." He maintained a positive outlook toward the value of life, however, and wrote many Waka poems praising the importance of life (Sakai 1993, 35–38).

In ancient Japan, according to its mythology, disease was understood as a punishment and/or curse of *kami* (shinbatsu or tatari). Disease was blamed on the influence of evil spirits. The ancient Japanese believed that there were various *kami* (god) and evil spirits that possessed living human being and caused different types of disease. People depended on prayers by having special ceremonial events to avoid disease or to recover good health (Fujikawa [1904] 1941, 5–8).

IV. THE INFLUENCE OF BUDDHISM IN MEDICINE

When Buddhism was introduced to Japan around the sixth century, it was used as a tool to control power struggles and establish the political hegemony of the ruling class. People believed that widespread epidemic diseases, famines, and political disorders were caused by traditional gods who were angry because the people had accepted Buddhism. Various incantations were performed to calm the spirits and Buddha by having official prayer rituals as well as intensive reading of sacred scriptures. This historical event led to the establishment of various festivals in Shinto shrines and Buddhist temples. Many of the amulets sold today at shrines and temples, which are thought to protect followers from evil and offer good fortune, can be traced back to this time (Sakai 2002, 40–41).

Buddhism, Confucianism, and Taoism had enormous impact on Japanese political, cultural, social, and religious life. Japanese medicine and medical practitioners received a unique blend of ethics from these Chinese influences via Korea. As early as 602, a prominent Korean Buddhist monk, Kwalluk, brought to Japan a series of books on diverse subjects, including astronomy, medicine, and magic (Fujikawa [1904] 1941, 19). From that time, with the active support from the Yamato government ruled by Ohkimi (The name of the Japanese sovereign before the term of Emperor was adopted) in the Nara area during fourth to seventh century, Chinese medicine then was spread rapidly throughout Japan by Korean and Chinese physicians, pharmacologists, and Buddhist priests, who utilized their medical knowledge for healing as a part of their religious activities.

Many Japanese physicians were especially interested in the medical theories of the Chinese scholar Sun Ssu-mo (Simiao) (c. 581–c. 682) (see Chapter 21). His work signaled a shift away from magico-religious concepts of disease toward a more secular conception. Sun Ssu-mo emphasized that medicine needed to be a combination of the prevention and healing of disease with a concern for "ethical behavior." According to this concept of disease, the body is not the possession of the individual but is a gift from one's parents and one's health depends on the harmonious interaction of *yin* (negative) and *yang* (positive) principles. Thus, it was one's filial duty to sustain one's health by maintaining harmony with the environment, inasmuch as disease and will were believed to arise from imbalance at the physiological, psychological, or cosmological level.

Chinese medicine also encouraged acupuncture (*shin or hari*), moxa, or moxibustion (*kyu*, set on key acupuncture points and burned slowly), the application of plants as counterirritants, and herbal medicine. Generally speaking, Buddhist priests took care of sick common people. In particular, *Kango-so* (Buddhist priests for the care of the sick) were respected as the merciful care givers. In 723, the *Seyakuin* (Dispensary) was established in the grounds of *Kofukuji* Temple, literally translated as The Temple of Flourishing Happiness in Kyoto. Significantly, Buddhist leaders in Japan also affirmed that what one learned from the Chinese medical-ethical tradition was in complete harmony with the fundamental Buddhist principle of compassion, which requires the act of giving, caring and serving for other persons. In keeping with this principle, Prince Regent Shotoku (573–621) built a temple, providing an asylum, a hospital, and a dispensary on the temple grounds (Sakai 2002, 36).

Following his example, pious monarchs and aristocrats sponsored other medical charities. In the face of this rapid development and use of Chinese medicine, the Emperor Daido in 808 issued an order to keep a record of the Japanese local and traditional folk medicine. The book titled, *Daido Ruijyuho, The Collected Medical Documents of Daido era*, was edited based on this survey. The only existing edition of this book, however, is from the *Edo* era (1603–1867), which is believed to offer only fragments of the original documentation (Fujikawa [1904] 1941, 50–53). Therefore, today, we do not have this valuable book in its entirety, which is said to have contained ideas about physicians' code of behavior. If the same text in the *Edo* edition appeared in the original book, this would be the first physician's code of ethics written in Japanese.

In the ninth century, Japanese medicine developed closer ties with Buddhism. Several public service agencies were set up, based on the Buddhist notion of benevolence for the poor and the sick. Empress Komyo (701–760), who is known to have converted to Buddhism, established *Seyakuin* (Pharmaceutical Institute). Legend says that Empress Komyo helped to bathe the back of a female patient who had a severe skin disease involving pus. This patient turned out to be *Amida* (Buddha)

(Sakai 2002, 40–42). This story illustrates the belief that medical services should be provided by upper class people, including members of the imperial family, to help treat the sick from lower classes or commoners. In this way, medicine came to be looked upon as an expression of benevolence. This meant that healing should come as merciful behavior from the top, usually physicians with knowledge and experience, down to patients suffering from illness, thus establishing a very hierarchical system.

Buddhist scripture arrived in at the beginning of the sixth century, bringing with it new medical knowledge and medical technology that transformed ancient Japanese medicine. Although these were applied clinically, the synthesis of the new religion and medicine led to the evolution of the essential spirit of Japanese medical ethics.

V. ACCEPTANCE OF CHINESE MEDICINE

Although the existence of Japanese folk medicine, *Dento Igaku* (traditional medicine), is recognized, the unique system of medical discourse in Japan has its roots mainly in Chinese medicine, which was transferred from China approximately the sixth century. As outlined in the, the importation of Buddhism from China had a significant impact on traditional Japanese folk medicine. In 701, *Ishitsurei* (Medicine and Disease Law) became the first law relating to medical services in Japan. It was part of *Taiho-Ritsuryo* (The Great Treasure of Legal Code) and emulated the Chinese Tang Legal Code, which is a compilation of administrative laws in various sections, such as the appointment of bureaucrats, examination, defense, and medicine and disease. This first Japanese medical code established a unified system and bureaucratic structure for medical service. This law remained effective throughout the 400-year history of the *Heian* era (794–1191) (Fujikawa [1904] 1941, 29).

Although the social system established by *Taiho Ritsuryo* was completely demolished at the time of the *Kamakura* era in the beginning of the twelfth century, the *Ishitsurei* (Medicine and Disease Law) remained in effect and was not replaced until the Meiji Restoration in 1868. The central-government system of Japan was completely reorganized by the newly enacted *Taiho-Ritsuryo*. Medical services were nationalized and all physicians were hired by the government. The law sanctioned not only the term of study and requirements for becoming a physician, but also the placement and status of physicians. All of these legal and administrative systems had their origins in China's model such as Tang Legal Code. Major medical books edited and published in ninth-century Japan can trace their roots to Chinese and Korean medical books such as *Huang-ti nei ching* (The Yellow Emperor's Classic of Internal Medicine), *Shen-nung pen tsao ching* (*Materia Medica of*

Shen-nung), *Shan han lun* (*Treatise on Shan han, a typhoid-like acute febrile disease*), and *Chin kuei yao lueh* (*Important Prescriptions Worth Treasuring in the Golden Chamber*). For example, *Shen-nung pen tsao ching* outlined three specific categories of physicians in the upper, middle, and lower classes, ranked according to technical maturity and level of medical performance by each physician. These medical classics became the source and basis for Japanese medical practice and medical ethics.

Although very few physicians qualified to practice under *Ishitsurei* (Medicine and Disease Law), Japanese physicians were eager to study Chinese medicine. They learned that *Yin* represented the shadow, dark, cold, wet, negative, passive, chronic side of the universe and *Yang* represented the sunny, bright, hot, dry, positive, active, acute side but that neither is absolute because *Yin* and *Yang* are relative notions. Therefore, if a person developed a cold and had symptoms of high fever and a severe headache, the patient should be treated as being in a *Yang* state. If another person developed a cold and had no remarkable symptoms or complaints except a slight loss of appetite, the patient may be treated as being in a *Yin* state. In this way, physicians began to incorporate fundamental ideas such as *Yin* and *Yang* in their clinical discourse (Otsuka 1976, 323).

One of the most important medical documents written during the *Heian* era is the oldest extant Japanese medical encyclopedia titled *Ishimpo* (The Medicine's Heart and Method). This medical encyclopedia was composed of thirty volumes dealing with various aspects of medical knowledge, including prescribing drugs, herbal lore, hygiene, acupuncture, moxibustion, alchemy, magic, directions for sexual life, and regimen. It was written and compiled by Yasuyori Tanba, who quoted from many original Chinese medical texts and presented the work to the Emperor Enyu in 984. Yasuyori Tanba clearly framed medical ethics in relation to religion, by combining aspects of both Buddhism and Confucianism and quoting original resources in China. In the preface of the encyclopedia, Tanba writes that medicine "should be performed in the spirit of *Taiji-Sokuin* (the great mercy of Buddha and the loving kindness of Confucian teaching)." He also lists ethical principles for physicians to follow (Tanba [1984] 1991, 5–7):

> Physicians should disregard difference with the patient's social status, such as rich or poor, enemy or foe, good or bad, wise or fool, urban or rural.
>
> Physicians should be ready to accept patients without any discrimination and with a hearty spirit of parental affection.
>
> Physicians should have great sympathy with the suffering of patients, as if it were physician's own.
>
> Physicians are obliged to visit patients for the purpose of healing regardless of distance, day or night, cold or hot weather, thirst or hunger, or even fatigue.
>
> Physicians should not look around too much when visiting the patient's home and should not enjoy themselves excessively, even if they are provided delicious meals and fine music.
>
> Physicians should not talk and laugh too much, or have any quarrels, or preach, or argue amongst themselves about right and wrong treatment, or seek fame, or accuse other physicians of wrongdoing, or show off.
>
> It is fatal for physicians to think that they can do everything they want.

Although the original copy of *Ishimpo* might have been lost, one of the copies was stored in the Imperial court, and later, circa 1573, this copy was given to the Nakarai family by the Emperor. Several other copies were kept in specific Buddhist temples such as Nin Na Ji Temple, and there were at least forty three different handwritten copies, which have been circulated among the limited circles of physicians (Sugitatsu 1984, 108).

Ishimpo is an extraordinarily valuable store of ancient Chinese medical works, containing more than 200 medical sources in *Han*, *Sui*, and *Tang* dynasties, most of which are completely lost in China today. In subsequent years, it was reprinted by the *Tokugawa* Feudal Government around the end of Edo era in 1854 (Kimura 1994, 2).

VI. PHYSICIAN'S ETHICS FROM THE *AZUCHI MOMOYAMA* ERA TO THE END OF THE *EDO* ERA

Japan's first encounter with Western medicine in the sixteenth century is a pivotal moment in Japanese medical history. During the *Azuchi Momoyama* period European medicine arrived with Portuguese traders and Roman Catholic missionaries. By the mid-sixteenth century, Jesuit missionaries established clinics, hospitals, dispensaries, and leprosy sanatoria. One of the famous medical missionaries was Luis de Alameida from Portugal, a successful surgeon-turned-Jesuit. For the most part, European missionary–physicians admired the high quality of *kampo-ijutsu* (Chinese-style, mostly internal medicine) practiced at that time in Japan. Their contribution was mainly to new techniques of surgery, which were badly needed in the war-torn nation.

The Jesuits terminated their medical activities in Japan approximately 1560. Afterward, Japanese physicians trained by European missionary–physicians carried on their work until the feudal regime ordered the extermination of all traces of Catholic missionary influence in the mid-seventeenth century. Although the tradition of *Namban* (literally, "Southern Barbarian") medicine was short-lived, its scientific approach, coupled with an altruistic spirit and ethical imperative, left a significant imprint on the history of Japanese social welfare, medicine, and medical ethics (Ebisawa 1944, 258–68, 373–79).

In the early seventeenth century, the *Tokugawa* Shogunate closed Japan to foreigners. Only a small Dutch trading post in Nagasaki remained open. In reality, contact with foreigners was prohibited and the influence of Dutch medicine remained very minor until the end of the Edo era. Traditional Japanese and Chinese medicine, however, continued to flourish during this period.

During the *Tokugawa* period (1603–1867), as a result of the regime's support of Neo-Confucianism, Japanese medicine abandoned its Buddhist underpinnings and sought a new foundation in Neo-Confucian metaphysics, physics, psychology, and ethics. Under Neo-Confucian influence, *ido* (the way or ethics of medicine) was summed up in the phrase *i wa jin nari* (the practice of medicine is a benevolent art). The first systematic treatises on medical ethics written in Japan were the *Ibyo-ryogan* (Thoughts on both Medicine and Disease) and the *Ibyo-moando*, (The Questions and Answers on Medicine and Disease) by Takenaka Tsuan (Fujikawa [1904] 1941, 630).

Kaibara Ekiken's (1630–1714) *Yojokun* (Teaching on the Care of Life) was published in 1713 and this book became one of the most well read, popular books for teaching of health care among the Japanese (Kaibara [1713a] 1961). About that time, a group called *Gosei-ha* (School of Later Centuries) emerged from among the physicians of *Kampo-i* (Chinese style medicine) and became influential as they sought and taught an intricate fusion of medicine with Neo-Confucian philosophy.

One of the most influential works by *Gosei-ha* on health care was *Yojokun* mentioned previously. As a Neo-Confucian scholar, Kaibara wrote widely on various subjects for the edification of people in all walks of life. His lifelong dedication to the cause of health care can be observed through his writing:

> Medicine is the practice of humanitarianism. Its purpose should be to help others with benevolence and love. One must not think of one's own interests but should save and help the people who were created by Heaven and Earth. (Kaibara [1713a] 1961b, 124)

This represents the view that human beings are created by the union of Heaven and Earth, that is, the parents. Because medicine is an art that can make the difference between life and death, it is a profession of utmost importance. This means that physicians must be culturally and intellectually accomplished. Kaibara urged physicians to be conversant with the best medical books, to think logically and precisely, to acquire important theories, and to practice "lifelong education." He proposed an ideal image of the physician as one who excels in qualities of character and scholarship, in contrast to the "inferior physician," who serves his own interests rather than saving others.

In volume 6 of his book, Kaibara lists several requirements for the physician which can be summarized as follows:

1. Have a high goal in life;
2. Be cautious;
3. Acquire scholarship of wide scope;
4. Make the profession of medicine a full-time pursuit;
5. Be thirsty for new and ever greater knowledge;
6. Be humble;
7. Be clean at all times;
8. Be magnanimous. (Kaibara [1713a] 1961b, 116–36)

Toward the end of the Edo era, when restrictions were eased on foreign goods, Japanese physicians sought out texts on Western medicine, training themselves in *Rangaku* (Dutch methodology and practice). Among the texts available through the Dutch trading was Christoph Wilhelm Hufeland's *Enchiridion Medicum* (Medical Handbook) (1836). It was translated from German into Dutch by Hermann H. Hageman (1838) and became influential among The *Ranpo-I* (The Dutch School Physicians).

An 1849 translation of *Ikai* (Medical Admonition) by Seikyo Sugita is based on Hufeland's chapter on the responsibilities of physicians and asserts that physicians have a duty to take care of all patients regardless of their social or economic status. This was widely read and accepted by Japanese physicians (Sugimoto 1992, 5–10). A thirty-volume translation of Hufeland's writing, completed in 1861 by Koan Ogata, is an important work because it established Western medicine more firmly among Japanese physicians. *Rangaku*, meaning "Dutch Studies," including medical studies, flourished after the end of the self-imposed isolation of Japan. Toward the end of the *Edo* era in 1867, these "Dutch Studies" became the main source of Western medical knowledge in Japan (Sakai 1984, 94–99).

VII. MODERNIZATION OF JAPAN AND JAPANESE MEDICINE

In 1868, feudal samurai in *han* (local provinces), such as Satsuma, Choshu, Tosa, and Hizen, initiated the restoration of political power to Emperor Meiji after the *Tokugawa* Shogunate's reign of 264 years (1603–1867). Confucian ethical teachings, dominant among the samurai during the *Tokugawa* shogunate, were integrated into *Kyoiku Chokugo* (the educational Edict of the Emperor, 1890) as the basis for moral teaching in the elementary school curriculum. These classes were compulsory and this edict was abolished only after World War II in 1948. Confucian ethics, as embodied in this edict, attributes great mercy and benevolence to the emperor and affirms the importance of virtues such as loyalty to the emperor, as the head of the "state-family," and filial piety or respect for parents. This edict also emphasized the importance of brotherhood and sisterhood, obedience to law and maintenance of order, the necessity of education, and devotion to the state (exemplified by men of service). *Jiyuu-minken undo* or grass roots movements for liberty and civil rights in the political process were increasingly popular but were suppressed by the emperor's proclamation of the Meiji constitution in 1889, which consolidated political power in the hands of the emperor and established the Diet (Parliament) in his name (Kimura 2004, 1706).

Modern Japanese medical ethics cannot be isolated from this social and political milieu. The strong paternalistic nature of Japanese medical practice is the natural outcome of Confucian teaching of the filial piety, which calls for respect for the master and views the authority of the master as a source of unquestionable wisdom and truth.

As Japan opened to the West the Dutch ceased to be the sole source of Western culture. This process of modernizing Japan began in the second half of the nineteenth and continued into the twentieth century. It was aided by *oyatoi gaikokujin* (foreign advisers) from Western countries who were hired by the Japanese government to provide advice about developing industry, education, government, finance, science, technology, and medicine (Sakai 1998, 137–57). Seeking a model for modernization, Japan adapted the German approach because of the success and progress of German science and technology as well as the similarity of the authoritarian political system established under the Prussian Kaiser to its own under the Emperor. Acceptance of Western medicine, particularly German, guided the development of Japanese policy on medical administration and education and set the course for the future (Oshima 1983, 223–28).

By the end of the nineteenth century the legacy of authoritarianism had far-reaching effects on Japanese medical education and practice. This legacy, combined with the Confucian self-righteousness in rendering benevolence to the patient, undermined the development of any notion of patients' rights. Research became the main interest at many university hospitals, and patients who presented interesting cases were treated as research material. All of these influences can be seen in the *Isei* (seventy-six guidelines for medical administration) drafted by Sensai Nagayo in 1874. *Waho* (traditional Japanese medicine) and *kanpo* (traditional Chinese medicine) fell out of the medical mainstream after the adoption of *Isei*. Despite this modernization, acupuncture and moxibustion remained part of folk medicine and enjoyed widespread support among the public (Otsuka 1984, 334–38).

VIII. RECENT DEVELOPMENTS OF MEDICAL ETHICS

In 1951, the Japan Medical Association (JMA) issued a statement on physicians' ethics. This action ushered in a new era for Japanese medical practice and signaled a return to the prewar state of medical ethics. Article I of the statement explicitly reaffirmed the fundamental and central place of the ancient principle of *jin* (Confucius notion of loving-kindness). This notion of benevolence in Confucian teaching in medical practice was reconfirmed and it asserted that physicians, as the elite of society, must embody the spirit of *jin* (Kimura 1991, 236–39). This mandated the physician to always consider the welfare of the patient as well as the benefit of treatment. Further, in cooperation with other professionals, it called upon physicians to take the initiative in social reform and, as ethically oriented people, exercise great self-discipline.

In 1968, a series of consultations and presentations by scholars on ethical issues in medicine was held under the direction of Dr. Taro Takemi, then president of the JMA, in an attempt to update the 1951 statement. The publication of *Ishi Rinri Ronshu* (Collected Papers of Physician's Ethics) (1968) was the outcome of this research; however, no work was done to write a new ethical code. During his 25-year tenure, Takemi developed an interdisciplinary study project titled "Raifu Saiensu no Shinpo (Progress of Life Sciences)" which focused attention on bioethical issues such as the allocation of medical resources, ethical implications of high-tech medicine, and physician–patient relationships. The professional orientation of this study excluded the lay public for many years. This autonomy and authoritative decision making by the medical community continued to exclude patients from the process until recent years.

In April 2000, the JMA officially adopted the physician's new code of ethics due to the internal and external reasons mainly caused by the continuous occurrence of the cases of medical malpractice and the need for disciplinary self-control mechanism based on the criteria of new ethics code. The following is the contents of this new ethics code:

1. Physicians must commit themselves to lifelong learning, in order to acquire medical knowledge and technology and thus to contribute to the progress and development of medical science.
2. Physicians must maintain their professional dignity and responsibility, acquire general knowledge, and cultivate their character.
3. Physicians should respect those who require medical service, show kindness toward them, and explain medical treatment, in order to earn the confidence and trust of patients.
4. Physicians must respect each other and provide medical service by cooperating with other health care professionals.
5. Physicians must recognize the public role of medical service, by contributing to society through their medical works and by obeying legal rules and orders.

6. Physicians should not provide medical care primarily for profit or financial gain. (Japanese Medical Association 2000)

Faced with new challenges in the development of medicine and the emerging concern by patients' interest groups, medical ethics has become the a topic not only for professional medical groups, such as the JMA, but also has emerged as an area of major concern to the public. Since the beginning of the 1980s, the Japanese bioethics movement has had an enormous impact in challenging traditional, paternalistic Japanese medical ethics and questioning establishment values in the medical profession (Kimura 1987b, 267–72).

IX. CONCLUSION

One of the most eminent Japanese medical historians, Dr. Yu Fujikawa (1865–1940) mentioned in his book *Ishin* (Medical Admonition) in 1935 that physicians are bound by special obligations and responsibilities and must develop a special ethical consciousness in their daily practice (Kimura 1987b).

The development of new biomedical ethics in Japan has just begun. It is not simply the responsibility of the medical professional to establish ethical standards but is the mutual responsibility of patients and physicians to implement new ethics codes in our historical, cultural, and social context as we have analyzed. The national policy for the Japanese health care system calls out health for all by saying "Daredemo, Dokodemo, Itsudemo." These three key words mean equal access to health care by "anybody, anywhere and at any time" (Government of Japan, Ministry of Health, Labor and Welfare 2003, 268–85). We believe that this unique shared health policy in the framework of Japanese egalitarian health care ethics was the outcome of efforts by many Japanese people including those in the medical profession for many years.

The accomplishment of Japanese bioethics during these 20 years focusing on the patients' rights and the equal opportunity for all patients to be cared by our national health care service has been our basic departure point for the new image of medical ethics beyond our traditional medical paternalism (Kimura 1997, 137–38, 1998, 200).

CHAPTER 23

THE DISCOURSES OF PRACTITIONERS IN ANCIENT EUROPE

Heinrich von Staden

I. INTRODUCTION

From the earliest surviving Greek literary texts – the *Iliad* and *Odyssey* – moral value terms appear in characterizations of physicians, of their activities, of their relations to patients, and of their attitudes. As in many spheres of Greek culture, so too in the ancient Greeks' uses of these value terms a considerable heterogeneity of rival views becomes visible. The absence of centralized control over physicians in Greece, the lack of any licensing and of formal professional sanctions, and the aggressive competitiveness and adversariality that marked much of ancient Greek culture all contributed to the diversity of views held not only by, but also about physicians. Whereas some Greeks, for example, agreed with the Homeric hero Idomeneus that "a healer (*iatrós*) is a man worth many men, [since he knows how] to cut out arrows and to sprinkle gentle drugs on [wounds]" (*Iliad* 11. 514–15), others depicted physicians as greedy, unscrupulous charlatans who collected fees by impressing patients and onlookers with ostentatious displays that merely veiled their ignorance and incompetence. It is impossible to do justice to this diversity of ancient views within the scope of this chapter; the reader therefore would be well advised to keep in mind that only a few conspicuous strands in Greek medical ethics are singled out for consideration here.

II. HIPPOCRATIC TEXTS AND THEIR CORE CONCEPTS

At the center of many ancient reflections on medical ethics stood Hippocrates, whose historicity is not in doubt but whose own views remain elusive. More than sixty extant works now known as "the Hippocratic Corpus" or "the Hippocratic writings" (Littré 1839–1861; Hippocrates 1923a, 1923b, 1928, 1931, 1988a, 1988b, 1991, 1995) were attributed to Hippocrates already in antiquity, but they were written over a period of several centuries by a variety of authors who display divergent, at times even contradictory, theoretical and clinical commitments. Most of these treatises seem to date to the years 440–330 BCE, but some may have been composed as late as the early years of the Roman Empire. Some of these works deal with technical subjects without much reference to questions of an ethical or deontological nature, but others attempt to distinguish between praiseworthy, responsible, expert practitioners and those whose conduct is reprehensible. In these contexts numerous concepts, observations, and reflections that are significant for the purposes of this volume appear.

Central to the self-understanding of many Hippocratic physicians are the concepts *dóxa* ("reputation," "what one seems to be to others") and *téchné*. In the Corpus, *téchné*

352

tends to refer to a result-oriented, professional medical expertise and a practice in full accordance with this expertise. A mastery of the *téchné*, whose servant he is, sets apart the praiseworthy physician from the reprehensible one and, in most cases, not only secures the desired therapeutic result but does so in morally and professionally laudable ways. Once the medical *téchné* has been fully mastered, it becomes an internalized body of expert knowledge that the physician – including the itinerant healer – can put into practice wherever he sees patients. The *téchné* acts both as a constant, stable lodestar and as an internal censor and judge, informing the physician what to do and, equally significantly, warning him what not to do. The Hippocratic terms of strong reproach accordingly include *átechnos*, "lacking in *téchné*."

Among the factors depicted as motivating the Hippocratic healer, a frequent complement to this responsibility to one's *téchné* is the need for external social approbation, as is evident in the recurrent emphasis on the importance of reputation (*dóxa*). The relative insecurity of medicine within the social order partly accounts for the overt preoccupation with reputation, and likewise for the defensive and often polemical tone with which some Hippocratic writers stake out the claims of their "new," "nonmagical" medicine. Several Hippocratic treatises also explicitly link their valorization of accurate prognosis to the need for a good reputation among lay people.

III. THE HIPPOCRATIC OATH

It is noteworthy that both of these central concepts, *téchné* and reputation (*dóxa*), play an important role in the most famous of ancient medical texts with an ethical content, the *Oath* attributed to Hippocrates (Littré 1839–1861, 4:610–33; Hippocrates 1923a, 289–301; Edelstein 1967, 3–65; see Susruta Oath, chapter 20). *Téchné* – to refer to what the oath-taker knows, teaches, practices, guards "in a pure and holy way," and lives from – makes four significant appearances in the *Oath*, and "being held in good repute (*doxazómenos*)" among all human beings for time eternal is held out as a principal reward for fulfilling the oath.

The authorship, date, and historical context of this brief but enormously influential text remain as controversial as the interpretation of a number of its central concepts and clauses (Deichgräber 1983; Edelstein 1967; Jouanna 1998, 1999, 50–52, 128–31; Lichtenthaeler 1984; Nutton 1996b; Rütten 1994; Smith 1996). Furthermore, several versions of the *Oath* were attributed to Hippocrates in antiquity. A plausible case, however, can be made for dating its canonical, most famous version to the late fifth or early fourth century BCE, and for locating it in a period when a relatively closed, clan-based medical apprenticeship began to yield to a more open and accessible system of apprenticeship, usually with a single physician–teacher, who charged some pupils a fee. Immediately after the

opening invocation of three generations of Greek healing gods and then of "all the gods as well as goddesses," for example, the oath-taker swears "to regard him who has taught me this *téchné* [of medicine] as equal to my parents and to share, in partnership, my livelihood with him and to give him a share when he is in need of necessities." Like the oath-taker's promise to judge his teacher's offspring "equal to my male siblings" and "to teach them this [medical] *téchné*, should they desire to learn it, without fee and written covenant," the reference to a teacher who is not a parent points to such an expansion of apprenticeship beyond the immediate clan. Yet, the analogies he evokes, notably to treat his teacher *like* a parent and his teacher's offspring *like* his brothers, suggest that, even as new historical circumstances began to transform access to medical training, the earlier clan-based transmission of professional medical expertise remained the model for relations between teachers and students – at least in the circle(s) in which the *Oath* was produced and used. Furthermore, transmission within the family itself continued to shape professional deontological acculturation.

From this socio-pedagogic deontological context, the *Oath* turns to a series of positive and negative sworn promises concerning the practice of medicine. The first of these is to use regimen for the benefit of the ill but to avoid causing them harm or injustice. This solemn undertaking is consonant with a famous principle enunciated in the Hippocratic treatise *Epidemics*, Book I: "As to diseases, practise two things: to benefit or not to harm" (Hippocrates 1923a, 11). In this respect, the *Oath* therefore is not at odds with other Hippocratic writers. Indeed, a remarkable range of Hippocratic and other ancient medical authors explicitly comment on the need to avoid iatrogenic harm. Some confess that they had committed errors of commission or omission that led to the worsening of a patient's condition and even to his or her death. Examples occur in the Hippocratic treatises *Epidemics* V. 27 (Hippocrates [1962] 1994, 179) *Epidemics* VII. 123 (Hippocrates [1962] 1994, 415), *On Wounds in the Head* 19 (Hippocrates 1928, 43–45), *On Fractures* 36 (Hippocrates 1928, 181–3), *On Joints* 12 (Hippocrates 1928, 228–231), *On Affections* 13 (Hippocrates 1988a, 23–25), and *On Diseases* I. 8 (Hippocrates 1988a, 115–19). A strong, widely diffused awareness that even the best-intentioned and most skillful medical intervention could, and often did, cause a patient irreparable harm undoubtedly was in part responsible for the emphasis on avoidance of harm, which in turn led to the recurrent Hippocratic endorsement of the principle of nonintervention in incurable cases. Like iatrogenesis, incurability is a remarkably prominent theme in the Hippocratic Corpus, and it often is accompanied by explicit reflection on the limits of the medical *téchné* and of human cognition (Amundsen 1996, 30–49; von Staden 1990). This recurrent Hippocratic reflection on the limitations of medicine and of its practitioners is also visible in the

Oath, especially in its emphatic repetition of the restrictive phrase "in accordance with my ability and my judgment." It is also reflected in the threefold definition of medicine in *On the Art* (Hippocrates 1923b, 3:193–95): to deliver those who are ill completely from their sufferings; to blunt the vehemence of diseases; and not to treat those who have been vanquished by their diseases.

The Hippocratic oath-taker's next two promises are among the most controversial sentences in ancient Greek medicine: "And I will not give a drug that is deadly to anyone if [or 'when' or 'although'] asked [for it], nor will I suggest the way to such a counsel. And, likewise, I will not give a woman a destructive pessary." The first sentence does not specify who is envisioned as requesting "a drug that is deadly" from the oath-taker. It could, for example, be a patient, his or her kin, an incurable patient's close friend, someone's enemy or rival, a fellow-practitioner, a doctor's assistant, or a king or ruler with evil intent. One, therefore, would be ill-advised to interpret this promise restrictively, as merely abjuring active euthanasia by means of lethal drugs; rather, the oath-taker gives a much more comprehensive assurance that *nobody* will ever be handed a deadly drug by him, and that he will give *nobody* advice concerning such drugs. The rich ancient lore about the poisoning of adversaries and rivals, the occasional use of poison as a means of suicide (Rütten 1997, 68–91), and the ancients' early awareness of the potentially harmful effects of certain natural substances used as simple drugs or as ingredients in compound drugs (for example, hemlock, opium, mandrake, and henbane), confirm that physicians knew only too well that part of their formidable pharmacological arsenal could be put to harmful and even fatal use. Here such use is forsworn, again motivated by the overarching principle of not harming anyone.

The sworn promise not to give a woman "a destructive pessary" seems to abjure the prescription of any abortive suppository. Already in antiquity some readers, such as Theodorus Priscianus and Scribonius Largus read it this way. Soranus of Ephesus perhaps interpreted this sentence as prohibiting all abortions, but it should not be overlooked that Soranus proceeds to describe a variety of methods of therapeutic abortion. (Burguière, Gourevitch, and Malinas 1988–1994, 1:XCVII–C and 59–65; Temkin 1956, 62–68; Mudry 1997; Rütten 1996b, 1997, 91–98). The recurrent ancient recognition that abortive suppositories could be dangerous to the health or life of a woman may have been one of the factors that contributed to the inclusion of this sentence in the *Oath*. It should not be overlooked that many abortifacients, both in the form of vaginal suppositories and of other kinds, are described and prescribed by Greek medical writers from the Hippocratic Corpus to later antiquity. There is ample evidence that women used a variety of early-stage abortifacients as well as contraceptives with impunity throughout Greco-Roman antiquity (see Riddle 1992; Dixon 1988;

Hopkins 1965–1966; Nardi 1971). Greek sacred laws at times depict voluntary abortion or involuntary miscarriage as a source of religious pollution, but giving birth, dying, sexual intercourse, menstruation, and other natural bodily processes likewise were regarded as sources of pollution that required purification and temporary exclusion from sacred precincts (Parker 1983; von Staden 1992a, 1992b). These laws therefore do not necessarily signal a condemnation of abortion on moral grounds. Furthermore, the Hippocratic writings make no explicit reference to these religious views. The inclusion of numerous abortifacients in the doctor's pharmacological arsenal suggest that at least some Hippocratics also dispensed such drugs, as did numerous later Greek physicians. Moreover, the Hippocratics – unlike, for example, Aristotle, some Stoic philosophers, several early Christian writers, and Galen – do not seem to have participated in the ancient debate about whether the fetus is a "living being," about when the embryo acquires soul (*psyché*), and so on. In view of these larger contexts too, it might be prudent to take the *Oath*'s relatively narrow forswearing of a "destructive pessary" or abortive suppository at face value. Regardless of how one resolves this hermeneutic challenge, here too the more fundamental principle of not harming is at work.

At the structural center of the *Oath* stands a remarkable undertaking: "In a pure and holy way I will guard my life and my *téchné.*" The Greek words for "pure" (*hagnôs*), "holy" (*hosís*), and "life" (*bíos*) suggest that the oath-taker here offers a profoundly moral pledge that covers not only his professional conduct but also his life as a whole, and hence his private, personal conduct too (von Staden 1996a, 1997). He commits himself under oath to a way of life ("my *bios*") that will be free of any personal moral defilement (*hagnôs*) that might cause a rupture in his relations with the gods and, at the same time, free of offense to the gods in his interactions with the profane or secular sphere (*hosís*). The same commitment explicitly covers his practice of his professional expertise ("my *téchné*"). The professional and the personal, the public and the private, the religious and the secular are therefore comprehensively covered by the same sworn commitment to preserve them unremittingly "in a pure and holy way." Although much of Hippocratic ethics and deontology concerns professional conduct, this section of the *Oath* reflects a view shared by physicians and lay persons – a view also visible in decrees honoring physicians, in funerary inscriptions, and in subsequent Greco-Roman medical writings (von Staden 1997) – namely, that professional competence and moral character both are essential to the efficacious, successful, and ethical practice of medicine.

Three further features of the *Oath* merit brief mention. First is the famous sentence, "I will not cut, [and] certainly not those suffering from stone." It has puzzled numerous readers, especially in view of the extensive descriptions of surgical procedures elsewhere in the Hippocratic Corpus (as in other Greek and Latin medical writings). If, however, the sentence in the *Oath* is read as referring only to lithotomy, it would be consonant with the undertaking to bring no harm to the ill, inasmuch as lithotomy was recognized in antiquity to entail very high risks for the patient.

Second, the oath-taker undertakes to refrain from "all voluntary and destructive injustice, especially from sexual acts, both upon women's bodies and upon men's, both of the free and of the slaves," whenever he enters any house. The *Oath* recognizes that the practice of medicine often entails forms of physical proximity and contact that are fraught with social and moral delicacy and peril, and it addresses these comprehensively: "*all* injustice," "women's bodies *and* men's," "the free *and* the slaves" (emphasis added). Like most of the oath-taker's other undertakings concerning the ill, this is a negative promise (i.e., not to do certain things), thus again illustrating the centrality of the principle of doing no harm to one's patients, which here is extended from medical intervention to the physician's personal conduct and social interactions. The mention of women and slaves in the *Oath* is not surprising, especially given the relative frequency with which Hippocratic works, including nongynecological works, refer to female patients. Although slaves are mentioned less frequently in the Corpus, the *Epidemics*, in particular, refer to both male and female slaves who were patients. The extant textual evidence suggests that at least some Hippocratic physicians tried to treat slaves and women with the same care as male patients. A remarkable passage in *On Diseases of Women* (1.62, in Littré 1839–1861, 8:126–27) also warns against the errors committed by male physicians who treat female patients as though their disorders are the same as those of male patients. The same passage emphasizes the strong sense of shame that prevents female patients from telling male physicians about their ailments, thus rendering the physician's task even more difficult.

Third, the final promise in the *Oath* again is to refrain from doing harmful things, even if it is formally cast as a positive statement: "And about whatever I may see or hear in treatment, or even without treatment, in the life of human beings – things that should not ever be blurted out outside – I will remain silent, holding such things to be unutterable [sacred, not to be divulged]."

Framed by two brief promises to act for the benefit of the ill, the oath-taker's broad range of negative undertakings, that is, to refrain from certain acts, suggests the extent to which Hippocratic medicine understood itself not only as a source of life-saving help but also as a potential source of multiple iatrogenic harm. Not only through his dietetic, pharmacological, and surgical interventions – all three kinds are mentioned in the *Oath* – but also by his sexual behavior and his verbal indiscretions the healer can cause enormous harm to patients and others. The practice of medicine is constantly fraught with physical, social, and moral perils for physician and patient alike, and it is this fundamental insight, rather than specific doctrines about, for example, abortion or euthanasia, that shaped most Hippocratic and other ancient reflections on the actions and conduct of healers.

IV. Related Hippocratic Texts

Several of the Hippocratic deontological treatises (notably *Precepts, Decorum, Law*, and the first chapter of *Physician*) reflect similar concerns, even if they address divergent issues and introduce many ideas and concepts not represented in the *Oath* (e.g., the appearance of the physician, his language, truthfulness, manner, and fees). Most of them were probably written in the Hellenistic period (i.e., the last three centuries BCE) or in the early years of the Roman Empire. Responsibility to one's *téchnē*, reputation (*dóxa*), and benefiting or not harming others remain important themes in these later Hippocratic texts. After advising the physician not to discuss fees with a patient at the outset, the author of *Precepts*, for example, explains that it might cause a patient's condition to deteriorate; furthermore, he adds, reputation is more important than profit (Chapter 4). He also recommends that doctors sometimes offer their services free of charge to those of lesser means and that they assist strangers who are in financial straits, for, he says, if love for human beings (*philanthropía*) is present, love of the *téchnē* (*philotechnía*) also is present (Chapter 6). The controversial word *philanthropía* and its cognates do not appear in pre-Hellenistic Hippocratic works, and even here it is not elevated beyond the immediate context to a central principle. Only when Romans in the first century began to use *humanitas*, and Galen in the second century *philanthropía*, to characterize Hippocrates as the ideal physician, did "humaneness" and "love of humanity" become valorized as a general moral principle for medical practice (see later; on philanthropy see Amundsen and Ferngren 1982).

V. Other Hellenistic Works

In other Hellenistic medical works, some of the emphases traced in the Hippocratic Corpus also emerge. According to a fragment attributed to Herophilus (the third-century BCE pioneer of systematic human dissection), for example, a perfect physician is "one who is capable of distinguishing the things that are possible from those that are not possible" (von Staden 1989, 126), thus again underscoring the limits of the medical *téchnē*. Herophilus' contemporary Erasistratus also seems to have reflected on its limits, distinguishing between the "scientific" and "conjectural" ("stochastic") parts of medicine and, significantly, including all of therapeutics and semiotics among the stochastic parts (Garofalo 1988, 70, fr.

32). To Erasistratus also is attributed the following view on the relation between character and competence:

> The most felicitous circumstance is whenever each of two things has come about, that the physician is both perfect in his professional expertise and best in his character. If, however, one of the two were to be missing, it is better to be a good man who is lacking in learning than to be a perfect, expert practitioner who has a bad character and is lacking in virtue. (pseudo-Soranus, *Medical Questions*, in Garofalo 1988, 70, fr. 31)

It has often been suggested that the Romans cared much more than the Greeks about the personal virtue of physicians, and that the Greeks insisted above all on the professional competence of doctors (for example, Edelstein 1967, 323–24, on the Greeks; and Gourevitch 1984, 436, on Romans vs. Greeks). The evidence from the Hippocratic Corpus, from Greek and Latin inscriptions of the Hellenistic period, and the Roman empire, as well as from non-Hippocratic Greek and Latin medical works, early and late, suggest that on this point, at least, a fairly continuous strand is visible in Greco-Roman medical and lay thought – one that makes both professional competence and personal moral conduct central to the definition of the good physician.

VI. ROMAN WORKS

Roman medical writers such as A. Cornelius Celsus and Scribonius Largus in the first century nevertheless display distinctively Roman voices, also in their reflections on ethical and deontological issues (Pigeaud 1997; Mudry 1997; von Staden 1996b). In the preface to his work on compound drugs Scribonius, for example, introduces influential concepts that had not been central or explicit in classical Hippocratic texts, even while he recognizes Hippocrates as "the founder of our profession" and echoes a number of Hippocratic ideas, including that medicine is a science "of healing, not of harming" (pref. 5; Sconocchia 1983, 2–3). Among the new concepts is *misericordia*, "compassion," "pity," and "tender-heartedness." Unless the mind of physicians "is full of compassion (*misericordia*) and humaneness (*humanitas*), in accordance with the wish of the profession itself," says Scribonius, "they should be hateful to all humans and gods" (pref. 3; Sconocchia 1983, 2). Further, he claims, "if medicine is not fully vigilant, with everyone of its parts, for helping those who are in physical distress, it does not provide the compassion which it promises human beings" (pref. 5; Sconocchia 1983, 3). It remains controversial whether and to what extent the Roman concept of *humanitas* renders the Greek term *philanthropía* ("love of humanity"). The novelty of Scribonius' overt emphasis on compassion – or more literally, having a heart (*cor*) capable of being moved to pity or sorrow

(*misereri*) for others or their misfortunes – as a central feature of the praiseworthy practice of medicine appears to be beyond dispute (Mudry 1997).

It is striking that Scribonius' older contemporary A. Cornelius Celsus, the Roman encyclopedist whose eight books on medicine (Celsus 1915; Spencer 1935–1938) represent the earliest extant, reasonably comprehensive account of medicine written in Latin, likewise views being "compassionate" (*misericors*) as a desirable quality in physicians (albeit more specifically in the context of surgery and with certain restrictions). A surgeon should be "compassionate" in such a way that he wishes to cure [the patient] whom he has accepted, but without being moved by the patient's cries and therefore becoming rushed or cutting less than is necessary. Although motivated by compassion, he should exercise his skills undistracted by any emotions triggered by the patient's cries (7 proem. 4; Spencer 1935–1938, 3:297).

In Celsus' report of the Hellenistic Empiricists' sharp criticisms of human vivisection on moral, epistemological, methodological, and therapeutic grounds, the good physician's *misericordia* (proem. 43; Spencer 1935–1938, 1:24) also is contrasted with the violent cruelty of the vivisectionists, but in this passage it is difficult to distinguish between Celsus' own views and the Empiricists.' It nevertheless is noteworthy that Celsus himself subsequently rejects human vivisection – but not human dissection – as cruel and superfluous (proem. 74; Spencer 1:41), and that not only human vivisection but also systematic human dissection are attested for only two ancient Greek physicians, Herophilus and Erasistratus (Garofalo 1988; von Staden 1989). Although Greeks from at least Aristotle to Galen conducted vivisectory experiments on animals, opening the human body, dead or alive, for the purpose of scientific investigation, was incompatible with religious sensibilities expressed in numerous ancient Greek sacred laws concerning pollution, purification, death, and cadavers (Parker 1983), and likewise with moral sensibilities to which certain philosophers and poets allude (von Staden 1992a). Even if the bodies belonged to condemned criminals, as in the case of Erasistratus' and Herophilus' vivisectory experiments, such forms of investigation were almost universally rejected.

The justification for vivisection reported by Celsus is, paradoxically, based on a fundamental tenet of Hippocratic ethics: the benefit of patients. The immediate purpose of vivisection was to observe in living subjects the parts which that has concealed, that is, their exact position, color, shape, size, arrangement, relative density, interconnections, projections, depressions, and so forth in their normal state, unaffected by war wounds or death. The ultimate justification was to seek remedies, through such vivisectory observations, for the benefit of innocent people of all times, present and future (Celsus 1935–1938, proem. 23–26; Spencer 1935–1938,

1, 14–15; Mudry 1982, 106–11; von Staden 1989, 144–48). It is not cruel, they argued, to seek benefits for innocent patients of all future ages in the sacrifice of very few criminals who have done harm to others. Despite its careful contrasts between the innocent and the guilty, between the benefits envisioned for patients and the harm done by criminals, between the many and the few, and between the brief present moments of vivisection and the remedies that will benefit all ages, this therapeutic justification convinced neither physicians nor lay persons and, judging by the extant evidence, human vivisection was never resumed in antiquity after Herophilus and Erasistratus.

VII. Galen

Perhaps the most influential reader, ancient or modern, of the Hippocratic writings was Galen. Thirteen of his extensive commentaries on Hippocratic treatises survive, and although none is devoted to a deontological treatise, they are remarkably attentive to Hippocratic ethical reflections (Manetti and Roselli 1994; Jouanna 1997). Fragments of a lost commentary on the Hippocratic *Oath* survive in a ninth-century Arabic translation (Rosenthal 1956) and, despite recurrent doubts about its authenticity, it appears to be a genuine work of Galen's. The extant fragments are, however, devoted mainly to the opening section of the *Oath* and therefore do not deal with most of the issues addressed previously herein. Along with Galen's treatise *That the best physician is also a philosopher* (Kühn [1821–1833] 1964, 1:53–63; Wenkebach 1932–1933), his commentaries offer rich evidence of Galen's transformative appropriations and expropriations of Hippocratic medical ethics.

Galen not only endorses a number of Hippocratic views discussed previously but also formalizes them as components of the method he adopts in his daily practice of medicine. In commenting on the phrase "to benefit or not to harm," for example, Galen remarks that at first he found it an insignificant, self-evident maxim unworthy of Hippocrates, but faced over and over with difficult therapeutic choices in his practice, and observing the unintended iatrogenic harm done by even distinguished physicians, he eventually recognized the profundity of the Hippocratic maxim and turned it into a methodological principle. Thus, whenever selecting a treatment for a given patient, he would never do anything without first having weighed carefully exactly (a) to what degree a given treatment might be useful for realizing his therapeutic goal, (b) to what degree said therapy might harm the patient, and (c) to what degree nonintervention – that is, not realizing the therapeutic goal – would harm the patient. He suggests that part of this consistently and meticulously applied method entailed eschewing remedies which, if they happened to fail, would do great harm to patients (Kühn [1821–1833] 1964, 17.1:148–49; Wenkebach and

Pfaff 1934, 76; Jouanna 1997, 215–17). The Hippocratic "maxim" thus is transformed by Galen into a therapeutic "method," whose steps are specified in detail.

An issue by which Galen seems to have been more vexed than the Hippocratics is the truthfulness of the physician, also in relation to his or her patients. Perhaps inspired by his strong philosophical training, Galen insisted that the ideal physician will always be guided by truthfulness and by the virtuous mean (i.e., avoiding excess and deficiency, also in deontological matters, including appearance, clothing, tone, and manner). Any deviations from this ideal that are motivated by the physician's self-interest are unacceptable. Reluctantly, he concedes that departures from the ideal might have to be tolerated if they are in the interest of the patient. Deviations from the mean might, for example, be necessary to please the patient and thus to improve the relation between physician and patient, and partial or total suppression of the diagnostic or prognostic truth might be required by the fragility, anxiety, or sensibility of a patient; indeed, despite the ideal of unwavering truthfulness, a physician might on occasion even be compelled to lie to a patient to avoid harming the patient's health (but without telling any "big lies," Galen insists: Kühn [1821–1833] 1964, 17.1:995–96; Wenkebach and Pfaff 1946, 115–16). Even in the latter case, however, the physician should tell the full truth to those taking care of the patient and should not fail to encourage the patient to adhere strictly to the doctor's prescriptions. Any deviations from the truth or from the mean thus have to meet two conditions to be acceptable: they must not harm the patient, and they must benefit the patient, especially by rendering him or her willing to adhere strictly to the prescribed course of therapy. Galen's insistence on the doctor's truthfulness thus becomes integrally linked to this appropriation of Hippocratic ethics.

Galen's valorization of truthfulness with one's patients are to some extent at odds with emphases in the postclassical Hippocratic deontological treatises. The author of *Decorum* (see Chapter 16), for example, recommends that the doctor should not say anything at all to patients about their present or future conditions, lest it cause a deterioration in their condition (Littré 1839–1861, 9:242; Hippocrates 1923b, 298–99). Galen nevertheless shares with this author too the classical Hippocratic commitment to the best interest of the patient as the overriding moral principle.

With the Hippocratic treatise *Precepts* Galen also has in common the overt rejection of material gain as a motive for practicing medicine and an emphasis on "love of human beings" (*philanthropía*) as the desired alternative. Indeed, Galen elevates "love of human beings" to a guiding principle and to an essential characteristic of the good physician and of the true *téchnē* of medicine. In these contexts too Galen tends to systematize scattered Hippocratic remarks in such a way as to construct Hippocrates as the ideal, coherent, unequaled representative of all these qualities: a companion and lover of the truth, a friend of moderation and of the mean, one whose will shows itself as contempt for wealth and love of hard work, loving other human beings while maintaining a well-ordered life of his own, one well versed in all branches of philosophy (through logic he always finds the right method, through "physics" the true nature of the body, and through ethics the afore-mentioned virtues). No such composite "ideal physician" appears in any Hippocratic treatise, but Galen repeatedly argues that it is this "Hippocrates" that physicians should emulate to reverse the decline suffered by medicine ever since Hippocrates' death. At least as influential as this Galenic construction of Hippocrates (Smith 1979) was Galen's explicit fusion of medicine and philosophy (Barnes 1991; Frede 1987, 223–98; Hankinson 1992, 1994, 1998; Jouanna 1997). He was far from the first physician to introduce philosophical perspectives into medicine, but his systematic, overt advocacy of a comprehensive integration of philosophy into medicine, like his massive attempt to demonstrate the compatibility of Platonic philosophy and Hippocratic medicine, was not only without precedent but also rich in its complex historical consequences. In his history of medicine Celsus claimed that scientific medicine at first had been part of philosophy (as represented by Presocratic philosophers, such as Pythagoras, Empedocles, and Democritus), but that the great Hippocrates then separated medicine from philosophy, thus transforming scientific medicine into an autonomous form of expertise (Spencer 1935–1938, 1:4–5). Galen, by contrast, reinvented Hippocrates as the first and greatest philosopher–physician who, as such, also represents the ethical ideal and model for all physicians.

VIII. CONCLUSION

The image of Hippocrates and the precepts of the Hippocratic *Oath* and related texts had an important influence on medical ethics in Europe and the Middle East from the ancient period onward. The *Oath* apparently committed those who swore it to a way of life that sought to responsibly manage the physical, social, and moral challenges of medical practice. The *Oath* should not be interpreted in isolation, but rather in the context of related Hippocratic texts that underscore professional competence and upright conduct to understanding what it meant to be a good physician. Subsequent writings in Greek and Latin continued to emphasize these themes (see also Chapter 24).

CHAPTER 24

THE DISCOURSES OF EUROPEAN PRACTITIONERS IN THE TRADITION OF THE HIPPOCRATIC TEXTS

Vivian Nutton

I. INTRODUCTION

To describe the ethical writings within the Hippocratic Corpus is far easier than to evaluate their use and influence over the centuries. There are two main reasons for this. First, our surviving ancient and medieval sources are so scattered that it is difficult to gain a coherent impression of developments over different centuries, cultures, and communities. Second, and far more significant for the historian of ethics, the very notion of Hippocratic morality has changed considerably over the centuries, both in the narrow sense of works written by or associated with Hippocrates, and in the wider sense of a system of medical ethics that appeals, in some way, to the very earliest days of Greek medicine for its values. Indeed, far from determining contemporary medical morality, the Hippocratic Oath, the major ethical text that has been presumed to have normative value, has been regularly adapted and interpreted to fit the concerns of the present (Hippocrates 1923a, 289–301; Nutton 1995, 1996a).

II. THE HIPPOCRATIC TEXTUAL TRADITION

It is important to realize at the outset that in Antiquity, and arguably until the nineteenth century, what Hippocrates was thought to have believed and written about matters ethical was not confined to the handful of deontological texts within our Hippocratic Corpus. Although it is likely that the Corpus was largely formed in Alexandria by 250 BCE, it was never a fixed body of writings. It neither contained everything believed to be by the historical Hippocrates nor, in its present form, is it confined to works written during his lifetime. Some later texts, notably *Decorum* and *Precepts*, once attached to this block of earlier material, were copied over the centuries as if they were part of the original Corpus (Edelstein 1967, 133–44, 328–30). Not every manuscript of Hippocrates, however, included every text from the Corpus, and it was not until 1526, with the first printed edition of the works of Hippocrates in Greek, that the Corpus took on the fixed form familiar today.

There were other writings that bore the name of Hippocrates that never entered our modern Hippocratic Corpus, although to their medieval copyists and readers they were just as authentic. One such text, the so-called *Testament of Hippocrates*,[1] from the first two centuries and originally written in Greek, but surviving also in Latin and Arabic, described "What the medical student ought to be like." He is to be of free birth and noble character, young, of medium stature, sturdy, capable in everything, sound in body and mind, resourceful, modest, brave, slow to anger, and full of energy. Besides these and many other personal qualities, he should not indulge in abuse, or have his hair close-cropped or too long. His nails, clothing, gait, should all be appropriate, and he should adjust the time and manner of his visit to the patient to suit each case.[2] In some redactions, he must also have had a preliminary training in grammar, astronomy, music, and geometry, but not in rhetoric, for this only leads to vaniloquence. Philosophy he will learn alongside medicine (Deichgräber 1970, 100).

Texts in Latin from the fifth or sixth centuries make similar claims to Hippocratic authority. Basing themselves on themes, hints, and statements from the Hippocratic Corpus, Galen, and Cassiodorus, they are sometimes ascribed in the manuscripts to Hippocrates, to a variety of classical authors, or to none (MacKinney 1952; Kibre 1985, 198, 232–33; Gālvao-Sobrino 1996). Although the *Oath* is mentioned or implied in several of these treatises, their relationship with any Greek original in the Hippocratic Corpus is somewhat remote. In one group of manuscripts, a version of the Hippocratic *Oath* is supplemented by a quotation from *Precepts*, and preceded by rules for the need for preliminary instruction in grammar, rhetoric, geometry, and astronomy (Mackinney 1952, 13–15). In another text, which is ascribed to Hippocrates only in late copies, the prospective medical student is given advice on how to visit the sick and the questions he should ask. In this document close parallels can be found with the *Medical Questions* of Rufus of Ephesus (fl. 110) and with statements in Galen, but direct copying from either source is unlikely.[3] Behind some of these texts lurks the practical advice of Galen. So, for example, in a letter ascribed to Hippocrates, Galen, or, more misleadingly, Isidore of Seville, the physician is warned always to read, shun indolence, and avoid quarrels and instead to praise the cures of others, because thereby one will obtain a better reputation. It is less clear whether the original version of this little guide contained the injunctions to refrain from getting involved with incurable or certainly fatal cases and to claim half the agreed fee at the outset, for "when the pain ceases, your services also cease."[4]

Later views on Hippocratic morality were not derived solely from writings that might be classified as ethical (Temkin 1991). The definition of medicine in *Breaths*, that the doctor sees terrible things, touches unpleasant things, and grieves himself at the sufferings of others, became commonplace in Greek moral, medical and theological literature (Jouanna 1998, 102). The Hippocratic *Letters* showed Hippocrates as the noble patriot, defending his native island against Athenian aggression, coming to the aid of Greece in time of plague, and refusing to treat the King of Persia, no matter how much he offered, because he was the enemy of Greece (Pinault 1992). That the last incident conflicted with other injunctions to offer medical aid to all in need does not seem to have troubled ancient commentators. Galen developed a few words in *Epidemics* VI (of uncertain meaning) into a long discourse on the theme

that the doctor's own behavior was an essential element in effective therapy. Whatever contributed to the well-being of the sick constituted good practice (Deichgräber 1970; Jouanna, 1997). His characterization of Hippocrates, "our guide to all that is good," as a philosopher, a lover of truth, even to the extent that he could admit his own errors, and a despiser of pomp and glory, also influenced later conceptions of what a doctor should be (Wenkebach 1932–33; Bachmann 1965; Brain 1977; Nutton 1993). They did not entirely obliterate the less favorable story that Hippocrates had burnt the temple of Asclepius to prevent others from deriving the same benefit as he had from the medical writings contained therein (Rütten 1993, 30).

The actual texts themselves underwent changes over time. Some were minor: archaic words or forms were replaced by more modern ones, or the pagan preamble to the *Oath* changed to one more suitable for Christians or Muslims (Jones 1924; Rütten 1996b, 70–71). Others were more substantial. One copyist removed all references to the teacher's dependents, and the Christian version of the *Oath* says nothing about any obligation to one's teachers. A complete sentence from the *Law* was missing from most manuscripts, and from all printed texts before 1996 (Jouanna 1996). Translation presents its own hazards of interpretation. Is the ban on cutting in the *Oath* to be understood as a ban on all surgery, or only on lithotomy (Rütten 1996b, 71–77)? Is the abortion clause a prohibition of only one method? A common English version, printed from at least the 1940s, adds to the lithotomy clause the phrase "even for patients to whom the disease is manifest," which is not justified by either the text or the context. Modern appeals to the *Oath* as representing long-established ethical values concentrate on three sections only, dealing with abortion, euthanasia (although the Greek has wider connotations), and secrecy, although the other sections have an equal claim to ancient authority (Carrick 1985).

III. THE HIPPOCRATIC OATH AND ITS PROGENY

There is no doubt that from at least 200 BCE, the *Oath* in particular was regarded as the creation of Hippocrates himself and as representative, in some way, of the medical profession, even if, like Cato the Elder and Pliny, some saw it only as an agreement by doctors to cheat their patients (Edelstein 1967, 3–64; Lichtenthaler 1984; von Staden 1996a). Nevertheless, whether it was ever sworn is hard to determine. Scribonius Largus's call, around 47, for a return to the *Oath* and the discipline it entailed, implies that it was not followed (Deichgräber 1950; Mudry 1997). Galen's commentary on it, of which approximately half survives in Arabic, concentrates on antiquarian learning, not ethics (Rosenthal 1956). Not until the fourth century do we find an author implying that it was being sworn by medical students, but, although late-Antique Alexandria would be a plausible place for such a ceremony, we are told merely that the Christian Caesarius did not swear (Nutton 1995, 520). The placing of the *Oath* at the very beginning of some early manuscripts containing the bulk of the Hippocratic Corpus does suggest that some copyists did see it as the first thing to be studied (Rütten 1993, 51–54).

The *Oath* was well known in the Muslim world, in medical as well as in ethical writers such as al-Ruhawi (see Chapter 17), and it may also have influenced the Hebrew *Oath* ascribed to Asaph (Bürgel 1966, 1970; Lieber 1984; Newmyer 1989). Whether it was ever administered is less certain. Ibn al-Ukhuwwa (d. 1329), in enumerating the duties of the market-inspector, advised him to begin his examination of the physician by making him swear the Hippocratic *Oath* and then questioning him about his instruments and his learning. Books like Ibn al-Ukhuwwa's, although widely read, were not backed by any law, and merely suggest what should ideally be done (Karmi 1981, 75).

IV. Taking the Hippocratic Oath

Medieval Western medical oaths, although they might include echoes of Hippocratic wording, pledged loyalty to university and authorities (Nolte 1981). Not until the humanist revival of the sixteenth century is there clear proof that anyone openly took the Hippocratic *Oath* (Rütten 1993, 37–49; 1996a). In 1558, the new statutes of Heidelberg demanded that the Dean of medicine should publicly affirm the *Oath* and promise to adhere to its provisions until the end of his period in office. At the same time, graduands at Jena, founded 1558, had to agree to carry out in medical practice "all that Hippocrates demands in his *Oath* and in *On the Physician*," a provision still included in the statutes of 1785 (Nolte 1981, 42, 50–51).

In 1771, John Morgan, speaking at the conferment of the first doctorate in medicine at the College of Philadelphia, declared that the *Oath* had been generally adopted in universities and medical schools. Morgan was not entirely right, for, both at Leiden and Edinburgh, the *Oath* was no longer sworn, even partly, and was replaced by a much vaguer affirmation (Nutton 1995, 552; 1996a, 36). Oaths in Germany, full of moral affirmations, contained, save at Jena, only allusions to Hippocrates. Morgan himself was against all oaths, however ancient: his college wished to bind its sons only by ties of honor and gratitude.

Others, however, continued to appeal to the past. The 1804 statutes of Montpellier, the *civitas vere Hippocratica*, enjoined the medical graduand to stand before a bust of Hippocrates, specially donated by the French government, recite the *Oath* in Latin, and promise, in the name of God (from 1872 the *Supreme Being*) to be faithful to the laws of man and of honor. Montpellier's example was

followed later by Paris, Strasbourg, and other French universities (Dulieu 1988a, 131–36). In the middle years of the nineteenth century, campaigners in the United States stressed the need for the *Oath*, or for something like it, to distinguish orthodox from nonorthodox practitioners: the former refrained from abortion, following Hippocratic precept (Smith 1996).

By the end of the nineteenth century in Britain and the United States, the actual taking of the Hippocratic *Oath* was seen as old fashioned in the extreme. From the 1920s onward, and, still more, after 1945, however, there has been a major return to the taking of an oath at the beginning or end of a medical course. Some medical schools use the Hippocratic *Oath* in translation; others a more modern one; many something that they consider Hippocratic, although it may not correspond to any precise Greek original. Appeal is regularly made to the Hippocratic *Oath* in newspapers and other media as an ultimate standard in ethics, although, often, this is coupled with demands for a new Hippocratic *Oath* that relates to modern circumstances. It is also invoked by medical practitioners themselves because it is thought to arise from within the profession and is not imposed by outsiders, whether the state or patients (Nutton 1996a; Smith 1996).

V. Conclusion

In all these developments, the name of Hippocrates is associated with a hoped-for standard of medical morality. It is used to validate a contemporary ethical view with reference to the past, usually from a conservative standpoint. Its connection with historical fact becomes almost irrelevant. The modern popularity of the Hippocratic *Oath* has come about at a time when most historians of ancient medicine, following Ludwig Edelstein's arguments, no longer believe that it was written by the historical Hippocrates or that many of its precepts were widely followed by the average Greek doctor of the fifth century BCE (Edelstein 1967, 3–64; Carrick 1985). Instead, it has become a symbol, legitimating modern ideals by an appeal to ancient, perhaps eternal, values. What these values are thought to be, and what is understood as Hippocratic, often differ. Even Nazi medical murderers believed that they were continuing to follow the way of Hippocrates, and became indignant when their interpretations of the Hippocratic *Oath* were rejected (Leven 1994).

In such circumstances, the history of the survival of Hippocratic morality becomes a history of medical ethics in itself. Whatever precision there once was in the term has either disappeared or has become so narrow that it applies to a handful of themes, abortion, euthanasia, and medical secrecy, regardless of the wider context of ancient Hippocratic medicine. It has passed beyond medical history to medical rhetoric.

NOTES

1. A small deontological text probably composed in the first two centuries, and ascribed to Hippocrates. Its original title in Greek may have been: "What should a medical student be like," but it soon became known as the *Testament* of Hippocrates (Deichgraber 1970). It largely abbreviates themes from elsewhere in the Hippocratic Corpus – the student should be intelligent, with clean hands and clothing, tactful, discreet, moderate, and self-controlled, all qualities that contribute to a successful relationship with the patient.

2. Deichgräber (1970, 88–107), arguing for a dependence on Galen (Jouanna 1992, 557), dates it somewhat earlier. My translation is based on the Greek text given by Deichgräber (1970, 97). Other versions are provided by Jones (1924, 59–60) and MacKinney (1952, 16–19, Document K). On the Arabic versions see Bürgel (1970) and Deichgräber (1970, 108–13), who also discusses a reworking of this treatise by Rhazes (d. 925). Kibre (1985) has no entry for this work, although she cites one manuscript of it, 92, as coming from *De arte*, and another, 198, under the heading *Precepta*.

3. See MacKinney (1952, 24) and Garzya (1996, 358–59). For the ascriptions to Hippocrates, see Kibre (1985, 198, 233). A later tract on the same topic, usually anonymous (Kibre 1985, 233), is Salernitan in origin and has links with Galen. See the apparatus to De Renzi (1865, 74–80).

4. See MacKinney (1952, 23) and Kibre (1985, 91–93) 148. Kibre cavalierly deals with the various short ethical texts translated by MacKinney as if they were part of the same work, and, amazingly, declares that they "coincide with the first two or three paragraphs of the Hippocratic *De arte*." The briefest of glances at this Greek tract shows the folly of this remark.

CHAPTER 25

THE DISCOURSES OF PRACTITIONERS IN THE NINTH-TO FOURTEENTH-CENTURY MIDDLE EAST[1]

Ursula Weisser

I. INTRODUCTION: MEDICINE IN MEDIEVAL ISLAM

At the beginning of the seventh century, the new religion of Islam was revealed to the prophet Muḥammad who subsequently succeeded in uniting the Bedouin tribes of the Arab peninsula under its banner. After his death in 632, his successors set out to conquer the neighboring countries and to convert their peoples to the Islamic faith. Approximately a century later, the Arab rule extended from the Pyrenees to the Indus. The syncretistic civilization that developed in this vast area was dominated by the religion and language of the ruling Arabs, but also integrated manifold traditions of the local populations, among them the highly developed Hellenistic sciences, as they were cultivated in the Near East before the advent of Islam. In the course of large-scale efforts to arabicize the ancient scientific heritage, almost the entire medical literature of the Greeks that had survived so far, notably the works of Galen of Pergamon (129–c. 216) and a selection of the Hippocratic Corpus, was translated into Arabic and thus became the basis of "professional" medicine in Islam. Furthermore, the doctors of Islam adopted from the Alexandrian school of late antiquity the "Galenic system," a systematic outline of the concepts of humoral medicine as exposed in the huge oeuvre of Galen. This system enabled Islamic physicians to assimilate the rich corpus of knowledge accumulated by their predecessors and organize it into those clearly arranged handbooks, which constitute one of the major accomplishments of medieval Islam.

In the period under consideration, roughly the ninth to fourteenth centuries, Greco-Arabic scientific medicine was widely accepted as a theoretical foundation of medical practice. In spite of its pagan origins and secular orientation, and in contrast to other "foreign" sciences, it seldom encountered hostility for religious reasons. Apologetic writings defending medicine's indispensability and legitimacy (Rosenthal [1969] 1990b) give the impression of literary exercises amply drawing upon pre-Islamic models rather than of attempts to fight off actual attacks threatening its existence. Representatives of Galenic medicine considered themselves the only real doctors, a judgment apparently shared by the majority of laymen at least in urban settings, although Galenic practitioners certainly were not the only group to offer health services. Various medical subcultures must have flourished in medieval Islam, as they did in other premodern societies, with regionally differing types of folk medicine and a wide spectrum of healers. Their major domains naturally were the rural areas, where professional physicians were hardly available. Regrettably we have little reliable information on alternative healing traditions, because our sources, being mainly written by physicians, are heavily biased against irregular practitioners such as empirics, old wives, and itinerant healers, who are indiscriminately defamed as quacks. These writers also abound with vivid descriptions of charlatans and their tricks, which make amusing reading but most probably exaggerate the problem (Rosenthal [1978] 1990c, 87–89). The desire of Galenic physicians to disassociate themselves from those much-despised rivals is often advanced as an essential motive behind their ethico-deontological discourse, on which the following analysis will focus.

II. The Medical Profession in Islam

1. State of Research

Attempts to apprehend the social reality of the practitioner in medieval Islam (Conrad 1985) have yielded rather unsatisfactory results because of the specialized nature and normative character of the majority of the sources available so far (Weisser 1991). Authors of medical textbooks or texts on medical conduct depict an ideal to be adhered to rather than actual practice, and the innumerable stories and anecdotes about the skill and wisdom of individual doctors in biographical works cannot be regarded as true images of life either, much less of the life of ordinary practitioners, because they naturally concentrate on physicians of distinction. Sporadic insights into the daily life of doctors and patients, which albeit may not be generalized without reservation, are provided by documents of the Jewish community of Cairo preserved in the local Geniza (Goitein 1967–93, 2:240–61; Isaacs 1994) and to a lesser degree by case histories transmitted in medical works (Álvarez Millán 1999, 2000), such as the well-known case records of the "Continens" (al-Ḥāwī) of al-Rāzī (Rhazes, d. 925), because they emphasize technical aspects of medical care (Meyerhof [1935] 1984a). Therefore, this chapter focuses on what was thought and written about the moral and professional conduct of physicians with only occasional hints to what they actually did.

2. Types of Practitioners

Galenic medicine was represented in the first place by the physician proper, a general practitioner with a certain formal education, who concentrated on the treatment of internal diseases by diet and medications and who, as a member of the scholarly class, could claim a respected social position. Also active in this field was the simple practitioner trained empirically in an apprenticeship to an experienced master, often his father, because medicine was a typical family profession. Lists of the medical personnel of hospitals and manuals for the market inspector (see later) further mention surgeons, oculists and bonesetters, practitioners with little or no formal learning,

who specialized in forms of surgical treatment, although surgery as well as ophthalmology were also practiced by learned doctors, who wrote their own textbooks. Surgical practitioners were supposed to be called in by the attending physician to perform operations under his supervision, but in actual fact those specialists would have worked primarily on their own account. The medical establishment also included certain paramedics, medical craftsmen who practiced methods of evacuation often performed preventively, namely, phlebotomists, cuppers, and scarificators. As the female sexual sphere was taboo to men, treatment of gynecological conditions and difficult labor was as a rule performed by female healers, midwives, and female assistants – according to the directions of the physician in charge, if we can believe the male authors of textbooks (Fischer-Kamel 1987, 30–54).

3. Religious Minorities

Medicine transcended religious boundaries. For Jews and Christians, the religious minorities tolerated by Islam, medicine offered an opportunity to pursue a profession of high prestige without abandoning their faith. Only seldom were they confronted with religious prejudice as, for instance, by the Andalusian Ibn ʿAbdūn (wrote c. 1100) who suspected Christian doctors of not caring for the health of Muslims or even to do them harm intentionally (1947, 128). Caliphs, princes, and high officials often chose non-Muslims as their personal doctors. As the original representatives of Greek medicine in the lands conquered by Islam these physicians played a major role in the early development of Islamic medicine and dominated the profession well into the ninth century. In later periods, they still practiced in comparatively large numbers in areas formerly under Christian rule – Christians predominating in Iraq, Syria, and Palestine, Jews in Egypt and North Africa (Toorawa 1994), whereas in the Iberian Peninsula both groups probably counterbalanced each other.

4. Patterns of Medical Education

The efficiency of medical treatment being rather modest at the time, the various types of healers mainly distinguished themselves by the extent of their formal education. Although surgical practitioners and paramedics were normally trained in an empirical way, the instruction of future physicians centered on reading medical texts (Leiser 1983; Dols 1984, 24–32). Even among "learned" physicians levels of education could differ considerably, because medical instruction was neither institutionalized nor regulated; there were no obligatory subjects or examinations. Medical classes were arranged for privately between a teacher and one or several students. Although great value was attached to studying with a personal teacher after the model of the Islamic religious sciences, where oral transmission was thought indispensable to guarantee the authenticity of traditions, medical self-study also occurred. Formal instruction did not include bedside teaching, but probably a good number of medical students would have sought to acquire clinical experience by working under an accomplished doctor or in hospitals, which normally recruited their medical staff from among the leading physicians of the town (Goitein 1967–1993, 2:250).

Because the association of Galenic medicine with the canon of secular sciences inherited from the Greeks remained rather close for some centuries, among the medical elite we occasionally meet with scholars of universal learning, whereas scientists who placed their main interest in fields without direct professional application sometimes earned their livelihood as practicing physicians. Up to the eleventh century, the paradigmatic doctor with broader scholarly ambitions was the physician–philosopher, whereas with the gradual Islamization of medicine this type was gradually superseded with the physician–jurist who taught medicine as well as religious law (Rosenthal [1978] 1990b, 490–91).

5. Control of the Medical Profession

The physicians of Islam did not constitute a unified professional group, nor did they form organized bodies comparable to the guilds of medieval Europe that would enforce minimum standards of practice. State surveillance virtually did not exist, except for certain provisions to protect the public against downright incompetence and fraud. In Syria and Egypt, areas formerly under Byzantine rule, the office of "archiatros" was apparently resumed by a state-appointed "chief of physicians," whose main function apparently was to issue licenses for medical practice – whether on professional or rather on administrative criteria, we do not know. In the great cities, the market inspector (muḥtasib – the institution is called ḥisba) who supervised public morals was charged with the control of the commercial conduct of crafts and trades, among them sellers of drugs and spices, as described in numerous manuals specifying the duties of this high official. That these duties should extend to the licensure of the healing professions as well was first mentioned in the twelfth century by the Aleppine al-Shayzarī (d. 1193), who included detailed information on the qualifications required of the different types of practitioners and paramedics in his ḥisba manual (1946, Chap. 36–37, trans. Meyerhof [1944] 1984c, 126–32), which was later copied extensively by the Egyptian Ibn al-Ukhuwwa (d. 1329) (1938, Chap. 44–45, trans. Levey 1963). According to al-Shayzarī, the muḥtasib should, in addition to checking instruments and further medical equipment, examine physicians, surgeons, and oculists applying for a license on their theoretical knowledge, albeit confining his questioning to the most elementary facts as laid down in prescribed textbooks (Karmi 1981, 69–77; Hamarneh 1964).

Historians tend to take this as evidence of a sort of obligatory state examination, although most of them agree that it may not have been enforced with much consequence. In fact, there is reason to doubt whether regulations to this effect were ever passed by state authorities. Not only do we lack independent information on actual examinations of medical applicants by state officials, it must also be noted that al-Shayzarī, who was a doctor himself, depended heavily on an earlier deontological work (see later), whose author in his turn referred to pre-Islamic practices he urged contemporary rulers to revive (Ruhāwī 1967b, 81–83, 87). Thus, it would appear that al-Shayzarī intended to renew his informant's plea for reforms rather than describe regulations in effect in his own time.

III. Medical Ethics and Deontology in Islam

1. Sources

Our Arabic sources normally discuss ethical issues in close connection with more practical aspects of medical policy and etiquette; so Martin Levey appropriately characterized them as accounts of "practical ethics" (in Ruhāwī 1967b, 8). In addition to chapters on the right conduct of the physician in comprehensive medical textbooks or books on medical specialties, such as the influential medical encyclopedia of al-Majūsī (Halyabbas, written c. 975) (al-Majūsī 1877, 1:8–9, 2:451–54) or the "*Ophthalmological Guide*" of the Andalusian oculist al-Ghāfiqī (twelfth century) (al-Ghāfiqī [1933] 1986, 17–20), Islamic physicians composed a number of monographs on medical deontology or specialized aspects thereof (Ullmann 1970, 223–27; see also Chapters 8, 17, 37).

Our main sources of information are so-called Mirrors for the Physician (Micheau 1993), namely, guides to professional success, as they were produced in Islam for various professions. The genre demanded a certain amount of literary refinement, rhetoric, and display of learning. Starting out from the well-known cliché of the alarming decline of the medical art and the intellectual and moral decay among contemporary physicians, their authors appeal to their fellow physicians to return to the virtues of the great past, but also address the ruler to remind him of his responsibility for the well-being of his subjects and implore him to improve the state of the art by inaugurating obligatory examinations and an effective control of medical practice. Three specimens are available in print so far. The first one was composed by Isḥāq ibn ʿAlī al-Ruhāwī (Ruhāwī 1967b), a Christian or Jew active in northern Iraq probably toward the end of the ninth century. The second one was completed in 1072 by the Christian doctor Ṣāʿid ibn al-Ḥasan (1968c), also from Iraq, and the last one was dedicated to the famous Sultan Saladin by his Jewish physician Ibn Jumayᶜ (d. 1198) (1983). Conspicuously, all of them were written by non-Muslims, as was a collection of deontological aphorisms preserved only in Hebrew, which was ascribed to a Jewish doctor of Kairouan, Isḥāq al-Isrāʾīlī (Isaac Judaeus, first half of the tenth century), but may be spurious (Bar Sela and Hoff 1962), whereas Ibn Buṭlān (d. 1066), the author of a highly amusing satire on ignorant and greedy doctors in the form of a literary session (1985), was a Christian.

The qualities of the knowledgeable, skilled, and reliable as opposed to the ignorant and selfish physician are the subject of treatises on the choice of a doctor written in imitation of Galens *"Examination of the Physician"* (1988), which has been preserved only in Arabic translation. They were addressing the layman who needed criteria for his choice of a devoted family doctor, which did not require any expert knowledge.[2] One of these books was composed by al-Rāzī (Iskandar 1960), one of the most universal and original scholars of Islam, who also devoted a chapter of his medical handbook dedicated to the prince al-Manṣūr (1987) to this topic (Iskandar 1960, 494–514) and wrote on other professional matters as well, such as on charlatans and how to expose them (Leiser 1983, 66–67; Steinschneider 1866). The best method of medical education was a major concern to the Egyptian chief of physicians Ibn Riḍwān (d. 1068) (Schacht and Meyerhof 1937, 20–28; Lyons 1961), who also wrote treatises on the dignity of medicine (Dietrich 1984, 1991) and on the happiness to be gained thereby (Ibn Riḍwān 1982).

2. The Impact of the Ancient Tradition on Medical Ethics in Islam

The discourse on the ethical conduct of the doctor and his bedside manners in Islam is pervaded by ancient motifs (Bürgel 1966, 343–47; Weisser 1997), so much so, that our "Mirrors for the Physician" can be characterized as veritable syntheses of ideas scattered over Greek medical literature, although ancient concepts were modified to a certain degree to fit into their new cultural context. The main sources of inspiration were works ascribed to Hippocrates (Haddad 1982, 127–30), particularly the *"Hippocratic Oath,"* the *"Law"* (see Chapter 23) and a pseudepigraphic *"Testament"* listing intellectual, moral, and physical requirements for the medical aspirant (see Chapter 24), which were reproduced conjointly in the *"History of Physicians"* of Ibn Abī Uṣaybiᶜa (Rosenthal 1975, 183–85). They were supplemented by other deontological texts as well as various maxims from more technical works like *"On Prognosis"* or the *"Epidemics."* A second source was the voluminous work of Galen, who not only provided the authoritative exegesis of Hippocrates, but also in many places pronounced his own ideal of the formation and professional conduct of the physician. Discussions about

the nature of medicine, its status and usefulness from the scholastic tradition of late antiquity, as set down in prolegomena of Alexandrian commentaries, were also revived in Islam, with authors following the traditional pattern rather closely, as for instance Ibn Hindū (d. 1019/20) in his *"Key to Medicine"* (1989), or just borrowing certain arguments from them.

IV. ASPECTS OF MEDICAL ETHICS IN ISLAM

In the absence of state regulations as well as professional organization, universally valid standards of medical conduct did not exist, not to mention an official code of ethics. The ethical discourse was conducted by a small group of conscientious physicians, who were concerned about the quality of medical care and the reputation of their profession and who sought to reinforce traditional values of the medical art by providing guidelines for individual professional behavior. These guidelines were largely common property of the medical elite. Because Islam adopted scientific medicine in a highly developed and dogmatically fixed state, the general issues of medical ethics were defined right from the beginning. In fact, individual authors accentuated them somewhat differently, but no clear evolution of ethical principles is discernible. In marked contrast to classical antiquity, the ethical discourse of Islam is not only based on philosophical ethics, but also grounded firmly in religious faith – particularly pronounced with al-Ruhāwī. Adaptations of traditional motifs to specifically Islamic tenets are comparatively rare, although the ancient tradition had already in late antiquity taken on a definite monotheistic orientation that provided a common basis for Muslim as well as Christian and Jewish physicians. So the Christian Ṣāᶜid (1968b, 71–73), for instance, could support his defense of medicine with extensive quotations from Muslim religious authorities.

1. The Hippocratic Oath

A major point of departure for ethical considerations was the Hippocratic Oath, together with its commentary ascribed to Galen (Rosenthal 1956) (see Chapter 23). Although the teaching contract in its first part, which reflects specific conditions of Hippocratic times, understandably received little attention or was reduced to exhortations to reverence and gratitude toward one's teacher, the rules concerning the doctor's behavior vis-à-vis his patient enjoyed a remarkable aftereffect. Many Arabic physicians recapitulated them in their textbooks, often rather freely (Majūsī 1877, 1:8–9, trans. Haddad 1982, 127–28; Ghāfiqī [1933] 1986, 17–18), or at least hinted at one or the other.

We have little evidence as to the exact role played by the Oath as a model of conduct in Islamic medical practice.[3] We may be certain that it was not sworn by all physicians, although the idea was advanced in the context of ḥisba. Al-Shayzarī demanded of the market inspector to extract the Hippocratic Oath from practitioners applying for a license (Meyerhof [1944] 1984c, 129; Karmi 1981, 75), a procedure which according to Arabic authors was customary in Greece or Byzantium (Stern 1962, 60). As stated before, however, it remains doubtful if there ever was an official regulation to this effect or, if this was the case, whether it received proper attention.

The original stipulations of the Oath were sometimes modified to adapt them to the Islamic cultural milieu (Biesterfeldt 1984, 18–19). Thus, the prohibition to advise women on abortives was supplemented by the exhortation not to inform men about contraceptives, although Islam, unlike Christianity, did not unconditionally forbid birth control (Musallam 1983, 10–22); perhaps, emphasis here was on the potential harmfulness of the drugs in question. The prohibition of hetero- as well as homosexual contacts with members of the patient's household on the other hand was modified according to the stricter sexual morality of Islam to the admonition to avert one's eyes from the women's quarters (Meyerhof [1944] 1984c, 129). Following the example of the Hippocratic "Testament," secrecy regarding the personal circumstances of clients was often interpreted as professional secrecy in a narrow sense and related specifically to the nature of the disease, which some patients would not even reveal to their closest relatives (Ghāfiqī [1933] 1986, 18). Hemorrhoids and uterine disorders were named as particularly shameful conditions (Ṣāʿid 1968b, 105–6). Finally, as the goals in life in Islamic society differed from those of the pagan Greeks, doctors did not expect "good repute among all men for all time" in return for their abiding with the precepts of the Oath, but hoped for a high position at the court and the reward of God in this life and the life to come (Ṣāʿid 1968b, 105).

2. Attributes and Qualifications of the Physician

The extensive catalogs in our sources of physical, intellectual, and moral qualities expected to guide the practitioner's private and professional conduct, as, for example, intelligence and assiduity, perfect health, neatness of appearance, and cultivated manners, absolute moral integrity, conscientiousness, and compassion and patience with difficult clients (e.g., Ruhāwī 1967, Chap. 15; Ṣāʿid 1968b, Chap. 3), are again compiled from ancient, chiefly Hippocratic and Galenic, *topoi* with a few modifications conditioned by their new cultural environment, such as the accentuation of firm belief in Almighty God and His prophets (Ruhāwī 1967b, 19–20). These virtues are contrasted with the vices of indolent, unscrupulous, and greedy doctors, who misspend their time ingratiating themselves to the rich and noble to participate in their

life of leisure and luxury and endanger the lives of their patients by ignorance and neglect. Because of the stereotyped character of these listings, it would be a futile venture to give references for all their details.

3. Talents, Character, and Demeanor

The ideal doctor should possess a well-proportioned, healthy body, sharp intellect and perfect character, faith in God and reverence for his teacher, exhibit exemplary conduct and moderation in every respect, veracity, circumspection and discretion as well as sympathy, compassion, generousness and patience in dealing with the sick and loyalty toward his colleagues. According to Ibn Riḍwān, it was the responsibility of medical teachers to accept only students of extraordinary talents and high moral standing (Ibn Riḍwān 1982, lines 8–17). Although all healing power is from God, the physician has to prove worthy of His blessing. The physician should show an extreme zeal for learning and be untiring in his efforts to extend his knowledge for the benefit of the sick, remembering the Hippocratic dictum that "the art is long."

The great importance attached to life-long learning as well as the pious attitude of doctors in Islam is appropriately exemplified by Ruhāwī's description of the doctor's daily routine (Ruhāwī 1967b, 54–55). After finishing his morning toilet and prayer, his first activity will be the study of books, first religious ones to improve his character, than medical ones to improve his learning. Then, after praying for God's assistance in his treatments, he will set out to visit his patients and on his return see those waiting for him in his office. Only after having completed his professional duties may he tend to his own needs by bathing and eating, then spend the evening in the company of scientific books – a reading list is supplied (p. 93) – and a glass of wine, before concluding his day with another prayer.

4. Directions for Medical Education

The curricula presented in deontological texts (Ruhāwī 1967b, Chap. 16; Ṣāʿid 1968b, Chap. 4), which were inspired by Galen's highly ambitious ideas, describe an ideal scarcely ever attained in reality. Presumably only the smaller part of medical aspirants engaged in extensive theoretical studies or even fulfilled Galen's demand that the complete doctor also be versed in sciences other than medicine. Apart from the art of logic regarded as fundamental for every scientific activity, the "mathematical" disciplines of arithmetic, geometry, astronomy, and music were recommended for propedeutic study (Ibn Riḍwān in Iskandar 1976, 253–54). One of the stereotypes of Islamic medical deontology is the preference of ancient classics to compendia of Arabic authors for teaching (Ibn Riḍwān 1982 Ibn Jumayʿ 1983, Sect. 79–85) in close accordance with the curriculum of the pre-Islamic Alexandrian school with its selection of Galenic and Hippocratic writings (Ibn Riḍwān in Iskandar 1976, 144–52, 257–58; Dols 1984, 27–29). In fact those much defamed compendia, which presented the essentials of medicine in a more comprehensive and systematic fashion, gradually supplanted the works of the ancients for most students and practitioners.

As to the body of knowledge considered indispensable for the physician, the basic concepts of the Galenic system ranked first (Ṣāʿid 1968b, 92–93). In addition, the physician was supposed to possess a thorough knowledge of the materia medica to be able to identify low-quality or adulterated drugs, because druggists were often suspected of fraudulent behavior (Ṣāʿid 1968b, 95–96, 138–41). Most authors agree that rich experience in diagnosis and therapy is necessary to make a perfect doctor. Yet, when considering the relative values of theoretical and practical education, they tend to favor an inexperienced doctor of extensive learning, who would be able to deduct therapies for conditions he has never encountered before from what he has read in books, over the empiric with little or no formal training, who would be at a loss when confronted with a disease unfamiliar to him (Rāzī 1987, 235–36).

5. The Physician vis-à-vis the Sick

The physician is burdened with greater responsibility than any other professional, because in medicine grave mistakes may be irreparable. Furthermore, he is charged with the health care of man, who is the most noble of creatures, being endowed with soul and intellect. Because these are affected by his physical condition, the physician is responsible for man's psychic and mental as well as his bodily well-being (al-Ghāfiqī [1933] 1986, 18; Ruhāwī 1967b, 43–44). In fact, Islamic physicians place some emphasis on psychosomatic aspects of disease (Bürgel 1973). For the Hippocratic doctor, nature herself performs the healing, the physician being but her minister assisting in her healing efforts. The monotheistic doctors of Islam, who believed in divine providence, regarded Almighty God as the ultimate cause behind nature (Ṣāʿid 1968b, 108) and looked upon themselves as instruments for the execution of the will of God (Rosenthal [1969] 1990b, 528–29).

6. Consultation

Discussions on the doctor's bedside manners and ethical attitude toward the sick were for the most part conventional, beginning with the great importance attached to a neat appearance, decent attire, and dignified behavior (Ruhāwī 1967b, 53–55, 92). Well-to-do clients used to call in the doctor, who was expected to visit them once a day, in severe cases more frequently, others went to see the doctor in his home or office. Prescribing by letters or through messengers without seeing the patient at all was common practice too (Goitein 1967–93, 2:255–56). Before the consultation, the physician was supposed to recall the progress of the case and consider further options of treatment. If his earlier judgments were not confirmed by his new findings, he should be ready to revise his therapy (Ṣāʿid 1968b, 97–98).

In his dealings with the sick (Ṣāʿid 1968b, 100–5; Ruhāwī 1967b, Chap. 7) the physician should comport himself calmly and gently, but without too much indulgence, listen to complaints attentively, explain his prescriptions repeatedly and pay regard to the patient's own wishes and sensitivities (Rāzī in Deichgräber 1970, 108–13). If the sick person gives the impression of poor comprehension, the doctor should refrain from informing him about his illness (Ruhāwī 1967b, Chap. 7). Because the patient's mental condition was supposed to affect his bodily state, the physician was advised to allow himself some time to encourage the sufferer and cheer him up. Much attention was paid to the efficient questioning of the patient, who, being inexperienced in the interpretation of symptoms, would be unable to give relevant information of his own accord or might even try to keep it to himself because of fear or shame. In medical treatment, the benefit of the sick should always rank first, following the Hippocratic maxim "either to help or not to harm" (Epidemics I, Chap. 11). This implied that the physician should administer, by all means, the mildest of remedies that would have the desired effect (Ṣāʿid 1968b, 103). Some authors advised against taking up dangerous or hopeless cases, occasionally with reference to the example of Hippocrates, in order not to be blamed for the possibly fatal outcome (Ṣāʿid 1968b, 102, 136). Especially in surgery (Abū l-Qāsim 1973, 6; Renaud 1935, 20), this would have been a wise policy in view of the inability to control wound infection.

7. Reactions to Noncompliance

Because the "object" of medical art is endowed with a will of its own, the doctor must be on his guard against imprudent behavior of his patient that might frustrate his efforts (Ibn Jumayʿ 1983, Sect. 56–68). Therefore, our sources agree with the well-known statement of Hippocrates that it is essential for the physician to secure the patient's cooperation in fighting the disease, for if the patient allies himself with the latter, the doctor will be fighting for a lost cause (Ruhāwī 1967b, 68–69). Noncompliance or intentional lying by the patient were generally considered sufficient justification to abandon the case, as were disobedience or neglect on the part of the patient's attendants (Ṣāʿid 1968b, 100–1). Al-Ruhāwī, who particularly stressed the necessity of a special "ethics of the patient" toward his doctor, devoted a considerable part of his book to discussing all sorts of impediments to the doctor's work by ignorant or even malevolent patients, relatives, attendants, and visitors and the former's duty to educate them on the appropriate behavior (Ruhāwī 1967b, Chap. 3–11, 14, 19).

8. Malpractice and Its Sanctions

Deontological texts emphasize that whatever quacks would make the public believe, medicine cannot work wonders nor avert death. As a fallible human, the physician for all his diligence is subject to errors and commits mistakes (Ṣāʿid 1968b, 134–35). Safeguarding against accusations of malpractice was a major incentive for developing the art of prognosis since Hippocratic times. We have no indication that a public penalty was imposed on mistreatment in Islam, although al-Ruhāwī recommended a system of surveillance and prosecution of malpractice allegedly in general use in Greece or Byzantium as a model for Islam: Doctors were ordained to prescribe only in the presence of relatives of the patient and to leave copies of their records and prescriptions with them. In case of a lethal outcome, a group of renowned physicians would scrutinize these materials, and if they decided on malpractice, the guilty doctor had to pay an adequate recompense (Ruhāwī 1967b, 87). There is no evidence that a similar system was actually instituted in Islam, although al-Shayzarī included the story in his ḥisba manual (Meyerhof [1944] 1990c, 128–29).

9. The Physician's Remuneration

Remuneration issues were a much-debated subject (Rosenthal 1978, 480–84; Biesterfeldt 1984). In medieval Islam, as anywhere else, medical practice was thought of as a rather lucrative activity – "among the arts the most useful, among the enterprises the most profitable" (Ibn Buṭlān 1985, 50), as an often-quoted saying went. The stereotyped reports on fabulous riches heaped upon successful court doctors by grateful caliphs and notables, however, may not have been accurate in every case (Rosenthal [1978] 1990c, 480–81). Greed for money as the principal motivation for entering the profession was unanimously condemned, but that the skillful physician is entitled to an adequate fee for his services was disputed only by a small minority of pious doctors who expressed aversion against making money from the charitable act of relieving the suffering from their ailments (Biesterfeldt 1984, 16–18).

As urban doctors were consulted by people from all ranks of the society (Goitein 1967–1993, 2:241–42), the prevailing opinion was to fix the fee in proportion to the circumstances of the individual client (Ṣāʿid 1968b, 101, 103); some doctors are even reported to have left its size to the patient's judgment (Renaud 1935, 20; Meyerhof [1938] 1984b, 445–46). This principle implied treatment of the destitute without recompense, even to donate medicines to them, if necessary (Ghāfiqī [1933] 1986, 18). This ethical precept in its universal application went beyond classical ancient standards. To treat the poor for heavenly reward had been enjoined on Jews and Christians as well, but received additional emphasis in Islam, as almsgiving constituted one of the five principal duties of Muslim believers. To increase their religious merits, doctors were even advised to attend to the needy poor before starting out to visit the rich (Ṣāʿid 1968b, 82). Most ordinary practitioners perhaps did not comply to these noble standards (Rosenthal 1978, 487–89; Dols 1984, 37–38), but several famous and appropriately rich physicians like the converted Christian Ibn Jazla (d. 1100) are expressly reported to have given free treatment on a large scale. Some doctors even took up jobs outside medicine to finance such charitable behavior (Biesterfeldt 1984, 18–19), although additional occupations were disapproved of by others on the ground that business would interfere with the challenging duties of the physician and his obligation to continuing pursuit of knowledge (Ruhāwī 1967b, 55, 94).

V. Conclusion

In medieval Islamic medicine, the high standards of professional conduct inherited from Hellenism were upheld and provided with strong religious overtones stressing the foundation of moral behavior in the belief in God and his commandments, a conviction shared by all doctors, whether Muslims or Christians or Jews. The directions established in theoretical discourse, however, for the lack of state regulations or professional organization retained the character of recommendations. How far the individual doctor was willing to transform theory into reality was left to his own discretion.

Notes

1. In the reference list, editions of the original Arabic texts are given along with translations into modern Western languages. For the convenience of readers without Arabic, references in the text are to translated versions, if available.

2. More comprehensive deontological works include chapters on this subject too (Ruhāwī 1967b, Chaps. 15–16; Ibn Jumayʿ 1983, Sect. 100–116, 123–50; Ibn Riḍwān in Iskandar 1976, 244).

3. One instance involved the famous Christian translator Ḥunain ibn Isḥāq (d. c. 873) (Strohmaier 1974), another the most prominent member of the Andalusian Zuhr family, Abū Marwān ibn Zuhr (d. 1161/62) (Faradj [1935] 1996, 53).

CHAPTER 26

THE DISCOURSES OF PRACTITIONERS IN MEDIEVAL AND RENAISSANCE EUROPE

Klaus Bergdolt

I. INTRODUCTION

Medieval and Renaissance medical ethics in Europe were influenced by an astonishing variety of factors, authors, and spiritual mainstreams. Although authoritative texts dealing with medical conduct have been handed down from antiquity and from Arabic and Byzantine sources, the origin of many medieval texts on medical ethics remains something of a mystery.

This chapter provides an account of medical ethics in Medieval and Renaissance Europe. Particular attention is paid to sources of influence and how they were transmuted in various historical contexts and conditions. These influences included the Hippocratic Oath, Christian moral theology and philosophy, and Arabic and Persian texts that were translated into Latin. The tension that these influences created, especially that between Christian and non-Christian sources, is one of the distinguishing features of medical ethics during the period addressed in this chapter. The chapter then turns to the content of texts on medical ethics during this period, including texts written by physicians and by laypersons. The influence of the Plague on medical ethics is also described.

II. THE INFLUENCE OF THE HIPPOCRATIC OATH

One of these sources was the Hippocratic Oath (see Chapters 23, 24), although it had played a subordinate role during the first Christian Millennium. Saint Gregory of Nazianzus (c. 330–389) had even praised his brother who had refused to swear the Oath (Gregory of Nazianzus 1908: Oratio VIII). Apart from a summary in the oldest German medical book from 790 (Lorsch Book of Drugs 1989, 2:27), an early written version had been preserved from the tenth century (Venice, Marciana Library, Codex Graecus 269, f. 12r) (Rütten 1993, 51f.; Nutton 1993, 24). In the eleventh century copies in a cruciform shape (as Vat. Urbinas Graecus 64, f. 116) demonstrate that the content of the Oath was compatible with the Christian tradition (Rütten 1993, 51–53).

Manuscripts like this presented the Oath, inserted in the very beginning of the *Corpus Hippocraticum*, as a kind of introduction to the texts following. Latin and Greek editions of the corpus were prepared, respectively, in 1525 by Marco Fabio Calvo (c. 1470–c. 1527) (Rütten, 1993, 60) and in 1526 by Francesco d'Asola (c. 1480–c. 1535) (Rütten 1993, 59). Girolamo Mercuriale

(1530–1606) edited in Venice the first Greek–Latin version (Mercuriale and Colombo 1588).

The Oath stresses the doctor's moral obligation to care also about a healthful way of life of his patient. It rejects active euthanasia and abortion. The vaginal method of abortion described was understood as one example of a prohibited act (*pars pro toto*). The text also prohibits sexual relations between physicians and patients or their relatives and calls for discretion and a reputable lifestyle of the physician. It admonishes the physician only to assist and never to harm the patient. It dissociates also medicine from surgery, with the latter regarded as a mere skill or craft.

In the sixteenth century, the Hippocratic corpus, including the Oath, experienced a revival. Many humanist and physicians conducted research on Hippocrates and the Hippocratic corpus. Among them were Johannes Reuchlin (1455–1522) (Reuchlin 1512), James Cornarius (1500–1558), whose complete edition of the Corpus Hippocaticum appeared in 1546 from the famed publisher Froben in Basel (Cornarius 1546), and Anutius Foesius (1528–1591), who translated Hippocratic texts into Latin (Foesius 1595). The complete works of Petrus Forestus (1522–1597), nearly completely based on the Corpus Hippocraticum, were (posthumously) published in 1653 (Forestus 1653). One of the ethical achievements of the "Dutch Hippocrates" was the explanation of suicide as a possible result of melancholic illness or depression. The earliest clear evidence that the Hippocratic Oath was taken by young physicians dates to the German university of Wittenberg (1508). Ingolstadt (1550) and Jena (1558) followed suit (Nutton 1995, 521, Rütten 1996c, 65). In 1570 the Swiss physician, Theodor Zwinger (1533–1588), adapted elements from the Hippocratic Oath to formulate the Basel Doctorate Oath (Nutton 1995, 521). In contrast to the relatively slow reception of the Oath itself, ethical admonitions and precepts from other texts in the *Corpus* were repeated or paraphrased in many medieval medical texts. The Hippocratic Precepts, for instance, included recommendations such as not to discuss fees before beginning medical treatment because of the possible negative effect on the patient (Hippocrates 1923b, 316f., Precepts 4) or to apply different fees to the rich and the poor (Hippocrates 1923b, 318f., Precepts 6; Lorsch book of drugs 1989, 2:25; Anonymus Salernitanus 1856, 176). The authority of Hippocrates also drew on theological works (Augustine 1957–1972, 2:138–43). Saint Jerome (c.347–419) regards the Hippocratic Oath as a conduct model even for clergymen (Jerome 1991, 224f.).

III. Christian Influence on European Medical Ethics

Following the founding of Montecassino abbey in Italy by St. Benedict in 529, most Christian physicians in the second half of the first millennium were monks. Their medical ethics was initially determined by the Fathers of the Church (see Chapters 12, 14). Many of these early theologians had opposed the Hippocratic and Galenic legacy. The main question for them was whether Christian monks should be allowed to apply "heathen medicine." Many Christian authors – ranging from Origen (c. 185–254) (Origenes 1968, 2:56f.: Contra Celsum 3, 24) to ascetics like the eremite Anthony (c. 252–c. 356) (Athanasius 1950) – did not attribute any importance to physical health, approaching objectively to Stoic positions (Temkin 1991, 135). The martyr Ignatius of Antioch (m.c. 110) regarded the Eucharist to be the real "antidote against death" (Fischer 1956 1:160f.: Letter to the Ephesians 20, 2). Saint Augustine (354–430) stressed the double aim of medicine, namely, "taking away vices and curing the (body's) nature." He emphasized the "new physician" who followed the example of Christ (*Christus Medicus*) as a spiritual protector and savior of souls (Augustine Patrologia Latina 38:846f.: Sermones 155, 10). Also Bishop Eusebius of Caesaerea (260–339) presents Jesus as an "excellent physician," who to cure the sick, examines what is repulsive, handles sores and bears pain himself for the sufferings of others. Eusebius encourages the Christians to lead a lifestyle similar to that of physicians (Eusebius [1926, 1932] 1992, 1994, 2:402f.: Ecclesiastical History X, 4).

In much the same way St. Jerome held out physicians as role models of the same discretion and composure for clerics (Jerome 1991, 224f.: Epistula 52). Pagan medical ethics, such as the Hippocratic Precepts, were generally known not only to Christian practitioners, but also to theologians. Eusebius mentioned a group of Christians who admired Euclid, Aristotle, and Galen (Eusebius [1926, 1932] 1992, 1994, 1:522f.: Ecclesiastical History V, 28), indicating the acceptability of non-Christian sources. A physician's behavior, work, and role were still valued according to Christian principles, but the influence of the heathen tradition was increasing. Tertullian (c. 150–c. 230) had already defended personal hygiene and bathing for the preservation of health (Tertullian 1961, 90: Apology 42). Influenced by the Christian tradition, Western medicine began to emphasize both bodily and spiritual aspects of medicine. Doctors and priests therefore had, still in the high Middle Ages, nearly a similar status in the house of the sick (Anonymus Salernitanus 1853, 74).

Hippocratic and Stoic currents joined with the model of Christ to create a new ideal of philanthropic medicine (Temkin 1991, 145). Origen had already favored a physician who strengthened and comforted the patient (Origenes 1968, 2:166f.: Contra Celsum 3, 74). Approximately a century and a half later, Gregory of Nyssa (c. 331–c. 394) held that "philanthropy is the way of life for all of you who practice the medical art" (Amundsen 1995a, 1519). Medical practitioners came to be regarded as mediators of God's will, who "alone heals the ill" (Cassiodor 1937, 78).

Following a tradition set by the Fathers of the Church, later theologians such as Cassiodorus (c. 495–580) and St. Gregory of Tours (538–594) were convinced that the success or failure of medical treatment lay entirely in God's hands. Most monk–physicians believed that acts of compassion (Matthew 25, 35–40) were more indicative of quality medical treatment than perfection of medical technique. Illness was thought to be either divine punishment or trial, the work of demons (to be cured by exorcism), or a way to glorify God (John 11, 3f). Illness was also seen as a way to follow Christ in his passion. Despite these beliefs, Christian practitioners had to perform their craft conscientiously. Medicine had to be decent and devoted to God, however, or it warranted severe punishment as indicated by the example of Simon Magus, recorded in the Acts of the Apostles (8, 4–25). Piety was linked to conscientiousness and a knowledge of drugs as indispensable to the Benedictine physician. According to the rules 36 and 37 of the order (Regula Benedicti 1992, 163–65), he was morally obligated to serve the ill and the weak, both young and old brethren. Patients also had to practice an "Ethics for the ill" – patience and acceptance of the fate God had visited upon them and not to make "excessive demands" on physicians and other caregivers (Regula Benedicti 1992, 163).

Cassiodorus accepted non-Christian medicine definitively for Christian monasteries. He even endorsed the inclusion of pagan medical texts in the libraries of the monks (Cassiodor 1937, 78). He also praised lay physicians: "You promise your doctors to hate injustice and to love purity (Cassiodor 1894, 192). Cassiodorus's views were challenged by such figures as St. Gregory of Tours, who doubted the efficiency of worldly physicians and recommended instead the help of the saints (Gregory of Tours 1988, 1:103f., 1:211f., 2:24f.: Historia Francorum II, 5, III, 36, V, 6). Yet the Lorsch book of drugs (1989, 2:25) defends practitioners by pointing out that Christ and such saints as Sts. Cosmas and Damien had also healed the ill.

Collecting fees was ethically suspect in a Christian context because it conflicted with the idea of *caritas* (caring). Tradition told that Cosmas and Damian had healed "without money" (*anargyroi*) (Bergdolt 1998, 121). Nonetheless, some monk–physicians appear to have received rewards for their services. Such behavior was later forbidden by the Second Lateran Council in 1139. This prohibition was reinforced by the regional synod of Tours in 1163, which went further and forbade monks and regular canons from practicing surgery (Amundsen 1978b, 22–30). Notwithstanding a series of prohibition documents preserved, most clergymen, as Amundsen pointed out, have not been hindered to exercise practical medicine (Amundsen 1978b, 40–43). The delicate relation of clergy and medicine was relaxed especially during the Renaissance.

For example, the Dane Nils Stensen (1626–1686), who was a Catholic priest and later a bishop, was also a famous anatomist (Scherz 1963). In this period, surgery and practical medicine no longer implied the odor of a dirty or wicked occupation.

Returning to the contrast between *caritas* and fees, the anonymous Lorsch monk attempted to reconcile the conflict by proposing a fee-scale based on the financial status of the patient (Lorsch book of drugs 1989, 2:25). In proposing this, he seems to have turned for inspiration to the Hippocratic Precepts (Hippocrates 1923b, 318f.: Precepts 6). The durability of the tension is evident even in Dante (1265–1321), who contrasts Taddeo Alderotti (1223–1303), a famous medical professor who worked for worldly gain, with St. Dominic (Dante 1956, 894–97: Divine Comedy, Paradise XII, 70–84).

Christian ideals also permeated the ethics of treatment. Remedies had to be compatible with Christian morals – fornication or masturbation or magic practices were forbidden. During the Carolingian period, physicians were required to use the inexpensive, indigenous medical herbs found in the fields and forests of the countryside (Lorsch book of drugs 1989, 2:25). Were the patient to die subsequently, this was regarded as God's decision, and the physician was not to be held responsible (Lorsch book of drugs 1989, 2:23). The physician – as a mediator – had the pretension to be paid for his work, endeavor, visit, or advice. In a tenth-century Brussels manuscript (MS 3701–15, f. 5–7) he is admonished to be amiable, humble, and benevolent. The good physician hopes in God who "restores sweetness, inspires sagacity, maintains remembrances in the heart, love in the soul, discipline in obeying." He is to be defined as "an opportune worker who renders aid in time of need" (McKinney [1952] 1977, 183f.).

Before starting to treat a case, twelfth- and thirteenth-century physicians in Salerno, Italy, were morally required to inquire whether the patient had confessed and received the Host, transubstantiated into the body of Christ, as an important "condition of health," for "more dignity than the body has the soul and its salvation" (Anonymus Salernitanus 1853, 74; 1856, 148). Many later medical statutes continued to be influenced by theology, for example, the "Ten questions about the state of medical doctors" (*Decem quaestiones de medicorum statu*) of an anonymous, late-fifteenth-century German author at Ingolstadt university (Anonymus 1978, 47 and 59f.). This Medical "decalogue" condemned the practice of demanding payment from incurables, invoking the traditional view that spiritual assistance was more important than medical help. It also suggested that clerics should not have to pay for medical treatment. The priority of spiritual concerns is reflected in the fact that a seriously ill patient had to confess, even if the admonition to do so by the doctor could shock or horrify him (Anonymus 1978, 58f.: Decem quaestiones VI).

IV. Scholastic Medicine after the Reception of Arabic and Persian Texts on Deontology

After the establishment of medical curricula in occidental universities beginning with Salerno (c. 1000), European medicine became more than ever oriented toward classical antiquity, but also to Arab–Persian authorities that had preserved much of the medical knowledge of the ancient world (see Chapters 17, 25). Previously little-known medical ethics texts from the East and from antiquity began to become known in the West as a result of Latin translations. The "Book to Almansor" by Rhazes (865–925), translated into Latin in Toledo during the twelfth century, contained a code of behavior for physicians, and castigated charlatans (Neuburger 1911, 2:173). These points were reiterated in the text "On the conditions in the medical profession, which cause most people to avoid the respectable physician" (Neuburger 1911, 2:173f.). This work condemned greed on the part of physicians, such as the practice of demanding payment before the patient was treated (a common accusation from the Hippocratic Precepts up until the eighteenth century) and the apparently widespread flattering of rich patients. It also called for a high standard of personal ethics in calling for a modest lifestyle, the observation of specific medical dietetics, and opposition to charlatans. The Flemish doctor Jan Yperman (c. 1270–c. 1330) refers, like many other colleagues, to the Arabian authority stressing that a good physician needs a certain charisma and a strong constitution. His appearance is pleasant and winning. He has, as the English surgeon John of Arderne (active toward the end of the fourteenth century) claims, beautiful hands and well-formed nails, without dirt and "blackness." His language is precise, his behavior excellent. He flees drunkenness and all excesses (Welborn [1938] 1977, 207f.).

In *The Physician's Guide*, translated in the twelfth century, Isaac Iudaeus (c. 900–955) warned against "know-it-all" physicians and demanded that doctors lead a noble, exemplary life, free from gluttony and other vices. He also held that there is no work more laudable than helping the sick poor for nothing. On the other hand, Isaac confirms: "The more you charge for your treatment, the more your reputation will grow" (Neuburger 1911, 2:177). A literature containing practical advice and admonitions became part of the didactic material taught in numerous universities and were included in the principles of several medico-surgical guilds. In 1231, emperor Frederic II established a curriculum of medical studies that included a standardized examination before admission to the profession (Heinisch

1968, 94, 97). His intent was to increase the confidence of his subjects in physicians' qualifications.

The influence of Arabic, Persian, and other non-Christian sources and ideas reawakened concerns about medicine's compatibility with Christianity. In the view of many intellectual critics "Arabic" was synonymous with "atheist" and "immoral." In this vein, it was often remarked, as in the Parisian medical faculty in the thirteenth century, *Ubi tres medici, duo athei* ("where there are three doctors, there are two atheists") (Bergdolt 1992, 44). Gilles de Corbeil (c. 1140–1224), physician to King Philip Augustus of France, contrasts the "parrots" of Aristotle and Averroes with an idealized "old master" of medicine, who was "honorable, religious, austere, law-abiding, discreet, and modest" (Gilles of Corbeil 1826, 122–24). Just as Cato had once condemned Greek medicine, some scholars and early humanists now criticized the Arabs and those European medical faculties who seemed to follow them slavishly.

V. Medical Ethics in Medieval Europe

1. Ethics of Doctors – Contemporary Critics and Descriptions

In addition to the literature written for the most part by doctors, an important source of moral standards and ideals applied to medicine and its practitioners is found in literary works written by nonphysicians. A distinctive feature of this literature is that nonprofessional norms for practice emerge from criticisms of medicine and its practitioners. This literature joins that written by physicians who wanted to improve the moral level of their profession.

A. Criticism of Physicians – Laymen and "Experts"

Some treatises of the period began to distinguish *sapientia* (wisdom) from *scientia* (science) (Bergdolt 1992, 67–76). Medicine, as pure science, is not a means of opening ways to salvation and purgation of the soul. In contrast, religion is strictly bound to wisdom, based on contemplation and recognition of God. So, in Petrarch's view, who hated Averroes as a "mad dog" (Bergdolt 1992, 27), the doctor's daily activity is partly a "mechanical art" and partly a "science" that by its very nature ruled out reflection on the soul and on God, the real aim of human existence. As such, medicine was therefore under suspicion of favoring atheism and Averroism. The Cistercian monk, Bernard of Clairvaux (c. 1090–1153), accused physicians of maintaining "life in this world" while neglecting eternal life (Bernard of Clairvaux 1994, 481: Sermones super Cantica Canticorum 30, 10). Nonetheless, there was an interesting mix of pagan, Islamic, and Christian ideas in the medical ethics of the period. Physicians were bound to respect the following "classic" rules: not to promulgate false theories, to treat the poor free of charge, to encourage the seriously ill to confess, not to favor any particular dealers of remedies, and not to administer abortifacients or perform active euthanasia (Bergdolt 1991).

The twelfth-century scholastic John of Salisbury (c. 1115/20–1180) criticized physicians for their greed ("get money as long as your patient is suffering"), their self-importance, and their tendency to use specialized terminology incomprehensible to the layperson (John of Salisbury 1855, 830f.). This accusation was later reiterated and expanded by John's Italian contemporary Guido of Arezzo (active in the twelfth century) and – undoubtedly with a greater influence – by Petrarch (1304–1374) (Bergdolt 1992, 41). Guido, a physician with a philosophical ambition, rebuked his colleagues who had studied in Salerno or Montpellier for their academic arrogance (Guido d'Arezzo 1984, 1:231)

Petrarch took up the rhetorical argument of John of Salisbury that killing was a part of the physicians' daily work, attacking their spiritual conservatism and rigidity. His "Invective against a medical doctor" (1352), based on an exchange of correspondence with the personal physician of Pope Clemens VI, reveals his general antischolastic and anti-Arabic sentiments. In this work, he accuses contemporary physicians of arrogance, incompetence, inadequate methodology, deliberate use of a technical language incomprehensible to the patient, godlessness, and sadism (Petrarca 1978, 25–98). Petrarch regarded medicine per se as immoral and claimed that it had nothing in common with ethics (*medicina nihil commune cum ethica*) (Petrarca 1978, 76). He opposes medieval scholastic traditions, idealizing the (alleged) ancient and early Christian ethical standard and referring to Cato, who had already derided physicians as wage-earning people (Bergdolt 1992, 38). A good physician was taciturn. He must be able to keep secrets according to Virgil who had declared medicine a "silent art" (Petrarca 1978, 80; Virgil 1965, 528: Aeneis XII, 397). Petrarch's accusations may have been exaggerated but certainly they give us an unfiltered impression of the scholastic physician's reputation.

These critiques remind the works of Gilles de Corbeil, Roger Bacon (c. 1219–1292), and Arnold of Villanova (c. 1260–1311). Bacon's *"About the Errors of Medical Doctors"* also criticized the poor quality of many then-contemporary drugs. The author claimed that alchemists and physicians often sold placebos, that physicians frequently held conflicting views, and that they were incapable of mixing or using "compound drugs and had no knowledge of medication or of treatment" (Withington 1924, 143). Bacon believed that physicians lacked both knowledge of the natural sciences and ethical maturity. He admits, however, that they have not had the same possibilities as other scientists to experiment "because of the dignity of the matter

they have to do with" (Withington 1924, 149). Lay criticism was, in this way, added to "professional" criticism.

Physicians often offered similar complaints. Arnald of Villanova reproached his colleagues: "Respect that the physician is cautious with his predictions and promises and never assures health because he would thereby claim a supernatural role and offend God. He should vow to work with conscience and diligence, to be unobtrusive during the visit, kind in dialogue and to empathize modestly and empathically with the patient" (Sigerist 1946, 141; Neuburger 1911, 2:398). Albertus de Zancariis (c. 1280–1348), a professor in Bologna, tried to outline some rules of conduct for medical doctors. A certain distance from the "plebs" seems advisable, but also a sensitive information of the patient about the seriousness of his illness. In this situation, telling the truth is not always necessary nor a proof of morality (Albertus de Zancariis 1914, 17).

In his *Antipocras* (Anti-Hippocrates), the physician Nicolas of Poland (active c. 1270) defended "popular" medicine, declaring that God had provided the people with inexpensive and sufficient medication in the simplest of substances, already available to them in nature. Nicolas praised the efficiency of the *vilia* (low and despised things like stones or worms) that possessed a "secret virtue" (*virtus sepulta*), and like the Lorsch monk, he exhorted man to humbly accept the healing power of God provided through nature (Eamon and Keil 1986).

Ethical texts of the time often reflected the guild interests of their physician authors. For example, with respect to fees, statute 23 of the *"Collegium"* of physicians of Milan, dating from the fourteenth century, says that the doctor is obligated to discontinue treatment if the patient is discovered to be a debtor of one of the doctor's colleagues. There is a large range of fees to be charged by members (6 to 16 soldi), and the really poor are to be cured "by love of God" that is, free of charge. The guild also protected its own. Younger or inexperienced doctors are to discuss the patient's care "secretly and clandestinely" with older colleagues (Belloni 1958, 609).

B. Surgical Ethics

The French professor and surgeon, Henri de Mondeville (c. 1260–1325), offered an ethics that was quite critical of then-current practices. He contrasts the honest surgeon with the second-rate surgeon who sells out his art to pander to the rich. He also attacks any movement toward "alternative medicine" (Mondeville 1892, 11–13). Henri protested against the concurrence of "barbers, seers, dealers, con-men, forgers, alchemists, whores, matchmakers, midwives, hags, Jews, and Saracens" and refused the "uneducated, primitive, ignorant surgeons" (Mondeville 1892, 65, 67). In a long sketch, he illustrated the differences between a good surgeon's and a bad surgeon's behavior at the patient's bedside. The bad surgeon allows even his apprentices to collect fees for the "master." Henri also claimed that successful treatment by bad surgeons depended mostly on the fraudulent (not to say psychological) qualities of the surgeon, rather than his skill. A Christian doctor sins if he does not conscientiously respect the rules of the art. Henri's criticisms had, however, limited effect. For example, the Florence Guild of Doctors, Apothecaries, and Grocers (*Arte degli Speziali*) admitted all persons in the city "who practice physic or surgery, set bones, and treat mouthes" (Park 1985, 17–22).

C. Caricature as a Source of Medical Ethics

Some of the most revealing literature for discerning the nonprofessional standards of some medical practitioners is the caricatures of doctors from this period. An important example is the (aforementioned) Salernitan text *"About the Appearance of the Medical Doctor to the Patient"* (Anonymus Salernitanus 1853, 74–80). The caricatures in this text illustrate unethical conduct. For example, physicians are portrayed as crepe hangers who solemnly deliver poor prognoses to become famous as prognosticators or saviors of their patients. They are also portrayed as being against gazing on a wife or daughter of the patient with lecherous eyes (*oculo cupido*), but for the wrong reason, namely not risking loss of confidence by the patient who would then be unwilling to pay the physician's high fees (Anonymus Salernitanus 1853, 75). These texts mix real aspects of practitioner's all day life with a kind of sarcasm and irony.

> When you go [to the patient] look at him with a neutral expression and avoid any voluptuary and conceited gesture. Those who greet you, regreet with modest voice. If you sit down with familiars . . . begin to speak modestly. If you take this into account, speak about the position of that region and praise what people say. . . . (Anonymus Salernitanus 1853, 75)

Strangely, in spite of all cynicism, the author also points out that the sick person should be asked whether he has confessed. This may imply that the passage is actually based on a real account of the everyday life of an influential group of physicians.

Widespread prejudices against the medical profession during the Middle Ages frequently revolved around such caricatures, which were stressed in the parodic poem, *"On the Customs of Doctors"* (Anonymus 1955). This work presents the typical behavior patterns of "bad" doctors, especially their avarice and greed. These sketches may have presented an amusing reflection on everyday behavior of many doctors and appears to be implicitly critical of them.

A more serious approach to dealing with patients is reflected in the work of St. Thomas Aquinas, who glorified the characteristics of the good doctor as one who cares about those who seem to be lost (Thomas Aquinas 1984, 334f.). Even more influential was his concept of the four "cardinal virtues," which was later integrated also into hospital and everyday medical life, as is shown in a French illustration circa 1482 (Henry 1482, f. 11v). Thomas holds that prudence (*prudentia*) is the most important of the cardinal virtues. He offers a fascinating ethical theory: Whoever does not respect prudence which is to be derived from *pro-videntia* ("looking forward," i.e., the ability to take into account the *results* of one's actions) runs the risk that the other cardinal virtues (temperance, justice, and bravery) will turn into vices (Thomas Aquinas 1984, 206–19). Thomas' cardinal virtues are reminiscent of a list of virtues articulated approximately a century earlier by the abbess and physician, Hildegard of Bingen (1098–1179). She had designed a system of virtues for the everyday life of people and for the medical profession. She demanded fear of God instead of the pursuit of glory, truthfulness instead of lying, justice instead of injustice, moderation instead of immoderation, devotion to God instead of magic practices, generosity instead of avarice, and self-control instead of enthusiasm (Hildegard 1998, 240f.).

Scholastic medicine and medical ethics reflect the tensions among Christian, pagan, and Arabic influences, between the duty of *caritas* and the practical demand of earning a living. In addition, there was a lay literature that through direct criticism and caricature reveals that physicians were judged by ethical standards that derive from sources external to the profession itself.

2. The Renaissance

A. General Admonitions

Renaissance medical ethics reflects, in the beginning, the same sources as in the Middle Ages. From the sixteenth century onward, medial ethics was more and more an integral part of the university medical school curriculum. Among the texts taught were the recently translated Hippocratic Oath (Rütten 1993, 37–54; 1997) and such newly rediscovered ancient authoritative texts as the Precepts (Hippocrates 1923a: Precepts) and "Rules of Adequate Behavior" (Hippocrates 1923b: Decorum). As in early Christendom, appeals to *philanthropia* (love of humans) were made to inculcate respect in *philotechnia* (love of the art) (Hippocrates 1923a, 318f.: Precept VI).

Medical ethics in that period typically addressed a variety of old topics. Physicians should demonstrate both friendliness and discretion in dress and manners (Hippocrates 1923a, 324–27: Precepts 9 and 10). Unlike the charlatan, the Hippocratic physician, as Renaissance doctors learned, should consult with colleagues in critical cases and be aware of his limits. Following St. Antoninus (1389–1459), a Dominican friar and Archbishop of

Florence (Curran 1995, 2323), a brutally honest approach to communicating diagnoses and prognoses to the dying was not seen as advisable, "because the condition of many patients subsequently worsened" (Hippocrates 1923b, 296–99: Decorum 16). We can also derive from the often-translated Hippocratic text "About the Doctor" (*De Medico*), that the physician was advised to enjoy good health, because a physician who cannot heal himself cannot expect to gain the confidence of his patients (Hippocrates 1923b, 310f.).

B. Care of the Sick Poor

The care of the sick poor was also an important topic in medical ethics. Most of the poor could not afford physicians' fees and were therefore treated by quacks or charismatic persons in villages and neighborhoods. These individuals often relied on "kitchen-recipes" (home remedies) or superstitious practices (Cook 1995, 1538). After the time of the Black Death (c. 1348), it became increasingly common that "city physicians" – who were employed by municipalities on a fixed salary – treated poor people and took charge of a type of public health service (Park 1992, 87ff.). Any Christian doctor was, as St. Antoninus wrote, obligated to treat the sick poor willingly and free-of-charge, and his patient had to strictly follow the physician's instructions in return (Curran 1995, 2323). The prominent Italian physician Gabriele Zerbi (c. 1445–1505) proposed the same procedure "in order to improve the reputation of the doctor" (Zerbi 1495, 339f.).

C. Abortion and Euthanasia

The "Penal Legislation" of Charles V of 1532 held that abortion was a serious crime. Martin Luther (1483–1546) and the early reformers judged that physicians who performed abortions were guilty of a serious crime. Such views were consonant with the tradition established by such figures as Regino of Pruemm (c. 840–915) and Albertus Magnus (c. 1193–1280) (Jerouschek 1988, 73, 77, 96f.). A wide variety of views were expressed however. Most Medieval and Renaissance doctors subscribed to the Aristotelian theory of the gradual development of the fetal soul. Saint Thomas Aquinas and St. Antoninus of Florence taught that a male or female fetus was not ensouled until the 40th, respectively, or the 80th day of gestation. Abortion seemed licit during this time period but not later in pregnancy. For Aquinas an abortion before that moment was explicitly not an act of murder (Jerouschek 1988, 98–101; Cahill 1995, 31). The Dominican John of Naples (c. 1280–c. 1337) allowed the termination of pregnancy in the case of an "unformed" fetus to save the mother's life (Cahill 1995, 31). The Prague physician Johannes Marcus (sixteenth century) regarded the fetus only as a "part of the mother," a position that permitted abortion throughout

pregnancy (Connery 1978, 12), whereas the Italian forensic physician Paulo Zacchia (1584–1659) pleaded for a very prudent and generous interpretation of the individual formation (Jerouschek 1988, 184f.) On the other hand doctors such as Thomas Fienus (1567–1631) proceeded from the assumption that the fetal soul was present nearly from the moment of conception, making abortion illicit (Connery 1978). The 1588 papal bull *Effraenatam* (of Sixtus V) completely damned any sort of contraception and assistance in abortions (Bergdolt 1998, 650; Cahill 1995, 31).

Actual practice displayed a similar variability. The fifteenth- and sixteenth-century rules governing apothecaries forbade dispensing abortifacients. In contrast, midwifery texts of this period and herbal books as those of Leonhart Fuchs 1543, Hieronymus Bock 1543, and Otto Brunfels 1531 dealt with abortions in detail (Heilmann 1973; Fuchs 1543: Register "Geburt fürdern"; Bock 1543, 452ff.: Register; Brunfels 1532). Abortions were, like a normal birth, indeed performed by midwives, or in a legal gray area by "wise women" or "specialized" laypersons (Labouvie 1998, 198). Compounding the problem was the inability of physicians of the Middle Ages and Renaissance to determine reliably the degree of development of the fetus.

Euthanasia and suicide were also condemned as ethically reprehensible during the Renaissance. Even the translation of Platonic texts accepting these practices could not diminish the fundamental Christian tenet of respect for human life. On a more philosophical level, St. Thomas More (1478–1535) in his *Utopia* contemplated suicide and active euthanasia in cases of extreme suffering (Morus 1981, 130f.). In the seventeenth century, Francis Bacon (1561–1626) used the word "euthanasia" to mean to good death. He distinguished between exterior euthanasia, the termination of physical life to relieve suffering, from interior euthanasia, the preparation of the soul for death. Bacon condoned both (Bacon 1858, 594f.). Later writers such as the German philanthropic author, Johann Valentin Adreae (1586–1654), in his *Christianopolis* (Town of Christians) of 1619, warns against exterior euthanasia as a kind of murder, arguing instead for the ideals of charity and spiritual help (Andreae 1975, 136f.).

D. Emergence of a Distinctive Literature of Medical Ethics

In during the sixteenth and seventeenth centuries, comprehensive original works on medical ethics appeared. These paraphrased ancient or medieval authors as well as construct new syntheses. Examples of this literature include "Precaution measures of doctors" (*De cautelis medicorum*) written by the aforementioned Gabriele Zerbi (Zerbi 1495), the "Popular Errors" (*Erreurs Populaires*) of the royal French physician Laurent Joubert (1529–1582) (Joubert 1578), the "Dialogue in five books" (*Dialogus libris quinque distinctus* 1557) of Iulius Alexandrinus (active in the middle of the sixteenth century), personal physician of the Emperor Ferdinand (Alexandrinus 1557), for whom the physician is a kind of God, bound to philanthropy and piety (Alexandrinus 1557, 194), and the *Medicus politicus* of the Portuguese physician Rodrigo de Castro (1546–1627) (Castro 1614), who holds that "the doctor is nothing more than a servant of the nature" (Castro 1614, 99). Zerbi carefully described an appropriate bedside procedure, in something close to a "check-list." He reminds us that the acceptance of the opinion of experienced colleagues was a Hippocratic virtue and, reflecting the perduring problem of incompetence, that physicians require, apart from all morals, a certain talent (Zerbi 1495, 336). This work became a basic source for many authors who wrote about medical ethics

Zerbi held that a conscientious physician never stops learning and practicing. He should not forget to "meditate" on his work, contemplating a possible "quality improvement" (Zerbi 1495, 338f.). Many of Zerbi's suggestions draw directly on the Hippocratic Oath. He often refers to the ancient authority ("as Hippocrates says in his Oath") to introduce such topics as abortifacients (*abortivum*), which, he notes, often tend to be ineffective ("an abortion drug has no effect") (Zerbi 1495, 339f.). Yet, in a departure from Hippocratic ethics, he recommends that the physician should stay with the patient in cases of serious illness (Zerbi 1495, 339). On the other hand, whenever a doctor realizes that the patient is moribund he should "flee as far as possible." Accompanying or comforting a dying person does not belong to the physician's task (Zerbi 1495, 340).

To preserve the physician's authority, urine should be analyzed only in the patient's absence. To protect patients, doctors should refrain from making thoughtless remarks in their presence (Zerbi 1495, 335). Women are to be treated in a correct manner (Zerbi 1495, 346). Doctors should exercise great care with prognosis and be aware of the possible psychological effects of their action on the patient's well-being. In certain situations, lies are allowed to limit the patient's anxiety (Zerbi 1495, 339).

The famous physician Paracelsus (1493–1541) described the physician's virtue as the "fourth pillar" of medicine (Braun 1988, 49). The true physician treats the sick "out of love for his neighbor," in contrast to the "wolf doctor," who only thinks of financial gain. Like Hippocrates and Zerbi, Paracelsus admonished physicians to discontinue treatment "when nature gives up." The good doctor is unobtrusive, respectful, and sensitive, feeling responsible before God. One of Paracelsus's guiding principles is nature itself, which is a basic column of a successful therapy (Paracelsus 1965–1969, 1:573f.). His contemporary, Ambroise Paré (1510–1590), declared that doctors and surgeons may reflect all they want but God himself will heal their patients. He tells us that active euthanasia was practiced on badly wounded soldiers

during his lifetime (Paré 1963, 35f.). The appearance of printed versions of medieval authors, such as Arnold of Villanova, Guido of Arezzo, or Gilles de Courbeil, led to the widespread reception of the ethical content of these works from the sixteenth century onward.

E. Anatomy and Postmortem Examination

In its early stages, during the fourteenth and fifteenth century anatomy was associated with a certain notoriety because the acquisition of corpses in illegal or quasi-illegal circumstances was not widely tolerated. This phenomenon, which represented a break with the traditional respect of the dead, was extremely complex, and postmortem examinations were typically restricted to the bodies of executed criminals. More and more theologians and legal specialists, such as the German Benedikt Carpzow (1595–1666), refused this popular idea of postmortem dissection as a "second execution" and explained that crime was neutralized by the death of the criminal (*morte crimen finitur*) (Pauser 1998, 529). Organizing corpses for dissection took place, as a rule, in a juridical grey area up to the eighteenth century.

The phenomenon of the anatomy theater, particularly those that had a section for the public to attend, which began (with a temporary stage) in Pisa (c. 1522), Pavia (c. 1522), Padua (c. 1540) and (with a permanent one) in Padua 1595, can best be explained by a typical Baroque vanity, in which splendor, art, and enthusiasm for this world fused with medieval *memento mori* (reminders of the dead) (Bonati 1994, Pauser 1998). In the early seventeenth century, the anatomical dissection even became the showpiece of a controversial spectacle, the central character in which was the human body. At such universities as Padua, Bologna, and Heidelberg, honorary guests joined the audience of students to watch the "show." Musical intervals were added to enhance the enjoyment of the postmortem examination (Bauer 2001, 173f.).

VI. MEDICAL ETHICS IN TIME OF PLAGUE

The plague epidemic of 1347/48, the Black Death, was the first to occur after the so-called Plague of Justinian (sixth and seventh century) and created a new challenge of medical ethics. The issue arose, with urgency, of whether it was permissible for physicians to abandon the sick and flee to safety. Doctors and surgeons were confronted with many moral questions. Considering the decreasing number of practitioners, was it laudable or reproachable if physicians felt the pulse of infected people with an averted face or analyzed the urine only from a distance, as affirmed by the Florentine historian Marchionne di Coppo (Marchionne di Coppo 1903, 230f.)? In fifty contemporary Italian sources of the 1348 plague, we find some physicians desperately trying to help their patients and others fleeing their office or ambulatory or turning to charlatan and magic practices (Bergdolt 1989). On the other hand, it was natural to take all imaginable precautions.

In the rules of the Colleges (*Collegia*) flight was usually damned. New members had to swear to these rules. The Colleges' leadership emphasized the importance of this rule for maintaining the public reputation of doctors (Bergdolt 1994, 176). The French physician Jean Jacobi (c. 1320–c. 1384) proposed a minimal code of ethics: physicians should stay and care for plague victims, while taking all imaginable precautions (Amundsen 1977, 411). Marchionne di Coppo suggests that some physicians stayed with their patients, when he notes that "pharmacists, doctors and gravediggers got rich" (Marchionne 1903, 230–232). A physician who worked unceasingly and without seeming to take his own well-being into account risked to be suspected of greed (Welborn [1938] 1977), especially by his colleagues, but he was also viewed with disdain if he fled from possible contagion.

In contrast, even Galen had once fled Rome during a great plague (Galen 1830, 19, 15). As late as 1666, Thomas Sydenham (1624–1689), the "English Hippocrates," did not regard flight from plague as contrary to professional ethics (Bergdolt 1994, 175). In some areas, it was controversial even to visit plague sufferers. Jaime d'Agremont (active in the middle of the fourteenth century), a physician from Lerida, Spain, recommended in 1348 that payment and reputation should be disregarded in times of plague because the risk of death was too great and all the treasures of the world had not been able to protect many colleagues from infection and death (Bergdolt 1994, 175). Caring about desperately ill patients was not regarded the task of physicians.

Practice displayed a similar variation. There were certainly examples of heroism. Christian charity and moral principles might have influenced many practitioners. Gentile da Foligno (c.1290–1348) died "as a hero" of plague, "after having too much cared about infected people"

in 1348 (Sudhoff 1912, 87). He was commemorated in Perugia and Foligno for his heroism. The author of the 1354 "Short summary of the Italian History" (*Breviarium Italicae Historiae*) refers to a physician who had bled him: "The blood spattered in his face. And he fell ill the same day and died the day after, whereas I could survive by God's mercy" (Anonymus 1730). A certain elite of physicians were also free to leave a city (without breaking any law of their profession or commune), if their universities wanted to move to plague-free "safe" areas. The cause of the plague was also subject to a theological discussion. In 1348 already the question arose of to what extent a physician was allowed to act against the consequences of a divine punishment. The Colleges, on the other hand, were often commissioned by the government to draw up emergency plans for times of plague, examples of which can be traced back to 1348 in some Italian communes (Bergdolt 1994, 51–75).

VII. Conclusion

Medical ethics in the late medieval and Renaissance periods was influenced by Hippocratic traditions, other ancient, non-Christian sources, Christian ideas of nature, disease, and charity, prudential considerations, practical experience, and calamities such as the plague. The early part of this period was dominated by Christian moral theology and philosophy. By the end of the period secular institutions such as the guilds and Colleges, and university medical faculties, began to develop and enforce new standards. Certain themes are recognizable throughout this period, such as philanthropy and the obligation to care for the sick poor, to become and remain competent, prohibitions of abortion and euthanasia, and a bedside morality that emphasized modesty of person, dress, manners, and speech. At the same time, serious controversy arose about such matters as the physician's obligation to remain and care for the sick during times of plague.

CHAPTER 27

THE DISCOURSES OF PRACTITIONERS IN SIXTEENTH-
AND SEVENTEENTH-CENTURY EUROPE

Andrew Wear

I. INTRODUCTION

Despite apparent similarities with modern medical ethics, the relationship between medicine and ethics was very different from that found in Western countries in the twenty-first century. A major factor was that no one group of practitioners achieved a monopoly or near monopoly on legitimacy. Ethics, therefore, served, among other purposes, as a weapon in the war of words between rivals in the medical marketplace. Traditional medical ethics were much in evidence especially in the writings of physicians who modeled themselves on classical authors, but, significantly, there also came into play more general ethical considerations drawn from Christianity, which had wide social currency and appeal.

The contexts within which medicine and ethics operated helped to shape the early modern relationship between medicine and ethics. Today, the role of the state is crucial. It supervises the practice of medicine directly and/or indirectly by giving to a particular group of practitioners the right to act as a profession and to police the actions of its members. State control of medicine usually involves a strong ethical component, for instance, concerning the actions of individual doctors and the use of new techniques and medicines. In early modern Europe, state control over medicine was weak, although not completely absent. The tribunals of the protomedicato[1] in Spain, parts of Italy and in Spanish America, as well as the city colleges of physicians and guilds of surgeons and apothecaries throughout Europe, were given by the state the right to license practitioners and to supervise medical practice. The colleges of physicians attempted to create a monopoly for their members, the "learned" or university-educated physicians, who up to the mid-seventeenth century were usually supporters of Galenic medicine. Like the colleges, the tribunals of the protomedicato, which were composed of learned physicians, also prosecuted empirics but sometimes accepted their existence by licensing them and their products (Lanning 1985, 14–19; Gentilcore 1994, 1995, 1998, 29–38, 60–64, 107; Pomata 1998, 1–13). Both the colleges of physicians and the tribunals of the protomedicato used the ethical injunction of doing no harm to the patient as a justification for their prosecuting activities. The level of supervision was patchy and limited, however, and did not prevent a medical marketplace of many different kinds of practitioner from continuing as it had from the Middle Ages (Park 1992, 80). Patients might initiate complaints against individual healers, but they were not convinced that unlicensed empirics, herbalists, astrologers, wise women, Paracelsian chemical physicians, and the many other types of practitioner were all dangerous or useless. At this time patients' views mattered, in part because they had a wide choice over who treated them and how. Unlike the situation in the later nineteenth century, the ethical–professional views of the early modern learned physicians, which they broadcast abroad, had limited currency and effect upon society at large.

The existence of a medical marketplace where fierce competition between practitioners was the norm is crucial for understanding the relationship of ethics and medicine. Because many empirics did not write books, our understanding of the subject tends to derive from the ethical writings of the learned physicians and their literate rivals, the Paracelsians[2] and the Helmontians.[3] The former look very familiar, inasmuch as they are based on Hippocratic texts and communicate some of the values that came to characterize professional medicine from the nineteenth century onward. Moreover, just as today's medicine is linked to science, which is often taken as the epitome of objective and reliable knowledge, so the medicine taught to the learned physician at universities was underpinned by the natural philosophy of the Greeks, especially of Aristotle. This was considered by large sections of Europe's educated classes to be the most certain and prestigious type of knowledge apart from religion. In addition, learned physicians organized themselves all over Europe into what can be termed proto-professional groupings, having some recognition from the state, setting out educational standards for entry and disciplining its members when they did not follow such traditional norms of etiquette as refraining from openly competing with each other and from bad mouthing colleagues (Park 1985, 19, 36–37). The combination of knowledge claims, state recognition, and professional organization produced an ethical stance that looks deceptively modern; however, the inability of the learned physicians, or any other group, to establish a monopoly of practice meant that their ethical discourses were essentially polemical. Despite their embrace of elevated ideals, at a practical level they served as aids in their competition for patients with other practitioners as well as arguments for the creation of a monopoly.

Early modern physicians were pushing for monopoly and were unable by a long way to achieve it. For instance, the English Crown established the College of Physicians of London in 1518. From its beginning through to the mid-seventeenth century, it was a bastion of learned Galenic medicine. Despite an Act of 1523 that gave the College the duty of examining all physicians throughout England, it was unable to do so. In practice it was limited to licensing physicians and prosecuting unlicensed practitioners in London and 7 miles around. In the seventeenth century, the College's powers were gradually eroded (Clark 1964–1966; Cook 1986). The state certainly had no interest in increasing them. Indeed, as in many of the other royal courts of Europe, empirics were at times given protection and encouragement by English rulers and by powerful noblemen (Wear 1993, 121–22).

The book-based medicine of the Paracelsians and then of the Helmontians rival that of the Galenic physicians.[4] Paracelsianism found establishment homes first in the courts of the German Protestant princes in the late sixteenth century, and then in the early seventeenth century at Montpellier university and in the Parisian royal court (Trevor-Roper 1990; Moran 1990). Paracelsian and Helmontian chemical physicians turned to Christianity for their ethics.

The role of religion in early modern medicine increases the sense of difference and distance between our own age and the early modern period. Christian knowledge then had even greater status and truth value than natural philosophy. Its claims to moral authority were complemented in the minds of orthodox theologians and some radical thinkers by its revelation of physical and hence medical truths. Religion not only provided ethical norms such as charity – largely unknown to the classical world – supplementing Hippocratic ethics; it also legitimized the knowledge and practice of Paracelsians and Helmontians, who were hostile to the "heathenish" medicine of Galen. Religion, moreover, offered another form of healing. Christ continued to be seen as the Great Healer, as he had from at least the early Middle Ages (Amundsen 1982; Ferngren 1992). Protestantism differed from Catholicism in its repudiation of the mediation of the Church through rituals such as anointing the sick with holy oil and the intercession of priests and saints on behalf of the sick. Despite the belief by Calvinists that the age of miracles was past, and that priests no longer possessed the gift of healing, they continued to believe, as did Catholics, that prayer and repentance were powerful medicines that brought healing from God and his Son (Wear 1985, 70–78; Wear 1996, 146–59). Christianity thus represented a distinctive source of ethics as it related to medicine and was a healing resource in its own right. It added to the diffuse and varied nature of early modern medicine and further limited the endeavor of the learned physicians to get their medicine and ethics accepted across society.

The context within which medicine operated in early modern Europe was thus clearly different from that of the twenty-first century. A medical marketplace existed where competition between practitioners was intense and unregulated or poorly regulated. Because there was no monopoly of practice, strident claims and counterclaims as to which group or individual had the best knowledge and most efficacious practice were prominent in the medical literature. This meant that ethical medicine was often equated with one's own safe medicine, while the medicine of one's opponents was attacked as dangerous and murderous. In the competitive commercial medical marketplace all medical knowledge except one's own was subject to critical scrutiny and to ethical comment. Nowadays, given the near monopoly of scientific professionalized medicine in western countries the scrutiny is largely brought to bear upon itself.

II. Traditional Medical Ethics in Early Modern Europe

Deontological rules of behavior, largely developed from Hippocratic texts such as *The Oath*, *Decorum*, and *The Law* together with an admixture of Christian ethics were associated with learned medicine (see Chapters 23, 24). Descriptions of the character of a proper doctor often repeated the Hippocratic texts. The rules of the city colleges of physicians, on the other hand, were less concerned with personal virtue and more with binding their members together, and creating a corporate identity able to withstand the competitive pressures of the marketplace. The statutes of the London College did lay down in a traditional manner that

> Neither for intreaty, nor rewards, nor on any other cause, shall you give Medicines which cause Abortion or Miscarriage, nor Poisons of any kind for destruction, or to an ill use; neither shall you teach them to any one, whom you suspect will abuse them. (Anonymous 1693, 83)

In a further statute, the ethical injunction not to harm patients is clearly mixed with the self-interested wish of the College to keep medical knowledge within its own ranks: "Let none teach the People Medicines, or tell their Names to Them (especially if they are Vehement Medicines, as Purgers, Opiats, or Sleeping Medicines, or which cause Abortion, Vomits, or any other of greater moment or danger) lest by the abuse of them the People be impaired" (Anonymous 1693, 159–60). The previous statute forbidding physicians, except in special circumstances, from undercutting each other reinforces the impression that economic as well as ethical concerns were at work.

The statutes also ordained that colleagues should not insult or denigrate each other, how a second opinion should be sought and a consultation be carried out. The preservation of the honor of the members of the College was important. The second opinion was to be sought without weakening the position of the first doctor, while in a consultation the senior physician had precedence. Above all, "discord" had to be avoided so that the "Art" was not prejudiced (Anonymous 1693, 148–52). Consultations were to be in private, carried out in Latin, with no-one breaking ranks in front of the sick:

> If they shall often meet to visit the same sick person, let none prescribe anything, nay let him not so much as hint what is to be done, before the sick or bystanders, before [until] with joyned councels in

private, it shall be concluded among the Phisicians themselves. (Anonymous 1693, 155)

In an echo of *The Oath's* injunction to physicians to keep their patients' secrets to themselves, the College enjoined its members: "The secrets of the Colledge you shall divulge to none, that is not of the Colledge." It also urged its members to put aside considerations arising from influence – "by Letters from great Men" – or from money, and to do all in their power "in all things in the Art of Phisick for the honour of the Colledge and the Publick good" (Anonymous 1693, 84). The College becomes, as it were, the focus of ethical behavior. This was already present in Hippocratic texts where loyalty to the art of medicine and to a particular group of practitioners was expected. Just as in *The Law* empirics were castigated, so the College forbad its members from working with empirics and ordered them to "persecute by all honest means the unlearned Empiricks and Impostors" (Anonymous 1693, 183–84). All these rules were designed to bolster the corporate identity of the College and its members in the eyes of the outside world, as well as damaging the opposition. Significantly, members of the College had to reveal, unlike empirics, their "Secrets or Arcanas" [secret medicines], (Anonymous 1693, 86–87). In other words, the rules of behavior, etiquette, or ethics that bound the members of the College together, were meant to create a united body of learned physicians who, in contrast to the empirics, shared values and knowledge, cooperated with fellow members, and when competing with each other did so according to set rules.

Guilds of surgeons were also influenced by the rules of etiquette and ethics of the learned physicians. From the Middle Ages there had been attempts to make surgery a learned craft, that is one based on knowledge of the medical and surgical texts of the ancients as well as on practical experience. In the Renaissance with the humanistic revival of classical medicine, there were renewed efforts to produce learned surgeons (Siraisi 1990, 162–86; Nutton 1985b). As part of this movement, the ethics and etiquette of the physicians were taken on board by the guilds of surgeons, which, in any case, in a manner common to guilds, had emphasized to its members the need for corporate cohesion and the sharing of knowledge of secrets among its members.

Ethical injunctions were also highly visible in advice books for practitioners and even more so in polemical works against empirics. Works such as Gabriele de Zerbi's, *De Cautelis Medicorum* (*Advice to Medical Men*; 1495?), Ioannes Siccus's, *De Optimo Medico* (*On the Best Physician*; 1551), Baptista Condrochius's, *De Christiana ac Tuta Medendi Ratione* (*On the Christian and Safe Way of Healing*; 1591), and Rodrigo de Castro's, *Medicus Politicus* (*The Political Physician*; 1614) (see Chapter 26), set out humanistic and Christian norms of behavior, which reiterated Hippocratic values and the

Christian virtue of charity. In addition, they gave advice on how best the physician should comport himself in the society in which he worked. For instance, the learned physician was instructed on how to maintain his social standing against his competitors and in the eyes of lower class patients, while exhibiting polite deference when treating rich upper class patients. Roger French has described how Gabriele de Zerbi, who held a number of teaching posts in philosophy and in medicine at Padua, Bologna, Rome, and Padua again between 1468 and 1494, advised the good physician not to be seen shopping for food as this would lower him in the eyes of the plebeians (see also Chapter 26). Zerbi's ethical good doctor kept his social distance from the lower classes and ensured that he was viewed by all as a successful doctor. He did not take on hopeless cases, or those involving children, pregnant women, and diseases of women, all of which presented difficulties. Establishing a reputation for safe and successful cures lay at the heart of a profitable medical career. Zerbi's further advice to go for quick cures confirms this. On the question of payment, Zerbi wrote, in the manner of traditional Christianity, that the physician should accept whatever the poor could afford and, for reputation's sake, treat the destitute for free. The rich, on the other hand, should be squeezed. Zerbi further advised that to avoid nonpayment, the doctor should request it when the patient was suffering most (French 1993, 74–76). Avoiding harm to one's ethical and also commercial reputation lay behind Zerbi's caution to seek a consultation in potentially fatal cases, so that the responsibility was shared. As in the statutes of the London College of Physicians the consultation had to prevent at all costs any sign of discord among the physicians (French 1993, 79).

Zerbi's good doctor was similar to all those in the advice books mentioned previously: he practiced the best medicine possible and hence the most ethically and commercially sensible. This medicine for the learned physicians was Galenic medicine that could only be learned through long study and was distinct from the other kinds of medicine present in the medical marketplace.

Learned physicians deployed ethical norms to convince prospective patients that the treatments of their rivals were dangerous or worthless. Therapeutic rationales were thus strongly linked to ethics. Galenic physicians claimed that their method of treatment was safer and more effective than all others. It was, they asserted, based on individualized treatment that took into account the humoral constitution of each patient (phlegmatic, melancholic, choleric, and sanguine), age, way of life, environment, and changing state while ill, as well as the disease (Bylebyl, 1991). The medicine of empirics, in contrast, was presented as disease centered rather than patient centered. Furthermore, Paracelsian and Helmontian medicine was self-consciously disease centered. The learned physicians' emphasis on the patient allowed them to state that they,

and not their rivals, gave proper attention and care to their patients. From there it was but a small step to go further and condemn their rivals for providing inappropriate or dangerous remedies to the individual patient. (Today, the position is reversed, and curing the disease rather than the patient is the norm for establishment, scientific medicine. It is "alternative medicine" that now claims to consider the patient as a whole; how this change came about involves the rise of commercial drug sellers in the later seventeenth century and eighteenth century, and in the nineteenth and twentieth centuries of the hospital, the laboratory, and the pharmaceutical companies and has had profound effects on modern medical ethics.) Across Europe, Galenic physicians attacked empirics for lacking their method of treating the individual patient. Uroscopists, especially, were singled out. To the learned physicians they represented the worst possible practice, as diagnosis and treatment were given merely by inspecting the urine and often without the patient being present. In Holland, for instance, Pieter Van Foreest (1522–1597), the town physician of Delft, the "Hippocrates of Holland," was deeply influenced by the Italian medical humanism of Giambatista da Monte who had published Galen's method of healing. In *his De Incerto Fallaci, Urinarum Iudicio* (1589), he contrasted the Galenic method with the practices of the uroscopists (Nutton 1996b), and his attack on the latter is full of ethical insults. As was typical of the learned physicians, Foreest did not embark on an extended ethical argument against the uroscopists but went for sharp and brief name-calling redolent of the social prejudices of the middling sorts. Van Foreest declared that:

> This kinde of people seemeth to have cast off not only all honesty, and sold themselves to worke all manner of wickednesse with greedinesse: but even to have denyed all Divinity and divine providence ... The *devill* likewise being a most cunning craftsmaster, makes choice of such uncleane and wicked persons, receiving them into his service, to the end hee may by their meanes more easily deceive and intrap others: as namely, a perfidious Jew, an apostate and runnagate Monke, an ignorant Parish priest, Vagabonds, cheating and cogging knaves, busie bodies, charming old wives with all the rest of such rakehell. (Hart 1623, 56–58)

Likewise, Johann Lange (1485–1565), a professor of medicine at Heidelberg, fulminated against "the ignorant and inexperienced crowd of philosophers, [which] seduced by old women's superstition and by the impostures and false appearance of knowledge of the Jews and pseudodoctors whose effrontery knows no bounds, thinks falsely ... that the natures of the illnesses can be discerned by a mere inspection of urine" (Langius 1589, 124).

The language of insult was a normal part of early modern disputation. Here the emphasis was on deceit, fraud, imposture, as well as the references to danger found in other passages. At a time when licensing and regulation were lax, recognition by a "credulous" public of the good, namely learned, doctor was seen as rare (Hart 1623, 47, 67). Also lying behind the insults was a genuine belief that the new purified Galenic medicine was better than the alternatives offered by the empirics.

In England, a number of physicians such as William Bullein, James Hart, John Cotta, and John Securis from the sixteenth to the early seventeenth century argued for a reformation of medicine in which all other types of practitioner would be eliminated, leaving the learned practitioners free to practice according to Galen's method. For instance, Securis, who practiced in Salisbury and had been taught in Paris by Sylvius, the ultraconservative Galenic physician and anatomist, set out in traditional fashion the characteristics of the good, in terms of knowledge, ethical practitioner and of his bad or ignorant, unethical rival. In his *A Detection and Querimonie of the Daily Enormities and Abuses Committed in Physic* (1566) Securis, in a typical Renaissance fashion, applied classical material drawn from the Hippocratic *Oath*, *Law*, and *Decorum* as well as Galenic works to his sixteenth century concerns. After enumerating the qualities that a physician needed to acquire and to retain a good reputation and so succeed in the struggle to exist in the medical marketplace (Securis 1566, Aviiʳ–Aviiᵛ), Securis turned to the education of a physician. This was what made a physician learned and able to apply a proper method of cure. After first citing *The Law* on the need for long study to become a physician, Securis wrote that before one could practice medicine knowledge had to be acquired of philosophy and of other university subjects such as grammar, logic, music, arithmetic, and geometry, as well as of anatomy, simple and compound medicines and the different human temperaments (Securis 1566, Aiiiᵛ, Aviᵛ–Aviiʳ). Learning produced good physicians. Without it, he asked, "what securitie and savegard is there in these sort of fellowes: which now a days almost in al places so rashly, so fondly and so wickedly do abuse the noble art and science of Phisicke." They, Securis wrote, would have answered that they had experience, English books of remedies, and that "some of us have a gifte of nature to heale many diseases" (Securis 1566, Aviiᵛ–Aviiiʳ). In reply, Securis implied that unlearned practitioners did not possess the method of healing that tailored remedies to the patient, instead they used the same remedy for all patients suffering the same disease. This point is worth emphasizing for it lies at the heart of the learned physicians' claims of bad practice by their opponents. Securis gave an example of what he meant:

> What though you have geven a medecine, as for example, a purgacion to purge fleame to any man in the winter, supposing that man to be somewhat aged, of a flegmaticke complexion, usynge muche

flegmaticke meates [foods] muche slepe and muche reste: and that the sayde purgation hath taken good effecte and wrought well, all this supposed: Let the lyke medecine be geven in the sommer to a man of an other complexion, of an other diete and of an other age: yea supposyng this, that it be geven to the selfe same man in the Sommer: Shall the same purgation (thinke you) take suche effecte and operation, as it dyd afore in the winter? No verely. (Securis 1566, Aviiᵛ–Aviiiʳ)

Lack of knowledge, their knowledge, justified to themselves and their readers the learned physicians' condemnation of their rivals. That knowledge was learned at the university, and money as well as a genuine belief in the value of a medical education underlay the construction of the studious and ethical physician. In a medical market where there were few or no educational entry requirements, the welding together of medical and moral worth with education gave added value to the investment in time and money that a university education represented.

Securis complained that it was "a great foly for us to bestow so much labor and study all our lyfe tyme in the scholes and universities ... and the greatest follye of all were, to procede in any degree in the Universities with our great coste and charges, when a syr John lacke latin, a pedler, a weaver, and oftentymes a presumptuous woman, shall take upon them (yea and are permytted) to mynyster Medicine to all menne, in every place and at all tymes" (Securis 1566, Biiᵛ). Securis's indignation was such that he returned to the subject, this time bringing the charge of harm to patients against his unlearned competitors, and yet his indignation at financial loss came before his allegation of harm. Commerce often foreshadowed ethics in the minds of the learned physicians.

> What doth it prevaile for us that be lerned to procede (as I saide) in any degree of maister, of batcheler, or doctor, and so to be allowed and have authoritie to use our science? When every man, woman, and chyld that lyst, may practise and use phisike (*idque impune*) [and that with impunity] as wel as we? And so, many tymes not only hinder and defraud us of our laufull stipende and gaynes: but (which is worst of all and to much to be lamented) shall put many in hasarde of their lyfe, yea and be the destruction of many. Is this tolerable? Will the magistrates alwayes wynke at this? Shall there never be no reformation for suche abuses? (Securis 1566, Biiiʳ)

The traditional corpus of what we consider as the origins of medical ethics belonged, as it were, to the learned physicians. It was part of the classical medicine that formed the basis of their medicine. The sense in the Hippocratic texts of beleaguered exclusivity, of group identity, of individual one-to-one interactions with patients, and the existence of a diverse medical marketplace was echoed in the concerns of the early modern learned physicians. Perhaps they were more organized, more aware of the possibilities of state protection, but the *longue durée* moved slowly and there were sufficient similarities between the two periods to make traditional medical ethics relevant for the learned physicians, especially as they were a group concerned with recreating the medicine of the ancients.

III. CHRISTIAN ETHICS IN MEDICINE

The literate opposition to the learned physicians, the Paracelsians and Helmontians, relied on Christian rather than classical ethics to establish their moral worth in the medical marketplace (see Chapters 12, 14). It is true that they retained Hippocrates as the father figure of medicine, while denigrating Galen as a wordy and logic-chopping scholastic who had perverted the bedside experience of Hippocrates. They often ignored such distinctions in their wholesale condemnation of ancient medicine however. They pointed out that it had been created by pagan physicians and was inappropriate for Christian nations (Pagel 1958, 56–58; Pagel 1982). A Christian medicine had to be compassionate and charitable in contrast to the expensive and uncharitable practice of the Galenic physicians, who were also suspected of atheism (Webster 1993, 72). Moreover, as both Paracelsus and van Helmont argued, the physician was born and not made, his knowledge came from divine enlightenment together with hard work in the laboratory. The learning of the ancients had to be discarded as worthless and dangerous (Wear 2000, 374–78). The new medicine was to be disease centered rather than patient centered, and chemical remedies were used rather than plant-based ones. The radical alternatives to Galenic medicine thus appeared to be incommensurable with it in both medical and religious, and hence, moral terms (although some attempts were made at a conciliation between Paracelsian and Galenic medicine).

The ethics of Paracelsian and Helmontian medicine were given concrete expression in a series of plans for medical reform that combined charity with concern not only for the individual sick poor but also for the sick poor as a group. Such a social perspective was signally lacking in the learned physicians, who only imitated their rivals in providing organized free consultations and treatment for the poor.

In France, the Montpellier-educated Paracelsian royal physician and sometime Huguenot, Théophraste Renaudot (1584–1653) established around 1630 in Paris the Bureau d'Adresse, which acted as an early labor exchange. It also listed those physicians, surgeons, and apothecaries who offered free medical treatment to the sick poor. In approximately 1632, the Bureau provided the poor with free medical consultations and treatment. The Bureau's own charitable physicians were Paracelsians and their remedies were largely chemical. In 1643, with the fall from power of Richelieu, Renaudot's patron, the Galenic-dominated Paris faculty of medicine finally had their wish fulfilled and Renaudot was forbidden from practicing medicine in Paris. He had, however, set a precedent and the Paris parlement forced the faculty to provide free consultations for the poor (Solomon 1972).

In England, as Charles Webster has shown, the puritan reformers found Paracelsianism congenial with its condemnation of pagan learning, its emphasis on divine illumination, and its stress on charity. The charitable physician was increasingly identified as the Paracelsian physician, although that physician could also be a clergyman trained in Paracelsian medicine. The perceived need was to make medicine freely available to the poor. The clergy represented a nationwide network of potential medical expertise. Moreover, the clergy would be naturally sympathetic to charitable medicine (Webster 1975, 246–323). Gabriel Plattes, for instance, in his utopian work, *Macaria* (1641), wrote that "the parson of every parish is a good physician," and that a minister could cure both the soul and the body (Webster 1975, 259). Such schemes did not come to fruition. The attacks on uncharitable Galenic physicians continued into the Restoration, however, and the example of Helmontian physicians and dissenting ministers staying on in London during the plague of 1665, while most of the Galenists fled, gave added point to the rhetoric. By the end of the century, partly because of the negative publicity thrown at them by their rivals, and partly because of competition from the apothecaries, the College of Physicians set up a dispensary for the poor that gave free advice and low-cost medicine (Clark 1964–6, 2, 431–47; Cook 1986, 233–35, 238–40).

The physician's Christian duty to provide charitable treatment for the poor was recognized in the medical ethics of the learned physicians. The accusation that physicians were not charitable not only drew medicine into politics and religion, it also helped, and here I am speculating, to create a possible new ethical norm for medicine. Charitable care of the sick poor had been largely a duty of the Church; in the early modern period that duty seems to be in the process of being transferred to medical practitioners as well as to the state. On the other hand, the possibility that the clergy could act as physicians can be taken as a recognition of the failure of physicians to be charitable. What was needed was a godly charitable medicine, staffed by people who were charitable. Clergy as physicians can also be interpreted as another example of the Protestant spiritualization of the world[5] (Wear 1985, 57). In Denmark, where Paracelsian medicine had taken root at the University of Copenhagen by the beginning of the seventeenth century, it was enacted that all who desired to become country parsons should be educated in human anatomy (Grell 1993a and personal communication). The aim was that parsons should know the handiwork of God better and also be better medical practitioners in isolated country areas.

The notion of charity is clearly a disputed one. This, of course, was the case more generally, as from the early sixteenth century the poor were being differentiated into the deserving and the undeserving, and both Luther and Calvin denied that good works, such as charity to the poor, were a means to salvation (Davis 1975; Jütte 1994). The medieval image of the needy poor favored of God was still evoked by Catholic and Protestant governments, by preachers and by radical medical writers to elicit charity from the better off; and, in the case of medical practitioners, preachers and radicals tried to instill in them the notion of a duty of charitable care. In England, for instance, Nicholas Culpeper, a supporter of the Parliamentary side and a radical quasi-Paracelsian astrological physician, wrote in 1649 that physicians would not come "to a poor mans house who is not able to give them their fee . . . and the poor Creature for whom Christ died must forfeit his life for want of money" (Culpeper 1649, Ai^v). Such rhetoric, and schemes that would extend medical help to the poor, together with a genre of books that addressed the issue of providing them with cheap remedies such as Paul Dubé's, *Le Médecin des Pauvres* (*The Physician of the Poor*, 1669), brought to the foreground for medicine the ethical imperative of charity to the poor. It is a moot point whether this imperative now forms one component of the ethical altruism of doing one's best for a patient, or whether in reality the medical profession in the succeeding centuries left the duty of providing financially for the care of the poor to the church and to the state.

IV. TERRITORIAL BOUNDARIES IN RELIGION AND MEDICINE

Religion was not only a polemical resource to be used in the competition between different groups of practitioners. Christianity was the most powerful ideology of the time; it justified wars, politics, and national and personal morality. An activity such as medicine that dealt with life and death and might seem to run counter to God's providence in punishing sinful humans with disease, had to arrive at an accommodation with religion. Such an accommodation was part of the moral licence that allowed physicians, surgeons, empirics, and others to practice in the first place. It is, therefore, part of the ethical system into which early modern medicine as a whole was placed, even though it may not appear relevant to modern medical ethics.

No early modern medical practitioner believed that Christianity was at odds per se with the practice of medicine. For instance, Laurent Joubert, a notable Protestant Montpellier doctor who became personal physician to Catherine de Medici and then to the king, in his *Erreurs Populaires* (*Popular Errors*, 1578, part 1; 1579, part 2)

referred, like many of his fellow physicians, to Ecclesiasticus 38.1: "Honour the physician with that honour that is due unto him . . . for the Lord hath created him" (Joubert [1578] 1989, 49). He did this when correcting:

> another kind of error, founded in pure superstition by some fools who think it is an offense against God if they call physicians to heal their ills, claiming that in doing so one is resisting and opposing the will of God, who is visiting them with an affliction for their own good. For by chastising the body, the soul is purged of its sins and they say . . . "God has given it [the illness] to me as it pleases Him, God will take it away when it shall please Him. Blessed be the name of God. Amen." They submit their healing entirely to the intercession of the saints in heaven, making vows, giving alms, and saying prayers. (Joubert [1578] 1989, 49)

Joubert's further response was the standard one, that as illness came from God so "also proceeds healing through the means He has established in nature, giving to plants and other creatures the power to drive out and destroy diseases." Such means were not to be disputed, to do otherwise would be to expect God to act miraculously. For, he asked, "is it not tempting God to expect to see what He will do against the order of nature?" (Joubert [1578] 1989, 49).

Such reasoning had been articulated centuries before, but it had not lost its force over time, and formed part of the traditional *modus vivendi* between religion and medicine (Amundsen 1982). The accommodation did not, in the eyes of clergymen, preclude them from healing, although physicians argued that they should keep to their calling (Wear 1996, 159–64). There were, however, territorial boundaries. There was general agreement that dying represented a sphere of influence that belonged to the clergy. Catholic and Protestant writers stated that when the physician knew that the patient was dying he should leave the bedside to the priest or minister – in France this was a legal requirement. To remain would, it was argued, be to take money under false pretences knowing that the case was hopeless. More importantly, dying lay in religion's domain. Culturally it was a religious rather than a medical enactment (Ariès 1983; Stannard 1977; Vovelle 1983; McManners 1981; Cressy 1997; Houlbrooke 1998). The dying person had to make his or her peace with relatives and friends and settle worldly affairs. The act of dying involved preparing oneself by meditation and prayer for the fight for one's soul, the psychomachy, that took place between God and the Devil over the bedside at a time when the individual was at his or her weakest and least able to resist the temptations of the Devil. In addition, the dying publicly prepared themselves for the journey to the next world and God's judgement through the aid of the Catholic sacraments or with the help of a Protestant minister (Wear 1987, 236–40). It was not until the mid-eighteenth century that physicians regularly began to manage dying with narcotic drugs. By that time, with increasing secularization, the need to remain rational to publicly act out "the good death" had lessened. In the sixteenth and seventeenth centuries, however, it was generally considered unethical for a physician to remain with the dying.

At the time of birth, in contrast, religion did not assert any monopoly. Across Europe there was a requirement that the midwife should have a good moral character. This was partly so that she did not connive at infanticide or at the substitution of one baby for another. Moreover, the midwife was sometimes used as an instrument of the Church or of the local authorities. She might give an emergency baptism. If the father was unknown, the midwife could ask the mother for his name at the time when she was most vulnerable, in the midst of giving birth (Harley 1994, 50–51). From the fifteenth century German cities, such as Nuremberg, Frankfurt, Munich, and Stuttgart, employed midwives, whose morality was certified by respectable, well-off women who as "honorable" or "sworn women" judged the character of each midwife, while physicians examined their skills (Wiesner-Hanks 1993). In England, bishops licensed midwives on the basis of testimonials that spoke of their moral worth as well as their skill (Evenden 2000, 24–49). As with death, but not to such an extent, birth was put into a moral setting, side by side with the medical context represented by the midwife's technical skill. Beyond pointing out the moral dimension to what for us today is a natural or medical occasion, it is difficult to write of a body of medical ethics addressed to midwives. Cities and individuals could dismiss a midwife for perceived poor performance, and certainly the men midwives, who were trying to take over in England the business of the midwives at the end of the seventeenth century and in the rest of Europe a century later, did not hesitate to create a catalogue of their supposed faults. Given the difficulty of proving harm in law there were few sanctions that could be exacted against malpractice by a midwife. Her reputation, however, which, just as for any other type of practitioner, was crucial for acquiring clients, could well suffer.

V. Harm to Patients

There were several ways in which harm to patients became an issue. Everyone agreed that patients should not be harmed, and, as we have seen, competing groups of practitioners accused each other of harmful or useless treatments. Given the lack of medical consensus the notion of harm in the modern legal sense of some act or acts that ran against the consensus of best medical practice hardly arose in the early modern period. What was usually at issue was obvious damage to the patient or failure of treatment,

although in subsequent polemical discussions or in legal proceedings a sectarian concept of best practice might be employed. For instance, Galenists argued that violent chemical purges used by Paracelsians and Helmontians constituted bad practice, and Helmontians in turn argued that bleeding was bad practice on the part of the Galenists.

In the early modern period, it was very difficult to know for certain whether harm to a patient was caused by a drug. Certainly, over the centuries certain plants such as hemlock were considered poisonous, whereas others such as white hellebore were used only with great caution. Mercury, which came to general prominence with the advent of the pox into Europe at the end of the fifteenth century and was also favored by Paracelsian physicians, was viewed even by its supporters as damaging to patients. Its fearsome side effects, among which were seas of sweat and loosening of the bones, were dreaded; however, mercury was often requested by patients who feared the disease more. There were no official bodies that assessed the risk posed by particular treatments or balanced the side effects of drugs against therapeutic effectiveness (Wear 2000, 265–74). The pharmacopoeias published by European cities in the sixteenth and seventeenth centuries gave standardized ingredients for drugs, and, depending on whether the authorities were favorable to Paracelsian remedies, chemical medicines might be included. They did not, however, assess relative risk. Contemporaries were aware of the possibilities of medical trials, and a few were performed on criminals, but there was no systematic development of the medical trial in this period (Wear 2000, 384–86).

Despite the apparent certainty in remedy books and in empirics' broadsheets that medicines were safe and effective, uncertainty was rife. It was created in a medical sense, not only by the lack of trials, but also by the use of many drugs at one time and/or by the taking of compound remedies composed of many ingredients that made it impossible to distinguish among the effects of the different plants, animals, and minerals that were used. Moreover, the individualized prescribing of the learned physicians, although not always adhered to, made it difficult to generalize about the safety or otherwise of a drug. The effects of medicines were also rendered uncertain by European cultural beliefs. In a society that considered an illness and its cure could come from God, the Devil and his witches, from the environment, food and lifestyle in general, from nature, or from the physician and his medicines, certainty about a cure was difficult to arrive at, especially if one was a patient. In the absence of clear notions of effectiveness and harm, only the crudest form of damage to a patient could be judged as malpractice. To avoid any imputation of damage or failure, physicians, as we have seen, were urged to avoid taking on potentially fatal or difficult cases or to seek safety in numbers in a consultation. Similarly, surgeons were enjoined to consult with and be overseen by senior colleagues in dangerous cases (Wear 2000, 237–38).

VI. COMMERCIAL MEDICAL ETHICS

At first sight it looks as if the traditional injunction not to harm the patient was a dead letter, except in so far as it was used by those in authority, usually the learned physicians, to prosecute empirics, chemical physicians, healing women, and other unlicensed practitioners. Patients often sought redress for failed or botched cures, and they sometimes received it. The basis for the redress was frequently a commercial one, and it is possible to argue that in the early modern period a commercial rather than a Hippocratic or professional medical ethics could have developed. Patients would contract with a practitioner to be cured. The contract was either oral or written and part of the money was paid up front, the rest on completion of the cure or in installments. The learned physicians usually tried to insist on a fee for each visit to a patient, and it was normally surgeons, barber-surgeons, apothecaries, and unlicensed practitioners who contracted with a patient to cure them. On July 5, 1639, for instance, the London College of Physicians heard the case brought by Dorothy Banton who

> complayned of Mr White apothecary... who had undertaken to cure her of an infirmity, but not performed. Hee received 40s[hillings], of her the first weeke and three poundes more hee was to have when the cure was finished. Like-wise for three powndes more hee was to cure her husband of his infirmities; and upon this agreement the husband of the saide Mrs Banton sealed a bond of so much money. But these parties Banton and his wife findinge themselves still unremedied refused to pay the rest of the monies. Here-upon White put the bond in suite and cast the poor man into prison wher hee remayned at the time of this complaynte. (College of Physicians n.d., 492–493, vol. 3, fol. 700b)

The College attempted to convince White to release Banton from his bond, but he refused. The College conceded that it "could not recall the bond," but put pressure on White: "hee is threatened to bee proceeded against as a [illegal] practizer for so many monthes as appeared hee gave her and her husband physicke" (College of Physicians, *Annals*, 493, vol. 3, fol. 700b).

Agnes Selbye, on the other hand, had more luck when in 1589 the court of the Barber-Surgeons Company of London deliberated on the complaint of:

> the wyfe of Richard Selbye of London Ironmonger plantyf against William Wyse, for that he cured not her housbonds leg as he promised he wolde have don, and yt is ordered that William Wyse shall repaye againe of the money which he received in parte of the bargayne made betwene them[,] and then was in the presence of this Courte payde unto Agnes the wyf of the above said Richard Selby six shillings and eight pence. (Young 1890, 327)

Gianna Pomata, who has written in depth on contracts between patients and practitioners, has shown that in medieval Europe such contracts were common and were often adjudicated in the civil courts (Pomata 1998, 30–33). In early modern Bologna (the focus of her study) the institution of the Protomedicato or medical magistracy that oversaw medical matters, by the end of the sixteenth century had taken over the power to decide on civil disputes relating to medical contracts and had the powers to make patients pay practitioners and to force practitioners to refund patients by confiscating property, if necessary (Pomata 1998, 52–54). As Pomata points out:

> These agreements denied two basic tenets of medical professionalism: first, that medical practitioners deserve to be paid because they are licensed members of the profession, and second, that payment does not depend on the patient's satisfaction. As medical ethics became increasingly shaped by the principles of professionalism, negotiating with patients was rejected by physicians as demeaning and unprofessional. (Pomata 1998, 46)

Certainly, by the later seventeenth century contracts were dying out (Pomata 1998, 140–71); however, before then we have a situation in which medicine is seen partly in commercial terms, analogous to services and goods rendered. The contractual model imposes obligations for both patient and practitioner. The patient becomes legally obliged to pay the practitioner and obey the practitioner otherwise the contract is void, while the practitioner has to accomplish what is promised in the contract. The patient has the right to have a say on a practitioner's performance, harm is certainly an issue but not so much as the question of success or failure. If contracting a cure, to use Pomata's phrase, had developed, it is likely that medical ethics would now be vastly different. Judging whether a doctor succeeded or failed would be central to the patient–doctor relationship. Perhaps we are now slowly reintroducing success as a formalized criterion of the good doctor. Data on surgeons' rates of success are being collected in Britain and the United States, and, like hospital mortality rates, are being increasingly publicized. The only area in medicine today in which the commercial contract centered around performance applies is in the pharmaceutical industry. In the early modern period, apothecaries with their origins in grocers and spicers companies and guilds were also viewed by patients and doctors as providers of goods that could be good or bad, and if the latter was the case redress was possible through contract law. What is interesting is that for a while some of the rest of medicine shared in their situation.

VII. ETHICAL CONUNDRUMS

This has been very much a chapter that has put ethics and medicine into a broad historical context, rather than focusing on the development of medical ethics per se. This can be justified on the grounds that much of classical medical ethics remained unchanged. There were some issues, however, around which there was consensus and others that aroused debate.

For instance, in surgery, the need for the patient's consent was taken for granted. The one-to-one commercial nature of the patient–surgeon transaction often centered around a contract helped to ensure this. So, too, did the surgeon's anxiety that he should not be blamed for a patient's disability or death after an operation. Surgical treatises repeatedly stressed the point that the dangers of an operation had to be fully discussed with a patient so that consent was fully informed. The religious imperative of preparing oneself for death, which in Roman Catholic countries was formerly structured through the institutional ritual of the sacraments, but which was no less intense in Protestant countries, gave added weight to the need for the patient to be fully informed before an operation (Wear 2000, 236–47). There was less explicit discussion concerning consent in the case of physical or internal medicine. The ability of patients to change practitioners and the unified medical culture of the time, in which lay people shared in medical knowledge and often made their own remedies, ensured that patients often held the upper hand in the patient–doctor relationship. So consent was usually not an issue, although this did not mean that the doctor necessarily kept the patient fully informed.

More debatable was whether doctors should flee in the face of plague (see Chapter 26). In Protestant Europe, Lutherans argued that physicians should stay and look after the community, whereas Calvinists took the position that the physician, like the magistrate, was a valuable member of the Commonwealth and should flee (Grell 1993b). At the end of the day the decision was a personal one.

Whether to lie to the patient was another topic of perennial debate. As Winfried Schleiner has shown, lying to cure melancholia, or lying not to alarm a patient and so worsen their condition was seen as allowable by Rodrigo de Castro and Paulus Zacchias. On the other hand, the need for the sick to know of approaching death and so prepare themselves for it as Christians was acknowledged by Baptista Condrochius (Schleiner 1995, 8–12, 27–28). Undoubtedly, Canon Law and the casuistic tradition of Catholic Europe helped to develop debate on medical ethics, as did the continental European medical forensic tradition in which physicians and surgeons gave expert opinions to the courts (Crawford, 1994). For instance, in his *Quaestiones Medico-Legales* (1621–1635), Zacchias, who was personal physician to Popes Innocent X and Alexander VII and Protomedicus to the Papal State, dealt with many cases that straddled the border between Canon Law and medicine. These included issues such as the viability of the fetus, the causes of fetal death, types of madness, poisoning, impotence, malingering, the use of torture, witchcraft, miracle cures, judgment of virginity, types of wounds, and so forth. Some of these topics had moral as well as medical components and gave a dialectical edge to Zacchias's discussions. It was a sin, he argued, to prescribe to the poor expensive remedies that would impoverish them (Zacchiae [1621–1635] 1651, 392). A doctor could take a fee, he concluded, for caring for a dying person. Zacchias also believed that a patient did not have to obey a physician in taking harsh and intolerable remedies, especially as remedies are only probably effective and not certainly so (Zacchiae [1621–1635] 1651, 629). Zacchias, nevertheless, saw most issues through the eyes of the learned physicians, he belonged to the establishment. So, in general, he deplored the disobedience of patients and attacked empirics for being full of errors and lacking reason (Zacchiae [1621–1635] 1651, 627, 402–3). As part of his medico-legal enquiries Zacchias also asked questions related to specific aspects of medical practice. For instance, could amputation of limbs be performed with a safe conscience when, although it was necessary, there was a risk of gangrene. Zacchias replied that it was better to leave the patient in God's hands than attempt such a treatment, which promised no ultimate safety and whose horror and pain was clearly most troubling (Zacchiae [1621–1635] 1651, 635). The mix of medical and legal reasoning, characteristic of much of the argument in modern medical ethics, is unmistakable.

There was no subject or discipline of medical ethics in the modern sense however. The range of topics in Zacchias' book indicates his medical, legal, religious, and forensic interests, which came together in Canon Law cases. Rodrigo de Castro, a Portuguese Jewish physician who practiced in Hamburg, wrote on an eclectic and idiosyncratic range of topics in his *Medicus Politicus*. Many were traditional to the learned physicians, some relate to ethics, to competitors, and to justifying and praising medicine. They include, for example, the view that physicians and medicine should be rational (i.e., Galenic) and that physicians should be and be said to be good and prudent. The empirical sects were refuted, the sects of the chemists "understood and rejected," and arguments raised against those who argue that neither medicine nor physicians are necessary to the republic. Castro devoted space to the status and nature of medicine and argued that medicine is from God and explained the passage from Ecclesiasticus. He compared the medical art with the arts of war and agriculture and with jurisprudence, and asked whether astrology is useful and necessary to the physician. He stated that the physician should be a surgeon, but that it was dishonorable for a doctor to be a perfume seller. Castro expanded on the origin and progress of the art of medicine, which authors should be in a physician's library, warned that doctors should avoid avarice and jealousy, cautioned concerning prognosis, and condemned uroscopy, and so forth. What we have here is best advice on being a proper doctor in a hostile environment. Ethics and medical ethics can be found in it, but the book is not really about either, it is rather a defense of learned medicine under the guise of, as its subtitle puts it, not only portraying the morals and virtues of good doctors but revealing also the frauds and impostures of bad ones. Perhaps that is what medical ethics is really about.

VIII. CONCLUSION

There were discussions of medical ethics in early modern Europe. These were largely based on classical texts and were deployed by a group confident of its learning but nervous of the competition that it faced in the medical market place. Ideals of propriety and proper behavior were shaped, therefore, by a realization that they needed to be such that they helped physicians to survive and hopefully flourish in a world that still did not automatically accept them. There was also debate about ethical controversies in medicine largely by members of the same group; however, the influence of Christianity on all areas of life including medicine, the lack of consensus on what is acceptable medicine, the poorly regulated state of medicine, all argue for taking a broader view, for studying the general relationship between ethics and medicine in this period. What one finds are partial trends and incomplete developments, very much like the medicine of the time, and unlike the nineteenth century picture when medical ethics and an increasingly confident and powerful professionalized medicine complemented each other.

If one uses hindsight, one could say that during this period there was a proto-medical ethics just as a section of medicine was at a proto-professional stage. Whether the prior existence of classical medical ethics contributed to the physicians trying to organize themselves into a profession is a moot question. Ethics were certainly used to instill a sense of group solidarity and to justify attempts at monopoly of practice, and economic necessity and social aspiration must have been major factors in the initial moves toward creating a profession, the intense competition faced by the learned physicians from other practitioners meant that economic survival rather than ethical injunctions would have been their primary concern. One should also bear in mind that this is a time of flux. Other types of medical ethics might have emerged to become dominant in later centuries, just as groups of practitioners other than the university-educated physicians might have

become dominant (and perhaps in a hidden process did, if one considers the way empirical drug-based medicine was to become integrated with established medicine).

NOTES

1. The institution of the *protomedicato* originated in medieval Spain. It was named after the royal physician or *protomedico* who headed the tribunal. By 1477, it had a clearly defined identity and was enjoined by Ferdinand and Isabella to examine and license all those who wanted to become physicians, surgeons, bonesetters, apothecaries, herbalists and any other men or women who wanted to practice medicine or engage in occupations related to medicine. Additionally, the *protomedicato*, which normally consisted of two physicians and surgeons, visited apothecaries' shops to assess the quality of their goods.

Spain exported the *protomedicato* to the New World. Mexico City appointed a *protomedicato* (or chief physician) as early as 1525 to examine practitioners. In 1570, the Spanish Crown sent Francisco Hernandez as *protomedicato* to regulate medicine for all of New Spain (Mexico). In Europe, it was only in Sardinia, which was under strong Spanish influence, that a strong centralized *protomedicato* was set up. In Naples, which was also under Spanish administration and influence, the powers of the *protomedicato* were more diffuse and consisted of collecting license fees and inspecting apothecaries' shops.

The *protomedicato* was not always a royal (usually Spanish) institution. In Bologna, the College of Medicine appointed the *protomedici* of the city and created the tribunal of the *protomedicato* early in the sixteenth century. Its judicial powers were granted by the city authorities. This recognition and authorization by the state gave the "learned" university-educated physicians who sat on the boards of the protomedicato and on the disciplinary committees of the city colleges of physicians, a sense of power and status. The regulatory reach of the colleges and the tribunals of the *protomedicato* was never very extensive; although in Spain the *protomedicato* was the most organized.

Moreover, state recognition was always conditional and often weak. It is, therefore, no surprise that in early modern Europe the learned physicians never achieved a monopoly of practice, despite having the notional mechanisms to regulate and licence practitioners.

2. Paracelsian practitioners were chemical physicians who believed that the body worked chemically and that disease should be treated with chemical remedies. They tended to pick and choose those parts of Paracelsus's philosophy that they found congenial (see Paracelsus). After his death, Paracelsus's views from the mid-sixteenth century onward first found a home at the courts of the German Protestant princes.

For instance, the Paracelsian physician Adam von Bodenstein was personal physician to Otto Heinrich, Duke of Neuberg and Elector Palatinate. Court physicians and their noble patrons took up Paracelsus' chemical experiments and magical ideas but not his radical social philosophy. At the beginning of the seventeenth century Paracelsian medicine became influential at the court of the French King Henri IV with the appointment of Joseph Duchesne as royal physician. Paracelsianism spread also to the university of Montpellier. In Paris, the Montpellier physician Théophraste Renaudot began to implement the Paracelsus's belief that medicine should be provided free to the poor as an act of charity.

The strongest expression of Paracelsus's radical Christian and social views, which stressed the imminent coming of Christ, a skepticism about any established Church (including Lutheranism), the need for charity to the poor and the paganism of classical medical writers, came from English political and medical writers before and during the Civil War period. English reformers were also attracted by Paracelsus's emphasis on the intense personal relationship between God and the chemist working in his laboratory. Paracelsus's chemist–physician searched for personal knowledge with God's help by investigating nature and by seeking out practical knowledge from miners and others. Similarly, English Protestants believed in a one-to-one relationship between themselves and God (unmediated by the Roman Catholic Church), and they also thought that manual experimentation would unlock the secrets of nature. Paracelsus's followers at this time, as well as offering their patients chemical remedies produced in the laboratory, stressed how Galenists were uncharitable to the poor, how their knowledge was unchristian and pagan, and how their medicines did not work. The medical ethics of Paracelsus and his followers, therefore, drew upon the body of general Christian ethics.

3. Helmontian practitioners were followers of the medical doctrines of Johannes Baptista van Helmont (1579–1644). Helmontians, like van Helmont himself, can be seen as following in the footsteps of Paracelsus. Like him they advocated a chemically based medicine to replace the humoral-qualitative medicine of Galen that was taught in the universities. They differed from Paracelsians in the details of their chemical theories (see van Helmont), however, and, even more than Paracelsus, they imbued their work with a Christian spirituality.

Helmontians never gained as much prominence as did Paracelsians, and their influence was shorter lived being most apparent in the second half of the seventeenth century. In 1665, in England, they tried to create a Society of Chemical Physicians, but they narrowly failed to do so, their initial support among the court of Charles I having dissipated. Helmontians such as George Thomson, George Starkey, and Marchamont Nedham, nevertheless, through their writings vigorously expounded their medicine.

Many of their points such as the pain and unsuccessfulness of Galenic medicine, its unchristian origins and its expense and lack of charity should have had, on the face of it, wide appeal. Yet, as they admitted, they could not get patients to change from the traditional Galenic therapies of bleeding, purging, and the use of herbal remedies to their chemical remedies. Together with the lack of an institutional base, the adherence of patients to traditional therapeutics largely, but not completely, accounts for the ultimate failure of Helmontians to establish themselves. Other factors included their inability to create a distinct identity that would separate themselves from other practitioners of chemical medicine in the eyes of patients, and their failure during a time of intellectual flux to establish their chemical theories as part of the "new philosophy" that was replacing Aristotelian natural philosophy. Instead Robert Boyle's chemical philosophy took the intellectual high ground.

In Continental Europe, a similar process took place with Helmontians being lost to view by the first decades of the eighteenth century. Nevertheless, Helmontians represent one of the potential paths that medical ethics could have taken. They united a highly developed sense of commercial drug making and selling with an intensely Christian ethic. They saw their chemical researches as enlightened by God and believed that it was their duty to offer charitable medical care for the poor. In the years immediately after they had left the scene what remained and flourished was the commercial sale of empirics' remedies.

4. Galen (d. 200/216 AD) was the great medical authority whose works were taught in the medieval universities alongside those of Hippocrates. In the Middle Ages, university-educated physicians together with some surgeons made themselves into a self-consciously "learned" group of practitioners. They saw themselves as the followers of Galen and they fashioned a distinct identity for themselves separate from the other practitioners of the medical market place (empirics, herbalists, astrologers, and wise-women, etc.). Their stress on Galenic theory and practice was redoubled where, in the Renaissance, new works of Galen were discovered and old ones subjected to the new humanist scholarship.

The humanist culture of the renaissance believed that the era of the Greeks and Romans was possessed of the best knowledge as well as the best literature, art, and architecture. Medical research for Galenic physicians like Giambatista Da Monte (1498–1552), professor of the practice of medicine at the Padua, the foremost university for medicine in the sixteenth century, consisted in retrieving in its purest and fullest forms the medical teachings of Galen. Scholarship was a form of research, odd though that might seem today. Galenists, like Galen himself, saw the value of experience. Da Monte was one of the first to provide his students with bedside teaching (at the Padua hospital). Similarly, Andreas Vesalius (1514–1564 AD) had helped in the humanist retrieval of a pure Galen, and he also took to heart Galen's admonition to observe for himself and contradicted many of Galen's anatomical observations in his *De Humani Corporis Fabrica (On the Fabric of the Human Body)* (1543). In other words, while there were diehard Galenists, there were also more flexible, independent-minded Galenists.

The majority of Galenic practitioners would have presented themselves as possessing a mix of book learning and experience. Their group identity was often bolstered by membership of a city college of physicians as well as a shared university experience. They saw themselves as following Galen who believed that the best physician used both reason and experience. They stressed that they could reason about illness and its treatment (giving reasons why a treatment worked) while empirics only used experience, in the belief that as a remedy had worked in the past, it should do so also in the future. As discussed in this chapter, the ethical stance of Galenic practitioners was based on Hippocratic texts and on Galen's commentaries on those texts.

5. I adapt the phrase from Christopher Hill's "spiritualisation of the household" (Hill 1964, 443–81).

CHAPTER 28

THE DISCOURSES OF PRACTITIONERS IN EIGHTEENTH-CENTURY
FRANCE AND GERMANY

Mary Lindemann

I. INTRODUCTION

Medical behavior in the eighteenth century differed from that of the twentieth century. Although some ethicists maintain that the integration of modern science into medicine in the 1700s wrought the crucial change, that perspective properly applies only to the century's closing decades. For most of the long eighteenth century (1650–1815) in Europe no scientific medicine as we today understand it existed. Whereas one might speak of medicine as a "proto-science" in the eighteenth century and earlier in the sense that physicians based their social status and cultural prestige on appeals to intellectually authoritative sources, the idea of subjecting medical theory to any sort of scientific assessment was still rudimentary. The conflict between what science *could* do and what medicine *should* do simply did not pertain to medical situations before the 1790s.

Thomas Percival introduced the phrase, "medical ethics," in 1803 (see Chapter 36). One might therefore contend that before the phrase the thing itself did not exist (see also Chapter 46). Certainly, the sharp division of "ethics" and other forms of proper medical conduct was not apparent before 1803. What we might be tempted to call "medical ethics" for most of the eighteenth century

approximated more closely a form of deontology or the science of duty or moral obligations than a modern ethical system. Any review of medical ethics in the eighteenth century, therefore, must take into account several sometimes seemingly disparate topics: the paradigmatic model of a good physician; medical "politicking;" concepts of morality, etiquette, and manners (often subsumed under the rubric of *politesse*, or professional demeanor); the influence of the Enlightenment and of the philanthropic plans and endeavors for widespread improvements the Enlightenment fostered; the rules governing the relationship among physicians, between physicians and other practitioners, and between practitioners and patients; and the sick role. There is also a rough chronological progression here from the older image of the good doctor to that of the improving physicians, enlightened medical men, and budding clinicians of the late eighteenth and early nineteenth centuries. Likewise, the qualities of the physician shift from those of the scholarly and theoretical knowledge that were so highly prized in the late seventeenth and early eighteenth centuries to the new empiricism that stamped the ideal physician of late century. With the Hippocratic revival beginning in midcentury, empiricism, once disdained as the mark of quackery, became a term used positively. Indeed, "[e]mpiricism was thus shifting dramatically from the camp of quackery into the domain of socially useful and experimentally-oriented science" (Brockliss and Jones 1997, 668).

II. THE GOOD PHYSICIAN

The virtues associated with the figure of the "good physician" altered over the course of the eighteenth century. Although many of the features observable in the early years, such as piety and learnedness, persisted, other more novel factors combined to bolster already existing tendencies and especially underscored the function of the physician as a prime contributor to the common good and as a promoter of human happiness through health reform. A mix of the general ethical conduct expected of all persons and the more specialized rules governing the exercise of a particular occupation always characterized medicine as much as it did law and theology. Here, we will want first to examine the older image of the good physician and then observe how the Enlightenment and a burgeoning market culture wrought modifications.

Christianity determined or at least greatly influenced many of the attributes the good physician was to exhibit. Even in the more secularized climate of the mid-to-late eighteenth century, patients expected their healers be good Christians or, even more narrowly, exhibit "right belief." Baptista Codronchius' work on *Christian and Certain Healing* (*De christiana, ac tuta medendi ratione*) (1591) rehearsed the duties and attributes of a Christian physician in ways that would remain familiar throughout the century, although they would begin to appear somewhat shopworn and perhaps even slightly quaint by the 1770s and 1780s. As did many of his contemporaries and successors, Codronchi described proper ethics by detailing the incorrect behavior of physicians. The list is an unsurprising one: a physician should not abandon his patient until the course of treatment was finished; he should not supply abortions, contraceptives, aphrodisiacs, or poisons; and he should treat the poor for free. Physicians were to be collegial in their relationships with their fellows, cooperative but distanced in their dealings with other practitioners, and decorous in their management of patients. Physicians should not wrangle with their colleagues or should they treat their patients disdainfully. Codronchi deemed a series of other faults sins: working with a Jewish physician; lying before a court or in a legal case; or envying another his large or especially prosperous practice (Fischer-Homburger 1998, 91–95).

In the seventeenth and early eighteenth centuries, religion sometimes meant confession, as Girolamo Bardi suggested in his work on the *Political-Catholic Physician* (*Medicus politico-catholicus*, 1644). By the closing decades of the eighteenth century, however, commentators less frequently tied religion to orthodox Christianity and moved toward a kind of deism or more universalized religiosity, as one

might expect to have happened as religious toleration, skepticism, and enlightened modes of thought made their way. The Würzburg physician, Friedrich von Hoven, in his "medical profession of faith" stressed the centrality of Christianity to a physician's civic and occupational persona. He, however, adhered to what he called the "original form of Christianity," that is, a set of moral teachings (*Sittenlehre*). Hoven, like many others at the end of the century, found this type of religiosity most useful and proper for a physician (Hoven [1840] 1984, 385). In 1783, Konrad Friedrich Uden in his *Medical Politics* (*Medizinische Politik*) pointed out that the "physician is neither Jew nor Christian, but rather a human being (*Mensch*)" (quoted in Fischer 1933, II:73).

Others such as the Jewish physician, Rodrigo de Castro, based ethics "less on the traditional rules of conduct than on what was humanely possible." In his *Political Physician* (*Medicus politicus*, 1614), Castro describes what might be best understood as advice to the physician as to how to regulate his practice (Eckart 1984; Fischer-Homburger 1989, 96–98; see Chapter 26). This mixture of moral rules with endeavors (conscious or not) to elevate the status and advance the position of the physician typified the eighteenth century as the model of the good physician fused with issues of boundary definition. The medical paragon therefore adhered to precepts that were not perfectly coterminous with the teachings of either Christianity or religion per se: a physician should be "philosophical;" free of superstition; learned (that is, theoretically trained); and discreet (that is, exercise professional confidentiality, the *Schweigepflicht*). Several eighteenth-century books propagated these precepts and wove them into a more or less coherent code of conduct for physicians: Ferdinand Karl Weinhart, *The Physician as Official* (*Medicus officiosus*, 1703); Johann Bohn, *On the Twin Offices of the Physician, Namely the Clinical and the Forensic* (*De officio medici duplici, clinici nimirum ac forensis*, 1704); and, most famously, Friedrich Hoffmann (1660–1742), *Political Physician* (*Medicus politicus*, 1738). All of these sought to unite private and public virtues while proffering hints as to how a physician should conduct his day-to-day affairs. Late in the seventeenth century, Samuel Sorbière penned his *Advice to A Young Physician* (*Avis a un ieune medecin*, 1672). Despite its rather polemical tone and rambling style, it explained how the young physician should "conduct himself in the practice of medicine." Sorbière warned against too frank and candid a manner. He cautioned the novice that he would be "ill-received by the unlearned" and have to tolerate "the foibles of the ignorant." Moreover, he advised his readers to embrace a certain degree of guile, for the physician had "more need for politics than any other professional" and thus he should be willing to serve up a "few doses of nonsense" to cultivate his patients (Pleadwell [1950] 1977, 246–53). For his own taste, Sorbière preferred a man who combined the following traits:

I want neither the chatterer ... nor the taciturn one who has no elegance of discourse whatever; nor him who finds only mirth in mishaps; nor him who always knits his brow; nor him who wears too fine apparel; nor him who comes wearing dirty linen, and who sets all the dogs of the house to barking; nor him who with perfumes of musk and ambergris makes the ladies faint when he approaches; nor him who chews tobacco, or who exhales some more villainous odor. I would desire my physician to have a sweet breath, ... I should take pleasure in seeing him with a well-composed countenance, a little pensive, suggesting anxiety over my illness, study me quite leisurely, speak to me amiably, propose remedies with honest assurance, and finally tell me diverting stories. I do not require of a physician that he never converse about anything except medicine, and I am very glad that without losing sight of that subject, he make some digressions into the news of the day, or about ancient history, or about such other matters which he knows I am interested in; and I desire greatly that he unfold with good grace some pleasant story to make me laugh. (quoted in Pleadwell [1950] 1977, 261–62)

Hoffmann, writing in 1738, listed 200 rules that would beget a pleasing "elegance of spirit" (*"élégance de l'esprit"*) and "professional demeanor" (*"politesse professionnelle"*) (Elaut 1958, 179). His long list of precepts is an excellent example of medical deontology as a science of obligations. According to Hoffmann, the physician should be modest and Christian in his conduct. He should not be an atheist, although he should also not engage in vigorous religious disputations. Above all he should be a philosopher and a learned man. "He should be moderate, silent, should write as he speaks and [be] orderly in his habits ... courageous and not fearful" (Eckart 1984, 222). These qualities were not only moral ones, they were also "clever devices" to help the physician, and especially the beginner, comport himself in a way that would win him respect, status, and trade. Yet, although business was important, Hoffmann's text never lost sight of the well-being of patients as the primary goal.

These precepts reflected the newer influences of natural law and the Enlightenment in the development of professional urbanity. Natural law theory made explicit the connection between what might be viewed merely as manners/demeanor (*politesse*) and morality. Thus the distinction that John Gregory drew between "ethics" and "etiquette" – the first based on "real moral sentiments" and the second on "merely pretended sentiments" – fails to convey how important style, representation, and self-fashioning were for the formation of a special physician identity (Baker, Porter, and Porter 1993, 93). Manners, speech, and dress assisted physicians in distinguishing themselves from other practitioners and in lifting them above their putative inferiors.

In rural areas and small communities, residents judged practitioners on a variety of issues. Extramedical aspects of their lives – property ownership, family relationships, their reputations as debtors or creditors, piety, bearing, attire, and mannerisms – determined medical choices. Sometimes, admittedly, currying favor could degenerate into toadying to social superiors, to flattering women (insincerely!), and even to bribing officials. The line dividing shrewdness from corruption was not always distinct. In addition, and especially in cities, courts, and around universities, or among the aristocracy and the *haute bourgeoisie*, a newer social style, but one still often linked to older concepts of learnedness, offered physicians (as well as lawyers) a way to assert their autonomy and their right to a special social rank and power. As Johanna Geyer-Kordesch explicates:

> The point of professional urbanity lies in the adherence to the principles of civic virtue, as defined by natural law theory, where the professions are ethically bound to advance communal good rather than private fortune. Doctors and lawyers were not primarily money makers. Secularized natural law retained the value of responsibility in office as an ethical good. (Geyer-Kordesch 1993, 135)

Thus, the duties of the physician came to be inextricably linked to the common good. He could garner significant authority and status from an assiduous promotion of the general welfare. Scrupulous attention to his private patients was important here, but so, too, was his active involvement in civic affairs. Such participation could be official – in the capacity of a *physicus* or medical officer of health, for instance – or private and philanthropic involving him in an array of charitable and beneficial projects as well as in medical and hygienic reform.

Changes within medicine itself also helped modify the picture of the ideal physician and his ethical conduct. As Hippocratic thought revived near midcentury, medical expertise shifted toward an empiric mode, under the influence of Baconian scientific method (see also Chapter 30). *Expérience* (experimentation or experience) became the only valid test of a practice, a medicine, or a treatment (Brockliss and Jones 1997, 668). The good physician was now supposed to rely not only on his theoretical training but increasingly on his accumulated wisdom. Physicians gained such an accretion of knowledge by walking the wards of hospitals and by undergoing a course of clinical instruction. The rise and dispersion of clinical teaching might have been expected to raise ethical considerations about what the twentieth century calls patients' rights and informed consent (anachronistic terms, of course, for earlier times). Yet, it seems that opposition to "clinical experimentation" on patients among physicians and even among the nonmedical laity was muted although not completely unknown. The new clinics and clinical practitioners viewed patients as the legitimate objects of medical trials that would eventually benefit all humankind. Yet, although little ethical debate among physicians about the propriety of using patients (and especially charity patients) as pedagogical raw materials can be found, patients were not simply reduced to guinea pigs. Some clinical innovators, such as Ernst Gottfried Baldinger in Göttingen, sought to inculcate in pupils respect for their patients, admonishing his students to be understanding and kind. Several factors, moreover, always reined in the tendency to experiment recklessly. Lay hospital administrators or nursing sisters often shielded patients from certain procedures and treatments. Patients at home or patients in hospitals did not necessarily regard themselves as the hapless pawns of the surgeon's or physician's will – they dismissed physicians and left hospitals. Physicians, therefore, overwhelmingly practiced what one historian has labeled "safe science" on hospital inmates and sought "to balance appropriate conservatism in practice – one does *not* experiment on patients – with a properly innovative spirit – one *does* experiment judiciously on patients – or how else would medicine advance?" (Lawrence 1996, 21).

The rising star of empiricism, however, also had implications for how the boundaries between different kinds of healers would be drawn. "Enlightened, socially useful medical ideas should, it was held, be allowed to permeate through the whole of society" and this also could encourage "a feeling that health maintenance could actually be harmed by the learned medical practitioner" (Brockliss and Jones 1997, 669). Thus, in, such a climate, the lines separating licit from illicit practices, or the standards that elevated physicians over others became harder to perceive and preserve.

III. Setting Boundaries

Medical ethics in the eighteenth century has often been portrayed as deeply entangled with the growing professionalization of physicians. Professionalization was, however, in its infancy and thus is of only limited utility in explaining eighteenth-century trends in medical ethics. Although there is no doubt that physicians tried to strengthen the divisions separating them from other practitioners and to claim for themselves some more elevated status (mostly on the basis of academic training), these efforts did not directly lead to standards that correspond to those we recognize as typifying the modern professions. Equally clear is that although perhaps in England physicians' status and income rose markedly (earning the century the somewhat misleading reputation of a "golden age"), the situation on the continent remained less auspicious. Von Hoven, who later in life headed the famous

Julius Hospital in Würzburg, related in his memoirs a fairly typical story of a long and penurious struggle in his early years to make ends meet and build up a practice. For each physician who, like von Hoven, succeeded, many others failed entirely or lived from a patchwork of employments of which medicine was only one and not necessarily the most important or profitable (Hoven 1984 [1840], 91; Lindemann 1996, 79–81, 134–39).

Achieving a good practice was for physicians and all other practitioners closely joined to a need to establish boundaries and have them respected. The conflict between medicine as an art or calling and medicine as a business and as a indicator of status and cultural authority plagued the eighteenth-century practitioner. Many doctors swayed uneasily between the poles of "medicus politicus" and "Machiavellus medicus" (Eckart 1984). Part of the tension arose from the fact that physicians in no way enjoyed a monopoly of medical practice, for patients were medically promiscuous and governments rarely protected doctors from competition. Physicians competed with licensed and authorized practitioners and with a horde of others for their customers.

Much of the ethical content of eighteenth-century medical writings, therefore, involved delineating the appropriate sphere of action for each type of healer. Lester King identified, for instance, "one major root" of our contemporary medical ethics in "the eighteenth-century problem of competition." (King 1958, 232). Throughout the eighteenth century, most continental practitioners – with the significant *exception* of physicians – were organized in guilds. This official division of tasks, known as corporatism, produced what has been called for France a "differentiated medical community," that is a community divided into several specific occupations, each with its characteristic rights and privileges, distinct fields of action, and proper means of defending its territory against the trespass of others. In most of central Europe, surgeons, barber-surgeons, and apothecaries enjoyed guild protection. Likewise in these areas, physicians had no corporate structure and did not act as gatekeepers to the profession as they did in France and England to some, albeit imperfect, degree. As medical colleges (*collegia medica*) came to be established during the course of the eighteenth century in many countries, they functioned as boards of health and habitually exercised the right to license practitioners. The eighteenth-century state guaranteed physicians no monopoly of practice, although in most places they were the only ones permitted to engage in internal medicine. Physicians were also, it should be noted, forbidden to violate the territories of other healers. The Germans called this encroachment *Pfuscherei*, a word borrowed from guild language to denote someone who worked without guild sanction. Gradually, however, and increasingly toward the end of the century, the term shifted to *Quacksalberei* which bore a stronger connotation of incompetence and not merely infringement. Similarly, the French spoke of *impéritie* or incapacity (Ramsey 1988, 18, 48).

Otherwise the boards of health had little to say about moral considerations or standards of conduct, although they might piously urge practitioners to work peacefully with one another (Huisman 1992, 427–29). For most of the eighteenth century neither the state nor medical groups saw much need to develop or enforce a code of ethics specially gauged for physicians who were expected "to ground their behavior in the larger and venerable discourse on manners (Fissel, 1993, 42). Medical ordinances or boards of health might sometimes drafted fee tables and this sort of regulation, too, served a ethical function. In some parts of France provincial or local governments fixed costs. For instance, in 1734 the *parlement* of Poitiers set fees for physicians in the city of Poitiers and mandated maximums (Ramsey 1988, 62). Of course, the assignment of appropriate charges sought to achieve several goals simultaneously: (1) to prevent gouging and the unfavorable public opinion that accompanied it; (2) to suggest the limits of fair prices; and (3) to provide a living wage for all practitioners and not only physicians.

New market forces also affected medical ethics profoundly. The growth of medical advertising and the quite amazing rise in the number and variety of medicines, nostrums, and cures thus made available to the public might have been expected to raise issues of appropriate conduct. The debate about the propriety of medical advertising was, however, complicated by the fact that learned practitioners and respectable medical men might publicize their remedies just as vigorously as the "quacks" they fiercely castigated. The French nonphysician, Jean Ailhaud, in the middle of the eighteenth century, advertised his purgative powders widely and was condemned by physicians and boards of health across the continent. Jean-Adrien Helvétius, court physician in France, also touted his medicines unashamedly and, by the 1720s, was selling over 100,000 doses annually. Thus the ethical debate about advertising and about whether a physician should be a businessman was an especially convoluted one. The simple fact that one advertised was not alone sufficient to earn the censure of learned medicine, although that tendency grew stronger in the late eighteenth century. If quacks were more likely to publicize their wares and puff their talents, a university-trained physician did not necessarily risk his reputation either with the public or his colleagues if he, too, employed new marketing techniques (Brockliss and Jones, 1997, 652–54, 731–34).

IV. PHILANTHROPY, IMPROVEMENT, AND REFORM

The eighteenth-century Enlightenment activated a series of broad movements directed toward the betterment of human society. In the larger forums for reform – in economics, morals, social life, and letters – physicians often assumed conspicuous positions. Ten percent of the members of provincial academies in France, for instance, were medical men. Reforms in the narrower arena of medical care, of course, linked most nicely to the progress of a new type of behavior for physicians that expected them to be engaged actively in furthering the general good. Moreover, "Enlightenment egalitarianism" helped fire "the zeal shown by eighteenth-century medical theorists . . . to expand the field of corporative medical practice into hitherto neglected areas" (Brockliss and Jones 1997, 391, 441). Improving the health of the people was intimately tied to the statist concern for a multitudinous and industrious population, but it was also a field in which physicians could fruitfully labor to amass cultural and social authority. The cultivation of human happiness in the eighteenth century almost always included provisions for bettering the physical condition of the people. In this way health became part of a political agenda. Physicians' duties to the state, or rather to the state's inhabitants, expanded correspondingly. During epidemics physicians were now expected to be on the spot, diligently working to combat the disease, battling on the front-line, so to speak. Flight, once a condoned option for physicians in the sixteenth or even seventeenth centuries (when *pestmeesters* or plague-surgeons temporarily replaced physicians) was no longer considered fitting. (Of course, not all physicians had pusillanimously fled in the face of epidemics.)

The concept of the enlightened physician remained "still an ideal" in the 1770s and 1780s, but it was an example that had worked its way into the thought and even actions of a whole generation (see also Chapter 30). The secretary of the French Royal Society of Medicine, Vicq d'Azur, published short biographies on Society members that described the new model physician in heroic terms. "Above all, they were presented as devoted friends of humanity: half were said to have met their deaths at the disease-face, fighting epidemics in the deepest countryside on the behalf of everyman" (Brockliss and Jones 1997, 475). In central Europe, Johann Peter Frank projected an analogous image of the physician as the ultimate self-sacrificing civil servant – the medical policeman – who was a true hygienic hero and sometimes martyr (Frank 1779–1827; Fischer 1933, vol. 2, 125–29).

Charitable work – in secular terms of advancing the common good and rescuing a portion of the population from unprofitable destitution – became a standard ethical accoutrement for an enlightened physician who aspired to honor, distinction, and affluence. The number of philanthropic projects for promoting the common good that physicians took up was large. A few examples suffice to show how the involvement of physicians in such tasks, where they often toiled alongside prominent community members, raised their status and helped them gain influence as promoters of the public good as well as allowing them to forge ties of friendship and mutual interest with wealthy and influential persons. Typical, although by no means unique, was the domiciliary care system set up in Hamburg in the 1760s and 1770s. Physicians volunteered to visit the poor in their dwellings free of charge and apothecaries promised to distribute medicines as cheaply as possible. Other plans of domiciliary care developed elsewhere, but such public initiatives on the part of physicians were not limited to either Germany or to visiting care. The concept of working for the needy, or participating in such public/private forms of poor relief, tightly wove itself into the self-image of the enlightened physician. (Fischer 1799).

Ethical problems, however, troubled schemes floated to extend medical care on a broad scale. Several initiatives in the eighteenth century intended to produce new kinds of medical practitioners: the *routiniers* or priest-doctors. The idea underlying all of them was to offer a level – admittedly a low level – of medical care to more people. Newly devised visiting care programs or programs of medical care connected to established systems of poor relief drew mixed reviews. Medical practitioners who were *not* involved often protested the effects such programs had on their clienteles. Many physician-critics insisted that *routiniers* often did more harm than good and strewed about misinformation. Others pointed out the dangers trained medical personnel – and especially doctors – ran when they engaged in these endeavors. Visiting care was, for example, sometimes held responsible for the untimely deaths of young and promising physicians who, in entering the hovels of the sick, contracted the infectious diseases that killed them. Physicians would be, it was maintained, better protected in hospitals. Here, too, the Christian and civic duty incumbent on medical practitioners to assist the needy and succor the ill conflicted with practitioners' own well-being, both physical and financial. All such activities exceeded the older, more casual dictum of *pro bono* work.

Another aspect of enlightenment involved the propagation of medical knowledge to "the people," a practice that also raised quasiethical issues. Advice literature is quite old, but like medical advertising it, too, multiplied under the banner of enlightenment. Health instructions proliferated like mushrooms. Some were written by physicians, such as Christian Friedrich Richter's *Short and Clear Instruction* (1705), William Buchan's *Domestic Medicine* (1769), or Samuel Tissot's *Advice to the People in General, With Regard to Their Health* (1761); some by those distrustful of learned medicine, such as John Wesley's *Primitive Physick* (1747); some by government officials in attempts to preserve community health, such as Bernard Faust's *Catechism of Health* (*Gesundheits-Katechismus*) (1794) that was introduced in schools in Hesse; and some circulated with the boxes of remedies the French state distributed.

Many physicians were deeply involved in shaping a broader program of popular medical enlightenment. They drafted health catechisms and agitated for the introduction of basic health information into schools and rural communities. Governments and clerics (Catholic and Protestants alike) often labored with an almost evangelical fervor in the task of composing and distributing popular health manuals. Among physicians and the medical press, however, opinion divided. Obviously, as the aforementioned list indicates, many physicians authored texts, writing them, of course, in the vernacular but also taking care to cast them in a manner and language familiar to the common people or at least accessible to an educated laity that would then act as a conduit flushing medical enlightenment out into the mainstream. Still many others felt that such efforts were naive, ill advised, and probably even dangerous. First, such literature was suspected of putting the razor in the monkey's hand, of doing greater harm than good. Second, by catering to a public that then embarked on self-doctoring, physicians were committing a form of mass suicide. The debate over the composition and distribution of medical enlightenment, therefore, had important ethical dimensions.

Likewise, the application of new techniques, therapies, or drugs begot novel ethical predicaments and stimulated ethical debate. The introduction of smallpox inoculation – one of the Enlightenment's most cherished goals – was the most contested of the eighteenth century. Several physicians began inoculating almost simultaneously on the Continent in the 1720s and 1730s. Inoculation in its early days was, in many respects, an experimental process: surgeons and physicians tried out different methods of "ingrafting" smallpox. One generally accepted technique was to make small, fairly deep gashes into the flesh of an arm or leg and then insert pustulous matter from an active case of smallpox into them. The inoculee then developed a true case of smallpox; hopefully, a mild one. Death rates from inoculation were indeed far lower than in natural cases.

Although opposition to smallpox inoculation was never insubstantial, historians have sometimes vastly exaggerated the range and virulence of resistance. Undeniably, the procedure raised a series of ethical questions. Popular antagonism reflected religious uneasiness about man's presumptuous interference with God's will. Some foes of inoculation insisted that smallpox was the result of original sin and thus an "inborn, rooted, and necessary evil" that children must experience. Lay people also based their hostility to the procedure on the quite sensible argument that inoculation could (and occasionally did) spread smallpox. Physicians frequently shared these more general concerns, but also raised additional objections. Although some medical men were warm, even passionate supporters of inoculation, others were less convinced of the medical benefits of the procedure. Some feared that inoculation could transmit other diseases, such as syphilis, gonorrhea, scurvy, and tumors; others doubted whether the immunity granted by inoculation was full and permanent (it was); and still others felt that it was unethical for a doctor to induce a disease intentionally even in a good cause for the end did not justify the means. Whereas many physicians and numerous prominent lay people, such as Voltaire, were fervent proponents of inoculation, other equally esteemed medical practitioners refused to accept the method. Anton de Haën in Vienna felt a case of smallpox effectively purged lethal poisons from the body and that, therefore, every child was better off for having contracted the disease naturally. Some physicians also doubted that the few then existing trials were sufficiently unambiguous to justify a blanket introduction of inoculation or to warrant having it mandated by the state.

Smallpox inoculation was only part of the far broader program of eighteenth-century experimentation that included self-experimentation, animal testing, and research on certain populations such as slaves, prisoners, and the poor. Although no protocols guided eighteenth-century experimenters, some generally accepted, rough-and-ready rules for how trials or *essais* should be conducted developed over the course of time. "Witnessing" was, Schiebinger observes, "an important part of the procedure," as were signed testimonials and certificates (Schiebinger, 2003; Maehle 1999a). Here, however, the weight of the ethical debate rested on determining the validity of experimental results rather than on the morality of using certain groups and individuals as test cases.

V. Practitioners and Patients

The relationship between practitioners and patients is perhaps the most elusive part of eighteenth-century medical ethics. By the end of the century, the image of the physician's role had modified in several ways. Although he was still expected to be erudite, the Enlightenment had emphasized the importance of a humane and sympathetic medicine as well as a learned one. Enlightenment humanitarianism therefore affected the ways in which the physician was to interact with the public and also the part the patient should assume.

Much has been written about the patient's role and the sick role. Talcott Parsons addressed the reciprocity inherent in the patient–doctor relationship. When ill, sick people are not expected to fulfill their normal social and economic obligations, but they are expected to desire a return to health and to comply with the directives of medical experts to secure that goal (Parsons 1951). In two influential articles, N. D. Jewson documented a shift from what he calls "bedside medicine," in which the patient controlled the medical consultation, to "hospital medicine," in which the patient was increasingly subordinated to a

medical authority, especially that of a physician (Jewson 1976). Even if that alteration was never quite so pronounced or unidirectional as Jewson suggests, the relationship between the patient and physician at the bedside clearly changed in the eighteenth century. In a time-honored way, physicians continued to lament the interference of family, kin, and neighbors in their consultations with patients. Patients, however, doggedly exerted their right and the right of their chosen friends and family members to take part in treatments. At least for most of the eighteenth century, physicians seemed to recognize that they held a fairly weak hand vis-à-vis their patients and that they were particularly disadvantaged in dealing with the well-to-do. Physicians, apparently, sometimes accepted the active way patients entered into their own cures and authors often advised their readers how to circumvent obstacles deftly. Moreover, it is ahistorical to cast the patient–practitioner encounter solely in the form of a power relationship. Patients and practitioners often collaborated and there is much evidence to suggest that physicians encouraged this teamwork and listened closely to patients' narratives (either oral or written). Physicians sometimes proved quite amenable to modifying courses of treatment at patients' bequests. A study of the gynecological cases of Johann Storch, who practiced in Erlangen at mid-century, revealed a world of concepts and expectations shared between a physician and his female patients. Fitting conduct involved respect for patients' insights and their "feelings," which meant here not their emotions so much as their visceral perceptions of what was wrong with them and of how their bodies functioned (Duden 1987). If that sensitivity tended to fade with the rise of pathological anatomy in the late century, it never disappeared entirely and remained pivotal in the interaction between patients and practitioners.

Eighteenth-century propriety dictated that practitioners tended to observe and listen more than touch and prod their patients (especially their female patients). A physician might palpate a hernia or feel a lump (even a breast lump), but rarely did he probe orifices (especially female ones) with an intrusive finger. As the century wore on, physicians – literally – approached their patients more closely. Samuel Vogel in outlining how to do a good examination pointed out the necessity of at least some hands-on experience and suggested ways in which this could proceed methodically and discreetly (von Vogel 1796). Authors sometimes emphasized that practitioners should carefully define unfamiliar or technical terms. Thus many tried to bridge the gap they perceived dividing them from their audiences. Joseph Gotthard enjoined physicians to converse with their patients in local dialects (if necessary) and select expressions that "do not alienate them." Part of this might be read as a condescending approach, but it also betokened a recognition that the obligation of a physician was didactic, pastoral, and beneficent as much as medical and that those functions remained, even at the end of the century, integral parts of correct conduct (Gotthard 1793, 60, 170).

Karl Uden in 1783 offered a fairly complete discussion of the behavior of the physician faced with a variety of patients: the socially superior; women (and especially "ladies"); children; and the elderly. The "first rule" was always to act "properly" and be "diligent," but Uden also acknowledged that certain circumstances – such as the size of a city or competing demands – meant that a physician often came into conflict with his conscience (Uden 1783, 231). Uden was no naïf: he knew that "the more important the patient, the more glory one garners" from his or her patronage. In attending women, the physician must always be chaste and circumspect; children must be "cleverly" as well as carefully doctored; and in cases of fevers, the physician had a duty to protect himself as much as possible (Uden 1783, 257, 262, 289, 298). In respect to payment, Uden exhibited a characteristic mixture of practicality and *noblesse oblige*. To strive for great profit was simply "disgraceful." Yet, Uden was very aware that as patients recovered their willingness to pay declined and the physician was well advised to select a good moment to discuss compensation. If it was "unseemly" for a physician to ask for payment in advance, it was even less appropriate to conclude a contract (as, he sneered, typified "charlatans, quacks, barber-surgeons, and bathmasters"). Still, it was not unreasonable to expect to be paid. Of course, the physician must not pick an inappropriate time or place or pester the patient's relatives or friends. Moreover the payment of a physician must be "honorable" (*ehrenvoll*) and not be regarded as a wage (*Tagelohn*). In short, the physician should not present a bill listing "items," such as visits, consultations by letter, and prescriptions, but rather should submit a simple statement of total costs. When a patient refused to pay, there was apparently little to be done if the physician wished to retain his position of moral superiority (Uden 1783, 315–18).

Interestingly enough, this idea of not working for "wages" or "under contract" may have become more widespread in the eighteenth century than it had been previously. Although we do not have a great deal of evidence for contractual relationships between physicians and patients, Gianna Pomata's research on Bologna reveals that throughout the sixteenth and seventeenth centuries, patients and healers commonly contracted for cures. These binding agreements formed part of an "ancient horizontal model of healing" in which patients and practitioners accorded – often in writing – on the terms and stipulated the length of a "cure." Only when the practitioner actually fulfilled the "promise of cure" was his fee due. By the end of the eighteenth century, as Uden's commentary nicely illustrates, such contracts ceded place to a newer position "that medical service should be remunerated irrespective of results" (Pomata 1998, xvii). This shift, then, Pomata interprets as being as critical to the advancement of modern professional dominance as were the implementation of medical technologies and the founding of professional interest groups.

VI. CONCLUSION

The eighteenth century, therefore, blended older precepts of ethics based on Christian values and the idea of a calling with newer attitudes engendered by economic and political realities and the advent of the Enlightenment. These newer forces affected the conduct of practitioners and patients alike and recast the relationship between practitioners, their clients, academic medicine, and market forces.

CHAPTER 29

THE DISCOURSES OF PRACTITIONERS IN EIGHTEENTH-CENTURY SPAIN

Diego Gracia

I. INTRODUCTION

In the year 1700, a member of the French Bourbon royal family ascended the Spanish throne, ending two centuries of Habsburg rule. This dynastic change was of vital importance for Spain because it placed eighteenth-century Spanish culture, including philosophy, medicine, and ethics, under French influence, inspiring in the second half of the eighteenth century a pro-Enlightenment elite to modernize all aspects of Spanish life and culture. Their challenge to traditional ideologies culminated in a collision between the traditionalists and the Enlightenment, the consequences of which remain visible even today.

This clash of ideologies sets the context in which a new philosophical approach to medicine arose, creating a literature that we would today characterize as "medical ethics." This chapter contrasts this new medical ethics, grounded in the experientially based medicine and championed by partisans of the Enlightenment, with the traditional, pre-Enlightenment texts of moral theology. Its final topic is medical etiquette, as explored in texts written by physicians.

II. THE VOICE OF THEOLOGIANS: MEDICINE AND MORALS

Roman Catholic cultures have traditionally reserved the analysis of the moral problems related with life and death, the use of the body, and sexuality to priests and theologians. What came to be called "medical ethics" was considered a part of moral theology. Catholic moral theology employed a mix of casuistry, Canon Law, and moral reasoning to address moral questions. Texts were not written to be read by physicians but by priests, who used them to evaluate behavior during the sacrament of confession, which required them to act as judges and impose penances. On questions of medical morality there was therefore no clear line between moral theology and Canon Law (see Chapters 12 and 14).

Casuistry was widespread in sixteenth- and seventeenth-century Spanish moral theology, especially among members of the Society of Jesus or Jesuits. The first great casuist was the Spanish Jesuit, Juan Azor (1535–1603). His *Institutionum Moralium* (*Institutes of Morals*) were published in Rome between 1600 and 1611 (Azor, 1603, 1607). Casuistry introduced a new approach to moral theology, in contrast to the methods used by Thomas Aquinas in his *Summa Theologica* (Thomas Aquinus 1951–1952). Aquinas grounded moral theology in an account of the virtues and the vices. Casuistic moral reasoning was more concerned with precepts than with abstract virtues. Following the precedents of the Ten Commandments and Sacraments, casuistry identified specific obligations that resolved ethically conflictual cases (Jonsen and Toulmin 1988, 154–55; Keenan and Shannon 1995). This focus on precepts, specific guides to behavior in specific circumstances, gave casuistry a strong juridical and canonical orientation.

Casuistry, which has frequently been characterized as "baroque morality," was the dominant method of moral theology during the seventeenth century. One of its most representative figures was Antonio de Escobar y Mendoza (1589–1669) (Escobar 1652–1663), who was strongly criticized by Pascal in their *Provincial Letters* (Pascal 1987, 89). Throughout this period there was a pitched battle between the different "moral systems." The system called "probabalism" appealed to the newly developed idea of mathematical probability, "mathematizing" classical moral and legal probabilism (Hacking 1975). One question that occupied theorists of probabalism was the level of probability needed to make a wise decision. The distinctive feature of probabalism is that it analyzed questions by weighing the opinions of authorities, rather than by assessing arguments independent of the authority of the persons who made them. Is it necessary to follow the most probable opinion? Is the opinion defended by the majority of the wise and clever the most appropriate? Alternatively, can an opinion be considered acceptable and prudent to follow, if it is maintained by a minority of wise people? Those who thought that it was prudent to follow the most probable opinion were called "probabiliorists" (from the Latin comparative). "Tutiorists" believed that only the most secure opinion should be followed, whereas "laxists," in contrast, held that all opinions defended by moralists can be followed, because at least they have an authority behind them.

These controversies influenced not only moral theology but also many treatises written by physicians. Pedro Leòn Gomez, a doctor who wrote a treatise about pulses, discusses the degree of probability that a medical opinion had to have to be considered morally acceptable. To start with, he discarded options that had very little probability, that is, laxisms, for "No matter how learned and good a doctor may be, he cannot follow the opinion of one only author when it opposes the common belief of others" (Gomez 1768, 82). His thesis is that one can only follow the most probable opinion because this is most probably the correct opinion. The doctor "must follow or inform of the most probable opinion regarding the precept, because there is no probable opinion (in other words, which can be followed without sinning) which

favours freedom" (Gomez 1768, 82). Regarding drugs, he holds: "Even though there may be some happy experiences of certain medicines, without the patient's appropriate knowledge it can't be understood that it will be positive for him [. . .] If there should be other medicines with which the patient would be cured with more security and celerity, doctors should never stop using them, without bothering heavily their conscience" (Gomez 1768, 80). In opposition to Gomez, Father Lorenzo Zambrano y Goizueta (Álvarez-Sierra 1963, 569), a member of the scientific society known as the Medical Union of Sevilla, anticipating the later development of clinical empiricism, considered it licit to follow an opinion based on experience, "even though it may be opposite to the common opinion of authorities" (Granjel 1979, 84).

Treatises on medicine and morals written during this period had a common structure. They first analyzed the moral obligations generated by the Ten Commandments of the Decalog. They would later consider the so-called six Church commandments of the Roman Catholic tradition (to keep the Sundays and Holy Days of obligation holy, by hearing Mass and resting from servile work; to keep the days of fasting and abstinence appointed by the Church; to go to confession at least once a year; to receive the Blessed Sacrament at least once a year and that at Easter or thereabouts; to contribute to the support of our pastors; not to marry within a certain degree of kindred nor to solemnize marriage at the forbidden times), and finally the moral problems related to the administration of the seven Sacraments. Matters of medical morality are addressed under the rubric of various of the Ten Commandments, including the fifth (Thou shall not kill), the sixth and the ninth (problems associated with reproduction and sexuality), the seventh (which prohibits theft, and therefore, excessive fees), and the eighth (not to lie, which implies an obligation not to reveal secrets). Medical morality is also addressed by certain Commandments of the Church, including the second (the duty of confession when life is in danger) and the fourth (fasting when requested by the Church). Medical morality also intersects with the administration of several Sacraments, including baptism (discussing the problems posed by spontaneously aborted fetuses and monsters or infants with anatomical deformities), marriage (marriage in the context of such physical impediments as impotence), confession and communion (especially when the patient's death is imminent), and extreme unction or last rites (which raises the question of the doctor's duty to step aside and allow the administration of the ultimate sacrament).

A paradigmatic example of the application of casuistry to medicine was Paolo Zacchia's (1584–1659) masterpiece, *Quaestiones Medico-Legales* (*Medica-Legal Questions*, Zacchia 1621–1625), which remained influential into the eighteenth century. Following the casuistic method, the book provides answers to hundreds of practical questions.

For instance, he analyzes the legal and ethical problems related to the doctor's fee, summarizing the opinions of his seventeenth-century colleagues, together with the answers supplied by law and ethics (Magyar 1997). In the eighteenth century important, casuistic manuals appeared, including *Embriologia Sacra* (*Sacred Embryology*) published in the year 1745 by Francesco Emanuello Cangiamila (1702–1763), which was translated into Spanish (Cangiamila 1774). The book is an obstetrics manual for the use of priests and doctors concerning the theological implications of the embryo in utero. It considers such questions as the justification of abortion, death in utero, Caesarean section, baptism of fetuses, and so forth. There is much discussion concerning the point at which the soul informs the embryo, that is, at what point the fetus becomes a person. Further evidence of the significance accorded to this work was that King Carlos III sent a Latin copy of it to all of the Spanish bishops, asking them to keep it present in the practice of their ministry and giving them the order "to put everything at their hand for preachers and priests to adopt its doctrine, regarding the enormous spiritual and corporal need and utility that could be found in this medical and theological knowledge being extended to small towns that often have no doctors, surgeons, or matrons, because of the lack of funds to establish a decent dotation" or endowment (Riesco 1848, 6).

The most important eighteenth-century Spanish treatise on medical morality was written by Antonio José Rodriguez (1703–1777), a self-taught Cistercian monk, who was neither a theologian nor a physician, but who was nonetheless enormously prolific. He wrote a four-volume treatise on the subject, titled *Nuevo aspecto de theologia medico-moral* (*New Perspectives of Medico-Moral Theology*) (Rodriguez 1742–1760). As a manual for confessors, it follows the order of Sacraments, although in the unsystematic fashion of a self-taught author. It addresses such questions as baptizing abortuses and deformed fetuses and the question of "nocturnal pollution." Another question addressed, which is recurrent in canonical literature, is whether the severity of an illness can excuse the faithful from the obligation to fast. It is indicative of the mindset of the era that fasting was treated by complete monographic studies throughout the century (Gomez 1744; Rodriguez 1748; Nieto de Piña 1779). In his analysis of specific problems, Rodriguez uses the logic of probabilism to order authors' opinions as true, probable, or improbable. For example, the Twenty-Fourth Paradox addresses paradoxes related to fasting under the title, "It is probable that it is improbable and offensive to maintain that those obligated not to eat meat have no other obligations to fast" (Rodriguez 1742–1760, Vol. 1. Paradoxa XXIV). Unlike the new Enlightenment ideals, the mentality displayed in Rodriguez's work is conservative and absolutist. He rejected Enlightenment ideals as hostile to Christianity and, therefore, repeatedly attacked

Hobbes, Locke, Diderot, Rousseau, and other Enlightenment thinkers (Abellán 1984, 155–56).

III. The Enlightenment: Fighting Superstition and Speculation and Promoting a New Empirically and Clinically Oriented Medicine

Spanish adherents of the Enlightenment challenged beliefs that they characterized as "superstition" and "speculation" in every sphere of Spanish culture, especially medicine. Popular medicine was seemingly full of groundless beliefs and superstitions, which needed to be replaced with scientifically grounded views of health and disease. Benito Jerónimo Feijoo (1676–1764), a Benedictine monk, devoted himself to achieving this goal. His huge literary production is brought together in the nine volumes of his *Teatro crítico universal* (*Universal Critical Theater*, Feijoo 1726–1740) and in five other volumes, *Cartas eruditas* (*Erudite Letters*, Feijoo 1742–1760). Others, such as Pedro Martín Martinez (1684–1734) challenged the remnants of the nonempirical Galenic scholastic tradition, proposing a new scepticism that he identified with the clinically oriented Hippocratic tradition.

> Assessing the shortcomings of syllogisms and humane discourses, some put everything in doubt. They permitted themselves to be convinced only by divine revelation, by observational experience of events in nature, or by first principles of reason in metaphysical considerations. We call such people *"reformed sceptics"* and I belong to this group. (Martinez 1730, 3)

The appeal to experience, rather than speculation, derived from the work of the English philosopher, John Locke (1632–1704), whose ideas were disseminated by Etienne Condillac's (1715–1780) *Essay about the Origin of Human Knowledge* (*Essai sur l'origine des connaissances humaines*, 1746) and *Treatise on the Sensations* (*Traité des sensations*, 1754). Locke's English ideas were thus filtered through French philosophes to influence Spanish intellectuals (Abellán 1981, 512–26), especially in medicine. Locke himself was a doctor and a personal friend of Thomas Sydenham (1624–1689), who invented the modern concept of disease and emphasized the role of clinical experience (Sydenham 1676). Clinical empiricism acquired great importance for Spanish doctors during the eighteenth century. The clinical empiricists envisioned a medicine grounded in experience, logic, and methodology, eschewing the traditional medicine of abstraction and a priori speculation that lacked an experiential base. The empiricists believed that it was essential to start from specific observations and to proceed from them inductively, following a disciplined analytical method. This method consisted in identifying clear and distinct elementary sensory impressions, from which complex ideas could be formed by combination, elaboration, and synthesis. The diagnosis of diseases was to become a rational process based on objective data. The identification of these data, the medical analogue of Locke and Condillac's primary sensations, required a rigorous, new Semiology that would, in turn, serve as the foundation of a new clinical medicine. In this new Enlightenment spirit, clinical empiricism was introduced into eighteenth-century Spanish medical education, changing the practice of medicine and its ethics.

The medical schools of the day were still wedded to nonempirical, dogmatic Hippocratic and Galenic traditions. The clinical empiricist revolution required a different environment. For this reason, pro-Enlightenment kings promoted new medical institutions outside universities (Peset and Peset 1974, 259–82). The two most influential were the Royal Colleges of Surgeons (founded in Cadiz (1748), Barcelona (1760), Madrid (1780), Palma de Mallorca (1790), Burgos (1799) and Santiago (1799)) and the Academies of Medicine (founded in Madrid (1732), Cartagena (1740), Jaen (1756), Malaga (1757), Barcelona (1770), and Cadiz (1785)).

IV. MEDICAL ETIQUETTE

It was generally understood and accepted in eighteenth-century Spain that treatises on the professional morals of physicians should be written by theologians, not by doctors. Doctors, nonetheless, addressed questions of urbanity and etiquette, that is, the proper of physicians during the exercise of their professional activities. The first rule of these medical treatises is always the same: physicians must be "good Christians." This means that the first obligation of a doctor, "above all of the rest," is to follow faithfully the precepts and norms established in the moral theology treatises, a prudent approach during an era in which the watchful eye of the Inquisition was ignored at one's peril.

The texts about urbanity and etiquette drew their precepts from Hippocratic texts, including the books titled *Physician* (Hippocrates 1923b, 311–13), *Decorum* (Hippocrates 1923b, 279–301) and *Precepts* (Hippocrates 1923a, 313–33), and chapter 38 of the book of Sirach (the Apocrypha), which addresses the physician's role and the moral regard with which physicians should be held. The Hippocratic ideal of a good physician dominates these texts, appearing regularly in all medical books of this period (see Chapters 23, 24). "The dignity of a physician requires that he should look healthy [. . .] He must be clean in person, well dressed, and anointed with sweet-smelling unguents that are not in any way suspicious."

He must "not only be silent, but also of a great regularity of life [. . .], gentleman of character, and being this he must be grave and kind to all" (Hippocrates 1923b, 311). These are the typical precepts of medical etiquette followed by the Spanish doctors. In any case, they introduce novelties, as the duty of telling the truth, except in some dangerous situations. Francisco Suárez de Rivera (1680–1754) (Suárez de Rivera 1729) provides the following suggestions to the literate surgeon: "To tell the truth, to do pilgrimage, to study continuously, to have many carefully selected books, and to be logical, and dialectic, and finally, to be philosophical and metaphysical." The good surgeon must also be a good observer of a disease's manifestations, following the great book of nature. "As real minister and interpreter of nature, you must read, reconsider and observe in the book of this lady" (Granjel 1979, 84–85).

Although Hippocratic ideals are present in surgical and medical treatises, they appear more explicitly in those concerned with behavior or ethics. Hippocratic thinking is the main focus of texts composed by Fernando Oxea (Oxea 1777), Pedro Leon Gomez (Gomez 1744, 1768), Juan de Adeva y Pacheco (Adeva 1753), and Antonio Pérez de Escobar (Pérez de Escobar 1788). All of them are concerned with the social prestige of the profession and the reputation of medicine. They also consider it necessary for professionals to be able to remain calm and respectful in every action. This was not easy in certain circumstances, as for example the situation in which several doctors have to give a diagnosis about one and the same patient, a contentious situation analyzed by Sebastian de Acuña in a separate treatise (Acuña 1746).

V. CONCLUSION

The eighteenth century was the period in which the ideals of Enlightenment appeared in the Spanish culture. They introduced a more secularized idea of the world, opposed to the traditional one, based on religious grounds. All the century was a continuous struggle between these two conceptions of life. In medicine, the clash took place between the old speculative medicine and the new clinical empiricism. In ethics, the struggle apposed obedience and paternalism to freedom and autonomy. This battle was waged in the specific field of medical ethics by priests and theologians, which monopolized the literature on moral matters related to medicine. Physicians were reduced to deal only with questions related to medical etiquette and the promotion of professional excellence, following the Hippocratic and Galenic traditions.

CHAPTER 30

THE DISCOURSES OF PRACTITIONERS IN EIGHTEENTH-CENTURY BRITAIN

Laurence B. McCullough

I. INTRODUCTION

The discourses of British practitioners in the early eighteenth century focused on relationships among practitioners, in response to the intensely competitive, entrepreneurial world of medicine at the time. This has been labeled "etiquette" in the history of medicine and bioethics literature, implying that the subject matter of this discourse was practitioners' behavior toward other practitioners, which was largely the case, and also implying that there was no intellectual content to it, which was not the case. There was indeed intellectual content to this discourse of medical morality, namely, an ethos of personal honor or self-regard. By the middle of the century a distinctive discourse about moral virtues of physicians begins to emerge in Scotland, at the medical school of the University of Edinburgh, to which was joined an embryonic philosophy of medicine, from Francis Bacon (1561–1626), and a discourse about the intellectual virtues of physicians. There was, however, no clear intellectual foundation for this discourse of the intellectual and moral virtues of physicians.

By the latter third of the century, a philosophically sophisticated discourse about medical morality emerged. A product of the Scottish Enlightenment, this medical ethics was grounded in an account of the intellectual and moral virtues required of physicians as professionals committed to a life of service to science and patients. Medical ethics – even though it did not yet have the name for itself that Thomas Percival (1740–1804) gave it in 1803 (see Chapters 1 and 36) – emerged in a philosophically sophisticated, clinically applicable fashion during the Scottish Enlightenment. This chapter provides an account of this remarkable and influential historical development, focusing on the work of the Scottish physician-ethicist, John Gregory (1724–1773), who wrote the first modern medical ethics in the English language.

II. MEDICAL PRACTICE, RESEARCH, AND EDUCATION IN EIGHTEENTH-CENTURY BRITAIN

The development of medical ethics in eighteenth-century Britain should be understood in the context of then-current medical practice, research, and education (Risse 1986; Porter and Porter 1989; Wear, Geyer-Kordesch, and French 1993). Medicine was not yet organized into a profession that was socially sanctioned and granted exclusive privileges of licensure and the economic security that physicians have experienced over the past century in developed countries, as a result of the creation of private insurance and government payment plans and, indeed, national health systems. Because there was no stable, accredited medical curriculum, medical education was not standardized. There were many practitioners, including university-trained physicians, apprentice-trained surgeons and apothecaries, "irregulars," or, less politely, "quacks." Not all physicians took a medical degree, there being no requirement of having a degree, for which universities charged separate fees. Some universities sold medical degrees or conferred them unearned. As a result, physicians who claimed a "regular" education as a way to distinguish themselves from "irregulars" or quacks often did not have a "regular" education themselves. Thus, it was not always clear who was entitled to call himself a physician or what fund of knowledge and skills were expected of physicians.

There was no single, accepted concept of health and disease, as there is now (health and disease are a function of the complex interaction of genes, proteins, and the environment), or an accepted classification of diseases (which we now do by organ systems). Indeed, there were almost as many concepts of health and disease, and of treatment for disease, as there were practitioners. Self-"physicking," or self-care, was common among the sick. Physicians usually came from the middle classes, and surgeons and apothecaries from still lower socioeconomic strata, with female midwives perhaps the lowest of all. Some irregulars became very successful, garnering considerable riches.

1. The Private Practice of Medicine

There were two settings in which physicians cared for the sick. The first was in the homes of the well-to-do, from higher social classes than the practitioners whose services they purchased. These wealthy gentlemen required physicians and other practitioners to compete for the lucrative market of caring for the well-to-do sick. In this crowded and fiercely competitive environment, physicians did what they could to stand out, including the adoption of peculiar dress (long coat and sword, for example), manners (especially the polite manners of a gentleman), and speech (to at least appear to be refined gentlemen themselves), publishing broadsides and even books in which they advanced their cutting edge theories of health and disease and touted their successes (a custom that still flourishes), and sometimes attacking their competitors, as we shall see later in this chapter (see also Chapter 36). The practice of medicine in this setting was intensely entrepreneurial, a marketplace in which failure to gain and hold market share occurred, followed by poverty, unless one had taken a richly dowered wife (Porter and Porter 1989; McCullough 1998a).

2. Medical Practice and Research in the Infirmaries

The second setting was the newly created Infirmaries. Some had a royal charter like the Royal Infirmary of Edinburgh, where Gregory practiced and taught medical students from the University of Edinburgh. These hospitals were created by wealthy individuals to provide free care for the men, women, and children who worked for them in coal fields, cotton mills, ship yards, and businesses that later became the Industrial Revolution. Employers had an understandable self-interest in maintaining a healthy work force of the worthy, sick poor. Some employers remained committed to the concept of paternalism in its old meaning, namely, the obligation of the powerful to care for those subordinate to their power, a medieval idea that was in its death throes by the middle of the eighteenth century. Wealthy individuals financed the Infirmaries through an annual subscription and used their charity, in part, to advance their own social and political standing. An uncertain and even unstable mix of self-interest and philanthropy thus shaped the organizational cultures of the infirmaries (Risse 1986).

Gaining admission to the infirmaries posed challenges to the working sick poor. First, one had to obtain a ticket of admission from one's employer, who was under no obligation (recall that paternalism was dying out) to provide one. Ticket in hand, one presented oneself for admission and was interviewed by astute laypersons (physicians were not entrusted by the benefactors with this important task) who sought to determine whether an applicant's condition was fatal or curable (in the modest sense that improvement in symptoms could be expected). The benefactors understood very well the long tradition from Hippocrates to Friedrich Hoffmann (1749) of physicians pronouncing dying patients incurable and abandoning them to their fate, so that the disease and not the physician would be counted as the cause of the subsequent death (see Chapters 23, 24, and 26). Low mortalities rates would advance the infirmary's – and trustees' – reputation and social standing. Benefactors therefore wanted a low morality rate for infirmaries, which was achieved through aggressively screening out and denying admission to those who were not expected to survive (Risse 1986).

Life for the sick in the infirmaries was highly regimented. Physicians, surgeons, and apothecaries volunteered their time in the hope that an appointment to the "faculty" of the Infirmary might increase their chances of success in their private practices. Physicians gained considerable power over the sick, as did the female staff (forerunners of modern nurses). No such power over the sick existed in private-practice setting. The sick poor sometimes referred to themselves as "inmates," reflecting the hierarchical organization of power that they experienced in exchange for receiving free care. Physicians, surgeons, and apothecaries did not check their competitive instincts at the door of the Infirmary, sometimes using their power over the sick poor to advance their own, rather than the sick person's interests (Risse 1986; McCullough 1998a).

Gregory reports on a significant abuse of the sick poor in the Royal Infirmary of Edinburgh on whose "faculty" he served from the mid-1760s until his death less than a decade later. Younger physicians, ambitious to establish a name for themselves as cutting-edge scientists to aid them in growing their private practices, would quickly pronounce the sick to be incurable. These ambitious physicians would do so, not to abandon these unfortunates to their fate, but to perform experiments on them, using the physician's own secret remedies and nostrums (McCullough 1998a).

3. The Crisis of Intellectual and Moral Trust

Both the well-to-do sick in their homes and the inmates of the infirmaries experienced a crisis of intellectual and moral trust regarding medical practitioners (Porter and Porter 1989). The intellectual crisis of trust resulted from the myriad concepts of medicine, health, and disease and treatments – often-secret remedies and nostrums – offered by practitioners. The sick had little or no basis to make reliable judgments about whether practitioners knew what they were talking about, or what they were doing. The moral crisis of trust resulted from well-founded concerns that the primary motivation of practitioners was their own economic advancement and, in the infirmary setting, the pursuit and use of power for reasons of self-interest rather than the benefit of the sick.

III. An Ethos of Personal Regard and Proper Manners

Starting in the early eighteenth century, the main focus of medical morality was on practitioner–practitioner relationships, which is no surprise given the overwhelmingly entrepreneurial nature of private medical practice. The main topics were how physicians should interact with each other and also with surgeons, apothecaries, and other colleagues and/or competitors. It is important to remember that there was then no stable, accepted pattern of behavior for such matters as consultation, as there is now. Our contemporary patterns are violated sometimes, but every physician knows that they are violations, such as stealing patients sent to one on referral by generalist colleagues. In eighteenth-century Britain, there were no such guidelines to manage the fierce competition among physicians, surgeons, and apothecaries.

One source of self-regulation was the statutes or rules of the Royal Colleges. The *Statuta Moralia* (moral laws) of the Royal College of Physicians of London, for example, addressed a number of aspects of these relationships:

> No colleague will accuse by name another either of ignorance, malpractice, wickedness or an ignominious crime; not heap public abuse [on a colleague]. (Clark 1964–1966, 1:414)

There is a reason for rules like this: the proscribed behavior was common. Physicians did not hesitate to take practitioner–practitioner disputes public. Public disputes also took the form of pamphlets and broadsides, also known as "flytes" (see Chapter 36). The discourse of these disputes appealed to what it meant to be a gentleman. "Gentleman" in this discourse meant someone with a university education. "Gentleman" also meant someone concerned primarily with personal honor and its jealous protection. This was an ethos of jealously guarded self-interest.

Manners loomed very large in this ethos of personal honor. One could be critical, as Gregory was later in the century (see later), of the ethos of self-interest as altogether inadequate to a life of service to science and patients that would improve medicine. This ethos of self-interest, however, also experienced a crisis from within as the age of manners began to come to an end during the middle decades of the eighteenth century (Fissell 1993). It became increasingly difficult to infer with confidence from good manners to good character. Manners could be purchased from manners coaches and put on, just as one put on a proper suit of clothes or upper-class social airs. The ethos of self-interest began to break down under its own weight, contributing to the moral crisis described previously.

IV. Intellectual and Other Moral Virtues of Physicians

In the middle decades of the eighteenth century in Britain emerged a discourse of the moral virtues of physicians as well as their intellectual virtues, in a series of short addresses given by members of the medical faculty in the University of Edinburgh. These were usually given just before medical students began their clinical experiences at the Royal Infirmary, and in the Edinburgh medical oath.

John Rutherford (1695–1779), later John Gregory's mentor and sponsor of his appointment to the Edinburgh medical faculty, gave short, preliminary lectures as early as 1750 (Rutherford 1750). Following Boerhaave, Rutherford defined medicine, as well as health and disease, reflecting the variability and instability of these concepts and consequent need to provide definitions. Rutherford distinguished between the quack and the true physician, namely, a physician committed to Baconian method in clinical practice and research. When the physician consistently displays the habits of mind of the Baconian scientist, Rutherford said, he counts as a "true physician." Rutherford also counseled his students to stay with incurable patients and not abandon them, in distinction to the views of Friedrich Hoffmann in his very influential *Medicus Politicus (The Politic Physician)* (1749) and the long Hippocratic tradition of declaring the dying incurable and abandoning them to their fate. Here there is an inkling of the life of service to patients. Rutherford's lectures are also important because he is one of the first to begin to use the word, "patient," instead of "the sick" (which translated the commonly used Latin word, *aegrotus*).

Robert Whytt (1716–1766), a pioneer of the modern specialty of neurology at Edinburgh, defined medicine, health, and disease, and also set out rules for the clinical management of patients (White n.d.). Whytt insisted on Baconian method as crucial for the proper clinical management of patients' problems. Whytt reflected the Baconian admonition to be open to information from all sources, when he calls for his students always to ask patients what they think the cause of their problem is (clinical advice that remains pertinent).

William Cullen (1710–1790), with whom Gregory shared the professorship of medicine at Edinburgh, commented briefly on the proper temperament for a physician to cultivate (Cullen 1768). Cullen defined medicine as "the art of preserving health and curing diseases" (Cullen n.d.), at a time in which "cure" meant any symptomatic improvement, not the elimination of underlying pathology. Cullen suggested that physicians do not need a temperament specific to physicians but they do require a proper, general temperament.

The Edinburgh tradition of brief, introductory lectures on medical practice made explicit appeal to Baconian philosophy of science and medicine as crucial for physicians to be competent; however, their authors did not elaborate on the intellectual bases of their moral views and recommendations. As we shall see, Gregory made an explicit appeal to the then-contemporary Scottish moral sense theory to provide a basis for his medical ethics that is missing in these lectures. Nonetheless, there emerged in the Edinburgh "ethics" lectures a sketch of the intellectual and moral virtues of physicians.

The medical school at Edinburgh administered an oath upon graduation that reflected this emerging discourse on the intellectual and moral virtues of physicians.

> To practice physic *cautiously, chastely, and honourably;* and faithfully to procure all things conducive to the bodies of the sick; and lastly, never, without great cause, to divulge anything that ought to be concealed, which may be heard or seen during professional attendance. To this oath let the deity be my witness. (Ryan 1831b, 50–51)

The cautious practice of medicine protects patients from iatrogenic harm and the chaste practice of medicine protects patients, especially female patients, from sexual abuse, both themes with deep roots in Hippocratic medical ethics (see Chapters 23 and 24) and real issues for the trust of female patients and their nervous husbands at the time (Porter 1987). "Honourably" reflects the ethos of self-interest; however, the next two provisions are clearly patient centered. This is a more robust discourse of moral virtues than is to be found in the Edinburgh lectures. It is interesting, in this respect, to note that Rutherford, White, Cullen, or Gregory for that matter made no mention of this oath in their ethics lectures. This may reflect the fact that, by this time, taking the Hippocratic Oath was beginning to fall out of favor (see Chapter 24). Like their lectures, though, the Edinburgh oath does not provide the basis or justification for these virtues.

V. JOHN GREGORY'S MEDICAL ETHICS

John Gregory provided an extensive account of the intellectual and moral virtues of physicians and based his account on the philosophy of medicine of Bacon and the moral philosophy of David Hume (1711–1776), respectively. Gregory presented and published his lectures in the spirit of the Scottish Enlightenment to reform medical practice, research, and education.

1. The Scottish Enlightenment and the Science of Man

One cannot hope to do justice to the complex accomplishments of the Scottish Enlightenment in a book chapter, much less one section of a book chapter. My goal, instead, will be to provide an overview of the main elements of the Scottish Enlightenment that shaped Gregory's medical ethics (Carter and Pittock 1987; Daiches 1986; Davies 1991; see also McCullough 1998a).

Lester Crocker (1991) has warned against attempts to provide a single, over-arching definition of "The Enlightenment," a period, roughly coincident with the eighteenth century. Rather, the phrase he says is best understood as an attempt to capture a cluster of related phenomena. The challenge of definition is compounded by the fact that there was no single "Enlightenment" in Europe and the Americas in the eighteenth century, but related national enlightenments with distinctive characteristics (Porter and Teich 1981). Nonetheless, I take the Enlightenment to be a period in which, wearied by religious wars as a way to settle differences in increasingly pluralistic societies, Western European thinkers developed a secular moral discourse in the sciences, arts, literature, and the emerging professions such as medicine. By "secular" I mean that these thinkers sought to develop discourses and social practices, the intellectual and moral authority of which anyone could accept or reject without appeal to theological or religious sources. In addition, no hostility to religious beliefs and practices was implied.

Authoritative discourses and social practices were understood to be the products of the rigorous functioning of faculties that all humans possessed: reason and instinct. Appeals to reason played a major role in European enlightenments, whereas instinct, as we shall see shortly, played a major role in the Scottish Enlightenment.

The Enlightenment spirit was skeptical, especially of received ideas and authorities. Enlightenment skepticism in Scotland became not just an intellectual but also a social habit with the goal of being constructive, not destructive. Skepticism in the social domain led to a commitment to reform, by improving the knowledge base and standards of practice of social institutions. This reform-mindedness was often centered in intellectual clubs dedicated to the improvement of all sorts of human activities, from agriculture (no small matter, given the periodic, sometimes severe, famines in Scotland) to music (avoid too much listening to fugues, because their mathematical nature suggests exaggerated powers of reason) – and medicine.

The Scottish Enlightenment emerged in the context of Scotland having lost its status as a separate state with the Act of Union of 1707, joining Scotland to England. Scots, nonetheless, retained a strong sense of national identity. To explain, and sustain, this sense of national identity, the concept of "fellow feeling" developed. Fellow feeling involved a natural, instinctive regard for the well-being of others, especially those who are vulnerable to misfortune and the abuse of power.

The phenomenon of fellow feeling became subject to study in the new, distinctively Enlightenment enterprise, the "science of man" (Porter 1990a, 12), which developed along Baconian lines: disciplined observation of natural phenomena, including the recognizable patterns of human attitudes and behaviors; skeptical and critical evaluation of authorities; careful formulation of hypotheses to explain observed phenomena; rigorous testing of hypotheses by observation and experiment; and careful assessment of the likelihood that a hypothesis was true of the world (Bacon [1620] 2000). Hypotheses concern mainly "principles" and their workings. By "principle" Baconian scientists meant a real, constitutive, causal element in things that explains their activity.

To explain the evidently natural, instinctual fellow feeling of Scots for one another – Hume notes that strong fellow feeling is plainly a distinctive feature of Scottish national character, in contrast to its weaker variant in English national character (Hume [1777] 1987) – Baconian scientists of man posited the social principle. Fellow feeling was understood as the effect of the social principle. The social principle was a real, constitutive element of human nature that causes and, therefore, explains the widespread – and highly valued – social phenomenon of fellow feeling.

Human nature was understood to comprise two main principles: instinct and reason. For Scottish Enlightenment thinkers, in sharp contrast to the French and German enlightenments, reason was understood to be the weaker of the two principles, a mere calculating machine that attuned means to ends. Ends worthy of our pursuit, however, were understood to be a function of instinct. The social principle was therefore attributed to instinct. Thus understood, the social principle was a natural regard for others that formed the wellspring of moral obligations to protect them, especially when they are vulnerable.

The social principle was understood in secular terms. One could become aware of the social principle and its causal functioning and effects simply by using one's disciplined powers of observation, following Baconian method. No appeal to transcendent reality was required. Because fellow feeling binds us all together and creates obligations to help others, especially when they are vulnerable or in distress, fellow feeling is compatible with and therefore not hostile to dominant Christian beliefs of the time in Scotland and could be explained scientifically, that is, independently of religious beliefs.

Another distinctive feature of the national enlightenments was the creation of societies or clubs for intellectual and practical pursuits (Porter 1990a). These social activities strengthened fellow feeling and also put it to work, to "relieve man's estate," in Bacon's apt phrase. The relief of man's estate meant the reduction of hunger, disease, injury, and death in the world – the mortality rate by age 16 in Scotland in the eighteenth century was approximately 60 percent – and making life less harsh, rough, and ill mannered. Scots thus set up societies and clubs dedicated to improving medicine, agriculture, music, and many other human undertakings.

One of these clubs was the Aberdeen Philosophical Society, which Gregory helped to found in 1758 with, among others, his cousin, Thomas Reid (1710–1796), himself later to become a major philosophical figure of the Scottish Enlightenment (Ulman 1990). Gregory made a number of presentations to the Society, in which he absorbed completely the Scottish, Baconian commitment to the account of human nature as comprising instinct and reason, with the former the seat of the social principle, and the latter the weaker, merely calculating principle. These presentations appeared as Gregory's first book, *A Comparative View of the State and Faculties of Man with those of the Animal World* (1765). This book gained him a considerable reputation as a leading man of letters and figure of the Scottish Enlightenment.

The meetings of the "Wise Club," as the Aberdeen Philosophical Society was also known, were devoted to many presentations on the social principle and related topics. The discussions of the social principle centered on Hume's *A Treatise of Human Nature* ([1739] 2000). Hume's *Treatise*, subtitled "An Attempt to Introduce the Experimental Method of Reasoning into Moral Subjects," was read in Aberdeen as a Baconian investigation into the science of morals. Hume provided a detailed account of the social principle in terms of what he called sympathy: a real, constitutive, causal principle of human nature that, when properly functioning, provided the grounds of moral behavior, judgment, and virtues. As *the* moral sense at the heart of a moral sense philosophy, sympathy was as powerful as any of the physical senses.

Humean sympathy involved a "double relation" of impressions and ideas. Impressions were the physical impressions of the world against the senses. Ideas were then routinely abstracted from impressions and were organized into coherent explanatory packages by reason and then tested by observational experience. Sympathy, as the double relation of impressions and ideas, worked as follows. One sees another person in pain. From this impression of pain in another person, one automatically forms the idea of pain in that person. This impression naturally leads to the idea of pain in oneself and thence to the impression of pain in oneself that is similar to the pain that the person originally observed is experiencing. One can indeed feel the pain of, or feel for, one's fellow human beings and also for nonhuman animals. After one experiences the pain of another person as one's own pain, one is naturally inclined to relieve them of their pain – primarily for their own sake, secondarily for one's own sake.

In his contributions to the Aberdeen Philosophical Society, Gregory endorsed Hume's principle of sympathy. Gregory emphasized that sympathy needs to be trained in each of us, so that it functions routinely and well. In his *Comparative View* and in his posthumously published *A Father's Legacy to his Daughters* (Gregory 1774), Gregory enriched Hume's account by emphasizing the virtues of women of learning and virtue – whom Gregory had met in the 1750s when he lived in London and attended the social gatherings of Elizabeth Monatgu's Bluestocking Circle (Myers 1990; McCullough 1998a; see also Chapter 18). For Gregory, women of learning and virtue became the moral exemplars of the virtues of sympathy. In arguing for this view, Gregory articulated what Rosemarie Tong calls feminine ethics – which is distinct from feminist ethics, with its emphasis on the exploitation of women and the need to correct such exploitation (Tong 1993).

In his feminine account of the virtues of sympathy, Gregory underscores the centrality of tenderness and steadiness. Tenderness means that one's heart and feelings are open to and automatically responsive to the pain, distress, and suffering of others, as well as their joy and happiness. Tenderness is the antidote to hard-heartedness. Steadiness means that one's sympathetic response to others is disciplined by a steady focus on the well-being of others, not one's immediate, potentially undisciplined response to them. Steadiness is the antidote to over-responding to the plight of others. Gregory deploys the principle of sympathy and its feminine virtues of tenderness and steadiness as the foundation of his medical ethics.

2. Gregory's Medical Ethics

Gregory was born into a distinguished family, sometimes referred to as the "Academic Gregories" (Stewart 1901). He was educated through college in Aberdeen. He then studied medicine in Edinburgh, and later Leiden, and was awarded an unearned medical degree from King's College in Aberdeen; he had not completed his medical studies at Leiden and undertook none at all at King's. He then lived in London, returning to Aberdeen in the 1750s to become professor of medicine at King's. Gregory was appointed to the medical faculty of the University of Edinburgh in 1766 and within a year he also began to give preliminary lectures on ethics before the students were admitted to rounds and lectures at the Royal Infirmary of Edinburgh (McCullough 1998a).

In 1770, these lectures appeared as *Observations on the Duties and Offices of a Physician, and on the Method of Prosecuting Enquiries in Philosophy* (Gregory [1770] 1998a). This title reveals Gregory's emphasis on both the duties or offices (from the Latin, *officium*) of physicians, and philosophy of medicine, that is, an account of the proper method for becoming a scientific and morally competent physician. Gregory set out to address both the intellectual and moral crisis of trust experienced by the sick. The intellectual disciplines of Baconian philosophy of medicine and Humean philosophical ethics were both required for medical ethics to address these deep crises of trust that only made the perils of sickness and injury worse (McCullough 1998a).

It was a common practice to allow one's lectures to appear first in print anonymously, to test public response to them. Should the response prove negative, the author could disavow the publication as a complimentary gesture of perhaps overly enthusiastic students or other admirers. Should the response prove positive, one could then take advantage of an opportunity to revise and expand the lectures and publish under one's own name. The *Observations* were very well received indeed; in fact, a copy was carried by Gregory's students back to the American colonies in the year they were published. He therefore followed *Observations* with his own *Lectures on the Duties and Qualifications of a Physician* in 1772 (Gregory [1772b] 1998b).

Gregory opened his *Lectures* with a Baconian definition of medicine that echoes and adds to Cullen's: "the art of preserving health, prolonging life, and of curing diseases" (Gregory [1772b] 1998b, 2). Gregory did not mean prolonging life at all costs. From his days as a medical student, Gregory understood and accepted the Baconian idea that medicine would always have limited powers to treat disease and prevent death and that expansion of these powers almost always involved iatrogenic risk (McCullough 1998a). That this is his mature view, as well, is plain later in the *Lectures*, when he adds to this definition, "making death easy" (Gregory [1772b] 1998b, 109). In this vein, Gregory also stated in the *Lectures* that it is the duty of physicians to continue to care for the dying, "to alleviate pain, and to smooth the avenues of death" (Gregory [1772b] 1998b, 35–36).

In the spirit of the Scottish Enlightenment, and with a deep debt to Bacon, Gregory's wrote medical ethics to reform medicine, to transform it from a largely entrepreneurial, self-interested trade into a profession in the moral sense of the term. Physicians should become, to use the more technical language of ethics that Gregory did not use, "fiduciaries" of their patients: physicians should commit themselves to becoming scientifically and clinically competent and to use their competence primarily to protect and to promote the health-related interests of patients rather than the physician's self-interest. Physicians will become competent, Gregory argued, by submitting to the intellectual discipline of Baconian science, which is based on careful observation and analysis of the results of natural or contrived experiments. These results produce hypotheses, of varying likelihood, about principles, the constitutive causes in things that produce and therefore explain the observed results. Baconian science requires physicians to develop their capacity to be "open to conviction" (a phrase Gregory used repeatedly, echoing Whytt), to revising or even abandoning hypotheses – explanations of disease and of treatments for disease – based on new evidence. To this end, physicians should cultivate the professional intellectual virtue of diffidence, an habitual willingness to call into question or set aside even one's most cherished beliefs and clinical practices if evidence – including evidence from the experience of the sick or from arch rivals – requires one to do so.

Physicians should also be open to, and promptly respond to alleviate, the pain, distress, and suffering of their patients. Gregory called this capacity "sympathy" and "humanity." Gregory used these terms interchangeably, as was sometimes done in Scottish moral sense philosophy concerning the basis of our obligations to each other.

> I come now to mention the moral qualities peculiarly required in the character of a physician. The chief of these is humanity; that sensibility of heart which makes us feel for the distresses of our fellow-creatures, and which, of consequence, incites us in the most powerful manner to relieve them. (Gregory [1772b] 1998b, 19)

Scholars of Gregory's medical ethics are in complete accord on Gregory's medical ethics as self-consciously philosophical. Lisbeth Haaksonssen (1997), Meinolfus Strätling (1997, 1998), and Laurence McCullough (1998a) agree that Gregory draws deeply on Bacon's philosophy of medicine. These scholars also agree that Gregory drew deeply on the Baconian science of morals, a subfield of the science of man in moral sense philosophy. Both of these sources, these scholars also agree, helped to shape the reformist character of Gregory's medical ethics.

There are, however, differences of interpretation among these scholars about the philosophical basis of Gregory's understanding and use of sympathy in his medical ethics. Haakonssen (1997) argues that Gregory was strongly influenced by Cicero's idea of a social office (*officium*) and its implied contractual duties. Haakonssen also emphasizes Gregory's debt to the philosophical ethics of his cousin, Thomas Reid, who draws a distinction between duty and self-interest and holds that duties have their origin in an implied contract. Haakonssen argues further that Gregory's understanding and use of the concept of sympathy have their origins in the moral sense philosophy generally, not in Hume.

Laurence McCullough (1998a) argues that Gregory's took his understanding and use of the concept of sympathy from the moral sense philosopher, David Hume, with whom Gregory was personally acquainted after he moved to Edinburgh. In a detailed examination of the manuscript sources, McCullough shows that in the 1760s, when Gregory and his cousin both helped to found and actively participated in the intellectual life of the Aberdeen Philosophical Society, Gregory's understanding of sympathy was already Humean and differed in significant ways from Reid's understanding. Meinolfus Strätling (1997, 1998) also argues that Gregory's primary intellectual debt is to Hume.

All of these scholarly interpretations of Gregory's medical ethics and his intellectual sources agree that sympathy motivates the physician to choose the response that will relieve the pain, distress, and suffering of patients. As a Scottish moral sense philosopher, Gregory held that sympathy or humanity provides a reliable basis for moral judgment and action, but only when this moral sense was properly developed and trained. That is, physicians need to cultivate moral virtues that make sympathy an everyday reality in their moral lives.

The intellectual virtue of physicians, diffidence, and the moral virtues of physicians, tenderness, and steadiness, both discipline self-interest into a systematically secondary place. Diffidence-based clinical judgment and reasoning will be free of the distorting bias of self-interest in money, reputation, and fame and therefore be intellectually trustworthy. Tenderness-based and steadiness-based clinical judgment and behavior will be free of distorting self-interest in understandable – but not acceptable – self-protection in response to others' pain, distress, and suffering and will therefore be morally trustworthy. Gregory's behavioral test for the true physician was that he will treat the high-born and low-born alike – a criterion of particular moral and practical force, given that Gregory had been appointed the King's Physician in Scotland. In effect, Gregory says, physicians should treat the poor the way they treat royalty and royalty the way they treat the poor, just as he himself (by implication) does. The inability to identify the patient's socioeconomic status from the physician's demeanor and behavior remains an excellent criterion for judging who is a true physician, someone who has cultivated his or her character on the basis of the virtues of diffidence, tenderness, and steadiness.

Gregory deployed these virtues in an account of the wide variety of topics in clinical ethics. These included maintaining confidentiality, especially with regard to female patients, prohibiting the sexual abuse of female patients, recognizing the role of the patient in diagnosing and treating disease as required by being "open to conviction" from any quarter, communicating bad news to patients, remaining with dying patients to provide palliative care and thus "smooth the avenues of death," being willing to acknowledge and rectify mistakes in patient care, proper decorum in dress and speech so that the physician does not create a false impression of being trustworthy, conducting consultations among practitioners in a patient-centered rather than self-interested fashion, forging links between medicine and surgery so that both can be improved for the benefit of patients, avoiding inebriation, and defending physicians against the charge that the study of Baconian scientific medicine requires physicians to become atheists (Gregory [1770] 1998a, [1772b] 1998b).

In his discussion of communicating bad news, that is, information about grave illness with a poor prognosis, Gregory held that this is the most "disagreeable duties in the profession" (Gregory [1772b] 1998b, 35). Physicians then (and now) wanted to avoid unpleasant duties because we all do, as a matter of understandable self-interest. A consistent feature of Gregory's medical ethics, however, is that the physician's self-interest should never become the determining factor of his clinical judgment and behavior. Thus, those who are gravely ill need to be informed, but not by the physician. Family members should always be given this information, with the implication (left unexpressed by Gregory) that they will communicate the bad news to the patient. The reader should note that Gregory's ethics of truth telling does not involve paternalism, that is, restricting the patient's autonomy for the benefit of the patient (Beauchamp and Childress 2001).

Gregory took up a crucial topic in research ethics, namely, the practice of ambitious physicians labeling patients in the Royal Infirmary as "incurable," to justify performing experiments on them, primarily for reasons of the physician's own self-interest.

In treating the Patients under my care I am only to give you my Common Practice, & only prescribe such Medicines as I have had experience of their good effects in similar cases. I know very well that it is a common opinion with many young Gentlemen, that the Physician who attends an Hospital should always try Experiments on the Patients; this I think contrary both to Justice & Humanity: I shall therefore give you my common Practice & not sport with the lives of poor people: I would not give any Person a Medicine that I would scruple to take myself. I shall always have in my Eye that moral precept, "Do as you would be done by." (Gregory 1771, 9)

As this passage makes clear, Gregory condemned this practice. As a good Baconian (and anticipating evidence-based medicine by two centuries), he insisted that physicians first employ standard remedies in the care of the sick. Only when these demonstrably fail is it permissible to perform experiments. These must be limited by the intellectual requirement of being well designed (e.g., testing simple rather than compound remedies to reliably identify agents) and by moral requirements not to exceed the bounds of sympathy, which Gregory in this context expresses in terms of the Golden Rule. Gregory here interprets the Golden Rule to prohibit "sporting" with the sick poor, that is, using them with no regard for their well-being and solely for self-interest in advancing one's reputation and market share. Doing so violated the requirements of sympathy. This may be the earliest example of research ethics in the history of medical ethics.

3. Gregory's Medical Ethics as Professional Medical Ethics

Claims that medicine became a profession at one point or another in its history are contentious among historians of medicine. This is also the case for claims about when medical ethics becomes professional ethics among historians of medical ethics. Nonetheless, there is a good case to be made that Gregory's medical ethics should be understood as professional medical ethics and, if so, the first in the history of the English-language literature. Allen Buchanan (1996) identifies five elements of an "ideal" conception of a profession: special practical knowledge; a commitment to preserve and improve that fund of knowledge and skill; a commitment to excellence in the practice of the profession; an "intrinsic and dominant" commitment to a life of service to others; and effective self-regulation by the professional group. The Baconian philosophy of medicine in Gregory's medical ethics satisfies the first three elements; his commitment to Humean sympathy makes a life of service to patients ethically obligatory, providing the fourth element. As to the fifth element, Gregory was skeptical about self-regulation, given the need of physicians to earn a living by their profession. Instead, he called for physicians to be accountable to a group of financially independent, scientifically sophisticated students of medicine (Gregory [1772b] 1998b). Given the modest nature of medical knowledge and clinical skills in Gregory's day, this would have been a practical means of professional accountability and therefore effective regulation. Gregory's proposal was not adopted until the recent advent of evidence-based medicine, in which physicians become accountable to physicians and non-physicians, such as biostatisticians and lay leadership of health care organizations, for the quality of patient care. As a conceptualization of medicine as a profession, Gregory's medical ethics satisfies four of the five elements of Buchanan's concept of a fiduciary profession committed to competence and excellence and using competence primarily for the benefit of patients and not for the physician's individual or the profession's collective self-interest. Gregory's conception lacks the feature of self-governance to fulfill what became the modern concept of a profession. It also lacks the concept of medicine as a public trust, which Percival (1803b) adds to the modern conception.

A central feature of Gregory's medical ethics was its reformist nature. Gregory's medical ethics reformed and improved the meaning of both "professional" and "gentleman." Physicians in his time regularly used the word "professional" to describe themselves, but did so with the self-interested goal of distinguishing themselves from surgeons, apothecaries, and irregulars who, presumably, did not know what they were doing. Gregory also used these words. Early in his *Lectures* Gregory used "profession" largely in the sense of an occupation. Later in this text, however, Gregory's gave to the words "profession" and "professional" a moral content, when he refers to medicine as a "liberal profession," by which he means medicine as a fiduciary profession (even though he does not use the word fiduciary).

> It is a physician's duty to do every thing in his power that is not criminal, to save the life of his patient, and to search for remedies from every source, and from every hand, however mean and contemptible. This, it may be said, is sacrificing the dignity and interests of the faculty. But, I am not here speaking of the private police of a corporation, or the little arts of craft. I am treating of the duties of a *liberal profession*, whose object is the life and health of the human species, a profession to be exercised by gentlemen of honour and ingenuous manners; the dignity of which can never be supported by means that are inconsistent with its ultimate object, and that only tend to increase the pride and fill the pockets of a few individuals. (Gregory [1772b] 1998b, 39–40)

Gregory reformed the meaning of "profession" in medicine, in two ways. First, he created the modern conceptual basis for the social role of being a fiduciary physician, rather than a mere practitioner or self-interested gentleman. Second, he created the modern conceptual basis of the social role of being a patient as a function of, and protected by, the intellectually and morally reliable social role of being a fiduciary physician. As a patient, a sick person who can indeed repose intellectual and moral trust in the physician or surgeon who is a "liberal" professional. It is instructive in this respect, that "patient" appeared regularly but not consistently in his texts. He continued to use "the sick," as well. The transition to the exclusive use of "patient" occurred in Percival's *Medical Ethics* (see Chapter 36).

As a professional medical ethics, Gregory's medical ethics should not be understood as a tool of internal self-regulation for the advancement of guild interests, as exemplified by the *Statuta Moralia* (moral statutes or rules) of the various colleges of physicians or surgeons. Gregory attacked this "corporation spirit." Professional medical ethics remained a tool for self-regulation (and as a basis for social regulation later), but primarily for the benefit of present patients and, through the advancement of medical science, future patients.

Gregory also transformed the meaning of the word "gentleman." Men tended to understand themselves to be gentlemen largely on the basis of social accomplishment, class, and acceptable (but potentially false) manners, rather than on the basis of true moral character (Fissell 1993). When they understood themselves as gentlemen on the basis of character, they tended to do so on the basis of *"amour propre,"* a prickly, fragile, easily offended self-regard – a false and unreliable understanding of character. As a good Humean moralist, Gregory held self-regard to be the wrong characterological basis for being a gentleman. The proper basis was sympathy and its virtues of tenderness and steadiness, the reliable bases of a true gentleman's "ingenuous manners." Thus, Gregory reformed the meaning of "gentleman" and did so in self-consciously and distinctly feminine ethical terms, to boot.

Critics of Gregory (and also of Percival, see Chapter 36) have claimed that his medical ethics is concerned with *intraprofessional* issues, such as consultations, fees, and so forth, not with substantive moral matters (Berlant 1975; Waddington 1984). That is, medical ethics is primarily etiquette, as Leake (1927) famously put it. If this criticism were to hold up, it would undermine any claim that Gregory's medical ethics counts as professional medical ethics in a morally meaningful sense. This criticism of the discourses of practitioners as merely etiquette, namely, self-interested concern with personal honor and protection of market share, fully applies to the discourses of physicians such as the *Statuta Moralia*. It does not, however, apply to the modern medical ethics of Gregory, as should by now be clear. Scholars, such as Robert Baker

(1993), have shown that this criticism cannot be applied to Percival and subsequent professional medical ethics.

4. Gregory's Medical Ethics as Enlightenment Medical Ethics

Gregory was self-consciously a member of the Scottish Enlightenment. He was fully committed to the Baconian goal of "relieving man's estate" by reducing mortality and morbidity, at a time when mortality, morbidity, and disability from disease and injury were frightfully high. Gregory's goal was to reduce mortality and morbidity, ever attentive to the limits of medicine and therefore to the unavoidable risk of making things worse in the name of making things better. Gregory, as a Scottish Enlightenment thinker, did not think much of reason's capacities – typically, he called it the weaker principle, when compared with the instinctual principle of sympathy – and therefore did not take the view that reason would equip medicine with the ability to subdue and therefore control nature. This so-called Baconian project was entirely alien to Gregory's thinking.

VI. THE INFLUENCE OF GREGORY'S MEDICAL ETHICS

Gregory's medical ethics had considerable influence in the English-speaking world and through translations into the major languages of continental Europe. Benjamin Rush attended the medical school in Edinburgh and Gregory's lectures on medical ethics. Rush took Gregory's ideas home with him to colonial America and incorporated them into his own writings on medical ethics, using Gregory's title of *Observations* to which is appended the following: *Accommodated to the Present State of Society and Manners in the United States* (Rush 1805; see also Chapters 31 and 36). A major difference between Rush and Gregory is Rush's emphasis on the religious basis of medical ethics (McCullough 1998a), an emphasis that persists into nineteenth-century American medical ethics, such as in the explicit appeal to religion as a basis for the first Code of Ethics of the American Medical Association in 1847 (see Chapter 36).

Gregory also had a direct influence on his own son, James (1753–1821), a physician who succeeded him as Professor of Medicine in the University of Edinburgh. James published an exposé of abuses of patients at the Royal Infirmary of Edinburgh (Gregory 1800). He based his ethical critique on the claim, derived from his father's medical ethics, that physicians should understand their primary duty to be acting in ways that benefit patients and not themselves. Like his father, without using the word, James Gregory invokes the core professional ethical concept of the physician as fiduciary of the patient. James Gregory then derives a "right" of patients that is the corollary

of this duty of physicians, the right to competent medical care that does not expose them to unnecessary danger. The physician's obligations should be enforced and the patient's rights should be protected by hospital managers. The experiments still continuing at the Royal Infirmary did not meet these standards of clinical and health care management ethics, James Gregory argued.

John Gregory's reformist spirit was adopted and sharpened by Thomas Beddoes (1760–1808), a Bristol, England, physician. Beddoes (1799, 1802, 1806) launched a vigorous attack on quackery, having concluded, according to Roy Porter (1993) that Gregory and, after him, Percival had not done enough on this score to reform and improve medicine. Beddoes thought entrepreneurial medicine a serious menace and its ethos should be replaced with an ethics based on competence and the "well being of individuals" (Beddoes 1799, 3). This conceptualization of the basis of physicians' obligations to their patients owes an obvious debt to Gregory's medical ethics.

Thomas Percival drew on diverse intellectual sources in preparing his *Medical Ethics* (1803). These included Gregory's language of the professional virtues of physicians, tenderness and steadiness, that Percival employs in the very first paragraph of his enormously influential text (see Chapter 36):

> Hospital physicians and surgeons should study, also, in their deportment, so to unite *tenderness* with *steadiness*, and *condescension* with *authority*, as to inspire the minds of their patients with gratitude, respect, and confidence. (Percival 1803b, 9)

Gregory's medical ethics was also translated in Spanish (Gregory 1803), French (Gregory 1787), Italian (Gregory 1789), and German (Gregory 1778). In Chapter 33 of this volume, Diego Gracia provides an account of the importance and influence on Spanish medical ethics of the nineteenth century of the Spanish-language translation. A detailed history of the influence of these continental European translations of Gregory's medical ethics has yet to be written. To this day, southern European and also Latin American medical ethics emphasizes the professional virtues more than ethical principles (see Chapters 40 and 42). To what extent this distinctive tradition in medical ethics has its roots in the Scottish Enlightenment medical ethics of John Gregory remains an interesting and open question.

VII. CONCLUSION

During the eighteenth century the discourses of medical morality of British practitioners underwent a fundamental shift, from a self-interested "gentlemanly" ethos of honor and "corporation spirit" or guild mentality (Gregory [1770] 1998a) to the first modern medical ethics in the English language. This modern medical ethics was the product of the Scottish Enlightenment, the work of the Scottish Enlightenment physician-ethicist, Dr. John Gregory. His work had immediate and important influence in both Britain and America and influenced American medical ethics well into the nineteenth century. His work also had important, although still little understood, influence on nineteenth-century French, German, Italian, and Spanish medical ethics well into the nineteenth century and perhaps even through the twentieth century on virtue-based European medical ethics. His concept of the sympathetic physician remains influential. Gregory understood medical ethics to require a robust philosophy of medicine joined to an equally robust philosophical ethics, thus anticipating a major methodological commitment of the bioethics movement. He also anticipated much of the agenda of clinical ethics and also provided an account of research ethics, perhaps the first in the English-language literature of medical ethics.

CHAPTER 31

THE DISCOURSES OF PRACTITIONERS IN EIGHTEENTH-CENTURY NORTH AMERICA

Chester R. Burns

I. INTRODUCTION

Those professing to be healers in North American towns during the 1700s inherited moral values associated with specific communities: families, merchants, churches, schools, vocational societies, hospitals, judges, and governing officials. The "governors" of towns and colonies embedded their values in laws adopted to regulate "healers" in each polity. The Massachusetts Bay Colony (1649) and the Provincial Assembly of New York (1760) adopted such laws. Judges and juries began assessing penalties for those convicted of "malpractice." In 1791, the Supreme Court of Connecticut awarded forty pounds to the husband of a woman who had died after a breast amputation performed by the defendant (Burns 1969a, 54). The regulations of a few hospitals, such as the Pennsylvania Hospital (1752) and the Williamsburg State Hospital (1773), began to exert directive influences. Societies of physicians transformed the ideals of individual consciences into rules that could be enforced. In its constitution adopted in 1766, for example, the New Jersey Medical Society forbade the use of secret remedies. Medical schools, beginning in Philadelphia in 1765 and in New York City in 1767, added their moral expectations for doctors. Churches wielded omnipotent influences in shaping moral values.

As commerce expanded, healers wanted monetary rewards for their services. Families struggled to reconcile competing moral claims as they chose the services of specific healers.

The moral values of these and other cultural communities shaped the personal conduct, healing practices, and civic participation of healers, although the influence of each community varied for individuals, regions, and decades (Bell 1975, 5–39; Christianson 1980, 1987; Cassedy 1991, 3–20; Reiss 2000, 1–58). This chapter provides an account of various ways that some of these moral values intersected in the careers of three healers: Cotton Mather (1663–1728), Benjamin Rush (1745–1813), and Martha Ballard (1735–1812).

II. PURITAN MEDICAL ETHICS

Protestant, Calvinist, and evangelical, New England Puritans believed that their God sent them to the New World to escape Catholic, Anglican, and British persecution and to create a perfect community of saints and disciples. God was the sovereign creator and omnipotent master of the universe who revealed his Will through the Bible. Because of Adam's pride, every human was born in sin. God determined which humans would be saved eternally and which would be damned. Each congregation admitted to full membership only those who experienced conversion, who believed that they had received God's grace. These persons became the community's visible saints because their good works and holy ways of life signified that they had received this grace. Because an individual could never be certain that salvation had occurred, though, a lifetime of struggle was necessary to combat sin and honor all of God's covenants about grace, works, and redemption (Flower and Murphey 1977, 3–14).

The dominant Puritan cleric in New England for more than 40 years, Cotton Mather struggled to reconcile these faith claims, the rich scholarly traditions of Western physicians, and his own observations about diseases experienced by Boston's families. Mather himself had suffered the deaths of two wives and thirteen of fifteen children – all from infectious diseases except for a son lost at sea (Silverman 1984, 179–83, 271–73, 387, 400–401). Mather's struggles are vividly depicted in his writings about medicine and medical ethics, and in his support of smallpox variation.

Puritan beliefs about sin and disease are portrayed in his book, *The Angel of Bethesda*. Adam's sin was "The Grand Cause of Sickness" and death (Mather 1972, 5). Subsequent sins of every individual repeat and renew this original sin. These sins are "*Naturally* the Cause of Sickness . . . What are *Sicknesses* but the *Rods*, wherewith GOD corrects His own offending Children?" (Mather 1972, 6). "*Diseases* may be *Love-tokens!*" that prompt an individual to reaffirm God's ultimate goodness in providing Jesus as the vehicle for forgiveness and atonement (Mather 1972, 7). "*None but CHRIST*" can cure a "*Sin-Sick SOUL.*" "*O Invalids*, I am leading you to your true *Aesculapius!*" concluded Mather, who enjoyed a social role as an authoritative healer (Mather 1972, 10).

Ever eager to connect the supernatural and natural forces of the universe, Mather's support of inoculation was a unique opportunity to affirm the goodness of God, the power of courageous conversion, and the importance of sharing healing responsibilities with medical professionals (Silverman 1984, 336–63). Although smallpox pus was tangible, its power to elicit salutary effects from "the invisible world" was awesome when introduced in small quantities by variation. Almost half of Boston's 12,000 citizens experienced smallpox in the epidemic of 1721; approximately 900 died. Yet, only two percent of those acquiring the disease by inoculation died, in contrast to twelve to fourteen percent of those acquiring the disease otherwise (Breen 1991, 333, 357).

With inoculation, Mather demonstrated a way that God healed and "saved" the bodies of those willing to take a risk with the "invisible world" – ample proof that those willing to take a risk with Jesus could be spiritually "saved" too. Like his apprentice-trained, apothecary-physician

comrade Zabdiel Boylston, doctors could do much good if they were willing to trust the "invisible world." Faithful patients and healers would experience and witness God's abundant grace (Breen 1991, 354–57). Mather's advocacy of smallpox variation profoundly influenced the moral choices of Boston's doctors. Even William Douglass, the university-educated physician who had vehemently opposed Mather in 1721, became a convert to this technique later.

Nonetheless, Mather's powerful influence on the development of North American medical ethics had begun a decade earlier. In *Bonifacius* published in 1710, Mather delineated specific ways that healers could be good Puritans and good doctors. Physicians should be "studious" and "inquisitive," eager to make "some addition to the treasures" of their profession (Mather [1710] 1966, 99). Physicians should relieve anxieties and mental disorders by offering "the *right thoughts of the righteous*, and the ways to a composure upon religious principles" (Mather [1710] 1966, 104). Doctors should not neglect the souls of their patients. "You may make your conversation with them, a *vehicle* for such *admonitions of piety* as may be most *needful* for them" (Mather [1710] 1966, 104). Doctors who treat the poor with charity and compassion can approximate "the greatest of all glories . . . an imitation of your admirable SAVIOUR" (Mather [1710] 1966, 101). Good Puritan doctors who attended a patient's body, mind, soul, and social circumstances could glorify God as they performed deeds of healing (Mather [1710] 1966, xi–xii; Silverman 1984, 232–6). Mather believed that skillful physicians should be honored as gifts of God and he labeled the combination of roles as doctor and cleric in the same person as an "angelical conjunction" (Mather [1710] 1972, 190–91; Watson 1991, 1).

Honoring Mather's expectations, more than 100 Puritan preacher-physicians practiced in New England during the seventeenth and eighteenth centuries. A doctor-minister who cared for bodily ails could easily attend spiritual maladies, doing twice as much good and thereby doubling one's saintly credit. These "angelical" healers also enjoyed the extra income from medical (sometimes surgical) practice (Watson 1991, 43–67, 133). By 1750, however, an increasing number of Harvard and Yale graduates were becoming physicians only, not pastors (Watson 1991, 69–73). Ministers were losing cultural preeminence as colonials accorded more moral authority to doctors and lawyers (Haber 1991, 15–87).

In August 1776, Samuel Mather, the third-generation pastor of the North Church in Boston, read the Declaration of Independence to his congregation. A new polity had emerged, one shaped by cultural ideals that assigned more value to the natural world than the supernatural one. Benjamin Franklin, Benjamin Rush, and other signers of this Declaration wanted political freedom from the British

Empire (Silverman 1984, 427; Goodman 1934, 56), professional freedom from British hierarchies (Haber 1991, 3–14; Shryock 1960, 1–43), and cultural freedom from Puritan theism (Mather [1710] 1966, ix).

III. PHILOSOPHICAL MEDICAL ETHICS

When 30-year-old Benjamin Rush signed the Declaration of Independence, he had been practicing and teaching medicine in Philadelphia for seven years. For Rush, professional honor and authority were rooted in the scientific and philosophical ideals of his mentors in Philadelphia and Edinburgh. As a medical student at Edinburgh, he listened to the introductory lectures of John Gregory, the first systematic moral philosopher of medicine in English-speaking countries (Rush 1948, 42; Haakonssen 1997, 190–95). Gregory championed the scientific inquiry of Baconian induction and experiment, and a few key moral virtues such as Hume's notion of sympathy (McCullough 1998a; Burns 2000; see also Chapter 30).

One month after returning from Europe in 1769, Rush was invited to teach chemistry to medical students at the College of Philadelphia where John Morgan and others had organized the first medical school in the British Colonies of North America (1765). Rush taught this subject for 20 years, a testament to his belief that an uneducated, unscientific physician could not be morally virtuous (Goodman 1934, 29–31, 129). In creating medical schools, Morgan, Rush, Samuel Bard and others institutionalized their moral values about education and the improvement of medical science (Postell 1958; Stookey 1962). Bard's commencement address to the first group of students graduating from the new medical school at King's College in New York City in 1769 was a concise sample of the philosophical medical ethics acquired by the American students in Edinburgh and systematically developed by Rush (Bard 1769; Langstaff 1942).

Neither Bard nor Rush believed that scientific expertise was sufficient for a physician's moral virtuosity. After Rush became a professor at the University of Pennsylvania (1792), he emulated Gregory and gave several introductory lectures on medical ethics in various courses between 1801 (Rush 1811) and 1812 (Rush 1818). They demonstrated Rush's systematic adaptation of Scottish moral philosophy and British medical ethics to the problems and challenges of New World medicine (Burns 1999a; Haakonssen 1997, 216–26; see also Chapter 30).

Piety, humanity, and patriotism were the dominant ideals of the Scottish moral philosophers and their intellectual heirs. Rush specified many ways that physicians could be pious, humane, and patriotic. He braided his injunctions into a fabric of duties, virtues, pleasures, and successes that any conscientious student could understand. He wanted these students to become scientific doctors who blended Christian charity, compassionate gentleness, and profound respect for the "common good" of their new polity. Fulfilling their moral duties to God, fellow humans, and communities would confirm the merit of eternally valid virtues, meet the high expectations assigned truly professional doctors, and assure beneficial and progressive outcomes for all. Rush wanted all physicians to be moral philosophers who deliberately married the practice of scientific medicine to a philosophically grounded medical ethics.

Rush's impact on the development of medical ethics in the United States was profound. As the teaching of moral philosophy spread throughout American colleges after 1800, Rush's philosophical medical ethics percolated in medical school commencement addresses, medical society orations, and codes of medical ethics adopted by groups of physicians who wanted authority as scientific and virtuous professionals (Smith 1956; Sloan 1971; Burns 1999a). Unlike Mather and Rush, however, many American healers during the 1700s were not university educated.

IV. POPULAR MEDICAL ETHICS

Throughout the eighteenth century, hundreds of natives and immigrants received health care from formally untrained persons like Martha Ballard. Between 1785 and 1812, Ballard assisted at least 816 parturient women who lived in Hallowell, Maine along a 10-mile stretch of the Kennebec River (Ulrich 1990, 5). She was summoned at any hour of the day or night; and she even walked through blizzards and fell from her horse during rainstorms as she hastened to help the settlers of a town whose population doubled during the 1790s (Ulrich 1990, 167). "God grant me strength to bear my toil and affliction," she prayed repeatedly (Ulrich 1990, 230).

Only one of her patients died during delivery; five died afterward. After one difficult delivery in 1800, Ballard wrote in her diary: "She had a Laborious illness but Blessed be God it terminated in safety. May shee and I ascribe the prais to the Great parent of the universe" (Ulrich 1990, 169). She witnessed only fourteen stillbirths and five infant deaths shortly after birth (Ulrich 1990, 170). She sought help from physicians only twice (Ulrich 1990, 180). She expected payment for her services and received shillings, notes of credit, and many household items.

In addition to midwifery, Ballard prescribed and prepared herbal concoctions, gave enemas, counted worms discharged by children, and cleaned and prepared bodies for burial. During the 4 months before her death, the 77-year-old Congregationalist made fourteen deliveries, sustained as always by family, friends, and faith in a good and powerful Providence (Ulrich 1990, 127, 300, 340).

V. CONCLUSION: MULTIPLE MORAL AUTHORITIES

In fashioning templates of moral values for daily decisions, Mather, Rush, and Ballard juggled competing imperatives from different sources. Rush did not dismiss religious values as an integral part of a physician's ethics, but, unlike Mather, he did not use Puritan ideals to assess the right and wrong of medical practices. Instead, the moral judgments of university professors and fellow doctors became the principal sources of the standards used by Rush to determine morally acceptable conduct for physicians. Martha Ballard was probably not acquainted with Gregory's medical ethics. Yet, a strong desire to relieve the distresses of parturient women and the diseases of their families — an example of Gregorian sympathy — wove the ethical threads in the caregiving services cooperatively performed by Ballard, neighborhood women, and local physicians in Hallowell's social web (Ulrich 1990, 97–98). Ballard's religious faith and her persistent service in "doing good" would have surely pleased Mather. Yet, her willingness to test folk remedies with her own observations was also congruent with the experiential component of both Puritan and Scottish legacies.

For all three, the tests of "lived experience" and "favorable outcome" superceded the moral claims of churches, past medical authorities, professional societies, and unenforceable licensure laws. Smallpox inoculation saved lives; this reality trumped any opposing moral claim, even one from a university-educated doctor such as Douglas. Because some of the herbal remedies of North American Indians relieved the miseries of disease, Mather and Rush prescribed them (Vogel 1970, 43–45, 64–65). As they fashioned their healer consciences in a new polity in a New World, all three assigned cultural primacy to the politically unfettered choices of each individual (Strottman 1999). All three cherished the same political freedom that gave each of their patients the moral right to choose a pastor-physician, an apprentice-trained doctor, a university-educated physician, a midwife, or a quack.

The multiple sources of moral authority that shaped the consciences of Mather, Rush, and Ballard also undergirded the moral struggles of their successors in subsequent centuries. Worthington Hooker's vision of medical morality was no cultural accident. The only North American physician to write a monograph on medical ethics in the nineteenth century, Hooker was a graduate of Harvard Medical School and a deacon in the Church of the United Society in New Haven. In *Physician and Patient* (1849), Hooker blended the eighteenth-century legacies of English Puritanism and Scottish moral philosophy in a systematic analysis that focused on the morally distinctive feature of the new American polity. Physicians and patients should voluntarily and reciprocally share responsibilities for determining the moral standards that should guide their expectations and interactions (Burns 1967, 1995).

CHAPTER 32

THE DISCOURSES OF PRACTITIONERS IN NINETEENTH-
AND TWENTIETH-CENTURY FRANCE

Robert A. Nye

I. INTRODUCTION

The great watershed in the development and practice of medical ethics in modern France was World War II. Prior to the war there was neither a legal nor informal *régime* of ethics that was uniformly enforced or voluntarily followed. Substantial disagreement existed about the nature of doctors' obligations to one another, their patients, and to the state. All this changed during the Vichy regime that ruled France between 1940 and 1944. On October 7, 1940, in line with the corporatist ideals of the regime, a government-controlled *Ordre des Médecins* was founded with authority over licensing, discipline, and many of the details of medical education and practice. The new *Ordre* was retained following the defeat of the Germans, but was allowed more autonomy, including the legal enforcement of a written code of professional ethics, adopted by statute in 1947. For the first time in the history of French medicine, all doctors had a legal obligation to follow a standard body of ethical doctrine. It took a bit longer, as we shall see, for ethical principles themselves to change, but it was a momentous development in the practical moral orientation of French medicine.

Between the reorganization of French medicine during the French Revolutionary era and the brief reign of Marshall Petain, French doctors did not have a reliable body of ethical guidance. Indeed, if words mean anything at all, French doctors had no ethics whatsoever, because the word "ethics" itself rarely figured in what we might now define as ethical reflection and practice (see Chapter 28). This does not mean that doctors acted without moral direction or constraint; rather, the moral outlook of medical professionals was determined by a patchwork of formal and informal standards that were in turn dependent on a number of social, economic, and political developments. These standards may be grouped into a few distinct categories: (1) a regime of criminal and civil law and evolving jurisprudence; (2) the emergence of a professional *deontology* that attempted to regulate intraprofessional relations; (3) state intervention in the medical marketplace. This chapter will examine each, in turn.

II. THE SOCIO-ECONOMIC CONTEXT OF THE MEDICAL PROFESSION

Developments within these categories were in turn reliant on a range of socio-economic and demographic factors that impinged variously on doctors and their patients. The doctor–patient ratio and the density of medicalization, which changed throughout the modern era, inspired doctors to pursue political and deontological strategies appropriate to the situation. Good and bad economic times, the number of practitioners graduating from the medical faculties, and the hierarchical situation within French medicine itself also influenced how medical professionals reflected on their tripartite obligations to colleagues, patients, and the state. New developments in medical technology and practice also influenced moral outlook, but less than one might think, even though the midpoint of our period was the classic period of "pasteurization" in France and elsewhere in the West.

Unfortunately for French medical professionals, the combination of socio-economic and legal–political developments that structured their working environment unfolded almost wholly beyond their control. They could not muster the numbers or power to influence the state, and, divided among themselves, could not act cooperatively in their own collective interest. The Revolutionary legal settlements abolished the old corporations, including those of surgeons and physicians, and forbade their legal reorganization in the name of individual liberty. Through its control of medical education and licensing, the state did give practitioners a *de jure* monopoly over the practice of medicine, and therefore provided, at least in theory, the legal grounds for the prosecution of charlatans, empirics, and other unofficial healers (Ramsey 1988). Napoleonic legislators and their successors, however, not only created a less well-educated cadre of practitioners called *officiers de santé*, who clustered in less remunerative practices in the countryside, but also contributed to the formation of a medical elite by creating committees of medical luminaries in Paris to oversee the administration of public hygiene, and by founding an Academy of Medicine that gathered useful knowledge and dispensed political advice to governments (Weisz 1995).

In addition to these legal and social obstacles to collective organization, medical men were positively attracted to a liberal model of medical practice that placed great value on the independence of the individual practitioner. As contemporary observers understood, in the course of the nineteenth century, the defense of professional autonomy was at once a claim on bourgeois social status and an article of faith in the sacral nature of a physician's personal and financial relationship with his client (Lapie 1905, 394; Thamin and Lapie 1903, 62). Collective action with other doctors smacked of the tactics of disenfranchised workers that many feared was likely to attract the attention and hence the intervention of the state. Because, in any case, medical practice provided a barely adequate income for the bulk of medical professionals throughout this era, any development that threatened their professional independence was anathema.

The reputations and incomes of medical professionals were also threatened by the formidable army of irregular healers that swarmed over the countryside competing with doctors for clients and fees. Although the empirics, magnetizers, wise women, and clerical healers posed the greatest threat to rural practitioners, alternative modes of healing were far more common, widespread, and persistent than was once thought (Faure 1993, 29–41; Ramsey 1999). The clients of these "charlatans" were not inclined to press charges against them, even when a cure went dreadfully wrong. The district prosecutors were not zealous to intervene; they deplored irregular practice, but getting witnesses was tricky, and empirics were often acquitted in jury trials (Galérant 1990, 66; Léonard 1981a, 12). Medical men themselves bore the burden and expense of bringing charges, but success was far from certain and the bad publicity of bringing legal action against local personalities often outweighed the advantages gained by removing a competitor.

Thus, the state refused to help physicians in the areas they most needed assistance, and blocked their collective organization. It made no effort to limit the supply of newly minted Doctors of Medicine in crowded medical markets, and, as the century progressed, it thrust new public health and welfare obligations on doctors without assuring proportional compensation. It is not surprising that medical professionals were deeply ambivalent about state intervention in medical affairs. One segment of the profession favored increasing state support to protect medical incomes and prerogatives and another preferred both medical individualism and professional autonomy over surrendering any of their liberty to practice medicine without restraint. These conflicts plagued the profession until the Vichy "solution" was imposed from without.

There was, however, one thing on which all practitioners agreed. Theirs was a noble profession with historic claims to high status and social utility; it was distinguished from other professions and trades by its disinterested, courageous, and honorable mission (Menière and Brouchoud 1860, 11–21). The sense of corporate identity and unity inspired by this conviction served as the foundation for the moral outlook and the practical orientation that constituted medical ethics *avant la lettre* in French medicine. In the absence of state support or internal unity, this moral stance became the chief means by which medical professionals asserted and defended their rights, distinguished themselves from illegal competitors, and grounded their claims for state protection. This essentially intraprofessional ethos also brought certain positive benefits for patients, but this consequence was not originally or primarily the inspiration for it. To a considerable degree, modern medical ethics has evolved from a moral outlook that was designed to compensate for the profession's historic impotence.

III. The Regime of Civil and Criminal Law

It will be useful to consider the historical evolution of these developments by analyzing the interrelated categories noted previously. The Napoleonic code appeared during the first decade of the nineteenth century; the code and the jurisprudence derived from it has provided the legal environment for medical practice in the modern era. The code provided penalties in criminal (arts. 319, 320) and civil law (arts. 1382, 1383) for personal harm and damage suits, and the prohibition of abortion (art. 317). Neither aggrieved patients nor public prosecutors resorted much to these statutes in the nineteenth century. Only after the turn of the century did particularly grave cases of medical negligence attract large penalties or cash settlements, not coincidentally at the point when medicine itself became more efficacious (Carvais 1986, 226–47).

The principal element of Napoleonic law that affected doctors was article 378 of the criminal code, the so-called medical secret. Whatever it later became, the measure was originally intended to assure private individuals of the discretion of medical professionals, including pharmacists and midwives, who had access to the intimate details of their lives and finances. The law applied especially to doctors who were inescapably privy to all matters of birth, death, legitimacy, disease, and the physical health and potency of prospective brides, grooms, and married couples (Muteau 1870, 245–49). In a society that passed on the overwhelming bulk of personal wealth through bloodlines, the physician was a privileged observer of the biological facts that underlay the transmission of family property and reputation.

To their credit, medical professionals had the good sense, over time, to transform this legal constraint into a moral obligation that reflected positively on them. What began as a sanction became not only a virtue peculiar to physicians, but also the "angular rock" of the relations of trust between doctor and patient, and thus the source of medical authority itself (Villey 1986, 7–8). The self-restraint and discretion imposed on doctors by the law became an aspect of the medical character, smoothing the path by which the doctor replaced the priest as the keeper of the secrets and the honor of families in the nineteenth century (Muteau 1870, xiv). As one of the authors of the popular "physiologies" of professional life put it in 1841, as the prestige of the priesthood declines, "the doctor has become, of necessity, the keeper of the mysteries of the marital bed and of intimate affections, the obliging confident of all human weaknesses, and, in protecting the honor of families he has elevated his profession by enabling the secret of the confessional to become the secret of medicine" (Roux [1841] 1982, 8).

Legal scholars have pointed out precisely this evolutionary development, denying the claims medical authors have sometimes made that it was the prior existence of medical discretion that prompted the adoption of the statute rather than the other way around (Thouvenin 1982, 11). Rather, the ethical commitment of doctors to the medical secret may be deduced from the jurispru-

dence on article 378 over the course of the nineteenth century, as doctors incorporated the sanction into professional practice. As Emile Garçon wrote, by the end of the nineteenth century the law had attained a social and general interest that transcended the original intent of the Napoleonic legislator. The law operated "less to protect the confidences of a particular individual than to guarantee a professional duty indispensable to everyone. This secret is thus absolute and of public significance" (Garçon 1956, 516–17). Recent critics have alleged that the medical secret has been more of a cover for medical mischief than a protection for patients, but there is no denying the evolution of the social meaning of the medical secret from legal sanction to moral duty (Hulot-Pietri 1989, 18).

By the end of the nineteenth century, doctors fully appreciated the supplementary moral benefits of adhering closely to the medical secret, so much so that they were reluctant to set it aside for important public health initiatives. Public hygiene laws in 1892 and 1902 required specific medical verification of victims of various contagious diseases. Doctors had ordinarily revealed such information in plague time, but the new laws were meant to apply to quotidien medical contacts and were fiercely resisted by rank and file doctors. Some refused to comply at all; their stubborn resistance was partially responsible for the fact that venereal disease and tuberculosis, which were regarded as possibly hereditary and "shameful" afflictions at this time, were not included among the reportable diseases (Villey 1986, 84–89). Even before World War I, and well into the interwar period, the medical secret served as the basis for opposing third-party payments from government agencies where these required describing the condition being treated for reimbursement (Perreau 1905, 1–3; Villey 1986, 93–94).

It seems likely that by the dawn of the twentieth century the medical secret may have been as useful in the defense of professional interests as it was for protecting patient confidentiality. This may explain why jurisprudence in 1885 that broadened the grounds of the offense to include responsibility even when there had been no intent to do harm was warmly received by professionals (Brouardel 1893b, 15–28). Nonetheless, there is no doubting that the obligation of keeping the medical secret stimulated ethical reflection, although invariably of a distinctly defensive, even negative kind. One of the most debated issues was whether a doctor was obliged to keep from an intended bride the knowledge that her husband-to-be suffered from a venereal infection. Hard-liners refused to compromise, others suggested vague or allusive warnings, and more than a few felt justified in warning future husbands about such dangers but not future wives (Brouardel 1893b, 42–63; Harsin 1989, 72–95). The medical secret experienced a brief moment of glory between 1940 and 1945 when it served as a justification for resisting German and Vichyite demands for the denunciation of traitors, but today the secret is "shared" by law with public health officials and special exceptions are rare (Portes 1954, 131–54). Even so, it is still regarded as an ethical cornerstone of medical practice (Ordre National des Médecins 1983). In view of the mutual attitude of *laissez-faire* that prevailed between medicine and the state in France until 1940, it would be too much to say that the state actively shaped the ethics of the profession, but the legal structure set up in the first decade of the nineteenth century did provide an environment of incentives and penalties that guided doctors in their everyday interaction with the public.

IV. Professional Medical Deontology

Perhaps the most important category bearing on the moral practices of French doctors has been a professional deontology. The term, if not the concept, is an invention of the British philosopher Jeremy Bentham, meaning literally the "science of duties." Historically, deontologies have been short on metaphysics and have consisted entirely of rules governing professional conduct. The concept has been very popular in France; even today, during the ascendancy of medical ethics, deontology is regarded by many doctors as a more reliable guide to professional comportment than ethical casuistry (Almeras and Pequignot 1996, 1–3). The present Ordre des Médecins presides over a statutory body of deontological rules, and its Council possesses the power to discipline and expel transgressors, but, in truth, the code also serves as a legal shield for those who follow it with adequate scrupulousness.

Although we tend to think of rules as written, the first published deontologies did not appear in France until the 1840s. Most of these were partial, local, and voluntary and dealt almost wholly with intraprofessional relations. The most successful ones regulated geographically discrete populations of professionals, but they were often rhetorically inflated and unenforceable guides to ideal behavior. Of course, the graduates of some medical schools swore a leave-taking oath that ostensibly bound them to good conduct, but until the twentieth century only Montpellier graduates swore a brief oath modeled loosely on the Hippocratic credo, promising, essentially, to "do no harm," and some of the newer medical faculties still did not have an oath in place as late as 1936 (Dulieu 1988b, 134–36).

Both oaths of allegiance and the codes that regulated the relations between men belong to a far older tradition in oral culture that reaches back to the European Middle Ages (see Chapters 24, 26). They originated in oaths of fealty and codes of honor that situated noblemen in a hierarchical, often military, corporate order in which they were also, nonetheless, peers (Neuschel 1989, 17–19; Nye 1993, 23–26). Guildsmen and members of the free professions in medieval and early modern towns modeled their

internal relations on these same codes, although they did not resort so frequently as did their noble superiors to the *point d'honneur* to resolve their differences (Lefèbvre 1991, 142–47). The ultimate guarantee of good corporate conduct was a man's personal honor, which moved him to honorable acts and inspired him to avoid shame. Thus, a company of honorable gentlemen did not need written rules or disciplinary councils because they held the conviction that probity, a grasp of the etiquette of masculine sociability, and the sentiment of loyalty were natural to the sort of man who was already, or destined to be, of their number (Nye 1995, 98–100).

The abolition of noble privilege in 1789 and the termination of the medieval corporations, including those of surgeons and physicians, did not bring an end to these practices; they put down new roots in the egalitarian soil of bourgeois social life in the form of *cercles*, clubs, and trade and professional associations uniting men of common occupational and educational interests. Honor was less concentrated in these new venues, but no less exigent that every man's behavior measure up to standards that would not bring dishonor to the group (Nye 1993; Reddy 1997; Harrison 1999). Some of these groups adopted written statutes to regulate admission and set out goals, but they were typically lacking in specific injunctions other than that members must observe the "rules of honor" in their relations with one another (Agulhon 1977, 40). The first medical deontologies grew out of a similar social cosmos.

Without associations or unity, medical men needed a crisis to provoke the first halting steps toward constructing a code of professional duties. That crisis began to build in the 1840s in the form of growing concern about an oversupply of medical personnel, growing competition for patients, and shrinking professional honoraria. Much of the impetus behind these concerns came from urban doctors; the ratio of medically trained individuals to population was far lower in the countryside (Sussman 1977, 293–99; Weisz 1979, 6–7). The chief targets of concern were illegal practitioners and the *officiers de santé*, the paramedical practitioners created in the post-Revolutionary era.

At the urging of a group of Parisian doctors, led by a Parisian practitioner and medical editor, Amédée Latour, a medical congress was convened in Paris in 1845. The organizers understood that they should couch their professional concerns about medical competition in terms that flattered the charitable and selfless nature of their work; thus they coupled their demands with assertions about respect for the medical secret, a commitment to free treatment of the poor, and the heroic behavior of doctors in plague time (Guillaume 1996, 49–55). The chief aims of the congress were to recommend that the government eliminate the *officiers de santé* and facilitate the organization of regional disciplinary councils. Staffed entirely by local medical men, the councils were to bring charlatans and illegals to the attention of the authorities and regulate the private and professional comportment of doctors, thus becoming "the safeguard of medical dignity" (Weisz 1979, 11). The government bill that emerged to meet this crisis was not well received, and foundered, in any event, in the wake of the 1848 revolution; however, the experience nourished the resolve of activists to press ahead with other organizational plans, and to develop deontologies that could bring greater order and discipline, and therefore greater public respect, to medical practice.

On the organizational front, at the instigation of Latour and others, an Association Générale des Médecins de France was formed in 1858. The Association had a limited legal scope, confined mostly to mutual aid activities, but within a few years had registered a majority of French practitioners. In succeeding years, a wave of medical publications – L'Union Médicale, Le Progrès Médicale, and Concours Médicale – began to appear that concerned themselves to a considerable extent with deontological matters (Léonard 1981b, 195–201). The most important deontological treatise to appear during this troubled period was Maxmilien Simon's Déontologie Médicale (1845), the first text to treat Bentham's concept in a particular professional context. Despite this genealogy Simon's thought owed much less to Bentham and the utilitarian tradition than to an ethical outlook inspired by a Christian social romanticism peculiar to the times.

Simon's text was almost completely *sui generis*. It arose out of unique circumstances and had no direct French successors. In his fervent generosity toward the "miserables" of society, Simon spoke of the "holy apostolat" of medicine, invoked the example of Christ as healer and solace, and counseled the physician to follow the Christian injunctions to practice charity among the poor (Simon 1845, 4, 10, 29, 257). As an adept of the "medicine of the passions" popular in the era, Simon believed that mental states could positively or negatively influence illness and that the optimistic convictions and comforting presence of the physician could have an ameliorating effect (Simon 1845, 205–21). He deplored the skepticism about greedy and ineffective doctors that was widespread in society and warned his colleagues that only exemplary generosity, courage, and compassion could reestablish their reputations as healers. There could be, he wrote, no "aristocracy of pain" in a democracy of suffering.

According to Simon, the good character of the physician helped him to resist all temptations and to respect the secrets of families. He worried about the twin materialisms of money and science that could undermine the sacramental aspects of the practitioner's duties to society, patients, and medical peers, but was confident that prudence, perseverance, and sympathy would suffice to protect each man

and the reputation of the profession as a whole against slander and skepticism. Simon's Catholic outlook inclined him against radical experimental treatments, euthanasia, abortion, and marriages contracted only for the gratifying of the passions (Simon 1845, 336–38, 453, 472). The religiously inflected ethical vision adumbrated in this extraordinary text faded in the course of the next 40 years as French doctors overwhelmingly embraced the materialistic, anticlerical outlook characteristic of the era, but many of the principles in Simon's book were perpetuated in a new discourse of secular humanism.

There was little ethical writing until the 1880s, when the first of a "second wave" of deontologies began to appear. The most authoritative of these was the lengthy article published by Amédée Dechambre in the *Dictionnaire encyclopédique des sciences médicales*, the standard medical reference work of the era. Deontology, he wrote, was a body of duties and rights, but these were grounded inescapably in the personal qualities of the medical practitioner, indeed in his character as a "man of honor." The delicate tasks and heavy responsibilities of the physician required personal honesty but also a willingness to risk "disgust, fatigue, and life itself" in the service of others (Dechambre 1882, 481, 488–89). A doctor's reputation for honesty and circumspection, his personal habits and modesty, were crucial, argued Dechambre, for forging relations of trust with patients, which then served as an important part of his therapeutic armamentarium. Dechambre believed, with most of his peers, that a patient's chance of cure depended on the natural authority of the physician, and he was not beneath suggesting that a superior education, including Latin and Greek, were splendid complements to his scientific know how (Dechambre 1882, 504–505). Discretion, honor, and personal distinction in a medical man not only appealed to clients, they served to mark the differences with charlatans and quacks, and enhanced the reputation and solidarity of the entire profession. Character was thus the foundation of successful individual medical practice and of the prosperity of medicine itself.

Dechambre was doubtful, however, that honorable character could be taught from codes alone. What was needed, he averred, was some form of collective discipline that would have the effect of remoralizing the profession. Dechambre appreciated the distaste many of his colleagues had for any collective action that vitiated the principle of free practice, but toothless local medical associations were not up to the task; disciplinary councils or commissions of surveillance were needed that would defend the "citadel of public health" by repressing defaults of "dignity and professional honorability" that undermined patient confidence in all medical men. If the "nobility" of the profession consisted in the virile courage and moral correction of individual professionals, then doctors themselves must assume responsibility for eliminating flawed and dishonorable brethren (Dechambre 1882, 520–24).

Dechambre also offered particular advice on clients, honoraria, and intraprofessional relations. Of clients, he has little good to say. We are still a long way here from modern notions of patient rights and the respect due to the human personality. In Dechambre's view, patients are skeptical of the medical arts but the easy dupes of clever charlatans. They are prejudiced, ignorant of natural processes, and prone to give themselves over to divine mercy or religious cures. Doubtful of success at the outset of treatment, they are ungrateful and niggardly following a full recovery. Doctors must learn forbearance at clients' passionate rages, mockery, hypochondria, malingering, or frailty in the face of disability or death (Dechambre 1882, 541–59).

Dechambre's advice with respect to collegial relations is mostly concerned with the issues of medical precedence, the etiquette of consultations and the collection of fees, the proper honoraria to charge for medical services, and admonitions against offering criticism of the medical opinion of colleagues. In all these considerations the patient's right to abandon or change practitioners is respected utterly; the doctor who is replaced must vanish silently and not second guess his successor. On the other hand, consultations between colleagues are never conducted in the patient's presence, lying to the patient for his own good is countenanced, and any doctor retains the right to refuse an uncooperative or capricious patient if he chooses. Considerable space is spent in this and most other nineteenth century deontologies on the etiquette of setting up or vacating a practice, avoiding the appearance of poaching a colleague's patients, and abstaining from medical advertising or publicity (Dechambre 1882, 560–75). Dechambre was punctilious about doctors' obligation to respect the medical secret and refuse abortions but he did not dwell at length on matters that, in the event, were forbidden by law.

The era from 1880 to 1905 brought numerous changes to medical practice, most of which increased the incentive among medical professionals to organize and implement self-regulation. Several pieces of social and welfare legislation, culminating in a law of 1902, required an unprecedented number of involuntary medical treatments, inspections, and certifications at low levels of remuneration. The rapid growth of Mutual Aid societies (2,000,000 members by 1900), and industrial medicine confronted doctors with huge collectivities able to negotiate lower medical fees for their clients (Guillaume 1996, 106–13). A law of 1892 did give doctors some competitive relief by finally abolishing the *officiers de santé*, but this was easily outweighed by surges of enrollments in medical schools at the end of the century and by the addition of four additional degree-granting institutions. There were 590 medical degrees granted in 1889 and 1,152 in 1901; according to Paul Brouardel, Dean of the Paris Medical School, there were 5,000 students enrolled in his faculty in 1902 (Brouardel 1893a, 14; Hildreth 1987, 56).

Doctors were far from united in their responses to these new conditions of practice. The medical elite, mostly clustered in Paris, had well-paying clients, consultancies, and lucrative official connections. The youngest doctors were often obliged to take salaried positions as Mutual Society or industrial doctors. In between, the vast bulk of practitioners found that medical incomes had stagnated at the level they had been in 1850, hardly more than the annual earnings of a small shopkeeper (D'Avenel 1907, 117–48); it was this group that provided the most fertile recruiting ground for medical organization and activism throughout this era. A new syndicalist organization, a Union des Syndicats Médicaux, was founded by Dr. Auguste Cézilly in 1881. This umbrella federation, which united town and departmental societies from all over France, achieved the right to engage in legal negotiations with insurers and the state in 1892 and had enrolled well over fifty percent of the 20,000 doctors in France by 1910 (Guillaume 1996, 120).

The explosion of medical syndicalization coincided with a kind of golden age of deontological writing and debate. A vast deontological congress was held in Paris in 1900 at which the grievances of the profession were aired. Competition from recent MDs and immigrant physicians and also from recent women graduates had intensified the medical "struggle for existence," and speaker after speaker demanded a regulatory apparatus for medicine akin to the *Ordre des Avocats* that would protect the honor of the profession by treating all doctors as peers subject to the same discipline. It was also at this time that the principle of the right of a patient to choose his own doctor became an article of faith to which the vast majority of doctors — increasingly confronted by the threat of bureaucracy and third party payments — could subscribe (*Comte Rendu de la Première Session de Congrès International de Médicine Professional* 1900, 631, 181, 358).

At the practical level local syndicates themselves undertook the task of disciplining medical professionals in their regions. There are records of the deontological statutes some of them adopted, urging members to be "loyal" and "courteous" to one another and proclaiming their commitment to the "cult of professional dignity." Although the syndicates had no power to discipline nonmembers, and only limited powers over their own *syndiqués*, they reserved the right to expel men who transgressed deontological rules or engaged in questionable behavior and urge collective shunning (Nye 1995, 104–105). In general, the codes applied the rule, "Don't do to your confrère what you would not want him to do to you," but they also took aim at state interference by raising doubts about the propriety of salaried medicine and fees set by third parties (Syndicat Médical de Lille et de la Région 1903, 17, 25–26).

These brief deontologies were based on a large body of lengthier treatises produced during this period of organizational effervescence. Medical authors typically presented their deontologies as necessary to the profession and secondarily useful to patients. Courtesy, adherence to the medical secret, and the acknowledgment of a "natural" precedence of rank or age between consultants guaranteed an orderly and discreet path toward diagnosis and treatment. Resistance to "collective" medicine and the "loyal" commitment to fair competition protected a patient's unfettered freedom of choice, and the profession's solidarity against illegals and malpractice minimized the dangers of unsafe care (Cassine 1896, 36–56; Grasset 1900a, 11–12).

An unsoiled character, courage, and honor were still the most important elements of effective medical practice (Juhel-Rénoy 1892, 33, 66; Grelletry 1900). These essentially masculine qualities also operated to distinguish Frenchmen from women and foreigners who lacked, as one writer put it, "a chivalrous sentiment, a native generosity, a universally acknowledged disinterestedness, all eminently French qualities" (Peinard 1894, 24). The character of the medical man ought to transcend both law and morality and attain the certainty and the intuitiveness of faith "not unlike religion itself" (Cassine 1896, 63; Morache 1901, 154). Accordingly, the deontologies of the era were skeptical of the virtues of the modern "scientific" curriculum introduced around the turn of the century. The classical curriculum formed character more surely, for, as Joseph Grasset wrote in 1900, "One may always question the scientific abilities of a doctor, but one ought never to contest his high moral qualities. We ought to take it as a point of departure that we are all absolutely equal on this terrain" (Grasset 1900a, 21). The medical nationalism and antimodernism of French medicine in the interwar years are prefigured clearly here (Guillaume 1996, 126).

The Union des Syndicats Médicaux lasted until 1929 when it reinvented itself as the Confédération des Syndicats Médicales Français. This reorganization was prompted by continuing concerns about medical overpopulation, a rise in cases of embarrassing medical insurance fraud, and increasing numbers of foreign doctors who had obtained French medical degrees and settled in France or had become naturalized citizens. The new organization rededicated itself to the syndicalist "Medical Charter" of 1927 that had affirmed its support of the "liberal" practice of medicine. By 1930, the Confederation could claim approximately 80 percent of French medical professionals as its own and seemed inexorably to be inclining toward greater centralization to assure its aims. There was little support within the rank and file, however, for a centralized disciplinary apparatus. Local practitioners did not want elite doctors in Paris second guessing their ethical behavior, or imposing on them a set of deontological rules that accorded ill with the conditions of regional medical practice.

V. STATE INTERVENTION IN THE MEDICAL MARKETPLACE

In 1929, the Confederation membership read in the organization's publication, *Médecin de France*, about a government initiative to sponsor an Ordre des Médecins if the Confederation could agree on a plan. The journal assured its readers that they had nothing to fear from the "confraternal" surveillance of their peers; on the contrary, by engaging in a great work of "professional and social morality," the scandals associated with false insurance claims and third-party revelations of the medical secret could be ended once and for all and the sacred regime of doctor–patient relations restored (*Médecin de France*, March 1, 1929, 140). It was not the "French doctor" who was at fault, but the undeterred "foreign invasion which is slowly covering the whole of French soil" (*Médecin de France*, March 15, 1929, 169); an Order of Doctors would have the capacity to deal with that and other problems of deontology.

Within weeks Paul Cibrie, the long-term editor of *Médecin de France*, announced the new plan. The Order would have the power to inscribe and reinscribe doctors in an official register of all French physicians. The organization would be departmental and elective, with the possibility of appeal to regional councils. The departmental councils would resolve professional conflicts, arbitrate disputes between doctors and third parties (patients and insurers), and address infractions of the official deontology. The plan would assure total medical autonomy, no publicity of proceedings, and no legal grounds for state intervention. As a bill slowly worked its way through the Chamber of Deputies, it was amended to give government a greater role, including the appointment of magistrates to regional appeals courts (Cibrie, *Médecin de France*, March 15, 1932, 259–61). Meanwhile, a commission established by the Confederation to write a deontology found resistance among many doctors to injunctions that were too specific and sanctions that were too harsh and administered too distantly from locales. The Confederation was never able to resolve the contradictions between the fierce independence of grassroots practitioners and the need for a uniform code that had the force of law. The bill for an *Ordre des Médecins* foundered in the Chamber of Deputies and the Confederation pursued other legislative solutions to its problems (Evleth 1995, 96–100).

This failure did not preclude the eventual publication of a deontology that had the general support of the membership or the continuation of a tradition of local deontological self-regulation. In 1936, the Confederation published a Code de Déontologie, the first document in the history of French medicine that could claim to express the ethical concerns and practices of the majority of the profession. It had no legal standing other than the force of "professional jurisdiction," but it successfully incorporated both long-standing intraprofessional traditions and recent practical concerns and was neither too detailed nor too abstract to serve as a guide for the average practitioner. As the direct ancestor of the first official code of the *Ordre des Médecins* of 1947, this code deserves analysis.

It comprises fifty-two articles, divided between general duties, duties owed to patients, to collectivities, colleagues, and a final section on honoraria. Article one established the principle that doctors must display honor and dignity in their professional and their private lives and respect the "honor and dignity of the medical corps," and article two affirmed the individual responsibility and independence of every practitioner (*Médecin de France* 1936, 947). These bedrock principles were supplemented by warnings about publicity, bogus titles, untested cures, and other tactics in the arsenal of charlatanry. An innovative section of the code proclaimed respect for the "human person" and warned against experimentation on patients; otherwise, it adopted the usual injunctions against too few or too frequent visits to the sick, a rigorous respect for confidentiality, and the complete liberty of the patient to choose his physician (*Médecin de France* 1936, 948–49).

The section on collectivities aimed at ensuring the independence of the doctor and patient's medical secrets in relation to mutual aid societies, insurers, or duties of medical inspection, but it is clear that these justifications were meant to discourage doctors from accepting fees from any collectivity that might have the effect of depressing medical honoraria for all practitioners. The lengthy section on honoraria was equally firm on the dangers of undercutting colleagues or accepting less than the *minima* decreed by the local medical syndicate (*Médecin de France* 1936, 950, 954); indeed, the medical ethicist Jean Bernard remembered the 1920s as a time when ethical concerns were all about money (Bernard 1994, 318). Finally, and not surprisingly, the section on confraternal duties was the longest and the most dependent on ancient traditions, outlining a standard body of intraprofessional etiquette that might have been taken from any regional syndical code (*Médecin de France* 1936, 951–53).

Even before the code of 1936 was adopted, there is abundant evidence throughout the 1920s and 1930s that deontological self-regulation continued to be a regular feature of local professional practice. All syndicates had a Family Council that reviewed charges against doctors accused of padding or falsifying insurance or reimbursement claims (Portes 1954, 91). In the Department of the Oise, the Council put a doctor on the "index" who engaged in such behavior, ensuring his professional ostracism by fellow syndicalists (*Bulletin du Syndicat des Médecins de l'Oise*, Jan., 1933, 12–13). The Oise Council also

mediated "differences" between colleagues; it was especially hard on specialists who consulted outside their own neighborhood or members of the syndicate who maintained professional relations with those on the "index" (*Bulletin*, May, 1933, 90–95; July, 1933, 135–36). As a doctor from the Saone et Loire Department wrote about such judgments: "We are responsible only for the morality of syndicalists. We have an independent relation to the state and the right to judge or not judge on our own" (*Bulletin des Syndicats et de l'Association des Médecins de Saone et Loire*, 3 April, 1923, 30–31). Syndicated surgeons also employed a deontological committee that concerned itself with "clandestine" fee-splitting and other shady tactics (*Bulletin du Syndicat des Chirurgiens Français*, 1933, June, 1933, 24–25), and it appears as though the Administrative Council of the Confederation occasionally heard appeals from departmental syndicates and resolved intradepartmental squabbles (*Médecin de France*, May 15, 1934, 361–65, 417).

The Confederation was dissolved by Vichy and reconstituted after the war, but it was restricted to protecting the collective financial interests of practitioners, whereas deontological regulation fell to the new *Ordre des Médecins* (Loncke and Laroze 1987, 82–84). The Code for the new *Ordre*, promulgated in 1947, closely resembled its syndicalist ancestor of 1936. There was the same conviction that the freedom of patients to choose, direct doctor–patient payment, and the doctor's independence from collective entanglements guaranteed the moral foundations of professional practice (*Médecin de France*, June, 1947, 1080). Intraprofessional duties, and medical responsibilities with respect to "social" medicine, as it was now called, were little changed. The section on duties toward patients, however, revealed the first signs of the inexorable evolution toward present-day deontologies in which professional duties toward patients have been transformed into the enumeration of patient rights (*Médecin de France*, June, 1947, 1082–86). This development was slow and halting throughout the 1950s; however, doctors fought a long rear-guard action defending their right to keep the truth about a patient's condition from him on therapeutic grounds (Weisz 1990, 145–61), but notions of patient rights gained considerable momentum with the appearance of new reproductive technologies and medical rationing.

VI. CONCLUSION

We know too little about the detailed history of ethical practices in French medicine to judge whether the informal intraprofessional deontologies and the celebration of good medical character that dominated medicine during the century and a half before 1947 were much benefit to patients. Certainly some of the principles cherished by nineteenth-century doctors have survived. French patients still have free choice of their physician and may be confident that practitioners will respect their confidentiality. The personal moral qualities that practitioners once took to be the soul of the physician have been replaced by a scientific and technical education that serves now as the chief criterion of professional competence.

As Jean Bernard has written, doctors were more respected when they were therapeutically inefficacious. The debut of medical efficacy has inflated patient expectations, desacralized doctors, and made medical responsibility the legal and moral basis of much of contemporary ethical reflection (Bernard 1994, 200, 318–19).

CHAPTER 33

THE DISCOURSES OF PRACTITIONERS IN NINETEENTH-
AND TWENTIETH-CENTURY SPAIN

Diego Gracia

I. INTRODUCTION

In Spain, the nineteenth century really began in 1808, with the War of Independence against Napoleon. Spaniards of every persuasion – enlightened, conservative, or traditionalist – came together in the fight against the Napoleonic invasion. Conservatives fought against the ideals of secularization and the democratic principles of the French Revolution of 1789. Enlightenment liberals, on the other hand, fought for the possibility of developing their own liberal and democratic state without foreign interference. Resistance reached a critical point in 1812 with the promulgation of Spain's first democratic Constitution. This constitution was an important moment in the history of political liberalism. Indeed, the current political sense of the term "liberal," originated in Spain during this time period. From there it spread to become a commonly used word in other languages (Abellán 1984, 56). The Constitution of 1812 also had an important impact on both the subsequent history of Spanish liberalism and constitutionalism in several other countries, including Italy, Portugal, and many Latin American countries.

Spanish liberalism was destined to have a tempestuous history because of the determined opposition of the aristocracy and the Church, which tried to retain traditional privileges, recalling with nostalgia the past national glories of the sixteenth and seventeenth centuries. The Roman Catholic clergy also rejected liberalism as an anti-Christian ideology. The consequence of all of this was a series of civil wars in 1833–1839, 1845–1849, 1872–1876, and 1936–1939. Not until the last third of the twentieth century did the modernizing ideology of the Cadiz Courts of 1810–1812 triumph in Spain.

II. THE NEW MEDICAL ETHICS
OF THE "IDÉOLOGUES"

During the second half of the eighteenth century, there was a radical confrontation in France between two ways of thinking and doing, one "pre-revolutionary" and the other "counter-revolutionary." The first assumed many of the empirical principles and methods described by Condillac (see Chapter 32). This spirit prevailed in the French Revolution of 1789 and attained its apogee in the first decades of the nineteenth century, under the generic name, *Idéologie*. Idéologie's goal was to replace the rationalism of the "old regime" with a new theory of knowledge and science. This new mindset was deeply influenced by the British empiricism of Locke and Hume, which had appeared, and not by chance, in the context of the industrial revolution.

The *Idéologues* movement exerted a strong influence on French medicine (Rosen 1946b, 328–29) and, eventually, on Spanish medicine. A physician, Pierre-Jean-Georges Cabanis (1757–1808), was one of the founders of this movement. The focus of his reformist zeal was medical education in revolutionary France. He used the analytical method of Condillac and the rules of sensualism (or observations grounded in sensory experience, *sensations*) to reform clinical education, rejecting both Galenic dogmatism and the rationalism of the so-called systematics (Cabanis 1816).

Translations and editions of the works of Condillac, Cabanis, and Destutt de Tracy were plentiful in Spain during the last decades of the eighteenth century and the first decades of the nineteenth century (Gracia 1980, 232–33). Legislators in the Cadiz Courts were deeply imbued with this mentality. In addition to applying the reforming ideals of the Idéologues to politics and education, they also applied them to medicine. Ethics served as an intermediary in this process, as the title of one of Cabanis's books, *Rapports du Physique et du Moral de l'Homme* (*The Relationship between The Physical and the Moral in Man*, Cabanis 1802) indicates. Medicine freed of its traditional intellectual vices was to provide the scientific basis for Condillac's method, making apparent the way in which human life can be properly organized. Similarly, once purged of its ancient intellectual shibboleths, ethics too would aim to perfect human nature. As Cabanis puts it, the fundamentals of the moral man derive from the physiological man. The same ideals were also embraced by the Spanish ideologists of the first half of the nineteenth century, as evident in the life and work of Prudencio Maria Pascual, a reformer interested in educating new generations in the art of the right thinking, or Logic, and the art of right doing, or Ethics, as ways of reaching the freedom and the virtue that give place to the happiness of men. He wrote two books titled *Arte de pensar y obrar bien* (Art of Right Thinking and Doing, D.P.M.P.M. 1820), and *Sistema de la Moral o La Teoría de los Deberes* (*Moral System, or the Theory of Duties*, Pascual 1821).

The titles of Cabanis's and Pascual's books exemplify the ideals of ideologist ethics. Putting aside metaphysical and speculative prejudices, they aimed to base morality on the firm and secure foundations of physiology and medicine. Morality thus becomes closely allied with medicine. The goal of the former is to promote the greatest degree of happiness and fulfilment in human life. This goal can only be reached by perfecting the physiological dimension of human life. Theirs was a teleological morality, designed to maximize human perfection and happiness. A group of teachers at Salamanca University wrote a Report in 1820 recommending the reorganization of education on ideologists' principles. "The study of physiological man is as necessary to the doctor as to the moralist," the Report states, "because by discovering both the secrets of its organization, and observing the phenomena of life, the doctor is able to recognize the

status of perfect health, while the moralist can understand the operations that compose the functions of intelligence and the determinations of will" (Abellán 1984, 186). It is not surprising that the authors of this Report were very influenced by the English utilitarian philosopher, Jeremy Bentham (1748–1832), or that the ideologists introduced Bentham's utilitarianism into Spain (Abellan 1984, 193–96). The Report's main author, Toribio Nuñez (1766–1834), compares morality with medicine in prefatory remarks to his *Sistema de ciencia social* (*Social Science System*, Núñez 1820), using such concepts as "moral Physiology" and "moral Pathology" (Abellán 1984, 194). "Moral pathology," he argues, stands in need of "political clinics" to regulate people's lives via legislation, government, and law. Physiological ethics no longer depended on theologians and priests, but on philosophers, educators, and physicians. Ethics had become secular. With this secularization the relationship between morality and medicine changed. Whereas morality had previously been the domain of theologians, it was now the province of physicians.

An institutional infrastructure supporting Ideologie was created in Spanish medicine at the end of the eighteenth century, when new chairs of "clinical medicine" or "empirical medicine" were created in Granada (1776), Valencia (1786), Madrid (1795), Salamanca (1799), and by a royal order in 1801 in all other universities. Clinical teaching was now conducted in hospitals. In 1827, these chairs of practical medicine were included in the new curriculum of the schools of medicine and surgery, soon thereafter called Institutes for Medical Sciences, and, after 1845, simply medical schools. From their origin these chairs of clinical medicine had three characteristics. First, they were dependent on French medicine and, in particular, the medical school of Paris. Second, they considered themselves defenders of the "Hippocratic tradition," which they understood as pure, empirical, clinical medicine. Third, they defended the analytical method, in which clinical experience and observation are used to analyze the patient's physical symptoms and signs – which explains the strong influence of the Cabanis program in Spain.

In this intellectual milieu, Félix Janer (1771–1865) produced his *Elementos de Moral Médica* (*Treatise on Moral Medicine*, Janer 1831). This book appeared in a second edition 16 years later (Janer 1847). He also wrote a manual of medical logic and methodology, *Preliminares Clínicos o Introducción a la Práctica de la Medicina* (*Clinical Preliminaries or Introduction to the Practice of Medicine*, Janer 1835). His work on ethics was clearly influenced by John Gregory's *Lectures on the Duties and Qualifications of a Physician* (Gregory [1772b] 1998b), which had been translated into Spanish in 1803 (Gregory 1803; see Chapters 18 and 30). This book is quoted no less than eleven times: one of them in the paragraph on "duty in acquainting a patient and his relations, of his situation." Janer reproduces the text in which Gregory asserts that telling the truth to the patient or to his family at the end of life, in desperate situations, is "to a man of a compassionate and feeling heart, [. . .] one of the most disagreeable duties in the profession: but it is indispensable. The manner of doing it, requires equal prudence and humanity. What should reconcile him the more easily to this painful office, is the reflection that, if the patient should recover, it will prove a joyful disappointment to his friends; and, if he die, it makes the shock more gentle" (Janer 1847, 172; McCullough 1998b, 175). Janer was an important figure, and a handwritten text of Jaime Salvá (1793–1855), who was also professor of medical ethics in the Faculty of Medicine of Madrid, repeats nearly every one of its concepts (Salvá, 1844; March Noguera 2001).

III. The Reaction

In the middle of the nineteenth century, Ideologie and secular medical ethics provoked a strong reaction. Absolutist governors systematically distrusted the new medical knowledge, which they considered prone to atheism and materialism (López Piñero 1964, 61). The widespread acceptance of empirical clinical practice and analytical methodologies of the ideologists made a frontal assault on the scientific and intellectual foundations of medicine unlikely to succeed however. Instead, critics of the new medicine focused on secular medical morality, urging a return to traditional religious medical morality. The existence of a contemporaneous European movement favoring neo-Scholastic philosophy helped to legitimate this conservative critique. A paradigmatic example of the theological critique of the ethics of the Ideologues can be found in the work of the Dominican friar called Ceferino González (1831–1894). The contrast is apparent in the section on ethics in his book *Filosofía Elemental* (*Elemental Philosophy*, González 1873). Here, he directly attacks the idea of any morality independent of Christian theology. His disciple, Juan Manuel Ortí y Lara (1826–1904), continued this critique in his *Ética o Principios de Filosofía Moral* (*Ethics, or Principles of Moral Philosophy*, Ortí y Lara 1853), written in the neo-Scholastic tradition. Both considered Idéologues as "materialists," and defended against them a "spiritualist" idea of man and morality. "Spiritualism" was one of the stances taken by nineteenth century intellectuals and physicians, who opposed the ideas of the French Enlightenment (including those of many Encyclopedists and Idéologues) as excessively "materialistic."

By the middle of the nineteenth century, the confrontation between the new and conservative ways of understanding medical ethics focused on what became known as the "Hippocratic question," that is, which approach was truer to the Hippocratic texts (see Chapters 23 and 24). Spiritualists criticized empiricists and Ideologues, identifying them as advocates of a way of thinking that was anti-Hippocratic. Pedro Mata (1811–1877) responded to the conservative critique in a speech to the Royal Academy of Medicine of Madrid (January 1859) on the subject, "Hippocrates and the Hippocratic Schools." Mata argued that the appeal to Hippocrates made by spiritualists had no sense (Mata 1859). Mata went on to defend clinical empiricism against the dogmatism of reactionary doctors and criticized the attempt to subordinate medicine and philosophy to theology: "That unfortunate reaction has been felt, first in the scope of philosophy, and there are people who dream about going back to the times in which the light of mankind (philosophy) was the *ancilla theologiae* (handmaiden of theology)." His diagnosis was corroborated when famous doctors defended a spiritualist Hippocratism. Especially prominent conservatives were Tomás Santero y Moreno (1817–1888) (Santero 1859) and Matias Nieto y Serrano (1813–1903) (Nieto Serrano 1860). As a result to this controversy, Mata published a very long book, *Doctrina Medico-Filosofica Española* (*Spanish Medical-Philosophical Doctrine*, Mata 1860). Years later, Mata wrote another book covering the subject of moral freedom (Mata 1868), to which Nieto Serrano answered (Nieto Serrano 1869).

The opposition to secular medical ethics continued well into the nineteenth century. Jose de Letamendi's (1828–1897) spiritualism drove him to religion and theology, which then dominated his understanding of medical ethics. A large section of the first volume of his *Curso de Clínica General* (*General Clinical Course*) addressed "professional ethics" (Letamendi 1894, 575–728). He does not take a casuistic approach; undoubtedly because he reserves this for theologians. Instead, he considers the professional obligations of doctors on the basis of the Hippocratic tradition, interpreted in terms of early nineteenth-century idealism and romanticism (Riera 1973).

IV. An Attempt at Synthesis: Medical Deontology

From 1477 until 1822, when it disappeared completely, the main institution in charge of the control and supervision of the professional activities of physicians was the Protomedical Tribunal (Iborra 1987; see also Chapter 27). Colleges of Physicians were not founded until the end of the nineteenth century. During this century, private associations of physicians were formed and the associations attempted to regulate the professional behavior of their members. The Health Act of 1855 established "Medical Juries," which were appointed in each province and attempted, but failed, to enforce physicians' professional obligations. Medical associations continued to be formed in the second half of the nineteenth century, continuing the effort to self-regulate and improve the social image and standing of physicians. In 1898, a Royal Decree created colleges of physicians in each province (Granjel 1984, 71–74). Physicians were obliged to belong to a provincial college, which had a "deontological procedure" to control the dignity of the profession, sanctioning the procedures opposed to the content of the Code of deontology.

Older concepts of medical morality and new concepts of medical ethics were subsumed under the new "medical deontology" (see Chapter 32). The term, "deontology," was introduced by Jeremy Bentham (1748–1832) during the first decades of the nineteenth century. His goal was to reach a synthesis between ethical and juridical norms, and therefore between ethics and law. In Spanish medicine, professional deontology became an attempt to use juridical procedures to govern professional conduct. To this end "Deontological Committees" were created within each provincial college and were charged with adjudicating charges of misconduct brought against the members. These committees reached judgments by comparing allegations to the sanction catalogs that were included in the Statutes of Medical Colleges. These sanctions went from the warning in the slightest faults to the expulsion from the College and the impossibility of continuing the practice of medicine. A Royal Decree of 1930 gave the Colleges the power to sanction professional misconduct. In 1934, Alonso Muñoyerro designed a code of medical deontology to be used in the St. Cosme and St. Damian brotherhoods (Alonso Muñoyerro 1934). In 1945, the first "Deontological Norms" were published, as an appendix to the "Regulations of the Organization of Colleges of Medicine," giving rise to the first Deontological Code of the Spanish medical profession. This code has been periodically updated.

Many commentaries have been written on the Deontological Code, mostly by theologians, analyzing the moral and deontological obligations of doctors (Alonso Muñoyerro 1934, 1940; Peiro 1944; Sobradillo 1950; Zalba and Bozal 1955; Peinador 1962; Herranz 1992). In 1941, the subject of Medical Deontology became part of the required curriculum of the medical schools in Madrid and Barcelona. After 1943, this requirement was extended to all medical schools in Spain (Peiró 1944, 7). The subject was never taken seriously by medical students and because of progressive loss of prestige it was deleted from the curriculum in the 1960s.

Professional deontology had its critics, including very prestigious physicians who publicly voiced their skepticism. One of the most significant critics was Gregorio Marañon (1887–1960), who published an important book in 1935, *Vocación y ética (Vocation and Ethics)*. Marañon's thesis is that medicine is mainly a vocational profession and this vocation creates a way of life and behavior and, therefore, an ethics. One who has the vocation of medicine will be able to fulfill one's moral obligations routinely, even if one has not been taught one's obligations in medical school (Marañón 1947).

V. CONCLUSION: FROM MEDICAL ETHICS TO BIOETHICS

The deontological model became problematic in the late twentieth century. Colleges of physicians and medical deontology flourished in the context of private-practice medicine. After 1942, when public health insurance for workers was mandated in Spain, doctors began to see themselves as public bureaucrats and deontological codes seemed increasingly less suited to their needs and interests.

Bioethics introduced a new style to medical ethics. Bioethics secularized moral reasoning about human life and health care, even as it supplanted the narrow professional concerns of medical deontology. Bioethics introduced a new approach to the analysis of moral conflicts in medicine and established new ways of promoting quality and excellence in professional conduct (see Chapters 38 and 40).

The development of bioethics in Spain since 1975 occurred at the same time as the instauration of political democracy. The bioethical literature published since that time reflects the influence of American bioethics as well as an attempt to mix this influence with European cultural and philosophical traditions. Spanish bioethics has certain traits similar to those of other Mediterranean countries and has sometimes been called "Latin bioethics" (Gracia 1995) or "Mediterranean bioethics" (Savignano 1995).

Ethics began 25 centuries ago in a Mediterranean country, using the language of virtues and vices. This has been since then the typical moral style of Latin culture (Gracia and Gracia 1995). Mediterranean people are more sensitive to virtues than to rights or principles. They prefer benevolence to autonomy, friendship to justice, excellence to rights (Gracia 1995, 205). This is the reason why human rights in general, and patient rights in particular, are interpreted in a way in which family values, for instance, can take priority in some conflicting situations over the individual ones (Spinsanti 1992).

In any case, bioethics has drastically promoted freedom and autonomy in moral decisions related with the use of the body and sexuality, and life and death. This was traditionally an exclusive matter of priests and theologians, which bioethics has secularized. This has been the origin of a big confrontation in Latin countries about the authority of secular mind in these kinds of questions, considered by many an exclusive competence of religious authorities, and more specifically of the Catholic church (Gracia 1996). Consequently, there are two different conceptions of ethics, one centered on freedom and autonomy and the other on authority and obedience.

During the 1980s, bioethics was perceived in Spain as a movement of liberation in questions related to life and death, and the body and sexuality (Gracia 1987, 1988). In the 1990s, important debates on justice in health care arose, and during the first years of the new century, reflection is being centered on ecology, environmentalism, sustainable development, the rights of future generations, and globalization. Bioethical reflection has shifted from the individual problems of the first years of the movement to others of broader and wider dimensions, with important social and political implications, and recently the interest is being centered in the new international and intergenerational problems. If, during the first years of the movement, bioethics was seen as the new face of the old medical ethics, today it is considered a way of reflection about the duties of life in general, and with human life, present and future, in particular. Proceeding this way, bioethics is doing nothing more than honoring its own name.

CHAPTER 34

THE DISCOURSES OF PRACTITIONERS IN NINETEENTH- AND TWENTIETH-CENTURY GERMANY

Andreas-Holger Maehle and Ulrich Tröhler

I. INTRODUCTION

This chapter provides a critical discussion and historical contextualization of German medical ethics texts and discourses between 1800 and World War II. It considers four main areas: medical deontology as expressed in doctors' writings and codes of conduct; professional discipline through medical tribunals; the impact of modern science on medical ethics; and the development of public debates on ethical issues such as euthanasia, abortion, and human experimentation.

II. MEDICAL DEONTOLOGY: FROM *SAVOIR FAIRE* TO PROFESSIONAL ETHICS

In the eighteenth century, university-trained German physicians were largely dependent for their income on a small, wealthy, and urban clientele (Lachmund and Stollberg 1995). The social status of these patients was often higher than that of the doctor. This "patronage relationship," the absence of professional organization, and competition from nonacademic healers, produced the so-called *savoir faire* (i.e., know-how) literature. Its central objectives were to provide young doctors with techniques of conduct that would enhance their reputation and help to disguise their insecurities in medical treatment,

of which they became increasingly aware. To cultivate their image, practitioners had to demonstrate their moral standing, namely, that they were ready to sacrifice their own comfort and pleasure, even their health and life. Such moral elevation aimed at distancing doctors from the mercenary behavior of quacks (Ritzmann 1999; see Chapter 28).

This kind of publication continued well into the nineteenth century, typically dealing with the triple relation of the doctor to patients, to colleagues, and to society at large. The strong position of the paying client implied that the relationship to patients was of prime concern. For many early nineteenth-century practitioners, however, the road to private patients was actually through making a name for themselves in funded practice for the poor (Huerkamp 1985). Therefore, one moral postulate was to treat patients equally, regardless of their social status. This was demanded, for example, by the Prussian royal physician Christoph Wilhelm Hufeland (1762–1836) in an article on "The Relationships of the Physician" (1806), which was later included as a chapter in the many editions and translations of his authoritative handbook of medicine up to the 1850s (Hufeland 1836).

Influenced by Kantian ethics, Hufeland stressed that the patient must be treated as an end in himself, not as a mere means of medical art or scientific experimentation.

Good intentions were of greater moral relevance in a medical action than successful outcomes. Therefore, a doctor had to try even risky treatments in serious diseases to save perhaps his patients' lives, regardless of the potential damage to his reputation if he failed. Dying patients must not be abandoned and their suffering must be relieved, but never must their lives be actively shortened. Using the slippery slope argument, Hufeland warned that once the doctor "transgresses this line" by deciding on life or death, it was only a matter of "gradual progression" to extend such value judgments to other cases, making the doctor the "most dangerous man in the state." Because Hufeland believed that fear of death shortened the patient's life, he was against truth telling in hopeless situations, even if the patient asked for it. Maintaining human life was for him the essence of being a doctor. Accordingly he also abhorred the killing of the fetus in the interest of the mother's health.

Fully aware of the costs of medicine, Hufeland made reduction of costs a moral duty toward the patient, and in the case of funded practice, to the state (Hufeland 1836). In his further considerations on the doctor's relation to the public, he emphasized the indispensability of confidentiality and advised, in the interest of keeping one's reputation, to stay out of party politics and to avoid the appearance of being greedy for financial gain. Reputation was also the key to Hufeland's rules for the relationship with colleagues, particularly in consultations. It was wrong to disparage or criticize colleagues in the presence of laypersons, and mistakes of colleagues had to be covered up – unless the patient's life was in danger.

Although these thoughts predominantly reflected Kantian deontological ethics, they also kept features of the consequentialist thinking of traditional *savoir faire*. Hufeland's medical handbook was highly successful. Its fourth English edition came out in 1855, its tenth German edition in 1857. Soon, however, serious criticism of *savoir faire* emerged. Even the traditionalist Göttingen professor of medicine Karl Friedrich Heinrich Marx (1796–1877) denounced the "miserable tricks" of doctors in attracting patients. Instead he tried to show that medicine was "a part of ethics" (Marx 1876, 29). This meant that the doctor had to reject certain wishes of patients, such as those for abortifacients, aphrodisiacs and favorable medical certificates because it was better to lose good relations and income than to degrade truth, self-esteem, and professional honor. The latter he considered to be more important than personal honor, and telling the truth could take precedence over keeping confidentiality (Marx 1876, 53–54, 65). This view of confidentiality was remarkable because doctors were punishable under the German Criminal Code of 1871 if they disclosed "private secrets" of a patient without authorization (Placzek 1909; Maehle 2002; Maehle 2003). On the question of euthanasia, Marx entirely agreed with Hufeland (Marx [1826] 1952). As a teacher of medi-

cal history himself, the Göttingen professor hoped that young doctors would learn about ethics through intense study of prominent physicians of the past (Marx 1874, 1876).

Marx wrote against the background of the trade ordinance of 1869, which defined medical practice as a trade that could be exercised by anyone (*Kurierfreiheit*). Merely the title, *Arzt* (i.e., doctor), was legally protected. Doctors reacted by trying to demarcate themselves even more strongly than before from nonacademic healers (the so-called *Kurpfuscher*) through the formation of professional medical societies. In 1873, 2 years after the foundation of the German Empire, many of these were organized in a national association, the *Deutscher Ärztevereinsbund*, which represented doctors' professional and economic interests. A constitutive feature of many medical societies was their codes of professional conduct (*Standesordnungen*), which were partly modeled on the code of ethics of the American Medical Association (1847), which, in turn, had been inspired by Thomas Percival's *Medical Ethics* of 1803. The codes of the Munich and Karlsruhe Societies became particularly influential (Brand 1977, 52).

The Munich Code (1875) kept the traditional tripartite structure of the doctor's duties to patients, to colleagues and the profession, and to society. It also added two sections about the duties of the patient and of the community toward the physician, respectively. Its paternalistic general idea was that respect for the doctor and compliance with his views and advice should compensate for sacrificing his own comfort and health. Conversely, the doctor was expected to follow any call for help, although this was not required in the trade ordinance (Ärztlicher, Bezirksverein München 1875). The Karlsruhe Code (Ärztlicher, Kreisverein Karlsruhe [1876] 1900, [1876] 1900) was dominated by the notion of the profession's dignity and honor. It regulated in detail intraprofessional issues, such as behavior in consultations, taking over a colleague's patients, and common policies regarding fees. It explicitly prohibited advertising of medical services as an offense against professional dignity (Ärztlicher, Kreisverein Karlsruhe 1876). This rule remained central to medical professional codes in Germany in the face of competition from nonacademic healers as well as within the profession right up to the period of National Socialist dictatorship, which, shrewdly enough, abolished the *Kurierfreiheit* of the liberal trade ordinance (Binder 2000).

III. The Organization of Professional Discipline

The disciplinary powers of the medical societies extended only to their own, voluntary members, who could be excluded in case of serious misconduct. Both the Munich and Karlsruhe Societies, for example, formed courts of arbitration, which took action if offenses against the professional code had occurred. The court proceedings were not public. Conflicts were to be settled within the boundaries of the Medical Society (Ärztlicher, Kreisverein Karlsruhe [1897] 1907). In 1889, the national meeting of German medical societies (Ärztetag) decided in Braunschweig to adopt "Principles of a Medical Professional Code" as a model for all member societies. Drawing upon the Munich and Karlsruhe codes, these "Principles" prohibited advertising (including misuse of specialist titles), announcement of free treatment, offering benefits to increase one's clientele, prescription of patent medicines of unknown composition ("secret remedies"), any attempts to intrude into a colleague's practice, public criticism of colleagues, and underbidding in making contracts with health insurers (Ärztetag 1889). This latter rule reflected the growing influence of the compulsory health and accident insurance schemes for workers, which had been introduced by Chancellor Otto von Bismarck (1815–1898) in 1883 and 1884, respectively. Although extending doctors' clientele, it also heightened competition for lucrative insurance contracts (Labisch 1997; Sauerteig 2002). The Braunschweig Ärztetag demanded further that all medical societies create tribunals (Ehrengerichte) to control behavior according to those principles. In fact by 1890, of the 352 medical societies of the German Reich, 135 had adopted a professional code and 194 had created a disciplinary tribunal (Maehle 1999b, 317).

In addition, state-authorized Chambers of Physicians (Ärztekammern) with compulsory membership were formed in several German states, beginning with Baden (1864) and the Kingdom of Saxony (1865), followed by Bavaria (1871), Hesse (1877), and Prussia (1887). The chambers gradually formed state-controlled medical courts of honor, invested with authority to punish professional misconduct of any doctor practicing in the respective district. Only state employees (e.g., university professors) and military doctors were exempt. They were subject to the disciplinary (i.e., not the criminal) jurisdiction of the state and the army, respectively. In vain, liberal medical politicians, such as Rudolf Virchow (1821–1902) and Paul Langerhans (1820–1909), opposed the granting of disciplinary powers to the chambers. Their arguments that explicit codes of professional conduct were superfluous and that the sanctions of separate medical disciplinary courts would be futile did not prevail in the contemporary climate of intense competition among practitioners. In fact the courts of honor, once created, became very busy, issuing warnings, reprimands, and fines. In the most serious cases of professional misconduct, doctors' active and passive voting rights to the chamber were withdrawn, and the verdict was published in the medical press. The chambers were not entitled, however, to withdraw a doctor's licence. Only the state authorities could do this, usually in cases of criminal convictions. It has been calculated that the Prussian medical courts of honor, formed by law

in 1899, dealt with three accusations per every hundred practitioners each year in the period leading up to World War I. Approximately one in three accusations, most of which were made by other doctors, resulted in punishment (Maehle 1999b, 322–24).

The issues brought before the courts of honor concerned predominantly intraprofessional competition that had been highlighted in the Braunschweig "Principles." As to the doctor–patient relationship, cases of sexual misconduct toward female patients were prominent. The rationale behind the courts' decisions, in which medical men and jurists cooperated as judges, was to determine whether a particular action of a doctor was in line with professional honor and dignity. Also his conduct outside medical practice was considered. The medical courts of some states, such as those of the Kingdom of Saxony, used a binding professional code for making decisions. Others, such as those of Prussia, decided without a binding code, but used precedents where possible (Maehle 1999b; Rabi 2002). In fact, the Prussian Court of Honor for Doctors (i.e., the appeals court in Berlin) regularly published its most important decisions, which filled five volumes by 1934 (Preussischer Ehrengerichtshof für Ärzte 1908–1934). In a way these decisions formed a new, detailed deontology.

In addition, writings on the doctor's duties in the tradition of Hufeland continued to be published, in particular when proposals to integrate ethics teaching into the medical curriculum were being debated in the 1890s. The Berlin medical historian Julius Pagel (1851–1912), for example, published a "Medical Deontology" for prospective practitioners (Pagel 1897), and the Wiesbaden physician Oswald Ziemssen fostered "The Ethics of the Doctor" as a medical teaching subject (Ziemssen 1899). In the deontological literature between 1900 and 1933, four subjects were treated regularly: doctors' fees, confidentiality, postgraduate training, and prognostics (see also Chapter 32). Other important topics included consultations, locum practice (standing in for another practitioner), qualities of a physician, and solidarity among doctors when contracting with health insurers (to protect the profession's economic interests). New issues raised by medical science were research on animals and informed consent to human experimentation and to autopsies (Schomerus 2001).

IV. THE IMPACT OF MEDICAL SCIENCE ON PROFESSIONAL ETHICS

The British Cruelty to Animals Act of 1876, the world's first law regulating experimentation on animals (see Chapter 48), had important repercussions in Germany. Following antivivisectionist agitation, the issue was debated in a few state parliaments as well as in the Reichstag. Although some physicians were sympathetic toward the antivivisectionist cause, the majority followed the lead of prominent medical scientists, such as Carl Ludwig (1816–1895),

Rudolf Heidenhain (1834–1897), and Rudolf Virchow, a member of both the Prussian Landtag and the Reichstag. They all defended animal experiments with the argument of potential utility for human health. An administrative decree of the Prussian Minister for Religious, Educational and Medical Affairs in 1885, which, moderately enough, demanded the use of anesthetics and experimentation on lower species where possible, was the only tangible result of those debates. It served subsequently as a model for other states of the German Reich, despite numerous anti-vivisectionist petitions (Tröhler and Maehle 1990). Only the animal protection law of the National Socialists, in 1933, created a license system for animal experimentation that was comparable to the British regulations (Maehle 1996; Eberstein 1999; see also Chapter 48).

Another basic method of modern medical science, human experimentation, likewise gave rise to some parliamentary debates following press reports about abuses (Elkeles 1996). As a concrete consequence, the Prussian Minister for Medical Affairs, in 1900, issued a directive concerning "medical interventions other than those for diagnostic, therapeutic, and immunization purposes," that is, for research unrelated to medical care. Addressed to the physicians in chief of all state hospitals, it required information and consent of the subjects and prohibited experiments on minors and other legally incompetent persons (Minister der Geistlichen, Unterrichts- und Medizinal-Angelegenheiten [1900] 1901). The directive found relatively little resonance in the daily and medical press. Whereas critics of orthodox medicine with leanings toward naturopathy complained that the regulations did not go far enough, medical scientists feared that their freedom of research was going to be restricted (Sauerteig 2000).

An exception among the medical commentators was the Berlin neurologist Albert Moll (1862–1939), who was involved in local professional politics and published a 650-page handbook of *Ärztliche Ethik* (Doctor's Ethics, Moll 1902; Maehle 2001). For Moll, nontherapeutic human experimentation without consent was a central ethical issue. He considered it a moral abuse. Quoting hundreds of examples from the scientific literature he doubted whether a ministerial directive would have any effect. He therefore demanded written consent to serious interventions. On the other hand, he criticized too restrictive regulations for minor procedures. He thus pleaded for more differentiated rules. Generally, Moll defined the doctor–patient relationship in legal terms, that is as a contract. Philosophical systems of morality, such as evolutionary ethics and utilitarianism, were in his view an unsuitable basis for medical ethics because of their questioning the doctor's essential role as a healer (Moll 1902, 7–10). Although Moll's work on ethics was reviewed in leading professional journals, such as *Deutsche Medizinische Wochenschrift* and *Münchener*

Medizinische Wochenschrift (Schomerus 2001), and may be seen from today's perspective as a milestone on the road from medical paternalism to patient autonomy, it had actually very little impact in its own day. Anyway, the Prussian Directive of 1900 did not cover therapeutic experimentation. This reflected the *"do-ut-des"* attitude of the state – and the experimenters – toward the lower class patients of the public hospitals on whom experiments were performed. A research collaborator of Paul Ehrlich (1854–1915), the psychiatrist Konrad Alt (1861–1922), was thus able to test a precursor substance of Salvarsan (history's first chemotherapeutic agent, against syphilis) on patients who where unfit to give consent because of their age or mental condition (Sauerteig 2000).

Yet, another strand in the history of informed consent arose from high-handed medical interventions. In response to surgical treatments without consent, a debate on the legal justification of operations and the relevance of patients' consent developed among German-speaking jurists in the 1890s. The traditional legal view that surgery was objectively physical injury or battery, which went unpunished through the patient's consent, was challenged by some experts in criminal law, such as Carl Stooss (1849–1934) and Richard Schmidt (1862–1944). They agreed with leading surgeons, such as Ottmar von Angerer (1850–1918) in Munich and Franz König (1832–1910) in Göttingen, who acknowledged that consent seeking was part of professional ethics, but were hostile toward the legal notion of surgical procedures as physical injury (Maehle 2000; Prüll and Sinn 2002). The German Supreme Court (*Reichsgericht*), however, had endorsed the traditional legal view with its decision in 1894 on a Hamburg case of medically indicated surgery on a child against her father's will. This decision stated that medical interventions were punishable as assault and battery, if the doctor could not derive his right to operate "from an existing contractual relation or the presumptive consent, the assumed brief of a duly legitimised person" (Reichsgericht 1894, 382). Subsequent decisions in similar cases by the Dresden High Court in 1899 and by the German Supreme Court in 1907, 1908, and 1911 cemented this legal doctrine (Maehle 2000). In 1912, the Supreme Court issued a further decision that gave guidance on the extent of required patient information before obtaining consent to surgical procedures. Although the amount of information had to be sufficient to make the consent legally valid, there was no "obligation of the doctor to draw the patient's attention to all disadvantageous consequences that might possibly follow from the recommended operation." Reflecting medical paternalism, the court pointed out that patients might become unduly worried through information about risks, which might endanger the success of the treatment (Reichsgericht 1912, 433–34).

Although the notion of patients' self-determination and rights over their own body was brought up in the legal debates on medical interventions, doctors were endorsed in their traditional view that decision making on treatment remained ultimately their own responsibility. An exception among medical interventions (broadly defined) remained vaccination against smallpox, which had been made compulsory in the German Reich by law in 1874. Only a very few physicians, typically with a background in naturopathy, campaigned with lay antivaccinationists against this law, chiefly because they feared health risks for the vaccinated (Maehle 1990a).

Post-mortem examination, another key feature of medical research and education since the 1850s, led to irreconcilable differences between cultural values in the population and the belief in scientific progress among doctors. Pathologists tried to educate the public about the medical usefulness of autopsies, rather than to ask relatives for consent in specific cases. Although the question of consent to post-mortem examinations remained legally unregulated, outright refusals were usually respected. There was a tendency among pathologists, however, to ignore the issue of consent. During the Revolution of 1918–1919, for example, the democratic Reich Ministry of Science instructed the Berlin Charité Hospital to respect persistent refusals of relatives to permit autopsy. Yet, the Berlin professor of pathology Otto Lubarsch (1860–1933) eagerly seized the opportunity to dissect dead street fighters in early 1919 without caring about relatives' consent. Despite several reminders from the Ministry demanding acknowledgment of its order, he went on performing autopsies without consent during the following years (Prüll 2000, 2004; Prüll and Sinn 2002).

V. Public Debate on Euthanasia, Abortion, and Human Experimentation

On the question of euthanasia, doctors generally continued to follow the line of Hufeland and Marx that palliative care of the dying was a medical duty, but that any active shortening of the patient's life was unacceptable. It was recognized that high doses of painkillers to relieve terminal suffering might inadvertently hasten the onset of death. Yet, around the turn of the century, a group of authors, most prominently among them the German champion of Darwinism, the zoologist Ernst Haeckel (1834–1919), advocated mercy killing of terminally ill patients on their own request. Even more radically, Haeckel suggested, in 1904, that involuntary euthanasia should be considered, with certain administrative safeguards, in cases of incurable mental illness. The background to this view was his utilitarian rationale that such patients were kept alive at great public expense without being useful to the community or even to themselves. He was, therefore, also in favor of the idea of killing severely handicapped newborns (Benzenhöfer 1999, 96–97). Haeckel's writings had a wide

circulation, among the general public, as well as among professionals.

In the same vein, the retired Leipzig professor of law Karl Binding (1841–1920) and the Freiburg professor of psychiatry Alfred Hoche (1865–1943) prepared a joint manuscript, which was eventually published in 1920 titled *Die Freigabe der Vernichtung lebensunwerten Lebens: Ihr Mass und ihre Form* (The Release of the Destruction of Life Unworthy of Life. Its Measure and Form), which caused much debate in legal and medical circles (Kircher 1986; Benzenhöfer 1999). They added a third group to the two categories of patients mentioned by Haeckel: persons who through severe illness or accident had lost consciousness for a lengthy period might be put to death. Binding proposed a detailed administrative procedure for this, insisting that in doubtful cases the doctor had to bear the risk of error. In the subsequent debates, German physicians opposed the suggestions of Binding and Hoche, fearing that the slippery slope would lead down to the killing of invalids of war and labor, the blind, the deaf mute, the tuberculous, and the cancerous. It was further argued that although the economic gains of such euthanasia were small, their moral costs would be immense. In 1921, the German *Ärztetag* rejected almost unanimously a motion for the "legal release" of the "destruction of life unworthy of life" (Benzenhöfer 1999, 107). Nevertheless, the debate on the value of human life continued, and those thoughts on euthanasia prepared the ideological ground for medical killing in the Nazi period (Burleigh 1994; Chapter 54).

Another old issue, which was passionately discussed anew in the 1920s, was that of abortion. In the growing urban centers of Germany, abortion was a reality of everyday life: it was estimated that hundreds of thousands of procedures were performed each year. Before World War I, doctors had opposed abortion because of their pronatalism and because it was illegal according to the German Criminal Code of 1871. The only exceptions were situations in which the fetus acutely endangered the mother's life. After the War, the medical discourse on abortion revealed profound divisions within the profession. The small Association of Socialist Doctors campaigned for legalization of abortion according to the Soviet model, chiefly for social and eugenic reasons. By contrast, the medical establishment, represented by the *Deutscher Ärztevereinsbund*, at a specific *Ärztetag* in 1925 opposed any proposals for reform of the legal prohibition of abortion. These doctors pointed to the morbidity and mortality associated with abortion and styled themselves as moral arbiters beyond party politics. The traditional ethos of the doctor as the protector of human life, as expressed by Hufeland, remained binding for them. Moreover, they feared promiscuity and a loss of family values. The tiny Federation of German Women Doctors (*Bund Deutscher Ärztinnen*) even more radically split into reformers, who argued for the self-determination of women, and conservatives. Although these were the publicly voiced views, it remains an open question what medical men and women thought and did privately about this issue. Doctors both reflected and shaped public opinion. In 1926, the law on abortion was amended, reducing punishment for the pregnant woman from penal servitude of up to 10 years to imprisonment between 1 day (!) and at most 5 years. A decision of the German Supreme Court in 1927 permitted therapeutic abortion performed by a doctor. The National Socialist government on the one hand reestablished the legal status of abortion of 1871, banning also advertisements for abortifacients and abortion services. On the other hand, it cynically introduced compulsory sterilization (1933) and abortion (1935) on eugenic grounds, irrespective of the traditional medical ethos (Usborne 1992; Dienel 1993; Gante 1993; Chapter 54).

The issue of human experimentation and the associated problem of patient autonomy were likewise kept alive in the Weimar Republic. Debates on compulsory treatment of syphilitic prostitutes with Salvarsan, to be performed by licensed medical practitioners, culminated in a law for the combat of venereal diseases in 1927. On the one hand, this law reduced the choice of therapeutic method and healer, but on the other hand it introduced the right of patients to refuse "dangerous treatment," which included Salvarsan (Sauerteig 2000). This discourse on patient information and consent has to be seen in the context of contemporary criticism of scientific medicine. It had been formulated since the turn of the century by champions of natural healing and led by the 1920s to the perception of a "crisis" within orthodox medicine. Agitation against human experiments flared up again. In 1928, the Social-Democratic medical politician Julius Moses (1868–1942) reported a number of "scandalous" trials on newborns and children to the Reichstag. Later, in the same year, the Berlin Chamber of Physicians issued a statement on human experimentation, which emphasized the duty to inform subjects about the purpose of the trial. By March 1930 the health authorities of the German Reich had prepared guidelines on new treatments and scientific experimentation on human beings. The debate then culminated with the introduction of BCG immunization (against tuberculosis) in Lübeck in 1930, which – probably due to contamination with a virulent strain – resulted in the death of 77 newborns (Hahn 1995; Bonah 2003). In early 1931, the Ministry of the Interior issued the completed new guidelines. They went beyond the Prussian Directive of 1900 by including also therapeutic trials, which had to be preceded by animal experiments. Information and consent of patients involved in therapeutic experiments was made compulsory. Moreover, doctors were required to consider carefully whether testing of new treatments on minors was really necessary. Experiments on dying patients were prohibited. Doctors were warned against exploiting the social situation of patients when recruiting test persons.

The responsibility for trials rested with the head of the medical institution in which they were conducted, rather than with the individual researcher. Last but not least, the guidelines required that young doctors be repeatedly advised on all these specific duties (Reichsminister des Innern 1931; Sauerteig 2000; see Chapter 49). These administrative rules lacked legal force however. There were no provisions for sanctions. In the end this "soft law" failed to prevent the atrocious human experiments in the concentration camps of Nazi Germany (Mitscherlich and Mielke 1962; Kanovitch 1998; see also Chapters 50 and 54).

VI. Conclusion

In the nineteenth and early twentieth centuries, German medical ethics underwent profound, and ultimately disastrous, changes. The first half of the nineteenth century saw the vanishing of medical *savoir faire*, which had primarily focused on the practitioner's reputation in the eyes of his paying patients. Some principles underlying a growing body of ethics in medicine, such as preservation of human life (including prohibition of abortion and of active euthanasia) and confidentiality, belonged in fact to the traditional Hippocratic ethos. Others, such as equal treatment, strict truthfulness, and seeing the patient as an end in himself, reflected Kantian moral philosophy. The professionalization of German doctors during the second half of the nineteenth century, the challenges of the liberal trade ordinance of 1869, and the introduction of health and accident insurances on a grand scale as of 1883, reduced medical ethics almost entirely to questions of honorable behavior in a climate of fierce competition for clients and insurance contracts. The professional disciplinary bodies, which were created and vested with state authority in this period, thus predominantly controlled, quite efficiently, the conduct of practitioners in relation to colleagues and the profession.

Whereas doctors were clearly proactive in this intraprofessional arena, they were largely reactive, even defensive, in the broader ethical debates raised by the impact of medical science and modern surgery toward the end of the nineteenth century. Responding to public opinion, jurists and politicians took the lead. Medical paternalism, which had evolved in the nineteenth century with the rise of hospital medicine backed by prestigious science, was challenged as information and consent began to be required in certain therapeutic and nontherapeutic situations. Although there was no public concept of autonomy in a modern sense, the notion of self-determination of the patient as a person gained prominence in the legal world, which started questioning the doctor in his decision making. Thus doctors had to accommodate to administrative regulations of animal and human experimentation and autopsies, and Supreme Court decisions on medical interventions, which, however they did not really need to care for in practice. Moreover, as the controversial issues of euthanasia and abortion revealed in the early twentieth century, if any unity of professional ethics had existed, it was dissolving under the influence of Social Darwinism, eugenics, neo-utilitarianism, and Socialism.

Thus, although the intraprofessional disciplinary control of collegiality continued to function on the eve of National Socialist dictatorship, medical ethics in relation to patients and society was in disarray. Many doctors were succumbing to the seductions of a biologistic totalitarianism instead. For those who became involved in the so-called mercy killing or "euthanasia," or in the horrendous human experiments of the Third Reich, the values of the traditional medical ethos as well as those fostered by the "new" nineteenth-century medical ethics had ceased to exist. Hufeland's early nineteenth-century prophecy that a doctor who judges the value of life will turn into the "most dangerous man in the state" had become reality.

ACKNOWLEDGMENTS

A.-H. Maehle would like to thank the Wellcome Trust, the British Council, and the University of Durham (Research Committee) for their support of his research into the history of medical ethics.

CHAPTER 35

THE DISCOURSES OF PRACTITIONERS IN EIGHTEENTH-TO TWENTIETH-CENTURY RUSSIA AND SOVIET UNION

Boleslav L. Lichterman and Mikhail Yarovinsky

I. INTRODUCTION

For historical and geographical reasons, medical ethics in Russia prior to the Revolution of 1917 has distinctive characteristics. As Peter Chaadaev wrote in 1829 "we lived and continue to live only to give a certain important lesson for generations to come which will be able to understand it; in any case, at the present moment we constitute a gap in a moral universe. I cannot but be amazed by this unusual emptiness and uniqueness of our social being" (Chadaaev 1906, 14).[1] For centuries Russia was a backward rural country. *Obshina* (community) was the basis of social life. One can track from this origin of the emergence to supremacy of the community over the individual, the state over the personality. Such terms as *sobornost* and *soviety* ("The Soviet power") are absent from other European languages (Makshantseva 2001, 112–19). Correlatively, one does not find a Russian analog for *privacy* – this term simply does not exist in the language.

Christianity was adopted in Russia in 988 in its Byzantine or Orthodox version. From the thirteenth to the fifteen centuries, Mongolian hordes occupied most of the country. These two factors contributed to a prolonged isolation of Russia from the mainstream of European civilization. Complicating matters further, from the fourteenth to the twentieth centuries, Russia was at war 329 of 525

years (Makshantseva 2001, 114). Under these circumstances the value attributed to human life was significantly eroded. Severe spiritual and political censorship hindered the development of secular philosophical thought. Original ethical works first appeared at the end of the nineteenth century (*Justification of Virtue* by Vladimir Solovjev). Given the dominance of censorship, political and philosophical ideas were often expressed using the Aesopian language of literature. As Alexander Hertzen wrote, "literature in people without political freedom is a sole tribune from the height of which they can hear the cry of their indignation and their conscience" (Hertzen 1956, 7:198). Problems of medical ethics were not dealt with in treatises but through literary works by such writers as Leo Tolstoy (*The Death of Ivan Iljich*) and Anton Chekhov (*Ward N6* and *Ionych*, etc.).

II. RUSSIAN MEDICINE AND HEALTH CARE PRIOR TO 1861

Monastic and other forms of church-sponsored medicine appeared in Russia after the adoption of Christianity. Quacks and folk healers were persecuted as the devil's agents. The first physicians were invited into Russia from Europe under the reign of Czar Ivan III. Anton the German (Anton Nemchin) is mentioned in Russian chronicles for the first time in 1483. After unsuccessful treatment of the Tatar prince, Karakach Ivan III delivered the physician to the son of the deceased prince and poor Anton was slaughtered by the Tatars "like a sheep" under the bridge of the Moscow river. In 1490, another foreign physician, Leon the Jew (Leon Zhidovin), arrived to Moscow from Venice. After the death of the elder son of Ivan III, whom Leon tried to cure, the latter was beheaded by the order of the Czar. During the sixteenth century the first Russian medical text appeared, the first pharmacy opened, and the first medico-legal examinations for licensure were administered (Lakhtin 1903, 445–51). In 1581, *Aptekarskii prikaz* (Drug Administration) became the first government body to supervise the activity of state-employed physicians and pharmacists. Ordinary people were treated by quacks.

At the turn of the eighteenth century Czar (and first Russian emperor) Peter the Great "cut through the window into Europe." This was the beginning of the Westernization and modernization of the patriarchal lifestyle of Russia. Hundreds of foreign specialists and consultants were invited into the country, including medical doctors. Under Peter's decree the first school for feldshers (physician's assistants) was created at the Moscow military hospital in 1707, under directorship of a Dutch physician, Nicolas Bidloo (c.1670–1735).

The first Russian university, which opened in Moscow in 1758, had a medical faculty. At the turn of the nineteenth century several charitable medical institutions were organized under the aegis of a special department headed by the widowed empress Maria Fedorovna (Houses for Widows, Houses for Orphans, St. Mary's hospitals in Moscow and St. Petersburg). The *Obshestvo sorevnovanija vrachebnykh i fizicheskikh nauk* (Society for Competition of Medical and Physical Sciences) aimed at medical education of both the lay public and physicians was established at Moscow University in 1804. Similar Societies were soon thereafter established in all seven university cities of Russia.

A lecture by the dean of medical faculty of Moscow University, Matvei Mudrov (1776–1831), is considered the first Russian publication on medical ethics. This lecture was delivered to medical students in October 1813 (on the occasion of the reopening the medical faculty after the Moscow University was looted by the Napoleon army in 1812 and entitled, "Slovo o blagochestii i nravstvennykh kachestvakh gippokratova vracha" ("A Word about Moral Qualities of a Hippocratic Physician") (Mudrov 1814). This talk consisted of excerpts of Hippocratic writings that were translated into Russian for the first time and some comments. According to Mudrov, Hippocrates learned from Scythians who are forefathers of Russians.

There appear to be no major differences between medical ethics in Russia and in other European states during the early nineteenth century because most medical practitioners in Russia were Europeans (See Chapters 32, 33, and 34). In 1835, Czar Nicolas I (1796–1855) issued a special decree aimed at increasing the number of Russian physicians. Under this Czar, Russia became isolated from Western Europe and the tradition of sending young scientists abroad for postgraduate training was interrupted for political reasons. After the French Revolution of 1848 almost all faculties of Moscow University were either closed or significantly reduced to suppress liberal political movements, with the exception of the medical faculty.[2] All graduates of medical faculty had to swear the so-called *Fakul'tetskoe obeschanie* ("Faculty Promise"), which was similar to that taken by graduate physicians in Western Europe.

Medical ethics at this time was intensely practiced, as illustrated by the life and work of Fedor Gaaz (1780–1853). Gaaz came to Russia from Germany in 1806 as a home physician of countess Repnina. For 23 years (from 1829 until his death), he worked as an administrator and physician-in-chief of Moscow prisons. He suggested a new construction of chains for criminals – they became longer and not so heavy. He also insisted on covering irons with cloth. His credo is engraved upon his tomb: "Hurry up to do good!" (Koni 1914).

III. ETHICAL PROBLEMS IN RUSSIAN MEDICINE FROM 1861 TO 1917

In 1855, Nikolas I committed suicide after Russia's defeat in the Crimean War. He was succeeded by a liberal Czar, Alexander II (1818–1881), who began what came to be known as the "epoch of Great Reforms."[3] *Krepostnoe pravo* (serfdom of peasants) was abolished in 1861. This change had a major impact, inasmuch as ninety percent of the country's population was rural. Many regions elected local self-governing councils or *zemstva*. Zemstva were in charge of local health care and started to hire medical doctors. This zemskaya medicine became a prototype for socialized health care in Russia. Zemskaya medicine was based upon the principles of free and accessible health care and preventive medicine. These principles were later adopted by Soviet health care. According to M. S. Uvarov, "yesterday's slaves treated with mistrust and suspicion everything that originated from their former lords – including the suspicion that doctors were poisoning the people" (Uvarov 1903). Cholera riots during the reign of Nikolas I and the killing of doctors during cholera epidemics in the 1890s serve as vivid examples of these attitudes. "Under such circumstances the Western European pattern of doctor–patient relationships [that is, the relationship between a vendor and a customer] would be difficult to imagine … There were vendors but customers were unlikely to come" (Uvarov 1903,144). Most zemskie physicians were idealists who viewed their work as a public duty. They shared the idea of caring for the people and a sense of indebtedness to the people. Initially, zemstva employed a "ride-around system," in which a physician lived in the town and his assistants (feldshers) lived in villages. The zemsky doctor would then regularly visit villages to consult patients. It was later decided to replace this approach with a stationary system, in which hospitals were built in the larger villages. Physicians lived in these villages and provided health care for free to the local community. Within five decades 175 hospitals with 42,500 beds had been opened (Strashun 1937, 14).[4] Zemstva paid doctors' salaries, irrespective of the number of patients treated.

A physician was also required to teach peasants to follow sanitary rules. Otherwise doctors' recommendations would have been mere formalities. According to Uvarov, "the ethics of zemskie physicians is very simple and has little difference from the ethics of public figures ... The absence of financial interest between a patient and a doctor radically simplifies their relationship." In his or her spare time a physician could be involved in private, fee-for-service practice. Municipal hospitals for the poor were also established on the basis of the principles of zemskaya medicine.

By the beginning of the twentieth century zemskaya medicine was viewed as an anachronism. Although the pattern elsewhere was for medicine to become increasingly specialized, a zemsky physician continued to combine surgeon, internist, obstetrician, ophthalmologist, and other specialists in one person. A majority of zemstva had one physician for every 25,000 to 30,000 people, who lived in areas as large as 25–30 km[2] without proper roads. Apart from working at the hospital (usually approximately 20 beds), a physician had to see between 80 and 100 ambulatory patients daily (up to 20,000 outpatient visits annually). With this patient load the zemsky physician would take as little as 2 to 3 minutes to examine a patient. He or she also had to travel to remote villages to deliver babies, fight epidemics, and supervise the sanitary conditions of fifteen to sixteen rural schools. The working day of a typical zemsky physician lasted for 10 hours.

Medical care was rather primitive. For example, surgery was limited to removal of superficial tumors, opening abscesses, and amputations. According to one contemporary witness, "in such situation the figure of zemsky physician – a specialist in all diseases – becomes truly a tragic one" (Slavskii 1911). The average salary of a zemsky doctor was insufficient (1,200–1,500 roubles a year, which comprised about half of the budget of middle class family in Germany) (Zhbankov 1911). In such circumstances many doctors were involved in private, fee-for-service practice.[5] The trend toward private practice provoked severe criticism from more idealistic colleagues. For example, in 1911, D. N. Zhbankov claimed that private practice undermines the foundations of zemstvo medicine, which is based upon the principle of equal treatment for all. He stressed that "the communal (*obshinnye*) foundations of Russian life, which came to the surface with zemstvo, revealed the evil and abnormality of private [medical]

practice" (Zhbankov 1911, 14). Patients' fees for medical care were condemned as "a tax on the misfortunes of a fellow creature." Two evils were thought to result from private practice – "the waste of time that belongs to society and the loss of trust of the population." Moreover, Zhbankov objected to any increase in a doctor's salary: "A workman for the poor and among the poor should not differ from the population from the material standpoint. Otherwise he will not be trusted and his activity will not be productive" (Zhbankov 1911, 19).[6] The Soviet regime would later agree with such views (see Chapter 55).

Ethical issues were widely discussed in the medical journals of the late nineteenth century. In just one year, 1894, more than sixty books and articles on medical ethics were published in Russia (Korotkikh 1989, 18). A weekly periodical *Vrach* ("Medical Doctor") was particularly influential. It was edited by professor V. A. Manassein (1841–1901), who was nicknamed "a knight of medical ethics." The objectives of this periodical were characterized by Manassein as follows:

> 1) to be a true mirror of everything that constitute a real progress in clinical medicine and hygiene; 2) to attract to a cooperative scientific work the maximum number of medical doctors from different regions of Russia; 3) to provide a constant critical, independent and impartial analysis of all aspects of education, daily life and practice of a medical doctor.

Manassein was strongly opposed to private practice: "The complete trust and purity of the relationship which are necessary to a doctor for treatment and to a patient for recovery will be impossible until doctor's labor would be paid by the society or the state" (cited by Korotkikh 1989, 33). In 1884, this periodical published a Russian translation of the "Ethical Code of the Warsaw Medical Society" (Warsaw at the time being part of the Russian Empire) (*Obyazannosti* 1884, 497–9). According to the editor's footnote, "if in future ethical codes for *all* Russian doctors are going to be elaborated, irrelevant paragraphs have to be modified." Two sections of the Code were severely criticized: a statement that a physician may breach confidentiality upon the demand of the authorities or when it is dictated by public interests (article 2) and the obligation of a physician to inform authorities about a case in which he learns about actual or planned criminal activity (article 73). Manassein called for absolute confidentiality in all circumstances.

An all-Russian ethical code was never formulated, perhaps because Russia lacked a national medical society. Local medical societies, however, adopted their own medical codes. For example, *Obshestvo vrachei Volynskoi gubernii* (Society of Physicians of Volyn' Region) adopted in 1885 "Rules of Mutual Relations of Physicians at a Patient's Bed" with detailed descriptions of doctor's behavior during consultations (*Pravila* 1886). *Obshestvo kievskikh vrachei*

(Society of Kiev Physicians) established a special commission that published a project of ethical codes of the society (Proekt 1889). It included obligation to provide free care to the colleagues and their families and prohibited self-advertising. Medical doctors should not give "certificates of efficiency of pharmaceuticals or mineral waters."

The *Sankt-Peterburgskoe Vrachebnoe Obshestvo Vzaimnoi Pomoshi* (Physicians' Society for Mutual Help of St. Petersburg) was established in 1890 for "moral mutual support and fostering of doctors' unity." Initially it was planned to be named as "Society for the Protection of Physicians' Rights." This Society organized regular meetings (*Tovarisheskie besedy* – Comrades' talks) to discuss public aspects of medical life. At the first meeting, held on December 18, 1900, Dr. Evgeny Botkin posed the following question: "Would it be reasonable and possible at all to form a code of medical ethics?" (Borisov 1902a, 28–38).[7] Botkin himself gave a positive answer because: (1) it would give us a chance to know the opinion of our colleagues about a particular article of the code; (2) would help medical doctors to gain the trust of the general public (because the public would learn what things doctors consider obligatory for themselves); and (3) "if other professionals have their own professional codes, it is particularly needed for medical doctors who often deal with abnormal people." Those who supported the Code advanced the following arguments: (1) an ethical code would assist in resolving difficult or complex cases; (2) it would constrain weak-willed colleagues; (3) it would offer the public a more realistic conception of medical practice. Opposing views were presented during the discussion that followed. These objections included the following: (1) because no code can cover all specific cases, codification poses the danger that what is not explicitly prohibited will be considered implicitly permissible; (2) such a code would hardly reconcile the public with the medical community; (3) medical ethics is being treated as a special subject when all the guidance that a doctor needs is a well-known commandment "to love one's neighbor as oneself"; and (4) one's moral instincts speak louder than volumes of ethical codes. One of the opponents, Peter Borisov, put his position in the following fashion: "We commit sins not because we do not know a code. Any code that we create could easily serve as a screen sheltering improper actions" (Borisov 1902a, 30). The question was put to a vote and the majority of those present voted in favor of the code of medical ethics.

The questions addressed at the next meeting were: "What is the significance of a code which determines the relations between medical doctors and between doctors and the public? And, should such code be obligatory or just have a moral significance?" It was decided that a code should be obligatory for members of the Physicians' Society for Mutual Help of St. Petersburg and have moral significance for nonmembers. Topics in medical ethics such

as a doctor's obligation to attend a patient upon his or her first request, confidentiality and how to behave oneself in consultations with other doctors were also discussed. The Society's by-laws included a Court of Honor "in order to solve misunderstandings between members and review accusations against members concerning deeds that are blameworthy and incompatible with doctors' dignity." The Court of Honor consisted of three members and two candidates who were elected for 1 year at the annual meeting of the society. Appeals to the Court of Honor were rare – there were only sixteen cases for the 10-year period from early 1890s until early 1900s (Fainshtein 1904, 65). According to Dr. Fainshtein, a critic, "A Court of honor cannot exist [in Russia], because we do not share similar views on doctors' ethics; this subject is not taught at the university and it is underdeveloped and only few doctors are participating in medical societies where they might have had a chance to learn more about ethics" (see also Chapter 34).

In 1902 the board of the Tver' branch of the Society approved "Regulations of Doctor's Ethics" (*Sankt-Peterburgskoe Vrachebnoe Obshestvo Vzaimnoi Pomoshi* 1903, no. 6:232–4). Similar "Regulations" were elaborated by the Uman' Society of Medical Doctors in 1903 (*Vrachebnaya* 1903, no. 8:485–8). In 1908, a "Deontology Codex of the Medical Chamber of Eastern Galicia" was translated into Russian from Esperanto (Deontologicheskii Kodex 1908) In his foreword, the translator, K. I. Shidlovsky, wrote that Russian doctors had not yet elaborated a systematic code of medical ethics. Professional corporate organizations similar to medical chambers of Western Europe were also nonexistent. Decisions of Courts of Referees were based "upon imperatives of conscience and life experience founded on general ethical principles." According to Shidlovsky,

> a sort of a chaos in problems of medical ethics has its deep historical roots, related to theRussian life-style, particularly due to the institute of public medicine. The latter gives to medical ethics a special character and complicates the whole issue. A Western-European medical doctor could hardly imagine the complexity of our relationships and interactions. Nevertheless, Russian doctors do have a necessity to regulate this problem. (. . .) As everybody knows, ethical codes regulate exclusively private medical practice. Our medical ethics is rooted in the social and public sphere and can not be kept within a narrow scheme of pure professionalism. (Deontologicheskii Kodex 1908, 646–8)

Even in the pre-revolutionary period, Marxist medical doctors opposed the corporate character of medical societies and rejected the idea of a Russian code of medical ethics (Chebotareva 1970). *Zapiski vracha* (*Confessions of a Physician*) by Vikenty Veresaev (Smidovich) (1867–1945) serves as a good example (Veresaev 1948).[8] Published in 1901 by a 33-year-old Marxist medical doctor who, like Chekhov, gave up his medical career and became a writer, this book was translated into major European languages (English, German, and French). The central themes of this book are the doctor–patient relationship and human experimentation.

This book provoked controversial reviews after its publication in a literary journal *Mir Bozhy*. The changing attitudes toward this book are reflected in various sources. The weekly medical periodical, *Vrach*, praised the talented young author and the truthfulness of many of his statements (Vrach 1901, 68). *Vrach (A Physician)* was a weekly medical periodical, launched in 1880 by Vyacheslav A. Manassein (1841–1901). From 1902 until 1918, it was published under the title *Russkii Vrach (A Russian Physician)*.

Later a reviewer in the same periodical accused Veresaev of evident exaggerations "that may only bring harm by dissemination of mistaken views in our society, which trusts quacks and medical doctors equally" (Vrach 1901, 258).[9] The president of the St. Petersburg Medico-Chirurgical Society, Prof. N. A.Vel'yaminov, delivered a speech at the annual meeting in which Veresaev was described as a person with "huge self-importance who is constantly in doubt about his knowledge and his power, indicating an evident egoism with evident nervous irritability. That is why this book is unhealthy" (Vel'yaminov 1901, 1529–30). The English translation was critically reviewed in the *British Medical Journal*. The anonymous reviewer wrote that "we find a Russian physician washing his dirty linen in public with every sensational accompaniment that is calculated to attract attention to the nasty business." Veresaev was accused of denigrating Russian medicine because problems of medical ethics should be discussed only among professionals. "The proper place for Veresaeff's 'Confessions' is not the drawing room-table, but the dustbin," concluded the review in the BMJ (Anonymous 1904, 1020–2).

In reply to his critics Veresaev published a pamphlet *Po povodu "Zapisok vracha:" otvet moim critikam (A Propos "Confessions of a Physician:" A Reply to My Critics)*. According to Veresaev, the relationship of medical science and patient's personality is a key issue:

> Ethical problems of our profession may not be settled by a tiny codex of professional ethics. Sadly, we should admit that our science does not have ethics yet. One cannot mean by ethics that special corporate doctors ethics which just regulates relationship between doctors and public and between doctors themselves. Ethics in a broad, philosophical sense is needed. Such ethics should cover in full the above indicated problem of the relationship between medical science and a living personality. (Veresaev 1903, 51)

Veresaev argues that a problem "of borders, beyond which interests of an individual might be sacrificed to the interests of science ... is not a specific problem of some special doctors' ethics but a great, eternal, fundamental problem of the relationship between personality and higher categories such as society, science, law etc." (Veresaev 1903, 53). As Veresaev writes, "narrow problems of medical practice *first and foremost* should be resolved from the philosophical standpoint" (Veresaev 1903, 54, emphasis original).

About this time the German physician, Albert Moll, published *Ärztliche Ethik (Doctors' Ethics)* (see chapter 34), which received mixed reviews in Russia. According to Petr Borisov, "the author did not find a solid foundation of doctors' ethics in any [philosophical] system and founded it upon everyday *practice*" (Borisov 1902b, 669–70, emphasis original). Another reviewer, N. G. Feinberg, was even more critical. He wrote that Moll erroneously applied the term, "ethics," to practical problems such as doctors' obligations to the public, to colleagues, and to the state: "All these problems might be covered by the teaching about *obligations* of a physician – by *medical deontology*" (Feinberg 1903, 304–13, emphasis original). Although deontology is based upon ethical grounds, it is not ethics. Ethics is a science about the laws of manifestation of moral feeling that is the same for all professions. Thus, the term, "doctors ethics," represents a logical contradiction.

There were two Russian translations of Moll's book. The Moscow edition was edited by V. Veresaev, who also wrote a critical preface (Moll 1904). Veresaev accused Moll of philistinism: "Everywhere, as soon as Moll goes beyond purely medical ethical matters, we can see a cautious, moderate, and prudent philistine, who is devoid of noble purpose, without a wide range of interests, whose only ideal is to earn a piece of bread for himself and his people." The chapter about the physician's private life was omitted in this edition because its sole interest, Veresaev claimed, is "to illustrate the bourgeois outlook of the modern, ordinary German physician." A St. Petersburg edition of Moll's book was translated with a commentary by Dr. Ya.L. Levinson and had a revealing subtitle: "For medical doctors and general public." As Levinson noted in his preface, "under the close links that exist between physicians and general public, mutual mistrust and misunderstanding might be removed only in case that *both sides* would be acquainted with their moral *rights and obligations*" (Moll 1903, V, emphasis original). That is why this edition has numerous footnotes informing the reader about Russian realities (zemstvo medicine, Russian laws related to medicine, the medical press, etc.) and all special terms were replaced by words in general use.

At the turn of the twentieth century, Russian society was deeply divided. The medical profession was no exception. On the one side were medical doctors who shared Marxist and populist ideas, known as *narodniki* (populists). Many zemskie physicians shared such views. The journal, *Obsh-estvennyi Vrach* (*A Public Physician*), was their mouthpiece. It condemned private-practice medicine and praised the ideas of socialized, state medicine. Nevertheless, physicians needed a certain degree of freedom, "because exact regulation of the methods of diagnosis and treatment would have sounded the death knell for medical science which is mainly experimental" (Velshtein 1911, 63). A similar criticism was later made by V. Ya. Danilevsky: "The substitution of moral duty based on principles of altruism common to all mankind by official duty will inevitably result in the belittling of moral foundations of the medical profession... Instead of internal freedom, a physician will feel external coercion which will lead to the physician's depersonalization without fail." (Danilevsky 1921, 396)

On the other side were conservative and nationalistic physicians such as A. I. Dubrovin (1855–1918) who edited an anti-Semitic periodical *Russkoe Znamya* (*Russian banner*). He was one of the leaders of *chernosotennogo* (*Black Hundred*) *Souza russkogo naroda* (*Union of Russian People*), an armed nationalistic group that fought against revolutionaries and organized pogroms. Dubrovin was executed by firing squad during the Civil War because of his "anti-Soviet activity."

Anti-Semitism was a state policy in Imperial Russia and affected medical education and the treatment of patients. It was officially recognized that only three percent of Jews who graduated from the high school could continue their education at the university (Strashun 1937, 25). Despite numerous obstacles the number of Jewish medical students had been increasing. For example, the number of Jewish medical students in Kiev had increased more than three-fold during the late 1800s (64 in 1874 to 217 in 1883). The Council of Kiev University appealed to the authorities to restrict the number of Jews to ten percent of those accepted to the university (Vrach 1884, 469). Jewish doctors could not become government employees, but could be private-practice practitioners. Even then, they were required to live in a special zone (the so-called *Cherta osedlosti* – the Pale of Settlement) and were forbidden to live in Moscow and St. Petersburg. The "News and views" section of a weekly periodical "Vrach" gives the following characteristic case: "Physician L. E. Brodsky from Kiev and his family departed to a dacha in Svyatoshin – a settlement where Jews were not allowed to live. Doctor Brodskii considered that his medical diploma would grant him the right to live everywhere, but the police evicted him as a Jew and sent him back to Kiev, and later did the same to his small children even though one had a high fever" (Vrach 1901, 1086). The same periodical reports that a consumptive blood-spitting patient was not admitted to the hospital because of his Jewish origin (Vrach 1901, 1431). Yet another example: "Someone K., a Jew, was admitted to the hospital in Khar'kov and spent there about a month

but was involuntarily discharged by order of local police before his course of treatment was completed. Moreover, the Justice of the Peace in Nakhichevan' sentenced K. to a fine of 5 rubles for leaving the Pale of Settlement" (Russkii Vrach 1902, 122). Physicians themselves often engaged in discrimination:

> A Crimean Jew applied to the city court of Simferopol' complaining against the city doctor of Karasubaz Kupresov. K. came to Kupresov with his sick child and asked for medical care. Dr. Kupresov (an opponent of Jews in principle) did not deliver any help but drove both father and child out, cursing them. When K made a remark about physicians' responsibilities, Dr. Kupresov called a policeman and demanded that K be arrested. Both father and son were taken into the custody where they were finally examined by Dr. Kupresov. The court found Kupresov guilty and sentenced him to a fine of 5 rubles. (Russkii Vrach 1903, 919)

Finally, another illustration: "A Jewish boy came to a Red Cross clinic requesting removal of a piece of match from his ear. A physician B. examined the boy and asked, what is his faith? I am Jewish, the boy replied. Well, in such case, go to your Jewish doctors, Dr. B. said and refused to give the child any help" (Russkii Vrach 1904, 597). There are countless examples of such discrimination from this period. It should therefore come as no surprise that many Jewish physicians shared Marxist views and later participated in the Revolution.

IV. CONCLUSION

Raisa Korotkikh observes that "it is hardly possible to give a definite answer to the question, What were the formal ethical views of medical doctors in pre-Revolutionary Russia?" (Korotkikh 1989, 20). How can one explain the absence of an all-Russian code of professional medical ethics during the period under consideration in this chapter?

Boris Petrov, for example, points out that the European medical deontology and medical ethics were formed exclusively within the medical profession (Petrov 1970). In contrast, Russian ideas about morality and medicine draw their inspiration from the influence of "progressive public figures and philosophers," such as Alexander Hertzen, Dmitry Pisarev, and Nikolai Chernyshevskii. Materialistic philosophers and popularizers also exerted a strong influence on the *narodniki* (populists) and therefore zemskaya medicine, which was closely related to this political movement. Russian medicine of this period cannot, however, be limited to zemskaya medicine, which by the turn of the twentieth century was in a deep crisis.

Another influence was Russian literature. As Raisa Korotkikh observed concerning this source of influence, the spiritual vacuum of Soviet medicine by the middle of the twentieth century might be explained by slackening impact of classic Russian literature. The following statement by Anton Chekhov is symptomatic: "A desire to serve the common weal should be absolutely the need of a soul, a condition of personal happiness; in case it comes from another source, from theoretical or other considerations, it is not true" (Chekhov 1987, 17:8).

Finally, medical morality was understood as the moral life in action. The following comment by the editor of *Vrach*, responding to a paper by H. F. A. Peypers dealing with unification of chairs of medical history and medical ethics, is illustrative: "Even without separate chairs these subjects were covered by our best professors, and medical ethics was taught not only in word but *in deed*" (Vrach 1901, no.44, emphasis original). The strong sense of social morality and the emphasis on morally exemplary action perhaps thwarted efforts to develop a formal, "bourgeois" all-Russian code of professional ethics.

Notes

1. By order of the Czar Nikolai I, the publisher of Chaadaev's letter was exiled to Ust'-Sysol'sk and the author was announced to be insane and had to be visited every week by a doctor and a police officer. As we can see, a tradition of claiming dissidents to be psychiatry cases has a long history.

2. About the time of Nicolas I. See Gershenzon (1911), Polievktov (1918), Bruce Lincoln (1978). For the Russian universities of that period, see Petrov (1998).

3. About the time of Alexander II, see Pirumova, Itenberg and Antonov (1990), Graham (1935), and Mosse ([1958] 1995). For University reform of that period, see Eimontova (1998).

4. Strashun (1937) notes that all medical institutions of the Russian Empire in 1914 comprised 175,600 beds.

5. According to the official report of the medical department of the Ministry of Internal Affairs the total number of medical doctors in Russia in 1881 was 14,488; of them 2,629 were private practitioners (18%). In 1907, these figures were 18,215 and 5,291 (29%), respectively.

6. As Zhbankov wrote earlier (1903, 101), the "patient's suffering and doctor's labor should not be brought to the market and become an issue of demand and supply; honorarium, private practice and all bargains between a patient and a physician must be eradicated, medical care should be provided free of charge" Leo Tolstoy in his article "On purpose of science and art" also wrote that true medical assistance will start only when a physician will provide it for free and will live among the working people in the same conditions (cited by Lobanov 1912, 35).

7. See also Vrach, 1901, 2:63–64.

8. There were eleven Russian editions of Veresaev's book during a 25-year period. A British edition is Veresaeff, V. 1904. *The Confessions of a Physician* (translated from Russian by S. Linden), London, Grant Richards. An American edition is Veresaev, V. V. 1916. *Memoirs of a Physician*, New York, Knopf. For a biography of Veresaev in English, see Raskin (1961).

9. See also comments in Vrach (1901), 14:459 and 16:528.

CHAPTER 36

THE DISCOURSES OF PRACTITIONERS IN NINETEENTH- AND TWENTIETH-CENTURY BRITAIN AND THE UNITED STATES

Robert B. Baker

I. CONCEIVING MODERN MEDICAL ETHICS: THE EDINBURGH REFORMERS

Six reformers collectively conceived of modern medical ethics in the English-speaking world. Five were physicians and Dissenters, that is, people who would not sign the Church of England's thirty-nine Articles of Faith. These Dissenters were a persecuted minority in England, officially excluded from all "official acts" that had a religious dimension, such as marriage and burial, or that required the swearing of official oaths – a prohibition that prevented them from holding public office, serving on a jury, or attending Cambridge or Oxford University (Haakonssen 1997, 94–6). Forced to seek a medical education outside of these elite universities, all five physician–reformers were affiliated with the University of Edinburgh. Listed in order of their birth the five physicians are: John Gregory (1724–1773) an Edinburgh University faculty member whose lectures on sympathy left an indelible imprint on Anglo-American medical morality (see Chapter 30); Samuel Bard (1742–1821) a New York physician, whose *Discourse on the Duties of A Physician* (Bard 1769) was the first published work on "medical ethics" by an Edinburgh reformer (see Chapter 31); Thomas Percival of Manchester, England, (1740–1804), who coined the

expression "medical ethics" in his eponymous work *Medical Ethics* (1803); Benjamin Rush, a Philadelphian (1745–1813) who attended Gregory's Edinburgh lectures and who would later (1809–1811) lecture American medical students at the University of Pennsylvania in the same vein (see Chapter 31); and, the lone Catholic dissenter in the group, Irish obstetrician and Edinburgh alumnus, Michael Ryan (1800–1841), the first person to style himself a professor of medical ethics (see Chapter 1). The sixth reformer, a nonphysician, is the Reverend Thomas Gisborne (1758–1846), an Englishman, a graduate of St. John's College, Oxford, an antislavery activist and an Evangelical clergyman, whose correspondence with Percival about an impending manuscript stimulated Percival to pen the first draft of *Medical Ethics* (Percival 1794, 1803).

II. THE QUALITIES OF A VIRTUOUS PHYSICIAN

The Edinburgh physician–reformers drew upon a conception of the virtues of medical practitioners that was formalized in a "Hippocratic Oath" signed by all Edinburgh medical students from 1731 to 1867 (Nutton 1995, 522). Michael Ryan's translation of the Latin-language oath follows.

To practice physic *cautiously, chastely, and honourably;* and faithfully to procure all things conducive to the health of the bodies of the sick; and lastly, never, without great cause, to divulge anything that ought to be concealed, which may be heard or seen during professional attendance. To this oath let the Deity be my witness. (Ryan 1832, 50–1)

Forty years later, in 1806, the Edinburgh alumni who founded the New York State medical society required a similar "Hippocratic" oath of their members.

I, A. B. do solemnly declare, That I will honestly, virtuously, and chastely, conduct myself in the practice of physic and surgery, with the privilege of exercising which profession I am now to be invested; and that I will, with fidelity and honour, do every thing in my power for the benefit of the sick committed to my care. (Walsh 1907)

The claim that the Edinburgh and New York oaths are "Hippocratic" might appear questionable to anyone familiar with the classical Oath (see Chapters 23 and 24). Like other cultural artifacts, however, oaths are influenced by the ethos of the greater society. In the eighteenth and nineteenth centuries, Anglo-American middle and upper classes aspired to the social status and lifestyle of ladies and gentlemen. In keeping with this trend, physicians' conception of ethics went upscale as well. Their ethical discourse tended to be framed in terms of virtues (i.e., praiseworthy character traits) and honor, and their negative correlatives, vices (deplorable character traits), and dishonor. Although the classical Hippocratic Oath mentioned some virtues (purity and holiness), it was primarily a list of obligations and prohibitions. To use the technical language of moral philosophy, the classical oath is a deontological ethic, an ethics of duty. To adapt the duty-oriented classical oath to eighteenth-century ideals of honor and virtue, the author(s) of the Edinburgh Oath had to translate its (deontological) language of obligatory and prohibited *actions* into a virtue ethic emphasizing *character traits*. Verbs denoting obligations and prohibitions thus had to be replaced by adjectives and adverbs designating character traits. The classic Oath's prohibition of actions sexually abusing the bodies of the sick, for example, was converted into the virtue of practicing physic "chastely." The core obligation to "use treatment to benefit the sick according to my ability and judgment, but never with a view to injury or wrong-doing" was similarly converted into a single cardinal virtue, fidelity (to the patient).

Reformulated Hippocratic virtues – chastity, fidelity, virtue and honor – permeate late eighteenth- and nineteenth-century Anglo-American medical discourse. They form an underlying conceptual and linguistic substrate shared by Edinburgh reformers, by establishment

Oxford-educated physicians, like Thomas Beddoes (1760–1808), and by the common run of less distinguished apothecaries, physicians, and surgeons. In their eulogies, epithets, and commendations, eighteenth- and nineteenth-century physicians from all strata of society alike praised liberal genteelness: beneficence ("benefiting the sick in one's care"), caution, chasteness, diligence, fidelity, temperance, and honesty as virtues. Correlatively, all ranks of physicians condemned such ungenteel and illiberal behavior as selfishness, rashness, forwardness, laziness, infidelity, intemperance, and dishonesty as vices. Hippocratic ethics was universally garbed in the language of gentlemanly virtue and honor.

III. Reform Ideals of Science and Sympathy

What differentiated the Edinburgh reformers from their contemporaries was their advocacy of science and sympathy. The reformers held that medical practice differed from other arts, trades, or occupations because medical practitioners had a *moral obligation* to practice scientifically. Medical practice was to be governed by what twentieth-century commentators would later characterize as "the research imperative." Physicians were thus perpetually obligated to "industriously cultivate every Opportunity of Improvement . . . [lest they] rashly tamper with the Lives of . . . Fellow Creatures" (Bard 1769, 14). This moral commitment to research derives from the thought of Francis Bacon (1561–1626, see Chapters 7, 18, and 30), patron philosopher of the Edinburgh reformers. The research imperative meant that virtuous practitioners should do more than simply earn a living by practicing what they had learned as students. As Bard explained in a graduation address delivered to the first class to graduate from Kings College (which later became Columbia University), "Do not . . . imagine that from this Time your studies are to cease . . . your whole Lives are one continued Series of Application and Improvement" (Bard 1769, 13). "Let it be your constant Aim" therefore to "inquir[e] into the Causes of . . . Diseases, and thence improving your Knowledge, and making further and useful Discoveries in the healing Art" (Bard 1769, 24; cf. Gisborne 1794a, 415).

The Edinburgh reformers also required virtuous practitioners to be *sympathetic* – a philosophical ideal of the Scottish Enlightenment (see Chapters 18 and 30). Before this, nothing in Anglo-American medico-moral tradition required a practitioner to do more than treat sickness. Sympathy required practitioners to extend treatment beyond efficacy so that it encompassed the *feelings* of the sick person and of that person's family – treatment was transformed into caring. Bard thus admonishes newly minted physicians that "it is your Duty not only to endeavour to preserve . . . Life, but to avoid wounding the Sensibility of a tender Parent, a distressed Wife, or an affectionate Child" (Bard 1769, 21). It is the singular accomplishment of Bard, Gregory, and later Edinburgh reformers that, even today, Anglo-American patients expect good medical practice to be scientific and regard it as morally deficient, however technically effective it may be at "preserving Life," if it does not reflect attention, sympathy, and tenderness to sick persons, their families and their friends.

IV. WHAT DID THE REFORMERS THINK THEY WERE REFORMING?

The reformers saw themselves as instilling new ideals of science and sympathy into a callous, complacent, feckless, and unscientific medicine. They believed that Anglo-American medicine was in danger of becoming a low-status, ungentlemanly trade whose aspirations for effectiveness and eminence were undermined by partisan rivalries and commercialization. Bard thus condemns "those little Arts of Cunning and Dissimulation, which to the Scandal of the Profession, have been but too frequent among us" (Bard 1769, 20). Ryan sounds a similar theme 6 decades later.

> Base and unprofessional and ungentlemanly behavior of late has characterized too many medical practitioners, and has debased and degraded the profession. The disputes and calumnies of medical men have been so frequent, so violent, so notorious of late, that the character of the profession is lowered in the estimation of the public to a degree unequal in the history of medicine. (Ryan 1831b, 54–55)

The reformers also believed that the dissension undermining the medical profession was a byproduct of the ethics of gentlemanly honor. The primary avenue of enforcing the ethics of gentlemanly honor, beyond an individual's own sense of propriety, was the threat that accusations of "ungenteel" conduct might lower one's status in the eyes of one's peers (who could censure or ostracize), one's patrons, one's institutional trustees, or one's private (fee-paying) patients. Practitioners thus had strong incentives either to behave honorably, or, failing that, to appear to have done so. They also had reason to defend themselves against accusations of dishonorable conduct.

Defending honor was particularly important because, as an ethics of character, the code of gentlemanly honor did not admit of degrees: one either was a gentleman, or one was not. Practitioners charged with dishonorable conduct thus felt a pressing need to fend off accusations. They often did so by flyting, that is, reestablishing their honorable status through verbal interchanges proclaiming the propriety of one's actions and one's honorableness, while attacking one's accusers' honorable intentions or gentlemanly status. Flytes were typically oral and brief, but they

were sometimes continued through an exchange of hostile letters, or a public interchange of accusatory pamphlets (a pamphlet war). In rare instances, flyting spilled over to lawsuits, or duels (see Harley 1990, 1993). It was these honor-protecting disputes – flytes, pamphlet wars, lawsuits and duels – that Ryan was condemning. Ironically, the very measures that individuals undertook to protect their individual honor as gentlemen were undermining honor of the profession as a whole.

V. THE BIRTH OF THE MEDICAL ETHICS PARADIGM: THE PERCIVALEAN REVOLUTION

By the end of the eighteenth century, it was becoming clear to reformers that affairs of gentlemanly honor imperiled public support and private patronage for the new scientific medicine forming in such collaborative endeavors as charity hospitals, medical schools, and public health departments. The incompatibility of the old individualistic ethics of gentlemanly honor and new collaborative scientific medicine was driven home to Percival in 1792. The trustees of the Manchester Infirmary (one of the larger hospitals in England) charged him with forming a committee to draft a code of conduct to end the flytes and pamphlet wars that threatened the Infirmary's ability to function (Pickstone and Butler 1984). In 1792, Percival's committee delivered this code; 2 years later Percival published a preliminary version of a general code of ethics for physicians and surgeons; he ultimately publishing the code in 1803, under a new title, *Medical Ethics* (see Chapter 18, and Pickstone 1993).

Medical Ethics differed from other works written by the Edinburgh reformers. Originating as a response to a real institutional crisis, it reformulated Edinburgh virtues in terms of practitioners' duties: specifically their duties to their patients, to fellow professionals, and to society (Baker 1993a). As one would expect of a code, the duties were presented as numbered articles, a format that forced restating Edinburgh virtues as specific duties. Thus the Edinburgh ideal that "temperance and sobriety are virtues peculiarly required in a physician" (Gregory [1770] 1998a, 107; [1772b] 1998b, 173) was codified as a duty specified in Article II, Chapter II of *Medical Ethics*: "The strictest *temperance* should be incumbent" (Percival, 1803b).

In some cases, reformulation was transformative. Reformulated in terms of duty, the virtue of sympathy became the obligation to respect the *"feelings* and *emotions* of patients no less than the symptoms of their diseases" (Percival, 1803b Chap. I, Art. III). This, in turn, was held to imply a correlative duty to respect a patient's emotional right to decline treatment, so that "extreme timidity [about an intervention] contraindicates its use [because] Even the prejudices of the sick are not to be contemned, or opposed with harshness" (Percival, 1803b Chap. I, Art. III). It is important to appreciate that in contrast to later bioethical formulations of the right to refuse treatment, Percival does *not* ground this right in Kantian notions of respect for persons' autonomy and their rational choices, but rather out of sympathy for patients' feelings. For Percival and other Edinburgh reformers persons were emotional as well as rational beings, respect for persons thus encompasses both the emotive and the rational dimensions of their nature.

As one would expect, given the nature of the institutional crisis that inspired it, many of duties enumerated in *Medical Ethics* deal with dispute resolution. Percival's strategy for dealing with disputes is stated out in the oft-quoted statement: "The *Esprit du Corps* is a principle of action founded in human nature . . . Every man who enters into a fraternity engages, by a tacit compact, not only to submit to the laws, but to promote the honour and interests of the association, so far as they are consistent with morality and the general good of mankind." Every practitioner is thus committed by a "tacit compact" to obey the collaboratively determined "laws" of the medical profession and to promote the profession's interests, insofar as they are moral. More specifically, individual practitioners are obligated to accept regulation by their peers through such "professional" mechanisms of collaborative decision making as rounds, committees, and through the peer adjudication of disputes (for details see Percival 1803b, Chap. I, Arts. X, XIII, XVIII, XIX, XXI; Chap. II, Arts. IV, V, VII–X, XXII–XXVII; Chap. III, Arts. I–V).

Percival also sought to replace the concept of the physician as "gentleman" with the new concept of the "medical professional," both to cement solidarity among physicians, surgeons, and apothecaries, and to undermine the conceptual source of flytes, the concept of gentlemanly honor. Earlier Edinburgh reformers had criticized the dispute-generating aspects of gentlemanly honor (Bard, 1769, 19–20; Gregory [1770] 1998a, 109; [1772], 176), but they had not sought to replace the key normative notion of "the gentleman" with the concept of "the professional." In their writings, and in all of Percival's pre-1803 publications, the term "profession" simply meant "occupation." In *Medical Ethics*, however, Percival deploys valorizing quotations from Bacon and Cicero to transform the concept of "profession" into something more than "occupation." In his usage – and in later Anglo-American usage – profession designated a collaboratively self-regulating occupation whose individual members are bound by a social compact to each other, to those they serve, and to the service of society in general (see Chapter 18).

Percival's *Medical Ethics* was thus revolutionary. It offered practitioners a new conception of themselves, a new way of thinking about their moral obligations and a new discourse in which these novel conceptions were parsed. A fundamental change in the way medical morality was conceptualized, justified, and enforced – a moral revolution – establishing the concepts of medical ethics and profes-

sional ethics was on offer. Yet intellectual revolutions, including scientific revolutions, conserve even as they transform (Cohen 1985). Thus, despite the transformative nature of Percival's conceptual revolution, the norms of conduct championed by earlier Edinburgh reformers are conserved, albeit reformulated as *professional* duties rather than as gentlemanly virtues.

It is the hallmark of any intellectual revolution that it generates new forms of discourse to encapsulate its conceptual innovations. Percival had to coin three expressions, new, not only to English, but novel in any language to express his revolutionary conception of medical morality: "medical ethics," "professional ethics," and "professional etiquette" (i.e., conduct requisite in dealings with fellow professionals [Percival 1803, Chap. III, Art. III; see discussion in Chapters 1 and 18]). The novelty of these usages allows historians to track the spread of Percival's ideas, that is, of the spread of the medical ethics revolution. One can thus track the appraisal of specific acts, such as "Pretending to Secrets, Panaceas, and Nostrums," that earlier reformers had condemned as "illiberal, dishonest, and inconsistent with your *Characters, as Gentlemen*" (Bard 1769, 20, emphasis added), with later versions of this condemnation as "disgraceful to *the profession*" (American Medical Association (AMA) [1848] 1999, Chap. II, Art. I. Secs. 3, 4; AMA, 1903, Chap. II, Sec. 8; AMA, 1912, Chap. II, Sec. 6). (See Chapter 18 for a more detailed discussion of the dissemination of Percival's concepts and discourse.)

Based on this linguistic evidence, it is clear that British and American medical morality began to diverge by mid-nineteenth century. For while Percival's conception of practitioners as professionals became equally prominent in both British and American usage by 1900, his concept of medical ethics had become commonplace only in American but not in British usage. After the mid-nineteenth century, American and British physicians thought about medical morality differently. In the light of this spilt, British and American medical ethics will be treated separately in the rest of this chapter.

VI. The British Approach to Professional Etiquette and Ethics: 1800–1946

At the beginning of the nineteenth century attempts to establish such collaborative medical enterprises as hospitals, medical schools, and public health departments were imperiled by an ethics of gentlemanly honor whose enforcement mechanisms undermined collaboration as well as patron and public funding. Had the challenge not been met, the growth of these institutions could have been stultified. Yet, British and America medicine responded to this challenge differently. Although aspects of the Edinburgh reform tradition were accepted in nineteenth-century British medicine, it was not until the second half of the twentieth century that Percival's conception of codified medical ethics had any impact in Britain – and then only in response to events across the channel: horror at medical complicity in the Holocaust. Hospitals adopted some of Percival's rules, but as hospital rules, not as "medical ethics." In general, Percival's *Medical Ethics* tended to be treated as a collection of helpful aphorisms (see Pickstone 1993, 162). To be sure, medical educators paid lip service to Edinburgh ideas of sympathy and science, but the specifics of the reform agenda – constraints on experimentation, patients' prerogatives, and so forth – were largely ignored. Dissenters, Catholics, and Celts (Irishmen, Scots), the reformers lacked the social authority essential to changing actual medical practices in their native country.

Protesting this situation, in 1827 an anonymous editor reissued *Medical Ethics*, with detailed footnotes contrasting practitioners' actual conduct with the ideals envisioned by Percival (Anonymous 1827a). A review in the reforming journal, *The Lancet*, approved the editor's "reflections on the corporate institutions of medicine and surgery" remarking, however, "that they somewhat disturb the gravity of Dr. Percival's aphorisms" (Anonymous 1827b, 696). Note the reviewer's choice of words "aphorisms," "profession" and his eschewal of "ethics." By the 1820s, Percival's conception of medicine as a profession had become commonplace in Britain; however, the neologisms he used in his aphorisms – medical ethics, professional ethics – rarely found there way into *The Lancet*, or into British medical discourse generally.

Later reformers, like Ryan, received a similarly mixed reception. *The Lancet* published a sarcastic review of Ryan's work in medical ethics and medical jurisprudence. The reviewer focused on Ryan's comments on "the propriety or impropriety of making clinical experiments with new remedies" (Anonymous 1831a, 141). Concern over experiments that exploited vulnerable populations was a recurring theme in the Edinburgh reform literature. Gregory had proposed a Golden Rule test: in conducting "dangerous Experiments . . . I would ask that man if he have done so to his Child, if he would not do it to his own Child, why should he indanger the lives of other people" (Gregory [1772] 1998, 249). Percival mandated a peer review panel that would preapprove "such trials" to see whether they were based on "sound reason . . . just analogy [and] well authenticated facts" (Percival 1803, Chap. I, Art. XII). Gisborne condemned "rash, hastily adopted . . . ignorant . . . careless . . . obstinate experimenters" who were all too willing to countenance the "death of an obscure, indigent, and quickly forgotten individual" (Gisborne 1794, 407, 408).

Continuing in this tradition, Ryan argued that "administering a dangerous medicine to gratify . . . zeal for science, to ascertain the comparative advantage or disadvantage of some new remedy . . . is . . . a breach of ethics . . . and a great breach of trust towards his patient. . . . [that] the profession [i.e., the Edinburgh reformers] . . . has always reprobated" (Ryan 1831a, 37). Ryan continued, "in this age . . . *all experiments are made upon inferior animals.*" *The Lancet* reviewer was scandalized. "Will it be believed that Dr. Ryan can be so ignorant, as to be unaware that to the experiments he repudiates are we indebted for the discovery of . . . the therapeutic effects of all our remedial agents? As to the performance of *therapeutic* experiments on *inferior* animals – such a thing is scarcely heard of." (Anonymous 1831a, 141). Ryan replied: "I am censured . . . for having stated the rule laid down by the profession [i.e., the reformers] . . . that dangerous experiments should not be made on the sick without their consent." "Perhaps in his zeal for science" the reviewer "would allow a few experiments to be made on himself . . . Or would he prefer the application of these things on the poor?" (Ryan 1831b, 224).

Responding in a later issue "on this worthless subject," *The Lancet* reviewer "appeal[ed] to our practical readers. How would they investigate the *curative* powers on any unknown substance? The obvious answer is, by its administration to persons in a state of disease, in minute and gradually increasing doses" (Anonymous 1831b, 225). Protecting the sick poor from zealous experimenters may have been a central concern to the Edinburgh reformers, but Ryan's specification of Percival's consent doctrine to human subjects experimentation was dismissed as "worthless" by *The Lancet* reviewer.

A year after this exchange, in 1832, the Provincial Medical and Surgical Association was founded, forming the basis of an organization that was reconstituted as the "British Medical Association" (BMA) in 1856. Although the organization's founder, Charles Hastings (1794–1866), favored formulation of a code of conduct (Morrice 2002, 15), no formal code was promulgated by the BMA during the nineteenth century – although there were efforts to draft such a code in the 1840s, 1850s, 1860s, and 1880s (Bartrip 1995a). Jukes Styrap (1815–1899) offered the BMA a thoughtfully updated version of Percival's code in 1882 (Bartrip 1995a; Styrap [1878] 1995).

Although Percival and Ryan had little impact on British medical practice, some Edinburgh reform ideals seeped into the mainstream. In an 1843 address to the entering class of students at St. Georges Hospital, London, for example, Sir Benjamin Collins Brodie (1783–1862), surgeon to Prince Albert and later President of the Royal Society, conveyed the gist of the nineteenth-century and early twentieth-century British conception of the good practitioner. "Good moral character is not less necessary to your advancement in the medical profession than skill and knowledge." Beyond "strict observance of the higher rules of morality," good practitioners must "feel and act as gentlemen." They "sympathize with others, and are careful not to hurt their feelings" (Brodie 1843, 30). The good British practitioner is thus the skillful, knowledgeable, sympathetic gentleman.

Because the Percivalean concept of codified professional medical ethics was almost entirely ignored, how did British medicine resolve the problems created by gentleman defending their honor? To a certain extent, they failed to control these behaviors. Protests over breaches of medical etiquette appeared regularly in the pages of *The Lancet* in 1830s and 1840s, and elsewhere through the early twentieth century (see Banks 1839; Anonymous 1878). They only diminish significantly in the latter part of the nineteenth century when British medicine turned to a traditional mechanism of social control: the power to censure, to expel, and to ostracize.

This power was asserted by the Royal College of Physicians (RCP), which was founded 1518 with a Royal mandate, that is, with governmental backing. The RCP had committees of censors and committees of the whole empowered to adjudicate conflicts and to censure, to expel, or to ostracize, any member whose conduct failed to meet their expectations for "decorous, honorable, erudite and virtuous" conduct (RCP 1772, 4, 15, 16). When the Provincial Medical and Surgical Association was founded in 1832 its local branches assumed similar powers – albeit without governmental authority – and the tradition was continued by the BMA.

The Medical Act of 1858 restored the imprimatur of semigovernmental authority to the tradition of "censors" monitoring the profession. The Act stated the conditions under which the government would recognize practitioners as registered – that is, as successfully completing a regular academic education. It also empowered a quasi-nongovernmental body, the General Medical Council (GMC), to "erase" or to "strike" names from the register. It was not illegal to practice without registration, as long as one laid no claim to being registered; however, because regulars were forbidden to consult with nonregistered practitioners, having one's name struck off the register effectively excluded a practitioner from such "regular" institutions as clinics, hospitals, medical schools, and medical societies (Bynum 1994, 179). More specifically, the GMC was empowered to erase a name from the register if a practitioner was convicted of a crime, or was "judged by the [GMC] to have been guilty of infamous conduct in any professional respect" (Smith 1995, 206). Formal accusations were considered by the GMC in a quasijuridical process. Following the precedent set by the BMA and its precursors, however, the GMC declined to draft any formal code specifying the forms of conduct that qualified as "infamous."

Before 1883, the GMC even refused to state *why* particular individuals had their name struck from the register (Smith, 1995, 207). After 1883, it began to issue notices explaining why a specific case was considered "infamous conduct in a professional respect." Gradually this list of explanations expanded into a system of "Warning Notices," which were ultimately published in medical journals and collected as a small pamphlet (Smith 1994, 1995). Nonetheless, when, in 1903, the GMC received a petition from 133 Scottish practitioners requesting formal guidance, so that they might anticipate what would constitute "infamous conduct," without actually committing a transgression, the GMC replied that they "have no power to legislate or to issue regulations binding upon the profession." Insofar as conduct is a function of honorable character, formal codes of conduct are useful *only* to persons who, having failed to attain the attributes of an honorable gentleman, nonetheless wish to pretend that they had. It was thus "not *desirable* to pass a resolution condemning any practice in general terms . . . for the profession" (Smith, 1995, 210, emphasis added; for an account of the GMC process by a Scottish physician, see Cronin [1937] 1965, 350–68). One consequence of the GMC's adamant insistence on the ethics of honor and its concomitant refusal to codify conduct for the profession was that, unlike the ethics committees of the AMA, the GMC never sought investigatory powers (see Chapter 61).

Around the same time, 1902, as part of a general reorganization, the BMA established a Central Ethics Committee (CEC) to address medico-ethical and medico-political problems (Morrice 2002, 17). Again, even though the head of the CEC, Robert Saundby (1849–1918) published codes of ethics (Saundby 1902, 1907), neither the CEC, nor the BMA – nor, to reiterate, the GMC – would officially accept any formal code of professional conduct, or acquire investigatory powers, until relatively recently. As a function of gentlemanly character, honor needed no codification, and was not subject to anticipatory investigation. Indeed, there were no official British guides to good (i.e., ethical) medical practice until the 1980s.

VII. AMERICAN APPROACHES TO MEDICAL ETHICS 1800–1946

The Edinburgh reform agenda may have been peripheral in Britain, but the American medical establishment embraced it. Unlike their British counterparts, the Americans turned to the "different publications of Gregory, Rush and Percival" for guidance (Association of Boston Physicians [1808] 1995, 41). Gregory's ideals were embraced wholeheartedly, as was Percival's eminently practical notion of formulating them in codes designed to control intrapractitioner relationships. In 1808, just 5 years after the publication of Percival's *Medical Ethics*, the Boston medical society adopted a "medical police" (Association of Boston Physicians [1808] 1995). This code employed Percival's justificatory concept of *"Esprit du Corps"* and borrowed heavily from those sections of *Medical Ethics* that dealt with regulating intrapractitioner conduct but ignored those that dealt with practitioner–patient relations. Percival's code format was thus adopted merely as a practical mechanism for controlling intrapractitioner strife.

Other American medical societies soon followed this precedent. Unlike the Boston physicians, their codes also dealt with patients. To do so they borrowed language and precepts from Gregory, not from Percival.

Until 1847, American practitioners had recourse to three major discourses of medical morality. They used the popular discourse of gentlemanly honor found in the 1806 New York Oath, which was especially prominent in flytes and pamphlet wars. Public lectures and formal codes tended toward Gregory's discourse of moral sentiments. Percivalean language on professionalism and duty tended to be restricted to codes of ethics. No one conception of medical morality was dominant until the founding of the AMA in 1847. With the foundation of the AMA, however, Percivalean conceptions of professional medical ethics became dominant. (For further discussion of pre-1847 American codes of medical ethics, see Chapter 18 and Baker 1999, 29–36.)

The process that led to the formation of the AMA was initiated in 1846 when Nathan Smith Davis (1817–1904), a recent medical school graduate dismayed by the inadequacies of his own education, persuaded the Medical Society of the State of New York to convene a national conference on this issue. The conference deadlocked. As it began to disband in failure, Isaac Hays (1796–1879), editor of the leading medical journal of the period, *The American Journal of the Medical Sciences*, asked Davis to endorse a proposal for a second national convention to establish a permanent national medical society. This society would be dedicated, not only to reforming medical education, but also to reforming American medical science and public health, and to establishing a common code of medical ethics for the profession. Davis agreed. When Hays put the proposal to the conference it passed unanimously (Baker 1999).

To prepare for the second national conference, committees were formed to draft a constitution and various proposals. A committee of seven, chaired by John Bell (1796–1872), was commissioned to draft a code of ethics. Hays served as the committee's secretary. It was not happenstance that Hays had proposed a code of ethics for the organization that was to become the AMA, nor that Bell was chosen to chair the drafting committee. Both had editorialized about the need for a national code of medical ethics in the journals they edited; moreover, two decades earlier, in 1823, both had collaborated in editing *Extracts from the Medical Ethics of Dr. Percival*, for the Philadelphia Kappa Lambda Society of Hippocrates, an ethics reform society. This edition of the Percival's code was the source of approximately two-thirds of the code of ethics "drafted" by the committee (Baker 1999, 28–9; see also Chapter 18).

The Code of Ethics that Bell and Hays put before the convention was based on the idea of reciprocal moral obligations – a tripartite social contract between physicians, and three other parties: their patients, the profession collectively, and the public at large (Baker 1993a; Bell [1847] 1999). As a statement of reciprocal obligations, the Code included two unusual sections: a section stipulating the obligations that patients had *to* their physicians, and a parallel section stating the obligations that the public had *to* the medical profession. In effect, these sections stated what physicians expected from patients and the public as a quid pro quo for their commitments to patients and the public (AMA [1848] 1999, Chap. I, Art. II, Chap. III, Art. II). For example, in exchange for physicians' commitment to preserve the "secrecy" of the information that their patients imparted to them (AMA [1848] 1999, Chap. I, Art. I, Sec. 2), patients were expected to reciprocate by "faithfully and unreservedly communicating to their physicians . . . never being afraid of thus making the physician his friend and adviser" (AMA [1847] 1999, Chap. I. Art. II, Sec. 4).

More conventionally, the Code obligated physicians to treat patients with attention, steadiness, humanity, delicacy, and "condescension," that is, to treat them as moral equals irrespective of their social status. It also forbade "abandon[ing] a patient because the case is deemed incurable" (AMA [1847] 1999, Chap. I, Art. I, Sec. 5). Patients' reciprocal obligations involved such things as not abandoning their physicians without "delar[ing their] reasons for so doing" (AMA [1847] 1999c. I, Art. II, Sec. 8).

The code was also a social contract between the profession as a whole, represented by the AMA, and its individual members, who agreed not to advertise, not to sell or prescribe secret nostrums, and not to consult with sectarian or "irregular" practitioners. The code definitively characterized "irregulars" as those whose practice was based on "an exclusive dogma, to the rejection of the accumulated experience of the profession, and of the aids actually furnished by anatomy, physiology, pathology and organic chemistry" – the reference to organic chemistry excluded homeopaths whose pharmacopoeia was based on principles incompatible with chemistry (AMA [1847] 1999, Chap. II, Art. IV, Sec. 1). Individual practitioners were also obligated to have recourse to the full range of Percivalean mechanisms for adjudicating and arbitrating disputes, to prevent public flytes, pamphlet wars, and duels.

Perhaps the most striking innovation in the 1847 Code was "the Duties of the Profession to the Public" and the reciprocal "Obligations of the Public to the Profession." The profession accepted a duty to serve the public's health by providing medical care for "individuals in indigent circumstances . . . cheerfully and freely" (AMA [1847] 1999, Art. I, Sec. 3). During epidemics, it was an AMA physician's "duty to face the danger, and to continue their labors for the alleviation of suffering, even at the jeopardy of their own lives" – no minor commitment in an era in which physicians were as subject to fatal infectious diseases as their patients (AMA [1847] 1999, Chap. III, Sec. 1).

Never before had physicians or medical organizations undertaken self-imposed duties as rigorous as those in the 1847 AMA Code. Yet, when the code was put to a vote, it passed unanimously. Lauded as a major reform in the medical and popular press, the 1847 Code was published in Berlin, Munich, Paris, and Vienna and provided a model for the codes of professional ethics that was emulated around the globe, including Canada, Germany, and Japan (Haller 1981, 237–8; Maehle 2002, 39; Roy and Williams 1995, 1633; see Chapters 22 and 34).

In 1855, the AMA proclaimed its code *binding* upon all allied societies and institutions, and their members. Thus all regular asylums, clinics, dispensaries, hospitals, medical schools, and medical societies in America were bound by the AMA's code of ethics. To implement the code affiliated societies tried to clean house by expelling members who performed abortions, who advertised, who publicly endorsed secret nostrums, who patented medicines or medical products, or who consulted with homeopaths and other irregular practitioners. The AMA also began a campaign to reform medical and premedical education by requiring extensive training in laboratory sciences and in hospital practice. By the first decades of the twentieth century, most of the reforms envisioned by the AMA's founders had been achieved. AMA lobbying had helped to persuade the federal government to found the U.S. Public Health Service in 1903, and the Food and Drug Administration in 1906 (Baker and Emanuel 2000) and after the publication of the Flexner Report (Flexner [1910] 1973), medical education required training in the basic sciences and hospital experience.

Ironically, the closer the AMA progressed toward its original goals, the greater the degree of dissent and rebellion within the organization. In 1882, the Medical Society of the State of New York, the very society that had initiated the chain of events leading to the formation of the AMA, withdrew from the AMA protesting that its "code of ethics" was an illiberal "etiquette" masquerading as ethics (Post 1883; Warner 1999). The New York society had been politically active throughout the 1870s and 1880s, lobbying to found a state board of health, to pass regulations protecting children's health, and to stiffen educational requirements for medical licensure. It had also lobbied against an 1872 law licensing homeopaths and to thwart antivivisection initiatives prohibiting experiments on animals (see Chapter 48 and Lederer 1995, 51–72).

The antivivisection initiative was narrowly defeated in the New York State legislature, but not the 1872 law licensing homeopaths. Mindful of the new licensure law, the New York society felt obliged to accept a homeopathic physician as a member. Society members began pressing the AMA's Code of Ethics on several other fronts

as well. In their zeal for public health legislation the New York Society proposed abolishing the legal protection of patient confidentiality, even though the AMA Code of Ethics expressly protected "the obligation of secrecy" (AMA [1847] 1999, Chap. I, Art. 1, Sec. 2).

In 1881, retiring President William Bailey (1825–1898) took it upon himself to criticize the very notion of a code of medical ethics. It is a "serious question, whether the society of medical men should not drop its written law of ethics entirely." These codes are "but an appendix to [the] real work and scope" of a medical society, whose primary functions are educational and intellectual. Bailey envisioned a generation of physicians who needed no formal system of ethics because "constant association with the sick and afflicted naturally develops their sympathetic nature" (Bailey 1881, 107, 110, 112).

Bailey's speech catalyzed the members of the New York Society to reconstitute their organization as a professional society that would serve as a forum for scientific discourse and for disseminating scientific knowledge but not as an ethics watchdog. Abraham Jacobi (1830–1919), Bailey's successor as President of the New York Society, endorsed a new code that permitted consultation with "all legally qualified practitioners of medicine" including homeopaths, but which did *not* address physicians' relations to their patients. By its silence on this subject, the new code failed to protect the patient's right to confidentiality.

The "New Code," as it came to be called, was attacked on two fronts. "No Coders" championed a return to an unwritten ethics of gentlemanly honor, especially on such questions "As to whether we should advertise in public" (Medical Society of the State of New York 1882, 26). Partisans of the "Old Code," on the other hand, condemned the New Code as an unprincipled collection of rules that protected physicians while ignoring the rights of patients. It "cannot properly be called a code; for a code should . . . contain [a] declaration of moral principles . . . which should govern us as a profession;" "nothing," for example, "is said in regard to confidential communications" (Medical Society of New York 1882, 29).

On February 7, 1882, the New York society officially adopted the New Code, setting in motion a complex chain of events culminating in the AMA's expulsion of the New York society and the concomitant exclusion of New Yorkers from the International Congress of Medicine that the AMA hosted in 1887. Although the *casus belli* in the Old/New/No-Code struggle was homeopathy, the deeper issue was the unwillingness of an elite group of New Yorkers, including some of the country's leading medical researchers and specialists, to submit themselves to constraints of a clinically oriented democratic organization (Warner 1991, 1999). They feared that ethical regulation would fetter "progress," in the form of sanitarian reform, scientific research, and specialty medicine;

moreover, many of the New Yorkers believed that public health medicine, or sanitary science, rendered "the period of individual health cobbling" obsolete (Jacobi, 1909, 88). As one delegate to the AMA's 1879 convention complained, the Old Code was a practical impediment to sanitary science because "physicians must sometimes serve in sanitary organizations with irregular practitioners of medicine, or they must refuse to give the public the benefit of their knowledge of, and skill in, sanitary science" (Hibbard 1879, 387).

The AMA code's constraint on advertising was also vexing specialists. The constraint had twin roots: in the ethics of gentlemanly honor, which abhorred all forms of commercial conduct, and the Edinburgh reformers' drive to create a medicine based on science rather than self-promotion. Yet, specialists needed to make the public and fellow practitioners aware of their specialty to practice. In principle, the issue was how to prohibit self-promotion without strangling specialty medicine. In practice, principles tended to become entangled with economic and other interests.

The issue came to a head in 1868 when the AMA expelled Julius Homberger (1839–1872), founding editor of the *American Journal of Ophthalmology*, for violating ethical constraints on advertising (AMA 1868, 1869, 19:25, 29). In 1869, the AMA forbade specialists to place advertisements in professional publications – rescinding this policy a year later, in 1870 (*Transactions of the American Medical Association* 1870, 21:39–40). Affronting the deepest sensibilities of specialists, the AMA also required them to identify their expertise as a "limitation." Thus, instead of identifying themselves as *experts* specializing in some area, such as ophthalmology, they were to be characterized as limitations on general practice. Ophthalmologists were "limited to diseases of the eye" (AMA 1868, 1869, 25:31).

In the 1870s, the specialists revolted. A delegate from New York proposed the "abolition of the Code of Ethics" (*Transactions of the American Medical Association* 1870, 21:39). By 1875, the cry for abolition was taken up from the President's podium by the most famous gynecologist of the day, J. Marion Sims (1813–1884). Lampooning defenders of the Code as "High Priests" of the "Holy of Holies" (Sims 1876, 96), Sims defended physicians' right to hold patents, to make money from medical innovations, and to prescribe secret nostrums. He proposed that Americans emulate the British ethic of gentlemanly honor. "Honorable men do not need [a code's] protection. Dishonorable men are not influenced by its edicts. We must educate the profession up to a higher law, the unwritten code regulating intercourse between gentlemen. This is the code that governs in England and France. The man that violates it is by common consent dropped out, ignored, and allowed to vegetate in isolation" (Sims 1876, 99).

Sims neglected to mention that he had been reprimanded by the New York Academy of Medicine for "self-advertizement." His comments about the use of the Code as "an engine of torture and oppression" by "men jealously, maliciously intent upon persecuting a fellow member, may distort . . . entering into a regular conspiracy to blacken character," may have been autobiographical (Sims 1876, 99; Barker-Benfield 1976, 97–8). Just 2 years earlier, in 1874, the AMA had condemned a researcher for violating its Code by treating human research subjects "inhumanely" (Lederer 1995, 8), so Simms might also have feared that he might be condemned for using unanesthetized female slaves as involuntary research subjects to perfect his most famous gynecological operation, repair of vesico-vaginal fistulae (Barker-Benfield 1976, 91–119).

A stew of issues congealed to unite sanitarians, scoundrels, specialists, and scientific researchers in an anticode alliance. In 1886, they formed an alternative Bailey-model, scientist-specialty national medical and scientific society, the Association of American Physicians (AAP). Its first President, Francis Delafield (1841–1915) proudly proclaimed the organization's rejection of "medical ethics" in his inaugural address (Delafield 1886, 16). No coders also purged existing societies, like the New York Academy of Medicine of codes of ethics, transforming them into Bailey-model professional societies that, to quote Jacobi, were to be committed *solely* to "The promotion of the Science and Art of Medicine" (Van Ingen 1949, 203–5). Because the AAP was the progenitor of America's major specialty colleges, which were founded during this period (Stevens 1999), specialty medicine thus inherited as its birthright an animus against professional ethical self-regulation and Bailey's presumption that professional competence alone assured moral integrity. American research and specialty medicine remained true to this birthright through the 1970s.

Despite a vigorous defense of the 1847 AMA Code by others in the profession (see, for example, Cathell 1898, 61–4), in 1903, AAP and New/No Code sympathizers seized control of the AMA, replacing its mandatory Code of Ethics with a purely advisory statement of the Principles of Medical Ethics (King 1983). To use some technical philosophical jargon, the 1903 principles were thought of in "positivist" terms; that is, they were principles posited without deeper moral grounding. Gregory and Bard, in contrast, had believed that they were explicating a morality inherent in the ethics of sympathy and the concept of being a physician. Percival, Bell, and Hays thought of professional ethics in terms of a social contract. The authors of the 1903 AMA Principles, however, believing their principles lacked moral grounding, regarded them as merely "suggestive and advisory . . . without definite reference to code or penalties," leaving "large discretionary powers . . . to state . . . societies" (AMA [1903] 1999, 335). The practical correlative of this positivist approach was that every American medical institution could follow its own moral compass.

More formally, the positivist vision of the AMA principles rendered social contractarian elements of the 1847 Code conceptually obsolete. Thus, all mention of the reciprocal duties of patients and the public were deleted from the 1903 Principles, as were all statements the patient's and the public's claims on the profession. One consequence of these deletions was that in a new section aptly titled *"The Limitations* of Gratuitous Service" the AMA abandoned its earlier commitment to "freely accord" medical care to "individuals in indigent circumstances" (AMA [1847] 1999, Chap. III, Art. I, Sec. 3), eliminating AMA members' obligation to provide free medical care to the poor – although such care was still morally permissible (AMA [1903] 1999 Chap. II, Art. VI, Sec. 1). In deference to the sanitarian origins of antiethics revolt, however, the Principles retain language about physicians' duty care for patients during epidemics, even at risk of their lives (AMA [1903] 1999, Chap. III, Sec. 2).

The 1903 Principles emerged from an ethos that looked back to ideals of gentlemanly honor, now reconceptualized as professional honor. It thus inherited a professional (i.e., gentlemanly) disdain for commerce. Reflecting this self-conception the Principles prohibited fee splitting, that is, commissions or "kickbacks" for referring patients to particular specialists or hospitals (AMA [1903] 1999, Chap. II, Art. VI, Sec. 4). More practically, in an accommodation with the pharmaceutical industry, patent medicines were distinguished from secret nostrums: doctors were forbidden to prescribe secret nostrums but prescribing patent medicines became permissible (AMA [1903] 1999, Chap. II, Art. I, Sec. 8).

In less than decade, problems began to surface. Although the Principles condemned fee splitting, because it freed members from following its advice, fee splitting scandals became commonplace. In response, in 1912, the AMA abandoned its positivist stance and found a moral underpinning for the Principles in "service to humanity" which rendered "financial gain . . . a subordinate consideration." The Percivalean ideal of professionalism was also resurrected to restore the right to prescribe and proscribe practitioners' conduct: "The practice of medicine is a profession. In choosing this profession an individual assumes an obligation to conduct himself in accord with its ideals" (AMA [1912] 1999, Chap. I, Sec. 1). To give this provision bite, a new body, the Council on Ethical and Judicial Affairs (CEJA) was empowered to recommend the expulsion of individuals found guilty of fee splitting and other unprofessional conduct (AMA, *Proceedings*: June 1912, 11, 45; June 1913, 12–16, 49; June, 1915, 12, 60, 61). Moreover, in keeping with their newly stated goal of service to humanity, the profession's obligation to provide gratuitous service to the poor was restored (AMA [1912] 1999, Chap. II, Art. VI, Sec. 1).

Despite the reforms of 1912, the AMA remained ambivalent about enforcing ethics standards. As originally constituted, CEJA was a passive body, lacking the authority to investigate professional misconduct. In 1924, however, it was empowered to investigate abuses of ethical standards and to recommend the expulsion of any "county society found to enroll so many . . . unethical, members as to render it impossible for that society to enforce the ethical standards of the medical profession" (AMA, *Proceedings*, June 1924, 21–22, 40). From this point onward, despite occasional decades of retreat, the AMA reasserted self-regulatory authority, especially with respect to fee splitting and related conflicts of interest. It actively campaigned against such manifest conflicts of interest as physician-owned or partially owned diagnostic laboratories, physician-owned healthcare appliance outlets, physician-owned hospitals, physician-owned home health agencies, and the more traditional abuses of fee splitting and accepting commissions or rebates for "steering" patients to specific commercial organizations and laboratories (Baker and Emanuel 2000).

During the earlier period of ambivalence about enforcing ethics standards, the AMA was confronted by a series of research scandals. Notorious abuses were paraded in the popular media and these, in turn, prompted proposals for governmental regulation, including a licensing system for scientific researchers seeking to experiment on human subjects (Gallinger [1900] 1995). Researchers, however, resisted governmental regulation, citing the nobility of the research imperative, even as they disowned notorious examples of impropriety by disparaging the researchers as "unbalanced." To defuse the situation, they proposed a regulatory mechanism more formal than professional honor but less constraining than government licensure: formal principles of research ethics promulgated and enforced by the AMA (Lederer 1995, 73–100).

Championing this proposal was Walter Bradford Cannon (1871–1945), Chairman of the Council for the Defense of Medical Research of the American Medical Association from its founding in 1908 to its dissolution in 1926. In 1909–1910, Cannon had defused an antivivisectionist campaign aimed at abolishing the use of animals in scientific research. His strategy was to persuade medical laboratories to voluntarily adopt standards for the humane treatment of animals used in research (Cannon 1909; Lederer 1995, 73). Five years later, when antivivisectionists campaigned against research on humans, Cannon's Council on the Defense of Research proposed a similar strategy. The AMA would promulgate principles of research ethics that would be enforced through a voluntary agreement by journal editors to require that all researchers "plainly state that the patient or his family were fully aware of and consented" to the experiment (AMA Committee on the Protection of Research 1914, 94; Lederer 1984, 391–97; 1995, 94–85).

In an editorial in the *Journal of the American Medical Association*, Cannon carefully distinguished experiments that might have value for patients from those whose primary value was to science. In both cases, he argued, it would be "a serious error," to conduct an experiment "without the consent of the person on whom it is tried." Such experiments violate the "fundamental right which any individual possesses . . . of controlling the uses to which his own body is put" (Cannon 1916, 1373).

Led by Simon Flexner (1863–1946), Director of Rockefeller Institute for Medical Research (founded in 1901) and editor of the *Journal of Experimental Medicine*, researchers subverted Cannon's efforts, forestalling a vote on Cannon's proposed principles of research ethics in the AMA's House of Delegates. Flexner's *Journal of Experimental Medicine* also scuttled efforts to require statements of informed consent as a precondition of publication in medical journals. During World War I, antivivisectionism lost public support and, as this external pressure declined, the movement to establish principles of research ethics lost impetus (Lederer 1995, 73–100).

VIII. BRITISH AND AMERICAN MEDICAL ETHICS, 1800–1945: A COMPARISON

By the end of the nineteenth century, American medicine had a fractured sense of medical morality. The AMA was propounding an ethics based loosely on Percivalean principles. Researchers and specialists rejected these principles, preferring instead an ethics of professional competence and honor. British medical morality had never fractured. Medical practitioners, sanitarians, specialists, and researchers all embraced common ideals of gentlemanly/professional honor (Porter 1995, 1553). They had little choice. The GMC could erase their names for any conduct considered "dishonorable." Yet, despite these differences, British and American medicine shared a common sense of professional misconduct. Practitioners were expelled from the AMA (Konold 1962) and affiliated societies (Baker 1995), for the same reasons they were expelled from the BMA (Morrice 2002), or had their names erased from the register by the GMC (Smith 1994). In both countries, practitioners were censured or expelled for the following reasons: abuse of alcohol or drugs; performing abortions; advertising, publishing testimonials for devices or remedies; soliciting patients; violating medical confidentiality; providing false certificates; claiming false qualifications; consulting or hiring unqualified, irregular, or sectarian practitioners or assistants; deprecating colleagues in public disputes; committing sexual offenses, or having intimate relations with patients; splitting fees; or extorting money from patients. They were also expelled for committing various crimes and misdemeanors ranging from petty larceny to murder to acts of bioterrorism (e.g., expelling an AMA member for "complicity with an attempt to poison the water of the Croton Reservoir, by which the city of New York is supplied with drinking water" (*Transactions of the American Medical Association* 1866, 16:35).

The AMA and BMA were similarly in accord in championing positive ideals of professional self-regulation against corporate, governmental, insurer, and trade union control – both supported major lobbying efforts against such initiatives as national health insurance. Moreover, unlike counterpart organizations in Germany and Scandinavia, neither the AMA nor the BMA supported state-sponsored eugenic initiatives such as the sterilization of those with mental disability. The U.S. Supreme Court may have ruled that "the principle that sustains compulsory vaccination is broad enough to cover cutting the Fallopian tubes" (*Buck v. Bell* 1927), but compulsory sterilization of patients with mental disability never obtained the moral imprimatur of the AMA and was declared unconstitutional in 1942 (*Skinner v. Oklahoma ex rel. Williamson* 1942).

Pre-1946 American and British medicine also shared another less laudable heritage: the racist and sexist proclivities of Anglo-American culture. Slavery had been legal in the British Empire until 1833. It was ended in the United States by Lincoln's Emancipation Proclamation of 1863 followed by the passage of the fourteenth amendment in 1866. Women were disenfranchised in Britain and in the United States until the second decade of the twentieth century. Full voting rights were not guaranteed to African Americans until the 1960s.

Denied full citizenship, black and women medical practitioners tended to acquire their medical expertise as irregulars. Prohibitions against consorting with irregulars thus served as a convenient cloak for the racist and sexist proclivities of medical men in the AMA and BMA. Black and women practitioners could not be admitted to the profession without a "regular" medical education. Despite walls of prejudice erected by educational institutions, some succeeded. The first African-American known to have acquired a medical degree from a regular medical college was James McCune Smith, who graduated from the University of Glasgow in 1837. In 1850, Harvard medical school admitted three African-American students, who were driven away by organized agitation and petitions by white medical students. In the same year, 1850, the single-sex Female Medical College of Pennsylvania (later the Woman's Medical College) was founded. In 1854 the Boston Medical Society, accepted as a member John V. DeGrasse (1825–1868), who had earned an M.D. from Bowdin College, becoming the first AMA-affiliated medical society to formally admit an African American.

The barriers against women were lowered in 1868 when the AMA's Committee on Ethics determined that gender was not grounds for exclusion from membership. Three years later, in 1871, on a vote of 83 to 26, the AMA House of Delegates admitted women to membership (Konold 1962, 23). In 1873, the BMA admitted its first woman member, Elizabeth Garrett Anderson (1836–1917) who was also the first British woman physician. The first female delegate to the AMA's national convention was Sarah Hackett Stevenson (1841–1909), Professor of Physiology and Histology at the Woman's Hospital Medical College, who attended the national convention in 1876 as a delegate from Illinois (*Transactions of the American Medical Association*. 1876, 27:66; Fishbein 1947, 91). She was made welcome at the AMA's national meeting by that year's president, J. Marion Sims who proclaimed, "if any woman [in] the medical profession makes such a reputation . . . as to be sent as a delegate . . . we are bound to receive her. And if any colored man should rise to the dignity of representing a [society] we must receive him as such" (Sims 1876, 93).

Despite Simms' words, the AMA was not accepting of "colored men" representing affiliated societies at national meetings. The issue had come to a head in national conventions from 1870 to 1873, during the reconstruction period in the aftermath of the American Civil War. In 1870 the AMA's national convention rejected the credentials of African-American representatives from the Freedman's Hospital of Washington D.C., the newly founded Howard Medical College (1868), and the National Medical Society of the District of Columbia. The nominal issue was the consultation clause prohibiting association with homeopaths and other irregular practitioners; however, because the same convention accepted the credentials of the Massachusetts medical society, which had also admitted homeopaths, the underlying issue was race. AMA President Nathan Smith Davis, a Northerner with strong Southern sympathies, strove to reunite the established all-white Southern medical societies into the AMA. Perhaps for that reason he became the leading opponent of recognizing the African-American delegates. Championing the admission of the African-American delegates was Alfred Stillé (1813–1900), a friend and ally of Hays, who had served on the committee that drafted the AMA's 1847 Code of Ethics. The African-American delegates were excluded on a roll call vote of 114 to 82. The issue was revisited in 1873 with similar results. In the face of continuing discrimination, African-American physicians founded alternative "mixed" or Negro state and local medical societies. A National Negro Medical Association was established in 1895.

Medical education remained separate and unequal through 1910, when there were seven negro medical schools and three women's medical schools. The Flexner report recommended coeducation for women, and quality but separate education for black men (Flexner 1910, 178–81). It thereby affirmed a pattern of institutional segregation for African-American physicians that persisted until the 1960s, when affirmative action and civil rights era litigation and laws turned organized medicine away from traditional patterns of gender and racial discrimination and segregation. A declaration of civil rights was

included in AMA's 1977 Principles of Medial Ethics (6.08). Nonetheless, discrimination against women and blacks lingered. It was not until the last decades of the century that the title, "doctor," was commonly associated with anyone other than a white male anywhere in the English-speaking world.

Although the regulars in the BMA and the AMA shared many common moral sensibilities – both were, for example, adamantly pro-life in the pre–World War II period, campaigning against abortion and against repeated initiatives to legalize euthanasia (Emanuel 1994, see Chapter 7) – differences in the legal frameworks of the two countries led them to express their values in different ways. Abortion at any stage of fetal development was a criminal offense in Britain from 1803 until 1967. Thus, when British practitioners declined to perform an abortion, when the CEC expelled an abortionist from the BMA, or when the GMC erased his name from the register, they were enforcing the law and ridding the profession of criminals. In contrast, for most of the nineteenth century, Americans, and American state laws, presumed that the fetus was *not* alive before quickening (i.e., the sensation of fetal movement, usually in the second trimester), and thus accepted first-trimester abortions as legitimate. U.S. law did not criminalize prequickening abortions until the 1870s. Before this, when American physicians declined to perform abortions they were acting on principles unsupported by either public opinion or by the law. Declining to perform an abortion thus meant loss of fees and, in all likelihood, loss of a fee-paying patient. It also cost the regulars marketshare because competitors, from homeopaths to midwives, openly advertised a willingness to perform abortions. The regulars' principled stance on prequickening abortion was thus uneconomic, impolitic, and unpopular (Mohr 1978).

Why, then, did American regulars oppose prequickening abortion? They did so, in part, as Percival's heirs. He had condemned "extinguish[ing] the first spark of life," as "a crime" (Percival, 1803, 79; Chap. IV, Sec. X; cited in Storer 1866a, 720; see Chapter 7). After the introduction of the stethoscope (1819), regular physicians could detect the heartbeat of a fetus well before quickening. In an era in which the heartbeat represented life, the stethoscope provided definitive evidence that quickening was not a valid indicator of human life. Hugh L. Hodge (1796–1873), Professor of Obstetrics at the University of Pennsylvania (1835–1863) and founding member of the AMA, lectured his medical students on their moral obligation to educate women on the "true" nature of prequickening abortion.

What, it may be asked, have the sensations of the mother to do with the vitality of the *child?* . . . Every practitioner of Obstetrics can bear witness that children live and move and thrive long before the mother is conscious of its existence. . . . how can a fetus be termed *inanimate* when it grows is nourished, and manifests all the phenomenon of life?... From the moment of conception it must be alive, for immediately it begins to be developed.... [In educating women about these facts] often, very often, must all the eloquence and all the authority of the practitioner be employed; often he must, as it were, grasp the conscience of his weak and erring patient, and let her know, in language not to be misunderstood, that she is responsible to her Creator for the life of the being within her... medical men, must be regarded as the guardians of the rights of *infants* [in utero as well as after birth] so that... criminal abortion be properly reprehended, and that women, in ever rank and condition of life may be sensible of the value of the embryo and ftus, and of the high responsibility which rests on the parents of every unborn infant. (Hodge [1839] 1964, Hodge 1872, emphasis added)

American obstetricians' antiabortion exhortations initially had little impact, except to alienate patients. By mid-nineteenth century, abortions were commonplace (Mohr 1978, 46–85). In 1857, on the recommendation of a Committee on Abortion organized and chaired by Boston physician Horatio Robinson Storer (1830–1922), the AMA's house of delegates decided to take action. It unanimously approved a resolution calling on medical societies to undertake an extensive lobbying campaign to criminalize prequickening abortion. Following up on this initiative, in 1864, the AMA declared that it would award a prize for the best "short and comprehensive tract, for circulation among females, for the purpose of enlightening them upon the criminality of physical evils of forced abortions" (Storer 1866a, 713). The award-winning essay, "The Criminality and Physical Evils of Forced Abortion," was written by Storer himself, and was immediately published as a popular pamphlet, *Why Not? A Book for Every Woman* (Storer 1866b).

Historian James Mohr credits Storer's committee, this pamphlet, and Storer's organization of "the vigorous efforts of American regular physicians" as "the single most important factor" leading to the criminalization of prequickening abortion throughout the United States (Mohr 1978, 157). Storer's pamphlet was influential because it was distributed during and after the civil war, when there was a felt need to "repopulate" a country devastated by fratricidal combat. It also changed the rhetoric of the antiabortion debate. Where Percival and Hodge emphasized the rights of the fetus, Storer focused on the impact of abortions on women's lives. He compiled data to show that abortion endangered women's lives and their health. "A larger proportion of women die during or in consequence of an abortion, than during or in consequence of childbed at the full term of pregnancy. A very large

proportion become confirmed invalids... The tendency towards serious, often fatal disease... is rendered much greater" (Storer 1866a, 724).

Persuaded by Storer's data, states criminalized prequickening abortion. Texas was one of the states in which Storer's data about the impact of abortion on maternal health formed part of the rationale for criminalizing abortion. Ironically, approximately a century later, in a landmark legal decision involving the Texas abortion law, *Roe v. Wade* (1973), the U.S. Supreme Court stood Storer's argument on its head. In striking down criminal abortion laws, the court held that since there was greater risk to a woman's health if she carried a fetus to full term than if she had a first or second trimester abortion, the state's interest in protecting maternal health, combined with a woman's right to privacy in her own body, outweighed the state's interest in protecting potential human life for a previable fetus (See Chapters 7 and 47; Dyer 1999; Luker 1984; Mohr 1978; Reagan 1997).

Differences in the legal-regulatory environment also affected the BMA's and AMA's stance on matters as seemingly different as their attitudes toward alternative medicine and confidentiality. Regulars in both countries disdained the former and embraced the latter. In both countries, sectarian schools offered a comprehensive alternative to regular medicine. Founded by charismatic figures, like Samuel Hahneman (1755–1843) or Samuel Thomson (1769–1843), alternative medicine distinguished itself by offering an astute critique of regular medicine and an alternative conception of illness and its treatment (Bynum and Porter 1987; Wolpe 1999). Leading regulars accepted the validity of sectarian critiques. "If the whole *materia medica*, as now used, could be sunk to the sea" Oliver Wendell Holmes, Sr. (1809–1894) observed, acknowledging the homeopathic critique of the regulars, "it would be all be better for mankind, and all the worst for the fishes" (Holmes 1891, 203). Nonetheless, Holmes and other leading regulars rejected sectarian medicine as resting on the unscientific ideas of charismatic founders, rather than on the cumulative, incremental findings of empirical science.

Although the leaders of both the AMA and the BMA defended orthodox medicine, attitudes toward homeopaths and other alternative practitioners differed. The British profession, secure in the knowledge that the Medical Act of 1858 had legally defined alternative schools as irregular, was relaxed about policing professional boundaries. The issue never became the focal point of organizational politics, as it did for the AMA. For the British, consultation with homeopaths was laughably "useless" not a heresy (Morrice 2002, 23). Lacking any privileging legal status, American medical practitioners zealously policed the boundaries of their profession, embracing a reactive conservative medical orthodoxy. Thus instead of rejecting homeopaths' condemnation of conventional therapy as "allopathic," that is, as designed to counter symptoms rather than underlying pathology, regulars embraced both the label "allopath" and the harmful therapies properly criticized by homeopaths. In 1864, for example, an AMA committee censured the Surgeon General of the U.S. Army "for a most grievous offence against the dignity, usefulness, and humanity of our profession." The "insult?" Removing calomel (mercury chloride) from the supply table of the army. In an evidence-based study, the Army had found that "medical pathology has proved the impropriety of the use of mercury." Holmes and other leaders lampooned the AMA's position, but it serves to underline the destructively conservative stance regular practitioners often took in their struggles with homeopathy (Report of Committee on Order No. 6 of the Surgeon General, 29–32; Holmes [1882, 1891] 2001; see Warner 1999; Wolpe 1999).

Differences in the laws of the two countries also affected their interpretation of traditional ethical precepts such as confidentiality. All major nineteenth-century Anglo-American codifications of medical morality contained confidentiality clauses (Percival 1803, Chap. I, Art. VI; AMA [1847] 1999; Chap. I Art. 1 Sec. 2; Styrap 1878, Chap. 1, Sec. 1, Rule 2; American Institute of Homeopathy 1888, Chap. I, Art. II, Sec. 4). Styrap's proposed BMA Code, however, waives "secrecy... under... very exceptional circumstances – as, for instance... pertinacious concealment of pregnancy after seduction, in which it would probably be the practitioner's duty to communicate his fears to a near relative of the patient" (Styrap 1878, Chap. 1 Sec.1, Rule 2). The BMA was itself divided on the nature of physicians' duties of confidentiality in cases of abortion, adultery, divorce, illegitimate pregnancy, and sexually transmitted diseases. Because a divided medical profession could not effectively assert a claim to privilege in law, British law recognized only a weak presumptive, easily overridden, right to confidentiality (Morrice 2002, 26). As late as 1971, the GMC supported a British physician who had disclosed to her parents a 16-year-old patient's request for contraceptives (GMC 1971, 79–80; Veatch 1981 141–3). In contrast, even the AMA's 1903 Principles – one of the low points in American professional self-regulation – state that "Secrecy [is] to Be Inviolate... except when [disclosure is] imperatively required by the laws of the state" (AMA [1903] 1999, Chap. I, Sec. 3). American state and federal law have tended to accommodate the AMA's unwavering insistence on a strong presumption of confidentiality.

These differences aside, however, until the mid-twentieth century, the unwritten medical morality of British regular practitioners and the formalized medical ethics of American regular practitioners were remarkably similar. Both shared the racial and gender biases of their societies and both embraced paternalistic pro-life moralities committed to an ideal of professionalism and

opposed to state or corporate control of medicine. In both countries, regulars prohibited advertising, abortion, and a variety of lesser offenses, and in neither country did professional medical ethics address the ethics of research on human subjects. This would change later in the twentieth century.

IX. British and American Medical Ethics 1946–2000

Between 1946 and 1948 events in four cities – Nuremberg, London, Chicago, and New York – changed the nature of Anglo-American medical ethics. In Nuremberg, American and British prosecutors tried German doctors and medical researchers for "war crimes and crimes against humanity." In New York, a committee chaired by Eleanor Roosevelt (1884–1962), scandalized by reports emanating from the Nuremberg trials, began to fashion the Universal Declaration of Human Rights (Baker 2001). In London, a BMA-sponsored conference convened to found a World Medical Association (WMA), conferees became preoccupied with the Nuremberg Trials. The WMA condemned Nazi era German researchers for "ignor[ing] the sanctity and importance of human life, exploiting human beings both as individuals and in mass ... betray[ing] the trust society had placed in them as a profession ... The care of the individual patient ceased to be the doctor's primary aim and the humanitarian purpose of medical science was subordinated to the needs of war" (WMA [1949] 1995, 1:7).

In Chicago, Andrew C. Ivy (1893–1978), scientific director of the Naval Medical Research Institute at Bethesda, Maryland and AMA observer at the Nuremberg trials, urged the AMA to adopt principles of research ethics that differentiated legitimate medical research from unethical (i.e., Nazi) research. Legitimate research on human subjects, Ivy argued, requires scientific validity, prior animal experimentation to establish that "the experiment [will] yield results for the good of society unprocurable by other means of study." Legitimacy also requires the "consent of the subject," who has "been informed of the hazards if any." Experiments, moreover, should be conducted by qualified researchers who "avoid all unnecessary suffering and injury," and who have "no *a priori* reason to believe that death or disabling injury will occur, except in such experiments, as those on Yellow Fever," where the experimenters served as subjects (Ivy 1946, 10).

In 1946, the AMA's House of Delegates adopted a version of Ivy's principles requiring the voluntary consent, prior animal experimentation, and proper medical supervision. These principles of research ethics – the first promulgated by any official body in the United States or Britain – were weaker than those proposed by Ivy. They did not require that the research subject's consent be informed, or that experiments be "for the good of society," or that they yield information "unprocurable by other means," or that they preclude the likelihood of unnecessary suffering, disability, or death.

Having secured the AMA's endorsement of some principles of research ethics, Ivy testified that the AMA principles formalized standards used in his own laboratory, in pre–Nazi Germany, and by "civilized" researchers everywhere. Although, as historians were later to point out, the claim that all civilized researchers accepted the precepts underlying the AMA principles stretched the truth to the breaking point, the Nuremberg Tribunal accepted Ivy's expert testimony as accurate (Harkness 1996a, 1998, Marrus 1999; Weindling 2001). On the advice of Colonel Leopold (Leo) Alexander (1905–1985), an expatriate Austrian-Jewish neurologist who served as war crimes investigator and advisor to the U.S. Secretary of War, the prosecution fleshed out Ivy's bare-bones principles. In its final judgment, the Nuremberg Tribunal, offering ten "basic principles" – later known as "the Nuremberg Code" – to justify condemning the Nazi researchers. The Nuremberg Code thus joined the AMA's principlist conception of medical ethics, to the nuanced detail provided by Alexander, and Ivy's ideal of basic universal civilized standards of ethical research. (See Chapters 34, 49, 50, 51, and 54; Alexander 1949a, 1949b; Annas and Grodin 1992, Baker 1998a, 1998b; Grodin 1992; Schmidt 2004. For a detailed analysis of the sources of each of the ten principles, see Weindling 2004, 357–8.)

Before 1945, there were no internationally recognized standards of research ethics and few formal research regulations of any kind. Within 3 years, horror at the Holocaust and the need to relegitimate medical research on human subjects had led to the creation of three differently conceived standards of research ethics: Principles issued by professional societies (the 1946 AMA Principles); universally agreed basic or fundamental principles (1947 Nuremberg Code); and human rights (1948 UN Declaration of Human Rights). Ironically, although all of these conceptions originated, in whole or in part, in Britain or American, *none* found their way into nonmilitary Anglo-American medical ethics until *after* it became embarrassingly evident that British and American researchers had conducted flagrantly unethical experiments on human subjects (see Chapters 49–51).

In the immediate postwar era the AMA and the BMA paid little attention to medical ethics, focusing instead on resisting national health insurance initiatives. The AMA was successful until 1965 and, even in defeat, succeeded in limiting national health insurance to seniors (Medicare) and the poor (Medicaid) – leaving a robust demographic of nonpoor adults and children for private medicine. The BMA was less successful. A National Health Service (NHS) was instituted in Britain in 1948. The establishment of the NHS reinforced the British proclivity to look to law and to the GMC to enforce professional standards. The

concept of medical ethics seemed otiose. Thus differences in cultural attitudes toward the relevance of medical ethics in Britain and American were exacerbated. The nature of these differences became evident in the responses to the research scandals that erupted in both countries in the mid-1960s.

Both the UK and the United States increased funding for medical research in the postwar era. Demand for human subjects increased concomitantly (Rothman 1991). Disdaining all codified forms of ethical constraint as necessary for Nazis, but unnecessary for civilized researchers – who would naturally conduct themselves honorably – researchers in both countries refused to acknowledge the Nuremberg Code. The AMA even forgot its own Principles of Research ethics, failing to incorporate them into a 1949 publication of its *Principles of Medical Ethics* (Beecher 1970, 221–2) or into its 1957 revised *Principles of Medical Ethics* (AMA 1957).

In both countries, however, researchers' ethics of honor proved insufficient to prevent abuses of human subjects, and, in both countries, whistle blowers ultimately called professional and public attention to this scandalous state of affairs. The two primary whistle blowers had served in the military medical corps of their respective countries; otherwise they were quite different. The British whistle blower, Maurice Pappworth (1910–1994), was the proverbial outsider. Denied an appointment as a hospital consultant in 1939 because "no Jew could ever be a gentleman" (Booth 1994) and denied membership in the Royal College of Physicians, Pappworth made a living tutoring those applying for positions denied to him. His first tutee was given the very hospital consultancy he had been denied. In contrast, Henry Knowles Beecher of Harvard Medical School (nee Harry Unangst, 1904–1976) was a consummate insider. A self-made gentleman who embraced the ethics of gentlemanly honor, he resisted the imposition of the Nuremberg Code on fellow researchers (Baker 1998, 253–5). Discovering that his fellow researchers were not acting honorably, however, Beecher informed the profession. From 1962 to 1970, Beecher and Pappworth publicized cases of abusive research in major hospitals and institutions (including NHS hospitals), conducted by leading researchers, funded by prestigious sources, and published in leading medical journals (Beecher 1966, 1970; Edelson 2000; Hazelgrove 2002; Pappworth 1967; Rothman 1991).

The medical professions of both countries reacted to the scandals as one does to any trauma: denial, anger, negotiation, and, ultimately, reluctant acceptance. Acceptance required new measures to regulate research. The way in which the new research regulations were conceived and enforced differed significantly in the two countries. In Britain, the national government controlled major sources of research funding through the Medical Research Council (MRC); it controlled licensing through the GMC; it controlled access to human subjects through the NHS. It was thus natural for the British to exert control administratively through these quasi-nongovernmental organizations (MRC 1963, Beecher 1970, 262) – although the BMA also issued research guidelines (BMA 1963; Beecher 1970, 268). An administrative-regulative model was thus cobbled together to resolve the problems of research ethics. This model, in turn, became the dominant British paradigm for addressing the biomedical problems that, in the United States, came to be conceived under the rubric "bioethics" (see Chapter 61). Through the end of the twentieth century medical ethics in Britain tended to be conceptualized in terms of an ethos of honor and a discourse of "the done thing," which was to be informed and enforced through governmental-administrative-regulatory model. Bioethical concepts and discourse, in contrast, tend to be marginalized as "Americanisms" (cf. Chapters 38 and 39).

X. The Bioethics Revolution: American Medical Ethics 1970–2000

America lacked Britain's institutional resources. It had no NHS to control access to patients. Despite the growing influence of the National Institutes of Health (founded 1930) in the 1970s the U.S. government had no mechanism comparable to the MRC through which it could authoritatively assert control over research, or even over research funding. Federal laws regulating research, moreover, would have been unprecedented. Self-regulatory codes might have been appropriate mechanisms of control, but America's principal code-issuing professional body, the AMA, had a history of ignoring principles of research ethics. Moreover, in 1957, on the 110th anniversary of adoption of its Code of Ethics, the AMA had adopted a new format for its code – articulation of a few basic principles (originally ten), supplemented by extensive commentary and advisory rulings on specific subjects (AMA [1957] 1999). In the process, the AMA virtually abdicated its regulatory responsibilities.

Before analyzing these code revisions, it is worth noting that in 1957, on its 110th anniversary, the AMA stood at the apex of its power. The AMA represented medicine to the public, to the press, to politicians, and to the medical profession itself. When the AMA reparsed the Principles, it spoke as the authoritative voice of the profession. This voice, however, proclaimed the Principles merely "standards by which a physician may determine the propriety of his conduct" (AMA [1957] 1999, 355–6). The expressions – "a physician," "his conduct" and the all too permissive, "may" – are personal, solipsistic, and, to reiterate, permissive. The wording is not inconsequential. The 1912 Principles assert the profession's *right* to regulate individual conduct, stating a physician's "obligation to conduct himself in accord with [*the profession's*] ideals;" in contrast, the 1957 Principles, merely affirm that

"Physicians should merit the confidence of patients." No mention is made of an obligation to conduct ones self in accordance with the profession's ideals of good conduct. The prerogative of interpreting professional standards had been deeded to each individual physician's own moral sensibilities.

The moral sensibilities of researchers were informed by an entrenched ethics of professional competence and honor that immunized them against feelings of shame or guilt with respect to issues considered secondary to the "research imperative" of improving medical science (Callahan 2003). True to their birthright, researchers and specialists rejected all suggestions about professional codes of research ethics and berated any notion of government regulation (Jonsen 1998, 90–8; Rothman 1991, 171–82).

The case of Sloan-Kettering researcher, Chester Southam, is illustrative. Southam's license to practice medicine had been suspended by New York State in 1965 because he had injected live cancers cells into thousands of patients *without informing them*. Nonetheless, in 1966, when the results of these experiments resulted in meaningful advances in understanding the nature of cancer, Southam was elected Vice-President, and, in 1967, President, of the American Association for Cancer Research (Katz 1972, 64–5). Research professionals saw nothing wrong with honoring research professionals whose work had been officially condemned as unethical.

The situation cried out for a new constellation of social controls and a new ethical paradigm strong enough to override the accepted ethos of professional competence, honor, and the research imperative. These controls and their justificatory paradigm emerged from an unlikely amalgam of bureaucrats, dissident intelligentsia, and concerned professionals. The alliance was forged in the 1960s and 1970s in the context of social ferment over civil rights, the Vietnam War, woman's rights, and other issues of social justice. A small group of intellectuals moved from protest politics to government commissions and hospital ethics committees (see, for example, Baker 2002b, Loewy 2002; Veatch 2002). Marshalling these forces were two "think tanks" founded by liberal Catholic intellectuals: The Hastings Center (founded in 1969 as the Institute for Society, Ethics and the Life Sciences in Hastings-on Hudson, New York) and the Kennedy Institute of Ethics (founded in 1971 as The Joseph and Rose Kennedy Center for the Study of Human Reproduction and Bioethics) at Georgetown University. Cofounding the former was Daniel Callahan, executive editor of the lay Roman Catholic journal, *Commonweal*, from 1961 to 1968; founding the latter was an Edinburgh University – educated Dutch Roman Catholic scientist André Hellegers (1911–1979), nicknamed "The Pope's Biologist." America's leading Roman Catholic family provided initial funding for The Kennedy Institute (Walters, 2003; Jonsen 1998, 22–24).

Like Jews and Blacks, before the Presidency of John F. Kennedy (1961–1963), Roman Catholics had been excluded from the mainstream of American social and political life. When, for example, Edmund Pellegrino (Director of the Kennedy Institute of Ethics, 1983–1988) applied to medical school "a letter from one Ivy League school complemented... his grades but declined his application stating that he would be 'happier with his own kind.'" Pellegrino's academic advisor told the young man that "Italians... were no more welcome than Jews in the major medical schools, and he might fare better if he changed his name. Pellegrino refused" (Geraghty, 2001). Like the nineteenth-century dissenters who created modern medical ethics, twentieth-century American Roman Catholics drew on their experience as a religious minority to critique the powerful in the name of the powerless – extending that critique to encompass the rights of patients and research subjects.

Although founded and often funded by Roman Catholics, the new bioethics think tanks catalyzed a dialogue among health care professionals, lawyers, philosophers, scientists, social scientists, and theologians from a variety of religions on such subjects as abortion, contraception, population growth, genetics, new biomedical technologies, and research on human subjects. This outreach effort was partially inspired and catalyzed by the theological ferment associated with Vatican Council II (1962–1965), which promoted an ecumenical dialogue between Catholics and theologians of other faiths about many subjects, including developments in biomedicine that became the substantive content of the new field of bioethics (Curran 2003).

As this interdisciplinary group engaged in a dialogue about biomedical subjects, they developed a multidisciplinary pidgin that began to coalesce into a discourse amalgamating concepts drawn from law, medicine, philosophy, social science, and theology with argumentative strategies drawn from analytic philosophy. This discourse became more public in the 1970s as it was disseminated in a literature indexed in the *Bibliography of Bioethics* (founded 1975 and edited by LeRoy Walters of the Kennedy Institute, Walters 2003), and encapsulated in *The Encyclopedia of Bioethics* (Reich 1978, 1995a) edited by Warren Reich (Reich 2003) of the Kennedy Institute of Ethics.

The discourse and conceptual frameworks of the newly emerging field of bioethics entered the public domain through well-publicized legal cases (such as the Karen Ann Quinlan case (*In re Quinlan* 1976) and through government reports issued by The National Commission for the Protection of Human Subject of Biomedical and Behavioral Research (1974–1978). In 1978, as it was ending its work, having drafted what evolved into the "common rule" regulating research involving human subjects conducted or funded by any U.S. government agency, the National Commission issued the *Belmont Report*. The *Report* stated that research on human subjects needed to be justified in terms of three "basic ethical principles.... respect for persons, beneficence, and justice" (National Commission 1978).

Commission reports generally serve as verbiage in which proposals are packaged in the process of becoming regulations. Like all packaging, they tend to be discarded after the goods have been delivered. The *Belmont Report* was unusual. It stated principles for regulatory proposals that had already been acted upon. On any "realistic" assessment, it should have been consigned to the dustbin of history. Instead, it became a seminal document for American research ethics.

To appreciate the significance of the *Belmont Report*, it is helpful to recall that for over 150 years no proposal or regulation had been able to hobble the research imperative. Ryan's proposal for obtaining the informed consent of research subjects had been dismissed as a "worthless subject" in *The Lancet* in 1831. Cannon's 1914–1916 informed consent initiatives were ignored or subverted. Ivy's 1946 proposals had been weakening and discarded. The Nuremberg Code was dismissed in the 1950s and 1960s, as were condemnations and regulatory initiatives throughout the 1960s and 1970s. The history of Anglo-American research ethics had been a cycle of scandal-induced regulatory initiatives temporarily embraced – only to be subverted or discarded as memories of scandal grew fainter.

Earlier reforms can be characterized as "naked norms," that is, regulations, moral precepts, or laws bereft of any comprehensive readily internalized justificatory framework. Without some guiding justificatory framework, the interpretation, specification, or application of naked norms tends to be legalistic, and is often perceived by researchers as arbitrary and capricious. More importantly, naked norms fail to be internalized and thus cannot be enforced by appeals to personal integrity, pride, peer pressure, guilt, or shame. Enforcement is external and dependent on such mechanisms as loss of privileges, fines, or other punishments. Absent internalization, it is all too easy for researchers to dismiss naked norms as unwarranted and intrusive assertions of power, as happened in the Southam case.

Research ethics reformers had never fashioned a robust conception of research ethics that encapsulated a *rationale* for treating certain forms of research as *unethical*. The three Belmont principles responded to this challenge. The principle of beneficence legitimated the research imperative, even as it required researchers to weigh the potential benefits of their research against the risks of harm to subjects and society. Tempering the principle of beneficence was the principle of respect for persons, which, for the first time, provided a readily grasped theoretical foundation for informed consent regulations. The third Belmont principle, justice, legitimated rules governing the selection of research subjects. This triad of principles forced researchers and research review committees (reconstituted as Institutional Review Boards, or "IRBs" in the United States) to reconceptualize experiments like Southam's as morally problematic, *not* because they circumvented some technicality about consent, but because, not informing subjects that they were being used as subjects, failed to give them the respect due them as persons. Even someone blinded by the research imperative could still recognize that it was wrong to be disrespectful of persons. (This account draws on staff member Tom Beauchamp's recollection of his discussions with Staff Director Michael Yesley; Beauchamp 2003, 21.)

The *Belmont Report's* influence was amplified significantly by the near simultaneous publication of *The Principles of Biomedical Ethics* by the philosopher-religious-studies-scholar team of Tom Beauchamp and James Childress (Beauchamp and Childress 1979). The *Principles* grew out of Beauchamp and Childress' collaboration in the Kennedy Institute of Ethics' Intensive Bioethics Course. As they explain in a 1976 prospectus to Oxford University Press, this "basic textbook in biomedical ethics . . . rather than [using the standard format of] presenting biomedical ethics as a series of topical problems," would use "principles to resolve moral problems that arise in cases," and then use "the cases, in turn" to "test the adequacy of principles" (Childress 2003, 48–9).

Deceptively similar to the Belmont principles, Beauchamp and Childress' principles number four: the principles of respect for autonomy (self-determination), beneficence, nonmaleficence (i.e., not harming), and justice. The significance of these principles lies not in their number or in their nuanced differences with the Belmont principles, but in their unifying conception. They apply to both clinical ethics *and* to research ethics. The principle of respect for autonomy thus offsets the principle of beneficence in the clinic and in doctors' offices, just as it does in the research laboratory. One-and-the-same principle thus applied to researchers like Southam and to Karen Ann Quinlan's physicians. Both were condemnable as "paternalists," that is, as those who presumed to impose their conception of beneficence on others, impermissibly overriding a person's own right to self-determination.

Textbooks are the overlooked arbitrators of what we believe we know. They are the primary vehicles for disseminating theories of all sorts. The textbook format of Beauchamp and Childress's *Principles* made it an excellent vehicle for disseminating the new bioethics discourse, as well as their own revolutionary new paradigm for understanding and analyzing issues in biomedicine. Easily and often conflated into a single view, "principlism," the Beauchamp and Childress/Belmont principles – and its attendant bioethics discourse and critique of paternalism – became the standard discourse employed to justify and legitimate a new regulatory infrastructure in

clinical and research ethics, and a new field of expertise – bioethics. The new regulatory infrastructure of hospital ethics committees and IRBs was recognized and encouraged by United States state courts (after *Quinlan*), by state legislatures, by funding bodies (the National Endowment for the Humanities, the NIH, the National Science Foundation, the Rockefeller Foundation) and by accrediting organizations (the Joint Commission on Accreditation of Healthcare Organizations) as mechanisms for assuring professional accountability. Lacking a centralized source of governmental authority over medical scientists and clinical medicine, American society had turned to a coalition of nonprofessional administrative and intellectual forces – bioethicists – to assert public accountability, in the laboratory, in the clinic, and in the public policy arena.

Just as the ascendancy of Percival's discourse of professional medical ethics tracked the advances of the medical ethics revolution, the ascendancy of bioethics discourse tracked the increasing acceptance of bioethics in America. A study of more than 52,000 articles and books on "genetic intervention, gene pool, gene therapy, or germ cells" by sociologist John Evans demonstrates that between 1959 and 1995 bioethical discourse had supplanted the originally dominant discourses of theology and science in discussions of ethics and public policy on these areas (Evans 2001). The dominance of the bioethics paradigm was firmly established in June of 1990, when the AMA supplemented its physician-oriented principles with a statement of patient's rights, the *Fundamental Elements of the Patient-Physician Relationship*. The *Fundamentals* open with an endorsement of the bioethical vision of medical decision making as a "collaborative effort between physician and patient" in which physicians "serve as their patients' advocates . . . by fostering [the following five] rights:" information, treatment refusal, respect and dignity, confidentiality, continuity of care, and the advocacy of her/his physician to ensure adequacy of care (AMA [1990] 1995, 360–61). Four years later, the AMA again endorsed the bioethics paradigm by invoking the principle of respect for autonomy as *the reason* for recognizing a patient's right to refuse life-sustaining treatments: "The principle of patient autonomy requires that physicians should respect the decision to forego life-sustaining treatment who possesses decision-making capacity" (AMA 1999, 2.20).

In the period between 1970 and 1990, American medical morality underwent a revolutionary transformation, a bioethics revolution that was similar in its impact to the earlier Percivalean medical ethics revolution of 1808 to 1848. In both cases, a new conception of ethics – expressed in a new, ultimately dominant, discourse – displaced an older conception, legitimizing new institutions and new configurations of power. Ironically, by embracing the bioethics revolution, the AMA had actually returned to a position that, in many ways, is close to its own Percivalean roots. (For a detailed discussion of the bioethics revolution see Chapter 38.)

XI. CONCLUSION

The history of nineteenth- and twentieth-century Anglo-American medical ethics can be told as a tale of moral ideals articulated by semiempowered spokespersons of disempowered groups – Dissenters, Jews, Roman Catholics – empathizing with others still more powerless. It can also be told as a tale of discrimination, exploitation, scandal, reform, revolution, and counter-revolution; or, as a tale of weak and ineffectual constraints hypocritically embraced for self-serving reasons, only to be abandoned whenever they proved inconvenient. Then again, it can be constructed as a tale of ultimately triumphant efforts to develop sophisticated mechanisms of ethical control, a tale of moral progress, complete with villains and heroes. Or it can be constructed as a tale of two cultures, sharing a common heritage, finding different, but parallel and equally effective solutions to problems created as medicine was transformed from a gentlemanly pursuit to a formal, ever more scientific profession, practiced in increasingly more complex institutions. However one constructs the tale, the ending remains open.

CHAPTER 37

THE DISCOURSES OF PRACTITIONERS IN THE MODERN AND CONTEMPORARY ISLAMIC MIDDLE EAST

Vardit Rispler-Chaim

I. INTRODUCTION

The Middle East is a variegated area of the world in its nationalities, religious groups, ethnicities, political regimes, and social structures. These are only a few of the elements responsible for the area's complex yet pivotal role in world history from ancient times to the present.

The religion of Islam, which originated in Mecca (in modern Saudi Arabia) at the end of the sixth century, is the most prevalent religion in the Middle East in terms of the number of its followers, the Muslims (see also Chapters 8, 17, and 25). Despite some significant diversity of ideological inclinations and theological perceptions among Muslims, several dogmatic elements, legal doctrines, and ethical boundaries can be seen as common denominators uniting Muslims all over the world. This chapter deals with common denominators in the wide field of Islamic medical ethics, especially those emanating from Middle Eastern contemporary Islamic sources and literature.

II. THE LITERATURE AND OTHER CHANNELS THROUGH WHICH ETHICS TRAVELS

The contemporary literature on medical ethics in Islam is for the most part written in Arabic. This literature has been accumulating since the second half of the twentieth century and has become abundant since the last decade of that century. Interest in medical subjects such as bedside manner, the role of the physicians in society and vis-à-vis their patients, pharmacology, and so forth, has been manifested through philosophical and legal books and treatises and in scientific professional manuals throughout the fourteen centuries of Islamic history (Ridwan 1984; Ullmann 1978). The current preoccupation with modern medical ethical dilemmas was forced upon Muslim ethicists, just as it has been forced on other religious and "secular" ethicists, by the rapid changes that medical knowledge and techniques have undergone, and by the efficient media vehicles that rapidly spread news about such advances.

Today only a few books are dedicated entirely to medical ethics in the Islamic world (Ghanem 1982; Ebrahim 1989; Krawietz 1991; Rispler-Chaim 1993; Al-Daqr 1997). Contemporary Islamic medical ethics, however, is typically conveyed in the form of an individual fatwa (judicial opinion) issued by a mufti (juris consult). A fatwa is usually issued in response to a supposedly real but sometimes hypothetical question addressed to the mufti by a Muslim man or woman, or by some governmental agency or officer. The fatwa provides the mufti the opportunity to state his (muftis are all male) learned opinion, and sometimes the regime's preferred policy on a given topic (Masud, Messick, and Powers 1996, 26–32).

There are many muftis but there is no central or chief mufti who can speak for the entire Islamic world. Muftis have undertaken many years of religious and legal training, and their fatwas are always predicated upon some of the venerated sources of Islamic law, such as the Qur'an and Prophetic Tradition (*Sunna*) or the legal scholarship of Muslim jurists embodied in the *fiqh* literature (Islamic law), which has ripened since the eighth century when Islamic law was created. In the face of modern dilemmas, the classical Islamic legal tools often prove insufficient, so muftis resort to the medical literature, or consult Muslim physicians, or simply appeal to common sense.

Fatwas vary in size and in the depth of the legal reasoning employed, depending on such factors as the personality and the political affiliation of the mufti, the nature of the prospective audience or readership, and the type of publication in which the fatwa appears. Most of the "medical" fatwas in recent years have been published either in fatwa collections associated with a particular mufti, for example, Shaltut (1966), ʿAbd al-Halim Mahmud (1986), Hasanayn Muhammad Makhluf (1952), Al-Shaʿrawi (1981), Yusuf al-Qaradawi (1987), and ʿAbd al-Aziz ibn Baz (1988), or with a council of muftis working under the auspices of one governmental body, such as Wizarat al-awqaf (the Ministry of Endowments) in Egypt. This ministry publishes annually a collection of fatwas by various muftis under the title *Al-Fatawa Al-Islamiyya*. Lajnat al-Fatawa (the Committee of Fatwas) attached to Al-Azhar Institute of Islamic scholarship and research in Egypt often publishes its fatwas in the periodical *Majallat al-Azhar*. Hayʾat Kibar al-Ulamaa (The Council of Greatest Religious Scholars) in Saudi Arabia is responsible for the multivolume collection *Majallat Al-Buhuth al-Islamiyya*. Many fatwas are first published in daily newspapers and in periodicals, as answers to questions from the public, before they are collected and published in book form. In recent years muftis have utilized the availability of radio and television to spread the message of their fatwas to illiterate populations and remote regions with limited or no access to printed material. The Internet has been employed, too, but is accessible only by the affluent and the educated. The written word, however, remains the primary vehicle for the dissemination and the "canonization" of medical ethics in the Islamic Middle East. This chapter draws mainly on these written sources.

III. The Main Muftis

A mufti's religious position, the nature of his relationship with the political regime, his personality, and his charisma are crucial for assessing the influence of his fatwas on medical ethics. In the Islamic Middle East, the muftis whose authority is most respected, and whose opinions are often sought or cited, are mainly, although not exclusively, from or associated with Egypt or Saudi Arabia, the two major centers of scholarship. Even muftis who reside in the same geographic zone, who belong to the same religious institute, and who are active at approximately the same time sometimes offer diverse opinions. This diversity mirrors the changing circumstances in the dynamics of medical science, different political trends, and the relative freedom of legal reasoning in Islam, especially when the classical sources of Islamic law on a given subject are silent.

The following are the leading muftis in the formulation of Islamic medical ethics in recent decades: Muhammad Rashid Rida (1865–1935), Hasanayn Muhammad Makhluf (1890–1990), Mahmud Shaltut (1893–1963), Abd Al-Halim Mahmud (1910–1978), ʿAbd Al-Aziz Ibn Baz (1912–1999), Yusuf Al-Qaradawi (1926–), Muhammad Mutawalli Al-Shaʾrawi (1911–1998), Jad Al-Haqq Ali Jad Al-Haqq (1917–1997), Muhammad Sayyid Tantawi (1928–), Mustafa Al-Zarqaʾ (1904–1998), Muhammad b. Salih Al-Uthaymin (1926–2001), and ʿAbd Allah b. Jibrin (1930–).

Many more muftis participate in the endeavor of issuing fatwas on an occasional basis. Their fatwas may be found from time to time in daily newspapers and periodicals published in various Arab states and even in collections carrying their names (Mannaʾ, al-Zarqaʾ, Kishk, and more). The muftis listed above are certainly well known and are held in high repute by Muslims all over the world as authorities on legal issues. They do not, however, always speak with one voice.

IV. Major Topics Covered

1. Abortion and Contraception

The most discussed medical ethical topics in the fatwas are abortion, family planning, and birth control (see also Chapter 8). Many lengthy fatwas exist on whether birth rates should be determined through medical intervention or left to divine guidance (*Al-Fatawa al-Islamiyya*, 7:2573–4; Shaltut 1966, 293–7; Al-Shaʾrawi 1981; Samiullah 1983, 5/7:15–19; Mahmud 1986, 2:284–5; Jad al-Haqq 29 Dec. 1980, 11 Feb. 1979; Al-ʾUthaymin 1995, 2:657–9; Tantawi 1996, 13; Mahmood 1977; Saqr 1996; Hayʾat Kibar al-Ulamaa 1994).

All legal attitudes toward abortion stem from the Islamic theory of embryology, according to which the fetus goes first through three stages of growth of 40 days each. Only at the end of this 120-day period does ensoulment take place. From the moment of ensoulment, the fetus is viewed as a whole human being entitled to legal rights (see Chapter 8). This renders the first 120 days of its life (approximately 4 months) a period in which the fetus is defined as a "potential human being" (*insan bil-quwwa*) not an "actual human being" (*insan bil-fiʾl*). Abortion may therefore be legitimized with relative ease during the first 120 days of pregnancy, if it is desired for certain justified reasons.

The living pregnant woman always has priority over the yet unborn. Thus, when the fetus endangers the pregnant woman's health, she always has a valid a reason to abort it, even beyond the 120-day limit. Living children also have priority. So, if the pregnant woman is still breast-feeding an infant from a recently completed pregnancy and the new pregnancy might spoil the taste of her milk, abortion of the fetus is permitted so as to save the living baby's source of nourishment, of survival. Abortion could be avoided, however, if the father could afford to hire a wet-nurse for the baby, to provide mother's milk for the baby instead of its biological mother's. Even with the existence of synthetic mother's milk products today, the principle of priority of the living over the unborn is sometimes evoked and a pregnancy may be terminated with the aim of ensuring a baby the 2 years of nursing, or the intimacy with its mother if not nursing, as inscribed in Qur'an (2, 233).

Among the other reasons that may justify abortion are the following: poor economic conditions of the parents, who may be unable to feed a larger number of mouths; the deteriorating mental health of the bread-winner in the family, who dreads the arrival of another child; a fetus diagnosed with a genetic disorder; and a fetus produced by rape or fornication. These rationales for abortion are still subjects of debate among the legal scholars, some of whom argue that the welfare of the family or any of its members should not take precedence over the prohibition against killing innocent life. Most muftis have determined that abortion should not be seen as a means of contraception. Legitimate killings in Islamic law are always viewed as punishment for certain grave crimes committed by a legally responsible adult Muslim. Yet, a fetus cannot be accused of a crime for which it deserves the death sentence. Other means of contraception are permitted under Islamic law so as to space pregnancies when both spouses agree, and especially to maintain the 2 years of "breast-feeding" as recommended by the Qur'an.

2. Family Planning

On the issue of family planning most muftis hold that birth control, if it means placing a limit through strict state laws on the number of children a couple may bear, is non-Islamic (al-Zarqa' 1999, 287–8), because it betrays the Divine wisdom that devised reproductive organs in males and females to bring to life more believers. Thus, while family planning (*tanzim al-nasl*) in the sense of spacing pregnancies, with or without contraceptives, is encouraged, birth control per se (*tahdid al-nasl*) is totally rejected. The use of contraceptives, as mentioned, is permitted by most muftis in analogy to coitus interruptus (*ʿazl*). It is related in early Islamic sources that *ʿazl* was tolerated by the Prophet Muhammad in the seventh century, albeit not recommended. Even with regard to the licitness of

coitus interruptus, the legal debates continue. Opponents still view this method of preventing the man's sperm from reaching the woman's ovum as having the same results as killing a fetus. Supporters rely on the theological principle that legally life does not start before 120 days of pregnancy. The muftis emphasize the need for proper education of the public to achieve the desired family planning with little resort to unjustified killing of innocent fetuses on the one hand, and in accordance with the Qur'anic message on the other.

In Egypt, more than elsewhere, the subject of abortion has been closely linked to demographic concerns, the problem of poverty, and the search for national economic growth. Over-population remains a significant problem (*Al-Ahram Weekly* Nov. 11, 1991, 12). Generally, abortions have not been permitted on humanitarian grounds. As a result, one in four or five pregnancies end in illegal abortion (Ragab 1981: 507–18).

By contrast, in Saudi Arabia Hay'at Kibar al-Ulama' asserted in 1994 that the demographic threat is only a hoax and a hypothesis, so no family planning is in order (1994, 430). They deemed the use of contraceptives a violation of the purpose of the woman's body, namely to bear children, a health hazard to her, and a cause of her ugliness. The two conflicting examples of Egypt and Saudi Arabia hint that medical ethics are sometimes echoes of socio-political discourses within countries or societies.

3. The Obligations of the Sick

Another subject that much preoccupies the muftis is how a Muslim should fulfill the Islamic commandments when he or she is sick. The main ethical dilemma concerns whether divine commandments should be given priority over a physician's recommendations. A number of ethical challenges arise. What type of physician should be trusted in general? Should the physician's authority be accepted only when implementing medical advice makes it impossible to fulfill a religious duty? For example, many questions are printed in daily newspapers as the time for the fast of Ramadan or the pilgrimage to Mecca approaches. Writers inquire whether certain health problems exempt one from performing ones duty to fast or to make a pilgrimage (Rispler-Chaim 1993, 50–61). Because religious duties are prescribed by Allah, how can a devout Muslim not perform his or her duty? Also, how can a physician, a human being, advise a patient – another human being – not to obey divine will? Most solutions that the muftis offer rely on the general principle "Necessities render the prohibited permissible" (*al-darurat tubih al-mahzurat*).[1] Saving life is a holy purpose in Islamic theology. Islamic religion also takes pride in the fact that Allah desires "ease" (*yusr*) for the believers, not "hardship" (*ʿusr*). As a result, whenever a religious duty cannot be fulfilled because of medical impediments, or whenever its fulfillment may jeopardize the health of a believer or cause damage to an already precarious state of health, the duty is to be waived. If the duty can only partially be performed, as, for example, in the case of broken limbs, which cannot be properly washed for prayer or bent as part of prayer, the sick should do whatever they can within the latitude provided by Islamic law in such circumstances. If the sick are unable to perform even parts of the duty, the law itself provides alternatives such as almsgiving, fasting, ritual sacrifices that the sick might still be able to perform. The advice of a "trustworthy physician,"[2] an important concept that has multiple applications, as explained below (Section V), in such cases provides the patient with assurance that the doctor's recommendation is clear of errors or bad intentions.

4. Assisted Reproduction

Assisted reproduction has been discussed by muftis since the 1980s, and includes in vitro fertilization, surrogate parenting, sperm and ovum donation, and ova transplantation. The main ethical reasoning about assisted reproduction is that if fertilization occurs using the husband's sperm and the wife's ovum, no breach of Shar'i norms occurs. If, however, the sperm comes from a donor, not the husband, or if it is a mixture of the donor's and the husband's, then fertilization of the wife's ovum is as sinful as fornication. In such cases, all the involved parties, including the physician, are subject to punishment if proven guilty. It is very hard to prove fornication in Islamic law, mainly because four witnesses to the act of penetration are required. It is as hard to prove unlawful artificial insemination. Several countries have, nevertheless, promulgated laws against artificial insemination by donor. Surrogate parenthood is forbidden as well because it also involves a third party besides a husband and a wife in the procreation process. Transplantation of reproductive organs is in principle permissible, but not the transplantation of testicles or ovaries, which are believed to carry the genetic code. This prohibition is meant to preserve the purity of genealogical lines (nasab), which is cherished by Islamic law and society.

5. Organ Donation and Transplantation

Many fatwas deal with organ donation and transplantation. Organ donation is generally considered a legitimate means of saving life. Organs should be donated and not sold to prevent the exploitation of poor donors by rich patients. Donations from the living are permissible if the donor is not risking his or her life and if the recipient of the organ has a good chance of recovery after the operation. Failure to meet either condition means that the operation comes close to suicide with respect to the donor, and to euthanasia with respect to the recipient. Both ways of ending a life are unacceptable in Islamic law.

In the case of cadaveric organs, the crucial issue is identifying the moment of death. Organs can only be harvested postmortem. Most contemporary muftis have accepted that the criteria for brain death identify the moment of death. This view marks a major break from the traditional cardiopulmonary criteria for determining when death has occurred. As in Western medicine, Muslims have stipulated that doctors who declare that the potential organ donor is dead should not be the same as those who will later perform transplantation. Another stipulation is that, prior to harvesting an organ from the dead, surgeons must always obtain written permission from the family of the deceased or use one prepared by the deceased himself or herself before death.

There are also debates about donations between Muslims and non-Muslims and whether the transplanted organ of a non-Muslim would defile the body of a Muslim recipient, or whether a Muslim's organ is contaminated when it is transplanted into a non-Muslim's body. The answer of the muftis is often that donations in both directions are permissible, because death somehow has a purifying influence over the human body and its organs. Humanitarian motives are also invoked to justify this practice.

When more than one patient is awaiting organ transplantation and only one organ is available, it is suggested that lots be drawn. Muslims worried about the fate of the donors' bodies on Resurrection Day are assured that Allah can easily gather their organs from wherever they may be found into their original bodies (Shaltut 1966, 325–9; Mahmud 1986, 2:245–6; Al-Qaradawi 1987, 562–3; Al-Sha'rawi 1981, 24–5; Mahmud 1996; Jad al-Haqq 1980, 9:3213–28; Saqr 1999, 134).

6. End-of-Life Care

In Islamic theology, Allah is understood to have the power to cure the sick at any time, even severely disabled people and the terminally ill. Furthermore, only Allah, who created life, may terminate life; it is not a privilege of any human being. No life is worthless. Recently the discourse on euthanasia has spread to questions of the quality of life of deformed fetuses and neonates, of unwanted fetuses, and of severely disabled adults (Rispler-Chaim 1999; Al-Daqr 1997; see also Chapter 8).

7. Definition and Determination of Death

During the closing decades of the twentieth century, debates in Islam over the definition of death and determining the moment of death were closely connected to the question of the legitimacy of euthanasia. Euthanasia in principle is viewed as interference with divine will and wisdom. No suffering justifies cutting short one's life because life is always to be seen as a gift from Allah.

8. Obligations to the Newly Dead

Obligations to the human cadaver have been analyzed in relation to cadaveric organ donation and also with regard to postmortem examination and their legitimacy, whether performed on deceased Muslims or non-Muslims. Postmortem examination involves certain elements that run counter to the Islamic requirements of a speedy burial, respect for the body of the deceased, and preserving it whole. Nevertheless, postmortem examination is on the whole deemed legitimate because it serves to verify the cause of death, an especially important consideration if the death of an individual is thought to be due to a criminal act. Postmortem examination is also regarded as essential for training new physicians in medical schools. The "public good" (*maslaha*) is evoked in this case to persuade people that Muslims as a society may benefit more than they are harmed by the outcomes of postmortem examination, although certain Islamic precepts may indeed be violated (Rispler-Chaim 1996).

9. Tobacco, Alcohol, and Dietary Restrictions

Fatwas on the hazards of smoking and the consumption of alcohol and pork appear sporadically. The last two are prohibited already in the Qur'an (Rispler-Chaim 1993). Smoking is reprehensible in Islam, an attitude supported by contemporary medical research. A few fatwas deal with mental health and psychotherapy. It is often recommended that following the Islamic path in worship, especially praying and fasting, has preventive and perhaps curative power against mental illness. A few scholars explain the appearance of mental illness as a result of abandonment of the Islamic lifestyle and religious duties (Al-Zayyin 1991; Atiyya Saqr in Minbar al-Islam May-June 1994, 84; the same mufti also in May 15, July 1996, 4, and 20–26 Jan. 1997, 6). Others muftis discuss medicines that contain ingredients unlawful for Muslims to consume, such as alcohol, pork, and blood, and whether in cases of emergency they may be taken or not. Usually the rule seems to be that when a life is in danger any substance that might save it is allowed.

10. Research with Animals and Humans

The muftis have addressed ethical questions concerning animal and human experiments. In humans, experimentation is allowed only on dying people, for whom the new medication or technique is a last resort, and with the approval of the sick person or his or her family. Regarding animals, Islamic law encourages care, never abuse or causing pain, and urges preserving their lives as much as possible. This allows some research to be performed with animal subjects.

11. Genetic Engineering and Cloning

Fatwas concerning genetic manipulation, engineering, and cloning have recently appeared and ethical reflection about these advances is therefore less well developed than for more recurring topics such as abortion. Although it is claimed that Muslims have been involved in perfecting the genetics of plants and animals for the benefit of humankind since the Middle Ages, human intervention is not allowed with regard to human cloning, except by a few Shi'i scholars. The latter maintain that human cloning does not interfere with Allah's creation, but involves only a new interpretation and application of scientific wisdom that Allah bestowed on man ages ago (Hathout 1990; *Al-Ahram Weekly* 11 July 1991; Atiyya Saqr in July 1994, 106; *Al-ʾAlam Al-Islami* 5–11 Aug. 1996, 14; 16–22 Dec. 1996, 13; Al-Harandi 1997; Salama 1997; Al-Tikriti 1981, 389–99; Rispler-Chaim 1998).

12. Topics Yet to Be Addressed

Some subjects known to preoccupy ethicists in the West have not yet been addressed in Islamic medical ethics. These include financial considerations, allocation of resources, and rationing resources when they are scarce, and the order of priorities that should or should not be followed in conditions of scarcity. Almost absent from Islamic medical ethics to date are questions of authority and paternalism, especially who should have the final say in the decision making – the political regime, the hospital, the patient's physician, or the patient and his or her family.

Literature on the field of pediatrics is sparse, with few works on the clinical management of neonates, premature infants, and the entire issue of the representation of children when choices have to be made regarding their well-being. The same lacunae can be found concerning medical problems of geriatric medicine and health care.

The muftis hardly ever refer to the planning and provision of health services as national and social goals, and whether these embody the duty of the modern state to its citizens, as is so typical of medical ethics in the West. They more often refer to medical ethics as concerned with an individual doctor caring for an individual patient. Only when society at large is threatened by an individual's state of health or by misconduct are private and the public domains linked. An example of this link can be found with regard to patients with human immunodeficiency virus infection and acquired immunodeficiency syndrome, who are not treated only as individuals but often as a social hazard, implying that they must have contracted the disease in sin. Another example is the objection to the establishment of sperm banks. These are outlawed, even though individuals might need them, because their services may lead to blurring of genealogical lines (*nasab*) – an intolerable phenomenon in any Islamic society.

V. The Doctor–Patient Relationship

The doctor–patient relationship everywhere is based on an unwritten, implicit contract. This is usually understood to mean that the doctor pledges to do his or her best to heal, cure, or relieve the patient of his or her maladies. At the same time the patient waives, at least temporarily, their rights to privacy and secrecy, as a necessary condition for the success of medical treatment. Medical interventions are inherently invasive of the patient's body or soul, or both, although the level of invasiveness may vary. One of the tasks of any system of medical ethics is to monitor this level of invasiveness, limiting it to what is necessary, so the dignity of the patient is protected see also Chapter 25).

Muslim ethicists have monitored this delicate balance between the patient's dignity and the doctor's treatment through the following measures: (1) ranking physicians according to their personal qualities and religious conduct; (2) assessment of the terms "privacy" and "secrecy" in an Islamic context; and (3) defining the legal responsibility of the physician.

1. Ranking Physicians

Many muftis stipulate in their legal advice that the physician possess certain personal qualities. This is even more strongly encouraged when the physician is consulted on matters related to the fulfillment of religious duties (such as justified exceptions to fasting during Ramadan, whether to embark on a potentially exhausting pilgrimage to Mecca, or even whether to perform the relatively easier five daily prayers). The muftis are often addressed by individuals suffering from temporary or permanent ailments, who inquire whether they ought to perform the duty or if they are exempt.

A system of ranking physicians has emerged from this discussion. A patient's first choice should be to consult an observant Muslim physician, a nonobservant Muslim physician as second choice, and only as a third choice a non-Muslim physician. The last option should be selected only in cases of emergencies and to save one's life. The justification for this ranking is that non-Muslim physicians may sometimes have the wrong motivations. They may advise Muslim patients unknowingly or even knowingly in ways that go against the letter and spirit of Islam. If a non-Muslim physician must be consulted, preference should be given to the selection of a God-fearing physician of another religion who actively practices his or her respective religion. The muftis taking this position seem to equate any piety with "moral conduct." Therefore, physicians who are God-fearing should be regarded as more trustworthy than other non-Muslim physicians because

their conduct will be guided by morality emanating from the scriptures they follow. This scriptural morality, it is assumed, will shape the physician's personal and professional ethics (Rispler-Chaim 1993).

In the Islamic law of evidence and of transactions, it is common to consider an eyewitness or partner as *ʿadl* (trustworthy) when that individual is a Muslim who is first of all religiously pious, and only then a speaker of truth and an honest person. This view comes into medical ethics as follows: a physician should first be obedient to God to be considered *ʿadl* or *thiqa* (reliable) by Muslim patients. Then he should be blessed with other good qualities such as forgiveness, love, moderation of temper, and being easy going, humble, not hasty, and fair to the poor and the rich (First International Conference on Islamic Medicine 1981). Because physicians are entrusted with considerable power over their patients, investigation into their personal morality prior to consulting them is ethically mandatory. In an emergency, by contrast, this caution is not required, because the aim of saving life overrides all other considerations.

2. Reassessment of the Terms "Privacy" and "Secrecy"

Two prohibitions that appear in the Islamic legal literature with regard to privacy and secrecy have considerable relevance to proper medical care. These are the prohibition against *khalwa* (seclusion) and against exposure of *ʿawra* (genitals, hidden parts of the body). *Khalwa* is defined as the seclusion of a man and a woman, or their being together by themselves in a room. Seclusion is permitted only to a man and a woman who are properly married, or who are forever prohibited from marrying one another because of their close blood relationship, namely father and daughter, siblings, and the like.

When *khalwa* is not permissible by law it is prohibited, as it is believed to lead to fornication (*zina*) then to the birth of illegitimate children and to social deterioration. Based on a famous Prophetic tradition, "when a man and a woman are unlawfully secluded in any place, the third present is the devil" (*shaytan*). This tradition teaches that any unlawful seclusion may bring about an immoral stumbling and therefore must be avoided. *Zina* is a major offense in Islamic law and is therefore severely punishable, by stoning to death of the married partner or flogging of the unmarried partner.

The doctor–patient relationship is replete with occasions of seclusion, as the doctor often needs to examine a patient or talk with her or him privately. Seclusion is more avoidable in psychotherapy or psychiatric treatment, in which physical examination does not routinely occur (Rispler-Chaim 1993, 64). At the same time, the confidentiality made possible by the intimacy of seclusion is often a key to the success of medical treatment

(Ibn Idris 1997, 53–5). Confidentiality concerns not only information conveyed orally from patient to doctor, but also visual and other data gathered through the doctor's examinations (see Section V.3 later for more in this topic).

The term ʿawra designates a person's most intimate organs, those that in principle should always be hidden from a stranger's eye: "strangers" are those with whom khalwa is prohibited (Rispler-Chaim 1993). In Islamic law the ʿawra of a woman implies her whole body except for the face, the palms of her hands, and her feet. The ʿawra of the man is the part from the navel to the knees. Considering these strict limits, one may justly wonder how at all a physician can examine a Muslim patient, man or woman.

The problematics of khalwa have commonly been solved in Islamic societies by encouraging women to be treated by female doctors and men by male doctors, whenever possible. In cases of emergency, when a physician of the same sex is not available, a physician of the opposite sex is allowed to examine and treat the patient, especially if that physician is held to be ʿadl and has a reputation for moral conduct and religious obedience, as explained above.

The presence of another woman or a nurse in the examination room is another acceptable method to mitigate what might otherwise be viewed as a prohibited khalwa (Elkadi 1976, 27–30). When saving life is at stake, however, the prohibitions of ʿawra and of khalwa are overlooked so that necessary intervention is not delayed (Rispler-Chaim 1993).

Privacy, as emphasized by the term ʿawra, requires that even organs that are not reproductive in the human body have to be covered because of their vulnerability and because they may provoke sexual temptation. According to the rules of the concealment of ʿawra, even a physician of the same sex as the patient should not expose a part of the patient's body that is not essential for the examination or treatment. Whenever the exposure of the body is required, all that remains is to trust the moral personality of the physician (Manna' 1990, 73). The good reputation of the physician in this regard is viewed as a valid guarantee that the rules of ʿawra and khalwa will be upheld and that the physician will not abuse the delicacy of the situation or the patient's trust.

3. Defining the Legal Responsibility of the Physician

According to a famous Prophetic tradition, "every sickness has its cure." It is the duty of physicians, therefore, to search for cures and metaphorically at least to mediate between Allah and the patient awaiting cure. The doctor is entrusted with the task of finding and delivering God's creativeness and the symbols of divine wisdom (cures and medications) for the benefit of human beings. The doctor must be loyal to Islamic doctrine and to the professional medical oath that he or she has taken. If a doctor does not fulfill this oath to the best of his or her ability a kaffara (monetary compensation) is in order, as is the case with any breach of oath in Islamic law (Rispler-Chaim 1993, 66–9).

It is understood that doctors may sometimes err. The Islamic legal literature, from its early formative period, devoted chapters to the doctor's liability, and they are titled daman al-tabib (doctors' liability). These chapters acknowledge the obligation to compensate patients injured or harmed by a physician's negligent treatment.

During the Middle Ages, circumcision and surgery were the most common, although not exclusive, fields of medical intervention wherein accidents occasionally occurred. Doctors had to pay daman (compensation) when they were responsible for damage. The legal principle was that if there was no crime, namely criminal intent, there was no punishment, unless specified by the written law (Al-Zuhayli 1989, 9:711). So, in practice, if negligence on the part of the physician could not be proven, malpractice charges would not be brought against him or her. This attitude was intended to encourage doctors to treat even the difficult medical cases, free of the fear of the prospect of malpractice charges. Today's muftis are not unanimous on this topic and debate whether compensation should come from the physicians' personal funds, from the hospital that hired him or her, from the doctors' union to which they belong, or from private insurance companies.

Medicine is classified as a fard kifaya (a communal duty) in Islamic law. This implies that the profession has to be staffed by a sufficient number of believers before the rest of the community is exempt from its responsibility to care for the sick. A sufficient number of physicians guarantees that the well-being of the community will be maintained. Under the ever-present threat of malpractice action it is realized that physicians cannot serve their communities properly. Therefore, in classical Islamic law only in cases where the doctor himself or herself has been negligent did he or she have to pay compensation out of his or her own funds. In all other cases, the state or its treasury (bayt al-mal) provided compensation instead of the physician doing so. For lay people, this is another reminder of the rule established by Islamic law of injuries that no human life is violable, and that any physical harm caused, even if unintentionally, entails compensation, namely blood money (diya), or one of its contemporary equivalents.

Before any surgical treatment the patient has to sign a consent or a refusal, which must be honored by the physician. The physician is always required to honor patients, to treat their bodies with care and respect, to be sensitive to their pains and needs, and to keep concealed the secrets entrusted to him or her. This rule must be followed unless a good reason to disclose a secret is furnished by court order or due to pressing public interest (Elkadi 1976).

Thus, although the doctor–patient relationship has its delicate aspects in any given culture, in Islamic societies, or when Muslim patients or doctors are involved, some special ethical concerns arise. The progress that has been achieved in "scientific" medicine in recent decades has not diminished the religiously based moral caution in the doctor–patient relationship. The relative secularism of the Western world, to which "scientific" medicine is often related, may have rendered this caution more urgent and indispensable for Muslims.

VI. SCIENTIFIC INFORMATION

The Arabic sources leave no doubt that the muftis are well informed about the scientific and technological advances of medicine. Sometimes the scientific ideas mentioned in the fatwas precede the actual practice of the time when the fatwa is issued. This may indicate that the muftis are informed by cutting-edge researchers, not only by practicing doctors. In the case of cloning, for example, the muftis are well aware of the process and the technique, but as regards human cloning they are ahead of their time in that they treat the ethics of human cloning as if it were an existing reality, not a futuristic forecast (Al-Harandi 1997, 80–98).

The same attitude emerges in the field of artificial insemination. Among other options the muftis discuss planting a fertilized ovum in the womb of an animal before retransplanting it in the womb of the woman, who will carry it until birth. In practice, as far as we know, this has not yet been tested and the moral dilemmas surrounding it have not been resolved (Rispler-Chaim 1993, 21–22).

Regarding more popular subjects such as contraceptives, the muftis are acquainted with the whole range of methods and devices that exist on the market, including their advantages and disadvantages (Al-Zubayr 1991, 261–80). They provide information similar to what can be gathered from popular medical manuals intended to serve the average layperson all over the world. Sometimes a famous Muslim physician is quoted as well to render the fatwa more authoritative from an Islamic point of view. Dr. Muhammad Ali Al-Bar (1981), the Saudi doctor who shows in his writings the adjustment of Qur'anic wisdom to the recent medical data, and Dr. al-Jamili (1987) are among the most respected and cited.

Scientific knowledge does not, however, go unchallenged. The muftis emphasize that the scientific knowledge assumed by physicians is limited and narrow compared with divine knowledge. Doctors' knowledge is occasionally wrong, and whenever it is true it is first made possible by Allah. This means that scientists never "discover" or "invent" in medicine – or in any other field of human endeavor. Physicians are only mediators between Allah and a patient in extending the cure that Allah has created. With regard to cloning, for example, it has been stressed that scientists only "recover" truths that Allah already placed in the world at its creation. More than being indicative of human advancement, these "recoveries" are rather proof that the human intellect is limited; that is why it has taken so long for humans to reach this level of comprehension that enables them to understand secrets such as cloning and the like (Al-Harandi 1997, 40–2).

God's knowledge and wisdom are prior to and wider than those of the physicians. Therefore, if the two seem to collide the fault must lie with physicians. A devout Muslim physician (ᶜadl), however, is surely able to settle such conflicts, because after all, medicine is also one of God's branches of knowledge (ᶜilm), and any apparent conflict is not a real one but derives from ignorance on the part of humans.

The response to this conflict can sometimes become complex. Consider sterilization, which is normally prohibited. Now consider surgical sterilization of a woman following three dangerous cesarean deliveries, to maintain her health. In this case, the mufti entrusted the decision to a reliable physician. The usual prohibition could be waived upon a physician's recommendation. In another case, a patient needed blood products during the days of Ramadan, and the doctor asked the prospective donors to break the fast on that day to provide a good blood transfusion. The dilemma was whether God's commandment to fast could be transgressed on the advice of a physician anxious for both the patient's and the donors' well-being. Eventually the final decision was entrusted to a reliable Muslim physician. In a recent fatwa the repair of a virgin's hymen after rape was labeled "permissible." A Muslim physician's testimony that the rape and injury had indeed occurred just hours before was required for the repair to be done (Wasil 1998). (Actually the Muslim physician was forced into performing a procedure that contains an element of deception and pretense against a future groom and possibly others in society, to rescue an unfortunate girl from being twice punished, that is, becoming a social outcast after having suffered the trauma of rape.)

All in all, medicine and the science that supports it are viewed as tools created by Allah to help human save life. This general ethical stance ensures that the conflict between Islamic dogma and physicians' recommendations is kept minimal. Even the obvious issue of conflict between the Shariᵃa and medical ethics over determination of the moment of death has been resolved to the satisfaction of both sides in most Islamic and Arab countries. For the purpose of organ harvesting, the "medical" definition of the moment of death has generally been adopted everywhere as the death of the brain stem. For burial rites, inheritance, and other purposes, however, the Shar'i definition of death, namely when breathing and heart activity cease, is the norm (Al-Daqr 1997).

In the debate over the legitimacy of postmortem examination, supporters rely on arguments related to the advancement of medical knowledge and the pursuit of justice, whereas opponents speak against the violation of the wholeness, hence the dignity, of the human cadaver. In fact postmortem examination has for the most part been legitimized. A semicompromise has been achieved in favor of Muslim medical students, who are supplied with cadavers of non-Muslims or of executed Muslim criminals. These examples illustrate the general view that science should be employed for the benefit of the Muslim public as long as it does not violate existing religious dogma; however, religious dogma is circumvented when an alternative interpretation for it can be furnished and the quality of a Muslim's life seems to gain.

VII. THE STATUS OF THE MUSLIM PHYSICIAN

The Muslim physician is in a way a "public officer" willingly accepted by the community as a necessary vehicle to provide health and well-being. This is evident from the fact that a physician can hardly ever be charged with criminal acts in medical care. The community owes respect to the physician, and the muftis allow trustworthy (ᶜadl) physicians to make decisions even at the expense of religious duties. In modern courts in Egypt, for example (ᶜAbd al-Hamid 1966; Shaham 1997, 312–15), but elsewhere too, the physician is a welcome consultant or an expert witness in most social issues. These include custody of minor children, abuse of women and children in marital disputes, and cases of a spouse's illness that is believed to jeopardize marital life and or sexual behavior. Sometimes the physician, equipped with the latest medical data, ends up fighting old dogma in the court. In this respect, the doctor brings modernity into traditional society. By means of cosmetic interventions the surgeon can improve a young woman's chances of winning a proper match, and by a sex change operation can help a suffering intersexual to be admitted into heterosexual society. The doctor is believed to be able to deliver a cure, hence extend human life and improve its quality. His or her opinion in certain cases is given priority over that of the mufti. In many cases the doctor's opinion is equal to that of the mufti. Muftis and doctors may collaborate on the compilation of popular medical books, wherein such words as "Islamic," "Qurʾan," or "Sharᶜi" are often part of the title (Al-Bar 1981; Al-Jamili 1987; Al-Zubayr 1991; etc.). In this way

both the religious and scientific domains are afforded due respect.

VIII. CONCLUSION

Although many topics discussed in bioethics in other countries are also discussed by Muslim ethicists, some topics that Muslims care about and Muslim ethicists address are unique to the Muslin world. These are always associated with Islamic law and religious lifestyle. The patient, the doctor, and the religious authorities must address these unique topics not only in Islamic states or Arab countries, but also in other countries wherein Muslims are a minority, and regardless of whether it is the patient, the doctor, or both who follow Islam. The solutions that Islamic medical ethicists provide are often pragmatic and workable for all milieux. Ignoring them, from a devout Muslim's point of view, would be considered disregard of the Islamic tradition and its moral code. The growing interest in the West in Islamic medical ethics is proof that a sincere attempt to overcome this ignorance is being made.

NOTES

1. This is a well-known and pragmatic principle in Islamic law since its early times, and is often applied to medical ethics by the muftis of today. What this principle implies is that medical situations or medical treatments, which would normally be forbidden by Islamic law (*mahzurat*), are tolerated and even approved by it if they can be shown to be saving life or indispensable to maintaining good health (*darurat*). It is under this principle that curative abortions, intake of medicines which involve alcoholic ingredients, plastic surgeries, organ donations from the living and the dead, post mortem examinations and many more controversial medical issues gained the legitimacy of Islamic law.

2. One of the most recurring considerations in Islamic medical ethics is the personality of the physician, or the moral conduct expected of him. In matters of prohibited seclusion between a doctor and a patient of opposite sexes, privacy, secrecy, taking decisions which seem to clash with Islamic dogma or law, deciding whether to save life or let die because medicine is unable to help, convincing a family to donate organs of a dear one and more, it is important that the physician be trustworthy. Usually this means that he or she is a devout Muslim with no immoral conduct recorded against them. Often the trustworthy physician follows the requirements of a trustworthy witness (ᶜadl) in Islamic law, that is being Muslim, responsible, sane, and with no criminal or immoral past. When a trustworthy physician is available, the patient gains peace of mind an assurance that he or she receives the best and indeed mandatory treatment.

PART VII

THE DISCOURSES OF BIOETHICS

CHAPTER 38

THE DISCOURSES OF BIOETHICS IN THE UNITED STATES

Albert R. Jonsen

I. INTRODUCTION

The word, "bioethics," was fashioned in 1970 by a biological scientist, Van Rensselaer Potter, to name his vision of a new conjunction of scientific knowledge and moral appreciation of the converging evolutionary understanding of humans in nature (Potter 1970).[1] Hardly had the word been uttered by its author than it was appropriated to identify a related but much narrower vision: the ethical analysis of a range of moral questions posed to medical practice by the advances in the biomedical sciences and technologies. In 1971, the Kennedy Institute of Ethics was founded at Georgetown University to pioneer the development of a new field of joint research that its the Institute's founder, Andre Hellegers (1911–1979), chose to call "bioethics," Warren Reich of the Institute began to plan *The Encyclopedia of Bioethics* in 1972, in which he defined bioethics as "the study of the ethical dimensions of medicine and the biological sciences" (Reich 1978, xix–xx; Reich 1995a). In 1974, Daniel Callahan, who founded the other major research institute in this new field, The Hastings Center, wrote an influential article entitled, "Bioethics as a Discipline" in which he suggested that this new field could develop itself into a unique discipline, using both the traditional methods of philosophical analysis and sensitivity to human emotion and to social and political influences

with which medicine was practiced (Callahan 1973). This emerging discipline should be designed to serve those who were faced with the crucial decisions that arise within medicine. Thus, within a few years, a neologism with indeterminate meaning became the focused name for an emerging field of study. That word, and the activity it designated, marks a boundary between the long tradition of medical ethics and a quite distinct approach to moral questions in medicine and science. That distinct approach took the form both of an academic discipline and as a style of public discourse that entered medical discussions and policy debates (Jonsen 1998).

II. CHALLENGES TO THE LONG TRADITION OF MEDICAL ETHICS

For many centuries, the practice of learned medicine has been associated with certain moral behaviors, qualities, and values. The dominant moral and religious notions in these cultures cast their light over the work of healing and, although these notions are diverse, the duties and decorum of physicians toward their patients are remarkably similar around the world. Moral maxims guide physicians who tried to perform their work in a moral manner: the moral physician was competent, dedicated, kept confidential what he learned about patients, and cared for the sick poor without charge. As healers gradually formed themselves into guilds and professions, questions about the relationships between practitioners and of economic rivalry also appeared on the agenda of medical ethics. Thus, although the language of medical propriety might differ from time to time and from culture to culture, it is not unreasonable to speak of a long tradition of medical ethics prevailing in many places over many centuries (Jonsen 2000).

At mid-twentieth century, this traditional medical morality encountered unprecedented problems. The conditions in which medicine was practiced had changed dramatically. Science had brought much more effective treatments. Many more persons had access to trained physicians and physicians became not only more educated and competent, but earned more money and social prestige than the profession had previously enjoyed. Old ideas about medical morality, particularly about the relationship with patients, were challenged by these new conditions.

Thomas Percival's *Medical Ethics* (1803), the first book to actually bear that title, came to be seen in England and America as a compendium of medical morality (see Chapters 18 and 36). The American Medical Association drew on it extensively when, in 1847, it produced its first *Code of Ethics* for American doctors (see Chapters 18 and 36). Its inadequacy for the sorts of problems confronting modern medicine was noted as early as 1927 however. In his edition of Percival, Dr. Chauncey Leake commented on the need for a deeper understanding of medical morality, based on explicit theories of moral philosophy;[2] only with a more philosophically grounded ethics could physicians confront the conditions that were, even then, dissolving the personal relationship of trust between doctors and their patients (Leake 1927). A quarter of a century later, Joseph Fletcher (1905–1991), Professor of Moral Theology at the Episcopal Divinity School, Cambridge, Massachusetts, authored a book, *Morals and Medicine*, that did utilize a vague form of an explicit philosophical theory of ethics, utilitarianism, to criticize and reformulate traditional medical morality on euthanasia, telling the truth to patients, abortion, and contraception (Fletcher 1954). Fletcher frankly discussed these issues, providing ethical arguments to support his often-controversial contentions. In addition, Fletcher was not himself a physician, whereas almost all of the voluminous writing on medical ethics had come from physicians themselves. *Morals and Medicine* was widely noted as a new direction in medical ethics.

III. THE AGENDA OF FLEDGLING FIELD OF BIOETHICS

1. Selection of Patients for Treatment with Scarce, Lifesaving Technologies

Advances in the biological sciences and in medical technology pushed these questions even harder. For example,

the invention of the artificial ventilator by Danish anesthesiologist, Bjorn Ibsen, in 1954, led another anesthesiologist, Dr. Bruno Haid, to ask Pope Pius XII to discuss ethical questions raised by the newly developed techniques for artificial support of respiration. The Pope responded with a lecture before an international gathering of anesthesiologists that repeated the old Catholic teaching that no one had a moral obligation to sustain life by use of "extraordinary means," applying that venerable doctrine to the new circumstances of ventilatory support. The Pope's reference to that doctrine revealed that the long tradition of Catholic moral theology had accumulated an articulate body of principles and a casuistry about medical ethics that could be relevant to quite modern problems (Kelly D. 1979). One of the instigators of bioethics in the United States, Dr. Henry Beecher (1904–1976) of Harvard University, was present at that papal audience. He realized that the Pope's words had a relevance for modern medicine beyond any denominational limits and would later cite them frequently, especially in the revolutionary report by a committee he chaired on the definition of death (Ad Hoc Committee of the Harvard Medical School 1968).

In 1961, Dr. Belding Scribner (1921–2003), Professor of Medicine at University of Washington, Seattle, invented the arteriovenous shunt, a simple device that made possible continued hemodialysis for patients with fatal kidney disease. It was immediately evident that more patients would need this new lifesaving technology than could be accommodated. A committee of laypersons was formed to select those patients who would be treated, and thus, live and those who would be rejected, only to die. It was extraordinary to hand over to a "God Committee" of non-physicians the power to choose which patients would live and which would die. A *LIFE* magazine article, appearing on November 21, 1962, vividly told the story of the God Committee (Alexander 1962). In the ensuing public debate, some philosophers and theologians became interested in the problem of selection for lifesaving procedures and a small literature began to appear on this topic. One of philosophy's major ethical theories, utilitarianism, was again brought to the debate. A philosopher advocated that the selection of patients should be made on the basis of social utility, assessed in light of the social worth of individuals as contributors to society (Rescher 1969). Several theologians responded that the inherent dignity of individuals required that judgments of social worth be repudiated and that selection should be made by random methods, such as lotteries (Childress 1970; Ramsey 1970b). Scholarly legal analysis sided with the theologians (Saunders and Dukeminier, 1968). Thus, the first major debate of the new bioethics was initiated.

The story of the invention of chronic dialysis was a dramatic social event that revealed how medicine's technology could pose previously unaskable questions about life and death. It was also the first example of involving laypersons as essential players in medical decision making.

It revealed that what had appeared to be medical decision making was actually the making of social policy. It was the first event to catch the attention of persons from academic ethics and intrigue them about life and death decision making. The public discussion of this event also initiated a public policy process that concluded with the passage of Federal legislation (1972) providing financial support for the treatment of end-stage renal disease by dialysis and transplantation. Thus, the case of chronic hemodialysis stimulated both the discipline and the discourse that was bioethics. The discipline profited from the articulate analysis of the problem by philosophers, theologians, and lawyers. The discourse advanced from media presentation to the formulation of public policy.

Americans, always fascinated by technology, were entranced by the rapid and widely publicized advances in medical treatment. The federal government was pouring funds into the growing National Institutes of Health, which distributed the money generously to research laboratories in medical schools, whose academic hospitals became centers of the innovative forms of care. Federal legislation also funded the expansion of community hospitals, which supplied themselves with the expanding array of new technologies. The invention of chronic hemodialysis, the advent of organ transplantation and other forms of previously rare and risky surgery on the heart and brain, the expansion of pharmacological therapy for conditions formerly almost untreatable, from cancer to schizophrenia, provided the American public with a constant array of "medical miracles." The prominence of problems raised by medical technology quickly captured the attention of the small group of scholars engaged in bioethical reflection. Thus, although Van Rennselaer Potter conceived of bioethics as a new discipline that would amply embrace the challenges of the human condition posed by its own evolutionary development and its place in the terrestrial and cosmic environments, the vision of those who actually inaugurated these reflections was focused on the clinical questions raised by medicine and medical science. Even the Hastings Center, which had opened with a similarly expansive scope (reflected in its formal name, Institute of Society, Ethics, and the Life Sciences), found itself pulled toward the medical and the biomedical. Bioethics contracted from the liberal invitation of Potter to consider the human condition to a narrower exploration of the world of doctors and patients. This had the effect of making American bioethics a philosophical revision of medical ethics. During the three decades of its development, American bioethics has lived largely in the medical world, although it constantly strains toward the wider world of environmental, population, industrial, and political ethics.

2. Research with Human Subjects

One of the earliest topics of bioethical experimentation was not a new technology itself, but rather the condition for creating those technologies. Medical progress requires experimentation and experimentation often requires human beings as its object. When experimental medicine was emerging in the first half of the nineteenth century, one of its pioneers, the French physiologist, Claude Bernard (1813–1878), declared "it is our duty and right to experiment on man, whenever it can save his life, cure him or gain him some personal benefit. The principle of medical and surgical morality, therefore, consists in never performing on man an experiment which might be harmful to him to any extent, even though the result might be highly advantageous to science, that is, to the health of others" (Bernard [1865] 1957, 101). This rigid rule was, however, unrealistic, for all experimentation is a journey into the unknown and poses some risk. Thus, as the century of experimental medicine moved on, the paradoxes of medical research with humans became increasingly apparent. After World War II, the horrors performed by Nazi physicians in concentration camps revealed how far uncontrolled experimentation could go. The Nuremberg Code (1947), drawn up in the course of the trial of those physicians, was widely acknowledged as the epitome of the ethics of experimentation with humans: medical research must be done only after free and informed consent of the subject and in light of a reasonable relation between risks and benefits (Annas and Grodin 1992; see Chapters 50 and 54). Although Americans could hardly believe that such things would happen here, they learned that, indeed, similar things did happen. In 1966, a distinguished medical researcher, Dr. Henry Beecher, published an analytic expose of abuse of human subjects of research in the country's most prestigious medical journal (Beecher 1966). In particular, a study initiated in 1931 by the Public Health Service, which still left 399 rural black males without treatment for syphilis, shocked the nation (Jones 1981, 1993).

The Federal Government, which funded so much biomedical research, had to assure that the research was not abusive to its subjects. In response, Congress established The National Commission for the Protection of Human Subjects of Biomedical and Behavioral Research (1974–1978) to develop the ethical principles that should guide research and to recommend rules and procedures to protect the rights and welfare of human subjects. During its 4-year tenure, the Commission issued specific regulations to govern the conduct of research and a statement of principle, *The Belmont Report*, which proposed that three principles should guide researchers: respect for persons, beneficence,[3] and justice. These principles entailed respectively, informed consent, the assessment of risk in relation to benefit, and the equitable selection of subjects for research (National Commission for the Protection of Human Subjects of Biomedical and Behavioral Research [1979] 1998). The Commission had called upon many philosophers and theologians for help in clarifying issues as it debated the ethics of research with children, with the mentally infirm, and with incarcerated persons. The thought of two scholars was particularly influential: Hans Jonas (1903–1993), a philosopher, and Jay Katz, a physician and professor of law, both of whom delved deeply into the complex relations between respect for individuals, consent, and the duty to contribute to scientific knowledge (Jonas 1969; Katz 1972). Again, bioethics manifested itself as discourse and discipline. The widespread public debates about abuses of experimental subjects was gradually shaped into legislation and regulation. The discipline was improved by scholarly analysis of concepts such as "free and uncoerced consent," and "research versus practice," and of the logic involved in arguing for the rights of research subjects in relation to the common good of society.

3. Human Genetics and Its Clinical Application

One of the most dramatic breakthroughs in the biological sciences was the announcement in 1956 that James Watson and James Crick had discerned the "secret" of life, the double helical structure of the DNA molecule. The possibility of learning the most basic lessons about how biological organisms developed, how defects entered that development, and how scientists might consciously modify that development, engendered great excitement. It engendered great concern as well, arousing memories of the ill-conceived eugenics that had entranced the nation for the first half of the century, promising improvement of the "stock" by controlled breeding and sterilization. A debate over these issues among scholars erupted in the mid-1960s. Philosophers and theologians endorsed the potential of these sciences to eradicate and alleviate disease but they questioned the wisdom of modifying human characteristics, for which few criteria of perfection exist. In particular, the prospect of cloning humans aroused vigorous debate. The scientific potential to modify the human genetic structure was named "genetic engineering" (President's Commission for the Study of Ethical Problems in Medicine and in Biomedical and Behavioral Research [1982] 1998b); however, the scientific prospects of modifying the human genome seemed still far in the future and these concerns abated somewhat in the 1970s. Their place was taken by another advance in modern genetics, the ability to test and screen for the presence of genetic diseases and conditions. Again, this was a great medical advantage but hidden within its techniques lay the potential for discrimination against persons who were discovered to have some genetic condition. Because few therapies were available to treat the conditions for which testing was available, the prospect of stigmatization, risk of loss of insurance and of work, were troubling. Intense study of the ethical implications of this important medical advance led to guidelines and legislation that defined

the permissible scope of screening programs. Just as the ethics of biomedical experimentation stressed the consent of the subject, so the ethics of genetic screening emphasized that programs of premarital and prenatal carrier screening be done with the knowledgeable consent of those screened (President's Commission for the Study of Ethical Problems in Medicine and in Biomedical and Behavioral Research [1983] 1998c). When the next major advances in genetics occurred, the ethical questions had already been formulated and were ready to be applied to the new endeavor, the mapping and sequencing of the human genome. When Congress provided vast funds for this project in 1989, it included as an integral part of the scientific research The Ethical, Legal and Social Implications Program, charged to review these implications and to fund academic research to illuminate them (Cook-Deegan 1994).

4. Organ Transplantation

Another dramatic moment in the progress of medicine came in 1968, when Dr. Christian Barnaard took the heart from a dead person and transplanted it into the chest of a living person, who lived for several months. The era of organ transplantation had begun in the early 1950s when kidney transplantation between genetically identical twins was successful; soon powerful drugs allowed transplantation between unrelated persons by controlling the process of immunological rejection. Physicians, exhilarated by the ability to save lives doomed by kidney failure, also realized that, to do so, they had to invade the body of a healthy person, seemingly violating the most ancient ethical maxim of medicine, "do no harm." Also, the obligation of persons to donate an organ to one in need was much debated. Scholars struggled to define the moral nature of the act whereby a part of one human would be used to save another. Finally, the ethical ideal of "donation" was extolled as the justification for placing one person at risk to save another (Fox and Swazey 1974; see also Chapter 62). It quickly became obvious that lifesaving organs were in short supply and that the problem of allocation that had troubled the Seattle dialysis program would be played out on a national stage (Task Force 1986). Bioethicists contributed to the design of public programs for organ procurement and distribution.

Heart transplantation, however, was the drama that propelled the ethical issues associated with that medical advance into public attention. The symbolic value of the heart as the center of human emotion led some persons to question the morality of transferring one person's heart into another person's body. The still imperfect understanding of the human immune system and the inadequacy of drugs to counter immunological rejection led to tragic disappointments. Heart transplantation, unlike renal transplant, required a new way of thinking about death, because the organ, which itself must be physiologically living, must be taken from a person who is already legally dead. From time immemorial, physicians had designated death as the moment when breathing and circulation of blood ceased. New formulations of this definition were attempted; most famous of these was the "Definition of Irreversible Coma: Report of the Ad Hoc Committee at Harvard Medical School to Examine the Definition of Brain Death" (Ad Hoc Committee of the Harvard Medical School 1968; see Chapter 63). This reformulation stressed the irreversible loss of the neurological activities of the brain. Many states enacted legislation to change their legal criteria for determining death. The Harvard criteria, however, were ambiguous and 13 years later, the newly appointed President's Commission for the Study of Ethical Problems in Medicine (1979–1982) issued a more careful definition, defining death as the cessation of all brain activity, including the brain stem (President's Commission for the Study of Ethical Problems in Medicine and in Biomedical and Behavioral Research [1981] 1998a). During the long debate over the redefinition of death, bioethicists argued both that the new definitions moved into dangerous territory, opening the possibilities of considering "dead" persons who retained biological life, and also that the definitions did not go far enough, considering as "alive" human beings who lacked all possibilities for human communication. Although the more conservative formulation of death became law throughout the United States, a valuable literature about the nature of death, of personhood, and of the obligation between persons enriched bioethics.

IV. The Agenda of the Mature Field of Bioethics

Selection of patients for life and death therapies, experimentation with human subjects, the eugenic and discriminatory potential of molecular biology, and the interpersonal complexities of organ transplantation, all occurring during the 1960s, were the topics that raised concerns among professionals and the public and that engaged the attention of philosophers, theologians, and legal scholars. These topics were on the first agenda for the nascent bioethics. During the decades of the 1970s and 1980s, other topics brought the field to a maturity of method and social organization.

1. Medical Care at the End of Life

Life-sustaining technologies, such as hemodialysis and respirators, both of which were developed at approximately the same time, have several effects. These technologies substitute for a damaged organ system, thus keeping alive a person who would otherwise have died. Usually, these technologies are used on a temporary basis,

but they can be used as a permanent support – even when vital organs have irreversibly failed. This sometimes leads to a second effect: supporting biological life when mental life is badly deteriorated or gone. It may also have the effect of prolonging inevitable death. These effects raise the question: under what conditions should we decline to initiate life support or decide to discontinue it? In 1973, a team of physicians who cared for immature newborn babies exposed their own practice of allowing such babies to die when their prognosis for healthy life was dim (Duff and Campbell 1973). Their article aroused surprise and anger among the public, although they reported a practice that was accepted by many other physicians who treated these severely ill babies.

Two years later, the story of 21-year-old Karen Ann Quinlan captured the attention of the nation. Brought to a hospital in coma, she lingered unconscious for months supported by a respirator. When her parents asked that the respirator be stopped, the hospital refused and the first legal case to deal with allowing a patient to die went to the Supreme Court of New Jersey. The Court determined that her parents had the authority to withdraw life support, offering a thoughtful analysis of this unprecedented problem (*In re Quinlan* 1976). Many similar cases have since arisen, one of them, the Case of Nancy Cruzan, was adjudicated by the United States Supreme Court. In essence, the Court affirmed the right of patients, and their surrogates, to refuse life support when recovery to health and consciousness was highly unlikely, provided there was some evidence that the patient would have chosen such a course (*Cruzan v. Director, Missouri Department of Health* 1990). Bioethicists followed these cases closely and often contributed to the formulation of moral arguments, usually as justification for allowing such patients to die. A substantial body of literature about the appropriate care of the dying was created (Veatch 1976). In the 1990s, the debate turned from the appropriate criteria for withholding and withdrawing life-sustaining treatments, to the even older question of euthanasia, asking whether physicians should be allowed to assist their hopelessly ill patients to commit suicide.

2. Assisted Reproduction

Human reproduction, long considered a process set immutably by nature, became the object of scientific manipulation in the late nineteenth century. The first successful artificial insemination by donor was performed in 1884 and not reported until 25 years later because those who performed it feared a negative public response. That anticipated response followed and has continued over each subsequent development in reproductive technology. The religious traditions of the Western world have definitive doctrinal positions on the matters of sexuality and reproduction, and these aspects of human life are surrounded by strong beliefs in public morality. The development of chemical contraceptives in the 1950s made possible a rational means of preventing birth, which contradicted some religious teachings, particularly those preached by the Roman Catholic church. Ironically, the science that contributed to this means of preventing birth also contributed to the new understandings of the physiology of fertility, making possible the conception of children for infertile couples. In 1979, two English physicians reported that they had fertilized a human ovum in a petri dish and introduced it into the womb of the woman who bore a baby named Louise Brown. This procedure, in vitro fertilization, made possible many other manipulations of the human embryo, all of which have been vigorously debated. In addition to yielding more than 100,000 births worldwide, the new forms of assisted reproduction have led to new forms of family, because a woman can now conceive a child without intercourse and a child can be conceived, borne, and born by a "committee" of progenitors, the contributors of sperm, eggs, and uteruses and those who have agreed to rear the child. Determining responsibilities among the members of this "committee" of progenitors and decisions about the use and disposal of embryos created by this procedure has been a constant topic of bioethical debate and legal regulation (Advisory Committee 1988).

3. Abortion and Embryo Research

The moral problem of abortion, long framed by the religious traditions of the United States as an absolute moral evil, broke into public debate with a 1973 decision of the Supreme Court, *Roe v. Wade*, which gave legal approval to medical abortions with very few restrictions (*Roe v. Wade* 1973). From the time of this decision, constant political debate has surrounded not only the question of abortion itself, but also many other issues that concern the human embryo and fetus. Experimental use of tissues from embryos and fetuses, which are of interest to researchers as potential sources of therapy for many diseases, has been stringently curtailed by federal law and regulation. Despite multiple reports from scientific bodies and ethics commissions that approve the cautious use of embryonic and fetal tissue, legislators, responding to conservative constituencies, have consistently repudiated this science. Indeed, even research into the medical procedures of assisted reproduction have been denied public funding, leading to the expansion of a widely used and desired medical practice without appropriate research into its scientific basis. The most heated public and political debates have surrounded the proposals to utilize embryonic stem cells for research aimed toward therapies for many diseased individuals. Questions of reproductive ethics have been among bioethics' most vividly debated but, strangely,

the debates have had very little influence on public policy.

4. Public Policy Development

The concern over the rights and welfare of humans who were experimental subjects in the many government-sponsored research projects prompted the Congressional establishment of the National Commission for the Protection of Human Subjects of Research in 1974. Concerns over the care of the dying, over genetics, and other issues led the Congress, in 1979, to continue the life of that Commission, with a new mandate and mostly different members, under the title, President's Commission for the Study of Ethical Problems in Medicine and in Biomedical and Behavioral Research. The National Commission worked for 4 years; the President's Commission for 3 years. Both produced substantial reports and recommended regulation and law. Above all, both provided a visible space for bioethics on the national scene and a forum for public debate. Following the expiration of the President's Commission in 1983, several other efforts to establish national bodies came to grief. Other, more limited, bodies were formed within the Department of Health and Human Services to deal with specific questions, such as organ transplantation and fetal and embryo research. In 1997, President Clinton appointed the National Bioethics Advisory Commission, which in subsequent years produced major studies of the ethics of cloning, stem cell research, and other current bioethical questions. The normal life of this Commission ended with the term of President Clinton. President Bush appointed a President's Council on Bioethics in 2001 with a broad mandate "to conduct fundamental inquiry into the human and moral significance of developments in biomedical and behavioral science and technology." The first task of this body was to formulate recommendations regarding the ethical issues associated with cloning and stem cell research.

5. Institutional Committees

During the 1970s and 1980s, scholars, Commissions, and committees put hard work into the concepts and arguments that surround all these issues. In so doing, they not only clarified the issues themselves, but also improved their own understanding of how to analyze and argue bioethical questions. Many scholars who had previously known of these issues only as observers or hardly at all were attracted to the study of these problems. They became the original bioethicists. In addition to the scholars, many other persons, professional and lay, became peripherally involved in bioethics. Government regulations about research with human subjects required that all research institutions have an Institutional Review Board

(IRB), charged with review and approval of all scientific proposals to use human subjects. Hundreds of these IRBs came into being and thousands of physicians, scientists, and others became familiar at first hand with the principles for ethical research, the regulations to protect subjects' welfare and rights and their application to particular cases. Similarly, hospitals began in the late 1970s to set up Ethics Committees to deal with the complex problems of deciding when life support should be discontinued for particular patients. These committees, which were advisory to physicians and to the institution, undertook to clarify policies about resuscitation and life support. Again, many persons who served on these committees became familiar with the language, concepts, and literature of bioethics. Around the country, conferences and courses were held and books and journals appeared for this new population of part-time "bioethicists."

V. BIOETHICS PROFESSIONALIZED

The professional bioethicists came principally from two disciplines with a long tradition of intellectual analysis of moral problems, theology and philosophy. The theologians were early participants in the discussion. Roman Catholics brought a venerable tradition of moral theology about medical care (Kelly 1979; McCormick 1988). Jewish scholars as well could draw on a rich wisdom about the sanctity of life[4] and care of personal health (Bleich and Rosner 1979). Protestant theology, although less endowed with historical teachings on these issues, came to the debates with a strong appreciation of the moral life in society (Verhey and Lammers 1993). Eminent theological scholars, such as James Gustafson, Paul Ramsey (1924–1988), Moishe Tendler, Richard McCormick (1922–2000), and Charles Curran, became frequent contributors to the debates. From the philosophical community, only recently awakened from almost purely theoretical concerns about moral language to the problems of practical life, came scholars such as Hans Jonas, Stephen Toulmin, Alasdair MacIntyre, Joel Feinberg, and Judith Jarvis Thompson. They contributed an acute sense of ethical analysis and a common vocabulary to the discussions. Within a short time, the theological voices became less doctrinal and denominational; the philosophical voices became less formally analytic. Despite the persistence of disciplinary origins, a common bioethical vernacular emerged and a new breed of scholars, fluent in that vernacular, became the full-time bioethicists. In recent years, those from a theological background have been urged to return to their religious roots and those from philosophy to become more rigorous in their analysis.

By the mid-1970s, a large volume of literature on these topics had been published, much of it written by philosophers and theologians. That decade began with a powerfully expressed, rigorously argued, and unabashedly contentious book, *Patient As Person*, by Princeton University theologian Paul Ramsey. This book took up the topics of that era, experimentation, genetic engineering, organ transplantation, and definition of death and the care of the dying and pursued a close ethical analysis, based on the fundamental ethical notion of fidelity between patient and physician. Ramsey's words in that book and on the many other bioethical topics he subsequently addressed, echoed through the emerging field of bioethics (Ramsey 1970a, 1970b). Several research centers, the Hastings Center (1969) and the Kennedy Institute at Georgetown University (1971) had been established. Professorships to study and teach these subjects had been opened at medical schools. Professors, as is their way, created curricula, wrote textbooks, and explored theoretical approaches to draw the classical disciplines that deal with morality, philosophy, and theology, together with the practical questions about the pursuit of science and the practice of medicine. Clearly, by the end of the 1970s, the neologism, "bioethics," described more than a vision: it designated a new a discipline, with a distinctive literature and all the panoply of courses and conferences that academic disciplines engender.

VI. BIOETHICS AS DISCIPLINE AND DISCOURSE

The discipline is not, however, unified by a single dominant theory or methodology. It reflects the circumstances of its evolution: questions about the ethical dimensions of science and medicine were raised and debated by a variety of commentators: scientists, physicians, and other health care professionals; lawyers, politicians, and public policy experts; social scientists; and philosophers and theologians. These highly interdisciplinary discussions brought considerations from every side into the debate. The two disciplines most familiar with the logic and rhetoric of ethics, moral philosophy, and moral theology, provided their skills to the debates and, in so doing, often shaped the desultory discussion, so common to ethical discourse, into formats with distinct definitions and logical arguments. They did not, however, submerge the interdisciplinary features in any single ethical theory. Even though some bioethicists, such as H. Tristram Engelhardt, Jr. (1996) and Robert Veatch (1981), have attempted to formulate overarching theories, the discipline welcomes a wide range of arguments, views, and methods. Moral questions are argued in terms of some rather consistent moral rules, such as "do no harm" and those rules are justified by reference to a general conception of personal and social welfare.

One rule in particular, respect for the autonomy of persons,[5] holds a particularly important place in bioethical argumentation. Its dominance can be attributed, perhaps, to the sorts of problems posed to the original bioethics, particularly the use of humans in research and the eugenic threats of the new genetics, both of which called for a strong defense of individual dignity and liberty. It is an idea certainly congenial to the profound individualism that marks American culture. It may also be the heritage of the peculiarly American philosophy, the Pragmatism of William James and John Dewey, that prizes the striving of free individuals to meet challenges and to create a richer life and a better world. James concluded a seminal lecture on the Moral Life with the imperative, "Invent some manner of realizing your own values" (James 1967). Whatever the source of the dominance of the principle of personal autonomy, it has exercised both a benign and a malign influence on bioethics. Its benign effect has been to overthrow the unjustifiable paternalism of physicians and the arrogance of scientists: decisions about what is best for a person ought to be made by the one whose life will be affected; decisions about the directions of scientific progress ought to be in the hands of the people whose future will be changed. The malign aspect of the dominance of autonomy lies in the neglect of social and communal dimensions of ethical problems. Bioethics has been less successful in dealing with issues of public welfare than in resolving the interpersonal problems of clinical medicine.

Bioethics, however, is not simply an academic discipline in which debates over method and theory absorb scholars' attention. It has, from the beginning, aimed toward the guidance of practices and policies. It is not speculative but practical moral philosophy (and, for that reason, some have suggested that its fundamental philosophical perspective is American pragmatism). Thus, in addition to the disciplinary dimensions of method and theory, bioethics is a form of discourse, promoting public debate over substantial questions and encouraging the formation of agreement and consensus about the ways to resolve those questions. The many Commissions and committees that have been established over the last three decades have carried on that discourse and it has spilled into the places where regulations are made and legislation written, as well as the places, such as hospitals and professional groups, that seek to guide their practitioners through complex problems. A special subset of bioethics, sometimes called "clinical ethics,"[6] focuses on the ways in which ethical considerations can be integrated into the decisions that doctors, other health care professionals, and patients must make in the daily provision of health care. The formal disciplinary arguments, found in the literature, contribute to that discourse, as does the advice of the scholarly bioethicists, but the wider discourse draws on the ingenuity and insight of many individuals whose moral conscience focuses on these questions. In the state of Oregon, for example, during the 1980s, a program called Oregon Health Decisions, engaged thousands of citizens in such discourse over health care priorities; their discussions informed the legislature of that state about the people's bioethical values.

The United States provided a name, "bioethics," for an activity that, during the 1970s and 1980s, was appearing throughout the world. Countries that had developed highly technological forms of health care and that fostered large programs of scientific research found themselves facing the same problems that American physicians and scientists had faced in the 1950s and 1960s. In other nations, where medical technology was not so advanced and health care was still beyond the reach of many persons, the study of bioethics concentrated on the allocation of resources and the problems of the preservation of health and the prevention of disease. International bodies, such as UNESCO and the European Union, became interested in the ethical questions arising in genetics and reproductive sciences. Wherever bioethics has become established, it bears the marks of the indigenous culture's ethos as well as the practical issues facing each nation. The International Association of Bioethics, which meets biennially in different nations, draws a large group of scholars to participate in an extremely varied program.

Thus, bioethics has become, in three decades, an international enterprise. The details of that enterprise in other nations are addressed in the other chapters in this section of the volume. Some topics are universal, whereas others represent local concerns. The philosophical and religious context of bioethical reflections differs from culture to culture. It is sometimes said that bioethics outside the United States too quickly adopted the questions and concepts of American bioethics, but it is now clear that bioethical reflection in different cultures is increasingly marked by the indigenous thought and beliefs of those cultures. American bioethics, perhaps more so than the bioethics of other nations, has evolved into a formal academic discipline. This evolution is due, most probably, to the sponsorship of bioethics teaching by American medical schools, which prompted the emergence of a professional class, a standard curriculum, and professional societies.

VII. CONCLUSION

In the quarter century since bioethics was born, it has established itself as an integral branch of practical or applied philosophy and as a valuable adjunct to health policy and medical practice. It has developed some methodologies for dealing with the questions to which it is devoted. Those questions touch the human condition so deeply that no final answers will ever be given, but continued examination remains necessary. New questions arise as versions of the old questions, as new technical possibilities emerge from science, and as new social arrangements appear. At the same time, the theoretical and methodological boundaries of bioethics are flexible and are constantly being expanded by the introduction of new topics and new approaches to analysis. The earlier interest in a broad ecological and environmental ethic is reappearing. Methodological insights from other disciplines, such as anthropology and economics, are becoming more prominent. Feminist and multiethnic perspectives on ethics are being integrated into the discussion of issues. American bioethics today is much better prepared intellectually to study these questions than it was in its infancy. Its task is to promote debate, contribute clarity to those debates, and to criticize simple solutions to complex issues.

NOTES

1. Bioethics is a form of academic and public discourse, using the methods of philosophical and theological ethics, as well as legal and sociological concepts, about the ethical problems associated with advances in science and technology in medicine and health care. In a broader sense, that discourse also includes environmental and ecological ethics.

2. Consequentialism and deontology are the two most general theories of moral obligation. Deontology designates those forms of ethical reasoning that depend on the existence of certain principles and rules of actions that ground moral obligation and from which specific duties can be deduced for particular action; consequentialism designates forms of ethical reasoning that propose that the moral quality of actions and decisions depends on the production of certain results that conform to a theory of the human good. Kantian moral philosophy is often characterized as classical deontology; utilitarianism is the most common form of consequentialism. This distinction leaves much to be desired.

3. Beneficence and nonmaleficence are two ethical principles that play a prominent role in bioethical reasoning. Beneficence (doing good) refers to the duty to act toward others in ways that better their condition; nonmaleficence refers to the duty to refrain from actions that cause harm to others. These principles are not only general principles of ethics but also play an important role in the traditional ethics of medicine that enjoined physicians to "be beneficial and do no harm" (Hippocrates, Epidemics I,). Beneficence also has a central place within utilitarian ethics, as directing the maximization of the greater good of the greater number, but this meaning is seldom associated with its use in bioethical discourse.

4. Sanctity of life is a concept rooted in the Judeo-Christian belief that all life is created by a benevolent God and continues under the providence of that God (Buddhism also maintains an analogous belief, as do many other religions). The ethical implications of this concept are the duty to protect life and to foster its positive growth. Consistent application of this belief would prohibit warfare, suicide, murder, abortion, capitol punishment, or allow them only under extreme circumstances. The concept is often not consistently applied however. Also, the concept has been divorced from its religious roots and, for many, has become a general and somewhat empty slogan to be applied to any cause. In some debates, such as that over euthanasia, sanctity of life is distinguished from quality of life, raising the question whether there is a duty to preserve a life that has lost desirable qualities.

5. Autonomy is a philosophical concept describing the scope of individual liberty of thought and action. The ethical principle of respect for autonomy instructs persons not to interfere with the thoughts and actions of other persons, except when those thoughts or actions cause harm to others. This principle is loosely based on the philosophical views of Immanuel Kant and John Stuart Mill but is strongly influenced by the American penchant for individual freedom. Many believe that American bioethics has relied too strongly and exclusively on this principle and encourage a stronger reliance on other principles and on other perspectives on ethics, such as communitarianism.

6. Clinical Ethics is a distinct activity within bioethics, consisting of consultation by persons trained in bioethics in the actual cases of moral perplexity that arise in the provision of medical care to patients. Clinical ethics employs forms of ethical reasoning that aim at practical and reasonable resolutions of problematic cases, such as casuistry.

CHAPTER 39

THE DISCOURSES OF BIOETHICS IN THE UNITED KINGDOM

Kenneth Boyd

I. INTRODUCTION

In 1963, "four lectures and a conference" on "issues raised through the practice of medicine" were organized by what became the London Medical Group (LMG). The subjects discussed are not recorded in the chronicle of the LMG's first 10 years (Shotter 1975a). By 1965, the LMG program comprised sixteen lectures, a conference, and study seminars on topics including abortion, sterilization, birth control, suicide, pain and the care of the dying, prolongation of life in unconscious patients, clinical experimentation, the hospital as a community, and the welfare state (Shotter 1975b). These were not yet described as "medical ethics," which was still commonly identified with professional etiquette. During the 1970s, however, it began to be established as a term also covering an increasing number of morally and politically problematic issues in health care. "Bioethics" was and still is used more rarely in Britain, and often for issues, especially ecological and environmental, not directly related to health care.

II. THE ERA OF TRUSTING ATTITUDES IN DOCTORS

Before the advent of LMG, many British doctors believed that medico-moral questions "should be discussed only

between medical colleagues – and *in camera*" (Shotter 1975b). Professional ethics was governed by the General Medical Council, a statutory but largely self-regulatory body created in 1858 (see Chapter 36), and since the turn of the century the British Medical Association (the doctors' trade union) had a Central Ethical Committee to advise it on the subject. Meanwhile the public, largely unaware of these arcane arrangements, on the whole was inclined to trust its doctors. It was assumed, mistakenly, that they had "taken the Hippocratic Oath," and that this covered all such matters.

This trusting attitude was encouraged by the medical, legal, and ecclesiastical establishments. In 1936, when a bill to legalize voluntary euthanasia in the case of uncontrollable terminal pain was introduced into the House of Lords, it was defeated by opponents led by the King's Physician and the Archbishop of Canterbury, who argued that such matters should be left to the discretion of doctors. Not until half a century later did the public become aware that the terminally ill King George V's death earlier in the same year had been hastened by a drug overdose administered by the same physician. In 1957, when a doctor who had treated an incurably but not terminally ill patient with increasing doses of opiates was brought to trial for her murder, he was acquitted on the judge's direction that a doctor "is entitled to do all that is proper and necessary to relieve pain and suffering even if the measures he takes may incidentally shorten life" (*R. v. Adams* 1957). In the same year, another judge ruled that a doctor was not negligent if he acted "in accordance with the practice accepted by a responsible body of medical men skilled in that particular art" (*R. v. Bolam* 1957), thereby establishing the British "professional" rather than "prudent patient" standard for such cases. In a 1930s case, the judge had even extended medical discretion to abortion, hitherto a criminal act for which a doctor could be struck off the medical register. Abortion, he ruled, was not illegal if it was performed because the doctor judged in good faith that the woman's physical and mental health, and hence her life, was in jeopardy (*R. v. Bourne* 1938).

The public trust in doctors was not noticeably undermined by the evidence of medical crimes revealed at the 1947 Nuremberg tribunal (see Chapter 54). Until the publication in 1967 of M. H. Pappworth's *Human Guinea Pigs* (Pappworth 1967), the claim that unethical medical research "could not happen here" was generally accepted. In 1963, the Medical Research Council (MRC), responding to the rapid post-war growth in clinical research, issued a statement on *Responsibility in Investigations on Human Subjects* (MRC 1953) that emphasized the importance of consent and of avoiding harm to subjects. It was not until a decade later, however, that hospital research ethics committees were set up to safeguard patients and healthy volunteers, and even then the system was and has remained nonstatutory. This tardy response reflected a rather different legacy of World War II (see Chapter 36).

III. Bioethics, the National Health Service, and the Church

The year 1963 saw the deaths not only of John F. Kennedy and Pope John XXIII, but also of Sir William Beverage, the wartime architect of the British Welfare State. If bioethics was a child of its time – a time of exciting new ideas that for many contemporaries the pope and president had symbolized, its British embodiment was shaped by Beverage's legacy. Deference to authority had been weakened by the wars and political disappointments of the twentieth century. The creation in 1948 of a National Health Service (NHS), promising cradle-to-grave health care as a universal entitlement, renewed public trust in what now literally were "its doctors." Doctors themselves, although initially wary or even hostile, rapidly came to share this sense of common ownership. For the rest of the century the NHS was to be a powerful symbol of national identity and social solidarity, eventually surviving even the ravages of Thatcherism economics in the 1980s, and perhaps being the rock on which they eventually foundered. In the austere (but still scientifically optimistic) postwar decades, many patients regarded NHS care less as a right than as something to be grateful for, and when scarce resources or

new technologies created difficult problems, professionals and the public alike hoped that these could be resolved by consensus and an appeal to the common good.

Although British bioethics was born in the NHS, its midwife was a much older national institution, the Church of England. In an address printed in the LMG's first Annual Report, the Archbishop of Canterbury, Michael Ramsay, emphasized the complementary roles of religion and medicine and the importance of cooperation between doctors and clergy. The Church's role, he argued, should not be confused with "faith healing," and clergy in training should "gain a real knowledge of the life and working of a hospital from within" and also a sound knowledge of psychiatry (Shotter 1975b). Such themes were characteristic of liberal theological and pastoral thinking in the postwar British churches, and especially the Student Christian Movement (SCM), the ecumenical arm of the churches in higher education.

In the early 1960s, the SCM commissioned the Reverend Andrew Mepham, a U.S.-trained physician and currently chaplain to an English psychiatric hospital, to investigate the needs of students in British medical schools. At this time, public trust in doctors' ethics was not matched by any very overt efforts to educate doctors in moral discrimination. Apart from the occasional exhortation by the Dean, or a lecture in forensic pathology on what was popularly known as the "rule of As" (prohibiting abortion, addiction, adultery, advertising, and association with unqualified practitioners) (Higgs 1997), medical ethics was not part of the curriculum. According to the widely held "osmosis" theory, medical students absorbed their ethics through their apprenticeship. In their preclinical years, more adventurous medical students might also absorb some elements of a liberal education from contact with other university faculties. An increasingly crowded scientific curriculum left ever less time for this.

IV. The London Medical Group

Mepham's survey did not focus directly on medical ethics but on the broader goals of medicine: "our medical schools spend untold effort to give the student all the skills and knowledge available in the conquest of disease. But our learning and concern for the diseased tissue seem to distract us from the care of the patient as a man." He recommended "an educational service" to deal with such issues, emphasizing that "clinical medical students must be seen as part of the hospital community and not primarily as members of a university" (Shotter 1975b). In response, the SCM commissioned one of its staff, the Reverend Edward Shotter, to implement these ideas in the London medical schools, and it was there that what became the LMG held its first lectures in 1963.

LMG was a highly efficient organization. Topics were chosen and meetings organized by a representative council of students from the twelve London medical schools, advised by a consultative council of senior academics. Although nursing and other disciplines were included, both councils were predominantly medical. As LMG director, Shotter was convinced that the enterprise would not succeed if it were not focused on clinical issues. In practice this approach proved attractive to nonmedical as well as medical audiences, and provided a nonpartisan platform for religious as well as other views. Contributors to its debates included, for example, the leading Anglican moral theologians Bishops Mortimer of Exeter and Ramsey of Durham, distinguished Roman Catholic and Orthodox physicians and theologians such as Dr. Jack Dominian and Archbishop Anthony Bloom, and Dr. Immanuel Jakobovits, British Chief Rabbi and author of the authoritative *Jewish Medical Ethics* (Jacobovits 1959; see Chapter 16).

By 1975, LMG, now independent of SCM, was annually organizing more than fifty lectures and symposia in the medical schools, and a national conference attended by several hundred participants. Similar medical groups were set up in most other British medical schools, and in one of these, Edinburgh, a program of research in medical ethics and education was underway (Boyd 1979; Thompson 1979). To coordinate these activities, which were the main focus of medical ethics in Britain at this time, a postgraduate Society for the Study of Medical Ethics (SSME), later the Institute of Medical Ethics (IME), was created and, also in 1975, the *Journal of Medical Ethics* was launched (Shotter 1988).

LMG's rapid expansion was undoubtedly fueled by the bioethical developments and debates of the 1960s and 1970s. *Matters of Life and Death*, a collection of LMG lectures published in 1970, discussed organ transplantation, the definition of death, the nature and management of terminal pain, and other aspects of death and bereavement, concluding with a paper by the leading moral theologian G. R. Dunstan, calling for the education of public opinion on such issues as an "essential step in the ethical refounding of our society" (Shotter 1970, 55). The paper on terminal pain was by a regular LMG lecturer, Dr. Cicely Saunders, pioneer of research-based palliative care and the hospice movement. Other LMG lecturers were equally well-known and often charismatic figures in their respective spheres. Dunstan and Saunders also contributed to *On Dying Well*, an influential 1975 Church of England report on euthanasia (Church Information Office 1975), and to *The Problem of Euthanasia*, papers from an LMG conference midway between two further unsuccessful attempts, in 1969 and 1976, to decriminalize voluntary euthanasia (Dunstan et al. 1972).

More successful legislative attempts liberalized the law on suicide (1961), abortion (1967), and homosexuality (1967). These topics were frequently discussed by

LMG, as were other current concerns including: oral contraception; population policy and the 1968 papal encyclical *Humanae Vitae*; *in vitro* fertilization, from the first laboratory success in 1969 to the first birth in 1978; research into genetic conditions and progress in antenatal diagnosis; clinical experimentation, especially after Pappworth's 1967 publication; issues in psychiatry such as electroconvulsive therapy, psychosurgery, mental health legislation, therapeutic communities and the radical theories of T. S. Szasz and R. D. Laing; new social scientific research into health care systems; medical communication with patients and the media; problems of health care teamwork and, increasingly, of the allocation of scarce resources (Shotter 1975a). The number of ethical issues raised by the practice of medicine was now growing so rapidly that the first (1977) edition of the *Dictionary of Medical Ethics* (edited by three vice-presidents of SSME – A. S. Duncan, G. R. Dunstan, and R. B. Welbourn) was soon superseded by a revised and enlarged edition of more than 450 pages (Duncan, Dunstan, and Welbourn 1981). Of its 148 contributors, most had addressed LMG or other medical groups on their subjects.

During the 1960s and 1970s, LMG and SSME sought to create not just a "talking shop" about issues in medical ethics, but also a sound academic base for research and teaching. From 1975, the *Journal of Medical Ethics*, deliberately designed as a specialist medical journal but with multidisciplinary authorship, began to provide this outlet (*Journal of Medical Ethics* 1975). Leading philosophers (including Dorothy Emmet, Anthony Flew, R. M. Hare, and R. S. Downie), theologians, social scientists, and lawyers, as well as nurses and doctors from most specialties, and from the United States and other countries as well as Britain, all contributed to its pages. Its first editor, A. V. Campbell, a lecturer in Christian Ethics from Edinburgh University, was the author of *Moral Dilemmas in Medicine*, the first British publication to interpret modern medical ethics in terms of traditional moral philosophy (Campbell 1972). Although deliberately aimed at a nonphilosophical readership – it derived from an innovative lecture course for nurses – Campbell's book reflected a more general turn toward practical ethics in British academic moral philosophy, which hitherto had been largely concerned with meta-ethical questions. His successor as editor (1981–2001), Raanan Gillon, a philosopher but also a practicing NHS general practitioner, was also to make a major philosophical contribution to critical thinking about moral issues raised by the practice of medicine, in particular as the leading British advocate and interpreter of Beauchamp and Childress's four principles approach (Beauchamp and Childress 1979; Gillon 1986; Gillon and Lloyd 1994). A further significant publishing development was the inauguration in 1984 of the *IME Bulletin*, which monitored current events in British bioethics and subsequently, under the continuing editorship of Dr. Richard Nicholson, became the independently published and widely read *Bulletin of Medical Ethics*.

V. Bioethics and Law

Academic lawyers too were now turning their attention to medical ethics. In 1980, Ian Kennedy, Reader in Law at King's College, London, used the British Broadcasting Corporation's prestigious Reith Lectures to mount a highly iconoclastic attack on medical paternalism. His lectures, titled *The Unmasking of Medicine* (Kennedy 1981), ruffled many feathers in the medical establishment but also helped awaken it from its dogmatic slumbers: in the 1980s and 1990s, the British Medical Association and the General Medical Council began to address the public as well as the profession on problematic aspects of medical ethics. During these decades, growing public interest in medical ethics was stimulated by the advent of human immunodeficiency virus infection and acquired immunodeficiency syndrome, which forced reexamination of many traditional assumptions and practices, and also by legislative and legal developments related to both the beginning and end of life. A Government *Inquiry into Human Fertilisation and Embryology* (Department of Health and Social Security 1984), chaired by the eminent philosopher Dame Mary Warnock, led to legislation in 1990 allowing research on embryos up to 14 days, but under the tight control of a new statutory Human Fertilisation and Embryology Authority. A series of widely publicized legal cases, concerned with selective treatment of neonates (*R. v. Arthur* 1981), euthanasia (*R. v. Cox* 1992), and withdrawal of artificial nutrition and hydration from patients in a persistent vegetative state (*R. v. Bland* 1993), culminated in a report from the House of Lords on *Medical Ethics* (House of Lords 1994), which reaffirmed the principle of double effect and rejected proposals for legalizing voluntary euthanasia.

Serious consideration of such proposals undoubtedly was influenced by awareness of developments in the Netherlands, and during the 1980s and 1990s medical ethics in the United Kingdom was increasingly in dialogue with its Continental European partners. Although Britain did not sign up to the Council of Europe's Convention on Human Rights and Biomedicine, European Union (EU) funding of research projects in bioethics greatly encouraged such cooperation, and EU legislation on issues related to medicine and human rights was to have important implications for English and Scottish law. The United Kingdom, for example, had made detailed provisions for regulating the use of animals in biomedical research under its 1986 Animals (Scientific Procedures) Act (see also Chapter 48). As noted previously, it had made no comparable statutory provision for ethical review of research with human subjects. By 2004, however, it was legally required to conform to an EU directive laying down uniform rules for the conduct of clinical trials in all member states (Europa 2001).

As legal and legislative involvement in medical ethics grew, and its subject matter became more complex and extensive, health professionals as well as lawyers began to seek relevant educational qualifications. In 1978, the London Society of Apothecaries inaugurated a Diploma in the Philosophy of Medicine, and in the same year Ian Kennedy, G. R. Dunstan, and other academics at King's College set up a Centre of Medical Law and Ethics, which from 1984 offered degree courses in medical ethics and law. Similar, mainly postgraduate, courses were soon to be offered by other universities. In 1983, Raanan Gillon, in cooperation with IME, had inaugurated an annual intensive short course on medical ethics, which over the years was to provide large numbers of doctors and nurses with a basic grounding in the subject. At an undergraduate level, a need for ethics teaching also was perceived, first in nursing and then in medical education. In response to a 1984 initiative by the General Medical Council, IME set up a working party on the subject, whose recommendations, in the *Pond Report on the Teaching of Medical Ethics* (Boyd 1987), had been generally implemented in medical schools by the late 1990s, when a national curriculum in medical ethics and law also was agreed (Ashcroft 1998). Leading universities with a strong research as well as teaching focus on medical ethics were soon to include Birmingham, Bristol, Edinburgh, Manchester, Preston, and London's King's and Imperial Colleges.

VI. Conclusion

By the end of the twentieth century, the IME was only one of many organizations active in the expanding field of British bioethics. A significant new development in the early 1990s, for example, was the creation of the Nuffield Council on Bioethics, perhaps the nearest the United Kingdom would come to a national ethics committee. By then IME's ambitions for medical ethics in the United Kingdom had been largely achieved. The subject was regularly discussed, taught, and increasingly researched in a great variety of British academic, professional, and institutional contexts, more often than not at the instigation of individuals who had first encountered it through the London and other medical groups or in the pages of the *Journal of Medical Ethics*.

CHAPTER 40

THE DISCOURSES OF BIOETHICS IN WESTERN EUROPE

Maurizio Mori

I. INTRODUCTION

This chapter addresses the development of bioethics in continental Western Europe, by which I mean the area including Portugal, Spain, France, Belgium, Switzerland, Germany, Austria, and Italy. Great Britain, Holland, and other Scandinavian countries as well as Greece, Cyprus, Turkey and all the other countries which until 1989 were in the Eastern block are not included: they have a different "culture." (The development of bioethics in Britain is addressed in Chapter 39 and in Eastern Europe in Chapter 41.)

At the beginning of the 1970s, in continental Europe, ethical issues in medicine were limited to a few topics attracting the concern of a restricted number of specialists who discussed them quietly. In approximately two decades this situation changed radically, and bioethical issues are now debated in public and even influence political elections.

To understand how such a change occurred, it is useful to distinguish two aspects: bioethics as a *cultural movement*, that is, as an emergence of some new ideas and spreading of new attitudes; and bioethics in an *institutional setting*, that is, as organizational resources that support the debate in the field, especially research centers and university curricula. These two aspects of bioethics are related but distinct:

institutions are supposed to produce ideas and influence the wider culture, but seldom does even a well-organized research center have a significant impact on culture. On the contrary, new ideas can get off the ground and influence society at large, quite independently of institutional support.

II. THE ORIGINS OF WESTERN EUROPEAN BIOETHICS

In Western Europe, bioethics began in the late 1970s and early 1980s as a cultural movement. A few (mainly young) scholars were attracted by moral debate that emerged in the United States and in other English-speaking countries. The interdisciplinary work done at the Hastings Center since the late 1960s was a practical model of research, and papers in "applied ethics" provided a conceptual style to imitate. Debates on abortion were illuminating; in continental Europe abortion's immorality was beyond discussion and one could at most think that it had to be legalized to soften back-street abortion tragedies. In the United States, scholars, such as Judith Jarvis Thomson (1971), Michael Tooley (1983), Mary Anne Warren ([1973] 1987), and Richard B. Brandt ([1972] 1974), claimed that abortion was *morally* permissible, and even a woman's basic freedom. The United States

490

Supreme Court's *Roe v. Wade* (1973) confirmed this trend (see Chapter 38). This court case shocked Europeans. The Quinlan decision in 1976 (*In re Quinlan*), living wills, and other advance directives based on the patient's autonomy (see Chapter 38) proved equally shocking to European sensibilities.

"Bioethics" became the new word used to identify a new "spirit of the age" concerning biomedical issues, the *Encyclopedia of Bioethics* (Reich 1978) its reference work, and its interdisciplinary methodology. Bioethics was conceived not as one component of a larger movement of critical reflection on health care (Reich 1978, xv–xxii), but as a set of related issues (mainly focusing on birth and death) with no clear systematic links to each other. As a branch of applied ethics, it appeared somewhat "external" to medical practice.

Bioethics did not receive a warm welcome by the cultural establishment. Philosophers, in particular, had negative reactions. In Great Britain, for example, the leading journal, *Philosophy*, devoted a critical editorial to the newly published *Encyclopedia of Bioethics*:

> Do we *need* an Encyclopedia of Bioethics? If so, can we afford to live without an Encyclopedia of Aesthetics, an Encyclopedia of Political Theology?... It would be unfair to the *Encyclopedia of Bioethics* to treat it as specially deserving the doubts and suspicions that its arrival may evoke. The judicious camel, seeking to account for a broken back, must spread the burden of responsibility among the straws. It is not the fault of... (the Editor in Chief) or of... (the sponsor) or of... (the publisher) that the big business of publishing is more and more conducted like Big Business, and that the products of the industry of philosophers and other scholars are increasingly presented and promoted as if they were industrial products. (Editorial 1979)

Thus, far from responding to a real philosophical or social need, bioethics was ridiculed as a new fashion created by Yankee imperialism. Not surprisingly, this view was agreed with by most Marxists, who, until 1989, had a significant influence in continental Europe. Other philosophers, joining the "continental tradition," opposed bioethics because it was regarded as a shabby consequence of English-speaking "analytic philosophy." Even some of the few analytic philosophers showed skepticism, fearing that applied ethics could undermine the is–ought divide. No warmer acceptance was received from medicine; bioethics was simply ignored. Most physicians perceived the new moral challenges as irrelevant issues or as something absurd. Coming from outside medicine and contravening traditional medical deontology, bioethics was viewed as an improper philosophical intrusion into another's field.

To respond to this depressing situation, the first task of bioethics was to gain intellectual respectability and to be accepted as a significant field of "scientific" inquiry. The institutions devoted to bioethical research founded in the 1970s and 1980s – Barcelona in 1975, Paris in 1980, Lovein in 1983, Rome in 1985, and Milan in 1989 – greatly contributed to this goal. Most of them have been established by Roman Catholics (influenced by the Kennedy Institute of Ethics at Georgetown University in the United States), and this fact was seen as further evidence that bioethics was a Trojan horse, used by Catholics to reintroduce natural law theories into secular legislation. Nonetheless, bioethical debate was a bracing and provocative intellectual experience. In the 1980s, bioethicists were rare birds struggling for survival and accreditation. Because medical technology appeared to be the new Moloch to be faced independently of ideological, religious, or disciplinary divisions, bioethics soon began to take on the appearance of an innovative field with a promising future.

III. First Bioethical Institutions in Western Europe

The first Western European country to start institutional bioethics was Spain, where, in 1975, the Jesuit obstetrician Francisco Abel founded a Research Center for Bioethics at the Faculty of Theology in Barcelona (which became an independent Institute in 1984). Bioethics also attracted the attention of the Spanish historian of medicine Diego Gracia, who distinguished a "Mediterranean bioethics," in which the doctor–patient relationship is informed by "medical phyla" and open to family cooperation, from a "North European bioethics," in which such a relation has an individualistic and contractual character. This view gained some favor, but is not the final word on the matter. Development of Spanish legislation since General Franco's death in 1975 seems to show that contractual individualism is influential even in Spain. In 1985, a new law permitting abortion was passed and, in 1988, the Spanish Parliament enacted the most liberal legislation on assisted reproduction in Europe.

Spain started first, but France has paid more attention to institutional bioethics. In 1980, a center for bioethics was founded at the Jesuit Faculty of Theology in Paris and became an independent department in 1985. In 1983, the President of the Republic, François Mitterand, formed a *Comité National d'Etique* (National Committee on Ethics), to provide advice to the government on bioethical issues. All of the great "spiritual families" of France are represented in the Committee, which is the major expression of French bioethics conceived as "the time for reflection." A distinctive "French way" of doing bioethics has emerged.

In Italy, bioethics started to receive institutional attention after the publication of *The Report of the Committee of Inquiry into Human Fertilisation and Embryology* by a government committee led by philosopher Dame Mary Warnock in 1984 (Department of Health and Social Security 1984). In that same year, the "Santosuosso Commission" (named for its chairman) was appointed in Italy to prepare a bill on assisted reproduction that was presented in 1986 and completely disregarded. In 1985, the Pope himself inaugurated the Center for Bioethics at the Catholic University of Rome, which is a most influential institution in Italy (and in the Vatican). According to Monsignor Elio Sgreccia, director of the Center, bioethics has to set solid barriers to techno-scientific advancement in biomedical matters, because not everything that is technically possible is ethically permissible (Sgreccia 1999, 2002). On the other hand, since 1983, in Milan, a private research center, *Politeia*, has actively promoted bioethical debate from an interdisciplinary perspective. In 1989, the late neurologist Renato Boeri founded in Milan the *Consulta di Bioetica* (Bioethics Supreme Committee), a private organization that soon spread all over Italy and that supports a secular view of bioethics as critical reflection on biomedical issues without a priori limits or barriers (Lecaldano 1999). This means that Italian bioethics has come to be characterized by a sharp opposition between Roman Catholic and non-Roman Catholic (including Protestant and Jewish) views. This situation continues and has not been weakened by the creation of a National Committee for Bioethics in 1990.

In Belgium bioethics was developed at various universities, mainly by G. Hottois and J. F. Malherbe. In 1990, a new "liberal" law on abortion was approved, and King Baldovin "abdicated" just for 1 day to allow the law to be enacted without his signature. In Switzerland attention was devoted to bioethics by some theologians (Roman Catholic and Protestant) as well as by some physicians, so that various topics have been considered by the Swiss Medical Association.

The development of bioethics in West Germany (before reunification) was completely different. Until the 1980s, bioethics received virtually no attention. There were several reasons for this difference. Some are historical and connected with the Nazi experience (see Chapter 54), which made words such as "euthanasia" taboo, words that literally could not be pronounced. Other reasons were legal. In Germany the embryo's life is protected by the Constitution and abortion is forbidden. There are semantic reasons. The term, "bioethics," was understood by Germans to mean, not the application of ethics to a special field, but a special ethical methodology supporting a sort of naturalistic and utilitarian ethics contrary to sanctity of life and human dignity. The German philosophical milieu was also dominated by the "continental approach" and from this methodological perspective it was easy to dismiss bioethics as a shallow product of "analytic philosophy." Finally, physicians did not support the new field

within medicine, and therefore, in the 1980s, bioethics had hardly any impact apart from a few university scholars such as Hans-Martin Sass, Kurt Bayertz, and D. Birnbacher. In the late 1990s the situation started to change and German bioethics began to register some significant developments.

IV. WESTERN EUROPEAN BIOETHICS IN THE 1990S

In the 1990s, the new spirit of bioethics in Europe had major effects on public policy. Three major areas were addressed: the doctor–patient relationship, human subjects research, and the definition of death and regulation of organ transplantation.

The first public-policy change concerned the doctor–patient relationship. Most European legislatures formally recognized informed consent and patient autonomy but, in spite of the law, paternalistic attitudes persisted in daily medical practice. Some important court decisions in Italy, as well as in Spain, favored patient autonomy. Further evidence can be traced in the emphasis placed on the issue by the European Convention of Bioethics (1997).

Bioethics also influenced the development of new regulations on experimentation with humans. In 1990, France and Spain approved new legislation protecting human subjects of research and established a network of "Ethics Committees" (or Institutional Review Boards) to oversee and regulate human subjects research. In 1991, the European Parliament approved the new rules for Good Clinical Practice. The issue of experiments on animals was hotly debated and in 1993 Italy approved a law allowing conscientious objection to participating in animal experiments.

Laws that defined death and regulated organ transplantation were passed in the 1990s. In 1994, Italy incorporated the definition of death in terms of brain death into a new law. New legislation regulating organ donation was passed in Spain in 1996, in Germany in 1997, and in Italy in 1999.

Notwithstanding these positive results, the bioethical debates of the 1990s in continental Europe reflected a sharp opposition between Roman Catholics and non-Roman Catholics. Although at first Catholics contributed to making bioethics a respectable field, the situation started to change after the publication of the Holy See Instruction, *Donum Vitae* (*Instruction on Respect for Human Life* (John Paul II 1987a), on assisted reproduction. Pope John Paul's encyclical, *Evangelium Vitae* (*The Gospel of Life*) (John Paul II 1995a, 1995b), confirmed that the Roman Catholic church endorses the absolute sanctity of human life. Debates on reproduction (mainly on the embryo) soon reflected the hardening Roman Catholic line (see Chapter 14). In Portugal, Catholics opposed a permissive law on abortion, which was defeated by a small margin in 1999. Catholics regularly protest against abortion pills, the use of which is slowly spreading in Europe. Nevertheless, various forms of assisted reproduction have been accepted in Belgium and Switzerland. In 1994, France approved a general law on the body that has to be revised. Italy passed legislation on assisted reproduction in 2004 that permits using assisted reproductive techniques (ART) for the formation and transfer of a maximum of three embryos at one time but, in response to Catholic pressure, prohibits embryo destruction and embryo storage.

The ongoing controversy between Roman Catholics and non-Roman Catholics, together with new problems concerning nurses' and other health care professionals' roles, together with debates on the allocation of scarce medical resources, have propelled a more general reflection on the goals of medicine and the meaning of health care. Although, in the 1980s, bioethics was concerned with single topics, such as abortion and euthanasia, the perspective has since widened to include more general issues in the philosophy of medicine and the nature of health. To date, however, this new trend of thinking has had little impact on public policy.

Two other subjects should be mentioned. The first is the Peter Singer affair in Germany and Austria, where he was effectively silenced at different occasions in the early 1990s (Singer 1993). These traumatic events raised lively debates on the limits of intellectual freedom and helped the growth of bioethics in academic circles. A more positive note concerns the work done in the 1990s by the Council of Europe that led to the *European Convention of Bioethics*, presented at Oviedo, Spain, on April 4, 1997 (Council of Europe 1997a, 1997b) – an important step in the process of the "harmonization of European legislation" on bioethics.

V. WESTERN EUROPEAN BIOETHICS SINCE 1997

The announcement of the birth of the first cloned sheep, Dolly, in February 1997 was a watershed event because it changed the nature of bioethical debate in Europe. Before Dolly bioethics was a fast-growing and flourishing academic field; after Dolly it became fashionable, attracting daily attention everywhere. Apart from its profound cultural impact, the cloning of Dolly opened a new era in biological research: research on stem cells and therapeutic cloning, together with less noticed but important advances in pharmacogenomics are changing the scene. The British acceptance of the Donaldson Report in August 2000 reframed the discussion over the embryo because it is not any longer limited to reproduction, but it involves possible new therapies (Department of Health 2000). Even though it has been its major supporter, France decided not to ratify the European Convention before having revised

its legislation on embryo experimentation (to circumvent the controversial prohibition stated in article 18). Belgium is still looking at future events and in Germany the issue of stem cells started new debates.

Italy paid a great deal of attention to stem cells and both the National Committee and the Dulbecco Report issued guidelines similar to those in the Donaldson Report. In the media, debates over new developments of stem cells research are mixed (and sometimes confused) with controversies over "mad cow" syndrome and genetically modified organisms, an issue on which the European Union enacted a new law on patenting of biotechnological products in 1998.

Much attention has been focused on end-of-life issues. Discussions intensified in the 1990s under the stimulus of pioneer Dutch experience, in which physician-assisted suicide and euthanasia under certain conditions is allowed (see Chapter 7 for a detailed discussion of the Dutch experience with euthanasia). Since 1997 concern for advance directives has become prominent. Everywhere in continental Europe there are associations promoting advance directives; in Germany and Spain even Roman Catholic bishops have proposed forms for advance directives. In Italy bills have been introduced in Parliament to grant legal sanction to such forms. Palliative medicine is quickly becoming normal practice and an integrated system is promoted by the National Health Service in Italy. Withdrawing artificial nutrition from patients in a persistent vegetative state is now being actively debated in various countries, and active euthanasia is a topic of daily discussion in all continental Europe. In 1999, the Swiss Medical Association recognized that a physician may respond to the request of a terminal patient for aid in dying, and assisted suicide is now permitted in Switzerland (see Chapter 7). In Italy and France bills have been proposed to legalize active euthanasia, but their future is uncertain. At the European level some people claim that voluntary euthanasia should be allowed as a consequence of human rights.

VI. CONCLUSION

At the beginning bioethics had to fight against a robust resistance but in less than two decades it has become widely accepted and practices in Western Europe. In general, bioethics offers a major reconsideration of the Catholic sanctity of life view and a source of new attitudes toward human biological life informed by an increasingly secular perspective. In this sense bioethics appears as a continuation of Enlightenment ways of thinking (see Chapters 26–32). Bioethics at a cultural level calls for renewal of social life and social institutions, even though institutional change appears slow and difficult to achieve. Resistance to change is a function of the recurrence in some European debates (especially legal ones) of "human dignity," an ambiguous notion that can be interpreted both in conservative and progressive senses. Sometimes, bioethics is accused of being a clerical (mainly Roman Catholic) instrument to prevent social change. In contrast, bioethics is charged with being too quick to accept uncritically scientific and technological innovation. Such debates are mixed up with more general reflections concerning European "identity," that is, questions about whether "Europe" refers to not one cultural entity but to quite different cultural experiences or refers to one cultural entity uniquely grounded in Christian values (as the Roman Catholic church claims). Bioethics in Western Europe thus finds itself at the often combustible interface of biomedical technology, on the one hand, and more general cultural themes, on the other, with distinct echoes of the controversies about the future European Constitution.

CHAPTER 41

THE DISCOURSES OF BIOETHICS IN POST-COMMUNIST EASTERN EUROPE

Eugenijus Gefenas

I. INTRODUCTION

The post-Communist period started with the collapse of the Eastern Block in the late 1980s. This period has been marked by intensive integration of Eastern and Western Europe and the consequent reduction of ideological boundaries among the different parts of Europe. The term, "bioethics," has come into increasing use in the region, as a result of international cooperation of academics and practitioners from Central and Eastern European countries with bioethics institutions and scholars in North America and Western Europe, as well as the expanding influence of bioethical activities of such international bodies as the Council of Europe, UNESCO, and European Commission.

It should be pointed out that Central and Eastern Europe embraces culturally and economically diverse countries. For example, some of them are still under an authoritarian rule and some others have to cope with the consequences of a recent civil war. In contrast to those mentioned, however, there are also so-called accession countries, which have been making a rapid transition to democratic self-rule and had begun to join the European Union in 2004 (and which, consequently, are often referred to as "new member states"). The diversity of conditions for the development of bioethics in these

different countries makes generalizing about them challenging. Nonetheless, it is possible to identify trends that are common to the majority of the countries in the region that result from their decades of exposure to Communist ideologies and practices.

This chapter begins with a critical evaluation of what has been usually regarded as "medical ethics" discourse in the countries of Central and Eastern Europe during the years of the Soviet rule. Then it discusses the institutionalization of bioethics in the region in the context of European integration and provides a critical analysis of recent bioethics developments in the European societies in transition. The chapter closes with a reflection on the issue of the distinctiveness of the discourses of bioethics in the post-Communist Eastern and Central Europe.

II. "SOVIET" VERSUS "UNDERGROUND" MEDICAL ETHICS

The main features of the discourses of bioethics in the post-Communist countries of Central and Eastern Europe must be understood in the content of the peculiarities of health care ethics during the years of Soviet rule, which was imposed upon the majority of the countries of the region after the World War II (see Chapters 55 and 56).

Soviet ideology informed all areas of health care. For example, during the Stalinist era of the 1930s and 1940s, a restrictive antiabortion policy aimed at expanding Soviet military power was implemented. In 1956, this policy was replaced by a liberal one, with the purpose of proving that women's rights were respected in Soviet countries (Kovács 1991). To justify a prohibition of euthanasia, Soviet ethicists deployed the "interests of the society" argument. A book, called *Medical Ethics and Deontology*, argued that euthanasia was unjustified because "human life does not ultimately belong to a particular human being but is an inseparable part of a web of social relationships" (Ivaniushkin 1983). Political abuse of psychiatry was probably the most extreme and degrading example of the ideological misuse of medicine by the Soviet regime. Such terms as "sluggish schizophrenia" were invented to justify the use of psychiatric institutions to restrict the freedom of those who criticized the Soviet regime and ideology.

These illustrative examples of the imposition of Soviet ideology on health care convey only a partial picture of medical ethics under Soviet rule. In totalitarian societies, officially prescribed norms and principles that are imposed upon professional activities must be distinguished from the ethical norms and values actually accepted and practiced by health care professionals. Identifying medical ethics exclusively with official ideology and ignoring the existence of an alternative, underground medical ethics leads to uncritical and simplistic interpretation of the discourses of medical ethics in Central and Eastern Europe during this period.

Unfortunately, an oversimplified reading of medical ethics during this period is rather common among Western commentators as well as some writers in the region. For example, medical ethics of the former socialist countries of Eastern Europe and especially the former Soviet Union has usually been identified with the statements taken from "The Oath of Soviet Physicians." A number of sections of the Oath have been presented as representative of medical ethics in the "former Eastern Block" during the Soviet period (Veatch 1997, 15). These passages include performing conscientious work "wherever the interests of the society will require it," "the conduct of all my actions according to the principles of the Communist morality," and keeping in mind the "high responsibility I have to my people and to the Soviet government."

It is true that all graduating medical students in the former Soviet Union took this Oath. It is equally true, however, that the passages from the Oath that are cited here, as well as Soviet ideology in general, were never taken seriously by the majority of health care professionals, nor by society at large. Physicians did not think in terms of "inseparable web of social relationship" when they treated their terminally ill patients and many psychiatrists did not follow either the theory or the practice

of Soviet psychiatry. Psychoanalysis, which was regarded as incompatible with Soviet ideology, was practiced as an underground activity in many countries of the region.

People were forced to live in the bifurcated world of official versus "underground" ideologies and to use "politically correct" ideological phrases, which in many circumstances were very different from their actual motivation and commitments. It would be very difficult to understand the rapid collapse of the Soviet regime in the 1990s, were we to believe that people living in a totalitarian state wholeheartedly and without any critical distance simply accepted the official ideology.

Consider one of the most ideologically charged issues, the allocation of scarce health care resources. The debate about distributive justice helps us to reconstruct an important aspect of Soviet bioethical discourse. The Soviet constitution entitled every citizen to "free and comprehensive" health care. Such a right reflected the official ideology of absolute egalitarianism applied to the field of health care and was based on the principle "to each according to his or her needs." The reality was, however, that the Soviet "nomenclatura," the Party elite responsible for running the country, and health care professionals, and their patients did not follow this fundamental principle of Soviet health care.

First, even during the "golden age" of the Soviet Empire (and certainly during its period of decline) the principle "to each according to his or her needs" served simply as an ideological cliché. Those who had the greatest health care needs – the mentally ill, the disabled, and the handicapped – found themselves at the bottom of the health care pile. They were usually kept in "special institutions," places isolated from the "egalitarian society" and well away from the sight of visiting foreigners.

In contrast, the Soviet nomenclatura always had access to elite clinics and hospitals that were not available to general public, much less to the most vulnerable segments of the population. In fact, this was the two-tiered health care system that was criticized by Soviet ideologists as a form of inequality in Western health care. Finally, black market medical services were always a part of Soviet health care. Tipping enabled those seeking health care to jump to the head of waiting lists or simply to be more confident that health care professionals would do their jobs properly (Gefenas 2001a).

This example illustrates the grotesque and hypocritical discrepancy between the officially declared principles of distributive justice and the reality of resource allocation in the former Easter Block countries. Paradoxically, the outcome of declaring free and equal access to comprehensive medical care was that the so-called Socialist countries never implemented the ideals of equality and solidarity to the extent that the majority of free market–oriented European societies did. Consider, for example, Nordic countries that, until very recently, had not been questioning the justifiability of their one-tier public health care system (Norheim 1995).

To sum up, such official principles of Soviet medical ethics as "the interests of the society," "promotion of Communist values," and the like were mere slogans used not only to restrict private initiative but also to shape the health care provider–patient relationship. The official ideology elaborated by some apologetic Soviet writers, however, was not actually followed or accepted by the majority of health care professionals. The actual mode of medical ethics in everyday health care was traditional Hippocratic ethics, based on an individualistic and paternalistic understanding of the physician–patient relationship (Veatch 1989b).

III. EUROPEAN INTEGRATION AND INSTITUTIONALIZATION OF BIOETHICS

Achieving political independence in the late 1980s and early 1990s meant a radical shift in socio-cultural life of the countries of Central and Eastern Europe. Political obstacles to bioethics as an academic discipline were abolished and all those from the region interested in the field were free to participate in international bioethics initiatives. In addition, such bodies as the Council of Europe Bioethics Committee, the European Commission, and UNESCO have actively expanded their bioethics activities in Central and Eastern Europe. An optimistic scenario for this process of transition would project a future in which the division of European bioethics into its "Eastern" and "Western" branches would become history. Supporting the optimistic scenario is the speedy implementation of international bioethics instruments in the countries of the region. For example, the Council of Europe Convention on Human Rights and Biomedicine (so-called Bioethics Convention) has been ratified more rapidly in European transition countries than in Western Europe. By November of 2002, the Convention was ratified by fifteen of forty-three member states of the Council of Europe. Nine of those fifteen countries represented the region of Central and Eastern Europe. Similarly, the additional protocol on the Prohibition of Cloning Human Beings was ratified by the same nine Central and Eastern European countries of a total thirteen ratifications (Council of Europe Steering Committee on Bioethics 2002). Moreover, in line with the main principles of Bioethics Convention, one fundamental feature of new health legislation in many countries of the region has been the replacement of traditional paternalism with the principle of informed consent, a powerful force for transforming the doctor–patient relationship.

Another feature of developing bioethics in the countries of the region has been intensive institutionalization of bioethics. For example, during the first few years of independence many countries established national bioethics bodies, hospital ethics committees (at least in their largest health care institutions), and developed an ethical review system for biomedical research similar to that functioning in Western Europe or North America. In addition, teaching of bioethics and modern medical ethics has been formally introduced into the curricula of universities and medical schools. These developments illustrate the transfer of the Western model of institutionalizing bioethics to the countries of the region. What has been developing in the West for decades has been adapted in Central and Eastern Europe in a few years time. Let us explicate the mentioned aspects of institutionalizing bioethics.

First, national bioethics bodies have been established in almost all Central and Eastern European countries invited to join European Union after the fall of the Soviet Union (so-called EU accession countries): Bulgaria, Czech Republic, Estonia, Hungary, Latvia, Lithuania, Poland, Romania, Slovak Republic, Slovenia.[1] The information about non-EU accession countries is more difficult to obtain, however, there are reports indicating the establishment of the national bioethics bodies in other post-Communist countries as well (Javashvili and Kiknadze 2000). Most often the national bioethics bodies are affiliated with the Ministries of Health and have a broad mandate to facilitate the development of bioethics in the countries through educational activities and the impact on biomedical legislation. In relatively small countries, national committees are also assigned more specific tasks, such as ethical approval of multicenter research protocols (Trontelj 2000). In some cases, special ethics bodies are established to monitor nation wide scientific projects, for example, the Ethics Committee of the Estonian Human Genome Project (Tikk and Parve 2000).

The second aspect of institutionalizing bioethics concerns the establishment of hospital (clinical) ethics committees. The existence of this type of ethics committee has been reported in many Central and Eastern European countries, to mention but few of them in Croatia, Estonia, Hungary, Lithuania, Rumania, and Slovakia (Blasszauer and Kismodi 2001; Gefenas 2001b; Segota 1999; Tikk and Parve 2000; Glasa 2000). In the Czech Republic, almost twenty local ethics committees at the largest hospitals were set up in the early 1990s, however, later on they were transformed into the bodies approving biomedical research protocols (Simek et al. 2000). This brings us to the third type of bioethics institution, namely, research ethics committees. This type of bioethics body has been the most uniform and developed one in the whole region of Central and Eastern European, most probably because procedural rules of ethical review and substantive principles of research ethics have been based on well-known and internationally accepted guidelines. These guidelines have been rapidly spread in Central and Eastern Europe since the late 1980s by the researchers involved in multicenter clinical trials. That is why the research ethics committees have been most often based at the university hospitals and are similar to the institutional review boards functioning in the United States (Trontelj 2000) rather than regional research ethics committees of the Scandinavian countries. For example, in Poland each medical school has its committee for research involving human subjects (Gorski and Zalewski 2000). In addition, many countries in the region also have a separate net of research ethics committees on laboratory animals.

Emerging teaching programs and courses on bioethics or modern medical ethics might be regarded as a background feature of institutionalizing bioethics in the region. These courses have been gradually introduced into the curricula of most of the medical schools and replaced the mentioned Marxist type of "medical ethics and deontology" taught before the 1990s. Removal of the political oppression to the Church was another factor influencing bioethics discourse in Central and Eastern Europe. As a consequence, in some countries the emergence of secular bioethics has been followed by religious perspective on bioethics. This process has been particularly active in the Roman Catholic–dominated countries where some universities and medical schools filled in the appearing vacuum of medical humanities with the courses of Catholic bioethics and medical ethics (see Chapter 40). The process of replacing the Marxist biomedical ethics with the alternatives has not always been, however, a smooth one. In some cases, the dominance of one particular religious perspective on bioethics could have been regarded as an obstacle to develop free and pluralistic bioethics discourse in the societies having a very short experience of democratic debate. On the other hand, the credibility of newly introduced programs was sometimes compromised because the teaching of bioethics would be done by the former lecturers of Marxist medical ethics.

It should be stressed that even if the programs or teaching courses on bioethics exist nowadays in many medical schools and some nonmedical institutions in Central and Eastern Europe, it is still quite difficult to collect reliable information about the content of the courses, about their share in the teaching curriculum, and about research projects in which the newly established institutions are involved. Rather few academic centers dealing with bioethics have created informative websites or, as institutional members, joined international organizations such as European Association of Centres for Medical Ethics (EACME).[2] It is the impression of the author, that even if bioethics is sometimes hosted by the faculties or institutes of philosophy, theology, or law,[3] the most widespread mode of practicing bioethics is the teaching courses on medical ethics or medical humanities affiliated with the medical or public health schools.[4] These

are, however, rather short courses, which do not usually exceed 40 class hours.

IV. CRITICAL EVALUATION OF BIOETHICS DEVELOPMENTS IN THE REGION

Even though the features of institutionalization and Euro-integration might be seen as a success story of developing bioethics in the post-Communist countries, a deeper analysis reveals the complexity of the process. We should not take for granted that the speedy process of establishing different bioethics institutions or ratifying international bioethics instruments reflects a genuine development of bioethical discourse in the region. The most important feature of such a discourse is that signing and ratifying the international conventions should be an outcome of informed societal debate reflecting public understanding and consensus. The question might be asked therefore, if the countries of Central and Eastern Europe adopted the Convention on Human Rights and Biomedicine more as a consequence of the mentioned type of public consultation or rather as an expression of a political will to integrate with Western Europe? Of course, it is not easy to find a simple answer to this question because it is difficult to define what the informed public debate really is. Comparing bioethics debate in different parts of Europe we might think that the reason why some Western European countries have been rather slow to ratify the Convention was most probably related to the fact that these countries have been very sensitive to the discrepancies between the provisions of the Convention and socio-cultural attitudes prevalent in their countries. For example, Germany has expressed concern that the Convention is too liberal (e.g., with respect to biomedical research with persons not able to consent), whereas, for the UK, the Convention seems to be too restrictive (e.g., with respect to research on human embryos).

The attempt to evaluate different bioethics institutions might also provoke some critical remarks. First, due to the lack of published material available, it is quite difficult to collect the information about actual functioning of national bioethics bodies and hospital ethics committees in Central and Eastern Europe. Second, even if these institutions should have been established following the legal provisions already implemented in the countries of the region, there are some doubts if health care professionals feel these bioethics bodies are really needed. For example, according to the Hungarian authors, it is likely that hospital ethics committees most often "nicely exist in paper but not in reality" (Blasszauer and Kismodi 2001). Somewhat similar observations have been also expressed about the performance of national bioethics bodies. As has been frankly admitted by Czech commentators, their Central Ethics Committee has not been a very prestigious body and neither the Ministers of Health, nor the ordinary doctors feel the necessity of the committee as an advisory body (Simek et al. 2000). That is why it seems the institutions mentioned need a further effort and impetus to become real facilitators of bioethics discourse in the region.

The reason why bioethics entities do not always meet a genuine need for their existence might be that they were "imported" from Western countries into the Central and Eastern European societies without taking into account that "medical ethics" still has quite a different meaning in different socio-cultural contexts. For example, in Central and Eastern Europe the activities of established bioethics institutions, especially hospital ethics committees, have had very different functions from their American counterparts, because of quite different interpretations of "medical ethics" prevalent in the countries of the region. As has been revealed by the study of hospital ethics committees in Lithuania, "medical ethics" is often conceptualized as a deontology of professional rules of conduct, which is not what modern medical ethics or bioethics means in the United States. The cases most often reported and dealt with by hospital ethics committees have usually not been difficult end-of-life decisions, refusals to accept life-saving interventions, or controversial cases of allocating scarce biomedical resources (the cases usually referred to American hospital ethics committees) but rather intraprofessional disputes among health care providers, conflicts between health care practitioners and patients in cases of negligent behavior, malpractice, or bribery (Gefenas 2001b).

To sum up, at least in some Central and Eastern European countries medical ethics is still perceived as a mixture of "legalistic deontology" (used to cope with managerial or legal health care delivery problems) (see Chapter 32) and traditional Hippocratic ethics (see Chapters 23 and 24). We might also call a combination of these features a "traditional medical deontology." If, however, we conceptualize bioethics as a critical reflection on moral values and norms directing the development of life sciences and, in particular, influencing the delivery of health care, we might end up with the skeptical conclusion that bioethics is still at the crossroad to find its place in the European transition societies. To facilitate the development of bioethics, teaching and research programs should be strengthened at universities and medical schools of the region. Much more intensive cooperation between Central and Eastern Europeans involved in bioethics would also be mostly needed. For this purpose the Central and Eastern Association of Bioethics (CEEAB) was established in 1999.

V. THE DISTINCTIVENESS OF BIOETHICS IN CENTRAL AND EASTERN EUROPE

It might be claimed that the development of bioethics in Central and Eastern Europe has not brought any

innovations to the field and simply repeats the story of Western bioethics. The term, "Western bioethics," when used to describe the main trends of developing bioethics in the countries of the region, is, however, a rather ambiguous concept. For example, the distinction has been made between the European and American approaches to bioethics. It has been argued that, despite political differences among European states, the health policy shared by Europeans is based on egalitarian values in contrast to a basically libertarian American approach (ten Have 1998). Is it really the case that emerging bioethics discourse in Central and Eastern Europe might be affiliated with a Western European approach?

This question arises because, in theory, both European national law and relevant international documents are based on an egalitarian model of resource allocation, although in practice the egalitarian principles of distributive justice are not followed in the countries of the region. For example, the Bioethics Convention, which has been signed by the majority of the Council of Europe countries and which is already binding in many European transition societies, explicitly refers to "equitable access to health care" (Council of Europe 1997a, 1997b). The package of health care services is strikingly different in different parts of Europe however. It could be claimed that, in most of the Central and Eastern European countries, the upper limit of an available health care package would probably not encompass the bottom portion of what is regarded as an "adequate" health care package in the affluent societies of Western Europe. This is understandable, given the fact that, on average, health care resources in the region amount to less than one tenth of the resources allocated to health care in most Western European countries (Gefenas 2001a).

What is even more worrying, however, is that egalitarian principles are not followed in the domestic health policies of many countries in the region. Recent data revealed that in Lithuania, households in the top 10 percent of income bracket spend twenty times more on health care than the bottom ten percent of households (Report on Human Social Development in Lithuania 1998). The economic and political reality in the region at present is that access to health care is very much a function of the ability to pay and therefore amounts to a libertarian type of health care, despite the fact that equitable access is still declared as a priority in the official health policy documents. Such a situation contrasts sharply with that in the more affluent societies of Western Europe, which to a significant extent provide their citizens with comprehensive and equitable access to health care. That is why the distinction between European bioethics as egalitarian and American bioethics as libertarian (Wulff 1998) is not strictly applicable to Central and Eastern European societies that are still in transition. The reality of access to health care is at least paradoxical in societies that have explicitly declared the principles of equality and solidarity as fundamental in all spheres of public life.

Another popular distinction between American and European bioethics is supposed to be related to the claim that Europeans reject the historical importance of autonomy in bioethics (Marshall, Thomasma, and Bergsma 1998). It should be stressed again that from the perspective of the countries of Central and Eastern Europe, respect for personal autonomy is to be regarded as a principle of paramount importance. It is understandable why many Western, especially European bioethicists are critical of a minimalist libertarian concept of personal autonomy and stress its limits for health care ethics. They represent the perspective of a society that now takes for granted that the principle of informed consent is not only enforced by legal documents but is also followed in everyday practice.

The situation in Central and Eastern Europe is quite different. The practice and culture of respect for personal autonomy are not yet integrated into decision making in health care (Thomsen et al. 1993), because the values and principles of free and democratic society were heavily suppressed during the decades of totalitarian regime. Respect for personal autonomy was regarded as secondary to the "best interests of the society" and, as emphasized previously, every act of self-determination was severely punished, indirectly enforcing paternalistic attitudes in health care. In this quite different political and social context, replacing traditional paternalism should be seen not only as a safeguard against abuse of patients' rights but also as part of a wider social and political effort to develop a broader understanding of the respect for persons. Ethical concerns about the limitations of a minimalist account of personal autonomy justifiably have less weight in bioethics in Central and Eastern Europe.

VI. CONCLUSION

The concepts, practices, and institutions of American and Western European bioethics cannot be directly transferred to the post-Communist societies of Central and Eastern Europe. The main task of bioethics for the region might be seen as developing a critical dialogue between the discourses of "Western bioethics" and a "traditional medical

deontology" still influential among health care practitioners in the post-Communist countries of the region. This is the way to develop bioethics that will be sensitive to the socio-cultural context of the region and thus avoid unnecessary and even unhelpful cross-cultural comparisons.

NOTES

1. Central Ethics Commission on Drug Trials of the Ministry of Health in Bulgaria, Central Ethics Committee at the Ministry of Health in Czech Republic, Estonian Council on Bioethics at the Ministry of Social Affairs, National Bioethics Commission in Hungary, Central Medical Ethics Committee of Latvia, Lithuanian Bioethics Committee, Bioethics Commissions at the Ministry of Health in Poland, National Bioethics Commission in Romania, National Ethics Committee in Slovak Republic, National Medical Ethics Committee in Slovenia. For updated lists of bioethics commissions and research ethics committees in accession states see the following websites:

http://ec.europa.eu/research/biosociety/bioethics/bioethics_ethics_en.htm

http://www.drze.de:80/links/Ethikkommissionen?la = en

http://www.privireal.org/content/rec/countries.php

2. As of the end of 2002 there were only two institutes from CEE in the list of EACME (www.eacmeb.com): the Department of Bioethics of the Institute of Behavioural Sciences at Semmelweis University of Medicine (Budapest, Hungary), and the Center for Bioethics at the Institute of Philosophy and Theology (Zagreb, Croatia).

3. There is, for example, a 2-year postgraduate course in Bioethics, Faculty of Law, Warsaw University (Poland); Center for Bioethics of the Department of Medical Sciences at the Institute for the History and Philosophy of Science, Croatian Academy of Sciences and Arts; Chair of Bioethics at the Catholic University of Lublin (Poland) and some others.

4. Such institutions include Institute for Medical Humanities at the First Faculty of Medicine and Institute of Medical Ethics and Nursing at the Third Faculty of Medicine (both at Charles University in Prague, Czech Republic), the above mentioned Department of Bioethics of the Institute of Behavioral Sciences at Semmelweis University of Medicine (Budapest, Hungary), the Department of Medical History and Ethics of the Institute of Public Health at Medical Faculty of Vilnius University (Lithuania), the Department for Ethics and Philosophy of Medicine of the Chair of Psychiatry at Medical Academy in Lodz, the Department of Philosophy and Bioethics at the Jagiellonian University Medical College (both in Poland), and many others.

CHAPTER 42

THE DISCOURSES OF BIOETHICS IN LATIN AMERICA

José Alberto Mainetti

I. INTRODUCTION

Bioethics was born in the United States (see Chapter 38) and with time adopted (and adapted) by other countries. Among the countries accepting bioethics were those in Latin America, the name given to a linguistic and cultural community encompassing South America, Central America, Mexico, and part of the Caribbean. Because bioethics is a discipline whose discourse flourished in a North American cultural tradition, it is natural to compare Latin American and North American biomedical ethics. Latin American bioethics has evolved over a period of 30 years, in three decade-long stages, commencing in the 1970s, reception, assimilation, and re-creation. As a pioneer of the process by which bioethics was institutionalized in Argentina, I cannot avoid some personal reference to my own experience, as a testifying witness (Mainetti 1987, 1990, 1995, 1996). Such an autobiographical narrative about the emergence of bioethics in Latin America can be justified by the comment of a well-known American bioethicist who said: "Identifying the origin of bioethics in the United States is a matter of some considerable controversy. But the Latin American bioethics story is to a large degree the story of one man" (Drane 1996).

II. RECEPTION OF BIOETHICS IN THE 1970s

The 1970s were the reception stage for bioethics in Latin America. "Reception" should not be understood as a formal introduction of the discipline because in the 1970s the term "bioethics" was not in current usage, even in the United States. Instead, "reception" refers to how the cultural and historical situation in the region made possible or impeded the inception of bioethics. The 1970s were characterized by reaction, either resistance or rejection, to this new movement by those who adhered to a traditional civic and professional ethos. As a liberal and secular morality, bioethics promoted patient autonomy, introducing the idea of the patient as a moral subject into medicine and emphasizing the patient's role as a rational and free agent, whose decisions are central to the therapeutic relationship. These ideas were alien to the old medical ethics still reigning in Latin America. At that time, Latin American medical ethics remained confessional, following the moral doctrine and authority of Roman Catholicism, and paternalistic (see Chapter 14 on Roman Catholicism). Physicians practice according to Max Weber's "domination role," in which the physician's authority is paramount and the patient's role is to submit to the physician's authority (Macklin and Luna 1996).

Initially, bioethics was perceived primarily as "made in the USA," an American approach appropriate to American-style medicine and health care. American ideas, moreover, were bound to meet resistance because Marxist, anti-American attitudes were deeply entrenched in Latin America. Bioethics could not just be transplanted into the Latin American context without taking into account cultural and political differences and the meaning that "bioethics" would consequently have to change in those particular societies.

Argentina pioneered the reception of bioethics in Latin America.

> The first Ibero-American Bioethics Program was established in Argentina at the Institute for Medical Humanities of the José María Mainetti Foundation (1969). Dr. José Alberto Mainetti founded the Institute in 1972 and played an important role in the early bioethics activities in the Region. Later, educational programs were developed through a Latin American School for Bioethics, under the direction of Juan Carlos Tealdi. Over the years many scholars from the United States have participated in this project. The Center has published the journal *Quirón* since 1970, and has produced several monographs on medical ethics. (Figueroa and Fuenzalida 1996, 613)

This Institute fostered Latin American bioethical studies, under the influence of the Spanish School of the History of Medicine, led by Pedro Laín Entralgo, the patriarch of Ibero-American medical humanism. Laín Entralgo's history of medicine provides a way toward a theory of medicine based on philosophical medical anthropology, which is inspired by European existential and hermeneutic philosophy. This intellectual movement created favorable conditions for the reception of the American medical humanities movement in Latin American bioethics.

The first decade of the Argentinean Institute for Medical Humanities records the reception stage of these disciplines, spurred in part by personal and institutional intercourse initiated with the physician and philosopher, H. Tristram Engelhardt, Jr., who was then at the Institute for the Medical Humanities of the University of Texas Medical Branch in Galveston, and the physician bioethicist, Edmund Pellegrino, who was Director of the influential Institute of Human Values in Medicine, based in Washington DC. This medical humanities connection explains why Argentina and Spain were the first countries to start bioethics in Latin America and Europe, respectively.

The medical humanities movement, in search of medical humanism, was much in tune with Laín Entralgo's medical anthropology, whose school of thought I joined, along with many other scholars in Latin America (Escobar 1996). The reception of bioethics as part of the theoretical perspective of the medical humanities therefore means to us a *critical* attitude in the sense of challenging hidden assumptions and value judgments in both medicine and bioethics. During the 1970s, "post-modern medicine" emerged as a critique of positivistic medical reasoning. This criticism was far reaching and affected the object, method, and end of medicine itself. That is, medicine was no longer a "normal science" in the Kuhnian sense but was in the midst of a moral revolution. A critical literature about medicine emerged, including Ivan Illich's famous *Medical Nemesis* (Illich 1976a, 1976b), Ian Kennedy's iconoclastic Reith lectures, *The Unmasking of Medicine* (Kennedy 1981), and the critical social analysis of capitalist medical power by American writers like Vicente Navarro (Navarro 1975; see also Chapter 39).

"Post-modern medicine" owes its relativism to its increasingly comprehensive, interpretive, and evaluative nature, in short, to its reflectiveness. The philosophy of medicine encompasses medical anthropology, epistemology, and axiology. The latter study would include bioethics in both its clinical and public health aspects. In this way, in Latin America we approached bioethics as the new humanist medical paradigm, and primarily an ethics "implied in" rather than "applied to" medicine, that is an ethics derived from the intrinsic axiology of the medical profession. Thus, in contrast to the American development of bioethics, which involved physicians, theologians, philosophers and lawyers, the Latin American protagonists of the discipline were mainly physicians and other health care professionals.

III. ASSIMILATION OF BIOETHICS IN THE 1980s

Assimilation marks the second stage in the development of bioethics in Latin America. The academic discipline and public discourse became institutionalized throughout the region and in this respect followed the American model. With the restoration of democracy and introduction in Latin America of new medical technologies, such as critical care, transplantation, and assisted reproduction, public and academic interest in bioethics expanded in the 1980s. Assimilation reflected American bioethics in two ways. First, increasing malpractice litigation in medical cases and the movement for patient's rights imitated factors that led to the birth of bioethics in the United States. Second, with the restoration of democracy came a renewed interest in moral and political philosophy, as well as ideological pluralism and consensus formation, which were then applied to medicine and became key components of the new bioethics, as in the United States (Lolas Stepke 2000a).

In 1980, the Mainetti Foundation launched a second stage of the institutionalization of bioethics, in two academic settings, the medical school and the philosophy department at the nearby La Plata National University. The postgraduate chair of medical humanities provides the opportunity for reflection on a philosophy of medicine as a post-Flexnerian philosophy of the art of healing, rather than a reductionist model. Flexner's model involved the old positivist medical paradigm of medicine restricted to applied natural sciences. Latin American bioethics rejected this approach and turned to a new humanist medical paradigm that employed the social sciences and humanities to develop a theory and practice of medicine. In the 1980s, we continued to assimilate bioethics into the present philosophy of medicine. The chair of philosophical anthropology introduced bioethics as a cultural phenomenon, that is, the conception of a biological revolution that transformed human nature, and a new civic morality about health care.

The late 1980s witnessed the blooming of bioethics centers, institutes, and professionals in the field around the region. The Instituto Colombiano de Estudios Bioéticos (Bogotá, Colombia) was founded in 1985, encouraged by the remarkable teaching of Alfonso Llano Escobar, S.J., from the Universidad Javeriana. In Venezuela, Dr. Augusto León C., who wrote a classical text on medical ethics in 1975, was responsible for the article on bioethics in Latin America found in the first edition of the *Encyclopedia of Bioethics* (Leon C. 1978). The Universidad Católica de Chile created a bioethics unit in the School of Medicine in 1988, and several physicians participated in this program, notably Drs. Alejandro Serani and Manuel Lavados. The Pontificia Universidad Católica de Rio Grande do Sul, in Porto Alegre, Brazil, established a postgraduate program in bioethics in 1988, headed by Joaquim Clotet, a philosopher from Barcelona, Spain.

A radical stage of bioethics assimilation followed the critical reception stage in Latin America. Latin American bioethics' radical nature goes beyond philosophy of medicine to become a philosophy of culture and technology, moving from metamedicine to metaethics in seeking a fundamental questioning of technoscience. The novelty and seriousness of the problems concerning life today shape a bioethical crisis of the technological era. In this vital and normative crisis three new themes appear to be interwoven: (1) the ecological catastrophe, (2) the biological revolution, and (3) the medicalization of life. Bioethics became possible as a result of far-reaching changes in our understanding of the human condition and our increasing ability to transform the human body. From its very beginning the Latin American road to bioethics has been a quest for the human, in the sense of a search for the basis of bioethics in philosophical anthropology centered in the new capacity to alter the body and to create an alternative morality (Drane 1996, 1999).

IV. THE RE-CREATION OF BIOETHICS IN THE 1990s

In the 1990s, a Latin American bioethics re-created itself in ways that incorporate the region's own intellectual and moral traditions. In most countries of the region the bioethics movement is organized in the three areas, academic (scientific research and higher education), health care (clinical and public health consultation, as in hospital ethics committees), and health policy (advisory services and recommendations to public authorities on normative and regulative issues). Concurrently with each nationwide bioethics network, regional associations have developed and propelled the Latin American bioethics movement forward. As a result, a distinctive regional ethical identity has developed into the Latin American bioethical model.

Founded in 1990, the Latin American School of Bioethics (ELABE) of the Mainetti Foundation is the first initiative of academic work in our area of cultural influence. This is a training program to create human resources for leadership of the discipline in the countries of participants' origin, while providing a forum for cultural and scientific exchange throughout the region. The International Course of Bioethics of the ELABE during the 1990s was chaired by prominent professors from the leading international centers of the discipline. The Centro Oncológico de Excelencia (Mainetti Foundation) launched the Federación Latinoamericana de Bioética in December 1991.

In 1990, James Drane of the United States was commissioned by the Pan American Health Organization (PAHO) to visit several countries in Latin America and to produce a report that reviewed the development of bioethics in Latin America. This influential report proposed several steps for the further regional development of the discipline (Drane and Fuenzalida 1991). In the same year, PAHO published a special issue on bioethics, edited by Susan Scholle Connor and Hernán Fuenzalida-Puelma, formally introducing bioethics in Latin America (Scholle and Fuenzalida 1990). This is the first collection in which early authors in the field address diverse topics and set out different perspectives on the discipline. Finally, PAHO, a pioneer among international health organizations, created the Regional Program on Bioethics (1994), whose headquarters is in Santiago de Chile, but whose activities are decentralized to serve all the member countries of PAHO. This program, designed to be a comprehensive policy in bioethics and its associate disciplines, is in a new stage, under the leadership of the outstanding scholar, Fernando Lolas Stepke's Programa Regional de Bioética (2000).

The re-creation stage reveals a third feature of Latin American bioethics, its global concern. Bioethics is encyclopedic by definition, etymologically "ethics of life" (and "life of ethics"), but not semantically circumscribed to the technological *bios* and the liberal *ethos* characteristic of the North American model. In contrast, the Latin American model emphasizes a human *bios* and a communitarian *ethos*. That is why bioethics is now more of a political movement or social reform movement than an academic discipline restricted to the domain of health care (see also Chapter 40). In Latin American bioethics, the principles of solidarity and justice play the central role that autonomy plays in North American bioethics. Thus, Latin American health policies embrace universal access to health care and stress distributive justice and equity in health resources allocation.

This is not the place for a survey of bioethical developments in different Latin American countries or for a review of the bioethical problems peculiar to the region. (Mainetti, Pis Diez and Tealdi, 1992; Tealdi, Pis Diez, and Esquisabel 1995). Bioethics has become a field of new challenges in Latin America. A seeming uniformity hides a rich, heterogeneous set of activities. Not only European and Christian influences, but also indigenous intellectual traditions are very important in the development of Latin American bioethics. It does not have its own philosophy, as Anglo-American bioethics is perceived to have, but it does have its own literature and narrative style. The particular historical setting, cultural ethos, and social reality of Latin America could infuse new life into the global bioethics community. In this sense, a symptom of the new times is the fact that the Second Congress of the International Association of Bioethics took place in Buenos Aires, Argentina, in 1994, and the Sixth Congress was held in Brasilia, Brazil, in 2002. A "new Brazilian bioethics" or "hard bioethics" began to flourish in recent years, and inspired by the country's contradictory social reality, explores alternative perspectives to traditional bioethical currents (Garrafa 2000).

V. CONCLUSION

This chapter has provided an account of the development of the incorporation of bioethics in Latin America over the past three decades, depicting this development in terms of three stages, reception, assimilation and re-creation. Bioethics first arrived as a foreigner and then underwent a cultural transformation. Transplanted to a land that was not its "natural" habitat, bioethics in Latin America has now taken on its own distinctive character and voice and has become a strong intellectual and political enterprise (Lolas Stepke 1994, 1998).

In comparison to the North American style of bioethics, Latin American bioethics takes a more theoretical and philosophical approach. As a search for a critical, radical and global bioethics, Latin American bioethics represents a global, "post-bioethical" age (Drane 1988; Spinsanti 1995). Although Latin American bioethics is far from being a unified theoretical system or a single coherent perspective, it represents the *ethica spes* (ethical hope) of the new millennium.

CHAPTER 43

THE DISCOURSES OF BIOETHICS IN EAST ASIA

Ruiping Fan and Jiro Nudeshima

I. INTRODUCTION

This chapter provides an account of the emergence of bioethics in China and Japan, both as a critique of their conventional medical ethics and as a movement within their medical ethics traditions. It addresses three main themes: (1) clinical decisions in the context of traditional physician paternalism, familism,[1] and contemporary patient self-determination, (2) attitudes toward new medical interventions based on advanced medical technologies, and (3) health care system reform. This chapter will use these themes as heuristic examples to explore the development of bioethics, the understanding of bioethics, and the interaction between bioethics and traditional medical ethics in China and Japan.

II. PHYSICIAN PATERNALISM, FAMILISM, AND PATIENT SELF-DETERMINATION

During 1966–1976, due to the totalitarian restriction of the so-called cultural revolution,[2] most Chinese scholars knew little of academic research in the humanities and social sciences made outside of mainland China. Only after China's new policy of reform and opening up in the late 1970s, Western (particularly American) bioethics, together with other contemporary Western inquiries such

as psychology, sociology, and philosophy of science, came to be noticed by Chinese academia. Since that time, increasing numbers of bioethical conferences and publications have occurred in China. A Chinese professional journal called *Medicine and Philosophy* was established in 1980, which dedicated a major portion of its each issue to articles regarding ethical issues in health care. The journal also covers translation of Western bioethical papers into Chinese. In 1988, the first monograph on bioethics in the Chinese language appeared in China (Qiu 1988).

In the early 1980s, many Chinese scholars misunderstood bioethics as a subject that specifically uses newly proposed ethical principles (such as Tom Beauchamp and James Childress's four principles: autonomy, beneficence, nonmaleficence, and justice (Beauchamp and Childress 1979, 2001)) to deal with the ethical issues arising from the application of advanced technologies in biomedical practice. At the same time they attempted to maintain their conventional Socialist principle of medical ethics, the so-called revolutionary humanism, to guide bioethical explorations. It did not take long for them to recognize that bioethical inquiries are not limited to the issues regarding high technologies. Bioethical concerns involve a much larger and broader social and ethical scope that cannot be severed from deep-rooted moral traditions. Significantly, they have recognized that both Beauchamp and Childress' principles and their Socialist principle are abstract and ambiguous, without being rooted in any deep moral or cultural tradition. They have started to reflect on the long-standing Chinese medical ethical traditions and contemporary Western liberal bioethics from a comparative perspective. The prominent event in this regard was the publication in 1998 of a new Chinese journal titled *International Journal of Chinese and Comparative Philosophy of Medicine* (first through Swets and Zeitlinger Publishers and then via Global Scholarly Publications), with its mission set for facilitating in-depth dialogue between China and the West regarding bioethical issues.

Ethical issues around physician paternalism, familism, and patient self-determination serve as heuristic examples in this regard. On the one hand, it is generally recognized that the physician is obliged to provide necessary information and obtain consent from the patient and the family before conducting a medical intervention. A Chinese book about the patient's rights has been popular (Qiu, Zhuo, and Feng 1996). On the other hand, more and more scholars have become aware of the cultural difference between Chinese and Westerners regarding the practice of informed consent (Fan 1997; Guo et al., 1998; Cui 1999). Although the practice of direct informed consent from the patient has been one of the revolutionary developments in Western medical practice since the 1980s and although the principle has clear merits in the West, its implementation in Chinese societies has encountered considerable difficulties and dilemmas. Under traditional Chinese familism, the patient is always taken to be a patient in the family. Medical decisions are thus made by the whole family for the patient (see Chapter 11). For instance, instead of seeking a signature directly from the patient for giving consent to a surgery, the Chinese way is to obtain a signature by a family representative on behalf of the whole family, including the patient himself or herself (Fan 1999). The Chinese understanding is that the patient is weak and uncomfortable and should be left to relax and rest, without the burden of having to explore the course of treatment with the physician. This practice is not taken to be depriving the patient of the right of self-determination. Rather, it is taken to be undertaking the fiduciary obligation of the family to care for an ill family member. Chinese do not want to change this practice to the direct informed consent. As a result, a current challenge for Chinese bioethics is how to find an appropriate way in which Chinese familism can be preserved in health care and at the same time reject physician paternalism.

In Japan, the ethical reconsideration of the medical setting and physician–patient relationship began in the 1970s and spread into reality and administration in the 1980s. Truth telling and terminal care, euthanasia, and organ transplantation were the key issues. Since 1982,

medical schools have started to set up institutional review boards called "ethics committees" to govern human subjects research. In 1984–1985 the Ministry of Health and Welfare for the first time set up an ad-hoc advisory committee for bioethical issues. In 1987, a Japanese Association of Bioethics was established (Kimura 1995; Yonemoto 1988).

The traditional Japanese moral system has been formed on a sophisticated net of familial and communitarian relationships. It is not grounded in one specific religious tradition: Shinto, Buddhism, or Confucianism (Yanakita 1970; see also Chapter 22). Given this religious array, Japan is quite different from China and Korea, both of which built up their societies primarily on Confucian values. In the traditional Japanese moral system, it was family members, not the patient himself or herself, who were told of a serious diagnosis and were consulted for next step choices, especially in the case of an end-stage disease. Hard decisions were made by physicians based on the families' wishes. In a moral sense, physician paternalism was based on familial decision making; however, such a traditional moral system has been changed. Through urbanization and the increase in nuclear families since 1960s, the tight bonds of large, extended families were weakened, sometimes even destroyed, in Japanese society. As a consequence, claiming that family decision making justifiably restricts individual self-determination in the medical setting (e.g., in withdrawing life-sustaining treatment in terminal care or determining to donate organs after death) is no longer persuasive (Nudeshima 1991).

Although the Ministry of Health provides physician licensure through the national examination, Japan does not have a medical professional body, comparable to the American Medical Association, that offers disciplinary codes of ethics for doctors. This may be the most striking difference between Japan and Western countries in medical ethics. Due to this difference, those professional guidelines that are promulgated concerning controversial medical procedures are not necessarily followed by all professionals. Thus, the Japanese public is not content to trust medical ethical issues in the hands of the medical profession (Nudeshima 1997).

In short, Japanese people find themselves unable to rely on either traditional "familism" or physician paternalism. On the other hand, they cannot live up to the newly emerged Western self-determination/self-responsibility ideology, because it is not strong enough yet (see Leflar 1996).

III. ATTITUDES TOWARD NEW MEDICAL TECHNOLOGIES

Although Chinese culture has no general objection to the use of new medical technologies, there has been controversy regarding what laws should be made to regulate new technologies, such as organ transplantation, critical care, and research using embryos. For instance, some argue that the process of organ donation and transplantation must be transparent to the public, whereas others believe confidentiality is necessary (Zhang 1996). Many advocate legalizing euthanasia and physician-assisted suicide, while quite a few are strongly opposed to it (Lo 1998; Dong and Wang 1998; Yu and Shi 1998). Finally, people disagree regarding what moral appeals, principles, or theories should be used to address the ethical dimensions of newly developed reproductive technologies and research, such as gene studies and human cloning. Should traditional moral values and visions be appealed to for direction? Or should a modern materialistic scientific view be the right measure for such issues (Chan 1998; Fan 1998)?

In Japan, both the medical profession and the general public hold an ethically inconsistent attitude toward new advanced medical technologies. A typical example is organ transplantation (see also Chapter 62). Since 1980, the fiercest Japanese bioethical controversy has been over whether to accept brain death criteria to determine that an individual patient has died (see also Chapter 63). This debate was linked to the issue of organ transplantation. In 1997, the Organ Transplant Act was finally enacted, but it permits the brain death criteria to be applied only to those who have consented to donate organs. For anyone else, the traditional cardiovascular criteria of death is applied. This legislation reflects the hesitation of many Japanese to let transplant surgeons remove organs from brain-dead patients. The Act has no articles regulating removal of organs and tissues from living persons, although the kidney and partial liver transplantations in Japan rely mostly on living donors. Legally, brain-dead patients are protected by rigorous restrictions on organ removal, whereas living persons are left unprotected.

Reproductive and regenerative technologies have also joined the bioethics agenda in Japan. Although human reproductive cloning is legally banned by the Human Cloning Regulation Act of 2000 and human embryonic stem cell research is regulated by administrative guidelines promulgated in 2001, other reproductive technologies, such as in vitro fertilization and microinjection of sperm into the oocyte, and other types of human embryo research are not regulated publicly. Japan would be the first among developed countries to authorize human embryonic stem cell research without any regulation on human embryo research at large. This reflects the fact that Japanese people are rather indifferent to the issue of the moral or legal status of human embryo (Nudeshima 2001).

These examples suggest that the Japanese notion of personhood is peculiar. It does not regard an embryo as a person although recognizing the brain dead as maintaining the status of a person. These contradictions are manifested in everyday case-by-case decisions. It is difficult to discern a consistent notion of personhood based on any established belief system.

IV. Reform of Health Care System

Bioethics brought intensive attention to the issues of justice in health care allocation, which has generally been overlooked by traditional medical ethics (see Chapter 38). Health care justice has become a focus of current Chinese bioethical studies. China has a population of approximately 1.2 billion, with very small health care expenditures. For instance, in 1995, the percentage of gross domestic product spent on health care was only 3.88 percent, with per capita spending approximately twelve US dollars. Up to the year 2000, approximately 15 percent of the population was covered by health services financed through public resources (since 2000 they have begun to share their medical care cost under a savings account under the current urban health care reform), whereas the rest, mostly farmers in the countryside, had to self-pay. This is to say, approximately 1 billion Chinese people do not have any health insurance, whether public or private. Many Western bioethicists argue for "equal health care" for everyone in a state. This sounds attractive and fair to the ears of many Chinese. On the other hand, Chinese bioethicists have recognized that equality may not be an appropriate ideal for Chinese health care reform. An urgent issue is: what ideal should be upheld to guide China's health care reform? Should it be the ideal of equal health care? Chinese bioethicists invite us to notice some basic facts in today's China: China includes areas of diverse geographical, social, and economic situations, and it displays a huge economic gap between urban and rural areas. Per capita income in 1995 was 500 US dollars in urban areas and approximately 200 U.S. dollars in rural areas. Average per capita health spending in 1995 was twenty U.S. dollars in urban areas and six U.S. dollars in rural areas. Surprisingly, per capita expense per day in the intensive care unit of Beijing Medical University teaching hospital was 200 US dollars. This is to say that the 1-day cost of the intensive care unit for one patient equals the 1-year income of a Chinese farmer. Thus, an appropriate policy for Chinese health care reform cannot be to emphasize developing high-technology medicine or expensive critical care for everyone; rather, it should emphasize disease prevention and the ordinary means of health promotion. More public health care resources should be invested in rural areas, and at the same time should not attempt to implement a policy of equalizing health care in different areas (Cong 1998; Du 1999; Luo 1999).

In Japan, most hospitals have been developed from small clinics since the late nineteenth century and are still privately managed today. In 1993, only 18 percent of the Japanese hospitals were publicly owned. On the other hand, there has been a national universal health insurance system since 1961. Hence, Japanese health care is privately supplied and publicly paid. This approach has provided the Japanese people with good access to high-quality health care (Ikegami and Campbell 1996).

In such a structure, the Japanese health care policy has long focused on prices paid by the national insurance for medical practices and drugs. This has always involved negotiations between health care providers (represented by the Japanese Medical Association) and health care payers (represented by the Ministry of Health). Health care reform has also focused on price reduction, especially for health care for the aged. Issues concerning new devices and technologies, even those that raise thorny ethical debates, such as organ transplantation, have usually been introduced through discussion of pricing decisions, rather than scientific assessment or ethical considerations (Hiroi 1996). In fact, the problem is that the Japanese health care system is not and cannot be controlled by either the government or the market. Consumer politics is very weak in Japan. So is the patient rights movement. This may be a disadvantage of the mixed public–private health care structure in which citizens as health care consumers have a very small role to play. This will continue to be an important topic for Japanese bioethics to explore.

NOTES

1. The family has a central place in the Confucian way of life. From the Confucian understanding, a normal human cannot exist alone – his true nature must be embodied in appropriate human relations, namely, in familial relations. Metaphysically, Confucian familism holds that ultimately the family exists as the primary human community. Morally, the fundamental Confucian virtue (*ren*) must be first and foremost exercised within the family. It cannot be practiced as an egalitarian requirement of love. Rather, *ren* requires love according to the nature of relationships. In practice, one must follow the Confucian guidelines of "love with distinction" or "love by gradation" regulated by the Confucian rituals. Simply put, one must love one's family members first and love them more than others. From the Confucian perspective of *ren*, it is improper for one to love a stranger as one's relative, or a remote relative as one would a close family member. In health care, Confucian familism advocates family responsibility (rather than individual responsibility) for every family member's health care, including a model of family-shared decision making for the patient.

2. The Great Proletarian Cultural Revolution (1966–1976) was instigated by the Chinese communist leader Mao Zedong (1893–1976) as his last effort to destroy all capitalist, feudalist, and revisionist trends in China. It was an extremely tragic period for the Chinese people and their civilization. The whole period was marked by the horrible events of social upheaval, personal vendettas, violence, massive youth movements, and extreme ideological pressure. Schools were closed. Scholars and students were sent to farms to work and be re-educated to get rid of bourgeois influences on them. Mao's power reached its apex during this period when a cult of personality was born in the symbolism of a little red book consisting of his quotations, ubiquitous buttons that bore his portrait, and statues edifying him that were raised near any buildings of social significance across the land. At the same time, all traditional values were ruthlessly attacked and historical relics destroyed (Confucius' tomb and temple included). A great number of intellectuals, celebrities, and others were persecuted and lost their lives. Its damage inflicted on Chinese civilization is unbelievable and unrecoverable.

CHAPTER 44

THE DISCOURSES OF BIOETHICS IN SOUTH ASIA

Katherine K. Young

I. INTRODUCTION

The region of South Asian includes India, Nepal, Sri Lanka, Pakistan, and Bangladesh. This chapter will focus on India and Sri Lanka to provide examples of the transition from traditional Hindu and Buddhist medical ethics, which once dominated the region to contemporary bioethics. Many of the topics of modern South Asian bioethics are foreshadowed in traditional medical ethics. These include an understanding of well-being that integrates body, mind, and environment (although the modern version focuses not just on the patient but also on patient's rights). Whereas autonomy had its precedent in concepts such as the law of karma, it was generally muted because of the group orientation of traditional South Asian societies; in the modern period, autonomy increases and with it choice and informed consent. The same might be said for privacy and confidentiality; we find precedents but they become emphasized in the modern period. Whereas regulation of physicians was a concern in the past, it has become even more so today. Because hierarchy prevailed in premodern societies, access and justice become important topics for modern bioethics.

Consciousness-raising about the importance of bioethics has occurred in part through international collaborations and forums concerned with improving health care and ethics in developing countries. The European Union has helped a hospital in Chennai, India, develop its ethics policies and several medical schools in Norway have helped establish ethics programs in Sri Lankan medical schools. The World Health Organization has been active in the region to develop research, teaching, and public awareness about bioethics as well as to establish a regional network of experts on the topic. It reports that discussions of health ethics have been influenced by the colonial legacy, which marginalized the traditional systems of medical ethics when modern, Western medicine was introduced. Today discussions of health ethics in the region have been fostered by Christian missionary medical schools, the World Bank, and others. Research ethics is somewhat developed; teaching medical ethics, which generally occurs in departments of forensic medicine and focuses on malpractice, is still in its infancy (Kasturiaratchi, Lie, and Seeberg 1999).

Nepal, for instance, which had little modern medicine before 1951 because the ruling regime was against it, developed an interest in bioethics alongside the development of democracy. The Nepal Medical Council Act in 1964 provided guidelines for the regulation of physicians;

these were updated in the Code of Ethics 1992, and from 1996 all physicians working in Nepal have had to sign an oath to follow the code. Because physicians were trained in Nepal only from 1978, ethical practice has depended in part on where their training occurred (India, the Soviet Union, Bangladesh, or Pakistan) (Adhikari 1999, 64). Current concerns include malpractice (false claims to titles, inappropriate advertisement, providing false certificates of health and disease for a fee, breaking a patient's confidentiality, illegal abortion, violation of laws, inappropriate fees, recommending treatments to patients who cannot afford them, and "giving information regarding infectious illness in a patient to family members or of an incurable illness to a patient") (Adhikari 1999, 68).

II. MEDICAL ETHICS AND BIOETHICS IN INDIA

Because Buddhism had died out in the land of its birth (and is found today only among a few groups that have converted to Buddhism in modern times), the discussion here will draw on the continuities and changes from traditional Hindu medical ethics and contemporary bioethical ethical reflections by Indians. Buddhism will be discussed in the next section, mainly with reference to Sri Lanka. The two main traditional Hindu medical texts used for this discussion are the *Caraka-saṃhitā* and the *Suśruta-saṃhitā*. The early strata of these (represented by the presumed authors Ātreya and Agniveśa) were written from the third century BCE but were probably built on earlier traditions of empirical medicine in the previous century. Both of these texts likely represented compendiums of schools rather than works by individuals (the word *caraka* literally means "wander" and *suśruta* means "well-heard" or "famous"), a point underscored by the fact that there are internal accounts about parts being lost or added. (This process was ongoing. A redaction of the *Caraka* was made by Dṛḍhabala in the fourth or fifth century CE, and one of the *Suśruta* was done by one Nāgārjuna, who added the sixth and last part of the text, before the sixth century).

After independence in 1947, health initiatives in India were introduced by several 5-year plans with the goal of health for everyone by 2000 through the primary health care approach. The Indian Central government is responsible for a national health policy and the coordination of state health departments. Now India has "one of the largest health care infrastructures in the world" (Verma et al. 1999, 21). In addition, central and state governments in India have been active in the development of family planning, medical education, and drug control (permission from the Drug Controller of India and after that from local ethics committees is needed for clinical trials of drugs developed in India or abroad, the exception being common traditional medicines) (Verma et al. 1999, 40). All this has had dramatic effects in bringing down

the birth rate, the death rate, and the infant mortality rate as well as increasing life expectancy (Verma et al. 1999, 20).

In the following section, the distinctions between traditional Hindu medical ethics and modern bioethics will be discussed with reference to the four principles of bioethics – nonmaleficence, beneficence, autonomy, and justice (Beauchamp and Childress 2001) – the regulation of physicians, and the status of the traditional medical system. (For discussion of Hinduism and abortion, contraception, reproductive technologies – in vitro fertilization, surrogacy, sex selection, cloning, organ transplantation, terminal care, pain relief, and euthanasia see Chapter 3.)

1. Nonmaleficence

Ahiṃsā, which literally means the desire to do no harm/killing (*hiṃsā*), is central to the ideal of nonmaleficence. The ideal of *ahiṃsā* developed only gradually in the history of Hinduism, mainly because killing animals in sacrifice (*yajña*) had been the very center of the ancient Vedic religion: that which upheld the cosmos, not to mention the livelihood of the *brāhmaṇa* priests. Only after critiques of Vedic animal sacrifice by Buddhists and Jains did nonviolence become a key value in some Hindu circles. It appears first, for instance, on Manu's list defining virtues/universal ethical principles (*sāmānya*) *dharma* (see Chapter 10), but even then, practice of sacrifice continued. To deal with this conflict between not killing and killing animals in the sacrificial context, sacrifice was first made an exception to the general principle of noninjury. Over the centuries, sacrifice itself was gradually eliminated in Vedic rituals (leaving other Vedic ingredients such as grains, ghee, and so forth) or the public Vedic sacrifice was replaced altogether by worship (offerings of fruits, flowers, and incense) in temples. In addition, the problem of the moral conflict between sacrificial killing and the common duty of nonkilling was resolved by internalization (meditation on sacrifice rather than its actual performance) or symbolic reinterpretation. Not killing or doing no harm became the moral bottom line. Avoiding evil was more important than doing good as with the Western injunction *primum non nocere*: first, do no harm. The importance of *ahiṃsā* came to be reflected in the elite Hindu predilection for vegetarianism. Exceptions to *ahiṃsā* were still made, however, for individual and communal self-defense as is true of many cultures. Another exception was consumption of meat for medicinal purposes. The practice of *ahiṃsā* became an important criterion to distinguish the true physician from the quack in the classical period. Today, *ahiṃsā* is a key category for one Hindu approach to ethics in general (there are other approaches such as the just war tradition) and medical ethics in particular, thanks to its historical importance and to Gandhi's promotion of it as a general principle during the struggle for Indian independence.

2. Beneficence

Traditional Hinduism placed *beneficence* not in the universal-eternal category of ethics but in the place-specific one (*viśeṣa*). The concept of the good, after all, had to be understood with positive content, which was dependent on a person's "place" defined by variables such as sex, age, caste/subcaste, and so forth, which give rise to specific norms of behavior (see Chapter 9). This might explain why modern ethicists have had difficulty assigning specific content to a "flourishing" life in the sense of universal, positive entitlements. Nevertheless, the concept of beneficence in the modern period in India has been changing to include positive entitlements by the state and affirmative action to improve the material conditions and opportunities for exploited groups This has included the ideal of universal access to health care (see the discussion of justice later).

3. Autonomy

The fact that the group – family (*kula*), subcaste (*jāti*), and caste (*varṇa*) – was primary in the classical Hindu social order suggests a communitarian ethics in which choice was determined by preexisting values and obligations to others within the group was most important. Social relations within these contexts were carefully regulated by minute rules (see the discussion of *viśeṣa-dharma* in Chapter 9). Of course, the system of hierarchy placed some groups at a disadvantage in power relations. Because of this group conformity and hierarchy, the boundaries of the ego were considered weak even within the intimate family (sometimes expressed by the fear of being alone). This fluidity was a matter of concern because it could destabilize health and well-being. If ordinary well-being were defined by a dialectic between constraining social rules and ego hunger for intimate bonding, extraordinary well-being was defined by the categorical removal of the individual from this system of ordinary life. This signaled renunciation and radical (spiritual) autonomy initiated by a rite of dying to the ordinary world and led to a pursuit of liberation within this life by a spiritual path (yoga).

Today governmental and international development projects are addressing the issue of empowerment and support for women and other disadvantaged groups. Sometimes this takes the form of pressure for human rights, but many Asian societies think that extreme notions of autonomy (agency, independence, and rationality that transform personal desires into intentions, acts, and effects), which are often adversarial in approach, belong to the Western value system. By contrast, they argue, Asian societies are based on a group orientation, consensus, responsibilities, and duties as well as religious values such as compassion and altruism. A classical precursor to the ideal of autonomy existed in the individual freedom presupposed by the law of karma. Although this freedom had to work within the constraints of socially prescribed duties, there was danger that conformist ideology, fatalism, and abusive hierarchy could, and for some, did prevail. Nevertheless, *Yajñavālkya-smṛti* (I.349, 351) warned that "fate is nothing but the human effort of past lives manifesting its effect" (cited in Dastidar 1987, 103), and so human effort (*puruṣakāra*) was of the utmost importance. Hindu ethics therefore has been a combination of communitarianism and autonomy perspectives. At its best, this could be described as healthy selfhood within family, society, and the spiritual telos of life. In the modern period, the interest in autonomy has grown, and with it more concern for patient's rights, truth telling, confidentiality, and privacy.

The traditional system was patient-oriented for the purposes of diagnosis (attention to the peculiarities of body, personality, diet, and circumstance) but the prevailing ethical orientation was paternalistic. Today paternalism is giving way in some circles to a patient-oriented medicine and ethic. In 1972, the Medical Council of India published a Code of Medical Ethics (hereafter referred to as "the 1972 Indian Code"), which functions like an oath at the time that physicians are registered. It states that physicians are to attend to the health of the patient as the first consideration and to support community health, especially the prevention of epidemics. Physicians are told, moreover, that they owe a duty in law toward their patients, whether or not there is any contract with the patient.

Patient-oriented medicine and ethics are closely related to issues of choice. Despite its emphasis on the group, choice is now accepted, for instance, as part of modern India's approach to family planning. When forced sterilization was attempted by Indira Gandhi's son Sanjay, her government was promptly thrown out of power. The Indian population is becoming increasingly savvy over concepts of rights. (For some restrictions on abortion and other reproductive choices see Chapter 3.)

Informed consent must be based on the physician's full disclosure of the risks and benefits of the treatment, its alternatives, and its rejection so that a reasoned assessment of all relevant information can be made. In addition, the patient must be competent and free from any pressure by others. Risk assessment and the balance of benefits and risks were rare in premodern Hindu medical ethics for two main reasons: (1) risk is largely a modern concept related to rapid technological change (and the need to assess and prevent "new" harms); and (2) conflicts in traditional Hindu ethics were generally resolved not by quantification but rather by ranking the items according to their merits (otherwise, an irresolvable moral dilemma was acknowledged). Nevertheless, there were some examples of risk assessment in the Āyurvedic (medical) texts (see Chapter 9 for a discussion of Āyurveda). An important one assessed the patient's prognosis from the perspective of the physician: what are the risks to a physician's professional reputation if the patient dies while under his care? In an age of quacks, physicians wanted success stories, which were the best kind of advertisement for their expertise. To determine if a disease were incurable, there was a detailed analysis of the signs of death. In *Caraka-saṃhitā*[1] *Indriyasthānam* (XII.43–61), for instance, there are twelve chapters devoted to a discussion of the signs (*ariṣṭas*) of imminent death consisting of physical changes: "affliction of *prāṇa* (vital breath); clouding of understanding; drainage of strength from limbs; cessation of movements; destruction of sensory faculties; impairment of consciousness; restlessness in the mind; affliction of the mind with fear; deprivation of memory, intellect, natural modesty (*hrī*), and lustre (*srī*) of the body; aggravation of *pāpmā* (diseases caused by sinful acts) . . . cruel dreams," and omens of various kinds.

Alternatively, physicians could treat the incurable if there were public knowledge that the disease was terminal and if the news would not cause a problem for the patient or the relatives: "A physician should not announce the imminence of death without being specially requested for that, even if he is aware of the onset of such bad prognostic signs. Even when specially requested, he should not say anything about the approaching death if such announcement is likely to result in the collapse of the patient or distress of others. The wise physician should however refrain from treating patients having signs of imminent death without making announcement of the approaching death" (*Caraka-saṃhitā Indriyasthānam* VII.43–61).

The refusal to inform the patient about terminal illness, however, would be against the Hindu virtue of truth telling (*satya*) with its underlying rule "tell no lie." It was usually second in the list of universal virtues (*sāmānya*) (see Chapter 9). This posed an apparent conflict between the universal duty to tell the truth and the idea that in the case of a dying person it might cause distress, and therefore harm, which was against the first universal virtue: *ahiṃsā* (literally, being without even *desire* to harm). A way to resolve this moral dilemma was to make the case of not telling the truth about dying an exception to the general rule that the truth must be told. Another way to resolve it, though, was to think about the negative rule form of the virtue: do not lie is not the same as "tell the truth," because one always has the option to keep quiet. Still, it could be argued that it was important for Hindu patients to know the nature of their disease and its prognosis so that they could prepare for death calmly because it is such an important time to influence destiny (see Chapter 9). Many modern, urban, educated Hindus have criticized paternalism and are eager to institute informed consent. For this

reason, they advocate a presumption in favor of full disclosure to the patient. Cultures and religions change as do people. As far as proxy decision making goes, modern Hindus would be inclined to leave decisions to other relatives. "Because of the prevalence of the joint family system, the drawing up of a will as such is not a significant element in Hindu law, but expressions concerning posthumous arrangements for oneself and their proper respect are attested to. Hence, proxy decision-making is eminently acceptable" (Sharma 2002, 5).

The 1972 Indian Code contains instructions for informed consent: "Before performing an operation obtain in writing the consent from the husband or wife, parent or guardian in the case of a minor, or the patient himself as the case may be. In an operation which may result in sterility the consent of both husband and wife is needed" (Item 18). Of course, there is no informed consent in India's underground practice of medicine (especially to obtain organs for international clients). The fact that husbands have been known to volunteer their wives multiplies the culpability (see Chapter 3). Regarding truth telling, the 1972 Indian Code says "the physician should neither exaggerate nor minimize the gravity of a patient's condition. He would assure himself that the patient, his relatives or his responsible friends have such knowledge of the patient's condition as will serve the best interests of the patient and the family" (Item 12).

Choice is a two-way street. Sometimes there is a conflict of values for physicians. It is striking that there is no conscientious objector status for modern Indian physicians: "refusing on religious grounds alone to give assistance in or conduct cases of sterility, birth control, craniotomies on living children, and therapeutic abortions when there is medical indication unless the medical practitioner feels himself/herself incompetent to do so" is not allowed (1972 Indian Code: Item 12).

According to modern reports in India, when the physician and the patient are of comparable status, the relationship between patients and their physicians develops an intimacy. Prakash Desai observes, "The family physician is drawn into an intimate orbit, made into a kind of honorary family member. The physician becomes a counselor and advisor, and a mutuality develops in which the doctor–patient relationship goes far beyond the consulting room" (Desai 1989, 83). Desai has also observed that some patients prefer to have faith in a physician's power to cure. Both these physician roles – confidant and curer – correspond to ancient notions of the Hindu *guru*. This helps to account for the continued overlap between the domains of medicine and religion in modern India.

Desai bemoans the lack of an Indian tradition of voluntarism to care for and serve others: "If institutions of caring and healing spring from the popular consciousness of the voluntary sector rather than from a total reliance on government sponsorship, the sense of ownership so achieved will lessen alienation between the institutions and their users. The government's task would then be public health and preventive medicine, and at the minimum clean drinking water" (Desai 1989, 117).

Closely related to the topic of autonomy are the topics of privacy and confidentiality. These are briefly discussed in the Āyurvedic texts (see Chapter 9). According to Desai, modern Indian clinics open onto main streets to provide easy access and advertising. Because Āyurvedic physicians take the history of patients, and even do most physical examinations with other patients nearby, there is little privacy or confidentiality. The same public exposure occurs in the wards of public, government-run hospitals (Desai 1989, 83) even though the 1972 Indian Code says that physicians are to protect the privacy of confidences or knowledge of defects in character unless the law requires otherwise or unless it is necessary to protect the health of another person from certain communicability of disease (the standard being how one would want another to act toward one's own family member).

Patient-oriented ethics has become more of a concern in specialty hospitals (which are run as private, nonprofit foundations) than in public or private (commercialized) hospitals. One such hospital in the voluntary sector is T. T. Krishnamacharya Hospital[2] in Chennai (Madras). A hospital famous throughout Asia, it was begun by Shanta Ranganathan, the widow of an industrialist who had died from alcoholism after several unsuccessful treatments in London. Besides programs to treat alcohol addiction, the hospital has programs for drug addiction. It charges a minimum rate to clients; it is supported by the state government social work department and the European Community and staffed by counselors with Masters degrees in relevant subjects.

The philosophy of this treatment center is client-centered. To counter the social opprobrium of addiction, clients are treated with dignity and respect. Attempts are made to improve their quality of life, and to explore personal problems through one-on-one counseling, group sessions, and family consultations. The success rate is forty-seven percent. The key book that guides the institution's philosophy is called *Alcoholism and Drug Dependency*. It discusses the problems of addiction, treatment, professional conduct, values, and spirituality – based in large part on the philosophy of Alcoholics Anonymous illustrated by Indian case histories (disguised to protect anonymity). In addition, the hospital has an outreach program. Although there was prohibition in the 1980s, this is no longer the case. As a result, the drinking of *arak* has been a problem in the villages of Tamilnadu. Whereas the men are usually the consumers, women have been the sellers. Teams of experts from T. T. Krishnamacharya Hospital go into the villages to encourage treatment.

The spiritual orientation of Alcoholics Anonymous and the drug rehabilitation programs contribute to this hospital's focus on ethics. The staff is chosen very carefully; there are background checks on character and integrity because of the person-centered approach. In addition, the institution is oriented to quality assurance through peer review for effectiveness, ethical standards, and so forth.

The hospital has a code of ethics.[3] It begins with a statement of minimum standards on access to treatment. All services are to be available irrespective of religion, caste, and political belief. In addition, services are available irrespective of the substance or method of abuse, the history of prior treatment, the patient's ability to pay, or the patient's employment status. Exclusion criteria for admission are to be clearly identified (medical or psychiatric) as are expulsion criteria (such as violence or substance abuse on the premises).

After stating that the primary obligation is to ensure the quality of services to clients and to deliver these services with maturity and responsibility, the code says that staff are: (1) to conduct themselves as mature individuals and provide positive role models by not using alcohol/tobacco/other drugs; (2) to respect clients by treating them with dignity; (3) to have no sexual relationship of any kind with the clients; (4) to use no physical restraint or corporal punishment for clients who are in normal physical or psychological condition and not to seclude the client under any conditions; (5) not to use or exploit the client for personal or institutional gains; (6) to recognize the best interest of the client and make referrals if necessary to other agencies or professionals; (7) to protect the clients' privacy by disallowing use of photographic, audio, video or other means of identification of the clients without prior informed consent; (8) to maintain all client information in the strictest confidence and to divulge it to another person or authority only with the client's consent; and (9) not to discriminate against a human immunodeficiency virus–acquired immunodeficiency syndrome (HIV–AIDS) patient regarding admission or treatment.

Clients' rights are next enumerated: (1) to have a supportive, drug-free environment; (2) to be given dignity, respect, and safety; (3) to be fully informed of the nature and content of the treatment as well as the risks and benefits to be expected of treatment; (4) being made aware of conditions and restrictions prescribed in the center before admission; (5) to wear one's own clothes in keeping with local customs and traditions; (6) to have contact with, and visits from, family or support persons while in treatment; (7) to have confidentiality of information regarding participation in the program and of all treatment records; (8) to have permission to get discharged from the program due to personal reasons at any time without physical or psychological harassment; and (9) to have access to the person-in-charge or management to air grievances and register complaints about the treatment or the staff.

This hospital now guides the state government on ethical issues.

Because patients come from several Indian religions – Hinduism, Islam, Christianity, and so forth – all the religious festivals are celebrated at the hospital, and the worship room has pictures of Hindu deities, Mecca, and Jesus. The generic Alcoholics Anonymous language of God (who gives strength, patience, support, opportunities, and friendship) is used to provide scope for religious pluralism. Because most of the patients are Hindus (Hindus being eighty percent of the Indian population), there is more emphasis on this religion. Counselors draw on their own general religious background. Passages from the *Bhagavad-gītā* and stories from Vedānta are read; meditation prayers by Dayananda Saraswati are offered; Upaniṣads are chanted each morning; Sai Baba bhajans are sung once a month; and on New Years the *Viṣṇusahasranāma* (the thousand names of God Viṣṇu) is chanted for a whole day by visitors from the neighborhood. In addition to the worship room, there is a room for doing yoga. A typical Hindu word is used for the celebration of recovery after a year: it is called "Rebirth" and is celebrated annually like a birthday. Counselors from various religions are all personally religious, and this is said to be connected to the hospital's interest in ethics.

4. Justice

Justice had its classical expression, once again, in the law of karma, which states that good acts will be rewarded and bad ones punished (see Chapter 9). The caveat is that these rewards and punishments, when they involve a major change of status, generally occur only in the next life. One expression of justice is access to medical care. According to the *Caraka-saṃhitā* (see Chapter 9), people are to have some knowledge of medicine for their own well-being and for protecting others. Physicians should be charitable, moreover, but do not have to treat the incurable or the terminally ill. According to *Suśruta-saṃhitā*, for instance, physicians should offer free treatment to brāhmaṇas, elders, preceptors, friends, the indigent, the honest, ascetics, the poor, and orphans. This same text argues that violent and evil people should not be treated. As for others, they are to pay according to capability (although high fees were a common problem and sometimes people could not afford to pay for the drugs) (see Chapter 20 for specific references).

In modern India, there are attempts to emphasize universal values (what traditionally was called *sāmānya-dharma* in Hinduism, see Chapter 9) and to remove those values that had once been based on caste and hierarchy (*viśeṣa-dharma*). This change of perspective is apparent, for instance, in the fact that the 1972 Indian Code pledges physicians to service of humanity and to provide access to medicine not based on consideration of religion, nationality, race, party politics, or social standing (with the proviso that they are not bound to treat each and everyone except in emergencies for the sake of humanity).

One modern study in the Punjab found that infants, young children, women, and those of lower social and economic status had less access to health care (Dunn 1976, 154). An "estimated 10,000 children die every day in India; 5,000 of which are due solely to malnutrition, [a rate]... among the highest in the world. About two-thirds of these are preventable through relatively inexpensive means, such as immunization, oral rehydration for diarrhea, a cleaner water and sanitation, use of iodized salt, and prompt medical attention" (Bilimoria and Sharma 1998, 264). Lifesaving drugs and immunization programs are rare among the rural population and the urban poor. Desai points out, "In matters of health and illness the problems facing most Hindus are those of a Third-World developing country – problems of adequate nutrition and basic medical care. India, with vast areas of remote villages, is divided by a lack of easy transportation. Not only is medical care inaccessible, it is far too expensive for the people to afford" (Desai 1989, 116). There are other problems:

> It can be observed that there is an over-production of doctors while nursing and other health personnel are not being produced in sufficient numbers. The distribution of doctors is also irrational. Most of the doctors are concentrated in hospitals located in urban areas and metropolitan cities while villages, hilly and tribal areas and urban slums lack their presence. The tendency among doctors for over-specialization and the emergence of high technology have not only resulted in increased cost of health, but have also undermined the humanistic aspect of medicine. The health care delivery system and the medical education system are not working in a complementary manner. (Verma et al. 1999, 23)

In addition, there is a high degree of malnutrition. This has particularly affected female children and women. According to Amartya Sen, "the mortality differential against women in Asia reflects quite a remarkable departure from what could be expected on the basis of biological potentials, given symmetric care... The higher mortality and morbidity of women vis-à-vis men in these countries reflect serious 'attainment inequality,' in addition to exhibiting extraordinary extents of 'shortfall inequality,' given the biological potential in the opposite direction" (Sen 1992, 123–4). The fact that Āyurvedic physicians traditionally were male may have discouraged women from seeking medical help. (The fact that there were strict rules to eliminate contact between the sexes outside the family circle may also have contributed to women's reluctance to seek medical help and discuss female biology.) This may be changing because some female *vaidyas* are now being trained in Āyurvedic colleges. Certainly there are now many women studying to become "cosmopolitan" (also called Western, allopathic, or biomedical) physicians. And urban, educated women are becoming less reticent about discussing their bodies. Nevertheless, the health care of women, children, and other marginal groups continues to be a major problem.

Access is related not just to concepts of fundamental rights and justice but also to funding. Even wealthy, Socialist societies have had ethical dilemmas over what aspects of health care governments should pay for (for instance, whether fertility treatments should be included). The problems that face poor, democratic societies are enormous and raise many ethical issues. What is a reasonable standard of care when countries do not have financial resources and who is to decide this? How should the common good be defined, and when should the common good take precedence over the individual good? What claim does health care have when there are other pressing common goods such as education? Is it ethical even to speak of a right to health care in developing societies? Choice may now be theoretically possible in some realms but not practically so. The reason is often funding.

Indian medicine today has been characterized as pluralistic – Āyurveda, Yūnānī, Western ("cosmopolitan"), and homeopathic (see Chapter 9). Should all these receive government funding, or are choices to be made and on what basis? Furthermore, even Western medicine is struggling with the issues now posed by "alternative" ("complementary") systems of medicines. How much does medicine framed with cultural and religious values or belief in the physician as guru–healer count in the healing process? There is also the problem that many Hindus refuse medical treatment because they think the disease was caused by a deity, who would be annoyed if the person went to a physician. This creates the ethical dilemma of whether the physician should force treatment (Kasturi-aratchi, Lie, and Seeberg 1999, 28).

Funding in turn raises other ethical issues. What should be the scope of disclosure of different kinds of treatments when there is severely limited resources? For instance, now that information is available on the Internet, should not new treatments be disclosed? How do decisions regarding disclosure contribute to public and private health?

In India, the health system consists of both public (free) and private (cost) services, hospitals, and dispensaries. It is generally acknowledged that the latter are superior (and comparable to health care in developed countries) but they are not accessible to the poor.

Government hospitals do provide health services of reasonably good quality but they are over-crowded, have long waiting lists, and often lack cleanliness and courtesy. Sick patients at times are refused admission in government hospitals due to lack of beds. Many a time doctors in these hospitals have to rely on the second or third line of therapy, as the best may not be affordable by the patient. The physicians thus constantly face the ethical dilemma in the choice of treatment and in the choice of the patient who should receive the available treatment. The limited number of beds and equipment in the intensive care unit, thus necessitating the doctor to select from among the many patients who may require these services, exemplify this situation. It is to the credit of doctors that in most cases they try to choose patients according to the medical needs. Many of them prefer to use the limited resources for those who have treatable disorders and a reasonable chance of full recovery without any handicap. On occasions, patients suffering from disorders where normal mental functions cannot be assured and who require very expensive treatment are . . . given only restricted or palliative treatment. This may appear unethical although there seems to be no other choice. (Verma et. al. 1999, 28)

With all this in mind, take the case of AIDS. At the turn of the millennium, this epidemic in India had infected more people than in any other country except South Africa. As elsewhere, transmission occurs through sex, contaminated needles, and blood transfusions. In India the disease is largely a heterosexual one (on account of migrant workers to cities resorting to infected women in the sex trade, becoming infected, and then transmitting the disease back to their wives when they periodically return home).

According to Ashok Rowkavi (who is the chair of the Humsafar Trust, which works with AIDS patients in Mumbai), it is impossible to fund drugs. Instead, his organization teaches hygiene and use of filtered water along with local herbal preparations and better diets. This approach is not good enough for the wealthy Indian businessman, Yusuf Hamied, who earned his Ph.D. in chemistry from Cambridge University at the age of 23 and now runs Cipla, a huge pharmaceutical started by his father. He took his ethical case for access to drugs to fight this apocalypse right to the door of the European Commission in Brussels (Specter 2001). Hamied warned in no uncertain terms that if the West was not willing to face its responsibility to help alleviate this suffering, then he would ignore the patents and make and disperse the drugs himself. Because his company had often pirated the molecular formulas of new drugs (he argues that only the process is patented, not the final product) and then sold them at a fraction of the cost, this threat to make AIDS medications accessible was not empty. Key drugs that might cost a patient $15,000 in the West, are now, thanks to him, available for $350. For most people with AIDS, however, the cost is still prohibitive. Furthermore, "in practice, many doctors are refusing to provide treatment to AIDS patients who test positive for HIV. Many doctors have the unfounded fear of contracting HIV if they treat such patients" (Verma et. al. 1999, 34). Purushottama Bilimoria and Renuka Sharma also report that physicians commonly refuse to attend to people diagnosed with AIDS (Bilimoria and Sharma 1998, 267).

The ethics of how to deal with access to medicine in an international plague is to the forefront of Western and United Nations discussions. It has been argued that to stop this epidemic, people need free tests and access to expensive treatments (as an inspiration "to change their behavior" (Specter 2001, 81). But who is to pay for all this?

> Discussing any price reductions of these drugs is meaningless in countries like India, where poverty is so acute that the government can't afford them. When I was in Delhi, for example, Indian officials were debating whether to add the hepatitis-B vaccine to their program for children – because it costs sixty-five cents a shot, and not ten cents, like other vaccines. How can you argue about whether it's worth spending fifty-five cents to save a life and then begin to talk about spending immense sums on an extremely complicated treatment for a disease that cannot be cured? (Specter 2001, 83)

There is a need for a vaccine rather than costly treatments, but "most pharmaceutical companies believe that they will have a hard time selling enough vaccine in places like Africa or India to recoup their research costs. An irony exists: research suffers because it is a global public good – and an extremely costly one – in which no single country has sufficient incentive to invest" (Specter 2001, 84).

Verma and his associates argue:

> In India, it is not always possible to follow the four principles, i.e. beneficence, non-maleficence, patient autonomy and justice in making ethical judgements. This is because the rapid growth in population has put a tremendous pressure on the resources needed to meet the basic needs of the people such as food, housing, education and health. It is not surprising, therefore, that in bio-ethical decisions, sanctity of life is deemed to be less important than the quality of life. This kind of judgement poses many ethical dilemmas for the people, which, in practice, are resolved in the context of cultural traditions interacting with socioeconomic considerations. There is also a tremendous amount of age-old faith, trust and respect in the Indian culture towards physicians. The doctor is often viewed as a demi-god and his decisions are taken as gospel truth without any doubt or misgivings. This imposes immense responsibility on the physician to maintain

an ethical, correct and honest approach in his dealings with his patients. (Verma et al. 1999, 27).

5. Regulating Physicians

The classical Hindu medical text *Caraka-saṃhitā* (composed beginning about the third century BCE with additional strata added over the following centuries) has an ethical code to govern the relationship between physicians and patients (see Chapter 20). Although short on specifics, it was believed that this would be a moral foundation for the practice of medicine. The law of karma stipulated, after all, that one was responsible for all one's actions and causing harm to others would create demerit and negatively influence one's own future in this life and others to come (see Chapter 9). The idea of doing good and producing merit was related to a benevolent paternalism, for physicians were to treat their patients as their own sons (*Suśruta-saṃhitā Sūtrasthana* XXV.23) and patients were to have obedience to their physician (*Caraka-saṃhitā Sūtrasthana* IX.8).

The 1972 Indian Code stipulates that when new medical students register, they must pledge to abide by this twelve page code. On graduation, medical students take the oath found in the *Caraka-saṃhitā*: "Not for self, not for the fulfillment of any worldly material, desire or gain, but solely for the good of suffering humanity, I will treat my patient and excel all [sic]" (Verma et al. 1999, 24; see also Chapter 20). The 1972 Indian Code addresses issues of second opinion (and the norms for informing patients of alternative diagnoses), conduct in consultation (including prevention of sexual misconduct), substitutions, record keeping, and conditions for advertisement. There is a strong statement against accepting gifts, bonuses, rebates, or other financial and professional benefits or to the granting of special privileges (such as procuring services or materials for diagnosis). Fees should be paid according to the amount announced when the service is rendered. The code alerts physicians to the fact that those who commit professional misconduct will be subject to disciplinary action (including debarment from the profession) by medical tribunals or duly appointed committees on ethical relations established by the Medical Council of India or the State Medical Councils according to the Indian Medical Council Act of 1956 or State Acts.

Despite this professional and governmental attempt to regulate physicians and despite the fact that they can now be sued for malpractice, there have been serious problems. In addition, there is a common perception in India that suing is futile for the ordinary person (both because of the cost and because physicians will protect each other). In part, this problem is related to a deep suspicion of government: "A most difficult problem is the lack of legitimization of secular life and institutions. There is a massive distrust of public institutions; for example, the systems dealing with justice" (Desai 1989, 117). A study by the World Health Organization suggests, however, that it is now easier to obtain redress for physician misconduct or negligence with the Consumer Protection Act of 1986 because there is no cost to file a case and complainants need only to appear before a tribunal; they do not need a lawyer. The Indian Medical Association did not like this development. The issue of whether physicians could be prosecuted under the Consumer Protection Act went to the Supreme Court, which argued that they could be (Verma et al. 1999, 32).

Bilimoria and Sharma argue that traditional medical ethics have eroded in modern India, especially under economic liberalization – foreign investments, selective international aid, and market forces – which has commercialized and medicalized the health care system, catering to the rich, and even further marginalizing the poor. Pointing the finger at the Medical Council of India, which ostensibly monitors physicians at the national and state levels, they argue that in point of fact the Medical Council has prevented more socially concerned physicians from being represented on its boards. As a result, "over the years, this led to the formation of independent monitoring and advocacy associations, such as the Medico-Friends Circle, Medical and Hospital Users' Association, the Bio-Medical Ethics Centre (based in a Catholic hospital), and most recently the Forum for Medical Ethics" (Bilimoria and Sharma 1998, 254).

But according to Bilimoria and Sharma, even these organizations have yet to develop serious ethical analysis. For instance, the Forum, a critic of the Medical Council, publishes the *Journal of the Forum of Medical Ethics*, which reviews current books on medical ethics, analyzes ethical issues, and so forth. It presents both premodern medical ethical codes such as Hindu, Islamic, and Hippocratic ones and contemporary bioethical guidelines from various countries and organizations. Once again, it offers no critical analysis of the types of ethical thinking involved or how to deal with ethical dilemmas and conflicts in real life. In other words, there is a major gap between precept and practice. It does blow the whistle, however, on some unethical practices in India, such as physicians who purposely misdiagnose patients and refer patients to others in their network (thereby collecting commissions) or sending them to a nursing home that they own, or recommending surgery only to remove organs for transplantation unknowingly from the patient. The latter scam continues in many Indian cities despite the Human Organ Transplant Bill of 1994, "which adopts 'brain stem death' and regulates retrieval of cadaveric organs, while making commercial transactions in organs an offence in law" (Bilimoria and Sharma 1998, 256; also see Chapter 3). In addition, unscrupulous physicians perform major operations on people who are about to die, and unscrupulous

business men set up high-tech diagnostic centers, but do not maintain the machinery (if broken it is kept on display for its symbolism of advanced technology). Bilimoria and Sharma point out that the Red Cross has noted the lack of bioethics in India (Bilimoria and Sharma 257; see Note 6). Finally, these scholars observe that even though India has tried to regulate foreign-based pharmaceutical corporations, they have not managed to control "the plethora of spurious, substandard, even prohibited and harmful drugs from circulating in the market. During outbreaks of epidemics, such as the recent scare of bubonic plague in Surat, unregistered drugs flooded the chemist stores which people bought without prescriptions over the counter" (Bilimoria and Sharma 1998, 257).

6. Well-being: Āyurveda as Transnational

The modern focus on well-being is a change from narrow views of twentieth-century medicine focused on technologies and drugs to a more holistic view of the person in his or her individuality on the one hand and context on the other. For many Indians, this approach appears as but an affirmation of their own ancient views of medicine that have stressed the continuum of body, mind, environment, and soul/spirit. Concepts of harmony and integration, they argue, are the very premises of Indian medicine.

Indian views on well-being and health are becoming popular in North America, part of the thirteen billion dollar "alternative"/"complementary" medicine industry. Āyurveda, which was introduced to American audiences in the 1980s, has been described as holistic because it is humanistic, client centered, relational, emotional, and spiritual. It does not view human beings as machines, and it is interested in prevention as well as cure. Critical of Western views, one recent article said that Western medicine "treats disease as one would fix a machine, mechanically, with minimal regard for the person as a whole . . . it tends to ignore the patient's lifestyle, minimize his mental state and dismiss his spiritual needs – and as a result misses relatively simple forms of prevention and effective treatment for conditions unsolvable by either drugs or surgery . . . these methods are low-tech low-cost and involve a more personal relationship between doctor and patient" (Rajan 1998, 2). The article refers to the United States government's Office of Alternative Medicine established in 1992 and speaks of practices, such as therapeutic touch, Āyurveda – especially as popularized in the West by Maharishi Mahesh Yogi (Transcendental Meditation) and Dr. Deepak Chopra – and the teaching of alternative medicine now in well-known, Western medical schools. Sita Reddy, reporting on her Ph.D. dissertation in medical sociology on Āyurveda, notes that it has been reshaped:

not only by aspects of American medical culture, but by millennial, heterodox elements of American religious culture, such as the loose cluster of beliefs and practices (for example, vibrations, energy, balance, harmony, self-control, responsibility, self-healing, and yoga) known as New Age Religion. Because New Age Ayurvedic practices occupy the ideological and statutory middle ground between medicine and metaphysicis, they face a unique professionalizing dilemma: whether to present themselves as healing religions or as practices branches of medicine. (Reddy 2002, 97)

Reddy suggests that the popularity of Āyurveda is related to "the changing nature of healing professions in postmodern, multicultural America (Reddy 2002, 98). Because it has not been licensed and even its herbal remedies have run into conflict with the regulations of the Food and Drug Administration, it has sought legitimacy through its links with religion. Religion's "constitutional guarantees of freedom [have] allowed it to circumvent professionalizing routes of licensing and regulation that were usually sought by strictly medical practices" (Reddy 2002, 102). As a result, its main sites of practice have been the health spas and ashrams (spiritual retreats) and its current focus is more on vegetarianism, special diets, and massage treatments than herbal remedies. The health aspects of yoga, long recognized in India, have contributed to the popularity of Indian traditional medicine in the West.

III. Medical Ethics and Bioethics in Sri Lanka

As in our discussion of India, medical ethics and bioethics in Sri Lanka will be compared on the following topics: the four principles of modern bioethics, regulating physicians, and Buddhist views of well-being in a transnational context. Our focus in this section will be on Sri Lanka, a South Asian country where Theravāda Buddhism is protected by the state (see the Constitution, Articles 7.1–3). The development of modern bioethics in Sri Lanka has benefited by collaboration between the Department of Psychological Medicine, University of Colombo, and the Center for Medical Ethics, University of Oslo and the Center for International Health at the University of Bergen (Norway) (1992–1996) (henceforth referred to as the Collaboration in Medical Ethics). Through this collaboration, a number of workshops were held in Sri Lanka, which brought together twenty to thirty key resource people in fields such as medicine, law, and sociology to study representative case studies. Topics included AIDS policies, distribution of health care resources, ethical aspects of resource allocation, ethical aspects of biomedical research, teaching of medical ethics, and so forth. A basic library on medical ethics was developed at the universities of Colombo and Peradeniya and study groups were held in different locations to develop a national policy on medical

bio-ethics (genetics, assisted reproductive technologies, informed consent, medical auditing, peer review, and so forth). As part of the collaboration, Sri Lanka physicians and academics participated in Norwegian programs.

From 1996, there has been:

a growing awareness of the need for international collaboration in this field, and a growing need for the development of expertise in topics of importance to developing nations. One obvious area of concern is the possibility that developing nations are exploited by researchers eager to carry out their research which may have been rejected for ethical reasons in their home countries. Another concern is that research that is important to the needs of developing countries is not carried out for a variety of reasons. There is an urgent need to create a program of education in the field of Medical Ethics with the aim of ensuring that the necessary expertise in this field exists in developing countries. The purpose of this planning proposal was to initiate a training program in Medical Ethics in the South Asian region (India, Bangladesh, Nepal, Bhutan, Thailand and Sri Lanka). ("Medical Ethics workshop in Peradeniya," 1)

A major source for bioethics in Sri Lanka is the World Health Organization's report "Health Ethics in Six SEAR Countries" (Kasturiaratchi, Reidar, and Seeberg 1999). After noting the various organizations that deal with medical ethics such as the Sri Lanka Medical Association and the Sri Lanka Medical Council as well as the Ministry of Health and the faculties of medicine in the universities, it observes that "there is much interest in the ethical aspects of medical profession among politicians and the general public. The subject also receives attention in the mass media" (Jayakody and Kasturiaratchi 1999, 76). The report notes that "in general, patient autonomy, beneficence, non-maleficent [sic] and issues relating to justice are of concern to many clinicians. Paternalism is however still a factor to reckon with. Additionally, there have been a few instances where doctors have been subjected to indictments. In most of these cases what has been at issue was professional misconduct… Role models and actual ethics learning in the continuing education programme are yet to be evolved systematically" (Jayakody and Kasturiaratchi 1999, 80). The report concludes by noting which ethical issues have caused the most discussion in Sri Lanka: abortion and contraception, HIV/AIDS, trade unionism among physicians, and patient's rights (Jayakody and Kasturiaratchi 1999, 82).

1. Nonmaleficence

As for nonmaleficence, this is based in the first precept of Buddhism, which is noninjury to living beings (ahiṃsā) (Florida 1994, Harvey 2000). This precept was traditionally formulated as follows: "Laying aside violence in respect of all beings, both those which are still and those which move … he should not kill a living creature, nor cause to kill, nor approve of others killing (*Sn* 394)" and "Abandoning onslaught on breathing beings, he abstains from this; without stick or sword, scrupulous, compassionate, trembling for the welfare of all living beings (*M.* 1345; cf. *D.* 1.4)" (cited by Harvey 2000, 69). There are some qualifications to this Buddhist concept of nonmaleficence. The killing must be intentional (on the part of both the person who orders the killing and the person who does the act); intent to injure, although counter to the spirit of the precept, does not fully break it by most accounts; and the precept applies to all sentient creatures, not just humans (although it is worse to kill a human than an animal or a plant) (Harvey 2000, 69). Because *ahimsā* appears first in the lists of precepts, it has been the most important. "Non-injury is the distinguishing mark of *Dhamma*" (*Mil.* 185, cited by Harvey 2000, 69). Thus, in Burma, whereas most lay people, when asked which is the most important precept, specify the one on sexual misconduct, they nevertheless agree that killing leads to the worst karmic results and that physical and verbal abuse is the most blameable behaviour" (Spiro, 1971: 101–3 cited by Harvey 2000, 69).

2. Beneficence

Florida links the Western idea of beneficence with compassion (*karuṇā*) and argues that it is fundamental to the Buddhist world view (Florida 1994, 112–13). In this context, he points to *upāya* as skill-in-means (see Chapter 10) and to the four states of mind (*brahmavihāras*: loving kindness, compassion, sympathetic joy, and equanimity). "In the Theravādin tradition, the Buddha is recorded as having said: 'Whoever, monks, would wait upon me … honour me … follow my advice, he should wait upon the sick' (*Vin.*1.302). Practical expressions of compassion … have traditionally included monks looking after orphans in monasteries, and the rich and rulers caring for the poor or setting up hospitals. In his *Rajaparikatha-ratnamala*, the great Mahāyāna master, Nagarjuna advised: 'Cause the blind, the sick, the lowly, [t]he protectorless, the wretched [a]nd the crippled equally to attain [f]ood and drink without interruption'" (*RPR.* 320 cited in Harvey 2000, 109). Harvey links the Mahāyāna idea of working for the welfare of the world (*sattvārtha-kriyā*), directly to the activities of modern "engaged" Buddhists (see later) who help people through medical and social services.

3. Autonomy

Turning to the principle of autonomy, Florida defines this as the ability to choose and plan one's own life, as long as it is consistent with one's responsibilities (Florida 1994, 109). He follows Ratanakul in locating the Buddhist equivalent to autonomy in the law of karma. Florida does not want to see autonomy detract from the idea of mutuality however. For some Buddhists, the concept of autonomy is alien to Buddhism because of its close links to the idea of a self. A key Buddhist doctrine is the idea of the no-self (Skt. *anātman*; Pāli, *anatta*). The individual is impermanent; there is no fixed self (see Chapter 10). This supports an ethic of selflessness (rather than one that values individuality and entitlement:

> (1) the right to 'individuation': to be treated not just as a human being but as a particular one, with all one's personal difference; (2) the right to 'acceptance:' to be taken as one is, good or bad; (3) the right to 'self-direction?' to autonomy and the making of one's own choices; (4) the right to impartial treatment. Buddhism has not traditionally expressed its ethics in terms of 'rights' … but more in terms of the appropriateness and benefit of treating others well. This is partly because no unchanging 'owner' of inalienable 'rights' is accepted, and because 'demanding rights' can lead to anger and greed if one is not careful. Nevertheless, the Buddhist perspective on how one should treat others provides analogues to the above four 'rights.' (Harvey 2000, 36 following Ninian Smart)

Sri Lanka, even though Buddhism is its state religion, still draws on modern Western ideas in its constitution. In the preamble, for example, is the phrase "Wherein the dignity of the individual shall be upheld through the guaranteeing of human rights and fundamental freedoms and the rule of law" (Constitution of Sri Lanka, Preamble, 1).

Classical Buddhist texts have also reflected on issues of truth telling. One step in the eight-fold path is called right speech (*sammā vācā*). It is defined as abstention from lying (even white lies out of compassion), telling malicious tales, and harsh and vain talk. According to *Aṅguttara-Nikāya* (X.176), speaking the truth is related to truth, reliability, and confidence. Words, moreover, should be gentle, soothing, loving, courteous, timely, factual, useful, well argued, and moderate (Govinda 1974, 68 following the translation of *Dhammapāda* by Ñāṇatiloka).

Although this passage is addressed to everyone, it is especially meaningful for physicians. The link between devotion to the truth and reliability is important. Right speech creates trust between physician and patient. The patient has confidence that the physician is not hiding any vital information. The fact that there should be no lie for one's own advantage or another's would directly counter the idea that physicians should not tell patients about their impending death whether to protect the reputation of the physicians or the mental peace of patients and their relatives. Finally, the fact that speech must be in accordance with the facts, gentle, courteous, and with the right timing is relevant for full disclosure spoken in an appropriate manner.

The dilemma created by the tradition of abandoning the patient/not telling the patient or his/her relatives about impending death and the injunction to tell the truth is resolved in one Mahāyāna Buddhist text. It is said that if the physician "knows the patient to be doomed, he will not say so to him, but exhort him to take refuge in the Three Jewels, to think of Buddha, Doctrine, and Community, to practice making offerings – explaining to him that his illness is due to evil committed in previous existences, and that he should be mindful of it as a painful retribution and make confession. And if the patient should be provoked at these words and abuse him with harsh speech, he will not respond at all, but not abandon the patient either" (*Upasakasīla-sūtra* T 1488:5, cited by Demiéville 1985, 46). It is important in this context to remember that Mahāyāna monastic rules stipulate that *bodhisattva*s (even the lower stages of the path) must care for anyone who is ill and failure to do so anywhere under any circumstance amounts to a misdeed (*Bodhisattvasamvara-vimśaka* 17d; also *Brahmajala-sūtra* T 1484:2:1005c, cited by Demiéville 1985, 43).

The modern Thai bioethicist Ratanakul extrapolates from the Buddhist precept that prohibits lying (one of the five precepts) (see Chapter 10) the idea that telling the truth in cases of terminal illness is a moral duty without exception. To do otherwise is cowardly, selfish, abusive of trust, and reveals a refusal to cope with the human condition. Prognosis must be communicated discreetly and with adequate time for the person to cope (Ratanakul 1988, 308). Shundo Taniguchi looks to the *Abhayarājakumāra-sutta* of the *Majjhima-nikāya* for a more technical approach to truth telling: all statements are to be evaluated based on whether they are true or false; beneficial (or harmless) or unbeneficial (or harmful); and pleasant or unpleasant. Only if statements are true and beneficial should they be made. If they are pleasant, they are freely made; if unpleasant, judiciously stated (Taniguchi 1987, 81; 1994, 53). Florida comments on truth or veracity and also links it to the precept about abstaining from false speech. He argues from this that a Buddhist physician must always tell the complete truth to a patient. He does observe, however, that Mahāyāna might acknowledge an exception because there is an incident in which the Buddha, by feigning his own death, tried to make some foolish people take an antidote when they were poisoned. This would be a case, Florida suggests, of legitimate deception (Florida 1994).

4. Justice

Although Ratanakul has argued that justice is a basic Buddhist concept, Florida disagrees (arguing that it does not appear in Buddhaghosa's *Visuddhimagga* and that even the modern scholar of Buddhist ethics Tachibana admits that it is virtually nowhere to be found in the tradition). Closely related to modern concepts of justice is egalitarianism but, according to Florida, this too is difficult to locate. Florida

points again to Buddhaghosa who said "the severity of the offence is a function of the amount of virtue that the victim has" (Florida 1994, 110). (There is another interpretation of this, however; those groups, whose norm is nonviolence, deserve special protection.) Traditional Buddhist societies were, after all, hierarchical (as were Western ones prior to the modern period). This might have affected, among other things, the access to health care.

Medical care came to be provided in the early Buddhist monasteries (because monastics, having no family, had to care for each other). When some monks and nuns started to care for the laity, a conflict arose over the fact that physician–monks and nuns were becoming wealthy and arrogant, which was against Buddhist monastic vows of poverty and humility. This led to Theravāda monasteries stopping the medical care of the laity (see Chapter 20). Mahāyāna Buddhism, however, had an extreme version of virtue ethics. (This might be termed an ethic of supererogation because of its extraordinary altruism, which takes the Buddhist value of *dāna* (gift) and *karuṇā* (compassion) to their logical conclusion: the compassionate gift of one's own life to save another (see Chapter 10). Although this might have had largely rhetorical and doctrinal value, it no doubt informed the general ethics of medicine (the free "gift" of care, the building of hospitals, and so forth) (see Chapter 20), which made medical care more accessible. As Asian societies today move toward or embrace democratic governments, equality and justice have become more important to their value systems.

> Thus, while appeals to generosity, non-attachment and compassion certainly are key persuaders for Buddhists in working for a more just society, this need not be at odds with an appeal to justice per se. Mavis Fenn has pointed out that, in the *Cakkavatti-sīhanāda Sutta*, there is no reference to poverty being karmically deserved, and that a king reacting to poverty with sporadic personal giving is seen as ineffective. A king must act more systematically and effectively by preventing poverty from becoming systemic (Fenn 1996: 107). Moreover, this and the *Kūṭadanta Sutta* express 'views that correspond to simple notions of social justice – everyone should have sufficient resources to care for themselves and others, and to make religious life possible – and the notion that these values should be incorporated into the political system.' (Fenn 1996, 108 cited by Harvey 2000, 202)

Nevertheless, ideas of distributive justice may be muted, says Harvey, by the idea that at least some poverty and some wealth are the results of karma.

Buddhism today is developing concepts of justice and egalitarianism through the movement called Socially Engaged Buddhism. This was begun in the early 1960s by the Vietnamese Zen monk Thich Nhat Hanh to respond both to Christian critiques of Buddhist indifference to the world and to the devastation of his country during the Vietnam War. He promoted an activist and lay-oriented religion to improve the material lives of ordinary people. Thinking about the bombing and monastic insularity, he comments: "after careful reflection, we decided to do both – to go out and help people and to do so in mindfulness. We called it engaged Buddhism. Mindfulness must be engaged. Once there is seeing, there must be acting... We must be aware of the real problems of the world. Then, with mindfulness, we will know what to do and what not to do to be of help" (cited by Rothberg 1998, 268).

In the modern period, Buddhist giving, compassion, and loving kindness have been emphasized to support the voluntary sector for societal improvement, including access to medicine. Donald Rothberg characterizes the movement this way: "A first sense of the term, often identified when one speaks of 'socially engaged Buddhism,' has come to cover a broad range of approaches, unified by the notion that Buddhist teachings and practices can be directly applied to participation in the social, political, economic, and ecological affairs of the nonmonastic world" (Rothberg 1998, 268). He elaborates on the many projects of socially engaged Buddhism in South and Southeast Asian Buddhism: peace, environmental, developmental, AIDS, and human rights projects. In this sense, the traditional concept of Buddhist ethics (*śīla*) (see Chapter 10) has been extended from interpersonal relations to governments and international relations. In addition, he notes that another connotation of engaged Buddhism is simply the Buddhism of everyday life in family and society (which in Vietnam meant taking Buddhism out of the monasteries to the laity).

It could be argued that the four principles of bioethics are not useful in understanding Buddhism or that scholars such as Florida have presented an erroneous perspective because they speak in the name of Buddhism in general (whereas Buddhism has many internal differences). Despite Florida's criticism of Ratanakul's lack of fidelity to the sources, Florida has introduced his own selection and interpretation to make the implied ethics of the texts suitable to modern bioethics. His emphasis on mutuality, compassion, and skill-in-means shows, for instance, a Mahāyāna preference. In his eagerness to lessen the hold of the Vinaya monastic precepts (some violations traditionally could result in excommunication from the monastery), he utilizes the concept of skill-in-means (*upāya*) and implies that the precepts can be left behind, calling them but "useful" tools – hardly a traditional approach on the level of everyday life (although Mahāyāna had introduced some flexibility) and one that Keown thinks mistakes Mahāyāna and Vajrayāna rhetoric for actual practice (see Chapter 10).

There have been other criticisms of the four principles from a Buddhist perspective. Ann Boyd, Ratanakul, and Attajenda Deepudong (1998, 34) have argued that there can be conflict among the four principles regarding what is "good" action in a particular context and whether these four offer the best matrix for applied ethics. They argue, moreover, that from a Buddhist perspective compassion goes beyond the four principles "because it is based on altruism rather than justice" and that at the existential level religion informs morality more than ethical principles do (Boyd, Ratanakul, and Deepudong 1998, 35).

With this more general discussion in mind, let us turn now to ethics on the ground in Sri Lanka. The Sri Lankan constitution guarantees equality before the law and protection against discriminated on the grounds of race, religion, language, caste, sex, political or other opinion, place of birth, or any one of such grounds. At the same time, it allows for affirmative action to protect or advance disadvantaged or underprivileged individuals or groups (Constitution of Sri Lanka, Article 11, Sections 1–2, 4). In other words, the government reserves the right to exercise affirmative action to bring about justice. The constitution goes on further to declare that the state shall secure a social order based on "the equitable distribution of the material resources of the community" to ensure "the realisation of adequate standard of living for all citizens and their families including adequate food, clothing, housing *and medical care*" (Constitution of Sri Lanka, Article 50, Section d, Numbers ii–v). Since independence, Sri Lanka's record on access to health care has been, in fact, good:

> Along with Costa Rica, China, Cuba and Indian state of Kerala, Sri Lanka has been long noted for its successful implementation of primary health care services... Today, fewer infants (18 per 1,000 births) are dying, compared with about 140 per 1,000 at independence in 1948. Far fewer mothers (3.6 per 10,000) are dying at childbirth, compared with around 155 per 10,000 in 1948. Some 85 percent of all births now take place in well-equipped rural maternity homes or in district or city hospitals. Polio was eradicated in 1994 and there have been no cases of diphtheria since 1993 .... Literacy rates are an astonishingly high – particularly for a South Asian country – 92.5 percent for men and 87.9 percent for women, according to 1995 figures. Sri Lanka also has the lowest population growth rate in Asia – only 1.4 percent per year... The successes were achieved mostly through a welfare model adopted at independence, which ensured an island-wide, state-paid health service and free education from kindergarten to university. ("Sri Lanka: Asia's Health Leader Faces 21st Century" 1997, 1)

There seems, however, to have been a set back by the twenty-first century. Food subsidies (such as free school midday meals) have been removed through World Bank pressure, which has increased malnutrition in the poor and anemia in pregnant women. There is a resurgence of some epidemics such as malaria, Japanese encephalitis, and dengue fever. There are fewer efforts to extend medical services to the rural regions. There is a shortage of drugs in the cities, and as a result, there has been a growth in private hospitals. All this is blamed on economic liberalization ("Sri Lanka: Asia's Health Leader Faces 21st Century" 1997, 2).

Like India, Sri Lanka has mobilized to try to obtain cheaper medicines from multinational pharmaceutical companies. It has joined with other developing nations and Médecins Sans Frontières (see the Doha Declaration on the TRIPS Agreement and Public Health issued in 2001 in Doha, Qatar, by the World Trade Organization Ministerial Conference) to argue that expensive medicines necessary for public health can be obtained from a maker of the generic drug (with royalties paid to the holder of the patent) and they can be imported, and resold in a country, without the consent of the patent holder (called compulsory licensing and parallel imports). Because Sri Lanka does not have the capacity to manufacture these generic drugs, it must obtain them from a country such as India that does. This request was before the World Trade Organization in 2002 (Balasubramanium 2001, 1). One important qualification was that India (and other countries with compulsory licenses) must comply with other provisions of the TRIPS Agreement.

Cheaper drugs are especially important for those suffering from AIDS. Already by 1987 there were laws (Regulation No. 473/22) requiring medical officers to report HIV/AIDS cases to health authorities. Although this was supposed to be confidential, there were few controls and news easily spread. Moreover, "[m]any people have reported being stigmatised and harassed, even inside hospitals, after their HIV status became known: the media have hounded patients... and their immediate family members have lost their jobs, their children have been deprived of schooling... Other reports of transgressions include minor health staff demanding money from people who had tested positive, threatening to disclose their HIV status to the community if they refused to pay. Problems do not only occur to people who get tested voluntarily; in addition, some hospital patients have been tested without their consent" ("Sexual Health Exchange no. 2000–1: Sri Lanka" 2000, 1). As a result, in the year 2000, out of 7000–8000 cases, only 300 have been reported, making it difficult to monitor the epidemic and develop policies. The Community Front for the Prevention of AIDS has been working since 1991 to improve confidentiality and human rights for AIDS victims in Sri Lanka and has recommended appropriate legislation to the Ministry of Health and Justice. As a result of the Collaboration in Medical Ethics with Norway, the Sri Lanka requirement for compulsory screening for HIV was eliminated.

5. Regulating Physicians

According to Jayakody and Kasturiaratchi, the Sri Lanka Medical Council has the legal right to take away the licenses of medical practitioners found guilty of malpractice, although this has been rarely done and people have criticized the council for being composed only of its member physicians who tend to protect each other. The Sri Lanka Medical Association (SLMA) has tried to educate physicians about malpractice and to examine ethical issues in the practice of medicine (Jayakody and Kasturiaratchi 1999, 76), but its regulations are old and weighted against the complainant ("Opinion: Grievances and the Medical Council" 2001, 1). In addition, critics have pointed to the fact that physicians use television chat shows for advertising their own practice or the products of companies for which they receive a kickback. They are bombarded with promotional literature and visits by representatives from large pharmaceutical companies along with "incentives" (Patient-centred Healthcare 2002, 1–2).

6. Buddhist Views of Well-being as Transnational

Unlike India, which has provided government support for Āyurveda as the traditional system of medicine, the Sri Lankan Medical Council has tried to mainstream Western medicine (called allopathy) and separate it from Āyurveda and other types of traditional medicine by insisting that practitioners of the traditional systems not be allowed into professional medical associations, that they not be allowed to use laboratory test facilities, and that they not be allowed to teach subjects such as pharmacy, physiology, and anatomy. This exclusivity has been criticized by supporters of traditional medicine. "As a recent writer mentioned, 'Is the free education afforded to allopaths, from kindergarten to post graduate training abroad, all at state expense, not allowed to be utilized for the betterment of the Sri Lankan public?'" This exclusivity is especially noted by health care workers in the diaspora who are aware of the growing popularity of alternative medicines in the West: "While developed countries are adopting alternative therapies as integral parts of NHS hospitals, it is ludicrous that developing countries like Sri Lanka are sticking to archaic ideas and rules... It would be in the interest of the people's health, if the SLMC keeps abreast of trends in developed countries instead of adopting an ostrich-like attitude" ("Opinion: Grievances and the Medical Council" 2001, 2). Traditional South Asian Buddhist views of well-being have become transnational mainly through the interest in meditation.

IV. CONCLUSION

Modern bioethics in South Asia has been informed by traditional medical ethics (Hindu and Buddhist), by Christian ethics in the colonial period, and by Western style constitutions at the time of independence. Just after independence, countries, such as India and Sri Lanka, put considerable resources into creating greater equality by improving the quality of life for the majority including medical care, a process enhanced by their Socialist policies. By the end of the 1990s, however, economic liberalization led to greater privatization of health care and this in turn took resources away from general public health. Many of the ethical issues faced by South Asian countries relate to the fact that they are third-world countries struggling with overpopulation and poverty. Others, however, relate to the fact that new technologies have made their way into the region along with the ethical dilemmas they engender.

Today, there is considerable consciousness raising about the need for bioethics. By the end of the twentieth century, there were international collaborations toward this end, the World Health Organization, the European Union, and individual countries such as Norway all making contributions (along with nongovernmental organizations). There have also been religious movements such as Socially Engaged Buddhism seeking to make religion more responsive to the needs and dilemmas of everyday life.

The four principles of bioethics (nonmaleficence, beneficence, autonomy, and justice) have been analyzed in the South Asian context with special reference to their antecedents in Hinduism and Buddhism, the prevailing religions of the region (aside from Islam from the medieval period). Nonmaleficence had strong antecedents in the concept on nonviolence, the key virtue/principle for both Hindus and Buddhists, and this has provided a basis for the modern principle "do no harm." The concept of beneficence for Hindus traditionally was particularized (defined by sex, stage of life, caste, and so forth) and took place largely within the extended family context, although charity was a value for all and a duty especially for the king; in the modern period the (secular) Indian government has taken responsibility for beneficence and has tried to universalize access to opportunities and goods through affirmative action policies. By contrast, Buddhists traditionally viewed beneficence through the values of compassion and giving, especially in the Mahayana tradition with its supererogatory ethic. Like India, Sri Lanka has taken active measures in the modern, postindependence period to share more equally the goods of society through government programs. Both Hinduism and Buddhism in the past shared the idea of the law of karma, which was related to autonomy, and both viewed autonomy as limited by group responsibilities. (Hinduism, however, has been more comfortable with the idea of autonomy because it has held to the ideal of a Self, whereas Buddhism has had the doctrine of no-Self.) In the modern period, autonomy has increased in India and Sri Lanka, the result of Western influence and internal reforms to strengthen the position of women and others. The increase in autonomy is reflected in the growing interest in patients' rights. Finally, both societies traditionally acknowledged hierarchy as an organizing principle of society (although they had different views of the order of the castes). Thus, justice as equal opportunity (and access to medical care for the poor, women, and children) has been the most radical change in the ethical principles. Now, however, the language of universal rights supersedes the concept of charity to the poor or support of religious people (ascetics and *brāhmaṇa*s in the case of Hinduism and monks and nuns in the case of Buddhism).

Regulation of physicians was certainly an ethical issue already in the classical period as specialization and professionalism took root; there were oaths, the cultivation of virtues, rules for decorum, and so forth promoted by the Hindu *sampradāya* or Buddhist monastery or king; nevertheless, paternalism was strong and encouraged by the concept of physician as guru or religious healer. Today, physicians continue to regulate themselves through professional organizations and the governments regulate them (as kings did in the past). Now, however, in both India and Sri Lanka there is more surveillance by the society at large, which wants greater accountability. One of the big tests facing the ethics of health care is the pandemic of AIDS. This has led to greater activism to obtain cheap drugs and to ensure the privacy of patients.

The status of traditional medical systems (and their ethics) today differs considerably between India and Sri Lanka. India has publicly embraced a pluralistic system since independence. Sri Lanka, by contrast, has supported only Western medicine. As a result, *Āyurveda* is becoming increasingly popular both in India and the West. The Buddhist contribution has been more by way of diet, meditation, and palliative care than by traditional medicine per se although both Hinduism and Buddhism have shared a traditional idea of health as harmony (body, environment, and cosmos).

NOTES

1. All citations from *Caraka-saṃhitā* follow the numbering system of R. K. Sharma and V. B. Dash (trans.): 1972, *Agniveśa's Caraka Saṃhitā*, Vol. 1 (*Sūtrasthāna*) and Vol. 2 (*Nidāna-sthāna, Vimāna-stāna, Śarīrsthana, Indriya-Sthāna*) (Sanskrit Text with English translation and Critical Exposition based on Cakrapāṇi Datta's *Āyurveda Dīpīka*, (Chowkhamba Sanskrit Series Office, Varanasi). All quotations are from these sources unless otherwise noted. (On occasion, I have offered my own translations.) All

citations of *Suśruta-saṃhita* are from K. K. Bhishagratna (trans.): 1963, *The Suśruta Saṃhitā*, 2 vols., (Chowkhamba Sanskrit Series Office, Varnasi). I have taken the liberty of eliminating sexist language in translations, where it is clear that the reference can be to both men and women.

2. The following discussion is based on my visit to T. T. Krishnamacharya Hospital, Chennai (December 2000), and interviews with Dr. Raymol Rachel Cherian, Ph.D. Director of Research, Shanthi Ranganathan, Honorary Secretary, counselor U. Kanakam, and Srinivasa Venkatachari. I would like to thank them for their effort and their loan of relevant materials. Also I thank McGill University, which made this research possible with a Humanities Travel Grant. And I would like to thank Ashok Chowgle, Mumbai, who facilitated my research in Mumbai, December 2000, and Ashok Rowkavi, Humsavar Trust, Mumbai, for taking the time to be interviewed.

3. The code is described in the document as a modified version of the CHASP (Community Health Accreditation and Standards Program) standards. I have presented it here with slight modification of wording.

CHAPTER 45

The Discourses of Bioethics in Sub-Saharan Africa

Angela Amondi Wasunna

I. Introduction

Ethics in the practice of medicine was not an alien concept in much of African history (see Chapter 19). Most African traditional healers had closely guarded codes of ethics, which were passed down from one generation to the next. Some of these codes embodied concepts found in the Hippocratic tradition such as confidentiality and privacy. Similarly, bioethics, broadly defined, is not an entirely new notion in Africa. Many African cultures understood the sacred interdependency among the health of individuals, communities, and ecological systems. It was a common belief that the morality of one's actions had consequences, positive or negative, on one's own health, the collective health of the populace, and the environment.

Godfrey Tangwa, an African philosopher–bioethicist asserts that African ethical and metaphysical ideas have over the ages been shaped and colored by its ecological, biological and cultural diversity. He argues that within the African world view, the distinction among plants, animals, and inanimate material, and between the sacred and the profane, matter and spirit, and the communal and the individual is a slim and flexible one. Similarly, metaphysical conceptions, ethics, customs, laws, and taboos form a single continuum (Tangwa 1999, 5).

A discussion of the "emergence" of bioethics in Africa is therefore slightly misleading because bioethics has always been a part of the African way of life. In reality, the emergence refers to the globalization of bioethics (Knowles 2001, 254). Although there are several developments that fall under the broad rubric of contemporary bioethics discourse in Africa, three seminal events lie at the fulcrum, namely, the emergence of human immunodeficiency virus/acquired immunodeficiency syndrome (HIV/AIDS) in Africa, the globalization of biomedical research, and the transfer of biotechnology to African countries.

II. The Emergence of HIV/AIDS in Africa

The first AIDS cases in Africa were reported in 1983. A few years prior, clinical epidemics of chronic, life-threatening enteropathic diseases ("slim disease"), cryptococcal meningitis, progressive Kaposi's sarcoma and esophageal candidiasis were seen in Rwanda, Tanzania, Uganda, Zaire, and Zambia (Quinn et al. 1986; Essex 1994). The earliest blood sample from Africa from which HIV has been recovered was from a possible AIDS patient in Zaire, tested in connection with a 1976 Ebola virus outbreak (Getchell et al. 1987; Myers and Korber 1992).

Since it was first reported, the disease has spread at an alarming rate in Africa. Today, the continent has the highest number of adults and children living with HIV in the world. The disease predominantly affects the heterosexual population and is defined by denial, confusion, stigma, and discrimination. Lack of proper leadership and the politicization of AIDS have also contributed to delayed responses to curb the spread of the disease.

More people in Africa are dying of AIDS than as victims of war, and the numbers are staggering. Of the 36 million adults and children in the world living with HIV/AIDS in 2000, more than 70 percent live in sub-Saharan Africa. Since the epidemic began, more than 17 million Africans have died, more than 3.7 million of them children. AIDS has orphaned an additional 12 million children. An estimated 8.8 percent of adults in Africa are infected with HIV/AIDS, and in the following seven countries, at least one adult in five is living with HIV: Botswana [with] the highest estimated adult infection rate – 36 percent, Swaziland, Zimbabwe, Lesotho, Zambia, South Africa, and Namibia (McGeary 2001, 48–9).

Over and above the personal suffering that accompanies HIV infection, the virus in sub-Saharan Africa is devastating entire communities and erasing years of social and economic progress that African countries had attained in the years after independence. The HIV/AIDS scourge in Africa has therefore been described as a "development crisis" because it profoundly disrupts the economic and social bases of families and entire nations (World Bank Report 1999, 12). Because of its nature and mode of transmission, the disease raises issues in the realms of medicine, public health, law, ethics, and human rights. Perhaps more importantly, the disease illustrates the close relationships between these disciplines and their collective importance in the fight against the pandemic.

One of the major problems arising from the HIV/AIDS epidemic was and remains discrimination. Because the mode of transmission of the disease in Africa is primarily sexual, there were real fears that infected people would be labeled as "immoral" or in some instances, "cursed" and subjected to discrimination (UNAIDS/UNFPA 2001, 16). These fears were realized, in part, because education about the disease was not prevalent. People were afraid to get tested because of the societal perceptions about not just receiving a positive test result, but also simply volunteering to be tested. Several African countries therefore perceived a need to assert the rights of infected individuals and accord them special protections. In 1994, in Dakar Senegal, nine African countries, namely, Central African Republic, Côte d'Ivoire, Ghana, Kenya, Rwanda, Senegal, South Africa, Uganda, and Zambia signed what has now become known as the *Dakar Declaration*.[1] This Declaration encompasses legal, human rights, and ethical principles and serves as a guide for societies on how to treat HIV-infected individuals. Among the principles espoused in the Declaration are:

Non-discrimination: That a person directly affected by the epidemic should remain an integral part of his or her community, with the right of equal access to work, housing, education and social services, with the right to marry, with freedom of movement, belief and association, with the right to counseling, care and treatment, justice and equality.

Confidentiality and privacy: That every person directly affected by the epidemic has a right to confidentiality and privacy. It can only be breached in exceptional circumstances.

Adaptation: That every person and community should change and adapt social and cultural conditions to the new challenges of the epidemic in order to respond effectively.

Sensitivity in language: That language should uphold human dignity, reflect inclusion, be gender sensitive, accurate and understandable. (United Nations Development Program 1994)

After the signing of this important Declaration, African delegates were encouraged to set up law, medicine, and ethics research and education centers in their respective countries.

Apart from the aspirational principles laid out in the Declaration, HIV/AIDS has brought several other ethical issues to the fore in Africa. For example, in the face of scarce resources, the questions being examined include access to essential drugs, priority setting, and the role played by intellectual property. It has been recognized that "alongside the need for resources, and for just and accountable choices within these resource constraints, there is a need for a regulatory environment for the practice of medicine and for the pharmaceutical and biotechnology industries in which the public interest remains paramount" (Raja and Wikler 2001, 4).

Another issue raised by HIV/AIDS, which has not received the prominence it deserves, is euthanasia. In many African countries, HIV/AIDS is putting a disproportionate care-taking burden on families. Most Africans describe their families to include extended family members and, traditionally, children are expected to care for their parents in their old age. AIDS in Africa affects the most productive members of the society, that is, those between the ages of 18 and 45. Because they are the driving economic force in their families, the loss of people in this age group usually has serious repercussions in the family life because the most vulnerable, those younger than 18 and the elderly, are left without their economic support system. Many HIV-infected people do not want to burden their elderly parents or relatives by making them take care of them as well as the children they leave behind. In some cases, an HIV/AIDS diagnosis leaves a feeling of complete hopelessness in many people because, without good health insurance or personal funds, there are not many health options available to the patient. The temptation to end one's life and avoid putting the burden of care on the family can be quite strong. In countries like South Africa with high rates of HIV infection, there has been a surge of requests for assisted suicide and it is worth examining the correlation, if any, between the increase of requests and the high rates of infection in that country (Editorial 2001).

III. THE GLOBALIZATION OF BIOMEDICAL RESEARCH

The last decade has seen a significant increase in international research in the developing world. The number of countries in which clinical investigators conducting drug research that is tracked by the United States Food and Drug Administration increased from twenty-eight in 1990 to seventy-nine to 1999. (Office of the Inspector General 2001, iii). To use AIDS as an example, such organizations as the International AIDS Vaccine Initiative are conducting HIV/AIDS research in more than twenty African countries, often in collaboration with foreign universities. The combination of the increased burden of disease in the developing world and the absence of affordable therapies and vaccines has raised the sensitivity of health professionals to issues of ethics and equity in international biomedical research. Foremost among the concerns are whether new treatments should be compared against Western standards of care or against existing local standards (Lansang and Crawley 2000, 777). Other issues include the question of whether communities will benefit from the research results and the perennial difficulty of obtaining informed consent in the developing world.

There has been much debate in the international arena about these issues, resulting in the revision of the Declaration of Helsinki (World Medical Association 1964, 2000) and the Council for International Organizations of Medical Sciences, *International Ethical Guidelines for Biomedical Research Involving Human Subjects* (Council for International Organizations of Medical Sciences 1993, 2002; see Chapters 50, 51). The Joint United Nations Programme on HIV/AIDS (UNAIDS) has also issued a guidance document titled *Ethical Considerations in HIV Vaccine Trials* (UNAIDS 2000). The thorny ethical issues raised by biomedical research in developing countries have been addressed by the UK-based Nuffield Council on Bioethics and in the U.S., by the National Bioethics Advisory Commission (NBAC), a Commission appointed by the President of the United States.

The NBAC Report titled *Ethical and Policy Issues in International Research: Clinical Trials in Developing Countries* made several recommendations including a requirement that all research in developing countries must address local health needs. Additionally, the Report stated that the foreign researchers and sponsors should involve representatives of the host/local community and potential participants throughout the design and implementation of the research. Furthermore, in the design of studies, the Report recommended that researchers must justify the use of placebo and, when possible, provide members of the control group with an established, effective treatment, regardless of local availability. The Commission also thought it was important for researchers and sponsors to make efforts to ensure access to benefits for study participants and the larger host community (National Bioethics Advisory Commission 2001, i–xv).

The Nuffield Discussion Paper titled, *The Ethics of Clinical Research in Developing Countries*, stated that developing countries ought to set their own national health priorities and that foreign-sponsored research that fell outside of these priorities had to be justified to appropriate ethics committees. The Nuffield Working Party emphasized the importance of capacity building of local expertise by foreign researchers and sponsors. On the thorny question of standard of care, the report concluded that the appropriate standard of care to be provided to members of a control group in a research project could only be defined in consultation with those who worked within the host country. The report recommended that wherever appropriate, participants in the control group had to be offered a universal standard of care for the disease being studied. Where it was inappropriate to offer such a standard, the Working Group felt that the minimum that should be offered was the best intervention currently available as part of the country's national public health system (Nuffield Council on Bioethics 2002, xv).

African countries are now taking steps to ensure that research within their borders is done in an ethical manner. For example, many countries are now developing local ethics committees, the equivalent of Institutional Review Boards, to review international and domestic research protocols. Two organizations have been taking the lead to build research ethics capacity in Africa, namely, the African Malaria Network Trust (AMANET) and the Pan African Bioethics Initiative (PABIN).[2] These organizations are important because their leadership and membership are composed (almost entirely) of Africans.

Since its founding in 1994, AMANET (formerly known as The African Malaria Vaccine Testing Network – AMVTN) has prioritized the promotion of ethics in all of its capacity-building endeavors. The organization conducts workshops for researchers whose agenda includes among other things, proper collaboration between foreign and local researchers, sensitivity to local culture particularly in the informed consent process, and fairness in the ownership, use, and access to research outputs.

The PABIN was formed as an offshoot of AMVTN in January 2001 in Lusaka, Zambia. PABIN recognizes that there is a need to develop an African approach to ethical dilemmas in health research. It was formed partly because the current ethical guidelines governing international research did not have much input from Africans. Further, the application of these guidelines in Africa was hampered by several factors including language barriers, political and civil conflicts, poor access to health care, and inadequate ethical review of research proposals. PABIN aims to develop biomedical research ethics standards that take the African experience into account, undertake constant review of those standards to suit changing times, and promote capacity building, development of ethics review mechanisms, and standard operating procedures.

IV. THE TRANSFER OF BIOTECHNOLOGY TO AFRICAN COUNTRIES

The Convention on Biological Diversity describes biotechnology as "any technological application that uses biological systems, living organisms, or derivatives thereof, to make or modify products or processes for specific use" (United Nations Environmental Program 1992). Using this definition, one can argue that Africans have been adept at traditional biotechnology for food or beverage production for centuries. Beer brewing, cheese making, and production of sour milk are obvious examples (Egwang 2001, 1); however, today, modern biotechnology (particularly in agriculture and medicine) is centered on the technology of genetic engineering or recombinant DNA.

Although, for years, biotechnology has been seen as a preoccupation of the West, recent debates revolving around the potential benefits of genetically modified crops and the potential of genomics to improve the health of the poor have directed the biotechnology debate to the developing world. Modern biotechnology involving genetic engineering and applied in agriculture and medicine raises number of social, economic, legal, and ethical questions. The main questions raised for new biotechnology applications include the following: If they can eradicate hunger, can they assure sustainable development? Will they affect biodiversity and the environment? Can they provide a disease-free world? Will they ensure a renewable resource economy? Most importantly, what is their contribution to sustainable development (Bhardwaj 2001, 1)?

A recent Report published by the Program in Applied Ethics and Biotechnology and the Canadian Program on Genomics and Global Health found that to answer these questions and to work toward greater equity in the developing world, the first step is to identify and prioritize the most important biotechnologies for those countries. The Report, titled *Top 10 Biotechnologies for Improving Health in Developing Countries*, also found that to dispel myths

surrounding the applicability and suitability of biotechnology, there was a need to promote scientific research within developing countries; build capacity among local scientists; strive toward consensus building among the various stakeholders such as government, researchers and industry; engage the public particularly on contentious issues; and finally, seek innovative financing mechanisms to harness biotechnology for benefit of health in developing countries (Program in Applied Ethics and Biotechnology 2002, 79–85).

A consensus seems to be emerging among African countries that biotechnology for developing countries in the future requires a change from the present commercially driven agenda to a more human development focus, combining "old" and "modern" biotechnological techniques for the improvements in the health and living conditions of the poor (Horst 2001, 1).

V. CONCLUSION

The global bioethics movement in Africa is growing. Ethics curricula are being developed in Cameroon for Francophone African universities under the guidance of the Cameroon Society of Bioethics. South Africa already has sophisticated bioethics courses that are offered at the graduate and doctoral levels at several universities. The South African Research Ethics Training Initiative (SARETI), for example, is a multidisciplinary, education and training program in health research ethics. The program is a collaborative effort of the University of Pretoria, the University of Natal, and the Bioethics Institute at the Johns Hopkins University's Bloomberg School of Public Health. On its web page, SARETI describes its main goal as building African capacity for the ethical review of health research, and strengthening Africa's institutional training capacity necessary to achieve and sustain this aim (SARETI 2002).

SARETI provides a variety of educational programs, varying from short workshops and short courses to full Masters programs. Course modules include public health; ethics and human rights; informed consent and research in vulnerable populations; and ethical issues in international collaborative health research. A similar graduate level program has been developed at the Bioethics Center, University of Cape Town South Africa. The main goal of this program is to develop sustainable multidisciplinary expertise in international research ethics and bioethics in southern Africa. These programs are largely funded by the Fogarty International Center of the United States National Institutes of Health.

International interest in African bioethics is likewise on the rise. African participation in international bioethics meetings and events is increasing although still sorely inadequate. Institutions such as the Hastings Center, Johns Hopkins University, and Harvard are initiating bioethics projects in Africa and facilitating educational visits by African scholars. For example, the Hastings Center's International Program is engaged in a collaborative project with the Kenya Medical Research Institute and others in East Africa to examine legal and ethical challenges faced by African doctors treating AIDS patients. The Hastings Center also has an International Visiting Scholars Program, which offers individuals from outside the United States and Canada the opportunity to pursue independent study of ethical problems in medicine, the life sciences, and the professions. Under this program, the Center has hosted African bioethics scholars from a variety of countries including Nigeria, South Africa, Cameroon, Kenya and Uganda (The Hastings Center 2002).

The Harvard School of Public Health runs an annual 5-day summer workshop titled *Ethical Issues in International Health Research*. The program is cosponsored by Tufts University School of Medicine, University of Natal School of Medicine, Instituto Nacional de Salud Publica, Sree Chitra Tirunal Institute for Medical Sciences and Technology, and the National Institutes of Health. The Harvard School of Public Health encourages scholars from the developing world to apply for the program and it provides scholarships for eligible participants from developing countries. Participants from several African countries including Nigeria and South Africa have attended the course so far (Program on Ethical Issues in International Health Research, Harvard School of Public Health 2002).

The Bloomberg School of Public Health and the Bioethics Institute at Johns Hopkins University in collaboration with the U.S. National Institutes of Health offer a 1-year training program for scientists from sub-Saharan Africa. Fellows in this program take courses in bioethics, research ethics, and international research ethics. They are also offered the opportunity to take other courses that might be of interest, such as health services research methods, epidemiology, and international health systems. The program awards the fellows a certificate of completion at the end of the year of intensive training. Fellows are expected to spend 6 months of the yearlong program engaged in independent bioethics research projects in their home countries (Bioethics Institute, Johns Hopkins University 2002).

Organizations like the International Association for Bioethics (IAB)[3] are recognizing the importance of non-Western bioethics perspectives and are encouraging the participation of more Africans in the activities of the Association. This is consistent with the IAB's goals to facilitate contacts and the exchange of information between those working in bioethics in different parts of the world. A former president of the IAB, Dr. Solomon Benatar is from South Africa (the first African to head the organization). A strong African presence on this international bioethics body serves as a firm endorsement and recognition of African bioethicists in the international arena (International Association for Bioethics 2002).

Finally, a bioethics journal dedicated to developing world issues began publication in May 2001. The journal, *Developing World Bioethics*, is based in South Africa and it is published as a companion journal to *BIOETHICS*. By its own description, the journal is dedicated exclusively to developing countries' issues and aims to provide case studies, teaching materials, news in brief, and peer-reviewed articles. One of the journal's two editors, Willem A. Landman, is a bioethicist in South Africa and the editorial board is mostly drawn from bioethics scholars in the developing world. Since its inception, the journal has covered bioethics issues ranging from HIV preventive vaccine research, to ethics and genetics and to social justice issues surrounding health care delivery in developing countries (*Developing World Bioethics* 2001).

These are all positive developments. Great challenges confront bioethics in Africa. This chapter has focused on three main developments. However, several other areas require attention. For example, the commercialization of human organs for transplantation remains a problem in many developing countries (Bihl 2001), the emergence of reproductive technologies in regulatory vacuums (Wasunna 2000a), debates surrounding female circumcision (Wasunna 2000b, 49), and end-of-life issues in the face on a growing elderly population (HelpAge 2000). Africans have a great deal to bring to the bioethics table. Their views, however, need to be taken seriously, and their inclusion and participation in major international decision-making efforts assured.

NOTES

1. The Dakar Declaration of 1994 was one of the first public statements from African countries on the importance of human rights in the context of HIV/AIDS. The main aim of the Declaration is to strengthen the capacity of African communities and nations to discuss and contend with complex HIV-related legal, ethical, and human rights issues. The Dakar Declaration was drafted and endorsed by participants at the Intercountry Consultation of the African Network on Ethics, Law and HIV, organized in Dakar, Senegal, from 27 June to 1st July 1994, by the UNDP HIV and Development Programme (Dakar and New York). Participants came from Central African Republic, Côte d'Ivoire, Ghana, Kenya, Rwanda, Senegal, South Africa, Uganda, Zambia, the WHO Global Programme on AIDS, the WHO Regional Office for Africa, the UNDP Management Development and Governance Division, the UNDP HIV and Development Project in Asia and the Pacific, the Asian and Latin American Networks on Law, Ethics and HIV, the African Council of AIDS Service Organizations (AFRIC-ASO), the Association of African Jurists (AJA), ENDA Tiers Monde, the Network of African People Living with HIV/AIDS (NAP+), the Organisation Pan-Africaine de Lutte contre le SIDA (OPALS), and ORSTOM. The Declaration affirms that any

action, whether personal, institutional, professional, or governmental, in response to the HIV epidemic, should be guided by the following principles:

The principle of responsibility: Every person, government, community, institution, private enterprise, and medium must be aware of his or her responsibility and must exercise it in an active and sustainable manner.

The principle of engagement: Every person is affected, directly or indirectly, and therefore should respond with commitment, concern, courage, and hope for the future.

The principle of partnership and consensus-building: All persons, couples, families, communities, and nations must work together with compassion to build and share a common vision. These partnerships must reflect and actively promote solidarity, inclusion, integration, dialogue, participation, and harmony.

The principle of empowerment: The empowerment of every person, but particularly women, the poor, the uneducated, and children, is essential and must guide all action. Empowerment requires recognition of the right to knowledge, information and technology, freedom of choice, and economic opportunity.

The principle of non-discrimination: Every person directly affected by the epidemic should remain an integral part of his or her community, with the right of equal access to work, housing, education and social services, with the right to marry, with freedom of movement, belief and association, with the right to counseling, care and treatment, justice and equality.

The principle of confidentiality and privacy: Every person directly affected by the epidemic has a right to confidentiality and privacy. It can only be breached in exceptional circumstances.

The principle of adaptation: Every person and community should change and adapt social and cultural conditions to the new challenges of the epidemic in order to respond effectively.

The principle of sensitivity in language: Language should uphold human dignity, reflect inclusion, be gender sensitive, accurate and understandable.

The interests of the research subjects or communities should be paramount. Research should be based on free and informed consent, be non-obtrusive and non-coercive,

and the results should be made available to the community for timely and appropriate action.

The principle of prohibition of mandatory HIV testing: HIV testing without consent should be prohibited. HIV testing should also not be a pre-requisite for access to work, travel or other services. http://www1.umn.edu/humanrts/instree/dakar.html (visited November 24, 2007)

2. The Pan-African Bioethics Initiative (PABIN) is a new pan-African organization dedicated to the development of bioethics in the context of African culture and practices. PABIN provides a forum for regular meetings and discussion on bioethics in Africa. The Initiative is dedicated to preserving and promoting African traditions in ethics and bioethics in Africa and within the international community. French and English are the working languages of PABIN. Membership to PABIN is open to all Africans or persons residing in Africa who share an interest in developing ethical review in Africa. Membership is encouraged from researchers, physicians, patients, and their organizations, sociologists, anthropologists, philosophers, members of religious community and bioethicists.

In many African countries, there is a limited awareness and understanding of the concepts underlying health and human rights, informed consent, confidentiality, and the research protocol review process. This makes Africa more prone to exploitation by pharmaceutical companies and other research sponsors who are able to conduct their research with a minimum of administrative and legal obstacles. PABIN therefore sees a need to promote local research review and monitoring for compliance to ethics principles and international guidelines. PABIN plans to conduct educational courses for members and potential members of research ethics committees in Africa. (http://www.pabin.org/About.aspx).

3. The International Association of Bioethics is an international organization for bioethics that has the following educational and scientific objectives: To facilitate contacts and the exchange of information between those working in bioethics in different parts of the world; To organize and promote international conferences in bioethics; To encourage the development of research and teaching in bioethics; and To uphold the value of free, open and reasoned discussion of issues in bioethics. More information can be found on the Association's website http://www.bioethics-international.org/iab-2.0/index.php?show=index (visited November 24, 2007).

Part VIII

Discourses on Medical Ethics and Society

A. Ethical and Legal Regulation of Medical Practice and Research

CHAPTER 46

The Medical Marketplace, the Patient, and the Absence of Medical Ethics in Early Modern Europe and North America

Mary E. Fissell

I. Introduction

From the Renaissance well into the nineteenth century, no ethics particular to medicine governed the patient–practitioner relationship in Europe and North America (see also Chapters 1 and 28). Although elite university-trained practitioners wrote treatises on topics that we now consider under the rubric of medical ethics, the day-to-day relationships between healers and the sick were shaped by two sets of more general social norms. First, the structure of early modern health care provision has been likened to a medical marketplace. In such a marketplace, medicine was a commodity like any other, and so medical interactions were largely structured by the rules of commercial interchange. Second, as in other social relations of the period, both patients and practitioners appreciated the mutual obligations of patronage and deference between people of different social groups. At times, the patient was the patron, and the practitioner a client, whereas at others these roles were reversed. From the seventeenth century, patients were sometimes understood as a group deserving of special protection due to their temporary or permanent disability.

II. The Medical Marketplace

Over the past two decades, historians have become interested in the rank-and-file of medical practitioners and in the experiences of patients rather than just the elite of medicine. As a result of this broader canvas, they have come to describe health care provision in early modern Europe and North America as a medical marketplace (see also Chapter 27). Three key features characterize this model. First, there was a huge array of people providing health care, both formally and informally. Second, patients picked and chose among health care providers quite freely. Third, the boundaries between patient and provider were quite porous; one might readily become the other.

A person who fell ill in 1500 or in 1800 almost always first sought medical treatment in a domestic context. He or she relied upon his or her own medical knowledge of healing plants and procedures, consulted manuscript or printed health guides, and asked family, neighbors, and friends for advice. Letters and diaries, as well as a sizeable number of domestic medical guides, provide us with glimpses of this medical world. Ralph Josselin, a seventeenth-century English clergyman who kept an extensive diary, mentions 762 instances of illness in his family, but in only 21 cases was a healer from outside the family circle consulted (Beier 1985, 117). Domestic medical guides consistently expected ordinary people to possess considerable medical knowledge; many provided recipes for remedies, omitting any guidance about diagnosis and assuming considerable familiarity with healing herbs.

When a sick person sought medical care outside the domestic context, he or she had a huge array from which to choose. Formerly, historians accepted a description of early modern medical practice formulated by elite practitioners themselves: Medicine was divided into regular practitioners, arrayed hierarchically as physicians, surgeons, and apothecaries, and irregular practitioners or quacks. From the patient's perspective, however, any such tidy divisions or hierarchies vanish. A panoply of providers offered a wealth of services. In German-speaking lands, bone setting was often performed by the town executioner; he who dismembered bodies was presumed to be able to reassemble them too. In France, a few enterprising peasants specialized in providing viper meat for a powerful and sought-after remedy. In the Netherlands, the Dutch Reform Church appointed *ziekentroosters*, or comforters of the sick, who offered both pastoral care and medical advice to the sick of the parish. In both Catholic and Protestant countries, religious healers flourished. In eighteenth-century France, for example, the shepherd known as the "Saint of Savières" cured hundreds with holy water, and in the North of England, Bridget Bostock healed the sick with her "fasting spittle."

Much to the disgust of the elite of medical practitioners, patients felt completely comfortable choosing among this wide array of health care providers. Even the poorest and least-educated people decided for themselves which practitioner to consult. In 1745, a stable boy in a village near Bologna decided that the local surgeon–apothecary could not help him: "knowing that I could not get well in his hands, I asked him what was due for his services, and I got rid of him" (Pomata 1998, 153). In eighteenth-century Germany, a day laborer named Otto consulted a miller when his son became feverish, because he had heard of the miller's reputation as a healer. When Otto brought his son's urine to the miller Claudiz, many other people were waiting to consult Claudiz as well. Although the drops sold by Claudiz seem to have helped the boy, he was sick a week later and this time, his father went to see a Dr. Schmidt (Lindemann 1996, 354). At the other end of the social spectrum, Mme. de Sevigné consulted the elite court physicians but also a Capucine empiric and an Italian abbé, and sought relief at spas (Brockliss and Jones 1997, 293–5). Patients may have also chosen practitioners or procedures for reasons considered illicit by the practitioner. In eighteenth-century England,

for example, surgeon–apothecaries worried that women sometimes sought inoculation for smallpox because it was believed to cause an abortion.

Finally, in the medical marketplace, the boundary between patients and practitioners was sometimes very hard to pin down. William Dyer, an eighteenth-century clerk in Bristol, England, sought occasional medical care from local practitioners, but he also got interested in electrical medicine, purchased an electrical machine, and healed many local people free of charge. The only other such electrical machine in the city was in the Infirmary (Barry 1985, 154). In Lancashire, evidence from manuscript remedy books shows families purchasing recipes for remedies, reselling the recipes to their neighbors, and even brewing medicines from the recipes and selling those (King and Weaver 2000, 195).

When we see these microhistories of patient choice, we can begin to understand the frustrations expressed by the elites of medicine. As physician Girolamo Mercurio moaned in 1603, "every measly surgeon, every little barber, every old woman wants to play the doctor (i.e., physician)" (Gentilcore 1998, 59). In books, such as John Securis, *A Detection and Querimonie of some of the Daily Enormities and Abuses Committed in Physic* (London, 1566); Laurent Joubert, *Erreurs Populaires au Fait de la Medicine* (Bordeaux, 1578); Johann Oberndörfer, *De Veri et Falsi Medici Agnitione Tractatus Brevis, in Theorematum Forma Conscriptus* (Lavingar, 1600); Girolamo (Scipione) Mercurio, *De Gli Errori Popolari d'Italia* (Venice, 1603), and John Cotta, *A Short Discoverie of the Unobserved Dangers of Several Sorts of Ignorant and Unconsiderate Practisers of Physicke in England* (London, 1612), university-trained practitioners rail against quacks and itinerants. Sometimes these diatribes have been understood as a kind of prototypical medical ethic, prescribing behavior appropriate to the ethical practitioner by describing its opposite (Wear 1993). Works such as these, however, may be better understood as interventions in a marketplace, attempts to explain to recalcitrant patients why learned medicine was better than its many competitors.

This brief portrait of medical practice as a marketplace must be tempered by an understanding of geographical and chronological change. From the patient's perspective, medicine may have been a very open market, but from the perspective of the state, health care was increasingly regulated. From the late Middle Ages, Italian cities appointed physicians and surgeons to provide care for their citizens; many German cities followed suit. All over Europe, regular medicine had a corporate structure derived from the medical guild. Surgeons and apothecaries in cities and towns were trained by apprenticeship and became members of their local colleges or corporations, which attempted to limit practice to members only. Physicians were university trained but also might belong to local colleges or corporations that carefully guarded their privileges.

The "medical marketplace" model was first used to describe the pattern of health care provision in early modern England (Cook 1986; see also Pelling 1987; Loudon 1986b). British North America was the least-regulated medical marketplace, lacking the guild-based corporate structures of Europe. France's medical world has been described as a largely corporative structure of orthodox practitioners with a "penumbra" of others, although other historians emphasize a more thoroughgoing economic model (Brockliss and Jones 1997; but see also Ramsey 1988). Relations between patients and practitioners in Italy were shaped by a market that included a sizeable number of charitable and religious healers and institutions (Gentilcore 1998; Pomata 1998; Park 1985). Health care provision in the German-speaking lands was a patchwork of corporate structures. Each locality had a somewhat different array of officially sanctioned practitioners, as well as a wide range of other health care providers (Lindemann 1996; Duden 1991).

As Mary Lindemann points out, older, guild-based corporate structures coexisted with newer commercial and consumer-driven medical enterprises. Many patients understood health care provision both within a moral economy derived from guild-based norms about suitable livelihoods and embraced newer consumer possibilities (Lindemann 1996, 181–2; see also Chapter 28). Lindemann's observation about the coexistence of older notions of social obligation with newer ones about health care as an item of consumption holds true for much of Europe and colonial North America. From a patient's perspective, however, the nuances of the multiform patterns of licensure, patenting, guilds, and other forms of official sanction documented by historians did not seem to matter very much. Patients simply did not pick and choose their health care providers according to these official designations (Gentilcore 1998; Fissell 1991; Lindemann 1996; Pomata 1998). In what follows, I therefore focus upon both the norms of behavior appropriate to market relations and those deriving from broader social relations because health care was rarely governed solely by market relations.

Broadly speaking, such medical regulation was strongest on the Continent, and weakest in colonial North America, with Britain somewhere in between. As patterns of medical and surgical training gradually shifted away from apprenticeship and toward the hospital, new forms of corporate identity linked regular practitioners together and gradually overwrote older distinctions between physic and surgery.

III. Social Relations: The Market

Because health care was structured in part as a marketplace, many of the precepts governing the relationships between patients and practitioners derived from more general understandings of appropriate behaviors around buying and selling (Crawford 2000). In the examples of patients' choices of practitioners cited previously, the details of the monetary transactions were often recorded: Otto paid the miller Claudiz 10 *groschen*; the Italian stable boy paid the surgeon–apothecary "what was due for his services." "Services" in this case refers to bloodletting and the provision of a medicine so nasty that the stable boy did not finish it.

According to Luis Garcia-Ballester, it was in the late Middle Ages that medical care became an item of exchange, a service rendered for which payment could be expected. He cites Thomas Aquinas in 1272 noting that the power of money is such that medicine had become an *ars ad pecuniam* (art for the sake of money). By 1320, the French surgeon Henri de Mondeville included "salary" as an intrinsic aspect of the doctor–patient relationship (Garcia-Ballester 1993, 49). De Mondeville defined the relationship as a contractual one, a model that continued to be employed for centuries, although the nature of that contract changed. For de Mondeville, mutual confidence between patient and practitioner depended upon the patient following the doctor's instruction and the patient paying the fee (Garcia-Ballester 1993, 51).

Three different models overlapped in the individual patient–doctor relationship, whereas others prevailed in settings where a municipal authority or institution employed a practitioner. First, as Gianna Pomata has observed, some patients and practitioners entered into a contract for a cure, explicitly agreeing that no fee was due to the practitioner unless the patient was healed satisfactorily. Second, patients often bought specific medicines or medical/surgical procedures from healers. In both of these models, ordinary market relations governed much of the conduct of the two parties. Finally, a patient might implicitly contract with a practitioner for the treatment of an ailment, the treatment to rest upon the practitioner's expert knowledge. This was not, however, the dominant model in the past. From the later Middle Ages, learned practitioners tried to persuade their patients that they were buying more than just pills and procedures, but theirs was an uphill battle. It was not until the later nineteenth century that the medical marketplace and the social relations it engendered gave way to a modern profession with a specific set of social prescriptions for the patient.

As Gianna Pomata has shown, patients in fifteenth and sixteenth century Italy entered into contracts with practitioners agreeing to pay a set amount if they were cured. So acceptable was this practice that the Protomedicato of Bologna (a council of the city's leading practitioners) defended contractual relationships even in the case of unorthodox healers. For example, in 1633, a butcher appealed to the protomedicato because he claimed to have healed a boy suffering from ringworm. The boy refused to pay the agreed-upon 50 silver piastres, claiming that he was not fully cured. Surprisingly, the Protomedicato upheld the butcher's rights, lowering his fee to 16 piastres because the agreement had not been put down in writing. Only secondarily did the city's leading doctors note that a butcher was not supposed to be practicing medicine, although their decision implicitly endorsed some kind of healing role for him. In the early seventeenth century, contracts for cure began to seem inappropriate for Italian physicians. Paolo Zacchia's *Questiones Medical-legales* (1621–1625) argued that it was beneath the dignity of doctors to bargain for a cure. Zacchia thought it undignified to even mention payment, preferring to understand medical fees as honoraria (Pomata 1998, 149).

The contract for cure died slowly, however. In seventeenth-century Virginia, practitioners contracted for cures, often with the local authority for the cure of a poor person. In 1658, a Dr. Waldron agreed to cure Francis Warren by Christmas or be paid nothing. John Toton contracted to cure Robert Prichard in a fortnight for 40 shillings (Blanton 1930, 246). Patients or their caretakers bargained over cures. When Humphrey Browning's servant Peter Wells got hurt in a fight, Browning bargained surgeon John Penny down to 3 pounds 10 shillings (from 5 pounds) for the cure. Many patients expected to pay only if they were healed, suggesting a kind of implicit contract, at least from the patient's perspective. For example, the well-known Rose case in England involved an apothecary suing a butcher who did not pay his bill because he did not feel better; countless other patients simply refused to pay their practitioners for what they considered inadequate treatment but never ended up in court (Cook 1990).

The most common model for practitioner–patient relations in early modern Europe was not the contract but the sale of specific procedures or medicines. Patients understood themselves to be buying specific goods more than a practitioner's expertise per se. Early modern medical bills are often minutely itemized, listing each specific procedure, visit, or medicine provided. Both highly educated, full-time practitioners and those healers who were much more occasional treated charging for advice very gingerly, albeit for somewhat different reasons. Those practitioners who were not officially sanctioned by local authorities often treated their medical practices as the sale of specific items, a custom sometimes enforced by patients as well other practitioners. For example, the widow Hagen in the eighteenth-century German village of Voightsdahlum sold teas and herbal remedies, much to the annoyance of the local physicus and the apothecary. Despite frequent complaints by these official practitioners, the widow was protected by her community although her remedies were not cheap. Once she began to try to charge for advice, however, her neighbors started to complain to the medical authorities and she was prosecuted (Lindemann 1996, 357). Lindemann makes the point that patients often

praised those practitioners who charged only for material things, not for advice or visits. She is correct to note that medical advice was much more slowly commodified than medical procedures, long being understood as a form of social exchange or gift rather than expertise for which payment was appropriate.

More generally, in a world in which domestic medicine was the norm, and knowledge of healing commonplace, patients did not understand themselves as buying advice so much as buying specific medicines or procedures. Practitioners, especially surgeons and apothecaries trained by apprenticeship, were analogous to other early modern tradesmen, selling specific items upon which their guild or company often held some form of limited monopoly. Even physicians were reluctant to charge fees for their expertise, preferring instead to itemize visits and procedures. In colonial Virginia, for example, John Clulo billed a patient for more than 1,000 pounds of tobacco, but next to the item "for my visitts paines and attendance" he listed no fee (Blanton 1930, 244). William Broderip, a very successful apothecary in Bristol, England, made no charge for attendance in the city and its immediate environs, writing "attendance what you please" on the bottom of his bills. For trips outside the locality, he charged 5 shillings, but he made his fortune from the medicines he sold, not from attendance (Loudon 1986, 70). Benjamin Rush, the noted American physician, understood the psychology of medical billing well. He gave advice to a young practitioner never to "insert trifling advice or services in a bill." Instead, "you can incorporate them with important matters such as pleurisy or the reduction of the bone" (Sydenham 1978, 130).

The ultimate expression of this form of medical relationship lies in fee bills, a feature of early American medicine. Fee bills, which listed medical procedures and the fees that should be charged for them, represent an attempt at standardization by practitioners in a crowded marketplace (Rosen 1946a). Although fee bills have been understood primarily from the perspective of the practitioner, they are also revealing about the nature of medical practice as construed by patients. They depict medical care as a commodity that could be itemized minutely, bought and sold as a potentially unrelated series of procedures. An 1815 fee bill from New York City details the costs of verbal advice, letter of advice, an ordinary visit, a consultation, a repeated visit, a night visit, a mileage charge, specific rates for trips to Staten Island and other locales (these to be doubled in winter or storm) before going on to list procedures such as cupping, bleeding, and the like. In the midst of the list of procedures, as if some specific episode was suddenly called to the list-maker's mind, there is stern warning that "visits in haste to be charged double" (Rosen 1946a, 3). Patients, or consumers, happily undercut fee bills, patronizing healers who charged less than the bills specified.

Patients in this medical marketplace wanted their health care providers to abide by the more general norms of buying and selling. For example, patients wanted to get the product they paid for and not some inferior substitute. In 1772, the barber Carlo Gavessi had to return 15 paoli to his patient Domenico Buldrini because the barber's potion was not the powerful secret remedy composed of "gold, air, and silver" as promised (Pomata 1998, 147). Conversely, patients worried that practitioners, especially apothecaries and physicians, might provide too-powerful medicines and poisons. Renaissance drama reflects a larger cultural obsession with poison, depicting practitioners as both able to heal and to kill. As the English translator of a German physician's antiquackery text explains, "neither the Patient, nor his Friends, shall be able to know whether in stead of a Soveraigne Medicine, far set, and dear bought, they receive rank poison" (Oberndörfer 1602, 18). Patent medicines, which became an increasingly important segment of the medical economy in the eighteenth century, very often came with special seals or marks that indicated to their buyers that this was the genuine item and not an imitation. Historians of Italian and English medicine have noted that lawsuits for malpractice were relatively rare in the early modern period. On the Continent, the tradition of Roman law, namely that a practitioner could not be criminally prosecuted for a patient's death resulting from incompetence or negligence, remained strong. Instead, patients sued for breach of contract or simply refused to pay for treatment they found unsatisfactory.

IV. Social Relations: Deference and Hierarchy

1. Patron and Client

Healing was not just structured by market relations. As Lindemann suggests, some aspects of medicine were slow to be commodified, and commercial transactions themselves were subject to more general social norms. In early modern Europe, society was often understood as a finely graded hierarchy, stretching from ruler to pauper, with each individual aware of his or her standing. In small face-to-face communities, such hierarchies were maintained through everyday encounters, gossip and memory providing reminders and reinforcement. In larger towns and cities, greater attention was paid to appearance as a guide to status. In this hierarchical understanding of social relations, higher and lower stations in life implied mutual obligations and responsibilities. Servants, for example, were supposed to obey their masters, but servants also expected to receive their masters' help and protection.

Medical care might be part of these mutual obligations rather than, or in addition to, being a commodity. Healing, after all, carried with it profound religious meanings, and was often a part of charitable provision. In some

of the contracts for cure in colonial Virginia mentioned previously, the contract was made between a healer and a parish vestry, as a form of charitable provision for a poor person. So too, Peter Wells could expect his master Humphrey Browning to provide him with surgical care for a wound received in a fight, even if that care was the object of hard bargaining between master and surgeon. This instance does not represent an early form of workman's compensation – fighting was hardly part of Wells's duties – but rather a much older conception of a master's responsibilities to his dependents.

More generally, charitable provision for the sick was an embodiment of these ideas about the obligations of rich to poor. Catholic countries were especially well endowed with such institutions. The city of Naples in 1616, for example, had eleven hospitals, as well as twenty-six other institutions that housed a total of 6,000 of the city's dependent poor, mostly women, children, and the aged (Gentilcore 1998, 125). Protestant Northern Europe was slower to develop hospital care for the sick, but here too, such institutions were understood as an expression of the social links between rich and poor. On the individual level, countless women and men provided health care for their poorer neighbors. A German miller healed cancers and fistulas with benedictions and herbs, but noted, "my income is such that it is not necessary to earn my living with healing" (Lindemann 1996, 359). Lady Grace Mildmay, a Tudor gentlewoman, spent part of every day reading medical books and making remedies so that she could treat her poorer neighbors as well as her family (Pollock 1993).

The hierarchical nature of social relations in early modern Europe structured the relationship between healers and clients in paradoxical ways. Sometimes, the client was superior to the healer and expected deference. Good manners were essential to a practitioner's success. As James Lucas advised the surgeon–apothecary in late eighteenth-century England, "Affability, and polite manners form a professional man for an easy admittance into the company of his superiors" (Lucas 1800, 80). Apprentices were taught to be polite and not overly familiar when they were serving in the shop of their master; a rude apprentice might lose the master an important patient (Fissell 1993).

2. Inventing the Patient as a Special Case

The patron–client relation might also run the other way in episodes of healing. In early modern Europe, patients began to be considered a special kind of dependent to whom practitioners and others owed certain kinds of support. As mentioned previously, institutions for the sick grew out of institutions for the poor, to whom Christian charity was due. Physicians had long treated some poor patients for free, construing their calling as a Christian vocation that included the obligation to treat those who could not pay (see Chapters 26 and 27).

When healing powers were considered god-given, patients and practitioners often understood the healing relationship as one of charity as well as, or instead of, in terms of a medical marketplace. Ann Stanley, for example, was a woman born deaf and mute who healed a range of complaints in eighteenth-century England. She advertised that it was "by divine favour" that she "had naturally an extraordinary genius and Conception" and claimed that she knew people's diseases at first sight. She construed her healing as "doing good" saying that she "takes none in hand for any reward but those she does good to" (Loudon 1986b, 17). Although it is possible to interpret her statement as a kind of implicit contract for cure by an itinerant practitioner, her emphasis upon doing good and the religious language she employs suggests that she understood her role in more complex ways.

Patients might understand themselves simultaneously as both participating in a medical market and in extramarket relations of dependency and obligation. Gianna Pomata recounts the story of Angelo Ratti, a seventeenth-century carpenter who clearly understood himself in both contexts. He suffered from "pains," and on the advice of a priest and a vintner, sought treatment from a soldier named Fanti, who specialized in mercurial treatments. Ratti signed a contract for cure with Fanti, but then thought the better of it and asked for his money back. When the soldier refused, Ratti drew upon relations of patronage; he sought advice from the noted physician and surgeon Antonio Valsalva and from the dean of the college of medicine, Giovan Battista Cingari. Both told him not to use the mercurial ointments lest he be poisoned. Ratti's next-door neighbor, a barber, went further and scolded him for his reckless behavior (Pomata 1998, 125–7). Ratti, a lowly carpenter, expected and received free medical advice from his superiors, who understood that their civic role as medical leaders implied an obligation to the city's poorer denizens.

Writers on the law began to discuss the sick as a special class of person in the seventeenth century. Collating and discussing civil and canon law, authors such as Tommaso Azzio, I. V. Bechmann, and G. Fichtner developed the concept of the "privilegia infermorum," or special role of the sick. The sick, for example, were exempt from judicial torture and they enjoyed unusual freedom in suing their enemies in any court regardless of jurisdictional prerogative. As Gianna Pomata illustrates, the privileges of the sick derive from a larger understanding of the relationship between superior and inferior. A father who denied medical treatment to his child lost guardianship over the child; a husband who refused his wife medical treatment lost his right to her dowry if she died from the illness.

Although the earliest writers on the privileges of the sick were Catholic, the more general tradition was followed in Protestant Europe as well. As suggested previously, in both Protestant and Catholic countries, hospital treatment for the poor was a part of a larger general response to dependency. The individual relationship of dependence between a master and servant took precedence over any more general charity however. Writers on the privilege infermorum stressed that a master had to provide medical care for his servants and should continue to pay their wages. Although the governors of English voluntary hospital were wholly responsible for hospital admissions in general – patients were only admitted if they had a note from a governor – they were forbidden to send their own servants to hospital. Instead, they were supposed to provide their servants with medical treatment themselves. New forms of charity were not intended to replace older sets of obligations.

Before the late nineteenth century, therefore, most of the ethical basis for the conduct of patients with their practitioners did not derive specifically from medicine. Rather, health care was sometimes a commodity, governed by the norms of commercial interactions, and sometimes a social obligation between people of different status. With the development of the Continental tradition of the privilegia infermorum, it might be said that an ethic peculiar to medicine was first articulated with reference to patients, not doctors. These privileges, however, do not represent the precursor to any modern notion of patients' right. Rather, they look back to older ideas about the vulnerabilities of the dependent.

V. CONCLUSION: THE FORCES OF CHANGE

Four large interrelated changes in medicine put an end to this old regime and created the circumstances in which modern concerns about the ethics of the patient–practitioner relationship took root. First, as medicine became increasingly professionalized in the later nineteenth century, it developed a stronger hierarchical array of practitioners. Although early modern physicians considered themselves superior to apothecaries and barber-surgeons, patients did not necessarily concur. In the modern world, however, the phlebotomist who draws blood for medical tests does so according to a physician's orders, and is trained and accredited in ways that make him or her part of a larger hierarchically organized health care system. When early modern people had blood let, they went to a barber-surgeon, often at their own instigation – indeed, early American popular health manuals even advised their readers how to let blood themselves. Although domestic medicine has always remained an important component of health care, and we currently see much growth in complementary medicine (or alternative healing), state and professional control of licensing has reduced the untidy panoply of the early modern medical marketplace to a more streamlined hierarchy of medical practice.

Second, as medical science developed, diagnosis and therapy became much more specialized forms of knowledge. As W. F. Bynum observed, in the eighteenth century, "The language of disease was more widely understood than it was to become" (Bynum 1980, 230). By the twentieth century, practitioner's knowledge and patient's knowledge differed greatly. This difference meant that patients could no longer pick and choose various procedures or interventions or practitioners as they once did. Rather than buying a procedure and some advice from a practitioner, patients were now buying expertise. That expertise provided a diagnosis and a course of treatment as well as affording entree into an ever-more-specialized array of health care providers.

Third, health care was increasingly provided in specialized settings rather than the patient's home. In the mid-nineteenth century, only the poor went into hospitals for medical treatment. As anesthesia and asepsis enabled the development of more sophisticated surgical procedures, and as hospitals recognized the financial potential of paying patients, the hospital became the central medical workplace (Rosenberg 1987). Childbirth became a hospital procedure in the 1920s and 1930s in North America, and death and dying became so in the 1950s (Leavitt 1986). By the 1960s, less than 1 percent of all patient–doctor contacts were house calls (Freidson 1961, 66–7). Europeans continue to be born and die at home in greater proportions than do Americans, but in general, the shift from home to hospital has been accompanied by an almost inevitable loss of patient autonomy (see Chapter 7).

Finally, the relative social position of doctors and patients shifted. In the early modern period, practitioners of all kinds were rarely social elites. Gentlemen did not work with their hands, and even university-trained physicians who largely eschewed manual labor were often of somewhat lower social status than their well-to-do patients. In some circumstances, as discussed previously, practitioners were superior to their patients – in hospitals, or in charitable encounters. In the twentieth century, however, two factors rendered this a more common type of relationship. First, physicians' incomes grew, especially in North America, to the point where medicine as an occupation became predominantly upper middle class. Second, with the advent of nationalized health services in European countries, a huge reservoir of poor and working people had new access to the care of a physician. Both the economic status of physicians and the average status of their patient population changed, resulting in a new imbalance in power between practitioner and patient.

All four of these developments made modern health care a world in which patients were less autonomous than they had been in earlier centuries. Of course, some early modern patients who lacked economic resources had surrendered a measure of autonomy in exchange for charitable health care in an institutional setting. Most early modern patients, navigating between health care as a commodity and health care as a social obligation, had greater control over most aspects of their medical treatment than patients do today. The central concerns of a bioethics of the patient–practitioner relationship – issues such as informed consent or confidentiality – were of little import before the twentieth century.

Chapter 47

The Legal and Quasilegal Regulation of Practitioners and Practice in the United States

Stephen R. Latham and James C. Mohr

I. Introduction

The quality of medical care is regulated in a number of different ways. Some forms of regulation seek to assure medical quality prospectively, by setting standards of entry into different spheres of medical practice. Some seek to assure quality retrospectively, by punishing, correcting, or weeding out practitioners who have proven themselves incompetent or unethical. Unregulated markets, of course, control for quality to some extent: on the prospective side, persons with substandard qualifications have a difficult time attracting customers in a competitive market; on the retrospective side, those who perform a service badly have a difficult time getting paid for it, and those who develop generally poor reputations are unable to hold their patients' custom. It is now commonplace to note that the market for health care services – plagued as it is by information deficits and agency problems – is not an efficient self-regulator. Market mechanisms must therefore be augmented by law: prospectively by licensure requirements and standards governing medical training, and retrospectively by license revocation proceedings, criminal prosecutions, and private medical malpractice suits. Today's medical practitioners must not only compete for patients and payers; they must also be licensed, be graduates of schools whose curricula meet national standards,

and be willing, if they err, to face the possibilities of malpractice liability, state licensing board investigation, professional discipline, and even criminal sanction.

It is therefore startling to recall that for most of the nearly 400 years since the first European physician landed on Virginia's shore, the market for physician services in the British North American colonies and subsequently in the United States remained essentially unregulated in any formal sense. Medical malpractice actions in their modern incarnation appeared in the middle decades of the nineteenth century. Neither enforceable educational standards nor effective licensing laws appeared prior to the early decades of the twentieth century. Meaningful professional discipline has appeared only in the last 20 years. Today, the regulation of practitioners and practice in the United States is a complicated and constantly evolving complex of interactions involving state governments, federal agencies, private market actors, and professional associations. It was not, however, always so. In this chapter, we briefly trace the historical development of those interactions.[1]

II. Colonial Beginnings

Medical practice in the British North American colonies went effectively unregulated from their founding in the early seventeenth century to the American Revolution. That lack of regulation cannot simply be credited to the fact that the colonies were too rural or too distant from the control of Mother England for medical regulation to be possible; from the sixteenth century on France and Spain strictly regulated their distant, rural colonial medical practices (Numbers 1987). British colonial settlers did not lack the imagination to conceive of domestic licensing and regulatory schemes on their own: several are on record as having been proposed and rejected, and some as having been adopted but left unenforced (Packard [1901] 1963; Shryock 1967). A number of theories – many as provocative as they are unprovable – have been advanced to explain this phenomenon. For example, scholars have noted that medical licensing in rural England had been administered from 1511 to 1643, with more or less attention, by Episcopal bishops. That licensing authority had been "disestablished," along with the ecclesiastical hierarchy itself, during Cromwell's Protectorate, and was then reinstated in 1660 (Numbers 1987). America's religious dissenters – including the substantial number of clerical practitioners of medicine – may have resisted medical licensure in part because of its association with the Established Church. Although probable, such surmises are difficult to prove.

Somewhat better documented was the traditional Anglo-American distrust of government and preference for self-reliance, local control, and horse sense over any orders or standards issued from afar. Continental European traditions of medical regulation, which extended back to the Italian city-states of the Renaissance, tended to emphasize the direct role of central authority. The rise of the continental nation-state was also marked by an increasing centralization of power including, by the nineteenth century, complete central control over medical education and the right to license medical practice. English traditions, in contrast, had always stressed professional self-regulation and local control. As early as the sixteenth century, parliament delegated the regulation of professional activity away to various local organizations including, as noted earlier, local bishops in the rural areas, and, in London, the Royal College of Physicians (1518), the London Company of Barber-Surgeons (1540), and the London Society of Apothecaries (1617).

In the colonies, there was virtually no control of medical practice until the late eighteenth century. Virginia passed a statute regulating physicians' fees in 1639, but saying nothing about who could or could not practice medicine, or to what standard. In 1649, Massachusetts passed a law – so vague as to be unenforceable – prohibiting anyone from practicing medicine without first obtaining the "advice and consent of such as are skillful in the same Art (if such may be had) or at least some of the wisest and gravest then present." Another Virginia fee statute of

1736 distinguished between medical degree-holders and others, but only to the extent of allowing degree-holders to charge higher fees. Only the inconsistent, informal and wholly private custom of medical apprenticeship – increasingly common after 1700 – offered some uneven enhancement and a degree of consistency to the quality of American medical practice.

Halting efforts to upgrade the quality of medical practice in British North America took place in the decades just prior to the American Revolution. New York City passed the colonies' first real medical practice act in 1760, which empowered a board of nonphysicians to grant licenses to practice in the city. The board had no effective disciplinary authority and no ability to prevent nonlicensed practitioners from plying their trade, but a license from the board did, at least, enhance a practitioner's status and thus in theory gave him a better chance at succeeding in the market. In 1765, John Morgan of Philadelphia established the first recognized medical school in the British North American colonies, but the Penn family proprietors would not accede to Morgan's request for licensing powers in North America similar to those afforded the Royal College in England. In the 1760s, New Jersey gave its medical society the authority to grant licenses, and in 1773 Connecticut followed suit.

The postwar years saw an explosion of medical regulatory activity. In 1781, the newly founded Massachusetts Medical Society was granted authority to give medical licenses; it was not until 1803, however – after public testing showed that Harvard graduates vastly outperformed others licensed by the Medical Society – that Massachusetts law was amended to grant licenses either to Society designees or to Harvard Medical graduates. (Thus arose the first formal role of medical education in licensure – 38 years after such a role was originally sought by John Morgan in Pennsylvania.) By 1815, most of the original thirteen states had established medical societies, and virtually every state in the union had one by 1830. In the years from 1790 to 1830, these state societies sought, and in many cases obtained, licensing authority. By 1830, of all the states in the Union, only Pennsylvania, Virginia, and North Carolina lacked some sort of licensing law. These varied enormously, but licensure normally required some sort of state or local testing by medical society members, certification by medical faculty members, or both.

In sum, at the close of the eighteenth century, there were some not-terribly-effectual efforts being made to develop prospective controls on the quality of physicians' care, both through the formation of professional medical associations and through the adoption of state licensure laws. Unfortunately, neither medical societies' self-regulatory efforts nor state licensure laws were to bear much fruit in the next century. Eighteenth-century

Americans were left to develop their own, predominantly retrospective, techniques for regulating medicine.

III. Nineteenth-Century Developments

1. The Failure of Professional Self-Regulation

As Chester Burns's pioneering work made clear, issues and problems of nineteenth-century medical ethics were neither well distinguished one from the other nor from broader issues of professional regulation (Burns 1969a). Nineteenth-century physicians interested in those intertwined professional issues faced several daunting problems. First, because the regulation of medicine was considered a state matter rather than a national matter, whatever they did had to be done state-by-state. Unlike their European counterparts, they could not promulgate general policy from a central or national authority. Second, the eighteenth century saw a proliferation of theories or "schools" of medical practice, each with its own state societies and medical faculties. Because state governments adamantly refused to grant licenses to some brands of practitioners – thereby necessarily excluding others – effective regulatory standards could not be imposed as a condition of practice. In a society in which anyone could practice his or her own brand of medicine, standards had either to be voluntary and hence unenforceable, or imposed universally, on all citizens alike, rather than just upon those who practiced medicine. Third, the host of diverse approaches to healing meant that physicians in many different circumstances did not agree among themselves on what was ethical and what was unethical. Even among those most concerned about regulating professional behavior, sharp disagreements arose over basic therapeutics, as well as inherently contentious social issues. Consequently, regulatory and quasiregulatory mechanisms emerged slowly and unevenly.

In 1800, for example, two-thirds of the people who earned their livings as physicians in the city of Philadelphia were neither members of the local medical society nor graduates of any medical school (Bell 1975, 6–19). The situation was similar in New York City, where intraprofessional struggles among the few physicians who did belong to medical societies or medical faculties created fierce animosities inside and outside the profession (Kett 1968). Attempts at meaningful self-regulation through medical societies made some limited headway in New England, where the New Hampshire Medical Society and the Boston Medical Society among others (and their respective successor organizations) tried repeatedly through the nineteenth century to draft regulatory rules (see, e.g., New Hampshire Medical Society 1822 and Boston Medical Association 1852). As the eighteenth century wore on, the New England medical societies took their efforts seriously enough to engender extremely nasty personal battles. As

elsewhere, however, the New Englanders were ultimately in the same situation as every other medical society: anyone who wished to do so could practice medicine in their states without their sanction, and they complained bitterly about their own impotence.

2. The Failure of Early Licensing Laws

The licensing laws enacted during and just after the colonial period were essentially unenforced and unenforceable. Formally trained physicians had been relatively rare in the former American colonies, especially outside the major cities. Many individuals combined a smattering of medical practice with other occupations that ranged from planter to clergyman, so it would have been difficult to know exactly who should be licensed (Minot 1881, Fitz 1895). Most importantly, citizens were not prepared to demand licensure from the friends and neighbors who helped them in times of illness, childbirth, or injury. The result was a sort of two-tiered system in which a handful of formally trained physicians claimed the sanction of a license, but their license meant little in a world where anyone else could also practice medicine without holding a license (Shryock 1967, 3–42).

Post-revolutionary efforts to license American physicians also ran contrary to emerging democratic ideologies. In response to the political egalitarianism and antimonopoly sentiments of the 1820s and 1830s, state legislatures in the 1840s actually repealed most of the licensing laws that existed. The regulations had in any case long since become dead letters. Some states went so far as to make explicit, in the words of the 1844 New York State legislature, the fact that anyone could legally "prescribe for or administer medicine or specifics, to or for the sick" (Wiley 1904, 102). By mid-century, physicians all across the new nation found themselves adrift as individual competitive agents, hustling for business in an overcrowded and completely unregulated market that included a wide spectrum of alternative and often antagonistic healers, trained and untrained, ranging typically from the woman down the lane who grew a few herbs in her garden to surgeons who had apprenticed in European hospitals.

William Wood, who later became Surgeon-General of the United States Navy, summarized the regulatory status of the country in 1849:

> It is well known, that all efforts to limit the exercise of the profession of medicine to those who have the abilities and acquirements essential to its proper understanding, have utterly failed; and ignorant and impudent pretenders, under a great variety of humbugging titles, come before the public with equal rights, and a better chance for popular favor, than the regular practitioner. The public, unfortunately, seems to consider all efforts to limit the practice

of medicine to those of scientific attainments, as the attempt of a sect to monopolize rights. (Wood 1849)

3. Regulation through the Criminal Law

With self-regulation and state licensing laws essentially dysfunctional in the United States, American professionals turned to another alternative: the criminal law. Perhaps the most ambitious and best-documented attempt of physicians to use state criminal codes to prescribe professional behavior and enforce what they regarded as responsible and ethical standards occurred in New York State. In 1823, the New York State Medical Society approved what was to that point the nation's most comprehensive draft of medical ethics. As in other states, however, their rules were patently unenforceable in a situation in which the vast majority of the people practicing medicine in New York did not belong to the state medical society in the first place and had no compelling reason to join. One of the medical society's most prominent members was Theodric Romeyn Beck, a young, capable, and professionally ambitious Albany physician and medical professor. The same year the medical society promulgated its ethical regulations, Beck published *Elements of Medical Jurisprudence*, a book that would dominate medico-legal discussion for a quarter of a century. Beck was deeply distressed by what he regarded as the unethical and unprofessional behavior of many health practitioners active in America's wide-open medical marketplace. He regarded many of those self-authorized healers as a threat to public safety, and he also saw them as a long-term obstacle to professional organization at a level he regarded as desirable.

Beck was elected president of the New York State Medical Society in 1827. An ideal opportunity to influence government policy arose that same year, when the New York legislature appointed a commission to revise the state's criminal code. At the head of the codification commission emerged a politically influential lawyer, John C. Spencer, who was a former college classmate and now a professional ally of Beck. Spencer allowed Beck, whose book had already given him an international reputation in medico-legal matters, to insert a host of proposed revisions into the commission's working draft in 1828. Although couched in the form of potential new crimes, Beck's proposals would be regarded today as medical regulations (Beck 1823). Typical of the kind of proposals he put forward was a section that would make "every person who shall perform any surgical operation, by which human life shall be destroyed or endangered, such as the amputation of a limb, or of the breast, trepanning, cutting for the stone, or for *hernia*" guilty of a misdemeanor, "unless it appear that the same was necessary for the preservation of life, or was advised, by at least two physicians."

According to the report of the revisers (in arguments that Beck himself supplied to the commission), that proposal was necessary because, "The rashness of many young practitioners in performing the most important surgical operations for the mere purpose of distinguishing themselves has been a subject of much complaint, and we are advised by old and experienced surgeons, that the loss of life occasioned by the practice, is alarming. The [proposed revision] furnishes the means of indemnity, by a consultation, or leaves the propriety of the operation to be determined by the testimony of competent men" (Beck 1836, 829–30). Caution in capital operations and consultation with recognized experts were, of course, cardinal principles of early ethical statements, including the manifesto drafted 5 years before by Beck's own New York State Medical Society. Another proposal in the draft code would have made the use of instruments in obstetrical deliveries illegal unless two other physicians agreed to their necessity. This new crime was suggested because Beck and others believed that the clumsy use of instruments by "ignorant" practitioners was needlessly killing neonates.

Legislators subsequently struck those two sections from the final version of the criminal code they passed in 1829, but several other sections like them survived to become New York state law in 1830. Among the quasi-regulatory ethical enforcement sections that survived were new crimes related both to the administration of poisons and to the performance of abortions after quickening.

New York was certainly not the only state in which attempts to enforce ethical standards of behavior upon physicians were ventured through criminal legislation. The trend was widespread throughout the nation during the 1830s and 1840s, and it sometimes produced laws that seem rather quaintly naive or even vaguely comical in retrospect. The 1834 session of the Ohio general assembly, for example, passed a law that made the sale of secret remedies that endangered life a misdemeanor (the sale of secret remedies that merely made patients sick was presumably acceptable, even though the champions of stronger ethical standards generally opposed secret remedies of any sort); declared attempted abortion a misdemeanor (without defining abortion); stated that deaths resulting from attempted abortions would be treated as felonies (a sort of indictment in advance; you can attempt an abortion if you know what you are doing, but if your patient dies, we will come after you); and created the new crime of prescribing medicine while drunk. That last provision reflected both the ragged levels of professionalism then extant in the state's healing business and the dim view of physician behavior taken by many concerned citizens and public officials.

Throughout the rest of the nineteenth century, state-level lawmakers continued their efforts to regulate the practice of medicine through the use of criminal codes.

Sanction for those efforts lay in the police powers of the state and in the government's duty to protect public safety (Novak 1996). As a practical matter, most of the proposed regulations appear to have been drafted not by concerned citizens, but by physicians interested in upgrading and regulating the practice of medicine. Put differently, influential members of the medical profession itself, especially those with professionalizing agendas, were using the police powers of the state to try to regulate the practice of medicine and enforce ethical standards and behaviors upon fellow healers that they could not enforce in other ways. Perhaps the best single example of this phenomenon in the nineteenth century was the gradual criminalization of abortion.

The termination of a pregnancy prior to quickening (the first perception of fetal movement by the mother, usually about the midpoint of gestation) was not illegal anywhere in the United States through the first three decades of the nineteenth century. Beginning in the 1830s, as the apparent incidence of abortion began to rise, a handful of medical professors began to question the importance of quickening as a stage in gestation, and hence began to wonder why the termination of a pregnancy prior to that event was ethically any different than the termination of a pregnancy after that event (see Chapters 7 and 36). The most prominent among those professors was T. R. Beck's brother, John B. Beck, who taught and practiced in New York City. Aided by Hugh Hodge at the University of Pennsylvania and others, John Beck began to campaign against the quickening doctrine, partly because it allowed him to highlight the emerging power of medical science and partly because it served to demarcate educationally oriented regular physicians from unscientific and unsavory irregular practitioners in an era when both groups had the same legal status. Through mid-century, however, their campaign made little progress.

In the 1850s the campaign to criminalize abortion at all points in pregnancy was picked up by Horatio Robinson Storer, who used the newly created American Medical Association (AMA) (1847) as his principal political vehicle. Beginning in the late 1860s, Storer and his allies around the country were able to persuade state legislatures to make the performance of abortion at any point in gestation a crime of some degree (although many states retained the quickening distinction in stipulating penalties). By the end of the century, organized medical pressure had succeeded in making abortion a felony in most American states. For every instance in which documentation exists, those criminal sanctions against abortion were inserted into state codes, included in omnibus medical bills or passed separately at the state level, either at the behest of individual AMA-type physicians or as the result of pressure from the state and local medical societies. This was not a wave of legislation that the public clamored for; it was a wave of legislation engineered by a subset of regular physicians whose commitment to science-based medicine coincided neatly with their professional aspirations in the medical marketplace and their access to policy makers (Mohr 1978).

4. The Rise of Malpractice

If the use of criminal law was the first recourse of those hoping to regulate medical standards and professional behavior in the wide-open, unruly, overcrowded, and entrepreneurial medical marketplace of nineteenth-century America, an expanded use of the courts became the second. Suits against physicians can be found in English law as early as the fifteenth century (Walton 1983). In his famous *Commentaries on the Laws of England*, published in 1768, Sir William Blackstone included under *mala praxis* (the phrase from which was derived the modern word malpractice), "Injuries . . . by the neglect or unskilful [sic] management of [a person's] physician, surgeon, or apothecary . . . because it breaks the trust which the party had placed in his physician, and tends to the patient's destruction" (Blackstone 1768). Nonetheless, actions for malpractice were rarely taken in the United States through the first third of the nineteenth century, and the vast majority of American lawyers would not have known how to draft an action for medical malpractice. Even at a theoretical level, the medico-legal concept of malpractice was so arcane and so unimportant in the United States that American writers on medical jurisprudence, including Beck himself, did not bother to mention medical malpractice through the first four decades of the nineteenth century (Mohr 1993).

That situation changed rather abruptly around 1840 for a host of reasons. Shifts in religious belief not only diminished fatalism (and hence the willingness of people to regard physical affliction as the act of God) but also increased evangelical hopes for human progress and well-being. Many people began to believe that the human condition could be improved, and Americans launched the nation's first exercise and diet campaigns. Flamboyant medical advertisements in the burgeoning newspapers of the day raised false and unrealistic expectations regarding the ability of physicians to deal with various maladies; consequently, when patients failed to improve, they began to hold their physicians accountable. Lawyers, themselves caught up in the same wide-open, unlicensed, and intensely competitive professional marketplace that physicians faced, saw in medical malpractice a potentially lucrative new field, which they began to subsidize (through the assumption of risk) by taking medical malpractice cases on a contingent fee basis. Finally, American courts during the 1830s and 1840s relaxed the old English rules of tort pleading, which had the intended effect of encouraging medical malpractice suits. The overall result was a burst of medical malpractice suits.

From 1840 to 1860, the number of malpractice cases carried to state appellate courts in the United States as a whole roared ahead 950 percent. The population rose approximately 85 percent during that same period, which suggests that the rate of medical malpractice suits appears to have jumped abruptly by a factor of roughly tenfold during the middle two decades of the nineteenth century (DeVille 1990). After more than 50 years of barely noticing malpractice on the medical horizon, medical journals suddenly became all but obsessed with the phenomenon. Almost overnight – at least by historical standards – malpractice actions had become the nation's principal method of quasiregulation in the medical field (Elwell 1860). A century and a half later, of course, malpractice litigation remains an important quasi-regulatory mechanism, even though the United States subsequently implemented direct, state-sanctioned medical licensing. Indeed, in the early decades of the twentieth century, at the same time licensing laws began to take effect, medical malpractice litigation as a mechanism of patient recourse was essentially institutionalized and underwritten by a vast – and at the time unprecedented – system of liability insurance (Mohr 2000).

Medical malpractice litigation is now generally regarded as a mechanism that allows the public to demand compensation from physicians who fall short of established standards in any given case. Indirectly, therefore, it exerts regulatory pressure from outside the profession upon all physicians collectively to remain on their toes. Although medical malpractice litigation had a similar function in the nineteenth century, like the use of criminal statutes, it also functioned as a mechanism whereby physicians attempted to regulate their profession and to drive rivals from the field. The record of nineteenth-century medical malpractice cases makes clear the large number of instances in which one physician was out to punish another, whom he (or more rarely she) regarded as behaving unethically or unprofessionally. Individual cases were usually (but not always) brought by patients, but patients were often urged to the bar by a professional enemy of the defendant. The issues at law, moreover, regularly involved all of the classic subjects of ethical debate within the profession itself: appropriate fees, proper consultations, disputed therapies, false or unsavory advertising, and levels of professional decorum (see, e.g., Lowell 1825).

Testimony in medical malpractice cases also highlighted a related question faced by all those attempting to regulate the professional behavior of physicians: What should be the responsibilities of physicians in legal proceedings in general, and how should physicians be made to fulfill those responsibilities? Many well-educated medico-legalists at the end of the eighteenth century and the beginning of the nineteenth centuries had envisioned a major role for physicians in civic affairs. In their view, American medical doctors should work with policy makers in the new republic to ensure both the literal and the metaphorical well-being of the body politic (an idea of public service that they adapted from what some physicians in Europe at that same time were calling "medical police"). It also followed that American medical doctors should work with the courts to ensure the highest standards of justice. Although the modern concept of the expert witness was just coming into standard practice in the United States early in the nineteenth century, many physicians saw great potential in that professional role.

Those early republican dreams proved more attractive in theory than in practice. In practice, American physicians did not agree upon underlying concepts of disease and health, much less on therapeutics, so they had a hard time speaking with a unified voice on public health or environmental protection issues. Because the American court system was unrelentingly adversarial, medical witnesses were not consulted about holistic truths as they might have been, at least in theory, in European courts. Instead, American physicians were put upon the stand to make specific points that favored one side or the other. Because the state refused to recognize any group of healers as more legitimate than any others, every person who claimed to be a physician could be recognized as a medical expert on the stand. All of that, in turn, made the medical profession look even more internally divided than it already was. Medical societies tried to ban testimony in certain types of cases, but a lucrative market in medical witnesses-for-hire had already developed by the middle of the nineteenth century.

To make matters worse, longstanding English legal precedents permitted state and local jurisdictions to command both the services and the testimony of individual physicians whenever officials considered such services and testimony germane to public well-being or public justice. But public officials did not have to remunerate the physicians whose expertise they chose to commandeer, and when they did offer compensation it was rarely at rates considered professionally appropriate by the nation's best educated and most prominent physicians. The result was an ironic situation in which the nation's physicians no longer welcomed the prospect of public service, they bristled at it. In the 1870s, a number of state medical societies brought test cases to their state supreme courts in an effort to secure professional standing and professional compensation for public service but they made little headway. The new post of medical examiner resolved some of the most acute problems in the last decades of the nineteenth century, but the power of the state to enlist medical services remains a thorny issue with a host of unresolved regulatory implications.

At the close of the nineteenth century the United States had relatively few prospective controls on medical quality: The national spirit of democratic egalitarianism prevented states from enforcing strict licensure laws or educational standards; and the public mistrust of "monopolizing" professionals, combined with the theoretical disarray of medical science itself, left little opportunity for organized medicine to step in with effective self-regulatory measures. Nonetheless, two new and potentially powerful retrospective regulatory tools had been developed: criminal sanctions for gross misconduct and quackery; and medical malpractice lawsuits for damages by injured patients. Importantly, both of these backward-looking regulatory tools were enlisted in physicians' continuing project to gain professional status and power – a project that would succeed dramatically, and would dominate both the regulation and the delivery of medical services for the bulk of the twentieth century.

IV. 1900–1965: THE VICTORY OF PROFESSIONALISM

Working through state medical societies and the AMA medical regulars (those physicians who were committed to a scientific approach, medical research, and science-based medical education in contrast to "sectarian" practitioners such as homeopaths, naturopaths, herbalists, Thomsonians, and so on; see Chapter 36) had spent the second half of the nineteenth century trying vainly to bring order to the American medical marketplace and pushing for regulatory licenses (Shryock 1967, 43–76). The AMA's very first meetings were devoted to reforms of medical education and to approving a code of medical ethics, which, among other things, demanded scientific practice (Baker et al. 1999). Although they acted in the name of public protection, it was that subset of science-and-education physicians, rather than the public, who pushed for regulations. Given the paucity of scientific evidence favoring the "regular" over the sectarian approaches to medicine in 1847 (the regulars still practiced bleeding and purging and were ignorant of germ theory, bacteriology, and antisepsis), the public might be forgiven suspicions about the monopolistic goals of the regulars, who were pushing for reforms designed to injure their "non-scientific" competitors.

The AMA made little progress toward regulatory reform until well after the Civil War. Although the public began to demand better-credentialed physicians around midcentury, it was the bacteriological revolution (beginning, arguably, with Oliver Wendell Holmes's 1843 paper on puerperal fever contagion), combined with such things as the development of effective anesthesia and antisepsis in surgery, that finally provided the regulars with a plausible case for privileging their approach to healing over other approaches. The organized regulars made that case again and again in state legislatures during the closing decades of the nineteenth century. By 1895, nearly all the separate states had once again established state medical boards with licensing power – although in many

cases these boards were established only after medical regulars compromised and agreed to form "mixed boards," which would license both regulars and sectarians (Rothstein 1985, 308–10).

Recognizing the power of publicity in an era noted for its reform-minded "muckraking," the increasingly influential AMA moved to eliminate some of the worst defects of the early medical boards. In the opening years of the twentieth century, the AMA's *Journal* published a series of articles that compared the medical board laws of different states and also revealed different states' pass rates for medical licensure applicants from different schools of medicine and states of residence. The embarrassment of public exposure – the revelation, for example, that states tended to grant licenses more easily to applicants born within their borders than to outsiders – increased uniformity and tended to raise standards (Stevens 1998, 63–74). Boards had very little power, however, to check the unlicensed practice of medicine, and remained relatively ineffectual for decades.

Publicity tactics were also used in the battle for medical school reform. From 1896, the AMA *Journal* began to publish data comparing educational standards at different medical schools. In 1906, the AMA's Council on Medical Education formalized a program of inspecting and issuing report cards on medical schools. Building on that Council's work, Abraham Flexner issued his famous 1910 survey of medical education in America (Flexner 1910). The Flexner Report ratified a process already underway that resulted in the closure of dozens of substandard medical schools and eventually in the standardization of medical school curricula according to AMA-promulgated criteria. The adoption of educational standards gave the first real teeth to state licensure laws. By 1925, forty-nine states required candidates for medical licensure to be graduates of a medical college, and forty-six would not accept degrees from schools with low grades from the AMA's Council (Stevens 1998, 68).

Licensure statutes around the country developed further during the first half of the twentieth century, flirting with but never achieving nationwide uniformity. In 1915, the AMA created the National Board of Medical Examiners, a professional self-regulatory organization that administered voluntary tests of medical competence. By 1932, forty-one states had accepted the National Board's test scores as measures of qualification for medical licensure. The 1930s also saw the promulgation of uniform standards for specialty certification by various national professional self-regulatory bodies, but states governments declined to adopt separate laws for licensing specialists as such.

By the mid-1960s, the regulatory structure governing American physicians had evolved into what Derbyshire termed the "professional order" (Derbyshire 1969). In that "order," public law – heavily influenced by professional associations – regulated the quality of physicians' care prospectively by setting educational standards, as well as testing standards for licensure and specialty certification. Although in theory, state licensing finally offered the states themselves a means of trying to enforce high and consistent standards of ethical and professional behavior, in practice the states never made much use of the threat of license revocation to achieve those ends. By the time medical licensing became effective in the United States – roughly in the period from 1920 to 1950 – long experience with ethical and professional regulation through other means, principally criminal law and civil malpractice suits, may have eroded the sense of regulatory urgency that might have accompanied licensure. For whatever reasons, state licenses soon appeared in practice to be nearly permanent; once obtained, they were all but impossible to lose. Although licensing laws set base-level educational standards for entry into medical practice and limited the total number of practitioners, those who held the licenses were conspicuously reluctant to regulate themselves in any formal way. Under most states' laws, responsibility for initiating postlicensure professional discipline was formally delegated to state medical (or their equivalent sectarian) societies. Formal state-level disciplinary actions referred from within the profession remained so notoriously rare that, at least until the 1980s, a case could be made that state licensure was primarily a form of professional exclusivity rather than of professional regulation. The state boards themselves were generally made up entirely of volunteer part-time physicians from local organized medicine, and they had part-time staff. Most state boards did not even have jurisdiction to hear complaints about physician incompetence or negligence, but could address only such issues as criminal misconduct, substance abuse, and impairment.

Professional discipline took place at the local level and out of the public eye. Local physician grievance committees, hospital medical staffs, and local professional associations often facilitated private agreements between physicians and their aggrieved patients (Ameringer 1999, 31, 37–8); only the most serious of these matters were ever referred to the state authority for official action. A number of issues regarding physician competence and negligence were handled even less formally: The peers of a marginally competent physician might stop referring complex cases to him, and manifestly incompetent physicians could be forced into early retirement. Although they were no doubt sometimes effective in protecting the public, these informal modes of professional self-regulation resulted in no public reporting or official sanction. They could therefore never be held publicly accountable to standards of consistency or fairness. Above all, there was no guarantee that any particular failure to render quality care would trigger the informal sanctioning process. As a consequence, the nineteenth-century innovations

in retrospective regulation – in particular, malpractice actions brought publicly by aggrieved patients – remain salient even to the present time as important modes of regulating medical quality. These have been augmented since the 1950s by lawsuits based in the developing doctrine of informed consent, which allows patients who are injured by medical treatment to sue physicians for damages if they were inadequately informed of the risks of undergoing treatment (Berg et al. 2001).

The lack of official medical board activity in supervising already-licensed physicians did not go unnoticed. In 1961, the AMA called for increased vigilance by state medical boards, and indeed some small progress in the direction of supervision was made during the 1960s. By that time, however, the seeds of the destruction of the professional order had already been sown.

V. The Decline of the Professional Order, 1965–2000

Two major legal developments, both at the federal level, slowly but completely destroyed the professional order. The first was the collective judicial decision, articulated gradually in a series of cases in the 1970s and 1980s, to apply the full force of federal and state antitrust law to the practice of medicine and hence to medical professional organizations. The second was the expansion and development of the federal Medicare and Medicaid programs after their initial passage in 1965.

1. Antitrust and State Board Authority

Prior to the 1970s, Americans generally believed that the nation's antitrust laws did not apply to the activities of the "learned professions." The antitrust laws, after all, had been developed and articulated in the field of industrial manufactures. Their strictures applied to "trade and commerce" – words that at the height of the professional order in both law and medicine seemed hardly to apply to professional practice. Professionals had fiduciary, not commercial, relationships with their clients and patients (not "customers"). According to the dominant scholarly view of professionalism, professionals' insulation from market forces – and their presumed innocence of market motivations – were essential to their ability to serve both their clients and the public interest, and the depth of their learning made it necessary for professional peers – rather than governments, on the one hand, or the laws of supply and demand on the other hand – to regulate the markets for their services. Thanks to these widely accepted assumptions, the ethical rules and professional self-regulatory actions of medical and legal associations had restricted competition, limited advertising, and excluded competitors from markets, all without drawing any serious attention from antitrust enforcers.

These comfortable assumptions were threatened first in the 1960s, when a wave of antiprofessional scholarship undermined and questioned the authority of professional self-regulators. The professional order truly began to unravel when a series of courts opined that professionals, like other businesspeople, were competitors in the marketplace, and ought to be granted no special privileges. In the wake of those opinions, federal authorities set about prosecuting the AMA and other professional associations and dismantling some of the means by which they had insulated regular medical practice from the rigors of the marketplace. Under terms of a 1980 judgment, for example, the AMA was prohibited from promulgating ethics rules that limited advertising or otherwise restricted competition.

Ultimately, however, private enforcement of antitrust laws, rather than governmental efforts, most thoroughly undermined the professional order. The threat of newly available antitrust lawsuits by aggrieved competitors effectively gutted local professional associations' ability to discipline their members through grievance committees and other informal peer-review actions. It became easy for a physician to allege anticompetitive motivation on the part of any local society, medical staff, or group of physicians that had disciplined him, denied him hospital privileges, or cut off his patient referrals. Local professional associations, to whom the state medical boards had effectively delegated informal medical discipline, froze, fearing both the costs of lawsuits and the prospect of treble damages if they lost. This opened a power vacuum, and put a great deal of political pressure on the state medical boards to bring reform, to recruit professional full-time staff, and to move into a much more active regulatory role.

This pressure was augmented by the various "medical malpractice crises," which developed around the country in the 1970s and 1980s. In various states, during those decades, the rates of malpractice claims grew alarmingly, and the availability of affordable medical malpractice liability insurance greatly decreased. The causes of the crises are obscure: perhaps the very real and dramatic increases in technical medical competence had created unrealistic expectations about medical outcomes; perhaps the cultural upheavals of the 1960s had left patients more willing to challenge professional authority; perhaps the dramatic increases in physician earnings had made them less sympathetic and more attractive targets for lawsuits. In any case, organized medicine called for "malpractice reform" to curb the perceived "overuse" of private-law actions against physicians. This, in turn, inevitably called attention to the lack of compensating patient protection through public medical discipline by state boards.

The state boards took up the challenge. Beginning in the 1970s, but particularly in the 1980s, state boards around the country "professionalized." They hired full-time staff, reduced the number of their physician members in favor of consumer representatives, obtained bigger budgets, obtained jurisdiction over physician-negligence and physician-competence matters and shifted their caseloads in those directions, and – most dramatically – greatly increased the total number of disciplinary actions they brought. On average, state boards prosecuted 685 percent more cases per annum in the period from 1986–1996 than in the period from 1963–1967 (1,245 per year as compared to 181). Critics are not uniformly delighted with the state boards' performance – Dr. Sidney Wolfe of Public Citizen estimates that each state board ought to be disciplining one percent of its practicing in-state physicians annually, and only about half a dozen states attained that level in 1999. But the shift away from the old profession-dominated system in the last two decades of the twentieth century was unmistakable.

Further changes in state-board practices are no doubt in the making. A number of states have been investigating the possibility of using state boards to regulate quality in the new, post-1993 world of corporate-managed medical care. The possibilities are intriguing: Can state boards, for example, supervise the activities of physicians who are working as medical directors of health maintenance organizations? Can a medical director who makes an improper denial of a claim for care have his or her license suspended, or do his or her activities as medical director fall outside the scope of the "practice of medicine" over which the boards have authority?

2. Federal Programs, Medical Inflation, and National Quality Control

The second important federal legal development that undermined the professional order was the passage in 1965 – over the protests of the organized medical profession – of the Medicare and Medicaid programs. In addition to enhancing access to medical care, these programs gave new legitimacy to health insurance and, above all, made the health care "business" profitable, which in turn drew significant commercial investment into the area. The burgeoning numbers of well-insured patients encouraged physician entrepreneurs to invest in health-related businesses; over time, this hurt their professional reputations and opened organized medicine to fresh charges of profiteering. The programs' initially generous cost-based and fee-for-service reimbursement schedules, coupled with the "moral hazard" problem of medical overutilization by patients who were not bearing the costs of the medical care they received, added considerably to an already high technology- and salary-driven rate of inflation. By the early 1970s, there was widespread worry about health care cost-control, particularly among large employers, who were purchasing health insurance as employee benefits, and the federal government, which was footing the lion's share of the Medicare and Medicaid bills (Starr 1982). Those concerns led to new, enhanced roles in medical cost and quality control for private insurers, who had to hold down costs to keep their employer-customers happy. Most importantly, these developments pressed the federal government into a new role: that of leading market participant, as distinguished from simply an external regulator. That new role married the government's historic desire to maintain a high quality of medical practice with a now direct and steeply rising concern about cost control.

The programs' preferred technique for meshing cost with quality control was Utilization Review (UR), the retrospective review of medical records to determine the adequacy, necessity, or propriety of treatment. In principle, UR could help keep program costs down (by discovering and weeding out unnecessary care) and assure that the programs were purchasing only quality care for their enrollees (by discovering and weeding out inappropriate or inadequate care). Whatever its potential benefits, however, UR – whether undertaken by private firms or by federal programs – helped end the professional order by subjecting physicians' medical judgment to regular second-guessing and to outside control.

Some limited procedures for utilization review were included in the original Medicare statute; Medicaid added UR provisions within 2 years of its inception. Medicare's UR programs eventually expanded and changed considerably over time. The first major effort of the government-as-market-participant to control both quality and cost was the establishment, in 1972, of the Professional Standards Review Organizations (PSROs). PSROs were conceived as local authorities, designed to articulate local standards of medical practice and to facilitate review of local physicians' records for compliance with those standards. Each PSRO governed a single area with a population of 350,000. Twenty-five percent of the physicians serving each area were supposed to serve on the area's PSRO; however, in an effort to seize control over standard setting from organized medicine, the PSRO statute specified that medical societies and medical society membership would have no role in determining which physicians served. PSRO physicians were supposed to set regional standards of care for physicians. Physicians practicing in the region would then be subject to retrospective review in light of those standards. The key question – and the one whichone, which eventually spelled the PSRO's downfall – was, who should conduct the retrospective quality-of-care review? The PSRO legislation required the PSROs to accept reviews done by hospital medical staffs and other local organizations. In practice, this meant that local medical hierarchies still determined what occurred at the crucial level of review, even though organized medicine per se had been barred from the process of standard setting. Provider organizations battled over

who should actually conduct the reviews. The American Hospital Association felt that hospitals should have sole authority to review because the AMA preferred to vest reviewing power in the hands of local medical societies. These battles, and the inability to make local review effective, kept the law from achieving its goal. In 1983, the Reagan administration introduced legislation that substituted Peer Review Organizations (PROs) for PSROs.

PROs were considerably more threatening to the professional order. They were statewide rather than regional. Contracts for offering PRO services to the federal programs could be held by physician groups, but could also be held by the insurance companies or data management firms that sometimes served as program administrators within each state – and the contracts had to be won and maintained through a process of competitive bidding. Unlike PSROs, PROs could not accept the retrospective reviews of other bodies; they had to engage in their own reviewing. Most importantly, they had authority to sanction inappropriate care. As Brennan and Berwick (1996) demonstrate, an early overemphasis on their disciplinary function led to tensions between the regulators and the regulated, and handicapped the PROs' ability to focus on quality improvement. Over time, however, the PROs obtained mandates to review consumer complaints about program physicians' care, and to conduct long-term quality-of-care studies; and they soft-peddled their disciplinary function. Their ability to have genuine impact on program medical quality– both by spotting instances of inappropriate care, and by prescribing better practices – has expanded, and may continue to do so.

3. Fraud Control as Quality Control

PROs are not the only entities that review program physicians' medical practices. The program administrators ("Carriers") in the several states are charged with weeding out fraudulent and abusive billing practices; so, too, are the Office of the Inspector General and the United States Justice Department. Their efforts to separate legitimate from illegitimate program billing sometimes bleed over into a disturbingly cost conscious and punitive sort of "quality review." The so-called Stark regulations (named for the Congressman, Peter Stark, D-California, who led legislative efforts resulting in the regulations), passed during the 1980s prohibited program physicians from making referrals to health facilities (such as laboratories, hospitals and imaging centers) in which they have an ownership or other financial interest. The "Anti-Kickback" regulations prohibit payments for referral for any program-reimbursable medical care. Both of these regulations were primarily designed to keep program costs down, by outlawing investment or payment arrangements that might give physicians a financial incentive to authorize unnecessary care. It is, of course, poor medicine to offer any patient unnecessary care. Yet, these regulations, aimed as they are at ability to structure delivery systems in certain ways, have arguably interfered with efficient business arrangements that might have allowed providers to deliver quality care to patients at reduced cost. Thus, these cost-control regulations are quality-control regulations as well, and their net impact on the quality of medical care remains difficult to ascertain.

In the latter 1990s, the federal government began an extraordinary campaign against fraud and abuse in the Medicare and Medicaid systems. One powerful weapon in this antifraud battle was the False Claims Act. Originally intended to allow the government to prosecute persons who falsely filed for Civil War service pensions, the False Claims Act provides an impressive $10,000 civil penalty for each fraudulent or abusive claim for payment made to the U.S. government – this, in addition to treble the amount actually claimed. The trouble lay in the law's very broad definition of "abuse:" Abuse occurs whenever a claim is filed that results in the government's making an improper payment. Thus, claims made for services actually provided, but not sufficiently documented, are abusive, and so are claims made for services which reviewers later decide were not medically necessary. In fact, one contemporary critic estimates that the vast majority of fraud and abuse prosecutions involve disputed claims of medical necessity, including questions of whether the medical necessity of a procedure was adequately documented. Consequently, the full force of federal authority is being mobilized to ensure that physicians make proper determinations of medical necessity and properly document those determinations. These antifraud enforcement actions sometimes have the unwelcome effect of preempting the prescribed administrative appeals pursuant to which determinations of medical necessity are supposed to be made. In addition, given the frighteningly large penalties and fees in question, some physicians settle antifraud claims rather than fight claims of medical necessity. There is also some fear that some physicians may resist supplying novel but medically justified care to avoid being caught on the wrong side of a reimbursement enforcement action.

VI. REGULATION OF MANAGED CARE: 1990–2000

Health Maintenance Organizations (HMOs) – the most recognizable form of managed care, with roots going back to the 1930s – were given an enormous boost by the Nixon administration's federal HMO regulations in the 1970s, and in some parts of the country HMOs have enjoyed significant market share for decades. It was the failure in 1993 of President Clinton's efforts to establish a national health insurance scheme that led to the nation's startlingly swift embrace of HMOs and other forms of managed care. The 1990s witnessed a stunningly rapid transformation of the American health care marketplace, characterized by a marked increase in the market share of managed-care health insurance arrangements, and by unprecedented industrywide consolidations: hospital mergers and chain formations, the growth of ever-larger physician practice groups, the establishment of national medical management firms, and the creation of large, regional, integrated delivery systems. Regulation of the managed-care industry – as distinct from regulation of individual physicians or hospitals – has become a national political priority, although apart from some state-level piecemeal efforts, little effective regulation is yet in place. Much of the proposed regulation concentrates on the perceived need to force participants in this newly competitive industry to concentrate on quality of care issues rather than simply on cost control and profitability. This is a new brand of regulation for medical practice – one that aims not at the physicians' work itself, but at the institutional conditions under which physicians do that work.

The front line of industry regulation is state HMO licensing authority. Although the original HMOs of the early 1970s were established under the standards of the Federal HMO Act, most contemporary HMOs and other managed-care organizations (MCOs) are licensed according to state standards only. Various states have attempted to ensure quality of care through controversial laws that mandate the benefits that MCOs must provide, that interfere with MCO staffing decisions, and that mandate certain levels of capitalization and advanced planning so that the bankruptcies of insufficiently capitalized or poorly designed MCOs do not disrupt patients' continuity of care.

States have been severely hampered, however, in their ability to regulate the daily operations of state-licensed MCOs. In 1974, Congress passed a law designed to ensure the sound fiscal management of employee benefits, including pension and health plans. The Employee Retirement Insurance Security Act (ERISA) sought to ensure cross-state uniformity in the standards governing companies' benefits management by preempting all state regulation "relating to" any employee benefit plan. An unforeseen side effect of this law was that it effectively prevented states from regulating health plans that were funded by firms as employee health benefits. Even some state tort-law suits against negligent health plans (those that, for example, fail adequately to supervise their affiliated physicians) have been deemed preempted by ERISA; so, too, have the more obvious efforts by states to mandate coverage levels. In recent years, a series of judicial holdings has chipped away at the "ERISA shield" in tort law, and a number of states have attempted to create legislation that would increase states' ability to regulate health plans in spite of ERISA.

Federal efforts to regulate quality in the managed-care realm have increased, both because of popular dissatisfaction with managed care and because Medicaid and Medicare have become more active in managed care. A large number of states have received federal waivers that allow them to enroll all of the Medicaid beneficiaries in HMOs. In addition, the new Medicare +Choice managed-care program, although it is off to a rocky start, seems likely to expand. Among the most important new Federal regulations are those that govern the types of financial incentives that managed-care plans can offer their physicians. These regulations are designed to limit the potential bad effects of strong financial incentives that reward physicians for cutting back on expensive care such as specialty referrals and hospital inpatient stays. The regulatory regime also establishes a means for gathering information on the effects of various kinds of financial incentives on the care that physicians offer.

Potentially, the most important federal regulation of managed-care quality is, at this writing, still hypothetical. Several versions of a "patients' rights bill" have been introduced, and while one has passed the House and another the Senate, neither has yet been made law. In 1998, however, the President's Advisory Commission on Consumer Protection and Quality in the Health Care Industry laid out the parameters of an eight-point health care consumers' bill of rights. A law comparable to either the House or the Senate bill mandating patients rights would impact managed care in a number of ways; its most direct impact on quality of care would flow from proposed provisions that would streamline appeals of denials of care and place those appeals in the hands of neutral arbitrators, and from provisions that might eliminate the ERISA block to state-level regulation.

VII. CONCLUSION

At the start of the new millennium, physicians' medical practice is regulated by a bewildering assortment of professional, governmental, and market-driven forces. State and professional authorities attempt to ensure quality of care prospectively by setting standards for medical education and licensure. State medical boards, federal authorities, private insurers, and aggrieved patients attempt to regulate quality of care retrospectively through medical licensure actions, UR and fraud enforcement, and the filing of medical malpractice claims. State and federal authorities attempt to influence the new corporate atmosphere in which physicians' care is given by regulating the operation of managed care. In the past decade we have heard proposals for the elimination of state licensure, and for the return of medical regulation to the states; for the nationalization of health care delivery, and for its total privatization; for the abolition of professional self-regulation and for its revival as a more patient-friendly alternative to managed care; for the abolition of private malpractice actions as costly and poorly targeted, and for their continuation as a necessary check on medical quality. It seems unlikely, however, that we will ever return to our utterly unregulated past – a condition that was, after all, at least partially dependent upon a lack of information about medical science, and therefore about the standards required for medical training and practice. We may take comfort in the fact that our bewildering array of regulations is at least in part a creature of our successes.

NOTE

1. We do not attempt to trace the regulatory history of hospitals, of nurses and other allied health professionals, or of the pharmaceutical industry.

CHAPTER 48

THE ETHICS OF EXPERIMENTING ON ANIMAL SUBJECTS

Andreas-Holger Maehle

I. INTRODUCTION

The question whether experiments on living animals can be morally justified is today a central issue in bioethics. Advocates of animal experimentation argue for the scientists' right to use animals in research by stressing the medical benefits that arise from this practice (Botting 1992; Paton 1993). In other words, they appeal to the reduction of human suffering as their basic argument – and sometimes also the reduction of animal suffering, through progress in veterinary medicine. Adversaries, on the other hand, emphasize the interest of animals in avoiding pain, an interest that animals share with human beings. These critics demand protection of animals, some of them claiming that we have to acknowledge animal rights just as we respect human rights (Taylor 1999). The source of this conflict lies in different evaluations of the human–animal relationship (Manning and Serpell 1994). It is a matter of debate whether there are characteristics that *principally* distinguish all human beings from all animals; if they exist, whether they are morally relevant; or, to put the question from the opposite perspective, whether there are certain features that are common to human beings and higher animals that oblige us to apply the principle of equality.

These questions are not new and widely differing answers have been given to them. The wider debate about the moral status of animals was often taken up in the context of medical experimentation on animals. The first section of this chapter will therefore provide an overview of the use of animals in research in Western medicine from antiquity to the twentieth century. The following two sections will analyze more closely the development of the ethical debate about this practice in Western European thought.

II. HISTORICAL DEVELOPMENT OF EXPERIMENTATION ON ANIMALS

Experimenting on living animals, or vivisection, is as old as Western medicine. The Hippocratic text *On the Heart*, written *circa* 300 BCE, describes the vivisection of animals such as pigs to study the movements of the chambers of the heart and to explore the mechanism of swallowing (Littré [1839–1861] 1962, 9:80–7). Such experimentation, however, was only rarely mentioned in the other Hippocratic writings, which reflected a type of medicine that was more based on observation of the patient and theorizing about the origin of symptoms. In Hellenistic Alexandria, in the third century BCE, the physicians Herophilos

(c. 330–250 BCE) and Erasistratos (c. 305–240 BCE) appear to have vivisected more frequently – not only animals but also, as persistent rumors had it, criminals who had been sentenced to death (von Staden 1989).

Animal vivisection was more systematically employed in Roman times by Galen of Pergamon (c. 130–210). He used vivisection to study the physiology of respiration, movements of the heart, particular functions of individual muscles, and patterns of paralysis resulting from cutting the spinal cord at different levels. In Galen, we also find the advice that the researcher should prefer study of those animals whose bodies resemble most closely those of human beings to make his observations transferable (Singer 1956, 153). He did in fact use apes for the study of anatomy, as the dissection of a human corpse was taboo for religious reasons during this period. He was reluctant to use apes for vivisection, however, warning against the unpleasant facial expressions of an ape that is being vivisected (Lyons and Towers 1962, 15). Instead, Galen used goats and pigs for this purpose. Animal vivisection posed a problem in antiquity, but apparently one more of aesthetics than of morality.

During the Middle Ages Galen's medical doctrines were highly regarded, but his experimental method fell into disuse. It was taken up again only in the sixteenth century, as part of a cultural movement that aimed at recreating and imitating admired models of antiquity. Renaissance anatomists such as Andreas Vesalius (1514–1564) and Realdo Colombo (1516–1559) supplemented their public dissections of human corpses with animal vivisections in the style of Galen (Vesalius [1543] 1964; Colombo [1559] 1983; French 1999). Often these were performed to demonstrate Galenic doctrines of physiology. Occasionally, however, something new was found. Colombo, for example, discovered pulmonary circulation (i.e., the circulation between heart and lungs) while vivisecting dogs (Colombo [1559] 1983). The major physiological discovery of the seventeenth century, William Harvey's (1578–1657) demonstration that blood circulated throughout the body, was based to a large extent on experimentation on living animals (Harvey [1628] 1928).

The insight that blood circulates around the whole body had two immediate consequences. First, intravenous injection was attempted, starting with an experiment by the English natural philosopher and architect Christopher Wren (1632–1723), who injected a solution of opium into the veins of a dog in 1656. Second, in the 1660s experimental blood transfusions from animal to animal and from animal to human were performed. These early transfusions and intravenous injections led to complications and both methods were abandoned, to be taken up again only in the nineteenth century (Buess 1946; Maluf 1954).

Animal trials were used systematically from the late seventeenth century onward to study the effects of poisons.

Animal experiments were also undertaken to explore the efficacy and mode of action of old and new drugs (Maehle 1999a; Bickel 2000). For the most part, animal experiments in the eighteenth and nineteenth centuries were conducted in physiology, which gradually emancipated itself from anatomy and became a distinct field. In hundreds of experiments on at least fifteen animal species the influential Göttingen professor Albrecht von Haller (1708–1777) established the sensibility of nerve fibers and the irritability (i.e., contractility) of muscle fibers as central phenomena of animal life. Haller did this by stimulating mechanically, chemically, or thermally the various body parts of vivisected animals (Haller 1756–1760; Maehle 1992). He required a large number of experiments, because he was well aware of the variability of experimental observations and the problem of artifacts. Multiple trials, he believed, would yield average results that approximate the truth more nearly than the results of few trials. In the course of the nineteenth-century experimental physiology, as well as pharmacology, both became part of the academic culture of medicine in Western countries. Consequently, animal experiments were performed routinely and on a large scale (Lesch 1984; Coleman and Holmes 1988; Rupke 1990a; Cunningham and Williams 1992, Parascandola 1992). Invasive procedures on animals were further facilitated by the discovery of effective methods of anesthesia from the mid-1840s onward. A mixture of alcohol, ether, and chloroform was commonly used to anesthetize experimental animals.

In the second half of the nineteenth century the new field of bacteriology also required animal experimentation as a standard procedure. The development of bacteriology was strongly influenced by the Berlin medical scientist Robert Koch (1843–1910), who is perhaps best remembered for his discovery of the bacteria that cause tuberculosis (1882) and cholera (1883). Bacteriological research into infectious diseases required the identification and isolation of the supposed pathogenic microorganism, its pure growth in a culture medium, and the inoculation of this pure material into healthy experimental animals. These animals were then expected to develop exactly that kind of disease in which the microorganism had been found in the first place (Brock 1999; Worboys 2000). Moreover, work on artificially infected animals in the 1890s led to the first therapeutic antitoxins against diphtheria and tetanus. The production of these antitoxins was subsequently industrialized. The nascent pharmaceutical industry also began to employ animal tests routinely. During the first half of the twentieth century the number of animals used in research grew exponentially, as has been shown for Britain (Paton 1993, 60). Many medical developments of the twentieth century are largely based on animal experiments, including vaccines, hormones, local anesthetics, vitamins, and many therapeutic agents, such as antibiotics, antihypertensives, psychopharmacology, immunosuppressants, and virostatic drugs (Botting 1992; Paton 1993; Weatherall 1990).

III. The Rise of Moral Debate About Animal Experimentation in Western Thought

What were the ethical implications and responses to the historical development of animal experimentation in Western Europe? To answer this question we need to go back at least to the sixteenth century, when an explicit argument in favor of experiments on living animals was formulated by Renaissance anatomists. Vivisection, they argued, is necessary to learn about the *functions* of the parts of the body; dissection of corpses alone is insufficient, because it teaches only the position and shape of the parts (Vesalius [1543] 1964, 658; Colombo [1559] 1983, 256). Moreover, because *human* vivisection, as was supposedly practiced by Herophilos and Erasistratos in ancient Alexandria, was now held to be a horrible crime and a deadly sin, anatomists of the period concluded that animals had to be used as substitutes (Maehle 1993). Although this argument seems straightforward, its proponents appeared to be ambivalent about the morality of their actions. Colombo, for example, although thrilled by the opportunity of gaining new knowledge through this method, repeatedly characterized his canine subjects as "poor" or "unhappy" (Colombo [1559] 1983, 259–61). Compassion with experimental animals, expressed by the researchers themselves, emerged as a psychological problem, although it did not really stop experimenters from performing vivisections (Guerrini 1989).

In the seventeenth century, however, scientific and moral arguments against animal experiments were articulated. Thinkers in the tradition of Pythagoras who believed in the transmigration of souls seem to have argued that vivisection of animals might hurt a reincarnated human soul (Severino 1645, 152; Heister 1728, 8, 12). A more important argument was that doctors who regularly performed animal vivisections might become so hardened or brutalized that they might extend their experiments to dying patients (Riolan 1653, preface). This point was based on the traditional view already held in antiquity that cruelty toward animals leads eventually to cruelty toward human beings. With Thomas Aquinas (c. 1225–1274) this view had also been introduced into Roman Catholic doctrine (Passmore 1975). In addition to these moral arguments, scientific objections were raised. Observations made on animals, it was claimed, were not transferable to human beings; and vivisection created artificial conditions in the animal's body that could not teach anything about normal physiology (Riolan 1653, 106; O'Meara 1665, 75, 78).

Yet, experimenters were able to come up with arguments to defend the use of animals as experimental subjects. These investigators appealed to the authority of Galen, who was still held in high esteem. They argued that recent discoveries, such as the circulation of blood, would have been impossible without experiments on animals (Boyle 1744, 1:465; Rolfinck 1656, 30–4). With reference to trials with drugs and poisons they emphasized their therapeutic and forensic utility. Moreover, they used the so-called *tu quoque* or "you too" argument, which is still common nowadays: people who accept the slaughtering of animals for the production of food or clothes, they said, are hypocrites if they criticize the researcher who uses animals for the sake of new knowledge (Wepfer 1695, 132, 134; Heister 1728, 12–14).

An argument from natural theology was also used: Animal vivisection served the study of the Book of Nature, in addition to the Book of Revelation (i.e., the Bible). This increased knowledge would in turn increase people's admiration for God the Creator (Willis 1664, dedication; Wolff 1709, 16–18). The use of animals for experiments was also justified in the more general context of then current concepts of the human–animal relationship. Theologians pointed to humans' God-given dominion over all animals according to Genesis 1:26–8, including the right to kill them for their meat (Genesis 9:2–3) (Thomas 1983).

Philosophers of the seventeenth century, such as Francis Bacon (1561–1626), argued that animal vivisection was necessary for the progress of medicine (Bacon 1974, 109). René Descartes (1596–1650) famously compared animals with clocks or automata, which operated without a rational soul. Some of his more radical followers concluded from this that animals were incapable of suffering pain and that their cries during vivisection were nothing else but the noises made by a machine (Descartes 1960, 90–7; Fontaine 1738, 2:52–3). Influential writers on natural law, such as Samuel von Pufendorf (1632–1694), argued that legal obligations could not exist between rational human beings and irrational animals, because the latter lack a concept of duty. The relationship between human beings and animals was rather comparable to the state of war between nations (Pufendorf 1744, 1:509–10).

During this period animals were treated without much compassion in everyday life, in hunting, and in popular blood sports, such as bear-baiting, dog fights, or cockfighting (Thomas 1983). Few people really cared about the use of animals in experiments. Obviously, this was a world in which human beings came first and an anthropocentric focus was the basis of many of the arguments that defended the everyday exploitation of animals.

Anthropocentrism became less radical during the Enlightenment period of the eighteenth century, as urban populations, especially, began to develop a new relationship to animals and keeping pets became increasingly popular. A famous example is that of the writer Samuel

Johnson (1709–1784), who was a fierce critic of animal experimentation and was said to feed his tomcat, Hodge, oysters (Maehle 1990a, 1990b; Ritvo 1987). The artist William Hogarth (1697–1764), in his popular series of prints *The Four Stages of Cruelty* (1751), reminded people of the old wisdom that a youthful animal torturer might end up later in life as a murderer (see Manning and Serpell 1994). Theologians, philosophers, and other writers now looked for reasons to be kind to animals. Such reasons could be found in the Old Testament, for example in Proverbs 12:10, which teaches that "the righteous man regards the life of his beast" (Young 1798). Philosophers argued against the followers of Descartes that animals did have sensitive, more or less rational, and even immortal souls – and should therefore be treated with respect (Winkler 1743). The concept of a "great chain of being," linking all creatures from the lowest insect up to the angels, questioned the traditional sharp metaphysical and moral distinction between rational human beings and irrational animals (Jenyns 1790, 3:179–95; Lovejoy 1964).

Philosophers also reconsidered the question of human obligations to animals. Immanuel Kant (1722–1804) believed that there were indirect duties to animals, based on individuals' duty to themselves not to undermine or eliminate their compassion for fellow human beings. This could happen, according to Kant, if one acquired a hardened attitude through callous behavior toward animals (Kant [1797] 1907, 442–3). Other thinkers, especially Jeremy Bentham (1748–1832), went further and postulated direct obligations to animals based on the notion of animal rights. Bentham's central argument was that the traditional criteria of rationality and capacity for language were not relevant in attributing rights to living beings. Instead the capacity to suffer was morally relevant and this capacity united human beings at least with the higher animals (Bentham [1789] 1970, 283).

IV. ANIMAL PROTECTION AND ANTIVIVISECTIONISM

In the early decades of the nineteenth century, sensitivity for the suffering of animals had grown to such an extent in Britain and some other Western countries that legislation for the protection of higher animals was deemed necessary (Turner 1980; Ritvo 1987; Tröhler and Maehle 1990). The British Cruelty to Animals Act of 1822 was the first statute to punish mistreatment of horses and cattle with fines or several weeks' imprisonment. Yet some states, for instance Prussia in its penal code of 1851, punished cruelty to animals only if it had occurred in public and had violated the feelings of bystanders. Obviously, this was based on the old view, expressed by Kant and others, that the mistreatment of animals posed a threat to human morality with regard to fellow humans. In 1824, the Society for the Prevention of Cruelty to Animals was founded in London

to collect funds for the enforcement of the new British animal protection law. Initially, the Society's efforts focused on the treatment of animals in agriculture and transport. In the second half of the nineteenth century, however, its attention was also directed to the use of vertebrates in experiments, especially the use of dogs and cats in experimental physiology (French 1975; see also Chapter 34).

Some experimenters responded quite early to those developments. The English physiologist Marshall Hall (1790–1857) suggested an ethical code for experimentation on animals as early as in 1831. His code aimed at a reduction of the numbers of animal experiments performed and at minimizing animal suffering. Lower species were to be preferred to higher ones, and repetitions of experiments were to be avoided as far as possible. Careful documentation and publication of experiments would help in achieving this (Hall 1831, 1–11). Other experimenters, however, were less concerned about animal protection. In 1863, the British journalist Frances Power Cobbe (1822–1904) launched the first modern press campaign against an animal researcher, the German physiologist Moritz Schiff (1823–1896), who then worked in Florence and subsequently in Geneva (Guarnieri 1990). Cobbe soon became the driving force in the British antivivisection movement. In 1875, the antivivisectionist Victoria Street Society was founded in London, which was supported by the aristocracy (Lord Shaftesbury acting as its first president) and prominent members of the legal profession and the clergy, such as Lord Chief Justice Coleridge and Cardinal Manning. This first society subsequently split into two influential umbrella organizations, the National Anti-Vivisection Society and the British Union for the Abolition of Vivisection (French 1975; Kean 1998). Antivivisectionist societies campaigning for the abolition of animal experimentation, or at least its restriction and control, were established a few years later also in Germany, Switzerland, Sweden, and the United States (Rupke 1990a).

It is sometimes assumed that Darwin's theory of evolution must have had something to do with these developments, through an emphasis on the kinship between human beings and higher animals. Although this argument was occasionally used (Grysanowsky 1897), Charles Darwin (1809–1882) himself was actually a poor witness for the antivivisectionist movement. Although he was against animal experiments motivated by pure curiosity, he supported what he called "real investigations on physiology." In 1881 he even wrote, in a letter to the *Times*, that someone who retarded the progress of physiology committed a crime against mankind (Darwin 1995, 288–9).

The Victorian vivisection debate gave rise to the first legal regulation of animal experimentation, the British Cruelty to Animals Act of 1876. Prussia followed with a ministerial decree in 1885 (see Chapter 34). As in Marshall Hall's earlier code, the rationale behind the

British legislation of 1876 was the reduction of animal experiments and of animal suffering. The requirement of anesthetizing the experimental animals wherever feasible was new. Moreover, the British law also required specific licenses for experiments on vertebrates, and the registration and inspection of animal laboratories. The penal regulations included fines up to 100 pounds or imprisonment up to 3 months.

At the center of the late-nineteenth-century debate was the question of the medical utility of animal experiments. Prominent doctors and scientists, such as James Paget (1814–1899), Richard Owen (1804–1892), and Rudolf Virchow (1821–1902), pointed to the reduction of human suffering through modern, experiment-based medicine, which counted more than the suffering of animals (Rupke 1990b). Antivivisectionists, on the other hand, continued to criticize animal experiments as cruel and useless, and as an expression of an increasingly materialistic view of the world (Rupke 1990b; Tröhler and Maehle 1990). Some medical critics claimed that the whole experimental approach was wrong: doctors should rather trust in the "healing power of nature" and the preventive power of hygiene (Grysanowsky 1897).

The philosopher Arthur Schopenhauer (1788–1860) urged universal compassion as the basis of morality generally. He fiercely attacked the Kantian doctrine of indirect obligations to animals, which, in Schopenhauer's view, originated from the traditional, Judeo-Christian conception of humans' relation to the animal world. Rather than using animals as means, Schopenhauer argued, people should respect the metaphysical identity of human beings and animals based on their common will to exist. Only very important and immediately useful animal experiments appeared acceptable to him (Schopenhauer 1947–50, 4:161–2, 214; 6:393–401). The composer Richard Wagner (1813–1883) was deeply impressed by Schopenhauer's views and joined the emerging German antivivisectionist movement. The circle around Wagner subsequently joined antivivisectionism to anti-Semitism in their thought, blaming a hardened "Jewish attitude" toward animals for their mistreatment (Thiery and Tröhler 1987).

In the 1890s, the former Eton teacher Henry Salt (1851–1939) revived Bentham's idea of animal rights by founding the Humanitarian League in London. Salt and his friends, among them the writer George Bernard Shaw (1856–1950), campaigned not only for the total abolition of animal experimentation, but for many other animal protection issues, such as the abolition of hunting, and for broader humane causes, such as abolition of the death penalty and of corporal punishment, for disarmament, and for a better treatment of the indigenous populations in the colonies (Salt 1894; Hendrick 1977). Salt's Humanitarian League illustrates how antivivisectionism became part of a broader reform movement. This phenomenon can also be observed in fin-de-siècle Germany,

where antivivisectionists tried to win allies among vegetarians, teetotallers, adherents of natural healing methods such as air and sun therapy, followers of homoeopathy, and among opponents of vaccination. Yet, antivivisectionist societies kept a distinct social profile, with strong support from the aristocracy (especially financially) and through high proportions of female membership. As many as 70 percent of the members of some British antivivisectionist societies and approximately 45 percent of their German counterparts were women (Tröhler and Maehle 1990; Elston 1990). Partly, this had to do with the tradition of charitable work of women, particularly of those from the higher social classes. Animal protection and, by extension, antivivisectionism broadly belonged to this kind of activity. Yet, antivivisectionist engagement was also seen as a road to emancipation (Lansbury 1985; Elston 1990). In the years leading up to World War I, the older type of animal-loving aristocratic lady gradually gave way to the new type of emancipated animal protectionist and campaigner for women's rights.

In Germany, the link between anti-Semitism and antivivisectionism became more prominent as the National Socialists came to power in 1933. Some antivivisectionist campaigners had high hopes for the Nazis, who swiftly banned kosher butchering in April 1933. Many believed that vivisection was soon to have the same fate. In fact on August 16, 1933, Hermann Göring (1893–1946), then president of Prussia, issued (per announcement on the radio) a decree that prohibited "vivisection of animals of any kind" and threatened transportation into a concentration camp as punishment. In subsequent discussions, however, scientists from universities and the pharmaceutical and chemical industries persuaded the Nazi leaders that experiments on animals were indispensable (Maehle 1996; Arluke and Sanders 1996). The National Socialist animal protection law of November 24, 1933 reflected the outcome of these discussions. Although forbidden in principle, animal experiments could be performed with a license of the Ministry of the Interior in special laboratories. Moreover, no restrictions were imposed on animal procedures for the production of vaccines, and for diagnostic and forensic purposes. The penal regulations, with fines or imprisonment up to 6 months, were not substantially harsher than those of the British Cruelty to Animals Act of 1876.

The current antivivisection movement originated in the mid-1970s, with philosopher Peter Singer's book *Animal Liberation* (first edition 1975) as its intellectual manifesto. By this time, several other Western countries had introduced legislation to regulate animal experimentation. In the United States, the Laboratory Animal Welfare Act had been passed in 1966 and amended in 1970. France regulated animal experiments under a specific decree issued in 1963. Whereas Italy still operated under its old Animal Protection Law (1931, amended 1941) dating back to Mussolini's dictatorship, the Federal Republic of Germany had replaced the Nazi law of 1933 by its new Animal Protection Law of 1972 (Hampson 1990). Although such legislation limited the conduct of animal experimentation to suitably qualified researchers and demanded the use of anesthetics wherever possible, it posed no major obstacles to the large-scale performance of animal studies, recognizing their potential medical benefits. Singer, by contrast, argued that the selfishness of human beings in relation to animals was as reprehensible as racism and sexism among human beings (Singer 1976). The term "speciesism" (the ethically unjustifiable preference for our species over another), which Singer used for this attitude, became popular with critics of animal experimentation, as did the concept of animal rights. American philosopher Tom Regan soon argued in detail that rights should be granted to animals and that this virtually precluded the use of animals as experimental subjects (Regan 1983). Antivivisectionism became more radical in Western countries such as the United States and Britain, with militant actions of animal rights campaigners against research institutions and researchers (see Pence 1995, 207–9; Paton 1993, 236–44).

Both Singer and Regan described themselves as heirs to the intellectual legacy of Henry Salt (Singer 1976, 227–8, 274, 295–6; Regan 1983, 400). In the German debate on an ethical treatment of animals, the philosopher Ursula Wolf revived Schopenhauer's concept of universal compassion with all living beings (Wolf 1988). Not only were

historical concepts revived in recent debates, but older argument forms and problems retained their relevance, including the question of medical utility, the reduction of animal suffering, the "you too" argument, and last but not least the transferability of experimental results from animals to humans. On the other hand, recent debates have been enriched by the increasing availability of alternative methods, such as experimentation on cells, tissue cultures and isolated organs, and computer modeling of biological processes (Smyth 1978). Some critics of animal experimentation believed that these methods would make trials on whole animals superfluous.

V. CONCLUSION

With the advent of genetic engineering and the creation of specific "animal models" for human diseases, for example, transgenic mice for cancer research (Bodmer 1992), the significance of experimentation on animals was once again emphasized. Research can be conducted in such engineered animal models that would be unsafe to conduct in human subjects. Genetic manipulation of living beings and the cloning of animals have since raised new ethical questions about human beings' right to intervene in such a profound way into nature (Rollin 1995; Wilkie and Graham 1998; Cooper 2002). Concern for experimental animals is now only one facet of a complex debate about our responsibility for the environment and about biotechnology's alleged violation of the integrity of beings.

CHAPTER 49

THE ETHICS OF EXPERIMENTING ON HUMAN SUBJECTS

Susan E. Lederer

I. INTRODUCTION

Experimentation on human beings may be as old as medicine itself. The search for new therapies – drugs, devices, and procedures – required that someone go first, some individual participate in the trial of an innovative treatment, and experience both the risks and benefits of that participation. Although these risks and benefits remain for research subjects, the norms governing research with human subjects, the understanding of the ethical responsibilities of investigators and the rights of research subjects has undergone a profound transformation over the course of the twentieth century. Once implicit and informal understandings of the limits of appropriate experimentation have become codified into federal regulations that require (in the United States) written and informed consent of participants and institutional review of the proposed research (see Chapter 50). Ethical issues in the use of human subjects remain (for example, the conduct of human research by Western investigators in developing countries, an issue intensified by the acquired immunodeficiency syndrome (AIDS) pandemic), but there are some legal protections for human subjects and more clearly defined responsibilities for individual researchers and their institutions (see Chapter 51).

Legal restrictions on the use of laboratory animals preceded legal protections for human subjects by decades or more (see Chapter 48). The moral status of animal experimentation remains, in many respects, more highly contested than human experimentation. In particular, the use of nonhuman primates in laboratory studies has been criticized in light of the declining numbers of these animals and also on the grounds of their genetic relatedness to human beings (especially true of "higher" primates like chimpanzees).

II. ANCIENT EXPERIMENTS

Since antiquity, physicians and others interested in the anatomical structure and function of the body have turned to both animal and human subjects (see Chapter 49). Around 500 BCE, Alcmaeon of Croton demonstrated the function of the optic nerve by cutting this structure in a living animal and observing its resulting blindness. In the fourth century BCE, Aristotle (384–322 BCE) referred to the mutilation of living animals to investigate their living functions. The Hippocratic author of the text *On The Heart* (c. 350 BCE) similarly recorded the results of experiments in which he cut the throat of a pig in the process of drinking colored water, so as to study the process of swallowing. In the second century, Galen of Pergamon

(c. 130–c. 200), the physician to the Roman emperor Marcus Aurelius (121–180), described extensive dissections on living animals. Although Galen made no mention of moral questions about animal experimentation, his work suggests that some aspects of the process fostered anxieties. He advised investigators interested in the exposure of the brain, for example, to use pigs or goats rather than apes, because one could "avoid seeing the unpleasing expression of the ape when it is being vivisected" (Tröhler and Maehle 1987, 15).

Cutting open living animals shed some light on structure and function. Using human bodies provided additional information about "the parts which nature previously has concealed" (von Staden 1989, 144). In the third century BCE, the Alexandrian physicians Herophilus (c. 335–280 BCE) and Erasistratos (c. 304–250 BCE) reportedly performed vivisection on living human beings sentenced to death by the authorities. Although dissection and vivisection of human beings remained rare in antiquity, the practice of using criminals was defended by the Roman writer Celsus in the second century. "Nor is it cruel," observed Celsus, "as most people maintain, that remedies for innocent people of all times should be sought in the sacrifice of people guilty of crimes, and of only a few people such as that" (von Staden 1989, 187). The use of criminal bodies was not limited to the Alexandrians. Galen also recorded how such rulers as Mithridates VI and Attalus III, intensely interested in toxic substances, tried out antidotes on convicted persons to determine their efficacy.

The systematic practice of animal experimentation and the use of prisoners' bodies was discontinued for nearly 1,000 years. Beginning in the fourteenth century, dissection as a means of teaching anatomy gained favor at universities such as Bologna to further the education of physicians and surgeons. In the sixteenth century, physician Andreas Vesalius (1514–1564) performed extensive public anatomical demonstrations on both living animals and executed humans. For this work, Vesalius, like other anatomists, relied on authorities to supply bodies of those who were executed for their crimes, as well as on the bodies of the poor who were to be buried at public expense. Vesalius's monumental *De fabrica humani corpori* ([1543] 1964) concludes with a chapter "on the dissection of living animals."

In the early seventeenth century, experimentation on living animals and human dissection became essential to the research program of experimentalists. William Harvey (1578–1657), as *de Motu Cordis* ([1628] 1928) makes clear, conducted extensive animal experiments and some human experiments as part of the demonstration of the circulation of the blood. With the founding of the Royal Society in 1660, public demonstrations of experimental manipulations on living animals were held. Robert Boyle (1627–1691), for example, subjected large numbers of animals to his "pneumatick engine," a receiver from which air was removed. He and his contemporaries expressed little concern for the animals they killed in their demonstrations.

In the 1640s, philosopher René Descartes (1596–1650) had argued that nonhuman animals, in fact, did not feel pain, inasmuch as pain existed only with understanding that such creatures lacked. Apparent responses to painful stimuli, Descartes argued, were purely mechanical responses. Although this Cartesian formulation of beast-machines was highly influential, descriptions of experiments on animals suggest that natural philosophers like Robert Hooke (1635–1703) did not discount the existence of animal pain. Instead they privileged the advancement of knowledge over animal suffering. Nonetheless, some individual experimenters and public observers expressed distaste at the experimental dismemberment of dogs and other animals (Guerrini 1989).

The virtuosi of the Royal Society also conducted some human experiments. Perhaps the most well known was the demonstration in the 1660s of blood transfusion between animals and humans. Rather than criminals, the human subjects selected for these experiments were the insane. In France physician Jean-Baptiste Denys (1640?–1704) performed the first animal–human transfusion on a "madman." Although the warden of Bedlam refused permission to have his patients take part in transfusion demonstrations, the English physician Richard Lower (1631–1691) was able to recruit an impecunious clergyman, Arthur Coga, "to suffer the experiment of transfusion to be tried upon himself for a guinea" (Birch 1756–1757, 215). Coga, whose brain was reportedly "a little too warm," received blood from a lamb in the presence of many spectators. In light of the apparent success of the procedure, Coga underwent a second transfusion. The spectacle of such animal–human transfusion produced no discussion about the morality of such experimentation. After some sensational failures, blood transfusion lost favor as a therapy until it was revived in the nineteenth century.

III. Slaves and Other Subjects

The socially marginal and the physically vulnerable were often pressed into service as subjects of human experimentation. In addition to criminals and the mad, physicians had access in slave-holding countries like the United States to the bodies of enslaved persons, especially African Americans, for experimentation. In the early nineteenth century, slave bodies were valuable commodities; sick and injured slaves represented lost value to owners, who were encouraged to seek professional care for their investments. Although Southern physicians like James Marion Sims (1813–1883) made much of the "cooperation" of the slave women on whom he operated, the nature of enslavement permitted men and women slaves few, if any, options.

In the 1840s, Sims used the bodies of slave women to develop a surgical procedure to repair vesico-vaginal fistula, a hole between the vagina and the bladder caused by the physical action of childbirth or medical instruments, which produced incontinence and constant irritation in women. After encountering several female slaves with the condition, Sims contracted with several slave owners to board the women at his expense while he sought a treatment. In an era before the widespread adoption of ether and chloroform, three slave women each underwent as many as thirty operations until Sims successfully used silver sutures to close the fistula in these women and restore them to active lives. Perhaps the best known of physicians experimenting on slave bodies (in part because he recorded his experiments for posterity), Sims was hardly unique (Sims [1884] 1968). In life, slaves acted as objects of experimentation and in death they served as subjects for dissection. Even after the emancipation of slaves in the 1860s, the practice of using black bodies as "material" persisted in the United States for decades (Savitt 1982).

The legal invisibility of African Americans made them vulnerable to experimenters. Other factors came into play when investigators depended on the cooperation of their subjects. In the 1820s, Army physician William Beaumont (1785–1853) provided medical treatment for a French-Canadian trapper shot in the abdomen. Unable to close the gaping hole in the wall of the stomach, Beaumont opted to take advantage of this unique circumstance to study digestion in the person of Alexis St. Martin (1794–1880). When St. Martin found many of these experiments uncomfortable, Beaumont, intent on his studies, was forced to seek ways to ensure the trapper's ongoing cooperation. He and St. Martin entered into a contractual arrangement in writing that ensured St. Martin's services. In exchange for payment, the trapper agreed to perform various physical duties and to serve when needed as the experimental subject. This arrangement and Beaumont's use of St. Martin's affliction prompted only praise for the physician and admiration of St. Martin's anatomy. Even St. Martin's discomfort was less important than the knowledge to be gained from his predicament. Despite St. Martin's repeated absences and his lack of cooperation, Beaumont persevered in his research. Even after his death, the trapper attracted medical interest; rumors that eminent clinician William Osler (1849–1919) wanted to acquire the body led his family to keep his corpse at home until it had decomposed so badly that it would no longer be attractive to physicians (Bliss 1999).

Beaumont resorted to compensating his research subject to gain access to St. Martin's unusual anatomy. One way to obviate reliance on the cooperation of subjects was the time-honored practice of self-experimentation or the use of the bodies of colleagues and students. In the early nineteenth century, medical students at the University of

Pennsylvania, for example, performed self-experiments in digestion and skin absorption. Some students inoculated their fellow students with chancre of syphilis to determine the mode of action of mercury, and tested the action of the heart remedy digitalis on the healthy body (Atwater 1978). The introduction of chloroform also followed self-experimentation by the Scottish physician James Simpson. Seeking a safer alternative to ether anesthesia, Simpson inhaled chloroform; when he awoke, he found himself lying on the floor (Altman 1998).

In the twentieth century, self-experimentation continued to play a significant role in medical discovery and demonstration. Before World War II, a number of medical researchers lost their lives in research-related activities. The "heroes and martyrs" of yellow fever included physician Jesse Lazear, nurse Clara Maas, Rockefeller researcher Hideyo Noguchi, and British physician Adrian Stokes, who succumbed to yellow fever as part of their research (Lederer 1995). In addition to these self-experiments, two extraordinary physicians performed self-experiments that revolutionized medical thinking and practice.

In 1929 Werner Forssmann (1904–1979), a young surgical resident in a small German hospital, disobeyed the explicit orders of his medical superior in the search for effective ways to introduce drugs into the heart. The doctor secretly anesthetized his left arm, made an incision into his skin, and inserted a needle into his left antecubital vein. Forssmann then introduced a urethral catheter into the vein toward his heart. To document the catheter placement, he proceeded to a basement x-ray room where, with the assistance of a nurse, he could visualize with the help of a fluoroscope the catheter in his body. In November 1929, he gained public attention when he published an article about his discovery. Forssman used rabbits and dogs to establish that heart catheterization using contrast dye was also a safe procedure, and continued his self-catheterization at least eight more times. In 1956, he shared the Nobel Prize with Drs. Andre Cournand (1895–1988) and Dickinson W. Richards (1895–1973), American physicians who developed his technique for clinical use. (Forssmann 1974).

In the 1980s Australian physician Barry Marshall turned to self-experimentation to demonstrate to his fellow physicians a new explanation for gastric ulcer and disease. He ingested the bacterium *helicobacter pylori*, developed stomach inflammation, and provided evidence that countered the conventional wisdom about stomach disease (Marshall 2002).

In addition to self-experimentation, physicians prompted by proximity and enthusiasm used their children, spouses, and neighbors as subjects. In 1774, when English farmer Benjamin Jesty attempted to inoculate his wife and sons against smallpox by using material taken from the udders of cows infected with cowpox, his neighbors labeled him an "inhuman brute" when his wife nearly lost her arm because of infection from the inoculation. No such criticism ensued, however, when two decades later English physician Edward Jenner (1749–1823) successfully used fluid from the arm of a dairymaid infected with cowpox to vaccinate a neighbor's 8-year-old child. To test the protective nature of this vaccination, Jenner inoculated the boy with pus taken from a patient ill with smallpox. In the United States, physician Benjamin Waterhouse (1754–1846) similarly vaccinated seven of his children with cowpox, and later challenged the immunity of three children by exposing them to active smallpox. Although critics assailed vaccination, there was little concern about using children in this manner. One notable exception was the smallpox immunization for the English royal children. In 1721, when variolation (inoculation with smallpox) was introduced into England, six prisoners at Newgate jail submitted to variolation before the royal children underwent the procedure. Promised freedom for their participation, one of the six was further persuaded to spend 6 weeks in close contact with a smallpox patient to test the efficacy of variolation. She did not develop the pox (Hopkins 1983).

IV. The Rise of the Humane Movement

In the first part of the nineteenth century, the plight of animals in the laboratory provoked more concern than experiments on patients and other human beings. Opposition to animal experimentation grew out of the larger animal protection movement in Britain, which was closely associated with such humanitarian reforms as antislavery, penal reform, and protection of child factory workers (see Chapter 48). The early targets of the English antivivisection movement included the French veterinary school at Alfort and French physiologists Claude Bernard (1813–1878) and his mentor Francois Magendie (1783–1855; French 1976).

Vivisection or experimentation on living animals was essential to the research programs conceived by the French physiologists. Bernard offered the most complete and systematic explanation for the importance of animal and human experimentation to the progress of knowledge. "Experiments," he wrote in 1865:

> must be made either on man or on animals. Now I think that physicians already make too many dangerous experiments on man, before carefully studying them on animals. I do not admit that is moral to try more or less dangerous or active remedies on patients in hospitals, without first experimenting with them on dogs; for I shall prove, further on, that results obtained on animals may all be conclusive for man when we know how to experiment properly. (Bernard [1865b, 1927] 1957a, 101)

Bernard's bold defense of animal and human experimentation and his record as an experimenter made him anathema to animal protectionists; his own wife and daughter publicly assailed his sacrifice of laboratory animals.

In Britain where the antivivisection movement first took hold, a Royal Commission was created in 1875 to investigate the cruelties of laboratory animal use. The following year Parliament passed the Cruelty to Animals Act, a sweeping set of regulations governing the use of animals in research and teaching (see Chapter 48). (The act was amended in 1986.) Although the effects of these restrictions on physiological research in Britain have been much debated, the Act clearly inspired antivivisectionists in nations outside Britain to attempt passage of similar laws (Turner 1980).

In Germany and Switzerland, the composer Richard Wagner (1813–1883) was among those who financially supported organizations opposed to animal experimentation. Although unable to achieve the British legislation, German antivivisectionists helped foster an increasingly hostile environment for science. Such German antivivisection periodicals as *Thier-und-Menschenfreund* (Animal and Human Friends) not only supported restrictions on kosher butchering but also called for action against the "Judaification of doctors" (Tröhler and Maehle 1987). In the 1930s the Nazi regime passed laws outlawing experimentation on any animals and included warnings that "persons who engage in vivisection of animals of any kind will be deported to a concentration camp" (Proctor 1988, 227). It is unclear whether these laws were ever enforced. Such protections for animals were not extended to the human inmates of concentration camps, such as Ravensbrueck, where Nazi doctors labeled the female research subjects given gas gangrene wounds "rabbit girls" (Arluke and Sanders 1996).

In the United States, the antivivisection movement was split between moderates, who allowed animal experimentation with restrictions, and extremists who refused to accept any medical knowledge gained from the "torture" of living animals. Both moderates and extremists agreed that unrestricted animal experimentation would lead to dangerous and unfounded experiments on human beings (Lederer 1995). In part, antivivisectionists took seriously the warning offered by defenders of medical research that any restrictions on animal experimentation would lead to dangerous trials on patients. Just as Claude Bernard had argued, American defenders of medical research insisted that experiments must be made on either animals or humans. These defenders, for the most part, male physicians and other professional men, accused the female-dominated antivivisection movement of privileging animals over humans (Lederer 1995).

The antivivisection movement in both the United States and Britain collected and published cases of "human vivisection," the use of unsuspecting men, women, and children in tests of new drugs or procedures unrelated to their individual benefit. Some of these cases make for grisly reading. In the first flush of enthusiasm for the germ theory of disease, researchers eagerly sought to establish the bacterial agent of disease. Lacking animal models, they turned to human beings: orphans, prostitutes, the insane, immigrants, and hospital patients. Reports of persons inoculated with the germs of leprosy, syphilis, gonorrhea, cancer, and yellow fever appeared in both the medical press and the popular press in the late nineteenth and twentieth centuries. American antivivisectionists pressed for federal and state legislation to protect human subjects (Lederer 1995).

The bacteriological revolution ushered in by such giants as Louis Pasteur (1822–1895) and Robert Koch (1843–1910) heralded great benefits to medicine often achieved by animal and human experimentation. In perhaps the best known experiment in the late nineteenth century Pasteur successfully inoculated a 10-year-old boy bitten by a rabid dog with his new rabies vaccine. The success of this daring experiment largely overshadowed Pasteur's departures from the accepted ethical practices of his day. Pasteur's own laboratory notebooks, as historian Gerald Geison compellingly argues, demonstrate that Pasteur had not completed the animal experiments he used as justification for treating the child. Instead, the French chemist had only just begun the "vaguely comparable" experiments in a series of dogs (Geison 1995).

Human experiments were also responsible for the much heralded successful demonstration that yellow fever was transmitted by Aedes mosquito, a discovery that contributed to the building of the Panama Canal. Unlike the case of rabies, researchers investigating yellow fever had no animal model in which to study the disease; human experiments were necessary. They were also dangerous. In light of the dangers, Walter Reed (1851–1902), who headed the United States Army Yellow Fever Board in 1900 in Cuba, introduced written agreements with the men who participated as his research subjects. These contracts, written in both English and Spanish, outlined the risks to participants, as well as the financial compensations, which were considerable. Following Reed's example, other Army investigators working in the Philippines in the 1910s similarly adopted written permission forms (translated into appropriate languages) for their research subjects (Lederer 1995).

The success of human experimentation and informal protections for human subjects, like written contracts, made legal restrictions on human experimentation appear unnecessary to many researchers. In 1916, when the American Medical Association (AMA) debated changing its code of ethics to include the necessity of consent for human experiments, the group decided that formal protections were not needed (see Chapter 36, Section VII).

In Germany, the Lübeck disaster involved the deaths of more than 70 children who received contaminated Calmette (BCG) vaccine against tuberculosis (Bonah 2002). This calamity prompted the Reichs Minister of the Interior in 1931 to issue Regulations on New Therapy and Human Experimentation, which, among other things, required prior consent from a research subject. These protections for children, the dying, and the "socially needy" were technically in force in Germany until 1945, but they did not safeguard men, women, and children from Nazi experimenters during the Second World War (Sass 1983; see also Chapters 50 and 54).

V. MEDICAL SCIENCE SERVES THE STATE

Even before the Nazi regime came to power in 1933, physicians and surgeons in Germany enlisted in National Socialist professional organizations in sizable numbers. Ultimately, nearly 45 percent of Germany's physicians would become members of the Nazi party. Doctors played an extraordinarily significant role in fashioning the medical politics of the Third Reich. They were essential to the success of such Nazi policies as the Genetic Health Courts, which ordered the compulsory sterilization of 350,000 people to prevent genetic disease, and the large-scale "euthanasia" programs in which some 200,000 mentally challenged individuals, chronically ill people, and others were killed. An estimated 1,000 people perished in the course of the medical experiments conducted in the concentration camps (Proctor 1999). These experiments have come to represent the most heinous medical crimes against humanity in the twentieth century (see Chapter 54).

At Dachau, Nazi doctors used Jewish prisoners to conduct studies on hypothermia (freezing and rewarming the body), exposure to the high altitudes experienced by German pilots, and drinking seawater. At Ravensbrueck, young Polish women were injected with gas gangrene bacteria and other pathogens, and then tested with new drugs and surgical treatments to reverse the effects. Other experiments included infecting Jewish children with hepatitis and performing liver punctures, famine studies on Soviet prisoners, experiments on female prisoners of the menstrual cycle, sterilization experiments involving x-rays and caustic chemicals, epidemic jaundice experiments, typhus studies, incendiary bomb studies, and the collection of Jewish skeletons and other body tissues (Annas and Grodin 1992).

Many of these hideous experiments became known only after the Allied victory at the prosecution by American authorities of 23 Nazi medical personnel at the Nuremberg Medical War Crimes Trials. In the action, *United States v. Karl Brandt et al*, seven of the indicted, including Brandt, Hitler's personal physician, received the death sentence, and five were sentenced to life imprisonment (commuted to 15 or 20 years). More than that, the trial produced one of the most recognized documents in twentieth-century medical history, the ten rules of permissible human experimentation that have come to be known as the Nuremberg Code.

At the trial, American physiologist Andrew C. Ivy (1893–1978) served as the AMA's advisor to the American prosecution team. Aware that the German defense attorneys would compare the conduct of Nazi doctors to American experiments conducted in prisons and to the exclusion of African-American physicians from the AMA, Ivy worked to develop the rules regarding permissible human experiments. Ivy orchestrated, in addition, the AMA's adoption of three requirements for ethical human experimentation: the voluntary consent of the subject, the need for prior animal experimentation, and the requirement of proper medical supervision. These requirements, passed with little discussion by the AMA's House of Delegates in December, 1946, were cited in the successful prosecution of the Nazi doctors (Weindling 2001; see also Chapter 36, Section IX).

American medical research conducted during the war years, 1941 to 1945, did not often meet the standards identified by Ivy and cited by the Nuremberg judges. American military personnel, for example, participated in large-scale, clandestine tests of such warfare agents as mustard gas and nuclear weapons (Pechura and Rall 1993). American investigators also violated the first requirement for voluntary consent, when they used populations unable to exercise consent, including orphans and mentally ill and mentally retarded individuals. Using prisoners in research was more problematic. Whereas some argued that incarceration in prison did not permit voluntary consent, American investigators like Ivy maintained that prisoners were not coerced into research participation (Harkness 1996a, 1996b diss.). Such infamous prisoners as the convicted murderer Nathan Leopold argued that participation in wartime human experiments involving malaria enabled him to express his patriotism (Leopold 1958). Researchers, sponsored by the Office of Scientific Research and Development used several institutionalized populations orphans, conscientious objectors, and the mentally ill – for the study of diseases like dysentery, typhoid, hepatitis, malaria, influenza, and venereal diseases.

Research participation often posed considerable risks to participants. Investigators and their institutions tended to be more concerned about possible lawsuits in the case of bad outcomes than about moral issues. In 1942, for example, Harvard University officials rejected as too costly indemnification insurance for the blood substitutes experiments overseen by chemist Edwin Cohn (1892–1953). When a Massachusetts prisoner died after receiving a bovine blood substitute, they were concerned for the research program's continuation. The prisoner's mother accepted the posthumous pardon granted her son, and the burial expenses were charged to Cohn's research grant (Harkness 1996b, diss.).

VI. Aftermath of the Nuremberg Code

Medical research in the years after the Nuremberg tribunal was conducted under the shadow of the Nazi doctors. "The whiff of the concentration camp" came to represent the extreme, the brutal, and the fiendish. Despite the fact that for many physicians, the Nuremberg Code, in the words of psychiatrist Jay Katz (1922–), seemed like a "good code for barbarians," the judgment at Nuremberg prompted the World Medical Association (WMA) to formulate a code of ethics regarding human experimentation (Advisory Committee on Human Radiation Experiments 1996, 86). Founded in 1947 by physicians from countries invaded by the Nazis and doctors from many Allied nations, the WMA struggled for over two decades to realize workable and meaningful guidelines for human experimentation. In 1964, stimulated in part by the thalidomide tragedies in Canada and Western Europe, the World Medical Assembly in Helsinki formally adopted a set of guidelines for clinical research. Although representatives from Britain and France had argued for restrictions on using children and prisoners as research subjects, the Declaration of Helsinki, reflecting its American supporters, contained no explicit rules regarding these populations (Lederer 2004). Unlike the Nuremberg Code, which made the voluntary consent of the subject absolutely essential to permissible human experimentation, the Declaration of Helsinki authorized proxy consent, thereby making experimentation on children and other populations possible (McNeill 1993). Since 1964, the Declaration of Helsinki has undergone several revisions. In the face of a growing number of controlled clinical trials conducted by Western nations in resource-poor nations, considerable controversy has arisen over how trials should be conducted (the use of placebo controls, the best proven treatment versus the highest attainable treatment given economic constraints). Although the Declaration continues to be regarded as influential in guiding clinical research, it is no longer the only set of international guidelines. In 1993, the Council for International Organizations of Medical Sciences developed the International Ethical Guidelines for Biomedical Research involving Human Subjects (Levine 1999; Chapters 50 and 51).

During the 1960s influential and disturbing reports of widespread abuses of human subjects alarmed many observers. In Great Britain physician Maurice Pappworth (1910–1994) published an essay, later lengthened into a book, identifying dangerous investigations on unsuspecting patients, including experimental cardiac catheterizations performed on pregnant women, x-ray tests on newborn infants, and drug studies on hospital patients (Pappworth 1967a, 1967b). In the United States, Harvard anesthesiologist Henry K. Beecher (1904–1976) startled the medical community in 1966 when he described the twenty-two cases of ethically questionable research in mainstream American institutions (Rothman 1991). Unlike Pappworth, Beecher did not provide names and citations to the experiments, but some of his examples would become synonymous with research abuse (Hazelgrove 2002). Chief among these were the Willowbrook hepatitis studies conducted by pediatrician Saul Krugman (1911–1995) and the injection of live cancer cells into elderly, demented patients at the Jewish Chronic Disease Hospital (Faden and Beauchamp 1986). In response to these and other scandals the Public Health Service promulgated guidelines for human subjects use in 1966, two decades after the Nuremberg Code (McCarthy 1994).

In the United States the revelations about abuses of retarded children and the elderly were quickly followed by the news that the United States government had conducted a 40-year study of untreated syphilis in African-American men in rural Alabama. The so-called Tuskegee Syphilis Study began in 1932 under the auspices of the Public Health Service, and formally ended in 1972. From Congressional hearings, newspaper reports, and scathing editorial cartoons, Americans learned about the active deception of indigent Black farmers deceived into thinking they were receiving treatment for "bad blood" (Jones 1981, 1993). Outrage over this study continues to the present day and has been identified as critical to understanding African Americans' mistrust of the health care system, clinical trials, and AIDS research (Reverby 2000).

Public dismay over the Tuskegee Study and other abuses of human subjects helped ensure passage in the United States of the National Research Act in 1974. This legislation required institutions receiving federal dollars to create institutional review boards to oversee all proposals involving the use of human subjects and individual investigators to obtain written informed consent from research participants. The Act further mandated the creation of a National Commission for the Protection of Human Subjects of Biomedical and Behavioral Research (1974–1978), which issued the influential Belmont Report in 1978. The cardinal ethical principles, outlined in the Belmont Report, of respect for persons, beneficence, and justice remain influential in thinking about human experimentation.

Concern for justice, for example, and the recognition that women and minorities had been underrepresented in clinical research and thereby less likely to benefit from

the knowledge gained in clinical trials of new drugs and procedures prompted changes in the conduct of research in the United States. In 1993 the National Institutes of Health Revitalization Act legislated the inclusion of women and minorities in clinical research, although the progress reports of this legislation remain uncertain (Mastroianni, Faden, and Federman 1994).

In 1994, Americans were startled by reports in the popular press of Cold War human radiation experiments in the United States. Although such reports had surfaced previously, notably in 1986 when Congressman Edward J. Markey held public hearings, journalist Eileen Welsome linked names and faces of American citizens to secret wartime experiments involving the injection of plutonium into 18 people (Moreno 2000). A presidential-appointed Advisory Committee on Human Radiation Experiment spent 18 months reconstructing the history of the plutonium injections and some 4,000 other experiments involving radiation in the years between 1944 and 1974 (Advisory Committee on Human Radiation Experiments 1996). In 1995 President William Clinton offered these American "nuclear guinea pigs" a formal apology. Financial settlements have been reached with some of the experimental subjects or the surviving families (Welsome 1999). In 1997 a quarter of a century after the ending of the Tuskegee Syphilis Study, President Clinton invited the surviving participants of the study – men now in their nineties – and their families to the White House for an apology for the government's role in the Study (Reverby 2000).

VII. CONCLUSION

In the 1990s, the National Institutes of Health's Office for the Protection from Research Risks temporarily sanctioned a number of prominent academic medical institutions for violating the rights of research subjects and the failure to follow regulations relating to research risk. The publicity surrounding the deaths of two research volunteers – Jesse Gelsinger, an 18-year-old man, who died in 1999 in gene transfer trials at the University of Pennsylvania and Ellen Roche, a 24-year-old laboratory technician at Johns Hopkins University School of Medicine who died in a 2001 asthma study – brought renewed attention and concern about the protection of human research subjects. In addition to these domestic concerns, the conduct of AIDS research in the developing world has prompted controversial comparisons to the Tuskegee Syphilis Study, which exploited the economic situation of the participants to advance medical knowledge (Fairchild and Bayer 1999).

Over the course of the twentieth century, the nature and extent of protections for the human subjects of biomedical and behavioral research has expanded. Although there has been greater protection for research subjects and significantly more attention to the moral dimensions of human research, the search for appropriate guidelines and oversight continues. Experiments, the French physiologist Claude Bernard cautioned his readers in 1865, must be made either on man or on animals. In the twenty-first century, most researchers would argue that both are necessary features of continuing progress in the biomedical sciences. The efforts to ensure the safety, well-being, and moral standing of the subjects of biomedical research – human and animal – are likely to remain morally problematic in the decades to come.

CHAPTER 50

THE HISTORICAL DEVELOPMENT OF INTERNATIONAL CODES OF ETHICS FOR HUMAN SUBJECTS RESEARCH

Ulrich Tröhler

I. INTRODUCTION

Experiments on humans have been conducted since antiquity. The practices enjoyed a resurgence in the seventeenth century, becoming even more prevalent from the mid-eighteenth century onward (Howard-Jones 1982; Lederer 1995; Rothman 1995; see Chapter 49). The reasons for this renaissance were manifold, cultural, and medical. To stay within medicine: The discovery of the circulation of blood in the first half of the seventeenth century prompted physiological studies, including the intravenous application of traditional drugs. Effects of new drugs began to be tested in various ways in the eighteenth century (Maehle 1999a) and, about the same time, new surgical procedures were comparatively evaluated (Tröhler 2000a; Chalmers et al. 2003). Perhaps the most prominent of these early modern trials were those involving inoculation for smallpox, a series of experiments in preventive medicine implemented throughout Europe (Rusnock 2002). During this period no distinction was made between nontherapeutic studies aimed at understanding bodily functions in health and disease, and therapeutic studies testing (new) diagnostic, preventive, or therapeutic interventions relative to professional care. This chapter examines the history of the perception of the ethical dimensions of human experimentation and the origins of its regulation through international ethics codes.

II. "FOR THE PUBLIC GOOD": LITTLE REGULATION OF HUMAN EXPERIMENTATION PRIOR TO WORLD WAR II

Under the *ancien régime*, doctors had little difficulty finding patient–subjects with whom to work. Hierarchical societies with impoverished lower social orders were filled with people who could be commanded or paid to undergo experimental procedures, even if they did not understand them. Accordingly, in the early 1660s the effect of transfusion of the "good" blood of a lamb was tested in Paris on an insane patient, whose "bad blood" was evacuated by copious venesection and who was paid for this rational therapeutic trial. It proved to be dangerous, provoking angry moral concerns and prompting the Paris Parliament to prohibit such experiments in the future (Starr 1998). In the second half of the eighteenth century, there are reports of trials of new methods of lithotomy, amputation, wound treatment, and of operations for cataracts conducted on military pensioners and even on soldiers wounded on the battlefield.

566

New methodical concepts of eighteenth-century empiricism also prompted comparative clinical trials of the effectiveness of scurvy preventatives and of various drugs used against different types of fevers in groups of sailors. These trials raised ethical concerns. Some army surgeons saw no problem in allocating soldiers to groups to discover whether the mortality associated with amputation was lower if limbs were amputated immediately after the injury or when the intervention was delayed for a few days. Rational arguments existing for both. Others hesitated. When discussing a study of delayed versus immediate amputation during the Napoleonic Wars, the British Army Surgeon, George James Guthrie, had scruples even though he reported "success" with immediate amputation. He felt that he was not "authorized to commit murder for the sake of experiment" (Guthrie 1815, 39). So, despite his theoretical insight into the epistemic preferability of conducting prospective comparative studies and the unique opportunities afforded a commanding military surgeon to enforce them, Guthrie relied on retrospective analysis of his casebooks.

Another military surgeon, Charles McLean, took a radically different position. According to him, "reluctance to try experiments with the lives of men" constituted an ethical double standard because it wrongly presumed that "the practice of medicine, in its conjectural state, were anything else, than a continued series of experiments, upon the lives of our fellow creatures" (McLean 1817–1818, 2:500–94). McLean's position, however, was a minority view, whereas Guthrie represented the widespread opinion that those participating in research themselves "should benefit from the trials to which they were subjected and that they must not be put in danger for the sake of scientific curiosity" (Maehle 1999a, 268–9). Indeed, 50 years earlier, the naval surgeon James Lind had reacted in exactly that way to an experiment ordered by the Admiralty, but the case had ended quite differently. When starting a trial of the "malt-wort," Lind acknowledged the "murmur and disgust" when withholding vegetables from patients with scurvy at Haslar Hospital (because of their believing that the fresh fruit would improve their condition) and stopped it. But the Admiralty ordered it to be taken up at sea "where it was expected that patients would cheerfully submit" (Macbride 1764, 174–75). It is noteworthy that despite the climate of ethical awareness, there was no mention of the notion that subjects should consent to the experimentation. The prerogatives of status and power were omnipresent, particularly in the military but probably in civilian institutions as well.

Researchers sought ways to circumvent the risks involved in a trial with new methods. In 1804, James Currie observed that because "it would be unjustifiable to neglect for the sake of experiment any means of safety," his cold water bathing would be "superadded" to the tra-

ditional fever treatment – in other words, he used what today is called an add-on design (Currie 1804, 408). Currie's superaddition presumed, of course, that traditional venesection or bleeding was safe.

These early discussions of risk and safety, and the notion of presumed sacrifice "for the sake of experiment," illustrate the ambiguity of the notion of "experiment." Most eighteenth-century doctors understood "experiment" in the everyday sense, that is, a trial with unknown – yet nonetheless hoped for – results. For some this meant an intervention under well-controlled conditions and circumstances with respect to the selection of patients, the treatment(s) given, *and* the particular care with which the patients were attended. When Charles McLean remarked that he could not see much difference between an "experiment" with uncertain outcome and routine clinical practice, he was implying a distinction between traditional treatments on a merely conjectural basis, and those treatments the safety and efficacy of which had been properly established by controlled experiment. At the time, however, this distinction was hardly appreciated by doctors or by the public (Tröhler 2000a).

The debate over the meaning and ethics of research intensified in the nineteenth century, as the ethos of increasing scientific knowledge as a basis for progress became prevalent also in medicine. Further safeguards against inflicting damage to humans "for the sake of experiment" were sought, including prior work on animals and/or on the researchers themselves. There is evidence that these safeguards were actually used (Tröhler and Maehle 1990; Altman 1998). Animal experiments had been reintroduced since the seventeenth century, despite the sometimes-contested transferability of results to humans (Maehle and Tröhler 1990). In the nineteenth century, new surgical treatments, such as ovariectomy, nephrectomy, and thyroidectomy, were tested on animals before being used on human patients (Tröhler 1993). Self-experimentation played a role in the history of inhalation anesthesia. Because of the said ethos and/or insistence on surgery as a "last hope," however, other "first operations" tended to be performed directly on patients. A case in point was the first successful heart suture by Ludwig Rehn of Frankfurt in 1896, in a paradigmatic instance of a "last hope" emergency (Tröhler 1998). After the success of vaccination against smallpox and with the rise of microbiology in the nineteenth century, preventive and therapeutic measures against infectious diseases tended to be tried directly on patients because of the absence of animal disease models, or to advance medicine faster. The latter was the case with, for instance, Louis Pasteur's antirabies serum and his German competitor Robert Koch's tuberculosis treatment with *Tuberkulin* (tuberculin) (Geison 1995; Gradmann 2001). The former ultimately proved to be a success, the latter rapidly proved to be a failure.

Clearly, during this period no canonical rules protected participants, or for that matter, the public, against possible abuses. There was no consensus about the type of evidence deemed sufficient for an innovation to be considered safe enough for general introduction (Sauerteig 2000). The need for experimentation was stressed as indispensable, given the high priority of advancing medicine (Maio 2002b). Yet such influential works as the many editions and translations of Claude Bernard's *Introduction à l'Etude de la Médecine Expérimentale* ("An Introduction to the Study of Experimental Medicine" [1865] 1949) and lesser texts of the same kind offered no explicit section on the ethics of (human) research. Instead, Bernard reaffirmed the traditional limit of "never performing on man an experiment which might be harmful to him to any extent, even though the result might be highly advantageous to science, i.e. to the health of others" (Bernard [1865] 1949, 101). More stringent strictures had actually been laid down by the eighteenth-century British inventors of professional medical ethics, John Gregory and Thomas Percival. In dealing with ethical issues inherent in human experimentation, the former provided extended discussions (McCullough 1998a, 246–50), and the latter stated rules requiring both their usefulness "for the public good," provided they were scrupulously and conscientiously performed and vetted through a process of prior peer review (Tröhler 2000a, 130; Baker 1993a, 205; see Chapter 30 and Chapter 36, Section VI).

Although these early medical moralists were concerned to protect participants, they did not attempt to do so by appealing to the concept of informed consent (Rothman 1998). The whole subject was conspicuously absent from British and German deontological literature until the end of World War II – with a few exceptions (Schomerus 2001, Chapter 36, Section VI). Moreover the professional courts of honor of these two countries ignored the subject of research generally, except in cases of what we would today call "severe abuse" (Smith 1994; Maehle 1999b; Rabi 2002). One major exception was Albert Moll of Berlin (1862–1939). He was no man of the establishment. Rather, as a practicing neurologist he was interested in sexual medicine and sexual reform. In his 650-page *Aerztliche Ethik* ("Doctors' Ethics" 1902), he listed 600 cases of nontherapeutic research, published in the medical press, that he considered unethical because of positive damage inflicted, unclear or blatantly useless scope, bad design and, most notably, absence of any information and/or consent by the patient-subjects (Moll 1902).

The notion of informing a patient and obtaining consent prior to an experiment existed before World War I, but in legal rather than medical circles (Maehle 2000). The only English commentator to argue for a moral duty of informed consent, Michael Ryan (1800–1841), did so in the context of a book on medical jurisprudence. As early as 1830, English law held that a physician would "be obliged to provide compensation for any injury that might arise from adopting a new method of treatment" if consent had not been given for experimentation (Perley et al. 1992, 150). From the middle of the nineteenth century, there were isolated criminal trials in France, Germany, Norway, and Austria. Doctors were condemned, mildly, for having omitted to seek informed consent and for the lack of therapeutic use in nontherapeutic experiments. In the view of the judges, this meant that these physicians had committed physical assaults on patients.

In 1899, Albert Neisser, professor of dermatology and venereology at the University of Breslau (and discoverer of the gonorrhea bacillus), was condemned by the Royal Prussian Disciplinary Court. This was a special court for civil servants, that is, neither an ordinary criminal court nor a professional court of honor. Neisser had injected cell-free serum from syphilitic patients into eighteen prostitutes, some of whom were minors, without informing them or obtaining their consent, to test whether this might provide immunity against contraction of syphilis. This and similar cases ignited a campaign in the liberal press over the medical abuse of the poor, part of a larger campaign against the moral double standard employed by the wealthy. The press coverage set off public and parliamentary debates.

After the Neisser trial, in December 1900, the Prussian Minister of Religious, Educational and Medical Affairs issued a specific *Anweisung an die Vorsteher der Kliniken, Polikliniken und sonstigen Krankenanstalten* ("Directive to the Directors of State Clinics," Minister der Geistlichen 1901). Addressed to all physicians-in-chief of state clinics in the country, the *Directive* excluded all research not related to diagnostic, therapeutic, or immunization procedures on minors and otherwise not legally fully competent persons and unless the patient–subject had not unambiguously consented after pertinent explanation of possible adverse effects. The fulfillment of these conditions and the circumstances of the study had to be documented in the patient's record. This Directive was the world's first explicit administrative regulation for human research, but its requirements concerned only nontherapeutic studies. Patients in public hospitals were expected to be grateful to contribute to new methods of treatment and diagnostics (Elkeles 1996).

A generation later, in 1931, after World War I and the turmoil of its aftermath, formal research standards were again elaborated in Germany in *Richtlinien für neuartige Heilbehandlung und für die Vornahme wissenschaftlicher Versuche am Menschen* ("Guidelines for Innovative Therapies and Performing Scientific Experiments in Humans," Vollmann and Winau 1996). These regulations, issued by the Imperial Minister of Justice, distinguished explicitly between therapeutic and nontherapeutic research. Without exception, nontherapeutic studies could be conducted only with the subject's informed consent. Therapeutic research, however, was possible without consent in a medical emergency and if deemed in the patient's best interest. These categorizations were open for interpretation by the researchers. Built on the foundations laid by the 1900 *Directives*, the *Guidelines* developed risk–benefit assessment and a series of further prerequisites and obligations. Like their precursors, however, these regulations, too, were administrative, and had no standing in criminal law. Their practical significance must remain open. Some researchers may have acted cautiously as did Paul Ehrlich when trying his *Salvarsan*, the world's first chemotherapeutic agent, around 1910, above all to avoid public scandal (Sauerteig 2000). Although they were never revoked, the *Guidelines* were completely ignored during the period of National Socialism.

III. "Never Again": Regulations in the Post–World War II Phase

In Nuremberg, in 1946, in the aftermath of World War II, twenty-three medical researchers (twenty of whom were physicians) were indicted for "crimes against humanity." Fifteen were found guilty and seven were hung (including four physicians), but the true legacies of the trial were the revelations of abhorrent research practices, and the ten principles of researcher conduct propounded by the judges, which came to be known as the *Nuremberg Code* (Deutsch 1998; see Chapters 49 and 54). Because the Nuremberg Trial was based on several official declarations of the Allies regarding the post-war pursuit of war crimes (e.g., London 1942; Moscow 1943), the *Nuremberg Code*, effectively constituted a document of public international law (Arnold and Sprumont 1998). There was, however, no corresponding international institution to control its application or to prosecute violations. Apart from immediate attempts by the U.S. government and the World Medical Association (WMA) to implement it in military and clinical contexts, respectively (Baker 1998c), it had no great practical impact for some two decades (Herranz 1998; Hazelgrove 2002; see also Chapters 49 and 51, and Chapter 36, Section IX). Yet the Code became the foundation on which all international research standards would be constructed because of its insistence on prospective informed, voluntary consent from subjects with decision-making capacity, on the balance of risk and chance, on the right of the subject to quit the experiment and because of its legal status, as the cornerstone of international law with reference to medicine (Schuster 1997; Drinan 1992; see Chapter 51).

Ironically, the subfloor supporting these foundations were the German regulations of 1900 and 1931, reconstructed in terms of an American tradition of principles medical ethics. The contents of the *Code* rest on testimony and memoranda from two American physicians, Andrew C. Ivy, a representative of the American Medical Association (AMA), and Leo Alexander, a psychiatrist who treated war-crime victims. Both were familiar with the German regulations and drew on them extensively in recommending research principles to the court (Baker 1998c; Grodin 1992). Thus the attention to nonmaleficence, beneficence, and autonomy, and to prior animal if not self-experimentation was taken over.

The *Code* was stricter, however, in that it did not distinguish between types of research. Implicitly, it did not allow any research on noncompetent subjects (patients, children) because of the compulsory informed consent obligation. Also it stipulated the right of the subject to quit the experiment when continuation seems to him/her to be impossible. The responsibility was nontransferable and lay with the researcher – inclusive the assurance of the ethical qualities of the subject's consent; whereas the German regulations opting for a hierarchical model had laid the responsibility with the head of department. The 1931 *Guidelines* had, however, been more extensive in other respects: They explicitly excluded the exploitation of social and economic needs and research on dying persons, they requested the respect of the subjects' dignity in publications, a written research plan, and they stipulated an investigator's responsibility in teaching research ethics. These points were neither taken up in the Code nor in the first WMA documents (see Chapter 51; Vollmann and Winau 1996).

The Nuremberg trial had publicly exposed abuses of modern medicine. It had also shown that the medical profession lacked a written *charta*, a statement of principles professing its traditional ethos, which had been deemed self-understood and sufficient. In this situation, when the newly founded United Nations and the Red Cross prepared international covenants containing articles on human research (Tröhler 2002), the WMA was founded in 1947. It immediately became very active with respect to morality in medicine. As early as 1948, it issued the *Declaration of Geneva*, a modern version of the Hippocratic Oath, and a year later an *International Code of Medical Ethics*. Both contained passages that had a bearing on human experimentation. The *Oath* stipulated that "even under threat... I will not use my medical knowledge contrary to the laws of humanity" – on which the Nuremberg Code had been based. The *International Code* warned against damaging patients' interests when "providing medical care which might have the effect of weakening the physical and mental condition of the patient," for instance, when doing so without therapeutic needs in human experiments (WMA [1948] 1995a; WMA [1949] 1995b). In 1954, the WMA, following an initiative by the Dutch delegates, issued specific *Principles for Those in Research and Experimentation*. Designed to implement the *Nuremberg Code* and to allow research in certain conditions, such as in unconscious and psychiatric patients and in children, by introducing the notion of surrogate consent. Although

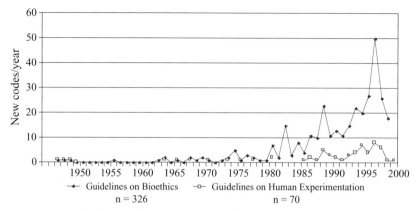

50.1. International Ethics Codes 1947–2000. *Note:* The number of international ethics codes (i.e., guidelines, recommendations, resolutions, conventions) issued by Inter-Governmental (IGO) and Non-Governmental Organizations (NGO) as well as miscellaneous international texts published each year (from 1947 to 2000) is represented. Each amended version of a given code was counted individually. Drawn from data collected by S. Fluss, 1999, and my own research. N = total number of codes in the respective category.

stressing informed consent, it otherwise remained somewhat vague referring to "strict adherence to the general rules of respect of the individual" without outlining inadmissible risks (WMA [1954] 1995c).

Although the Public Health Council of the Netherlands elaborated much stricter guidelines, massive resistance in the research community prevented the implementation of these Principles, even in the United States and Germany. Also, elsewhere they were seen as an unnecessary hindrance of research and progress, as abuses were attributed to (Nazi) criminals only (Baker 1998c; Winslade and Krause 1998, Maio 2000). The *Principles* are practically forgotten today. Sev Fluss does not mention them in his so far most comprehensive listing of international guidelines on bioethics (Fluss 1999). These documents, issued around 1950, started what was to become a movement of codification of ethical standards in various health care fields.

IV. INTERNATIONAL CODES OF ETHICS: A NEW PHENOMENON

When in the 1950s and 1960s, due to public concern, human research came again under scrutiny, nationally prominent bodies such as the British Medical Research Council (1953), the Harvard Medical School (1961), the British Medical Association, and again the Medical Research Council (1962) circulated appropriate memoranda and issued ethics guidelines (Medical Research Council 1953; Hazelgrove 2002). In 1964, after a preparation time of 4 years, the WMA *Principles* were reformulated under the title of *Recommendations Guiding Physicians in Biomedical Research Involving Subjects*. This document, now known as the WMA *Declaration of Helsinki* (I), was an example of the attempt at internationalizing the already ongoing national regulation of moral issues in a variety of

health care fields (Tröhler 2002). Both intergovernmental and nongovernmental organizations authored such documents. The latter did so partly to prevent the enactment of criminal or legislative measures in a field that doctors considered their own (Arnold and Sprumont 1998).

The phenomenon is illustrated in Figure 50.1. It shows the international guidelines, declarations, recommendations, and so forth, henceforth to be summarized by the term *ethics codes*, issued annually between 1947 and 2000. So far, the total number, according to the listing by Fluss, amounts to 326 versions. Eleven Inter-Governmental Organizations (IGOs) ranging from the United Nations (1966) and its suborganizations (UNESCO, WHO, UNAIDS), via, for example, the Council of Europe, the European Union, the Organization of African Unity to the World Labor Organization (1999) have issued 107 such codes. Thirty-six non-governmental organizations (NGOs), starting with the WMA (1948) and including, to name just a few, Amnesty International, the Council for International Organizations of Medical Sciences (CIOMS), the European Forum of Good Clinical Practice (EFGCP), the International Council of Nurses, the Human Genome Organization to the International Bar Association (2000) – have produced 186 documents, the Governmental Entity of the Vatican six, and miscellaneous bodies more than twenty (Fluss 1999). The number of national codes can only be guessed. The Swiss Academy of Medical Sciences alone has published twenty-nine versions in more than fifteen fields since 1969 including five versions of three codes relating to human experimentation (Tröhler 1999; Swiss Academy of Medical Sciences 2001).

It lies beyond the scope of this chapter to analyze the contents of this enormous amount of source material (see for this purpose Brody 1998, Schaupp 1993, Veatch 1995), but one can suggest some of the reasons for the growth of codification. One may distinguish internal, scientific, and external socio-cultural factors. Taboos were being broken in a number of fields. In reproductive medicine, for instance, Louise Brown, the first apparently healthy baby stemming from in vitro fertilization was born in the United Kingdom in 1978. In 1985, a pregnancy was brought to full term by a surrogate mother; in 1990 the ova of aborted fetuses were marketed; 1998 was marked by the successful cloning of Dolly the sheep and, in 2000, the national parliament engaged in a serious discussion of human "therapeutic" cloning (and finished by approving it). All that happened in a single country, the United Kingdom. The availability of life-sustaining measures was also a prerequisite for the criteria of brain death, which was sometimes discussed in relation to organ transplantation (Schöne-Seifert 1999). Xenotransplantation and tissue engineering most recently have brought about an array of moral issues. Modern genetics, too, has touched the roots of society as well as of health care policies during the last 25 years (Tröhler 2000b).

The one factor both common and essential to all these developments was human experimentation. Indeed, one-fifth of all international codes have dealt with human experimentation, more and more NGOs and IGOs having become active in related moral concerns in the 1990s (Figure 2), because the delegation of their regulation to the researchers (subsidiarity) has proved inadequate by further research scandals, particularly in Germany and the United States (Baker 1998). Governments have intervened increasingly and in various ways in a previously intramedical field (Winslade and Krause 1998); France became the first country, in 1983, to establish, by presidential decree, a national bioethics committee as a consultation body, *Comité Consultatif National d'Ethique de la Médecine et des Sciences de la Vie* (National Consultative Committee on the Ethics of Medicine and the Life Sciences). It proposed moral norms and practical recommendations that "contaminated" subsequent laws, such as, the Laws of Bioethics (lois de bioéthique) of 1994, including also a regulation of human experimentation (Mathieu 1998). This political process soon became internationalized, and IGO involvement reflects the growing attention of international legislative bodies.

Indeed, the Council of Europe and later the European Commission (EC) have developed a series of initiatives with respect to human experimentation (Figure 50.2; see Chapter 51). It is a little known fact that there is actually a European Commissioner of Health and Consumer Protection and that decision making on EC health programs has hitherto not been transparent. Recently it has been recognized that it is important, democratically speaking, that NGOs, such as the International Alliance of Patients' Organizations also be represented (van der Zeijden 2000). Indeed, moral issues in medicine have been increasingly seen from the perspective of moral rights.

Just as there are civil rights, human rights, or consumer rights, rights of minorities and of "vulnerables," such as the mentally ill, the elderly, the physically handicapped, children, home inmates, and prisoners, there are indeed patients' rights. The "rights approach" toward moral issues also takes account of race and gender. It can further be related to the new ecology, and the women's and students' movements of the 1960s, which the patients' rights movement can be seen as continuing. Altogether these movements are an expression of deep socio-cultural changes in the Western world. The basic document behind all of them was the Universal Declaration of Human Rights by the UN General Assembly in 1948. This was followed by the European Human Rights Convention signed in 1950 in the frame of the Council of Europe in Rome, and to which forty-eight states have since adhered. The latter is important in that it entailed, in 1952, the establishment of the European Human Rights Court in Strasbourg. This Court developed an unforeseeably dynamic and expansive jurisdiction that is increasingly being used. It is noticeable that, in the 1990s, in addition to the notion of human rights, the more vague (and corruptible) one of "human dignity" has increasingly come in the foreground, marking yet another cultural shift (Macklin 2003).

The next section will attempt a typology of the international ethics codes resulting from these scientific and cultural developments. It will focus on the reasons for and the mechanisms involved in their genesis by looking closer at two typical examples of codes regarding human experimentation from the perspective of an NGO and an IGO, respectively, to show their specific features.

V. The WMA Declarations of Helsinki I–VI

One type of code illustrates the traditional approach to regulating moral issues in medicine in that it endorses the paternalistic ethos of the health care professions fostering individual patients' beneficence as defined by professionals. This type can be exemplified by the WMA's *Declaration of Geneva*, its *International Code of Medical Ethics* and its approach to human experimentation from the *Principles* (1954) via the first (1964) through the most recent versions (2000, with clarifications in 2002 and 2004) of the *Declaration of Helsinki* (versions I and VI). Rather than to protect the freedom and the rights of the patient–subject, as the human rights type of code would, Helsinki I was designed to allow a continuation of human research. The rights that had been so firmly pronounced at Nuremberg were "eroded down to a conditional prerogative of the clinician researcher" (Schaupp 1993; Baker 1998c, 322). This setback in terms of contents was somewhat corrected in the amended versions (Helsinki II–V; 1975 in Tokyo, 1983 in Venice, 1989 in Hong Kong and 1994 in Somerset West). The Tokyo amendment (Helsinki II), for

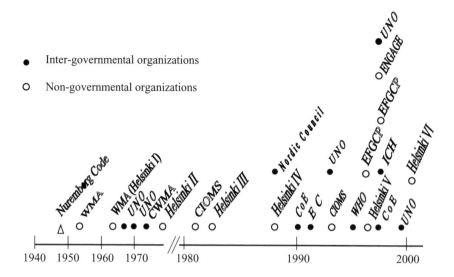

Notes:

1 25 (versions of) international codes (guidelines, recommendations) regulating human experimentation are listed in order of the dates of publication. Drawn from data collected by Fluss, 1999, and my own research.

2 The UN codes (Resolutions) deal only in part with human experimentation. Further explanations are contained in the text.

Abbreviations

WMA	World Medical Association
CWMA	Commonwealth Medical Association
CoE	Council of Europe
EC	European Commission
UNO	United Nations (Resolution on Human Rights and Bioethics)
CIOMS	Council for International Organizations of Medical Sciences
WHO	World Health Organization
EFGP	European Forum for Good Clinical Practice
ENGAGE	European Network of Good Clinical Practice (GCP) Auditors and Other GCP Experts
ICH	International Conference on Harmonization of Technical Requirements for Registration of Pharmaceuticals for Human Use

50.2. International Ethics Codes on Human Experimentation.

instance, introduced the concept of review by an appropriate ethics committee (or Institutional Review Board, IRB) prior to the onset of a project. Although versions II–V of the Declaration reendorsed the Nuremberg principles, they still allowed researchers greater freedom from compulsory consent obligations (Baker 1998; Winslade and Krause 1998). Furthermore, the personal, nontransferable responsibility of the researcher to assure the ethical quality of the patient-subjects' consent, and the right to leave the experiment if their personal condition seems to demand it, were not incorporated in any of the versions of the Helsinki *Declaration* (Herranz 1998).

In this context, it must be stressed that the WMA, as a private organization, represents the vested interests of the constituent national professional organizations (one per member country only). Its general assembly has so far voted seventy-six ethics codes, that is declarations, statements, recommendations, and resolutions, most of which are virtually unknown – as for instance the Declaration of Lisbon on Patients' Rights (1981, updated 1995; Fluss 1999). They have no legal force per se; however, such "soft law" may become "hard law" when integrated in legal documents. The WMA has no democratic legitimation either, for only part of a country's doctors are actually represented: The number of national delegates voting at the general assembly depends on the number announced to pay the membership fee to the WMA. This number is arbitrary in that it depends on the financial commitment a national professional organization is willing to make. The *Bundesärztekammer* (German Chamber of

Physicians and Surgeons), for instance, pays for some 30 percent of its members, which equals ten votes in the WMA general assembly, whereas the United States has twelve votes and France seven. The Netherlands did not pay for some time and Switzerland once left the WMA and both countries therefore temporarily had no vote (Doppelfeld 2000b). The British Medical Association resigned in the 1970s to protest against the admission of South Africa. It was readmitted in 1994. In that year, the total WMA membership was sixty-four; in 2001 it was seventy-one countries (Bulletin of Medical Ethics 1994, 2001).

It is not clear how and by whom the early WMA's ethics codes were formulated (Doppelfeld 2000b). Certainly, they do not follow a consistent philosophical concept of ethics. Rather they reflect, in essence, compromises arrived at strictly among doctors. One exception has been the draft for a new version of the Declaration (Helsinki VI) by Yale bioethicist Robert Levine (1999). Although the amended versions II–V corresponded, in terms of patient protection, to a gradual rebirth of the Nuremberg Code from the mid-1970s to the mid-1990s, Levine's proposal seemed to reflect a tendency toward deregulation in view of commercial interests in new biotechnologies (Angell 2000; Weatherall 2000; Tröhler 2000b). Also, in the first consultation process among affiliated medical associations in the history of the WMA, it generated a controversial debate as to whether human research should put the interests of research subjects first or if it should be allowed to yield more social benefit by getting clear-cut answers from science. This might imply, for example, the liberal use of placebo control groups at the price of again reducing rights of the individual patient–subject (Brennan 1999; Levine 1999; Klinkhammer 2000). This would be in disagreement with a number of codes on human experimentation issued by other NGOs and by nonprofessional IGOs such as the Council of Europe (see later). Such a hierarchy of values calls to mind the eighteenth and nineteenth centuries.

The amendments to Helsinki V (1994) finally voted by the WMA General Assembly (Helsinki VI, Edinburgh 2000) abolished the distinction between nontherapeutic and clinical research, returning therewith to the protective strictness of the Nuremberg Code. On the one hand, in justifying clinical research by its potential prophylactic, diagnostic, or therapeutic value "to the patient," Helsinki VI dropped these last three words (as in the Nuremberg Code, too), reflecting the intertwining of societal and industrial interests with clinical research. On the other hand, it stipulates the obligation of adequately informing potential patient-subjects of the sources of funding, possible conflicts of interest of the researcher, and his institutional affiliations (WMA 2000 §22). Helsinki VI was no longer termed *Recommendations Guiding Physicians*, but *Ethical*

Principles for Medical Research. Part of the ongoing debate on this latest revision is to be accounted for by the meaning of this change of status, partly by concerns about research access, particularly in developing countries. A subsequent note of clarification, published by the WMA Council only (2001), illustrates the now contestably legitimated presumption of the WMA's leadership in setting universal standards for human research (British Medical Journal 2001).

VI. The Council of Europe and Its Ethics Codes

Ethics codes adopted by IGOs do not have this problem of legitimacy. The Council of Europe, for instance, has a long-standing profile in matters of human rights, particularly in relation to medicine and biology. Its Parliamentary Assembly voted a Recommendation and Resolution on the Rights of the Sick and Dying in 1976 followed by one on the Situation of the Mentally Ill in 1977 and an additional eleven recommendations followed through 1999. The Committee of Ministers has voted twenty-one Resolutions, Recommendations, and Protocols through the end of the twentieth century (Fluss 1999). All these represent the "rights-type" approach to moral issues in medicine.

In 1978, after a series of experiments conducted at Stanford University in the United States demonstrated the practical possibility of genetic engineering and after the birth of Louise Joy Brown, the first human conceived by in vitro fertilization (IVF) on July 25, 1978, the ministers of justice of EU member states created the *Comité ad hoc des experts en bioéthique* (CAHBI, "Ad hoc Committee of Experts in Bioethics"). Each member state had one vote, whereas the number of delegates (usually academics and/or civil servants) was open-ended, depending on a state's political and financial commitment. CAHBI worked many years on a *Convention on Human Artificial Procreation*, which at the end fell through because of the uncompromising attitude of one member country, Liechtenstein. It was finally published as *Principles* by CAHBI in 1989.

As problematic ethical fields in medicine were increasingly being debated in some of the member states, the Ministers of Justice in 1990 replaced the CAHBI by a standing *Steering Committee on Bioethics* (Comité Directeur pour la Bioéthique, CDBI). Again, all forty-eight member states are represented with one vote, and Canada, the Holy See, the International Federation of Scientific Societies, Israel, and the United States have observer status. The CDBI has installed task forces working on specific fields such as organ transplantation and human genetics. Its main task, however, as decided by the ministers has been the elaboration of a convention on ethical issues in medicine and biology. It was to propound patient rights, such as informed consent in human research and in daily medical practice. There was also the idea of bringing some order in the array of national and international codes.

The committee of ministers soon realized that informed consent was too restrictive an issue and insisted on including human rights and human dignity issues. This led to a change in the title, which now reads accordingly: *Convention for the Protection of Human Rights and Dignity of the Human Being with Regard to the Application of Biology and Medicine* or shortened to Convention on Human Rights and Biomedicine (CHRBM). Thus, in terms of contents, the document is a hybrid. A philosophically sound system could not be implemented; however, as noted previously, human rights also represent a type of approach to ethics. The *Convention* was drafted according to the customary technique for arriving at such international documents: They end up as compromises, sometimes willingly formulated in an abstract, even incomprehensible manner – which does not, in the end, serve the legal order. In the specific case of the CHRBM Convention, the work of the CDBI was not very efficient, because many of the sixty to eighty delegates were neither particularly knowledgeable in international law nor in human rights issues and, as usual, the various legal systems had to be taken into account. Many points necessitated tough negotiations and the readiness to compromise (Reusser 2002). The Convention was finally modeled upon that on human rights. There are core paragraphs furnished with comments to help the interpretation and additional protocols allowing a rapid taking up of new issues. The political nature of this document can be seen in the proviso that any country having already its own legal regulations for a given issue need not follow the convention with this respect. In consequence, some countries introduced laws prior to signing or ratifying the Convention (Council of Europe 1997a, 1997b).

After a first draft had gone through the process of national hearings the final version was voted in December 1996 by the Committee of Ministers and presented for signature by governments and ratification according to national constitutions. By the end of the twentieth century, thirty-one countries have signed and seventeen have ratified the Convention, which means that it is in effect among the latter and they must take appropriate legal measures (Council of Europe 2000). The national hearings were a new feature. Previous international conventions had been drawn up without this additional democratic instrument. The hearing evidenced serious concerns in Germany about research on persons who are not able to consent when such research is not in their interest but in that of the population they represent.

VII. CONCLUSION

Human experimentation is an example of a very slowly recognized ethical need in Western experimental medicine, namely the need for patient–subject protection. Some moral issues surrounding experimental medicine, such as the obligation to avoid infliction of damage "for the sake of experiment" and the postulate of "benefit for the patient," were discussed by members of the profession in the eighteenth century. These discussions, however, were often misguided because of a failure to distinguish between appropriately and inappropriately designed experiments and no experiments at all. Although a legal tradition evolved at the national level before 1900, and on an international level after the *Nuremberg Code* of 1947, the legislation was feckless and the Code was endorsed in very few places and had virtually no impact on the research community, even in the United States. The WMA responded with its vaguely protective 1954 *Principles*, strengthening these principles only 10 years later by issuing the "paternalistic" *Declaration of Helsinki* (I) in reaction to serious abuses, such as the thalidomide case (Kirk 1999). This step served to protect research by preventing governmental regulation. Another decade later, with the updated Helsinki Declarations II–VI, patient protection was gradually improved as the twentieth century drew to a close.

Additional protection for human subjects was also offered by the "human rights and human dignity" IGO codes, most particularly of the CHRB of the Council of Europe; however, the latter also reflects societal and economic interests. Nonetheless, in view of a new spate of research scandals in the 1990s and the possibility of exporting research to third-world countries (Lurie and Wolfe 1997), the WMA's *Declaration of Helsinki* and many other international "soft law" ethics codes seem to be becoming less irrelevant. The issue is not so much one of legal status but of whether codes and laws reflect contemporary thought by addressing conflicts perceived by the public and offer realistic means of solving them.

Incontestably, however, the "soft law" codes offer some positive features compared with laws and international conventions, namely specificity and flexibility. Their legitimacy, unlike that of democratically enacted laws, is, however, problematic (Matthieu 1998), as the example of the WMA codes has shown. The process of genesis is important and should at least be transparent, which has not always been the case with the WMA codes.

The issue of international regulations raises the question of ethics and culture, not only regarding the universality of conflicts, but also the means of solving them, for instance, via informed consent and other principles that are not ubiquitously recognized. If the purpose of an NGO code or an IGO document is to contribute to a basis for legal liability, the prospects are mixed. The history of research on human subjects over the past 50 years is one of continuous abuses, despite the existence of such codes. The future looks more optimistic with respect to codes fostering patient rights and human dignity in daily medical practice and in research (Reusser 2000).

Ethics codes can serve to articulate idealistic aspirations. They can play the role of emblematic symbols (Smith 1996; Leven 1997), "express fundamental values, such as respect for persons and scientific integrity . . . set standards for moral criticism of medical practices or policies that may violate the rights of human subjects" (Winslade and Krause 1998, 140). Their general nature can also dramatize the need for national and international documents with binding authority (Perley et al. 1992). Of course, they can also serve as moral cover-ups (see Chapter 57). Finally, and not least, codes may serve as teaching aids. With legislation intervening in an ever more detailed way in all these matters, as shown in this chapter, it is important to preserve the advantages that codes offer, whatever their legal status, in order that "Hippocrates" not *hypocrisia* reign in human experimentation.

CHAPTER 51

INTERNATIONAL ETHICS OF HUMAN SUBJECTS RESEARCH IN THE LATE TWENTIETH CENTURY

Baruch A. Brody

I. INTRODUCTION

The development of codes of research ethics is described in Chapter 50. This chapter will focus on an analysis of the content of four official codes of research ethics from transnational governmental and legal authorities and from transnational medical organizations, rather than on codes developed by groups of private individuals and scholars. These documents have exerted and continue to exert considerable influence on both research ethics and the conduct of research involving human subjects. The emphasis in this analysis will be on codes concerning research on human subjects in general with occasional reference to issues involving special classes of subjects.

II. THE NUREMBERG CODE

As described in Chapters 34, 36, 50, 53, and 54, in the immediate aftermath of World War II, a series of military tribunals were convened to pass judgment on those Germans accused of war crimes and atrocities, including medical war crimes. In its final judgment concerning the medical war crimes, the Nuremberg War Crimes Tribunal asserted, "all agree, however, that certain basic principles must be observed in order to satisfy moral, ethical and legal concepts."(Katz 1972, 305) It then listed ten basic

principles, most having to do with risks and benefits. Principle One, the principle of voluntary informed consent, is widely viewed, however, as the *Nuremberg Code's* most important contribution:

The voluntary consent of the human subject is absolutely essential. This means that the person involved should have legal capacity to give consent; should be so situated as to be able to exercise free power of choice, without the intervention of any element of force, fraud, deceit, duress, over-reaching, or other ulterior form of constraint or coercion; and should have sufficient knowledge and comprehension of the elements of the subject matter involved as to enable him to make an understanding and enlightened decision. This latter element requires that before the acceptance of an affirmative decision by the experimental subject there should be made known to him the nature, duration, and purposes of the experiment; the method and means by which it is to be conducted; all inconveniences and hazards reasonably to be expected; and the effects on his health and person which may possibly come from his participation in the experiment. The duty and responsibility for ascertaining the quality of the consent rests upon each individual who initiates, directs, or engages in the experiment. It is a personal duty and responsibility which may not be delegated to another with impunity. (Katz 1972, 305)

This is a very strong requirement. It requires (1) voluntary, (2) informed (3) prospective consent from (4) subjects with legal capacity, with (5) the quality of that consent being ascertained by the experimenter himself. Moreover, there is a full discussion of what information must be provided to the potential subject before his consent is accepted.

Where did this requirement come from? There has been much historical discussion about this question (Annas and Grodin 1992). A general consensus has emerged that although there were precedents, the court was primarily influenced by two of its expert witnesses, Andrew Ivy and Leo Alexander. Ironically, the most explicit precedents for this requirement come from pre-Nazi Germany. In 1900, the responsible Prussian ministry required that research not be conducted on minors or others who are incompetent, but only on someone who has "declared unequivocally that he consents to the intervention" after "a proper explanation of the adverse consequences that may result from the intervention." A later 1931 Reich Health Council Circular modified this requirement to allow for proxy consent by legal representatives for innovative therapies, but otherwise maintained the same strict requirements on all forms of research (Grodin 1992, 127–9; see Chapter 50).

III. THE DECLARATION OF HELSINKI

Perhaps the most influential international code of research ethics after the *Nuremberg Code* is the *Declaration of Helsinki*, first adopted by the World Medical Association (WMA) in 1964 at its Eighteenth Assembly in Helsinki, and modified on several occasions since then. The origins of this effort and the sources upon which it drew are discussed in Chapters 49 and 50.

What is often forgotten is that the WMA had already addressed some of the issues in a 1954 "Resolution on Human Experimentation" (McNeill 1993, 44–5). The 1954 Resolution required the researcher to explain to the potential subject the nature of the research, the reasons for it, and the risks. In the case of experimentation involving healthy subjects, this explanation would be the basis of informed and free consent by the subjects. In the case of experimentation involving sick subjects, consent could be given by the subjects or their next of kin. In drawing this distinction, the World Medical Assembly began to allow for proxy consent in some cases. This permissive approach was continued in the *Declaration of Helsinki*. This differentiated its approach to the issue of informed consent from the requirement of informed consent in the *Nuremberg Code*.

One of the most important contributions of the *Declaration of Helsinki* was an additional protection, first introduced in its second version, the 1975 modification of the *Declaration*:

> The design and performance of each experimental procedure involving human subjects should be clearly formulated in an experimental protocol which should be transmitted to a specially appointed independent committee for consideration, comment and guidance. (Annas and Grodin 1992, 334)

This component of independent review has become widely accepted throughout the world, in large measure because of the influence of the *Declaration of Helsinki*, but its relation to the *Nuremberg Code's* requirement of informed consent has not been adequately understood. Since Helsinki, we have a system in which there are two separate protections of the rights and interests of research subjects; subjects protect themselves through the informed consent process and they are further protected by the independent review. Normally, each of these protective processes is necessary for the licitness of research, and only the satisfaction of both is sufficient for the licitness of research.

There is another feature of the *Declaration of Helsinki* that should be noted. Having enunciated its basic principles, the *Declaration* goes on to differentiate "clinical research" (defined as "medical research combined with professional care) from nonclinical, nontherapeutic research, providing extra principles governing each. The most important of these are the principle that clinicians must be free to use new diagnostic and therapeutic measures they judge to be appropriate (even outside a research setting) and the principle that "in any medical study, every patient-including those of a control group, if any-should be assured of the best proven diagnostic and therapeutic method. This does not exclude the use of inert placebo in studies where no proven diagnostic or therapeutic method exists." This principle has recently been a subject of great controversy, centering around the issue of whether it rightfully prohibits placebo-controlled trials when there is a proven intervention, but one which would not anyway be available to the research subjects (Brody 2002).

In many of the latter national and transnational codes (Brody 1998, 126–8), this distinction between types of research became the basis for requiring different levels of protection for the subjects. Subjects in nontherapeutic research, especially if they were incapable of giving consent, could be exposed to fewer risks and were afforded more protections in the informed consent. This whole distinction, however, has come under criticism in recent years, in part because much supposedly therapeutic research involves interventions, which turn out not to be therapeutic and in part because the control group receives no therapeutic interventions.

The *Declaration of Helsinki* has undergone many revisions over the years. The latest major revision was adopted in October 2000 (WMA 2000), although notes clarifying certain passages were added in 2002 and 2004.

> The first Declaration of Helsinki adopted by the World Medical Association in 1964 was one of the first attempts to transform reactions to the atrocities committed in the name of biomedical research during the Nazi period into preventive measures with a full global perspective. The second version, released in 1975, was rewritten from an observation point closer to active clinical science. The resulting impact on biomedical science was obvious within a few years. The requirement to establish research ethics committees made research ethics visible, not only among scientists but also in society at large. At the same time, biomedical research expanded toward society in epidemiology and toward basic life processes in molecular biology. Further extension took place geographically with an increasing globalization of research results and multinational research projects. Consequently, a thorough revision of the 1975 version has been necessary for some years, not to change its fundamental principles, but to account for the expanded scope of biomedical research. A new version should still serve the original aim: to balance the protection of, and respect for, research patients and healthy volunteers with the necessary freedom of research to facilitate scientific progress as a public good. (Riis 2000, 3045)

The latest revision reorganized the document, eliminating the separate section on nontherapeutic research. It added requirements of disclosures of potential conflicts of interest to the independent review board, to potential subjects, and to readers of resulting publications. It affirmed an obligation to provide subjects in clinical trials access to the best treatment identified in the study. It reemphasized an opposition to the use of subjects unable to consent unless their participation is absolutely necessary. Finally, it seemed to reiterate the earlier opposition to placebo-controlled trials when a proven therapy is available, even if it would not ordinarily be available to the population from which the subjects are drawn. These last two provisions have been criticized by many (Forster, Emanuel, and Grady 2001).

IV. THE CIOMS–WHO GUIDELINES FOR MEDICAL RESEARCH INVOLVING HUMAN SUBJECTS

The Council of International Organizations of Medical Sciences (CIOMS), in collaboration with the World Health Organization (WHO), produced an important set of guidelines in 1982 and modified them in 1993 (CIOMS 1993) There are a number of features of these guidelines that constitute their distinctive contribution to research ethics, a contribution that might well be characterized as raising difficult issues rather than resolving them. Many of these features are related to the fundamental purpose of the CIOMS effort, which was to "to indicate how the ethical principles that should guide the conduct of biomedical research involving human subjects, as set forth in the Declaration of Helsinki, could be effectively applied, particularly in developing countries, given their socioeconomic circumstances, laws and regulations, and executive and administrative arrangements" (CIOMS 1993, Background).

The first feature is a change in attitude toward the ethical issues raised by research involving human subjects. Instead of just protecting the rights and interests of subjects, these guidelines also emphasize the promotion of the positive goods produced by:

> The Guidelines must now strike a balance between the paramount ethical concern for vigilance in protecting the rights and welfare of research subjects and an ethical responsibility to advance the good of societies and of research subjects, which earlier international guidelines and declarations did not take into consideration research. (CIOMS 1993, Introduction)

The most important practical implication of this changing attitude is the greater support in these *Guidelines* for the inclusion in research of groups that have traditionally been excluded from research to protect them (children and women of childbearing potential). Still, the *Guidelines* are often equivocal on just how much involvement of these subjects is appropriate. Thus, in discussing research involving children, the *Guidelines* still say:

> Children should not be subjects of research that might equally well be carried out on adults. However, their participation is indispensable for research on diseases of childhood and conditions to which children are particularly susceptible. (CIOMS 1993, discussion of guideline 7)

So children should not be enrolled in trials to test promising new therapies of conditions that adults are equally susceptible to having, even if this means denying access to promising new therapies to pediatric subjects. Precisely the opposite, however, is asserted later on in the *Guidelines* in discussing access to new acquired immunodeficiency syndrome (AIDS) therapies: " . . . [they] should be made equally available to members of vulnerable populations, particularly when no superior or equivalent approaches to therapy are available" (discussion of guideline 12).

The second feature is a complex and important discussion of cultural variability and universal ethical principles. The CIOMS *Guidelines* recognize that many of the traditional rules of research ethics will have less meaning in some cultural contexts. This may be particularly true of the requirement to obtain individual informed consent from subjects in societies in which important decisions are normally made by cultural/societal leaders. The tension raised by such cases is well reflected in the discussion of research in underdeveloped countries (CIOMS 1993, guideline 11): "Investigators must respect the ethical standards of their own countries and the cultural expectations of societies in which research is undertaken, unless this implies a violation of a transcending moral rule." They are further reflected in the analysis of informed consent later in that same discussion:

> For example, where individuals are not sufficiently aware of the implications of participation to give adequately informed consent, the decision on whether to consent should be elicited through a reliable intermediary such as a trusted community leader. In some mechanisms other mechanisms may be more suitable. However consent is obtained, all individuals must be clearly told that their participation is entirely voluntary, and that they are free to refuse to participate or to withdraw their participation at any time without loss of any entitlement. This means that the mechanisms used to supplement consent that cannot meet the standards set forth in this document should not be regarded as replacements or substitutes for informed consent. (CIOMS 1993, guideline 11)

The third related feature is the *Guidelines'* discussion of the international components of research, especially research by first world researchers working with third world subjects. The concern expressed in the *Guidelines* is that such subjects and the countries in which they live may be vulnerable to exploitation. A number of standards are put forward (CIOMS 1993, guideline 11) by way of minimizing this concern: (1) the research protocols should be reviewed by independent review committees both in the sponsoring country and in the host country, with the host country committee being particularly responsible for ensuring that they relate to the health needs of the host country and that they are performed in a culturally sensitive fashion; (2) the research must be responsive to the health needs of the host country; and (3) most crucially, "the initiating agency should provide assurances that any products developed through such research will be made reasonably available to residents of the host community or country at the completion of successful testing ... Consideration should be given to whether the initiating agency should agree to continue to maintain health services and facilities established for purposes of

the study in the host country after the research has been completed." This third requirement, because of its economic implications, has become particularly controversial in recent debates about AIDS-related research in third world countries (Brody 2002). It is related to analogous requirements in the latest version of the Declaration of Helsinki.

V. Guidelines for Good Clinical Practice of the International Conference on Harmonization

The International Conference on Harmonisation (ICH) is a joint effort of the drug/device regulatory agencies of the European Union, Japan, and the United States.

> Harmonisation of regulatory requirements was pioneered by the European Community, in the 1980s, as the EC (now the European Union) moved towards the development of a single market for pharmaceuticals. The success achieved in Europe demonstrated that harmonisation was feasible. At the same time there were bilateral discussions between Europe, Japan and the US on possibilities for harmonisation. It was, however, at the WHO Conference of Drug Regulatory Authorities (ICDRA), in Paris, in 1989, that specific plans for action began to materialise. Soon afterwards, the authorities approached IFPMA to discuss a joint regulatory-industry initiative on international harmonisation, and ICH was conceived. The birth of ICH took place at a meeting in April 1990, hosted by the EFPIA in Brussels. Representatives of the regulatory agencies and industry associations of Europe, Japan and the USA met, primarily, to plan an International Conference but the meeting also discussed the wider implications and terms of reference of ICH. The ICH Steering Committee which was established at that meeting has since met at least twice a year, with the location rotating between the three regions. (ICH 1996)

The goal of the ICH is to develop unified standards that will facilitate the international approval process for new drugs and devices. In May 1996, it finalized one of its standards, its *Guidelines for Good Clinical Practice*. This standard is intended (ICH, 1996) to provide "public assurance that the rights, safety and well-being of trial subjects are being protected," as well as that "the clinical trial data are credible." These *Guidelines* draw upon earlier guidelines from the involved countries, as well as those from Australia, Canada, the Nordic countries, and the WHO.

The new component in the *Guidelines*, building on the *Good Clinical Practice Guidelines* already in place, is the stress on the ethical responsibilities of the sponsor of the research as well as of the investigator performing the research. The sponsor is "an individual, company, institution or organization which takes responsibility for the initiation, management, and/or financing of a clinical trial" (ICH 1996, 1.53). This may sometimes be an individual investigator, but in a world of expensive clinical research designed to prove the safety and effectiveness of a new drug or device, so that it can be approved by a regulatory agency for distribution and sale, this will usually be a company that hopes to manufacture/distribute the approved product. As these ethical standards were developed by agencies that regularly interact with such sponsors of research, it is not surprising that these are the standards that most address the ethical responsibilities of the sponsor.

The sponsor's ethical responsibilities are many. These include: (1) choosing appropriately qualified trial design personnel, medical consultants, investigators, and trial management personnel; (2) considering establishing an independent data monitoring committee to do interim assessments of the trial and its data; (3) properly manufacturing and distributing investigational products; (4) reporting adverse events; (5) confirming that the protocol has been appropriately reviewed and approved by an institutional review board (IRB); and (6) ensuring that the trial is appropriately monitored by qualified monitors. It is this last responsibility that is particularly important.

Among other responsibilities, the sponsor-appointed monitor must ensure that the protocol is being followed and that "written informed consent was obtained before each subject's participation in the trial" (ICH 1993, part V). As a result of these requirements on sponsor, both the investigator and the sponsor are now required to ensure that subjects are protected by the dual protections of independent review and informed consent.

VI. CONCLUSION

It is probably never wise to write any history as a linear progression. Nevertheless, just such progress seems to have occurred in the development of international standards of research ethics. The *Nuremberg Code* gave us the requirement of informed consent and the *Helsinki Declaration* gave us the requirement of independent review. CIOMS taught us the need to be culturally sensitive while still insisting on universal standards, and the ICH formalized these universal standards and imposed them upon sponsors of research as well as investigators. There are few clearer instances of steady ethical progress. Each of the documents added further protections of the interests and rights of research subjects and each raised new ethical issues to be resolved. The remaining challenge is to ensure that this progress is realized in the actual conduct of research.

B. Medical Ethics, Imperialism, and the Nation-State

CHAPTER 52

COLONIALISM, IMPERIALISM, AND THE HISTORY OF LATIN AMERICAN MEDICAL ETHICS

Juan Carlos Tealdi

I. INTRODUCTION

America's conquest by Spaniards – *la Conquista* – took more than six decades, from discovery in 1492 to the execution of the Araucanian rebel, *cacique* Caupolicán, in 1557. During this period, the Spanish engaged in a political and legal debate over the status of new lands as property, which was accompanied by a philosophical and theological debate over the justification of war to take Spanish possession of the territories and the moral status of the indigenous population. Overlaying this was an even more sophisticated argument about the ontological reasons concerning whether indigenous peoples had dominion over themselves and, thus, were not to be enslaved. These discussions occurred contemporaneously with two devastating events, the radical and rapid depopulation of indigenous peoples in the Americas known as the "Americas' demographic catastrophe," and the near simultaneous depopulation of many African tribes as their people were enslaved to facilitate the economic exploitation of the "New World." After their military and political conquest of Latin America, with its maleficent consequences, the Spaniards introduced sanitary measures and hospital developments to provide health services to the population as an expression of the Christian virtue of charity. Spanish colonialism in Latin America emerged

from the conquest and is a complex social and moral phenomenon.

During the nineteenth century, European intellectual influence changed colonial medical ethics, as Latin American physicians, emulating the unification of medical art with the scientific experimental method practiced in Britain, France, and Germany, found a new source of intellectual and moral authority. Latin American medical ethics found a new justification for its paternalism, although a political tradition of individual autonomy was introduced in those countries that modeled themselves on liberal democracies. During the twentieth century, medical ethics based on codes of ethical rules for physicians controlled by national medical associations turned from deontological physician-centered ethics to a human rights or a communitarian approach and to the interdisciplinary field of bioethics. Moral problems for medicine were replaced by communitarian moral demands to a right to health care, and moral obligations of physicians were replaced by an interdisciplinary responsibility in bioethical problems. The purpose of this chapter is to explore the following questions: What kind of relationship, if any, is it possible to find between the regional history in its several phases and that of medical ethics? Are there any present conditions in the Latin-American ethos that could be related to this history? Both these important questions refer to the subsequent development of colonialism and imperialism in Latin America (Acosta [1590] 1962; Clavijero [1781] 1976; Cortés [1522] 1976; Díaz del Castillo [1632] 1976; Sahagún [1582] 1975).

II. 1492–1557: WHEN WORLDS COLLIDE: CIVILIZATION, BARBARISM, AND THE MORAL STATUS OF INDIGENOUS PEOPLES

Columbus's first ceremony on his landfall was to take possession of the new lands on behalf of the Spanish monarchs (Colón [1492–1506] 1982, 30). The legitimacy of a claim or right to take this possession of lands in America was found in the legal thesis of the just appropriation by Christian monarchs of all newly discovered lands belonging to non-Christian princes. A Papal bull by Pope Nicholas V in 1455 gave Portugal the right to conquer pagans and reduce them to slavery in new territories to be discovered in Western Africa. In 1493, at the Spanish Catholic monarchs' request, Pope Alexander VI signed five bulls granting the same rights to Spain in America. Finally, by the Tordesillas Treaty in 1494, Portugal and Spain agreed to divide the Atlantic Ocean into two regions for exploration and acquiring property. The Portuguese claimed a right to part of the new world, Brazil; Spain claimed the remainder.

The political and juridical justification for America's conquest was criticized by Spanish theologians, especially Francisco de Vitoria ([1539] 1974) and Bartolomé de las Casas (las Casas [1552] 1977). They argued that Europeans did not respect the freedom of the indigenous populations and that the Pope did not have any power on secular questions related to the moral status of pagan peoples. Referring to St. Augustine and St. Thomas Aquinas, they held that natural law was the foundation for the origin of states and the legitimacy of the political power of pagan princes. As a consequence, the morality of just war applied to them. Just war theory demands justification for war, including conquest, known as *jus ad bellum*. Just war theory also requires that war be conducted according to ethical standards, known as *jus in bello*. Vitoria opposed the royal counselors' argument that Spaniards had the right to reduce American Indians by force, analogously to the case of Africa. Vitoria argued first, that Spain could have legitimate government over the new territories only if Spain acted for the good of the indigenous population, not merely for Spanish profit and, second, that the administration of the colonies should last only so long as the indigenous population remained in a barbarian, that is,, uncivilized, condition. This beneficence-based argument was buttressed by an autonomy-based argument that rejected the claim of the "natives' voluntary election" of Spanish dominion on the following grounds: the failure of the indigenous population to understand Spanish proposals for government of them, coercion by

armed force, and the lack of capacity of indigenous governors to make decisions about having new princes without the consent of their own people. As a consequence of that debate, the Catholic Queen Isabella authorized in 1501 the introduction of Black slaves into Spanish America and after 1518 there was large-scale trade in African slaves after the prohibition of American indigenous slavery in 1512 by the Theologians Council from Burgos.

This "African turn" marks an important difference in American and African colonization by Europeans but at the same time underscores their affinity and justifications given for them at the time. In the political philosophy of fifteenth-century Europe, powerful and organized kingdoms had the right to conduct diplomatic relationships. Because African natives were living in a barbaric state, they were not legal persons and so could justifiably be reduced to slavery. With the prohibition of the enslavement of the American indigenous peoples, the colonial Latin America population became a mixture of Indian servants, Black slaves, and white proprietors.

As the populations from these three continents came into contact with each other they exchanged infectious diseases. Smallpox, measles, leprosy, and tuberculosis were introduced by Spaniards into the indigenous population; yellow fever, anquilostomiasis, and dengue fever were introduced by Black slaves into the indigenous population and Spanish colonists; and, so some historians argue, syphilis was introduced by Spaniards into the indigenous population. The first quarantine was ordered in 1519 in Santo Domingo to prevent a smallpox epidemic, a catastrophic disease for the indigenous population with a ninety percent mortality rate. This catastrophe was repeated in the Colombian epidemics of 1558, 1564, and 1587. The American indigenous population was also devastated by smallpox and influenza epidemics. It is estimated that in Central Mexico the indigenous population was reduced from twenty-three and a half million in 1519 to one million in 1605 (Sánchez Albornoz [1973] 1977, 60–71). It would take four centuries for the Latin America population to grow back to sixty million, the estimated population on the day of discovery at the end of the fifteenth century.

At the same time, the increasingly active Black slave trade devastated many African tribes. From the sixteenth to the nineteenth centuries, half of the ten million Black slaves taken from Angola, Congo, the Slave Coast, and other African regions were shipped to Latin America, one third of the five million to Spanish territories and two-thirds to Brazil. This double demographic catastrophe had an impact everywhere, including on medical ethics. In the physician–patient relationship, some of the sick, African Black slaves and American Indian servants, were not persons, whereas others, the European white conquerors, were persons. The whole community and the health services in Latin America would be organized along racial and ethnic lines that reflected these differences.

III. 1557–1810: Colonial Medical Ethics During Spanish and Portuguese Administration: Christian Virtues and Beneficence for a New World

The colonial period in Latin America lasted from the end of conquest in 1557 to the beginning of the revolutionary movements for independence in 1810. There were two essential characteristics of colonial medicine: the beneficence-oriented political and administrative regulation of hospitals, *protomedicatos*, and medical educational institutions, on the one hand, and the virtue-oriented contributions to health care by different religious orders, on the other. In 1541, Charles V decreed that there had to be hospitals to care for the sick poor and practice Christian charity in all Spanish and Indian towns in *Nueva España* (New Spain) (Landa [1560] 1973). The first hospital in America was *San Nicolás de Bari* in Santo Domingo, founded in 1503, and the first hospital founded in Mexico in 1521 by Cortés, what has today become the *Hospital de Jesús*. By 1550 there were hospitals in Mexico, Panama, Cuba, Puerto Rico, Guatemala, Peru, and also in Brazil. It is possible to identify almost forty hospitals in Mexico alone during the sixteenth century. There were hospitals for indigenous and Black people, for smallpox and leprosy, for mental disorders and maternity. A health system was thus developed in Latin America, colonial medicine of this period, like its European counterpart, had little more than care and comfort to offer the sick (Guerra 1972, 347–50). This marks an important difference with the English colonies, where there were no permanent medical institutions until the middle of the eighteenth century, with the creation of Philadelphia and New York hospitals. From the early colonial period, medical practice in Latin America was regulated by a superior medical authority known as *Protomedicato* (see also Chapters 27 and 29). This was a council of physicians presided over by a chief physician, the Protomédico, who was obliged to live where the Court of Justice, the *Audiencia*, was located. The *Protomedicato* was charged with the tasks of examining physicians and regulating medical practice. The first *Protomedicato* was created in 1477 by the Catholic monarchs Ferdinand of Aragon and Isabella of Castile. Later, Charles V ordered medical, surgical, and pharmacological practices in America to be regulated as they were in Spain. In 1542, the *Protomedicato* was regulated by the "New Laws of the Indies" that Philip II would formalize in 1570. The entire body of Indies legislation would be compiled in 1680 (Carlos II 1680). *Protomedicatos* were created in Mexico and Peru (1570) and then in Cuba (1634), Nueva Granada (c. 1640), Buenos Aires (1776), and Santiago

de Chile (1786). These councils examined physicians, commissioned them to work, informed Spain about the number of both Spanish and indigenous physicians, controlled apothecaries, inspected ships to order quarantines and took other sanitary actions as deemed necessary. Protomédicos were also charged to gather information about trees, plants, herbs, and seeds in the region and to identify their medical uses by Spanish or indigenous people. Francisco Hernández, the first protomédico in Mexico, described nearly 4,000 types of plants used by natives. This marks another difference from English and French colonies in America, where medical regulation did not occur until the end of eighteenth century.

Colonial medical education in Latin America was based on the educational programs of the universities in Salamanca, Valladolid, and Alcalá de Henares (Felipe IV 1640, 1:299–309). The first institution to teach medicine in the region during the colonial period and the best example of this education was *Real y Pontificia Universidad de México* (Royal and Pontifical University of Mexico), founded in 1551. To earn a doctoral degree, students first had to complete study in the humanities and then take a 4-year program studying Hippocrates, Galen, and Avicenna, followed by practical clinical experience with a graduate physician and the preparation of a thesis. Chairs of Anatomy, Surgery, Method with Therapeutics, Astrology, and Mathematics were created in the seventeenth century. After 1645, students were required to make anatomical dissections. Chairs of Practical Anatomy, Physiology, Surgical Technique, Clinics and Legal Medicine were introduced in the eighteenth century. About ten physicians were graduated each year. Despite even greater challenges in establishing centers of medical education, other Latin American universities also taught medicine, including Peru (1551), Bogotá, Colombia (1639), Guatemala (1676), Quito, Ecuador (1693), La Habana, Cuba (1726), Santiago de Chile (1756), and Caracas, Venezuela (1763). These developments in medical education mark yet another difference from the English colonial territories, in which the first school of medicine was created in Philadelphia only in 1765 (Guerra 1972, 350–4).

The study of medical ethics was legally mandated. This subject of study combined Hippocratic ethics and moral theology. For example, physicians were ethically obligated to warn patients about the need for confession, especially in cases of acute, life-threatening diseases because, it was then thought, the cure of the body sometimes resulted from the cure of the soul. Medical education was intrinsically aristocratic and thus medicine was inherently elitist: To be a student in any university it was necessary to prove nobility and "clean blood," that is, one was not mixed race but of pure European origin (Felipe IV 1640, 1:40–2). Colonial medical ethics in Latin America was thus Hippocratic, religiously canonical, and aristocratic but also based on clear requirements of mastering theoretical knowledge and acquiring practical experience.

Religious orders played an essential role in the care of the sick through hospitals, churches, and convents. After its foundation in Granada in 1537, the Order *Hermanos Hospitalarios de San Juan de Dios* (Hospitaler Brothers of St. John of God) began to work in America. The Order *Hermanos de la Caridad de San Hipólito* (Brothers of the Heart of St. Hipolitus) was created at San Hipólito Hospital, founded in Mexico in 1567. Pedro de Bethancourt created the Order of Bethlemitas from *Nuestra Señora de Belén* (Notre Dame of Bethlehem) Hospital, founded in Guatemala in 1657. Most of the hospitals in Latin America had a religious origin and administration. Given the calamitous health events noted previously, especially epidemics, and given the still primitive scientific and technical medical knowledge brought from Europe, the Christian virtues of faith, hope, and charity, as well as compassion, fortitude, and temperance were of paramount importance for the care of the sick. The discourse of Christian charity motivated care for the sick and relief of their suffering and at the same time was open to a syncretism between Indian religions and Catholic faith.

IV. 1810–1898: IMPERIAL MEDICAL ETHICS IN THE NINETEENTH CENTURY EUROPEAN INFLUENCES, AND THE BEGINNING OF THE ERA OF RESPECT FOR AUTONOMOUS CHOICE

Starting in 1810, many independence movements arose in Latin America as a consequence of the political instability in Spain. These successively resulted in new independent nations with liberal constitutions. These constitutions abolished the slave trade, ending three centuries of slavery. They also embraced French-inspired, liberal-romantic social conceptions of freedom of speech, free trade and commerce, private property, freedom of thought and religious ideas for all citizens. Medical ethics was influenced by these important developments and must be understood in light of them. At the same time, however, it is possible to discern the beginnings of major changes in the practice of medicine resulting from changes in medical education.

Slaves were emancipated in all Latin American countries during the nineteenth century but this process took almost 75 years to complete. Many of the Spanish countries abolished slavery during the first half of the century, but it is not surprising that the last countries to do so were Cuba (1880) and Brazil (1888), because the slave trade was more intense in these two countries than anywhere else in Latin America. The social conception of autonomy in Latin America is rooted in this cultural background and political and social changes in different countries have modified this conception (Ianni 1976).

Whereas the new liberal Latin American countries closed the shameful chapter of African slavery in the region, something different happened with the American Indian servants and with their gradual replacement by "mestizos" (people of mixed Indian and European origin) in some places. A major effort to understand this change appeared in the influential book, *Facundo* (Sarmiento [1845] 1969), by Domingo Faustino Sarmiento (1811–1888), an Argentinean president, general, educator, and writer. In Sarmiento's book, if the fifteenth-century clash between "civilization" and "barbarism: was that of powerful European and Asian kingdoms against primitive African tribes, the nineteenth-century challenge was that of civilized European industrial and urban political concepts against the barbaric Spanish feudal and rural mentality. American indigenous or *mestizo* servants working in rural areas had to be transformed into industrial workers in the urban factories or be replaced by European white immigrants. This form of capitalist development in Latin America would, however, take a path different from that of the old English and French colonies such as the United States and Canada. Because of three centuries of Spanish rule and its Roman juridical system, with indigenous and Catholic religious traditions, social and economic disparities and population structure, the Latin American ethos of social change during industrialization would again be quite different (Abellán 1972; Biagini 1989).

The end of Spanish and Portuguese colonial administrations, based largely on gold and silver mining and *latifundia* (i.e., extensive cultivation of sugar, cacao, coffee, cotton, and bananas on plantations using Black slaves and Indian servants), was associated with the beginning of English and French European imperialism in Latin America (Galeano 1981). *Latifundia*, with its cheap labor force, poverty, and environmental exploitation continued into the nineteenth century. The new processes of urban concentration, although worldwide, were proportionally greater in the less developed regions of Latin America with the result that cities became an illusory salvation, marked by chaos and misery for many. The main American colonial industry of gold and silver mining stimulated and founded European capitalism but goods coming into America were only about one-fifth the value of exports. Seriously unbalanced trade became a constant in the region. In the nineteenth century, the diverse industrial production achieved by those countries that had begun to meet domestic consumption was undermined by the British and French doctrine and practice of free trade, which aimed at introducing European manufactured goods in place of locally produced goods. As a result, local industries could not compete without protection and the role of Latin countries as raw-material exporters was consolidated (Tealdi 1993).

Health conditions in Latin America at the beginning of the nineteenth century can be described in the same terms as the epidemiology of the period of conquest: high mortality from smallpox and other infectious diseases, lung disease among miners, and famine (Humboldt [1808] 1978, V:44–50). The European industrialization model was not all bad; it also supported the British sanitation movement and the development of public hygiene as a discipline. These movements succeeded in changing medical practices in many Latin countries. After Jenner's discovery of immunity by smallpox virus (1798), vaccination was begun in North America and in Latin America. In 1881, the Cuban physician Carlos Finlay presented his thesis on yellow fever transmission at the Academy of Sciences in La Habana.

Medicine in Latin America gradually became a more scientific field of practice. Medical morality consequently took a turn toward a distinctive paternalism in which scientific competence supported claims to both intellectual and moral authority of practitioners over the sick. The old charity-based health system was changing. In 1884, Bismarck introduced a new collective national health system in Germany that was adopted in different European countries and that came to be applied in Latin America. The administrative control of medicine by a feudal institution such as the *Protomedicato* was replaced by the new self-regulatory medical societies modeled on the British Medical Association (1836), the American Medical Association (1847), and the Association Générale de Médecins de France (1858).

Reflecting these transformations, medical education became a major beneficiary of reformation of the traditional requirements of the Spanish colonial model (García 1972). In 1800, the *Protomedicato* in Buenos Aires initiated this tendency by taking the Edinburgh University Program as a model. In 1808 the *Real Colegio de Medicina y Cirugía de San Fernando* (Royal College of Medicine and Surgery of St. Ferdinand) in Peru also reformed its medical education program, taking the Paris and Leiden universities programs as models. These new models of nineteenth-century medical education were characterized by small numbers of medical students as compared with the following century, increased numbers of professors and teaching hours, and the emergence of medical specialties and research institutes as leaders of medical progress.

A new European and North American influence made itself felt in medical ethics. The Edinburgh medical education model assumed in Buenos Aires was founded in John Gregory's (1724–1773) virtue ethics for physicians (Gregory [1772b] 1998b; see also Chapters 18, 30, and 36). Thomas Percival's (1740–1804) *Medical Ethics* (Percival 1803, 1803b) was also influential. The old Christian and aristocratic morality was refined as a result of their influence; at the same time their impact, as extended through the 1847 Code of Ethics of the American Medical Association (see Chapter 36), was also more democratic. Although it took until the twentieth century for

formal codes of medical ethics to appear in Latin America, colonial medical ethics was definitively transformed during this period. The major features of this transformation include the introduction of the liberal conception of individual autonomy, the population's growing tendency to urban concentration, the scientific development of medicine and public health, and the medical education reform adopting new codes of ethics for physicians.

V. 1898–2000: IMPERIAL MEDICAL ETHICS IN THE TWENTIETH CENTURY AND HUMAN RIGHTS: FROM PAN AMERICANISM TO GLOBALIZATION

Medical ethics in Latin America during the twentieth century continued to be influenced by social, political, and cultural factors in the region, as Latin American medical ethics had been since the period of discovery. At the same time, the international development of medicine and public health was followed by the transition from deontological medical ethics to the bioethical movement in the 1980s (see Chapter 42). European imperialism yielded to a new United States' imperialism in the region, ideologically founded on the American president James Monroe's doctrine of 1823 that rejected European intervention in America, Central America, and the Caribbean. Until World War I, Latin America became a theater for the expansionist influence of the United States, from the American military interventions and protectorates of 1846 in Mexico to 1915 in Haiti. This growing military and political control, exercised over many decades, was challenged by rural and urban guerrilla movements during the 1960s. In response to these political and military movements, dictatorships were subsequently induced, tolerated, and even supported by the United States. Unusually strong violations of human rights involved physicians as participants in many cases (Riquelme 1995). The 1980s opened the way for the emergence of democracy in many of these countries and bioethical issues began to be discussed in a more politically open and tolerant context.

During the twentieth century the political and juridical general evolution of democracy in Latin America confronted many challenges. At the beginning of the nineteenth century, the abolition of torture and slavery were the two main political ideas for new Latin American nations. The protection of human rights, including the right to health in the region, would become the main political concern at the end of the twentieth century (Fuenzalida-Puelma and Connor 1989). In 1969 the *American Convention on Human Rights (Pacto de San José de Costa Rica)* was signed creating the Inter-American Court on Human Rights, the most relevant regional institution. In Argentina, where Sarmiento proposed his ideas on liberal civilization and where paradoxically in 1984 the National Commission on Disappeared People (Argentina 1984) said "Never More" to violations of human rights, a new, reformed Constitution in 1994 gave constitutional status to most of the international conventions for the protection of human rights. This example illustrates the pattern of imperialism in the region: from repeated violations of human rights by imperial powers to revolutions in Latin American countries and the subsequent emergences of a political discourse, and increasing reality of human rights.

Latin American economics during the past century has continued to be based on an imbalance in trade, *latifundia*, and a cheap labor force, poverty, and consequent environmental damage in the largest ecological reserve in the world – as discussed in Rio Summit on Environment (United Nations 1992). During the early decades of the twentieth century, the processes of industrialization stimulated immigration and the development of a social class of industrial workers. The triple ethnological structure of colonial times became a diversified population of indigenous peoples and *mestizos*, Blacks and *mulattos* (people of mixed Black and white origin), white immigrants and *criollos* (people of European white origin born in Latin America). The social structure remained characterized by a large population of rural and industrial workers living in poverty, an usually small percentage of urban middle class, and a small wealthy population (10 percent) that controlled more than their proportion of wealth (35–50 percent) (Banco Mundial 1993, 302–3). Under globalization, a new regional phenomenon would be that of increasing numbers of unemployed people. As a consequence of these multiple and complex political, social, and economical changes, there was also religious change. Roman Catholicism, the main regional religion, even if conservative and orthodox in its leadership in many countries of the region, saw the emergence of a "Third World Church" and the "Option for the Poor" as movements closely related to the problems of the economically, socially, and politically disadvantaged. Archbishop Oscar Romero's assassination in El Salvador in 1980 became emblematic of the divorce between imperialist ideology and religiously led, local defense of human rights, as it had been 500 years before in Las Casas and Vitoria.

The theory and practice of Latin American medical ethics could not escape the influence of this changing social, political, and cultural reality. The entire conception of the life cycle, the physician–patient relationship, and the state responsibility in public health policies became rooted in an emerging communitarian ethos (Navarro [1976] 1978, 27–109). That history, however, developed many differences among Latin American countries in the ethnological structure and the population distribution by

age, living areas, income, life expectancy, epidemiological profile, and many others characteristics for a pluralist ethos. This communitarian medical ethics was institutionalized in the new Pan American Sanitary Office (subsequently the Pan American Health Organization or PAHO), which was created in 1902 and built on the public health advances of the nineteenth century. Governed by the General Assembly of Ministers of Health of all countries in the region, including the United States and Canada, this international administrative body has become a kind of modern version for the regional administrative health control like that of the old colonial *Protomedicato*. For nine decades, medical ethics at this institution was conceived in the traditional beneficence-oriented conception. At the end of the 1980s, the organization recognized bioethical advances in the field (Fuenzalida-Puelma and Connor 1989) and opened a regional program of bioethics.

VI. CONCLUSION

Latin American medical ethics has turned from deontology to bioethics (see also chapter 42). In 1916, under the influence of Grasset's deontology (Grasset 1900), a very influential Latin American code of medical ethics written by Luis Razetti was approved in Venezuela (Razetti [1916] 1963). Subsequently, similar national codes were adopted in different Latin American countries (Leon C. 1978). Deontological medical ethics was centered in professional conduct as in the old tradition from Hippocrates to Gregory and Percival (Mainetti 1995). During the century's last decade, however, a bioethical understanding was increasingly incorporated in medical ethics (Tealdi, Pis Diez, and Esquisabel 1995). This change opened the possibility of thinking about the history of medical ethics as a particular vision of the history of moral ideas in the region. The physicians' internal point of view in deontological approach to medical ethics changed to a more comprehensive analysis of health and disease, and life and death issues for the community as a whole.

As a 500-year cycle of medical ethos and ethics has concluded in Latin America, it is possible to find a moral lesson in history. Today there still are ethical problems with respect to life and identity, integrity and liberty, and health and welfare as human values, in a region with very extreme inequities. The need for justice in the history of imperialism and colonialism in Latin America changed the community approach to ethics. It is possible to imagine a new change in medical ethics, in times of globalization, if bioethics could open a critical dialogue on human values in the region.

CHAPTER 53

JAPANESE DOCTORS' EXPERIMENTATION, 1932–1945, AND MEDICAL ETHICS

Jing-Bao Nie, Takashi Tsuchiya, and Lun Li

I. INTRODUCTION

Although the notorious Nazi doctors are an archetype of the dark and evil side of modern medicine, the Nuremberg Trials have brought most criminals to justice and the ten principles formulated in the *Nuremberg Code*, a founding document of contemporary medical ethics, and in particular the principle of consent, is still guiding ethical medical research and practice (see Chapters 49–51 and 54). Unfortunately, there exists an Asian counterpart of Nazi medicine: Japanese doctors inhumanly experimented on human subjects in East Asia, mainly in China, from the early 1930s to the end of World War II. The experiments performed by Nazis and those undertaken by Japanese doctors are similar in that both involved the intentional killing, torture, and harm of human beings in the name of national interests, science, and medicine. Even more unfortunately, as a result of complex political and historical factors, including an American cover-up, Japanese denials, and the relative silence and nonaction of two Chinese governments, Japanese medical atrocities are far less publicized than those conducted by the Nazi doctors. Until very recently, medical ethicists – international, Japanese, and Chinese included – have ignored Japanese doctors' inhuman experimentation and its ethical challenges. The purpose of this chapter is to provide a brief

account of Japanese doctors' wartime experimentation and the aftermath, and then, to address ethical issues raised by this disturbing history.

II. THE FORGOTTEN MEDICAL ATROCITIES

Before and during World War II, Japan, a world power despite her relatively small size, invaded China, the Philippines, and several other East Asian countries, occupying territory in the name of building up "A New Order in East Asia" and "The East Asiatic Co-Prosperity Sphere." A Fascist alliance was formed with Germany and Italy. Japan was a signatory to the 1925 Geneva Convention that created a clear ban on biological and chemical warfare. Between 1932 and 1945, however, the Japanese Army established extensive biological warfare programs in China and elsewhere. These programs included Unit 731 in Pingfang (near Harbin) and its branches (in Mudanjiang, Linkow, Sunyu, Hailar, Dalian), Unit 100 in Changchun, Unit 1855 in Beijing, Unit 1644 in Nanjing, Unit 8604 in Guangzhou and Hong Kong, and Unit 9420 in Singapore.

These programs, run by the Japanese army under the guise of disease prevention and water supply programs, were actually "factories of death," in which Japanese doctors conducted a great number of vivisections and other barbarous experiments on human beings. Ishii Shiro,

589

holding the rank of a Lieutenant General in the Army Medical Service at the end of the war, was a specialist in bacteria-related fields and the major leader of Japanese biological warfare. Ishii called human experimentation the "secret of the secrets" in the empire of manufacturing bacteriological weapons. Japanese doctors' murderous experiments included:

- Intentionally infecting healthy men and women with such diseases as plague, anthrax, cholera, and typhoid, either by injection or aspiration, or forcing them or deceiving them into eating foods and drinks laced with specific germs.
- Vivisection and dissection of these infected men and women to investigate the natural progression of various infectious diseases.
- Frostbite experiments in which human beings were forced to endure freezing and subfreezing conditions for long periods of time and to be defrosted for investigating human physiological and pathological reactions to low temperatures and to test experimental antifrostbite methods or techniques.
- Forcible exposure of men and women to explosions of bombs containing infectious bacteria to test the effectiveness of biological bombs and other weapons.
- Experiments on the responses and tolerance of the human body to extreme conditions such as airtight chambers and high-voltage electrical shocks.
- Forcing healthy people to engage in sexual intercourse with individuals who had had venereal diseases such as syphilis.
- Other experiments that can, at best, be described as callous abuse, because their results were completely predictable such as bleeding the subjects to death, replacing subjects' blood with horse blood, and injecting horse urine into the kidneys.

Thousands of people, mostly civilians, were killed in factories of death and even more died in the Japanese army's bacteriological warfare. People were sent to Unit 731 and other programs on "special consignment" (as it was called) by the Japanese Gendarmerie to be experimented upon, tortured, and murdered. Mostly these human subjects were Chinese but they also included Russians, Koreans, and possibly some Americans and Europeans. Most were healthy men, women, and children, and even a 3-day-old baby. The individuals in Japanese doctors' experimentation were not seen as human beings or even as animals, but merely as "experimental materials." They were actually called "*maruta*" in Japanese, which translates as "logs of wood." In Unit 731 alone, no less than 600 people (two or three per day) were killed a year by Japanese physicians and medical scientists between 1939 and 1945 (The Khabarovsk Trial Materials 1950, 57). The Japanese army conducted biological warfare not only in battles but also in cities, towns, and

villages throughout China, including Ningbo in Zhejiang Province and Changde in Hunan Province. Thousands of civilians, including the elderly and children, men and women, died or were injured by human-induced infectious diseases.

It should be noted that human experimentation was far from limited to those "factories of death" and to the purpose of developing effective bacteriological and chemical weapons. At the hospitals and clinics in Japan-occupied areas, Japanese doctors and scientists also engaged in extensive human experimentation and other forms of medical atrocities. For instance, vivisection of healthy people or patients – babies, adolescents, and pregnant women included – was systematically conducted for practicing surgical skills of various operations, for training newly recruited surgeons, for teaching junior medical professionals about human anatomy and pathology, for making scientific and medical specimens, and even simply for fun.

Japanese experimentation and other medical atrocities from 1932–1945 were comparable or worse, if evils can be compared, to those committed by the Nazi doctors. Japanese doctors, however, never faced the equivalent of the Nuremberg Trials. The U.S. government made a deal with Ishii in the name of national security: they gave Ishii and his men immunity in exchange for data from their human experiments. As a consequence of the American cover-up (Harris 2004), the subject was never put on the agenda of the 1946–1948 war crimes trials conducted by the U.S.-led International Military Tribunal for the Far East in Tokyo. For whatever reasons, even those convicted of war crimes at the Khabarovsk Trial in the former Soviet Union and the military courts of People's Republic of China received remarkably lenient punishment. In general, far from being prosecuted or dishonored, the Japanese physicians and researchers who perpetrated these crimes, including Ishii himself, were protected by the Japanese and U.S. governments. Using knowledge they gained through human experiments in the "factories of death," in postwar Japan many of these doctors were able to promote their careers as respected medical researchers and administrators such as senior members of the Japanese National Institute of Health (NIH) and medical schools (Williams and Wallace 1989, 289). For instance, Yoshimura Hisato, who directed frostbite experiments including freezing people to death in Unit 731, became president of the Kyoto Prefectural Medical College, received one of Japan's highest honor (the Order of the Rising Star, third class), and even became president of Kobe Women's University.

Naito Ryoichi, who was Ishii's right-hand, became head of the Green Cross Company. This company is at the center of the Green Cross scandal, an infamous case. In the 1980s alone, some 500 individuals died of human immunodeficiency virus (HIV) complications due to having received infected blood supplied by the Green Cross

Company. Still more people have been dying of HIV or hepatitis C today.

The biological warfare programs are considered "forgotten atrocities" but not because they were unknown in Japan or China. Indeed, Japanese bacteriological warfare and inhuman experiments conducted during World War II have always been an "open secret." The basic facts were remarkably well established in the Khabarovsk Trial, although, unfortunately, in the political environment of the Cold War the evidence and conclusions of this trial have been totally ignored and dismissed as Communist propaganda in the West (Nie 2004b). The former soldiers of Ishii's units who came back from China started to confess and give personal testimony beginning in the 1950s, although, unfortunately again, they were largely regarded as having been brainwashed by Communists.

It should be pointed out that, ever since the early 1980s, more and more authentic archival documents, personal testimonies by former soldiers and victims or their relatives, detailed journalist investigations, and systematic historical studies in Japanese, Chinese, and English have accumulated providing ironclad evidence about a varieties of Japanese war crimes (see Chinese Central Archive et al. 1989; Guo 1997; Fujiii 1997; Morimura [1981, 1982] 1985; Tsuneishi 1981, 1994, 1995; Powell 1981; Williams and Wallace 1989; Gold 1996; Harris 1994).

On September 22, 1999, 67 years after the war crimes started and 54 years after the end of World War II, the Tokyo District Court, in response to a suit filed by the families of several Chinese victims, officially acknowledged the fact of the medical atrocities at Unit 731. Their findings were arrived at after hearing considerable testimony from witnesses, including former soldiers of Unit 731. The Court, however, denied these victims compensation. On August 27, 2002, in another judgment, the Court acknowledged that the Japanese Imperial Army waged banned germ warfare on Chinese civilians during the war, but again declined again to award compensation. On April 18, 2005, Tokyo High Court rejected an appeal for compensation by ten Chinese survivors (and their relatives) of Japanese germ warfare experiments and the Nanjing massacre.

Japanese biological warfare programs and human experiments are likely to remain "forgotten atrocities." Instead of facing the past seriously, the Japanese government has adopted the "Policy of three nos" to the war and to war crimes: no admission of aggression; no repentance and apology; and no compensation to victims. The U.S. government has never formally admitted or apologized for covering-up these war crimes conducted by Japanese doctors. Even the Chinese Nationalist and Communist governments have displayed ambiguous attitudes toward these medical atrocities and never rigorously pursued justice in the international community on behalf of the murdered Chinese people. Furthermore, far from seriously

taking up the ethical challenges of those atrocities, East Asian and international medical ethicists have long been silent on the subject.

III. CHALLENGES FOR MEDICAL ETHICS

We need to understand these wartime experiments, not only out of respect for the thousands killed in the "Eastern Auschwitz" and the consequent biological warfare unleashed on civilian populations, and not only for the historical justice, but also because these forgotten atrocities raise a number of perennial ethical problems that are crucial for many theoretical and practical issues in contemporary medical ethics. International as well as East Asian medical ethicists, however, have paid little attention to these atrocities in more than half a century. Even in Japan and China, through the end of the twentieth century, the subject has been treated as having little relevance to contemporary science, medicine, and medical ethics (Nie 2001a).

In Japan, the issue of "human experimentation" became taboo in the medical profession after the end of World War II, in part because many researchers who were personally involved in these experiments became prominent professors, deans, and presidents of medical schools. The essential role of the ethics of human experimentation was thus underdeveloped in discussions, publications, and teaching about medical ethics. This failure to confront history permits most Japanese to regard "human experimentation" as a barbarism performed only by mad doctors in the militaristic past, distancing it from research performed by normal doctors in enlightened and peaceful postwar Japan. They thus avoid reflection on the ethics of human experimentation in the military or in medicine generally. In fact, many cases of abuse of human subjects of research have been reported in Japan since the end of World War II. Yet, because of the lack of historical reflection, a framework for critically discussing and evaluating human experimentation is absent in the discourse of Japanese medical ethics. Medical ethicists have seldom explored the principles that should guide and regulate human subjects research (Tsuchiya 2003).

As of the early twenty-first century, still no systematic ethical studies on the medical atrocities have ever been published in China. Because medical ethics is a required course in almost all medical schools in mainland China, there are dozens of medical ethics textbooks. Yet, the subject is rarely discussed, even mentioned, in these textbooks. Officially, Japanese doctors' experimentation, as the Pinfang Unit 731 Museum shows, has been mainly used as material for the national and local education of patriotism. This subject recently became very visible in the Chinese media; however, it was treated more or less as the atrocities of some Japanese "devils" against Chinese people in wartime, thus having no relevance to medicine and medical ethics in contemporary China. In other words, nationalism is so far the dominant Chinese perspective in viewing this major event in twentieth century (Nie 2001a, 2004b).

As the last century approached its end, finally a group of international bioethicists started to make serious efforts to analyze ethical issues related to the Japanese wartime experiments and their relevance to contemporary medical ethic and medicine.[1] Although still preliminary in general and comprising mostly commentaries, the discussions so far on the ethics of Japanese doctors' wartime experimentation have touched a range of important theoretical and practical issues. The questions that have been raised and discussed include: What historical, socio-cultural and medical environments had led to the establishment of factories of death and prevented doctors from resisting (Tsuchiya 2000)? What challenges do those atrocities pose for medical ethics today in East Asian and especially in China (Nie 2001a)? How to learn from the past in light of similar German experience (Döring 2001)? Why should we bring up the past atrocities at the first place (Chen 2001)? Can the argument that "it was wartime" justify the atrocities and failure to bring the doctors to justice (Thomas 2003a, 2003b)? Does serious study of the subject lead to Japan bashing (Leavitt 2003; Nie 2003a)? What are East Asian values and culture and their relationship to ethics (Döring 2001; Nie 2001a, 2003b)? Why have Americans been so ambiguous in judging cruel human experimentation (Sass 2003)? What should the U.S. government do to repair the historical injustice it caused by covering up the atrocities (Nie 2004b)?

How could the Eastern version of "medical killing" have happened? There are at least five possible explanations. First, Japan was then a militarist country, and most Japanese people believed that everything was justifiable if it was done for the sake of the emperor and for victory in the war. Second, at the time most Japanese had deep and widespread prejudice against Chinese and people of other ethnicities, which was often embedded in eugenic and racist ideologies. A third factor was the fear of Communism, which had taken root in China. Persons who were regarded as Communists were arrested and tortured even in the Japanese homeland. Fourth, the doctors justified their murder by insisting that the subjects were suspected Communist spies or resisters and would be executed anyway. Fifth, researchers tended to lose sight of their common humanity with their subjects, as a result of medical atrocities being performed behind closed doors. The Japanese Government had completely hidden the laboratories from the public because the government recognized that international society would condemn Japan severely if such barbarity were to become widely known. As a result, researchers gradually seemed to become unworried about the constraints of normal medical ethics; integrity as a self-regulating mechanism failed (Tsuchiya 2000).

Except at army hospitals, most of the doctors who performed human experiments and vivisections were academic researchers who had been professors at leading Japanese medical schools and who were only temporarily employed by the Japanese army. Why did they participate? First, in fact, they responded to the prevailing pressure from a Fascistic society. Researchers would be branded as traitors if they refused to cooperate with the military. Yet, they did not really try to resist, even when they knew what they would be assigned to do in China. Second, Japanese medical schools were very authoritarian and hierarchical in structure at the time, such that researchers may have felt that they could not refuse their senior professors' orders without abandoning their academic careers. (This is still the case even today.) To get enough research equipment in wartime, professors had made deals with Ishii and promised to send their best disciples to his units. Third, Ishii's factories were comparatively "luxurious" and thus attractive for researchers. The annual budget of Unit 731 was extremely large (approximately eighty-six million dollars at present value), the salary of researchers was considerably high, and the food served there was said to be excellent. Moreover, insofar as it related to military medicine, research could be done essentially without restrictions. Finally, the factories provided Japanese doctors with the opportunity to observe patients and diseases that they could hardly ever observe in the Japanese homeland. The research possibilities were invaluable (Tsuchiya 2000).

For some scholars (Tsuchiya 2000; Morioka 2000; Chen 2001), East Asian values that are based on Confucianism and prevail in Japan, such as respecting superiors, should be blamed for the medical atrocities. For others (Döring 2001, Nie 2001, 2002, 2003b), Japanese doctors' atrocities violate not only human values in general, and not only Western ethical norms, but also East Asian ethical traditions and concepts, including Japanese and Chinese moral principles and ideals. In particular, when medicine became a slave of nationalism and imperialism in the Japanese death factories, it clearly violated the moral norm of "medicine as the art of humanity" (ren), a crucial concept of East Asian medical ethics with ancient roots in Confucianism. Those Japanese doctors seemed to be aware of their violation of medical ethics, Asian medical ethics obviously included. In his last pleas at the Khabarovsk trial in 1949, Kajitsuka Ryuji, a Doctor of Medical Sciences and Chief of the Medical Administration of the Kwantung Army, admitted that participating in preparation of bacteriological weapons is against the "sacred duty" of a physician:

> I began to study medicine in order to improve the protection of public health, to work for the benefit of mankind. I think it shameful to myself that, I, a physician, a member of a humane profession,

instead of performing my sacred duty, the duty of a medical man, took a different path, the path of preparing to conduct bacteriological warfare, in which bacilli are used as weapons. (The Khbarovsk trial materials 1950, 518)

Therefore, it was certain political environments, rather than East Asian cultural and moral tradition, that have brought about the atrocities and the unfortunate aftermaths (Nie 2003b).

Very often, Japanese researchers who participated in the atrocities are viewed as "devils" or "not human beings" (*guizhi* or *bushiren* in Chinese, *akuma* in Japanese). In other words, they are not "us." This seems to be the major intellectual reason that no serious and systematic study on the topic has yet appeared in Chinese medical ethics. To see the significance of studying Japanese doctors' human experimentation for medicine, science, and medical ethics today, it is crucial to overcome this way of thinking. Japanese doctors involved in wartime experiments should be treated not as somehow nonhuman or devils or monsters or beasts, but as fellow human beings, although cruel ones and militarists. Most of these Japanese doctors were *normal* medical researchers and professionals, who became involved in extraordinary and inhumane crimes against humanity. In their hands, medicine and science were transformed into killing machines. The crucial lesson that we should learn from both the Nazi and Japanese doctors' atrocities is that dehumanization constitutes one of the moral and psychological bases that permitted Nazi and Japanese doctors to participate in mass murder without much resistance (Nie 2001a, 2003b). To recognize our fellow human beings – victims and victimizers alike – as human beings thus will help to prevent the similar human-made tragedies from happening again.

As history demonstrates again and again, state and collective violence are the most destructive form of human violence. Japanese doctors' inhuman experiments constitute one of the worst examples of collective violence supported by the state. This is not simply a case of Japanese versus Chinese, but a form of inhuman treatment of some human beings by other human beings. State and collective violence exists in many places of this world, most strikingly in the twentieth century. Conceptualizing the Japanese doctors' human experimentation atrocities as an incident of state and collective violence can help us better understand the phenomenon of collective violence against humanity in general. For instance, although cases of state and collective violence happened in twentieth-century China (e.g., Japanese doctors' atrocities and violence of the "Red Guards" and students against teachers in the Cultural Revolution) they differ in socio-historical contexts and even in nature; however, they nonetheless, display some striking and frightening common features. They were conducted in the name of the good and even

of the holy. They occurred when there was no freedom of discussion and press. They involved the active participation of ordinary people who collaborated to accomplish extraordinary collective violence, treating other fellow human beings as nonhumans. They were facilitated by the state and its bureaucracies (Nie 2001a, 2005a).

Reflecting on the Japanese doctors' inhuman experimentation and its aftermath, "what has been sacrificed for the state and the national interests are the lives of thousands of people. So has justice. So has humanity" (Nie 2002c, s6). Historically speaking, Japanese doctors' human experimentation would not have been possible without the popularity of nationalism in Japanese society and medicine at that time. Whereas they brought the Nazi doctors to trials, U.S. officials made a deal with Japanese doctors in the name of national security or national interests. Chinese Communists officials justified their lenient treatment to Japanese war criminals by the overall interests of China as a state and country, and even by world peace. As a result, "to remain ethical, medicine should always examine nationalism and the various claims of the state made in the name of national interests. This lesson itself is not new at all. The issue is whether humankind has ever really learnt the lesson" (Nie 2002c, s6).

Obviously, Japanese wartime medical atrocities challenge the practice and theories of international bioethics today in many ways. Not only should the Japanese government apologize and compensate for the war and all war crimes, the U.S. government also ought to apologize and compensate for covering up the medical atrocities in exchange for the data of human experiments. For this cover-up not only trampled morality but, legally speaking, constitutes complicity (after the fact), a punishable offense in the common law tradition (Nie 2004b). Meanwhile, in addition to prohibiting unethical medical research and practice, contemporary international declarations or codes on human rights and medical ethics should include a special clause clearly banning any kind of complicity with respect to unethical research, both before and after the fact (Nie 2004b). For cross-cultural bioethics, Japanese atrocities raise issues about medicine, society, and ethics in this age of globalization and about the necessity and possibility of common human values and a universal medical ethics despite the great diversity of cultures.

IV. Conclusion

More than 60 years ago, some Japanese doctors perpetrated medical atrocities on Chinese and people of other ethnicities for the purpose of developing biological weapons and other reasons. Justice was never done and it is no longer possible to do it sufficiently. A great number of historical, political, cultural, and moral issues have been raised from the atrocities, but, in spite of some initial efforts, indepth and systematic ethical studies are still not available. If we do not take seriously the challenges of Japanese doctors' wartime inhuman experimentation, we and our children may be doomed to suffer from the similar atrocities. Not only those atrocities in the past but also the cases of abusing patients' dignity and rights in a variety of names in contemporary Japan, China, the United States, and other places in the world, all indicate that the task is still daunting for bioethics, together with humankind, to guard medicine as an art of humanity ("renshu," in the term of East Asian medical ethics), rather than allow it to be the means of inhumanity.

Note

1. In 1997, from a medical ethics perspective, Chinese doctor Yuan-fang Chen and Japanese-American obstetrician Yasuo Ishida published a commentary on and book review, respectively, of the first edition of the American historian Sheldon Harris' important book *Factories of Death* (Chen 1997, Ishida 1997). In 2001, an article by Takashi Tsuchiya, a Japanese philosopher, together with a commentary by another Japanese scholar Masahiro Morioka, appeared in the *Eubios Journal of Asian and International Bioethics* (EJAIB), an English periodical (freely available on internet) edited in Japan (Tsuchiya 2001a; Morioka 2001). This has stimulated a series of discussions in *EJAIB* by scholars from Japan, China, Israel, Germany, and New Zealand (Nie 2001a; Leavitt 2001; Döring 2001; Chen 2001; Tsuchiya 2003; Sass 2003; Thomas 2003a, 2003b; Leavitt 2001, 2003; Nie 2003a). Together with Tsuchiya, Jing-Bao Nie, an overseas Chinese scholar, organized a panel on the lessons of the medical atrocities for international research ethics and cross-cultural bioethics at the fourth annual meeting of the American Society for Bioethics and Humanities held in Nashville, Tennessee in October 2001. In addition to contributions to *EJAIB*, Nie also published his research results on the subject in *The Lancet*, *Journal of Bioethical Inquiry* (the new official periodical of Australasian Bioethics Association), and a German project on "human rights, culture and violence" (Nie 2002, 2004a, 2005a). He has given several public speeches in China, including in Hong Kong, and presented papers at several professional conferences including the 7th World Congress of International Association of Bioethics in Sydney in 2004 (Nie 2003b, 2004b). Sponsored by a research grant from the Royal Society of New Zealand, Nie is currently writing a monograph on the socio-cultural and ethical dimensions of Japanese wartime medical atrocities and coediting (with Japanese studies scholar Nanyan Guo and American medical anthropologist Arthur Kleinman) a volume of essays from a perspective of international comparisons by a group of scholars from different countries and various disciplines. Recently, Nie and Korean historian of science and bioethicist Sang-yong Song organized a symposium for the 22nd International Congress of History of Medicine held in Beijing in July 2005.

CHAPTER 54

Medical Ethics and Nazism

Ulf Schmidt

I. Introduction

Medicine under National Socialism raises profound questions about medical and research ethics. How was it possible that men and women sworn to the Hippocratic tradition of *nihil nocere* (to do no harm), trained as professionals in one of the most advanced scientific cultures, could disregard the dignity of human beings, ignore principles of informed consent, beneficence, and care and commit crimes of previously unseen proportions? Did they know that they were committing a crime, and how did they sanction their role? The history of medicine under Nazism strongly conflicts with traditional views and expectations of professional medical conduct, and thus needs to be assessed in its specific ideological and cultural context. The complexities surrounding these issues are an integral part of a wider political history of medicine and history of ideas. How do ideological and political formations shape the understanding of ethics and the code of conduct of the medical profession? How can we explain that most of the doctors did not value the life of the individual higher than their duty toward the state, the community, the party, or the *Führer*?

This chapter provides a contextualized and cross-cultural account of Nazi medicine and political ideology and discusses the extent to which medical ethics was shaped by racial theories and politics. Key ideological concepts of National Socialism such as its deeply rooted racism, racial hygiene,[1] the concept of the *Volkskörper* (body politic), and anti-Semitism need to be addressed. I will explore how these different senses and types of ideology shaped the understanding of medical ethics in Germany, and discuss the extent to which the relations of practitioners to patients and to the state were understood within defined ideological contexts. Medicine under Nazism was not only paramount in constructing major elements of Nazi ideology, but doctors also played an active and leading role in turning these ideas into reality in all areas of health and racial policy. An aggressive and powerful state introduced, administered, and sanctioned these policies. It was the concurrence of ideologies and destructive forces of German medicine and Nazism that led to some of the worst acts of recent human history (Schmidt 2002, 2004).

The various degrees of complicity of medical science in Nazi crime and the complexity of "Fascist" medicine in general make it difficult to identify the specific character of medicine under National Socialism. One of the more influential factors was a significant shift in perspective from the emphasis on the care and cure of the individual and the community to the "treatment" of the body politic, the *Volkskörper*, as a whole. Public health initiatives of the late 1920s and 1930s were geared toward improving the health of the nation, whereby the role of the individual was understood in terms of the contribution and "value" to the state. The individual not only had the right to adequate medical facilities, but the duty to preserve his or her health for the greater good of the community and the race. Medical ethicists and doctors came to regard "health" as the highest good; as early as 1920 one of the country's leading medical ethicists, Emil Abderhalden, declared, "Let us learn to see that we are a part in the greater whole, of a *Volk* and even more so of mankind" (Frewer 2000, 116).

The ideological and political position of German doctors, their *Weltanschauung* (world view), so to speak, may be summarized as follows: their essential point of reference was normative and holistic rather than individualistic. It was holistic because the central importance in their value system was the whole, and the individual human subject was neglected and/or subordinated under the whole (Hastedt 1998, 21ff.). It was also normative because it was a position of what *should* be done rather than of *is*. Their health activism was constant, dynamic, and multidimensional: the aim a social and racial utopia. German medicine incorporated a whole range of holistic positions, which at different times and in different situations assumed moral priority. Holistic concepts such as the community, the *Volk*, the race, the nation, the idea of National Socialism, mankind, and so forth, were of fundamental importance in initiating and sanctioning Nazi health policies. Such positions, as soon as one believed them to be normative, required almost constant action to turn a world how it *should be* into a world of present day reality, a world that in the end had nothing to do with any aesthetic or ancient ideal. Doctors saw themselves as men of action (*Tatmenschen*). They called for a revaluation of all values.

Nazism reveals a fundamental break with Judeo-Christian ethics, an attack against a traditional belief system based on altruism and compassion. German doctors and many Nazis replaced human responses such as sympathy and respect for the dignity of human life with hardness and rigidity. Hardness, not the "weakness" of compassion, characterized their relation and responses to other humans, and also toward themselves (Glover 1999, 317–97). Hardness was seen as a form of self-discipline; this included advocacy of hardness and the demand for sacrifice from others. Hitler saw himself as the "hardest man the German nation has had for many decades, perhaps centuries." In the notorious Commissar Order he directed his soldiers to wage war in Russia with "unprecedented, unmerciful, and unrelenting hardness." Hans Frank, head of the General Government (Poland), told his staff to arm themselves "against all feelings of sympathy" as a precondition of exterminating the Jews. Reinhard Heydrich said that Germans "must be as hard as granite, otherwise the work of our Führer will perish" (Glover 1999, 343ff.).

After the war, observers characterized Hitler's doctor, Karl Brandt, as a "cold and unapproachable intelligence." Hardness was one of the key defenses against allowing bleak reality to enter one's mind, deliberately cultivated to enable thousands to follow the visionary redeemer on his genocidal path. Overcoming feelings of sympathy and respect for their victims was central in making Nazi policies possible.

Nazi medical ethics can only be understood in its historical, socio-political, and cultural context (see Chapter 34). We need to look at the relation between medical conduct and certain policies, organizations, or individuals. The crucial shift from ethical positions concerned with the well-being of the individual to biologistic ethics aimed at purifying the race was far from clear cut. It was an uneven and twisted process that was rooted in nineteenth-century social Darwinism and the racial hygiene movement. Ideas about the biological survival of the race shaped the formation of a generative collective ethic (*generative Kollektivethik*[2]), which placed the role of the community above the interest of the individual. Concepts such as "Any Benefit for the Community Comes Before Any Benefit for the Individual" (*Gemeinnutz geht vor Eigennutz*) or "Eugenics as the Highest Form of Ethics" (*Eugenik als höchste Ethik*) became characteristic of medical scientists, who from the end of World War I promoted these positions in journals such as *Ethik* (Ethics) (Frewer 2000). In opposition to what they perceived as "false humanitarianism," leading medical ethicists called for the sterilization of the "unfit" and "valueless" members of society, and drew attention to the economic burden of those in institutional care. Their voices did not fall on deaf ears; those with far more radical ideas took them up and incorporated them in their hodgepodge of political ideology (Mosse 1964).

In 1926, Hitler wrote in *Mein Kampf*: "The process of cleansing our 'Kultur' will have to be applied in practically all spheres . . . The right to personal freedom comes second in importance to the duty of maintaining the race" (Hitler [1926] 1939, 216). These ideas epitomized Nazi thinking as well as they did right wing and *völkisch* ideology during the Weimar Republic. Hitler's ideas were anything but new or original, but they were truly radical, in expression and in intention:

Only after such measures have been put in practice can a medical campaign against this scourge [race mixing, homosexuals, venereal diseases, prostitution etc.] begin with some hope of success. But here again half-measures will be valueless. Far-reaching and important decisions will have to be made. It would be doing things by halves if incurables were given the opportunity of infecting one healthy person after another. This would be that kind of humanitarianism which would allow hundreds to perish in order to save the suffering of one individual.

The demand that it should be made impossible for defective people to continue to propagate defective offspring is a demand that is based on most reasonable grounds [and means in its methodical implementation the most humane act of mankind] [The English translation differs at this point from the German text. I have translated this passage so that it is closer to the German original: 'und bedeutet in ihrer planmäßigen Durchführung die humanste Tat der Menschheit'; Hitler 1936, 279; also Hitler [1926] 1939, 216]. Unhappy and undeserved suffering in millions of cases will be spared, with the result that there will be a gradual improvement in national health. (Hitler [1926] 1939, 216)

Hitler's demand for cleansing the *Volk* of unwanted elements, placing the race, state, and the community before the rights and integrity of the individual, all this became reality after 1933 with such breathtaking speed that even those advocating such measures before had difficulties in grasping its implications.

II. Racial Hygiene

The well-established importance of the racial hygiene movement in shaping German medicine and ideology stresses the complex amalgam of social, racial, and utopian ideas that were so attractive to the scientific and professional elite. These ideas neither originated in Germany, nor were they confined or unique to Germany alone; they were part and parcel of a broad movement about the inequality of mankind, nurtured by scientists of international renown, who alleged that the human race would degenerate unless man himself took the initiative and corrected the inevitable path into the biological abyss (see Chapter 59).

In Europe it was not until the mid-nineteenth century that the problem of race, race mixing, and race improvement figured predominantly in the writings of scholars who attempted to find solutions for the social ills of modern society. Charles Darwin's publication of the *Origin of Species* in 1859 marked a watershed in the development of biologically determined theories of society, in which he stressed principles such as "natural selection" and the "survival of the fittest." Darwin's work allowed scholars to apply the concept of natural selection and variation in the animal world, leading ultimately to evolution, to human society. Zoologists and natural philosophers such as Ernst Haeckel (1834–1919) projected the concept of the "struggle for existence" onto society, and argued that there were two forms of selection; although man's struggle for survival determined natural selection, there was also "artificial selection," the active process of "weeding out" the weak and potentially burdensome members of society. To bolster his argument, Haeckel referred to the Spartans,

who apparently had killed their weak, ill, or handicapped newborn (see also Schwartz 1996, 152–4). By the 1860s the English scientist Francis Galton, a cousin of Darwin, had come up with a new theory to improve the inherited conditions of a race to the highest ideal, a concept for which he coined the term "national eugenics"[3] in 1883 (Schmuhl 1987, 30). Most of these theories had certain factors in common: the transference and application of evolutionary biology and cell theory to modern society and state government. In practice, they established key elements of social Darwinism. Social ills of society were transformed into and perceived as illnesses of society as a whole.

In Germany, Darwin's ideas fell on less fertile soil. Scientists stressed the growing malaise of industrial capitalism, and the advent of revolutionary political movements. The struggle for existence alone, social Darwinists argued, was insufficient to cope with social and health problems of modern society, or to prevent mankind from sliding into biological degeneracy. They called for state-interventionist measures to avoid political turmoil and social chaos, in effect combining their criticism of modern civilization with "cultural pessimism" (*Kulturpessimismus*). In 1895 Germany's leading proponent Alfred Ploetz warned against counterselective forces such as war, inbreeding, alcohol, and venereal disease, which would lead to racial degeneration. All medical care for "the weak," he argued, was to be suspended, because it apparently resulted in the procreation of those who otherwise would not have survived, and thus damaged the quality of the people's germ plasm. His racial and social utopia stressed artificial selection by strengthening the best in society, but likewise called for Spartan methods of child murder to improve the race (Schwartz 1996, 1998; Schmuhl 1997).

Racial hygiene, the German derivative of eugenics, became the country's credo for improving the human race. In 1904 Ploetz founded the Journal of Racial and Social Biology (*Archiv für Rassen und Gesellschaftsbiologie*). A year later he established the Society for Racial Hygiene to promote his racial utopia in countries such as America, which he saw as a "bold leader in the realm of eugenics" (Kühl 1994, 13; see Chapter 59). America became a welcoming example for advocating eugenics at home. Membership of the Society increased in the 1910s and 1920s, including physicians, industrialists, and health zealots. By 1910, the Swedish *Sällskap för Rashygien* became the first foreign affiliate. Concerns for this generation of racial hygienists differed quite significantly from those during the Nazi period; up until the early 1920s, racial and social hygienists warned against a declining birth rate and a high infant mortality rate.

The process of industrialization, urbanization, and population growth placed the need for changes in the health and social security system high on the political agenda. Reforms in medical education toward greater specialization together with the expansion in the hospital system transformed institutional care, cure, and control, while redefining doctor–patient relationships. In reaction to frictions with state-employed health experts and professional challenges from healers and so-called quackery, a number of professional organizations were founded. By 1900, for example, the Association of German Doctors was established as one of the pillars representing the interests of the profession. Rechristened as *Hartmannbund* in 1923 after its founder Hermann Hartmann, these medical networks became powerful bodies in shaping the formation of professional codes of conduct.

At the end of World War I, tensions erupted in almost all spheres of society. Unemployment, political unrest, and hyperinflation fueled debates about the allocation of scarce resources in the welfare system (Kersting 1996; Walter 1996). Experts tried to stem the crisis by advocating institutional reforms in the hospital sector. The discrepancy between technical and scientific innovations, on the one hand, and pressing issues over poverty, health, and disease, on the other, widened the gap between the socio-political and medical ideals and daily reality in Weimar Germany. The erosion of liberal values during the Depression led to a further radicalization of medical views on racial hygiene. Throughout the political spectrum and professional elites, a call for sterilizing those with hereditary defects grew louder.

Although thousands of physicians had to flee from acts of discrimination and terror after 1933, German doctors were not pawns in the hands of the Nazis; they were willing collaborators who voluntarily initiated, ordered, abetted, or took a consenting part in introducing Nazi policies. The institutionalization of racial hygiene as a scientific discipline happened long before the Nazis came to power. Most racial hygiene institutes were established before 1933. The Kaiser-Wilhelm Institute for Genealogy in Munich, for example, was created in 1919 and headed by the racial psychiatrist Ernst Rüdin (Weber 1993); the Kaiser-Wilhelm Institute for Anthropology, Human Heredity and Eugenics in Berlin was founded in 1927 and directed by Eugen Fischer. Both institutions shaped the values of medical practitioners and would later train Nazi doctors. Without the aggressive and militarist nature of Hitler's state, however, racial hygiene would probably have remained impotent, replaced by advances in genetic research, and reduced to one of many currents of medical ideology.

Medicine under Nazism, though, cannot be understood as a simple suppressor/oppressor model. Recent work highlights a substantial amount of sophisticated research undertaken during the Nazi era. German epidemiological studies were among the most progressive works in the world (Proctor 1999). It is important to stress the Janus-faced nature of German medicine, with herbal medicine and progressive cancer research, on the

one hand, and compulsory sterilization, "euthanasia,"[4] and criminal experiments, on the other. The Nazis promoted a healthy diet, launched an aggressive antitobacco campaign, supported the production of nutritious bread, informed women about breast self-examination, and introduced radiological examinations to reduce the rate of breast cancer in the population. Nazi medicine, however, was meant for "different portions" of society – the good one for the German people, the other for what propagandists saw as "useless eaters."

III. STERILIZATION POLICIES

German doctors embraced holistic concepts and political parties that promoted the health of the *Volkskörper* and the ideal of the racial state (Burleigh and Wippermann 1991). Significantly, the medical profession had among the highest percentage of National Socialist German Workers Party or *Nationalsozialistische Deutsche Arbeiterpartei* (NSDAP) membership (Kater 1989). Following the Nazi takeover of power, medical organizations, research institutions, and universities were geared toward implementing a racially based public health policy. Thousands of Jewish doctors and scientists were forced to resign and emigrate, making room for other, often younger physicians to fill their positions. Careerism, various degrees of opportunism, and blatant ignorance were among the more common features explaining their attitude (Hubenstorf 1987; Kröhner 1989; Ash and Söllner 1996). On the whole the medical profession turned a blind eye toward widespread discrimination and state-sanctioned terror. Many believed that in times of national upheaval a certain degree of injustice was acceptable, justifying blemishes by pointing toward the "achievements" in public health and employment.

The Nazis were the first to introduce racial hygiene on a national scale. By 1933, the Law to Prevent Hereditarily Ill Offspring was introduced as one of the cornerstones of Nazi population and racial policy.[5] This law, which became known as the Sterilization Law, was a fundamental violation of individual autonomy and the right of procreation. It legalized compulsory sterilization for a wide range of alleged hereditary illnesses: congenital feeble-mindedness, schizophrenia, manic depressive illness, hereditary epilepsy, Huntington's chorea, hereditary blindness, hereditary deafness, serious physical malformation, and severe alcoholism. Eventually an estimated 350,000 to 400,000 persons were affected by this law.

Doctors applauded the Law and its implicit message. From now on they had reason to believe that they were the custodians of the health of the German people, the guardians monitoring the *Volkskörper*, ready to strike at and eliminate all "cancerous elements" from the national community (Proctor 1999). For the leading racial hygienist, Fritz Lenz, the Führer was simply the "Doctor of the

German people"; as early as 1917 Lenz had called for "The Renewal of Ethics," arguing that "man must locate himself within the larger organic unity – the unity from which he came and to which he may aspire to contribute" (Lenz [1917] 1933; Proctor 1988, 59ff.). For Lenz and many medical leaders this became "the absolute value of race," one on which all other values depended. National Socialism, unlike Marxism, Lenz argued in 1931, was applied biology. Physicians had been the professional vanguard advocating racial hygiene; now the political framework invited them to transform an ideology of inequality into a policy of exclusion and expulsion. In 1933, Lenz declared, "It is the will of the Führer, that the demands of racial hygiene should be put into practice, without delay" (Proctor 1988, 46).

Nazi physicians offered their services in establishing a comprehensive system to cleanse the nation's germ plasma, for example, by setting up an elaborate apparatus of laws and procedures and by serving on 181 Hereditary Health Courts and Appellate Hereditary Health Courts in 1934 (Proctor 1988, 102f.). Research into hereditary defects and the practical application of sterilization to thousands of men and women rapidly developed into a medical industry, from supply companies offering sterilization equipment to film producers making training films about the latest surgical techniques for male and female sterilization (Schmidt 2002). Students of medicine wrote more than 180 doctoral dissertations on the topic of sterilization (Proctor 1988, 108–9). Although individual doctors struggled to stay clear of the cycle of complicity, sometimes even voicing mild forms of protest, the profession, as a whole, initiated, supported, and conducted the government's racial program with relentless vigor. This program was not "ordered from above." It was introduced "from below," by the active collaboration of physicians. Driven by a remorseless health activism their degree of ignorance of the ethical implications for doctor–patient relationships and the nature of German medicine can hardly be overemphasized.

Sterilizing the mentally defective was only the first step in the regime's campaign to improve the race; ultimately there would emerge more radical solutions. While discussions on the Sterilization Law were under way, Hitler contemplated killing handicapped children and adults, but abandoned the idea because of potential opposition from the Church (Burleigh 1994, 97). During cross-examination at the 1947 Nuremberg Doctors' Trial,[6] Karl Brandt, Hitler's personal physician, confirmed that such ideas were also discussed in 1935, long before the "euthanasia" program[7] started. In the same year the regime implemented the notorious Nuremberg Race Laws that excluded Jews from citizenship and prohibited marriages and sexual relations between Jews and non-Jews. Although both laws marked a clear shift from positive to negative eugenics, the major attack on medical ethics

and professional codes of practice had begun shortly after World War I.

IV. "Euthanasia" and Medical Ethics

In 1920, the lawyer Karl Binding (1841–1920) and the psychiatrist Alfred E. Hoche (1865–1943) published their tract *Permission for the Destruction of Life Unworthy of Life* (Burleigh 1994, 15–22). The book was by far the most important contribution to the debate on "euthanasia" in Germany and significantly shaped discussions about medical ethics and the elimination of allegedly inferior individuals in the 1920s and 1930s. Their positivistic theory was a combination of legal norms and medical arguments that granted the state fundamental rights while overriding the rights of individuals. The traditional moral belief system that advocated care and compassion for the weak and unproductive was radically called into question. The book was written in the wake of World War I; readers were asked to compare the "battlefields littered with thousands of dead youth," with asylum inmates, who were seen as "not absolutely worthless, but actual existences of negative value" (Binding and Hoche 1920, 27).

World War I devalued individual life and shifted attention to the "survival" of the nation and the race. Binding and Hoche saw the handicapped as "life unworthy of life," who placed an extra burden on the financially weakened welfare system. Their life was seen as "useless;" their death would apparently not create "the smallest gap." Questions of consent seem to have been only of academic interest, presuming that the person dying was unconscious in most cases. Medical and legal ethics were nevertheless at the center of Binding's argument. They ask readers whether there is "human life which has so far forfeited the character of something entitled to enjoy the protection of the law, that its prolongation represents a perpetual loss of value, both for its bearer and for society as a whole" (Binding and Hoche 1920, 27). Both authors brushed aside the possibility of error; although Binding observed that "one more or less hardly counts in the balance," and Hoche claimed that there was "one hundred per cent certainty in selection" (Burleigh 1994, 18f.). The language and content of the book laid bare the authors' disregard for human rights and respect for human life and human dignity.

Although the book prompted heated debates among experts, the majority denounced involuntary "euthanasia" as murder. Most feared that it would undermine existing humanitarian and ethical values of care and cure. Others were anxious that the debate on "euthanasia" could poison fragile postwar doctor–patient relationships, and tarnish the image of medical institutions. By and large the medical profession was opposed to the book. Although many favored eugenic sterilization, killing patients was different. Binding's assumption that the mentally ill had no will to live, nor to die, and that their lives were pointless, was mostly seen as unacceptable. In 1921, the German medical profession rejected a proposal to legitimize the "destruction of life unworthy of life."

The debate, however, continued. In 1925, Ewald Meltzer (1869–1940), the director of the Katharinen-hof asylum in Saxony, comprehensively researched the issue of "euthanasia" by conducting opinion polls. He concluded that in certain cases permission for assisted suicide should be granted, but that the killing of patients was and should remain prohibited. He rejected the claim that the mentally ill had lost all elements of human personality, and stressed instead their capacity and desire to enjoy life. Sparta's practice of infanticide was dismissed as an historical aberration. Meltzer wrongly believed that parents would not consent to the killing of their children (some parents later petitioned to Hitler to have their child killed). Legalizing the killing of patients also undermined the public trust in mental institutions. He also warned about the slippery slope, "because soon there would be no limit above that" (Meltzer 1925, 62f.).

Assuming that any future legislation would require the parents' consent, Meltzer conducted what must have been the first opinion poll about euthanasia. Parents were asked whether one should shorten the life of their child, if experts had established that it was suffering from incurable illness. The results were a surprise: of 200 people polled, 162 responded. Of these, 119 (73%) said yes and 43 (27%) said no. Among those who said no, many said they would consent, if the state or the law would wish them to do so. Most of those who responded negatively did so because of strong emotional bonds or from ethical or religious convictions. Many wished that they would not be informed, hoping that the child would be "painlessly put to sleep" (Staatsarchiv Nürnberg, KV-Verteidigung, Handakten, No. 20, Fröschmann). Others argued that one should disguise the cause of death: "If one would say that [the child] has died of this or that illness, everyone would be happy" (Staatsarchiv Nürnberg, KV-Verteidigung, Handakten, No. 20, Fröschmann). The answers show that by the mid-1920s ordinary German parents would consent to have their handicapped children killed if the authorities felt it was right. Military defeat, the Treaty of Versailles, reparation demands, and hyperinflation had left the country with a vulnerable moral fiber; calls to reshape the traditional moral belief system were linked with ideas of nationalism, economic expediency, and racial improvement.

Before Hitler started the "euthanasia" operation he commissioned a report that was largely based on Meltzer's survey (Burleigh 1994, 98f.). The report recommended that the parents or relatives would not be asked for permission, that the program be implemented by doctors and nurses (which was meant as a safety mechanism), and that the relatives be given false causes of death. Several times the Dictator, who seems to have taken many of these issues to

heart, also attempted to introduce a law on "euthanasia," but postponed the plan after his advisors had stressed the various legal, moral, religious, and foreign policy problems involved. It was only then that Hitler authorized the killing of the handicapped as a top-secret operation.

The "euthanasia" program began in the summer of 1939 with the killing of the most defenseless and vulnerable populations, namely, children. Whereas scholars have argued in the past that the actual killing of one of the first children started between autumn 1938 and spring 1939, new research shows that this view cannot be upheld and that the beginning of the program was later than previously assumed, namely in the summer of 1939 (Schmidt 1999a). This shift in chronology raises a series of important conceptual and interpretative issues about the mechanisms of decision making at the highest levels of Hitler's government.

How were Hitler's wishes actually transformed, communicated, and introduced as concrete policy measures at a fundamental juncture of the Third Reich – 6 weeks before the outbreak of World War II? Recent work stresses the context of one of the first children, Gerhard Herbert Kretschmar, and how this triggered Hitler's decision to entrust his personal physician, Karl Brandt, and the head of the Chancellery of the Führer, Philipp Bouhler, with organizing the "euthanasia" program (Schmidt 1999a, 2000a). Both were "charged with the responsibility of enlarging the powers of specific physicians, designated by name, so that patients who, on the basis of human judgement, are considered incurable, can be granted mercy death after the most careful assessment of their condition" (Burleigh 1994, 112; Friedlander 1995, 67). When in 1941 the first phase of the program came to an end, more than 70,000 handicapped people had been killed; the experience gathered in this operation served to set up the subsequent killing structures in the East.

It is important to stress that the dynamics of war and the process of "cumulative radicalization" of the regime was essential in triggering some of the worst medical crimes. Research in recent years has not only stressed the link between the "euthanasia" program and the Final Solution. It has also reassessed the extent to which the killing of handicapped people is closely intertwined with the outbreak of war (Friedlander 1995; Schmidt 1999a, 2000a). The fundamental rationale of the "euthanasia" program was economic; it was a wartime measure to free bed-space and save on food rationing and materials (Burleigh 1994). To let the mentally ill and other "useless eaters" starve became official state-sanctioned policy after racial propaganda (by means of films, radio, and press) had stigmatized them as "life unworthy of life" (Roth 1985; Rost 1987; Schmidt 2002). Bombing raids and the need for hospital-space served as arguments to transfer and subsequently kill the infirm and elderly unless they could prove their ability to work. Killing the handicapped was also seen as a practical step toward purifying the body politic, to balance the death of "valuable" members of society in times of war, that is, soldiers, with the elimination of "ballast existences" (Platen-Hallermund [1948] 1998, 34f.).

Nazi doctors believed that delivering the patient from pain at all cost was the doctor's task, even if the patient was afterward dead. When the first gassing of mental patients occurred in January 1940, leading officials stressed that only medically trained personnel should carry out the killings, according to the motto, "The syringe belongs in the hand of the doctor" (Klee 1985, 112). In their world view the murder of tens of thousands was a medical operations. When asked after the war why they had used gas, Hitler's doctor, Karl Brandt, prided himself on having found such an effective method of killing: "This is just one case where major jumps are being made in medical history" (Friedlander 1995, 86).

The erosion of Brandt's and many other physicians' moral identity in the years prior and throughout the Nazi period partly explains such a distorted view. Whereas physicians generally perceive the preservation of life as their prime goal, death had become a core value in their overall belief system. The death of the weakling, the frail, and incurable sick was believed to be of intrinsic value for the greater good. Their death not only "delivered" them from suffering, but freed society from a financial, emotional, and even aesthetic burden. A whole set of social problems – homosexuality, gypsies, Jews, crime, alcoholism, prostitution, the handicapped, and so forth – were transformed into surgical problems. Like "surgeons of the *Volk*," as Karl Brandt stressed, Nazi physicians believed that they were "cutting out" the "infected" and "unhealthy" elements of the social organism. Medical imagery was central to Nazi ideology; the Jews and "undesirables" were stigmatized as a "cancer" of the German people, as "parasites" infecting the living organism. To gas an entire people was seen as a measure of "pest-control," the process of "delousing" as a powerful euphemism to camouflage genocide.

German doctors understood their primary obligation to be owed to the state and the race. At the same time they thought that the state took moral responsibility away from them, if experiments on humans, for instance, ended fatally (Moreno 2000, 72f.). Adopting the philosophy of Hegel, the state was seen as a "person" with its own destiny.

V. Human Experimentation

The use of prisoner populations for human experimentation in concentration camps marked the logical extension of an ideology based on inequality, superior and inferior races, and valuable and valueless members of society. Camp inmates figured at the lowest level of the scale. The possibility that the death of hundreds of human beings might improve the chance of survival of one German

aviator was seen as sufficient reason to sanction medicalized murder. In November 1942, Himmler attacked the critics of concentration camp experiments: "In these 'Christian medical circles', the standpoint is being taken that a young German aviator should be allowed to risk his life, but that the life of a criminal – who is not drafted into military service – is too sacred, and one should not stain oneself with this guilt" (Padfield 1995, 375). Any religious or moral objections had to be overcome so that Germany could pursue its expansionist policies.

The Nazi plan to exterminate whole peoples in Europe made life in concentration camps a cheap commodity, one that could be easily exploited for human experimentation. Most of the camp experiments were linked to Germany's war effort; physicians like the notorious Sigmund Rascher conducted cold water experiments at Dachau to test the survival time for German fighter pilots shot down over the English Channel, and to establish what kinds of protective clothing and rewarming methods were most effective. Other prisoners were placed in pressure chambers to see how the body would react when pilots had to bail out at high altitude, and to document their survival rates. At Auschwitz physicians experimented with mass sterilizations by means of X-rays to find out whether it would be possible to sterilize two to three million Jews earmarked as slave laborers. In 1943, Carl Clauberg prided himself on having developed a method that allowed the sterilization of 1,000 women per day. In Ravensbrück, Karl Gebhardt and Fritz Fischer performed sulphonamide drug experiments to prove that the drugs *could not* prevent (sometimes) fatal gas gangrene infections (Schmidt 2004, 2005); in Buchenwald and Dachau prisoners were infected with typhus and malaria, in others maltreated with biological and chemical warfare agents (Annas and Grodin 1992, 94–104). Despite irrefutable evidence, all twenty-three defendants at the Nuremberg Doctors' Trial pleaded not guilty (Schmidt 2004).

Although the issues underlying some of the experiments may have been relevant, and in a few instances may have resulted in useful information (i.e., in the rediscovery of a Russian rewarming method from 1880, or the development of the ejector seat) neither the experimental methods nor the execution of the experiments fulfilled the most basic standards of scientific inquiry, and of human experimentation, in particular. In all cases prisoners were used for experiments without giving informed and voluntary consent. There is no case reported in which the experimental subject was at liberty to withdraw. Often the experiments were performed by unqualified medical personnel, haphazardly, and under appalling conditions. Most of the experiments were conducted with unnecessary suffering and generally no safeguards were taken to protect the subjects from severe and multiple injuries, mutilations, disability, or death. Sometimes the death of the subject was part of the experimental set up. All of the subjects experienced extreme pain and almost all of those who are still alive are suffering from physical injuries and psychological scars. In 1945, after reading a statistic in the report on hypothermia experiments, the American war crimes investigator Leo Alexander concluded: "This table is certainly the briefest and most laconic confession of seven murders in existence!" (Alexander 1945, 52; also Schmidt 2001c). To stress the utility as opposed to the inherent criminality of the experiments, or to use and cite Nazi medical data without indicating its origin, overlooks the suffering of those whose human rights and lives were violated.

For Nazi doctors, the life of the individual had only biological value. Starting with the assumption that all actions needed to be directed toward improving the biological quality of the community, physicians lost sight of the individual person. The individual became meaningless. At Nuremberg Brandt stated:

> for the individual the event [i.e. the experiment] remains senseless, in the same vein as my action as a doctor seems to be, if one looks at it from an isolated perspective. The meaning lies deeper; the meaning is the motivating factor which is directed towards the community. Have I become guilty for the benefit of the community, I will shoulder it for the benefit of the community.

How can there be any meaning for the person, if he or she is killed? Of course there is no sense, unless we consider the death of a person to be meaningful, as a kind of "sacrifice." Taking the Nazis' value system to its logical end, this was exactly the case. They believed that the death of the defective or "valueless" person would improve the quality of the race. An idealized view of "sacrifice" (in the German language the word *Opfer* means both "sacrifice" and "victim") may have enabled Nazi physicians to believe that they had acted morally and responsibly. When in 1941 a ship sank and hundreds of people died, the malariologist Klaus Schilling said: "If we were allowed to sacrifice the same number of people who have just died in vain, there would soon be no disease which could not be conquered" (Klee 1997, 124). One year later he put his idea into practice at Dachau.

Most doctors involved in the experiments, and indicted in the Nuremberg and other postwar trials, claimed that German medical practice, on the whole, did not differ substantially from that of Allied medicine (Schmidt 2004). The defense team submitted evidence of American human experiments on prison inmates and conscientious objectors. One embarrassing example was evidence of large-scale malaria experiments on 800 American prisoners, many of them Black, who had been selected from various Federal penitentiaries. Human experiments had been conducted with malaria tropica, one of the most dangerous of the malaria strains, to aid the war effort in Southeast Asia. In June 1945, the magazine *Life* gave the story wide publicity, prompting one defendant to allege that "a certain number of fatalities had to be taken into account from the start when infecting eight hundred people with malaria" (Dörner and Ebbinghaus 1999, 2569). Further evidence of poison experiments on condemned prisoners in other countries, or cholera and plague experiments on children, raised considerable doubts regarding the research practices of Allied medical researchers.

Complicating the issue was the fact that there existed no international consensus among doctors about the use of humans in experimental research. Without clear and written research guidelines, the defense argued, there could be no violation of medical ethics standards. According to the principle *nullum crimen sine lege scripta, certa, praevia* (no crime without prior written, certain, law) there was allegedly no crime. The prosecution could show, however, that German doctors had violated their own laws and regulations. A research ethic including informed and voluntary consent in human experimentation was not only recognized and debated in Germany since the turn of the century, but was also laid down in a number of state directives and guidelines (Elkeles 1985; Vollman and Winau 1996).

As early as 1891 the Prussian Ministry of the Interior had issued a regulation that ensured that tuberculin would "in no case be used against the patients' will" for the treatment of tuberculosis. Seven years later, the Albert Neisser case caused a public furor when it was discovered that he had infected prostitutes with syphilis. He had neither informed them about the risks involved, nor had he obtained their consent. Although the medical profession closed ranks, some doctors stressed the need for informed consent, among them Albert Moll, a Berlin psychiatrist and advocate of medical ethics. In 1902, Moll published his book *Ärztliche Ethik* (Physician Ethics), which chronicled 600 cases of unethical research on humans (Moll 1902). In 1900, hospital and clinic directors had already been advised that research on humans was prohibited "if the human subject was a minor or not competent for other reasons" or had not given unambiguous and informed consent (Vollman and Winau 1996, 1446).

At the end of the 1920s, a series of unethical and fatal experiments on children prompted public debate about medical ethics standards and the reform of the German penal code (Frewer 2000, 139–45). In 1930–1931, the Reich Health Council therefore issued the "Regulations Concerning New Therapy and Human Experimentation"[8] (Sass 1983; Grodin 1992; see Chapters 34, 49, and 50). The directives were among the most comprehensive research rules by any standard at the time. Some elements were even stricter and more elaborate than the principles of the Nuremberg Code.[9] Contentious issues such as individual autonomy, beneficence, informed voluntary consent, or therapeutic and nontherapeutic research were formulated to protect the rights and dignity of patients. Thus, ironically, Germany was one of the few countries that by the 1930s had introduced state directives aimed at protecting human subjects in clinical research. The directives were especially aimed to protect vulnerable groups of society, for example, the handicapped and children. Significantly, they were the first victims of the Nazi racial program.

The discrepancy between existing codes of medical practice and actual behavior in German medical practice raises the question about the almost nonexistent effect of formal ethics regulations in Germany. It also raises the fundamental issue of medical training and ethics education (Schmidt 2002). The general disregard for ethical issues and patient rights in medicine ranged from overt violations of human and civil rights by concentration camp physicians to more sophisticated forms of circumvention or mere formal obedience. It also could become visible in ordinary doctor–patient relationships and medical paternalism, in daily medical examinations and tests, in medical records or use of discriminatory language, and also in medical films (Schmidt 2002). The handicapped, the sick, and frail no longer enjoyed the same degree of respect and sympathy as their fellow healthy Aryan citizens; tolerance and behavior toward a human being became dependent on whether the person was seen as a "valuable" member of society or rather a burden and a threat to the health of the nation. For the pragmatic Nuremberg prosecutors the issue was simpler: any use of involuntary subjects in a medical experiment constituted a crime, one that resulted in death, a crime of murder. Fifteen of the defendants were found guilty of war crimes and crimes against humanity (Schmidt 2004).

After 1945, many Nazi physicians argued that they had acted on higher authority; they saw themselves as courageous and obedient soldiers, as "the sons of Germany," anxious not to bring shame on their country. Sometimes it was the superior, the colleague (*Stabsarzt*), whom one had to obey, or the imperative was a national emergency. In most cases, either holistic concepts or a kind of superego was taking moral responsibility away from the doctors. Their own conscience was not questioned; individual moral decisions almost never seemed to have taken place. To resist an order or circumvent its execution seemed to be unthinkable for most; they were unable to say, "I do not want this any more, I am not continuing with this any more." Their willingness to judge any kind of higher authority as more important than the lives of humans explains in part why Nazism had such a profound impact on medical ethics and race relations. What is more, the doctors' inability to relate to the victims of Nazi crimes meant an inability to relate to victims generally. They had lost, as Ralf Giordano once said, "their human orientation" (Giordano 1987, 29–40).

VI. The Nuremberg Code and its Legacy

As an immediate reaction to Nazi medical crimes, and to distinguish between criminal physical injury, on the

one hand, and permissible research on humans, on the other, the Nuremberg judges felt the need to establish a catalogue of ten principles that would protect the rights of experimental subjects and other vulnerable groups in the future. These principles are laid down in the so-called Nuremberg Code (Schmidt 2001a, 2004; see Chapter 50). The Nazi Doctors' Trial was the first of twelve subsequent American military tribunals. The judges were all American nationals. The trial was nonetheless based on international law, which had been outlined in the "London Agreement on the Punishment of the Major War Criminals of the European Axis" in 1945. This meant that the judgment – and thus the Code – was *de jure* international in character, although, in practice, the world medical community largely ignored the legal nature of the Code, stressing and criticizing instead its relevance for medical ethics (Arnold and Sprumont 1997). The Nuremberg Code was clearly the first *international* medical ethics code.

The Tribunal acknowledged that scientists justified human experiments on the basis that they yield results for the good of human society that could not be produced by other means of study. There were, however, "certain basic principles," which, according to the judges, had to be observed to "satisfy moral, ethical *and* legal concepts," thus emphasizing that the rules of the Code would have legal status. The Code was an attempt to codify these "basic principles," and, at the same time, allow research on humans to be continued. The judges concluded that the ten principles had "much more frequently [been] honoured in their breach than in their observance." Experiments had been conducted in "complete disregard of international conventions, the laws and customs of war [and] the general principles of criminal laws of all civilised nations." The Code is an impressive document that states in a robust and uncompromising fashion that the rights and integrity of the research subject must be protected at all times. Of the ten provisions two were designed to protect the rights of subjects of human experiments, and eight to protect their welfare. The one provision that is perhaps best known is the first requirement, which says:

> The voluntary consent of the human subject is absolutely essential. This means that the person involved should have legal capacity to give consent; should be so situated as to be able to exercise free power of choice, without the intervention of any element of force, fraud, deceit, duress, overreaching, or other ulterior form of constraint or coercion; and should have sufficient knowledge and comprehension of the elements of the subject matter involved as to enable him to make an understanding and enlightened decision. (Dörner and Ebbinghaus 1999, pp. 11374–5)

Whatever the immediate effects of the Nuremberg Code, which for the first decade were mostly seen as "a good code for barbarians but an unnecessary code for ordinary physician-scientists" (Katz 1992, 228; 1996, 1663), it had major implications for contemporary medical ethics and ethics regulations. The principles laid down in the Code have been embodied, in one form or another, in various national and international conventions regulating the use of human subjects in biomedical research, for example, in Article 7 of the International Covenant on Civil and Political Rights, which states that "no one shall be subjected without his free consent to medical or scientific experimentation" (Perley et al. 1992, 153). Moreover, the Code was influential in shaping the four Geneva Conventions of 1949, which provide for some basic protection against criminal experiments on humans in times of war (see Chapter 50). During the Cold War the U.S. military also confirmed the legal validity of the Nuremberg Code in a top-secret memorandum, "Use of Human Volunteers in Experimental Research" (see Chapter 57). Since then the Code has also served many times as a point of reference in civilian tort actions involving nontherapeutic experiments.

For ethics regulations issued by professional medical bodies, in particular by the World Medical Association (WMA; see Chapter 50), we need to consider their origins and objectives. Founded in 1946, the WMA only alluded to Nazi medical crimes during its First Annual Meeting in Paris in 1947. A new physicians' oath was to promote the health of humanity; this was followed by discussions over "principles of social security," which were formulated to protect the welfare and economic interests of physicians themselves. It was not until 1954 that a "Resolution on Human Experimentation" was adopted by the WMA; these principles were less comprehensive and far reaching than those of the Code. Following new revelations of unethical human experiments in America in the early 1960, the WMA's Medical Ethics Committee produced a draft code of ethics on human experimentation. Four years later the final version of the code was adopted by the 18th World Medical Assembly, known as the "Declaration of Helsinki,"[10] or Helsinki I. In it a fundamental shift had occurred, from the rights of patients and the legal protections of human subjects in experimental research to the protection of patient welfare through physicians' duty and responsibility. It was a shift away from the essential requirement of informed consent. The 1964 Declaration of Helsinki states that the doctor "should, if at all possible, consistent with the patient's psychology" obtain the patient's freely given consent. It thus weakened the importance of informed consent as outlined in the Code, and reintroduced it with a more paternalistic value system of the traditional doctor–patient relationship (Annas and Grodin 1999, 304).

The Helsinki Declaration enabled the international medical community to regain control over human experimentation (see Chapters 50 and 51). Doctors and health experts had come to realize that professional ethics regulations and ethics committees could function as tools to preempt unwanted interference into research practices by state authorities. Those found in breach of ethics regulations did not have to fear any other sanctions than those enforced by their own professional peers. Developments have shown, however, that professional codes alone, whether national or international ones, are insufficient for an ever-more complex and global research culture. Yet, experts do everything but agree on the right balance among professional, judicial, and educational procedures that need to be in place to prevent doctors from violating the rights and lives of humans. It does appear to be the physicians' conscience and respect for the rights and dignity of individual human lives, inculcated in years of training and practice, together with a sense of social justice and care for the community, which may, ultimately, function as the best safeguard against human and civil rights violations in medical science.

The effects of Nazism on ethics and moral values in human society also led to the Universal Declaration of Human Rights by the United Nations in 1948 (Mann et al. 1999, 453–7), which marked the first time that the human being appeared as a category on the horizon of international law. The Nuremberg Code and the Universal Declaration not only established that it was the human being who was ultimately responsible for his or her actions, and not the state or any other higher authority or ideology, but that the human being was also granted protection through human rights. What was not fully accomplished, however, was the link: the protection of human beings enjoying human rights from human beings violating human rights. This will only be achieved once the international community has established global civil rights (*Weltbürgerrecht*), which are advocated, for example, by philosophers such as Jürgen Habermas. It may also be necessary, at one point, to create global patient rights (*Weltpatientenrecht*), as well as an agency that can establish whether these rights were violated, and, if necessary, enforce sanctions against the perpetrators. As Benjamin B. Ferencz, an international human rights lawyer and one of the Nuremberg prosecutors at the time, points out: "The true sovereign of international law . . . is the human being; only his or her protection matters."

Recent developments in international law, including, in particular, the creation of the International Criminal Court (ICC) in The Hague in the Netherlands, are pointing in this direction. Experts have also raised the prospect of an International Medical Tribunal (Annas and Grodin 1999), where cases of maltreatment could be heard, monitored, registered, judged, or even punished. It is possible that this Tribunal could fall within the purview of the ICC. Consequently, the violation of patient rights could be examined by groups of experts and sentences enforced transnationally. Such stringent and global policies appear to be needed as we move further into the twenty-first century in which the family of humans faces ever greater challenges in a more unstable and conflict-ridden world (see Chapter 51).

VII. CONCLUSION

Medicine under Nazism has shown that it is vital to work toward an international patient, civil, and human rights law that can be enforced independently of or in tandem with national legislative bodies. It would mean that the individual – the patient – would at last become the subject of medical research and practice, protected by international law against professional, economic, or institutional interests. This would also mean that some lessons may have been learned from Nazism and it destructive effects on medical ethics and moral values. As one of the Nuremberg prosecutors put it, "the wrongs in Nazi Germany were so calculated, so malignant, and so devastating, that civilization cannot tolerate their being ignored because it cannot survive their being repeated." This remains as true today as it does for our future.

NOTES

1. The terms "race hygiene" and "racial hygiene" included not only the meaning of the term "eugenics," which in German and English all referred to the improvement of human hereditary qualities, but also policies to increase the national population. From the beginning German racial hygiene placed a greater emphasis on negative eugenic measures than was the case in the Anglo-American and Scandinavian context. One of the leading proponents and founders of the German racial hygiene movement was Alfred Ploetz, who, in 1895, warned against counterselective forces such as inbreeding, sexually transmitted diseases, alcohol, and war, which apparently damaged the nation's hereditary stock. In 1904, Ploetz founded the *Archiv für Rassen- und Gesellschaftsbiologie* (Journal of Racial and Social Biology). One year later, in 1905, he founded the *Gesellschaft für Rassenhygiene* (Society for Racial Hygiene) together with other members of the racial hygiene movement. Membership of the society included Agnes Bluhm, Gerhard Hauptmann, Erwin Bauer, and Alfred Grotjahn. Ernst Haeckel was an honorary member. By 1910 the Swedish *Sällskap för Rashygien* became the first foreign affiliate. Concerns for this generation of racial hygienists differed quite significantly from those during the Nazi period; up until the early 1920s, racial and social hygienists warned against a declining birth rate and a high infant mortality rate. Although racial hygienists placed no, or little significance on "euthanasia" as a means of racial improvement, the establishment of racial hygiene as an academic discipline, most notably through the foundation of the Kaiser-Wilhelm Institute for Anthropology, Human Heredity and Eugenics in 1927, provided euthanasia advocates with a platform to campaign for the elimination of "life unworthy of life." The central importance that the Nazi regime placed upon racial hygiene as part of its genocidal policies totally discredited the discipline in the eyes of the Western world. As a result, no serious attempts have been made to resurrect the concept of racial hygiene.

2. The concept of a "generative collective ethic" (generative *Kollektivethik*) placed the role of the community above the interest of the individual. The concept was applied throughout the Weimar Republic and thereafter by medical scientists such as Emil Abderhalden, who promoted this positions in journals such as *Ethik*. The idea of a "generative collective ethic" fit well with Nazi racial policies in which holistic concepts such as the community, the *Volk*, the race, the nation, or the idea of National Socialism were seen as of greater importance than the life of the individual.

3. In 1883, the English scientist Francis Galton coined the term "eugenics" (from the Greek word *eugenes* – "wellborn") to establish the science of the biological improvement of human kind. Eugenics and racial hygiene, the specific German derivative of eugenics, were part of a broad movement about the inequality of mankind, nurtured by scientists of international renown, who alleged that the human race would degenerate unless man himself would take the initiative and correct the inevitable path into the biological abyss. Eugenics cut across the party-political and confessional spectrum and attracted Socialists and Social Democrats, as well as conservatives, racial anthropologists, Catholics, Protestants, anti-Semites and health zealots. Eugenics encompassed both positive and negative measures. Positive eugenics included support for families of "valuable hereditary stock" and incentives to have many children. Negative eugenics included sterilization legislation, marriage prohibition, and other forms of birth control such as abortion. To determine racial differences, eugenicists studied physical, psychological, cultural, religious, and social differences. Advocates of eugenics applied evolutionary biology and cell theory to modern society and state government and thus, in effect, established key elements of social Darwinism. The social ills of society were being perceived as illnesses of the body politic (*Volkskörper*). The tendency of the eugenics movement to create a hierarchy of valuable and less valuable races and groups of society provided a powerful intellectual basis for scientific racism. By the end of World War II eugenics was discredited because of its association and connection with Nazi racial policies that were aimed at improving the Aryan race and the extermination of the European Jewry. Recent years has seen a revival of eugenic ideas, which has been prompted by advances in biomedical and genetic research.

4. Euthanasia is the act of killing someone when there is sound and convincing proof, and on the basis of his or her distressing physical and mental condition, that this is believed to be in the person's own interest. Throughout the centuries the issue of euthanasia has been a contentious one that has concerned not only the medical and legal professions but also the Church and state governments. Those arguing against euthanasia often refer to the Hippocratic Oath, which states that the doctor should "give no deadly medicine to anyone if asked," yet the original Greek wording is ambiguous and can mean that the doctor should not become a party to murder by poison. Different forms of euthanasia need to be distinguished: Voluntary euthanasia is being performed at the request of the person himself. The boundaries between voluntary euthanasia and assisted suicide are blurred and not always easy to separate. Involuntary euthanasia is killing someone in disregard of his or her will. Involuntary euthanasia needs to be distinguished from

nonvoluntary euthanasia, which is the act of killing someone on the assumption that this is in the persons' interest, but when the person is not in a position to express his or her views on the matter. It is the latter form of euthanasia that is the most contentious one. Key figures in the debates on euthanasia in the 20th century were Karl Binding and Alfred Hoche, who in the 1920s argued for the killing of "lives unworthy of life." Their arguments provided National Socialists with a rationale to implement the "euthanasia" program during World War II, Today the issue of euthanasia is part of an ongoing public and academic discourse that is concerned about the quality of life, as well as with the role of autonomy and human rights in modern society.

5. One of the cornerstones of Nazi population and racial policy was the Law to Prevent Hereditarily Ill Offspring, also called Sterilization Law. Since the turn of the twentieth century a number of North American states had introduced sterilization legislation on a voluntary basis. German racial hygienists saw America as a bold leader in the realm of eugenics and used the American model to promote negative eugenic measures at home. The Nazi regime was the first government to introduce racial hygiene on a national scale and on a compulsory basis. The Sterilization Law was presented to the cabinet on 14 July 1933. To circumvent any opposition and safeguard the on-going negotiations between the Catholic Church and the Nazi government, the Law was published on 26 July 1933, 6 days after the Vatican had signed the Concordat with the new regime. The Sterilization Law came into force on 1 January 1934. The Law was a fundamental violation of individual autonomy and the right of procreation. It legalized compulsory sterilization for a wide range of alleged hereditary illnesses: congenital feeble-mindedness, schizophrenia, manic depressive illness, hereditary epilepsy, Huntington's chorea, hereditary blindness, hereditary deafness, serious physical malformation, and severe alcoholism. To underpin the Law's legal basis the government established 181 Hereditary Health Courts and Appellate Hereditary Health Courts in 1934. The Law targeted "ballast-existences," "useless-eaters," "inferior-work-shy," and those "inferior" but fit for work. Most of its hereditary diagnoses were, in fact, social ones. Reports sent by medical officers to the health authorities were part of a state-sanctioned program to register and monitor those with hereditary illnesses. Details of the private and public life of patients assigned for sterilization often provided Hereditary Health Courts with information to extend sterilization proceedings against the relatives of the patient. Most decisions to sterilize patients were made against their will. Between 1933 and 1945 approximately 400,000 men and women were compulsorily sterilized.

6. The Nuremberg Doctors' Trial was the first of the subsequent twelve Nuremberg war crimes trials that were established by the American military authorities after the conclusion of the trial of the major war criminals by the International Military Tribunal (IMT) at the beginning of October 1946. Its official title was United States of America versus Karl Brandt et al. (Case I). The trial was established on the basis of Control Counsel Law No. 10, which granted each of the major Allies the right to try war criminals in their zone of occupation before an appropriate tribunal. Law No. 10 obviated the necessity for a second international trial after frictions between the Allied powers had become increasingly apparent at the dawn of the Cold War. All twelve subsequent Nuremberg trials, which involved a total of 184 defendants, were therefore American trials, rather than four-power trials. In early 1946, the lawyer Telford Taylor became the head of the Subsequent Proceedings Division in the Office of Chief of Counsel for the Prosecution of Axis Criminality; he was thus in charge of prosecuting war criminals. Andrew Ivy, vice president of the University of Illinois and professor of physiology, as well as Leo Alexander, an Austrian-Jewish émigré psychiatrist and medical war crimes investigator, were appointed as medical experts for the U.S. prosecution. Both played a significant role in the origins of the Nuremberg Code. On 25 October 1946, the day that the Doctors' Trial was established, General Lucius Clay, Military Governor of the U.S. zone of occupation, appointed Walter Beals, Justice of the Supreme Court of the state of Washington, Harold L. Sebring, Justice of the Supreme Court of Florida, Johnson T. Crawford, former Justice of the Oklahoma District Court in Ada, and Victor C. Swearingen, alternate member and former Assistant Attorney General of Michigan, as designated Judges of Military Tribunal I. On the same day the United States charged twenty doctors, among them Hitler's personal escort physician Karl Brandt, and three bureaucrats with a common design or conspiracy, with war crimes, crimes against humanity, and membership in organization declared criminal by the IMT. The defendants were charged in particular with criminal experiments in the concentration camps of Dachau, Sachsenhausen, Natzweiler, Ravensbrück, and Buchenwald. Several of the defendants were also charged with murder, torture, and maltreatment of people who were not related to medical experiments, for example with the killing of the handicapped in the "euthanasia" program. All of the twenty-three defendants pleaded not guilty. The trial lasted 139 days. Fifteen of the twenty-three defendants were found guilty of war crimes and crimes against humanity. On 20 August 1947 seven of them were sentenced to death by hanging: Karl Brandt, Victor Brack, Wolfram Sievers, Karl Gebhardt, Waldemar Hoven, Joachim Mrugowsky, and Rudolf Brandt. In June 1948 the sentences against the seven defendants were executed at Landsberg prison. Five of the defendants were sentenced to life imprisonment, later commuted to 15 or 20 years. Herta Oberheuser, the only women on trial, was sentenced to 20 years imprisonment, but released in the mid-1950s. As part of the judgment, the Nuremberg judges issued a ten-point medical ethics' code on human experimentation that became known as the Nuremberg Code. Throughout the Cold War period, however, the Code was given relatively little consideration by the Anglo-American research community and was mostly seen as "A Good Code for Barbarians," which would apply to German medical scientists, but not to the Western scientific establishment. The Code is nevertheless seen by some scholars as a landmark in modern biomedical research ethics that established the principle of informed, voluntary consent as part of international law.

7. The Nazi "euthanasia" program stands for the systematic murder of tens of thousands of handicapped children and adults during World War II. The program started in the summer of 1939 with the killing of handicapped children. In the autumn of 1939 Hitler commissioned his escort physician, Karl Brandt, and the Chief of the Chancellery of the Führer, Philipp Bouhler, with the organization and implementation of the euthanasia

program. The euthanasia program and the Final Solution were intricately connected in that the former provided personnel and vital technical expertise for the latter. The murder of handicapped children and adults was also closely intertwined with the outbreak of war. As early as 1935, Hitler had indicated that he intended to "eliminate incurable handicapped people" during a war because he anticipated less resistance from the Church and the general public. The Nazi euthanasia program had both a racial and socio-economic rationale. The regime believed that the killing of handicapped would free urgently needed bed space and save on food rationing for German soldiers and civilians. To let the mentally ill starve became official state-sanctioned policy after racial propaganda (by means of films, radio, and press) had stigmatized them as "life unworthy of life." At the same time Hitler thought that the killing of the handicapped would purify the German body politic (*Volkskörper*), and thus balance the death of racially "valuable" members of society in times of war, that is, soldiers, with the elimination of "useless eaters" and "ballast existences." The program was conducted primarily in five killing centers (Bernburg, Brandenburg, Grafeneck, Hadamar, and Sonnenstein) of which four were in use at any one time. Active and passive resistance to the euthanasia program came primarily from the Church and charitable organizations, most notably from Bishop Clemens August Graf von Galen from Münster, as well as from the general public, which became increasingly concerned about the suspicious death of relatives and friends. Although Hitler had ordered the program to be conducted in total secrecy, rumors about the killings were spreading throughout the population. After the official stop of the euthanasia program in August 1941, the program continued on a more decentralized level throughout the Reich until the end of the war.

8. At the end of the 1920s, a series of unethical, and in some cases fatal experiments on children prompted public debate in Weimar Germany about medical ethics' standards and the reform of the German penal code. In February 1931 the Reich Ministry of the Interior therefore issued the "Regulations Concerning New Therapy and Human Experimentation." The directives were among the most comprehensive research rules by any standard at the time. Some elements were even more elaborate than the principles of the Nuremberg Code. Contentious issues such as individual autonomy, beneficence, voluntary consent, and therapeutic and nontherapeutic research were formulated to protect the rights and dignity of patients. Thus, remarkably, Germany was one of the few countries that by the 1930s had introduced state directives for the protection of human subjects in clinical research. The guidelines were especially aimed to protect the vulnerable groups of society, for example, the handicapped and children. Significantly, they were the first victims of the Nazi euthanasia program. The German ethics' guidelines from the 1930s are a poignant example that ethics' codes and other professional regulations are insufficient in themselves to protect patients against serious bodily harm, disability, and death.

9. As part of the judgement in the Nuremberg Doctors' Trial, which lasted from December 1946 until August 1947, the judges issued a ten-point medical ethics' code that laid down the human rights of patient-subjects and the duties of physician-researchers for experiments on humans. The aim of the Code was to find a solution to resolve one of the most fundamental conflicts in human experimentation: to balance the need for the advancement of medical science for the benefit of human society with the right of the individual to personal inviolability, autonomy, and self-determination. According to the judges, not all, but only "certain types" of experiments on humans conformed to the ethics of the medical profession in the civilized world. Human experimentation needed to remain within "reasonably well-defined bounds," they said. Unless "certain basic principles" were observed to "satisfy moral, ethical and legal concepts," experiments on humans were not permissible. The medical ethics code became known as the Nuremberg Code. The decision to include the Code into the judgment meant that, for the first time, written guidelines for permissible research on humans were incorporated into the canon of international law. This was a substantial achievement, irrespective of the limited effect that the Code had in the following decades for the protection of human and patient rights.

The Code established, for the first time, fundamental human rights in medicine, and placed the welfare of the patients into the foreground of medical practice. In the Nuremberg Code, neither medicine, nor science, nor society or any kind of collective or utilitarian ethics, have priority over the right of the individual to remain physically and psychologically unharmed. A person's right to self-determination and inviolability cannot be calculated against some fictitious need for medical progress, or any other claim that society and science may or may not have toward its citizens. In lucid and unambiguous language – something that cannot be taken for granted for most medical ethics' codes – the Code states that the rights and integrity of the research subjects have to be preserved at all times. Of the ten principles, two principles – one and nine – specifically refer to the protection and rights of the experimental subject, and principle eight to their well-being. Principle one of the Code has been of importance for the history of medical ethics that reaches far beyond Nuremberg. The principle links the experiment to the *voluntary consent* of the experimental subject. That means that the experiment can only be conducted after the "voluntary, personal consent" has been obtained, and only after the subject has been clearly informed in the best possible manner about the risk involved. The Code makes it unequivocally and categorically clear that the person involved in the experiment has to have the legal capacity to give a voluntary consent. Moreover, prior to obtaining consent, the exact nature, duration, and objective of the experiment, the applied methods and means as well as all potential implications of the experiment for the health of the person have to be made clear. The experimental subject has to have sufficient knowledge of and capacity to comprehend the subject matter to make an enlightened and informed decision. This was meant to protect unconscious and mentally handicapped persons or humans who, because of their specific illness, are unable to give voluntary consent. The Code made it clear that no experiments are legally and ethically permissible on the aforementioned patient groups. Since the late nineteenth century, the status of the voluntary consent principle was greatly enhanced as a central element of medical research. The Code, for the first time, transferred this principle as part of the Nuremberg judgment into international law.

Principle nine likewise deserves attention as another essential medical ethics' law: the right of the experimental person to terminate the experiment at any time. The principle was formulated as a right and not as a guideline, and thus constituted another legal precedent. These innovative patient rights were given further weight through the formulation of unequivocal duties of the physicians to act at all times responsibly toward the patient. The rights of the patient *do not* replace the duties of the physician as outlined in principles two to eight. A patient who has given his or her voluntary consent *cannot* be used for a random number of experiments; these experiments *cannot* violate professional medical ethics' standards because the patient had consented to the research. That is why, according to principle ten of the Code, it is the duty of the scientist in charge to terminate the experiment on his or her own initiative, and at any stage, if there is reason to believe that the continuation of the experiment would, in all probability, result in injury, disability, or death of the experimental subject.

The Nuremberg Code constitutes a particular, and in many ways unique, combination of human rights, which are part of international law, *and* the Hippocratic medical ethic. For the judges Hippocratic medical ethics were an important precondition to protect the welfare and lives of patients, but it appeared insufficient in protecting human lives in human experimentation. They realized that research subjects needed to have quite specific rights, if they were to be sufficiently protected from potential harm. That is why the conditions under which informed voluntary constant can be obtained in the Code are formulated in a much more comprehensive and legalistic fashion than in any other earlier medical ethics' codes. The principle of voluntary consent in the Code thus demands the status of an absolute, a priori principle. Moreover, the experimental subject is given the right to terminate the experiment at any time. The Nuremberg Code is therefore a legal code *and*, at the same time, a medical ethics code. That is the Code's particular strength. Yet it is also the profound weakness of many other ethics codes. They have no legal status whatsoever and are thus little more than "guidelines" that are interpreted and introduced by the respective expert group.

The judgment reflected a new case law to cover the legal issues that had arisen from this precedent. The judges believed in the creation of an international legal and professional framework that would empower those who had suffered harm to claim their rights against those who had violated them. The Nuremberg Code was in many ways a visionary and innovative medical ethics code. Its principles were designed to apply to all research involving human subjects. Even today, the Nuremberg Code has significant symbolic and, in many ways, an influential role in the field of medical politics, ethics, and law. It also serves as a major point of reference to assess whether or not scientists who conducted experimental research on humans complied with or violated medical ethics standards during the Cold War period.

There has been considerable debate about the origin and authorship of the Nuremberg Code. Scholars today agree that the Code was drafted and redrafted in stages before and throughout the Nuremberg Doctors' Trial. Among those involved in producing the material for the formulation of the Code were the two medical experts for the U.S. prosecution, Andrew Ivy and Leo Alexander, the head of the prosecution, Brigadier General Telford Taylor, and the four judges: Walter B. Beals, Harold L. Sebring, Johnson T. Crawford, and Victor C. Swearingen. Recent research seems to suggest that Sebring managed to assert his influence over the Tribunal in the field of medical ethics, and will, in all likelihood, have drafted a considerable part of the Code.

10. Following revelations of unethical human experiments in America in the 1950s and early 1960s, the Medical Ethics Committee of the World Medical Association (WMA) produced a draft code of ethics on human experimentation that was published in the fall of 1962. Two years later, the WMA officially adopted parts of the draft Code during the 18th World Medical Assembly in June 1964. The Code became known as the "Declaration of Helsinki." Important provisions of the draft Code were, however, deleted from the Declaration of Helsinki, for example, the prohibition to use prisoners of war in human experiments, whether military or civilian, or persons confined to prisons and mental institutions. The Declaration initiated an important shift in the quality of international medical ethics' codes, from the rights of patients and the protections of human subjects in experimental research to the protection of patient welfare through physicians' responsibility. The Declaration states that the doctor "should, if at all possible, consistent with the patient's psychology" obtain the patients' freely given consent. At the same time the personal, nontransferable, legal responsibility of the physician for his research subjects was deleted from the Declaration, as was the right of the subject to terminate the experiment at any time. The Declaration undermined the importance of the principle of informed consent as outlined in the Nuremberg Code, and reintroduced it with a more paternalistic value system of the traditional doctor–patient relationship. The Helsinki Declaration must be seen as a largely successful outcome of a campaign by the international medical community to supplant the Nuremberg Code with research regulations that were in line with modern biomedical research, and which reaffirmed and protected the position of the researcher. The Helsinki Declaration was one of many strategies by the medical profession to ensure that the level of legal liability – and indeed public embarrassment – of researchers and their institutions would be kept at a minimum at a time when civil liberty and human rights groups were exposing medical ethics' violations in the United States and elsewhere.

CHAPTER 55

MEDICAL ETHICS AND COMMUNISM IN THE SOVIET UNION

Boleslav L. Lichterman

I. INTRODUCTION

The year 1917 was a turning point in Russian and World history. Two revolutions occurred within that year. In February 1917 Czar Nicolas II abdicated the throne and Russia was proclaimed a republic. On October 25, 1917 (November 7th on the Gregorian calendar) power was seized by Bolsheviks, led by Lenin (Vladimir Ul'yanov) and Leo Trotsky (Leiba Bronshtein) under the slogans: "All power to the Soviets!" "Peace to the peoples!" "Land to the peasants!" and "Factories to the workers!"

Despite hunger, Civil War, and economic collapse, truly revolutionary changes were made in all spheres of life.[1] The *Narodny commissariat zdravookhranenija, RSFSR* (Ministry of Health of Russian Soviet Federal Socialist Republics) was established in 1918. An editorial in *The Journal of the American Medical Association* on Johannes Peter Frank (1745–1821) suggests that the best English translation of his term "medizinischen Polizey" is "public health by decrees" (Editorial 1967). That was exactly the way the Bolsheviks introduced the new system of public health – by decrees. Headed by Lenin's ally Nikolai Semashko (1874–1949),[2] the RSFSR issued decrees legalizing abortion (in 1920) and active euthanasia (physician-assisted suicide) (in 1922), becoming the first country in the world to legalize either.

For the 20-year period, from 1917 to 1937, the number of medical doctors increased fivefold. The Union of Soviet Socialist Republics (USSR) became the country with the second largest number of physicians in the world, second only to the United States.[3] Many medical doctors were women. Before the October Revolution of 1917 female doctors comprised approximately 10 percent of the total number of physicians. By 1937 their share had increased to almost half (Strashun 1937, 28).[4] In 1914 there were ten medical faculties at universities of the Russian Empire. By 1937 there were forty-nine medical schools, twelve dental schools, and nine pharmacy schools. The number of medical students totaled to 100,000 (Strashun 1937, 24). A system of postgraduate medical training was established.

At the same time, the economic situation for Russian physicians was poor. A medical doctor's average salary in 1928 was 99 rubles a month, whereas a bookkeeper's salary was 109 rubles and a manual industrial worker earned 126 rubles (Gekker 1928).[5] Physicians had to maintain a private practice and take on other jobs to make a living.

Statistical data indicate the hardships of the medical life: 16 percent of physicians died of accidental causes; 20 percent died of mental disorders and 44 percent died of heart attacks. Every fifth medical doctor regularly used narcotics (mostly morphine). The incidence of suicide was much higher than in the general population (1:28 compared with 1:1,200) (Koni 1928, 11). Cases of massacre and lynching of medical doctors increased. To halt violence against medical doctors, D. N. Zhbankov suggested the introduction of show-trials (Zhbankov 1927). These show-trials became routine in the 1920s and 1930s but they were aimed at those whom Stalin considered his political rivals, Trotskists, Bukharinists, and so forth. By that time the USSR had become a totalitarian state that controlled all spheres of life, including medicine. For example, the so-called *delo vrachei* (doctors' affair) was planned as a show-trial of a group of Jewish physicians accused of poisoning leaders of the Communist Party and Soviet government "on the orders of American imperialists." Only Stalin's death from a stroke on March 5, 1953 helped to stop this trial. Many Jewish physicians who were fired from their jobs were then allowed to return to work.

The share of expenses for health care in the state budget gradually diminished (6.6% of state budget in 1960 compared to 4.4% in 1986). Expenses for health care per capita also decreased (from 142.9 rubles in 1966 to 116.3 rubles in 1975). In 1986, only 70 percent of hospitals had central heating, 77 percent running water, 68 percent sewerage, and 38 percent hot water. The average salary of medical practitioners was comparatively one of the lowest in the country (135 rubles a month in 1986).[6] This was partly compensated by patients' presents and bribes or "tips" to the medical doctors (see also Chapter 56). At the same time the lion's share of the health care budget was spent on luxury hospitals and sanatoriums for *nomenklatura*, the Party and government elite and their families.

The Soviet system ceased to exist in December 1991, when the USSR collapsed; however, the old health care system survived almost unchanged.

II. SOVIET MEDICAL ETHICS

The very term, "Soviet medical ethics," is problematic. In the 1920s, when open discussion was still possible, some characterized "medical ethics" as "professional decency and honesty" (Lepukaln 1927, 379). Others denied the existence of professional medical ethics: "From our standpoint there might be only one ethics, the ethics of the honest Soviet citizen. Professional decency and honesty are very loose concepts" (Rafal'kes 1928, 147). This standpoint became dominant in ethical discourse about medical morality during the Soviet period. An anonymous writer in an obscure health care journal in 1928 wrote:

A notorious "professional ethics" was severely criticized because there should be one ethics for everybody – that is Marxist-Leninist ethics. Sometimes we simply forget that we live in workers Republic and first and foremost should serve their interests;

some of us has yet not changed the rotten charms of the pre-Revolutionary doctors ethics for principles of conscious and healthy community [. . .] We should truly to Sovietize ourselves and subordinate all our activity to the interests of the new community . . . Only such "ethics" would guarantee us a proper place in the chain of the whole Soviet system. (Anonymous 1928, 20)

This view was, almost literally, repeated by Semashko: "the first task of *the so-called doctor's ethics* is a political education of a medical doctor." If a physician "wants to work according to the guidance of the [Communist] party and [Soviet] government he will always find a correct pattern for his behavior" (Semashko 1945, 14).[7]

G. I. Dembo considered the so-called medical ethics to be a poor substitute for legal regulation: "Instead of proper legal norms, the scene is occupied by a substitute of poor quality, frozen, immobile common law norms that are named as 'doctors' ethics'"(Dembo 1930, 34). According to Dembo, with the development of medical professional law "the traditions of the so-called doctors' professional ethics are fading and growing pale and gradually degenerate into doctors' etiquette. The course of medical professional law is filled with content, whereas the course of doctors' professional ethics is dehydrated and dried out" (Dembo 1930, 37).[8] In this vein, an article on doctor's ethics in the first edition of Soviet medical encyclopedia states:

Principles of Soviet medicine solve the key problem in [medical] ethics – the problem of payment for doctor's care and advice. On the other hand new obligations of a physician emerged. When they are violated it should be seen as an unethical deed in situation of socialized medicine. For example the refusal of unemployed physicians in the cities to work in the countryside. (Bron 1928, 636)

In the 1930s, when the Stakhanovite movement aimed at increasing productivity became prominent,[9] there was an attempt to apply the Stakhanovite approach to medicine. A Leningrad urologist Dr. Barshtein wrote:

First and foremost we should completely eliminate the remnants of the so-called "doctors ethics" when it concerns human health and life, when dealing with criticism and self-criticism. Medical mistakes due to low qualification, haste, inattentiveness should be openly discussed at professional meetings of physicians and health care providers in order to stimulate the authors of such mistakes to get rid of their shortcomings as soon as possible. (Barshtein 1936, 10–11; see also Chebotareva 1970, 17)

"Ethics" was replaced by "deontology." The "deontological" period in Soviet medical ethics started with a booklet by Nikolai Petrov, *Voprosy khirurgicheskoi deontologii* ("Problems of surgical deontology") that appeared in several editions. According to Petrov, "while doctors ethics of the capitalist world mostly aimed at guarding the dignity and interests of physicians, medical . . . deontology of Socialist society mostly strives for improvement of patients' treatment" (Petrov 1956, 13). It was not clear, however, what the difference between deontology and medical ethics was (see also Chapter 32).

The first philosophical works on medical ethics were published in the 1960s as a result of *ottepel* ("the thaw" or a softening of a totalitarian regime after Stalin's death when some discussions in social sciences were allowed).[10] Several dissertations were also completed on the subject (Pozdnyakova 1965; Nikitina 1966).

For example, in her doctoral dissertation S. A. Pozdnyakova gives six principles of medical ethics: (1) humane attitudes toward patients (the patient's psychological well being should be protected); (2) the doctor's deeds should correspond to the social goals and tasks of medicine (for example, a physician has no right to participate in euthanasia and genocide because they contradict the social role of medicine); (3) advocacy for the physical and mental improvement of human beings (self-sacrifice and heroism should be the rule for doctor's behavior); (4) nondiscrimination, the obligation to help everyone independent of gender, race, nationality, religious beliefs etc.; (5) solidarity and mutual aid of colleagues; and (6) preservation of confidentiality (Pozdnyakova 1965, 14–15).

According to Chebotareva, the central principle of medical ethics is medical humanism. In this respect medical ethics is linked to psychotherapy (viewed as a special method of patient's reeducation). Every physician should be a psychotherapist and the success of psychotherapy directly depends on the level of moral development of a physician and his or her observance of norms of medical ethics (Chebotareva 1970, 60). The corporate spirit of professional ethics is characteristic of bourgeois society, whereas the Socialist society "does not need petty regulation of people's behavior" (Chebotareva 1970, 12). Any deontological rule should be in accordance with the general principles of Communist morality.

The Twenty-First Congress of the Communist Party of the Soviet Union took place in October 1961 and adopted *Programmu postroenija kommunizma* ("The Program of Building the Communism"), which included *Moral'nyi kodeks stroitelya kommunisma* ("The Moral Code of the Communism Builder"). Some months earlier the Sechenov Moscow Medical Institute Number 1 (now renamed the Sechenov Medical Academy) organized a discussion "On love of the medical profession" where the project of

"Torzhestvennogo obeshanija vracha" ("Solemn Oath of a Medical Doctor") was discussed (Meditsynsky Rabotnik 1961). This text resembles that of a moral code, when it declares, for example: "I promise . . . not to divulge information entrusted to me by patients *if such information does not pose a threat to society.* Together with [the Soviet] people I shall actively participate in the building of the Communist society" (emphasis added).

The Ministry of Health of the USSR allowed graduates of the Institute to take this Oath as an experiment (Kuz'min 1984). The First All-Union conference on problems of medical deontology in 1969 applied to the Ministry of Health to introduce "The Oath of a Soviet Physician" at all medical schools of USSR (see also Chapter 41). The experimental taking of the oath was approved by a special Decree of the Presidium of the Supreme of Soviet of the USSR (Soviet Parliament). In 1983 this text was supplemented by an obligation to fight for peace and against nuclear war. According to the Oath, private interests are secondary to public interests. For example, graduates of a medical school promised "to work conscientiously at places where public interests demand" (this refers to a system when graduates were often obliged to work 3 years after graduation in remote rural areas).

In the 1970s and 1980s, an enormous amount of literature on medical ethics and medical deontology (the terms were often synonymous) was published in USSR. Of more than 1,000 books, booklets, and articles, two-thirds were dedicated to deontology in different medical specialties (Korotkikh 1989, 69). As a rule, these works were written by medical doctors, based on their personal experience rather than a conceptual framework and did not address ethical problems in Soviet health care.[11] Despite this literature, 60 percent of the population was not satisfied by their medical practitioners (Korotkikh 1989, 309). According to a recent sociological survey 71 percent of Russians consider that it is impossible to get proper medical treatment and 62 percent were dissatisfied with the health care system (Izvestija 2003). It is telling that medical deontology was taught at Soviet medical schools as an optional subject.

III. TOPICS IN SOVIET MEDICAL ETHICS

Specific topics in Soviet medical ethics and concerning medical practice and research are worth separate consideration. The most important of these were confidentiality, informed consent, human experimentation, abortion, euthanasia, transplantation, and the abuse of psychiatry.

1. Confidentiality

Confidentiality in relation to medicine was never mentioned in pre-revolutionary Russian law (see Chapter 35).

According to the well-known lawyer, A. F. Koni, "when the obligation to maintain confidentiality contradicts the obligation to assist the court in finding the truth [Russian] law gives preference to the latter obligation. In the court the role of *a witness* pushes the role of *a physician* into the background" (Koni 1901). Thus, confidentiality was guarded "until the entrance to the court only" (Lublinsky 1930, 47). As M. Lakhtin stressed, "the physician's responsibilities are not restricted to his attitude towards his patients. He also has other, overriding obligations to the state and society" (Lakhtin 1903, 10). Russian Penal law did not punish breaches of confidentiality. As A. F. Koni wrote, "the view that disease was something shameful and needed to be concealed is mistaken" (Koni 1928, 13).

Soviet law continued the tradition of saying little about confidentiality. In a public debate on confidentiality Nikolai Semashko remarked, "Our goal is to abolish confidentiality completely. This results from our strong belief that "disease is not a disgrace but a misfortune" (cit. by Veresaev 1948, 466). Because the general population still endorsed confidentiality, however, it was thought worthwhile to preserve it to maintain patients' trust in their doctors. As Semashko noted, "when confidentiality is under the question, one thing is indisputable: collective interests are more important than individual interests" (Semashko 1945, 12). Osipov has correctly noted that "confidentiality, particularly in the Socialist state, is rather limited. Some people properly speak about medical tact instead of confidentiality" (Osipov 1930, 19). "Is the difficult problem of confidentiality – the only debated ethical question in medicine which exceeds the limits of professional ethics – solved? Surely, not," wrote K. P. Sulima in 1903 (Sulima 1903, 444). A century later this statement remains valid.

2. White Lies and Informed Consent

Confidentiality in Russian literature on medical ethics addressed not only the subject of confidential information *about* a patient but also the issue of whether information about an unfavorable diagnosis and prognosis should be given *to* a patient (Chebotareva 1970, 75). Protecting patients from psychological harm motivated concealing such information from them. A patient should not be deprived of hope. This is a "svyataja lozh" ("white lie" – literally "a sacred lie") as a founder of Russian internal medicine Sergey Botkin (1832–1889) phrased it. "The most sacred truth for a physician is to lie to a hopeless patient in order to relieve his last days and last sufferings, in order to leave him hope" – wrote Preobrazhensky several decades later (Preobrazhensky 1928, 312). The author uses such expression as "a ray of hope," which is a true "guiding star of life." Some authors, however, challenged the conventional wisdom on this subject. Koni doubted

that a physician's frankness might depress a patient: "Apart from the fact that fears about psychological injury are mostly conjectural, when a physician fails to mention the patient's dangerous condition or imminent death to the latter, the former takes upon himself the material and spiritual consequences of silence" (Koni 1928, 15). Physicians should not be *marchands d'esperance* (merchants of hope, to use the expression of French writer Prosper Merimée [1803–1870]). Patients' desire to learn the truth should be the ground for the physician's frankness; however, as in the case with his views on euthanasia (see later), Koni was in the minority.

The problem of informing patients was particularly acute in oncology. Nikolai Petrov recommended that physicians should avoid such terms as "cancer" and "sarcoma" and substitute for them such terms as "tumor," "ulcer," "infiltrate," and the like (Petrov 1956, 51). In order not to deprive a patient of hope and not to increase his or her suffering "one should never tell an incurable surgical patient that surgery is impossible; one should always inspire him with the idea that *surgery is not needed at the present moment*" (emphasis original) (Petrov 1956, 61). The argument that informing patients about unfavorable outcomes so that they might prepare a last will and testament, was rejected on the following grounds: "Elimination of private property makes the problem of not having a testament insignificant" (Chebotareva 1970, 79).

In the 1970s, there was renewed discussion about whether patients should be informed about a diagnosis of cancer. The majority, among whom was the director of All-Union Cancer Center in Moscow, Nikolai Blokhin, argued that a patient should be unaware of his or her diagnosis of cancer (Blokhin 1977). This was justified by humanistic (psychological and psychotherapeutic) reasons – because of the popular belief of incurability of cancer a patient might be depressed by such a diagnosis. There were cases when patients who learned their diagnosis committed suicide. A diagnosis might be insinuated, but only when a patient refused a recommendation of surgery. To shield patients from the psychological implications of the word "cancer" physicians should substitute it with such terms as "neoplasm," "blastoma," or "malignant ulcer." Forthright information about the diagnosis might be given to the patient's relatives but they, too, should be informed about the necessity of concealing the truth from the patient (Litvinenko 1977). The tactic of deceiving oncology patients is still prevalent among many Russian physicians.

The obligation to obtain the patient's consent for surgery was considered an ethical but not a legal requirement (Malis 1904). At the same time patient's consent does not make unnecessary (nonmedical) surgery lawful, which would lay a surgeon open to a criminal charge of physical damage.

Informed consent was discussed in 1910 at a special meeting of the St. Petersburg law society. Tregubov, a lawyer, claimed that surgery against a patient's will should be equated with physical damage. There followed a discussion in which a professor of pediatrics, K. A. Rauchfus, gave the following example. He was called in an emergency to a peasant's child suffering from diphtheria. A tracheotomy was urgently indicated put the child's parents refused permission for the procedure to be performed. Rauchfus reported that he then ordered his assistant and coachman to bind the parents and performed the tracheotomy.

"Did I commit a crime?" asked Rauchfus.

"According to our law, you committed not one but two crimes. You deprived the parents of freedom and caused physical damage to their child," Tregubov replied.

"And I performed such surgeries without taking the parents' preferences into consideration and I will do the same in the future!" Rauchfus exclaimed. (Cit. by Lublinsky 1930, 43)

A special governmental decree, issued December 1, 1924, stated that all surgical interventions required the patient's consent. For patients younger than 16, their parents' consent is required. Certain exceptions were allowed: when the patient is comatose or in emergencies and the child's parents are not available. It was not specified whether such consent had to be written or whether oral consent would suffice. Since the 1970s, patients' written consent for surgery has been required. As Chebotareva (referring to the above mentioned Rauchfus' story and cases in which Baptists who refused surgery died) noted, however, "an unconditional prohibition of surgery without consent contradicts the principles of Communist morality" (Chebotareva does not specify, but presumably because it is performed in the best interests of a patient although he or she may not realize it; this might be close to what is usually meant by humanism.) (Chebotareva 1970, 86).

3. Human Experimentation

Experiments on humans can be divided into two types. The first type involves experiments on healthy volunteers (nontherapeutic research). According to S. Girgolav, researchers may engage in auto-experimentation if necessary. Experiments upon nonmedical people, however, are intolerable (Girgolav, 1930). The second type of experiment includes investigation and approval of new surgical procedures and new drugs. In these cases, the patient's consent is obligatory. Scientific progress and possible benefit for subjects are necessary conditions for

such experiments; however, Grigolav mentions that in wartime the interests of individuals might be subordinate to research to improve outcomes for those with injuries or diseases.

Chebotareva also writes that one should avoid experimentation without patients' consent. This rule has one important exception: "In cases in which medical experimentation offers the only chance to save the patient's life, for example, in case of a clinical trial of a new drug, it would be permissible to conduct such experiments without consent" (Chebotareva 1970, 79). Chebotareva classifies such situations in the category of permissible involuntary treatment, such as vaccination. She denies the right of some religious groups to refuse vaccination.

4. Abortion

Abortions were prohibited in Imperial Russia;[12] however, criminal charges were seldom brought against women or physicians. For example, in 1906 in Russia fourteen persons were accused of performing abortions; eight were acquitted and six were sentenced (Grin 1914, 47). At approximately the same time (1914) the estimated number of abortions in Moscow alone was 10,000 (Gernet 1927). Vyacheslav Manassein (1841–1901) unconditionally condemned not only abortions but also contraception (cit. by Ivanyushkin 1998). Vikenty Veresaev shared this view and treated abortion as an act of homicide (Veresaev 1904, VII–VIII). At the beginning of the twentieth century the first articles and books defending a woman's right to control her own body were published in Russia. The Pirogov Medical Society suggested abolition of criminal sanctions for abortion in 1913. A year later the Congress of Russian section of International Union of Criminologists took the same position.

The debate about abortion continued through the period of World War I, the Civil War, and the October Revolution of 1917. Dr. Leibovich, a forensic expert from *Narkomzdrav* (Ministry of Health), was among the first to call for legalization of abortions in Soviet Russia by issuing a special report "Noveishy vzglyad na dopustimost' i nenakazuemost' abortov" ("A First Outlook on the Decriminalization of Abortion"). At the same time the *Narkomjust* (Ministry of Justice) sent an inquiry to *Narkomzdrav* about whether abortion is a crime and, if so, at what time: when contraceptives are used, when the fetus is formed, or during what month of pregnancy (cit. by Gens 1927). On November 18, 1920, Narkomzdrav and Narkomjust issued a joint decree that allowed abortions to be performed in medical establishments. This was perhaps the earliest decriminalization of abortion in the twentieth century. Predictions to the contrary notwithstanding, the birth rate remained unchanged but maternal mortality from criminal abortions decreased significantly. It was realized, however, that abortion was a harmful and dangerous measure for birthrate regulation. In 1923, contraceptives were legalized by a special circular of Narkomzdrav, which stated that the initiative in administering contraceptives should arise not from a doctor but from a woman (Gens 1929, 79). In 1936, by a special government decree, abortions were forbidden in the hope of increasing the birth rate. In 1955 abortions were again legalized by a parliamentary decree (ukaz Prezidiuma Verkhovnogo Soveta SSSR) (Romanovsky 2003).

5. Euthanasia

The Criminal Code of the Russian Soviet Republics of 1922 stated that causing death to relieve the unbearable suffering of a patient at that person's request should not be considered murder (cit. by Zil'ber 1998). Soviet Russia was thus the first state in the world to legalize euthanasia. Within a few months, however, this provision was rescinded to avoid abuse.

Koni, who was one of the advocates of euthanasia, argued, "Prolongation of life when every moment of it is accompanied by unbearable suffering . . . is in fact futile prolongation of suffering . . . Of course, suffering might be relieved by narcotics such as morphine, opium, etc., but these remedies lose their efficacy when used frequently . . . And isn't it equivalent to death to keep a patient in an unconscious and insensible state? That is why in cases in which there is no chance to end suffering completely without interrupting the thread of life it is ethically permissible for a physician to calm a patient forever" (Koni 1928, 16–17).

Koni also argued that several conditions must be fulfilled: (1) appropriate, conscious, and repeated request for merciful death must be made by the patient; (2) well-established impossibility of saving the patient's life, ratified in a collective decision in consultation with other physicians, following a written protocol; and (3) written notice should be provided to the office of the public prosecutor and a local representative of this office may be invited to help prepare the written protocol (Koni 1928, 17).

Because of the absence of modern acute health care, passive euthanasia (allowing patients to die) became a routine in many intensive care units during last decades. A distinction between causing death and allowing patients to die has been somewhat blurred. For example, it is enough to leave a patient in an unconscious state near the open window for a couple of hours in winter and then he or she will "naturally" die from pneumonia. Nursing is one of the main problems of health care in Russia.

Euthanasia was (and is) vigorously opposed in theory: "The intentional acceleration of a lethal outcome of a hopelessly ill patient on the grounds of a falsely understood humane consideration, namely, euthanasia, is inad-

missible from the standpoint of Soviet medicine" (El'shtein 1986, 368–71). At present, the problem of legalization of both passive and active euthanasia is a subject of hot debate in the popular and medical literature.

6. Transplantation

In 1924 Vladimir Filatov (1875–1956) – a surgeon and ophthalmologist – suggested a method of transplantation of cadaveric cornea. In 1937 Sovnarkom (Soviet Government) issued a special decree *O poryadke provedenija meditsynskikh operatsy* ("On Carrying Out Medical Operations"). In this decree Narkomzdrav (Ministry of Health) was given a right to set obligatory standards for all surgical interventions, including transplantation of cornea and organ transplantation. On December 1, 1937, Narkomzdrav adopted a special standard "On Use of Eyes of the Deceased for Transplantation of Cornea to the Blind." It was proclaimed, that:

> "Prior consent of relatives of the deceased for procurement of eyes of the cadavers who died in hospitals or were taken to a morgue is not required." (Cit. by Petrovsky 1988)

A cadaver was viewed as a public property which should used in public interests.[13] Relatives were not informed about organ procurement. Until 1992 forensic autopsy and procurement of cadaver organs were considered equivalent procedures.

The first heart transplantation was performed in USSR in 1969. The development of transplantation was impeded by the former Minister of Health of USSR, Boris Petrovsky, who fiercely opposed heart transplantation on ethical grounds and denied the concept of brain death. As one of his colleagues wrote "a physician should fight for patient's life up to its last minute, last breath, last beat of heart, using all of the technology of modern intensive care, and even after this, until biological death is declared" (Gulyaev 1970). There was also concern that the phrase, "incompatibility with life," often used in characterizations of "brain death," could be subject to an overly broad interpretation and therefore abused.

On the other hand, kidney transplantation using organs from cadaver donors became quite popular. In 1970s "Intertransplant" – a special program of exchange of cadaver organs between Soviet Block countries (USSR and Eastern Europe) – was developed within the framework of "Soviet ekonomicheskoi vzaimopomoshi" ("Council for Mutual Economic Aid"). It ceased to exist in 1990 due to disintegration of the Soviet political system.

A federal law regulating human transplantation ("O transplantatsii organov i (ili) tkanei cheloveka" – "On Transplantation of Human Organs and/or Tissues") was first adopted in December 1992. The law's first reading took place in June 1992. According to professor Anatoly

Dolbin who was one of the authors of this law there was a debate about which model of cadaver organ procurement should be adopted – "direct consent" or "presumed consent" (Dolbin 2003). The model of direct consent would require a lot of time and money (to create registration database, donor charts, etc.). On the other hand in Austria (where "presumed consent" model has already existed) the rate of procurement of cadaver kidneys was thirty-four per million, whereas in the United States ("direct consent" model) it was only twenty-four to twenty-five per million. So it was decided to adopt presumed consent model.

Since 1987, approximately 100 heart transplantations have been performed at the Institute of Transplantology in Moscow. There are approximately 500 cases of kidney transplantation in Russia annually; two thirds of them are done in Moscow. These are mostly cadaver kidneys because living organ donation by relatives is prohibited by law.

The main obstacles to the development of organ transplantation programs in Russia, apart from financial reasons, are the negative attitudes of intensive care specialists (many of them are not aware of the brain death concept) and of the lay public. A recent sociological survey indicated that only 20 percent of respondents would agree to donate their organs in case of their brain death. This means that replacement of the "presumed consent" by a "direct consent" model would have resulted in a five-fold decrease of organ procurement. According to Dolbin, the result of introduction of informed consent model into the law of the neighboring Ukraine was that transplantation programs in this republic have almost completely halted (Dolbin, 2003).

7. Abuse of Psychiatry

From the 1960s to the 1980s, there was a practice of declaring opponents of the regime, that is, political dissidents, insane. There was close cooperation between some leading psychiatrists and the secret police (KGB). The most frequent diagnosis was "*vyalotekushaya shizophrenija*" ("sluggish schizophrenia") invented by A. V. Snezhnevsky, a director of the Institute of Psychiatry in Moscow. This diagnosis allowed the authorities to isolate dissidents for years in mental hospitals where they underwent involuntary treatment.[14] Some of these psychiatrists now publish books on ethics in psychiatry, which is, at the very least, ironic. For example, the director of The Serbsky Institute of Forensic Psychiatry Tat'jana Dmitrieva claimed that psychiatrists labeled dissidents as psychotic for humanistic reasons to prevent them from being put into jail. It was much better, however, to stay in the Soviet jail for a limited period of time than practically endless incarceration at a special psychiatry unit with involuntary "treatment." Such practice has never been condemned by Russian medical community.

IV. CONCLUSION

When Bolsheviks seized power, the communal foundations of Russian life (the so-called *sobornost'* or solidarity) became apparent. The primacy of the *kollektiv* (or group) over an individual can be seen not only in involuntary organization of *kolkhozy* (collective farms that replaced individually owned farms) but also in attempts to eliminate confidentiality. A paternalistic model of the doctor–patient relationship in Russian medicine is evident in the denial that there is an obligation to inform patients about unfavorable diagnoses and prognoses. Even the right of medical ethics itself to exist was challenged, as reflected in the use of the term, "deontology," to describe medical ethics. The ideas of zemstvo medicine, such as universal access to health care and the condemnation of private practice, were put into practice under the Soviet regime.

Marxist phraseology had a purely rhetorical character and had a minimal impact on the actual practice of Soviet health care, and Marxist ideological taboos impeded research on the philosophical foundations of medical ethics. International codes of medical ethics were translated into Russian several decades after they had been adopted in other countries. Currently, Russia is being irreversibly, although at times painfully, integrated into the international community. With respect to the effects of this change on medical ethics, international ethical standards and their relation to traditional values should become an important issue for debate.

NOTES

1. According to Zhbankov in 1914–1922 "this country survived a *martyrology of Russian physicians*" For example, in 1918–1919, of 1,100 physicians in Petrograd 224 were infected with spotted fever and 48 of them died (Zhbankov 1928).

2. Semashko was a commissar (minister) of health of the Russian Federation from 1918 until 1930. He was close to Lenin and between 1901 and 1905 worked as a zemsky physician.

3. In the second half of the twentieth century, the USSR had more medical practitioners than any other country in the world. In 1986 there were 1,202,000 physicians and 3,227,000 nurses.

4. Currently, the majority of Russian medical doctors are women, which might be partly explain their low salaries.

5. Compared to the 1913 average salary of a physician comprised 13.8 percent in 1923 and 60–65 percent in 1928.

6. That was about 150 U.S. dollars according to official exchange rate of that period (90 kopeks for 1 USD). The black market value of the U.S. dollar achieved 5 rubles for 1 USD.

7. This article was reprinted in a slightly modified version under the title "Ob oblike sovetskogo vracha" (Semashko 1954). In this edition the following phrase precedes the aforementioned quotation: "Lenin and Stalin – these are ideals for Soviet physicians who should follow their example and teaching" (Semashko 1954, 250).

8. To confirm his standpoint Dembo quotes *Ärztliche Ethik* by Albert Moll, who also denied special doctors ethics.

9. The movement was named after A. G. Stakhanov (1905/1906–1977) – a face-worker at the Donbass mine who set a record for extraction of coal in 1935.

10. This period lasted from mid-1950s until the mid-1960s and was named after a novel "The Thaw" by Ilja Erenburg. The "thaw" gave way to the ideological "frosts" of the Brezhnev era and occupation of Czechoslovakia in 1968.

11. See, for example, a two-volume edition, "Deontologija v Meditsyne" ("Deontology in Medicine") (Petrovsky 1988).

12. Paragraph 1462 of Penal Code of Russian Empire prohibiting abortions (those who assisted abortions had to be jailed for 5–6 years and the woman who deliberately terminated her pregnancy had to be put in jail for 4–5 years) is placed under the section of murders (Svod zakonov Rossiiskoi imperii, kn.5, T.XV. Ulozhenie o nakazaniyakh ugolovnykh i ispravitel'nykh).

13. The State also claimed possession of living human beings – according to Lenin, "individual health is a public property" and as one popular song of the Soviet era says: *Ran'she dumai o Rodine, a potom o sebe* ("Think of your Motherland first, and only then – about yourself").

14. Some dissidents were indeed mentally ill, but it does not change the matter in principle.

CHAPTER 56

MEDICAL ETHICS AND COMMUNISM IN EASTERN EUROPE

Bela Blasszauer

I. INTRODUCTION

This chapter addresses ethical issues concerning Communism and medicine in Eastern Europe. From the perspective of the twenty-first century, just after the turn of the millennium, one can see that the radical political changes in 1989 and 1990, including the introduction of market economy and the rise of political and moral pluralism, have not solved many of the serious problems facing Eastern Europe. The region faces high unemployment, widespread crime and corruption, environmental pollution, abuse of power, and widespread poverty. Twelve years after the disappearance of Socialism Eastern European health care systems still suffer from many serious problems. These systems are under financed, their physical infrastructure is decaying, health care professionals and nonprofessionals are dramatically underpaid, and moral dilemmas and controversies increasingly accompany the daily work of physicians and nurses. These health care systems are also badly structured and organized. Corruption, waste, and chronic bankruptcy characterize them, and the elite do little to make the necessary changes. Yet, the dramatic increase in morbidity and mortality indicates that the situation is catastrophic. Citizens can no longer trust in their health care systems and they are therefore suffering from a severe moral crisis. Throughout Central

and Eastern Europe they seem to be, as a Russian author put it: "in a state of chaos and misery, in irreversible coma" (Yudin 1992, 5–6; see also Chapters 41 and 55).

II. MEDICINE UNDER COMMUNISM

During the Communist era (from the end of World War II until 1989 and 1990), all Soviet satellite countries claimed that the health care system was free, high quality, and accessible to all. All three claims are questionable. Although a free health care system was available everywhere in Eastern Europe and the Soviet Union, the practice of slipping cash-filled envelopes into physicians' pocket for the treatments they provided or were about to provide was (and still is) common. The practice of "tipping,"[1] or under-the-counter payment, has infiltrated every aspect of physician–patient relationship, casting into doubt the claim of free health care. Nevertheless, in most Communist countries, practically everybody appeared to get necessary health care. As soon as a little freedom of speech appeared in the 1980s, however, it became obvious that the morals of Socialism were in ruins, as was the Socialist economy. There were, of course, striking similarities in the functioning of the health care systems, as well as in the failures of reform attempts everywhere in the Soviet satellite countries.

Sociological and epidemiological surveys, however, documented a very poor general state of health in Eastern Europe. There were high mortality rates, many people with disabilities, and severely reduced life expectancies. Under Socialism, patients had one official right, the right to a free and high level of health care. Practically nothing was mentioned about other patients' rights, such as patient autonomy or informed consent. Issues such as euthanasia, acquired immunodeficiency syndrome (AIDS), and suicide were taboo (see also Chapter 55). It was simply presumed that a genuine member of Socialist society would not resort to suicide, unless that person had become mentally ill. Despite this belief, Hungary, for example, led the world's statistics in suicide – in almost all age categories. Until 1984 Hungary had led the world with 4,600 "successful" suicides annually. In the last one and a half decades, however, suicide has decreased by thirty per cent; thus, Hungary has dropped from the first place to the seventh place in the world's ranking. Nevertheless, Hungary still exceeds the average suicide rate of the European Union countries by two and a half times. At present 32 of every 1,000 people commit suicide. Considering the total population of Hungary, it means that 3,200 persons choose death annually (O.Z. 2002, 18).

As far as euthanasia was concerned, after a brief failed experiment with legalization in the early years of the Soviet Union (see Chapter 55), Communist countries prohibited the act. Patients were only killed under Capitalism, but not under Socialism, where the human being was held to be the highest value. Marxist philosophy and ethics, moreover, had practically nothing to say about death and dying. On the ownership of the body there was no question. The body, the organs, and everything else belonged to the "community," that is, those who held the power. As to informing patients and taking their decisions seriously, because Socialist states are inherently paternalistic (the proletariat needs to be led), patients received very little or no information about their conditions. Thus, the Medical Oath for the Hungarian university graduates of 1973 read:

> I swear by my honor that I shall always be loyal to the Constitution of the Hungarian People's Republic and to the working people. I shall respect my university and its teachers and shall behave worthy of my doctor's title. I swear that I will use my medical knowledge for the benefit of patients, and in case of a life threatening disease, if it is demanded by the public good, I will gently let the relatives of the patient (sic!) or other interested parties, know it in the right time. I shall keep the secrets of my patients, unless the law says otherwise. (Szilard 1973, 29–30)

Physicians were also unwilling to discuss diagnosis, prognosis, and intended therapy with the patient because of their characteristically negative judgment regarding their patients' medical knowledge and ability to make rational medical decisions (Blasszauer 1995b, 1598) and their isolation from the debates common in Western bioethics. In practice, physicians and health care institutions had no freedom to choose patients, and patients had no freedom to choose their doctors.

There was a strong medical establishment, largely made up of physicians who were members of the Communist Party or who enjoyed the favor of high Party officials. By the time the Communists established power in such Eastern European countries as Hungary (in 1948), approximately half of the physicians, approximately 4,500 in all, had joined the Party (Kovacs 1985, 69–82). The one-party system made certain that the vocabulary of the Communist ideology dominated health politics and policies, and individual careers were based mainly on loyalty to this ideology.

The level of the health care funding was determined by politicians. Even under Communist rule, there were limitations created by scarce resources. For example, the age limit for patients receiving hemodialysis was set at 55 years. In general, rationing was based on age. In Romania, the situation was perhaps worse than in other Communist countries. One author states:

> The situation of chronically ill patients was desperate. Drugs were mostly absent, even ordinary antibiotics; the investigation methods were sometimes rudimentary, intensive care usually limited to a simple perfusion and a candle. Patients were obliged to buy the drugs themselves. Transplants were a dream. Even renal dialysis was almost impossible: frequently patients were not accepted by the only dialysis unit in Bucharest. The elderly were forgotten. There were even plans to remove them from cities and send them to villages abandoned by the younger population. Under such circumstances, passive euthanasia was part of everyday medicine. (Maximilian 1991, 22–3)

Other Romanian authors also wrote about orphans with AIDS, and the mentally handicapped living in unspeakable circumstances.

Under Communism, there was gross abuse of psychiatry (see also Chapter 55). The abused victims of psychiatry were essentially those who were considered dangerous to the Communist regimes. Thau and Popescu-Prahovara identify the ideological excuse for psychiatric abuse that had been provided by the former Communist leader Nicole Ceauşescu in a speech to students in 1968:

> Undoubtedly comrades, no peasant, worker or intellectual could question the solidarity and the strength of Socialism in Romania. Only insane people could do that, and they will always exist. But

our socialist society could use a variety of means to deal with mad people, including the straight-jacket." (Thau and Popescu-Prahovara 1992, 13–16)

The Communists boasted from time to time that because of the "free," "high-level," and "accessible" health care system, even the worst Socialism was better than the best Capitalism. The truth is that the great majority of people, who did not have access to health care earlier in the pre-war Capitalist environment, were able to receive care under so-called Socialism. This access was, indeed, the most significant ethical achievement of the Communists.

III. Communist Ideology

Ideology, to put it in a simple way, comprises a belief in a certain way of life that is supposed to be superior to any other way of life and whose truth cannot be questioned. Viewed from the outside, however, Communism was an "ideology" in the sense of being a rhetoric that masked the reality of so-called Communist states, a rhetoric that served the needs of an elite and not of the people ("the proletariat"). Communist states had totalitarian forms of government, with different degrees of tolerance for dissent. Communist ideology was usually deployed in service of the self-interests of the elite, who maintained rigid control over the reins of power. Like Nazism, Communist ideology, in general, and Marxist morality in particular, could be interpreted in accordance with the taste, as well as the moral or political beliefs of top Party officials. Practically everything was considered "moral" as long as it brought the ideal world of Communism closer to realization.

Establishment of a Communist society was thus the primary goal of Marxist–Leninist ethics. Party leaders claimed to know infallibly how best to achieve this goal and coercively dictated this goal for everyone else. Behind these rules stood enormous state power acting through an extensive bureaucracy, much like the Fascist states. Political theoreticians presented a future-oriented ethics in which every desirable human goal was placed in the future state of Communism. These authoritarian systems, when coupled with state and medical paternalism, made moral pluralism in medical matters almost impossible.

Marxism originated from idealism but became one of the most successful manipulative mechanisms in the history of humanity. Its principal slogan was "the highest value in Socialism – the transitory stage to Communism – is the human being." Yet, ironically, it placed little value on individual human beings. In the 1980s, this very slogan gave critics of Communist society some room to question the system for failing to fill out this maxim with content. In everyday Socialist societies, only a few could experience

the reality of this otherwise attractive principle. In medical ethics, for example, the complete lack of patient rights could only be criticized on the ground of this often-repeated slogan (i.e., if the human being is so important, then why is his dignity or right to self-determination should not be respected?).

Marxists accused Capitalism of alienation and exploitation. Marxist morality was considered a form of ideology in the service of proletarian interests. Medical ethics could not be an exception to this tenet. Such essential features of traditional medical ethics as "the individual patient" or, in bioethics, "individual autonomy" were completely missing from Marxist vocabulary. Communism was defined and understood (although hardly believed) as a socio-economic system that will necessarily replace Capitalism. Communism is supposed to be a classless society in which all means of production are either in the public's interest or in the citizens' hands. Thus, there will be plenty of goods that will make it possible to realize the great principle of "from each according to his or her ability, to each according to his or her needs." Kolakowski, a well-known Marxist critic, says the following about the utilitarian way of reaching that utopian society:

> All repression, cruelties, armed invasions, etc. were justified if they were in the interest of the working class . . . Marx had shown that the decisive feature of the modern world was the struggle between the bourgeoisie and the proletariat, and that this was bound to end in the victory of the proletariat, a world-wide socialist state, and a classless society. (Kolakowski 1978, 1:216)

Nothing can illustrate better how an act on behalf of the dominating class (the proletariat) was justified, than the words of a Hungarian Marxist ethicist, who said the following in an official textbook published for college and university students:

> At times of pressure there maybe such deeds that are allowed (e.g., to spit on the friend during interrogation . . .) But every era has such deeds that can not be forgiven, even at the narrowest conditions of freedom (e.g., under no coercion may a person kill his own mother, *unless she becomes a traitor of the [working] class*). It means that the moral value of a deed doesn't only depend on itself, but on those circumstances too, in which an act is carried out. (Farkas 1978, 115, emphasis added).

IV. The Effects of Communist Ideology on Health Care

After World War II the glorification of Stalin, the Party, and the Soviet state began. The Stalinist type of Communist ideology had a tremendous effect on every aspect of life. Neither the member states of the Soviet Union, nor the Eastern European countries were the masters of their own destiny, because the leading role of the working class simply meant the dictatorship of the Party bureaucracy.

When viewing the whole health care sector, together with health care professionals, it is obvious that ideology played a significant role. Communist Party officials claimed that the working class was not only the dominating class, but the productive one as well. The health care "industry," together with its professionals, were considered nonproductive. Physicians, for example, were viewed as alien to Communism, not only for being nonproductive, but also for being outside of the working class and for still professing certain Capitalist values. One significant sign of this ideological view was the extremely low salary that the Party and state leadership established for physicians (as well as other health professionals). This was almost equal to the salary of semiskilled laborers. Therefore, it is hardly surprising that "tipping" became a prominent everyday practice in all Communist countries. Another example of physicians being an "alienated" class, or rather a low stratum of society, was that their title, "Doctor," was taken away for a couple of years. They had to be addressed as "comrades." Even today, the salaries of physicians in post-Communist countries are shamefully low, so is the salary of nurses. Nevertheless, some physicians could make up for their low pay by taking advantage of the "tipping" system. Not everyone, however, could supplement his or her salary in this way. The system favored those in "fashionable" specializations, who often made enough money through tips to live as well as their Western colleagues. Physicians who were not so fortunate in their choice of specialty, or who refused to accept tips, struggled for their daily survival.

There is a serious and impressive ethical debate in contemporary Eastern European medical ethics about "tipping" (money, material goods, or services and various favors given to physicians either voluntarily or on the basis of pressure, manipulation, or simple demand) (see Chapter 41). In fact, until the end of the 1980s, tipping was essentially the only "medical ethical" topic and "tipping" actually became a synonym for medical ethics. This practice radically affronted Communist ideology, because it contradicted the Party's claim of free health care for everybody. By focusing on the tipping debate, the authorities could ignore the existence of a great number of other ethical issues in medicine and health care. Arguments ranged from the meaning of tipping – for example, gratitude or bribery – to whom should be blamed for the practice, patients or physicians. Even today, many experts think that without this additional – often the main – source of income, the whole health care system would have collapsed. A Hungarian lawyer and ethicist wrote a book on tipping, while the Communists were still in power. Among other interesting things, he said the following:

Tips were calculated in the salary of physicians (even of nurses). The illegal tipping became semi-legal or legal through different interpretations. It spread so much that already in the 60s the concept of free health care was questioned. (Ádám 1986a, 1986b, 137)

According to this author, the Party and state authority silently legalized tipping by refusing to raise physicians' salaries. Another example of the irrational financial treatment of the "nonproductive" intelligentsia (including teachers) can be drawn from the former Soviet Union. Even in today's Russia, a bus driver makes four times the salary of a researcher in the Russian Academic Institute of Philosophy (Tichtchenko, Yudin 1992, 32–3). The "starvation" salary of physicians, nurses, teachers, or researchers – in the whole region – is an enduring legacy of Communism, as is the difference between the state-paid physicians and bus drivers. As far as tipping and combating tipping are concerned, the Pole Szawarski says the following:

> Commissions lack moral and professional authority . . . appearance in the Polish medical world of a peculiar and very ambiguous moral concept "the right to gratitude". According to this concept, if doctors have the right to gratitude – and many Polish doctors, particularly in the provinces, have no doubt that they do – then patients have a duty to show their gratitude to doctors in concrete ways. Whether gratitude should be expressed by a bunch of flowers, a box of chocolates, a bottle of brandy, or a bundle of bank-notes (preferably hard currency) is left to the patient. Another popular concept: patient also has the right to express gratitude . . . doctor has a duty to respect the patient's will and to accept the gift. (Szawarski 1987, 27–9)

One may conclude that Communist ideology can – at least partly – be blamed for the social position and low prestige of physicians, who were considered alienated, reactionaries, and nonproductive, and responsible for many of the ills of the health care system in Communist and post-Communist countries. An ideology that favored the proletariat and treated unfairly those who were not identified as members of this abstract community not only weakened the moral fiber of health care, but insinuated such false values as lies, subservience, and hypocrisy, and "the patient's right to express gratitude."

Besides status, prestige, and low salary, the medical profession could and can still be characterized as very much divided and working under a rigid, feudalistic hierarchy, which makes it impossible to achieve political unity for the purposes of improving medicine and physicians' economic circumstances. As in the larger society, general "norms" of behavior have won prominence, such as a self-serving invocation of solidarity and the permanent and cynical culture of lying and subservience. If, however, the end justifies the means, that is, everything is moral that brings Communism closer, then we should expect lying, dishonesty, egoism and other wicked behavior to become confused with genuine values. When immoral conduct becomes a daily norm at the top of a social hierarchy, then corruption spreads and affects all aspects of life, no matter how insignificant or trivial.

The Communist leadership launched endless programs and political campaigns against tipping. To ensure success, ethics committees were established. As with medical ethics in general, these so-called medical ethics committees were creatures of state ideology and power. Specifically, they were administered by the Physicians' and Health Care Workers Union. Their aim was to oversee the behavior of the medical profession and to condemn those who violated the rules of Socialist morals or its oath. These ethics committees were also supposed to protect those physicians who displayed proper conduct, but were falsely accused. In Hungary, for example, all these rules were codified in the Health Act of 1972. One may note that, according to this Act, physicians had to honor Socialist moral rules. Because these rules had not previously been codified, nobody knew what they were. Strangely, a "workers" union was to control medical ethics and to take disciplinary actions on ethical matters. Because union leaders were trusted Communists, the dominance of Party ideology was ensured. To no one's surprise, the national medical ethics committee consisted only of professors, hospital directors, and chief doctors loyal to the Party. The medical schools also had such committees, but it was not uncommon – neither is it today that no one knew who the members were, sometimes not even the members themselves! Even medical science could not escape from the ever-present domination of ideology. Szawarski says the following about this situation:

> In the sphere of practical life the all-embracing domination of ideology brought about a despotic control over all manifestations of scientific life. This control comprised serious restrictions on communication, scientific debate, and the possibility of foreign travel. Official censorship of all scientific publications and foreign mail became a standard routine. A respect for authority, a rejection of pluralism, a defensive attitude to the revealed truths, became the specific traits of the scientist in a totalitarian society. The most dangerous consequence of this approach was submission to political authorities in scientific matters. (Szawarski 1992)

V. Criticism and Revisionism

Many critics of the system, mainly the so-called revisionists, thought that "Socialism" could be given a "human face." Because the media had to be silent about social phenomena that disrupted the Socialist system, the impression given was that society was practically free of evil. By the 1980s – when individuals were allowed some freedom to speak out – it became obvious that both the Communist economy and the moral basis of Socialism had been eroded by poverty, alcoholism, suicide, corruption, abuse of power, a rising divorce rate, poor living standards of the intelligentsia, contra-selection (selecting leaders, e.g., chief doctors, professors, academicians, not on the basis of professional competence, but loyalty to the Communist Party) vandalism, bureaucracy, and subservience.

This criticism gradually undermined all the pieties of Communism. Critics existed in different numbers in various Communist countries. Lower levels of despotism correlated with higher numbers of critics. There were therefore many critics in Czechoslovakia, Poland, and Hungary, but very few in Romania and almost none in Albania. All the critics wanted some form of democratization, the end of repression, equality in the eyes of the law, and much more freedom for the press and for all other social institutions. They also wanted to abolish the special privileges enjoyed by the Party bureaucracy and those close to them. Among these privileges were such things as special shops, VIP hospitals and medical facilities, priorities in housing and obtaining cars, and hunting privileges. The revisionists originally appeared within the Party and were thus somewhat immune to persecution.

VI. Teaching Ethics and Medical Ethics

Some form of Marxist philosophy was taught in all universities. Marxist Ethics became a mandatory course, but was the least developed part of Marxist philosophy. In Hungary, for example, the teaching of ethics started only in 1962. The Central Committee's Agitation and Propaganda Committee of the Communist Party made a decision to introduce ethics into the curriculum. The real aim, however, was to change the ideological and political thinking of university students. Capitalism was ostracized for its alleged insincerity, injustice, hypocrisy, and other wickedness, whereas the utopian behavior of the Communist man was exemplified and glorified.

Although medical ethics had become a part of the teaching of general ethics in medical universities and health colleges, the ideas of autonomous professional ethics distinct from Marxist ideology were rejected. There were, however, attempts to establish a medical ethics based on Marxism–Leninism that would, therefore, be "scientific." Most likely no one knew what a Marxist–Leninist medical ethics meant, but it sounded good enough to be introduced into undergraduate courses and the medical curriculum as a part of Marxist Ethics. Communist authorities believed that medical ethics could also be used for ideological indoctrination of future physicians and nurses. After all, a totalitarian system forces people to accept its norms and ideology through manipulation, indoctrination, and terror.

How much time a school allocated to medical ethics largely depended on the person who was supposed to teach the general ethics of Marxism and Leninism. Besides ideological brain-washing, medical ethics in the Communist context dealt mainly with medical oaths (usually Hippocrates') and codes and existing laws. Philosophers and physicians taught medical ethics to medical and college students from the early 1960s. Ethics, as well as medical ethics, were taught in colleges and universities only by the departments of Marxism–Leninism. Nowhere in the Communist countries was the teaching of medical ethics nearly as formally established or officially supported as in the basic sciences. Medical ethicists received no training, nor was there any mechanism for formally recognizing them as "medical ethicists." It was generally thought (and still is in certain circles) that medical ethics was an exclusive domain of physicians and only medical knowledge and a bit of wisdom – that usually comes with aging – were all that was needed.

Critical medical ethics was – and largely is – unknown in Eastern Europe. There is no doubt that criticism can only exist in open, democratic societies, where discussing issues critically will not result in losing one's job or having to face retaliation. Thus, it is not surprising that medical ethics, even as it was developing, mainly attracted defenders of physicians rather than patients. Under Communism criticism was very uncommon. If it occurred at all, the critic usually had to follow an unwritten rule: ten lines of praise, one line of critical remarks. Such important issues as the ideal relationship between individual and society, the relative and absolute value of life, family planning, the care of the dying, the management of low-birthweight newborns, prenatal screening, who should make decisions and on what basis, the right to refuse treatment, issues concerning withholding or withdrawing treatments, and how society treats its most vulnerable members were hardly ever discussed. Neither were there workshops, public meetings, nor citizens' involvement in the ethical dimensions of health care policy.

In contrast, in the West, medical ethics under its new name, "bioethics," was a rapidly developing discipline and social movement. One only needs to look at some of the earlier editions of the *Hastings Center Report* or the *Journal of Medical Ethics* to see the rapid development of medical ethics all over the world – except in the Communist world, where all that occurred was the iteration of ineffective and empty rhetoric. Hardly anything in medical ethics happened in Communist countries. Even among those few publications that appeared on the subject, most addressed only trivial ethical problems, and some lacked any critical perspective whatsoever. In Communist Germany, for example, publications appeared praising the high moral standards of research (Tanneberger 1989, 9–10). One had

to wonder, however, to what moral standards medical research in Socialist society was held. Where were these standards written down? Were they better than those of the Helsinki Declaration? The former East Germany was not exactly known for its high standards of human rights or for its patient rights. There were many abuses, from the anabolic steroid treatment of athletes, to the shooting of people who tried to escape over the Berlin Wall or other border crossings to the West. This country was no exception to the general rule that the "the philosophy of medicine was so heavily burdened with the ideology, that it lost sight of its practical implications" (Beese 1991, 24).

Because the physician was the "captain of the ship," it was taken for granted that the patient's duty was to follow his or her orders. The Hungarian sociologist, Agnes Losonczi, described this situation well, when she stated that a sick person did not even have as many rights as the same person when he wanted to have his washing machine repaired (Losonczi 1986, 95). For example, no one asked the parents of seriously ill newborns about decisions regarding treatment or nontreatment of their child. A prominent Hungarian pediatrician stated the following after making a comprehensive survey of his colleagues:

> Paediatricians showed a strong paternalistic approach regarding the question of how life or death decisions should be made. They seemed to regard the treatment or non-treatment of defective newborn infants as a purely medical question, a medical decision which competent professionals alone can make. (Schultz 1992, 20–1)

Despite the "physician's silence," the Soviet Marxist ethicists claimed that there was a general rule concerning truth telling: "by and large one must be truthful to every patient, except in those cases when truthfulness cannot result in therapeutic utility" (Bakstanovszkij et al. 1978, 255).

Only in the 1990s – after the collapse of communism – was medical ethics acknowledged in most Central and East European countries as an independent discipline. Only in the twenty-first century, some years after the radical political changes that have occurred throughout Central and Eastern Europe, the teaching of medical ethics is encouraged in more progressive universities and colleges, and it is beginning to achieve a prominent place in the curriculum of some medical schools.

VII. THE CHANGING STATUS OF MEDICAL ETHICS

The beginning of radical change in the status and perspective of medical ethics took place when the East–West Conference on Medical Ethics was held at the Medical University of Pecs in Hungary in July of 1989, just before the collapse of the Communist system. This conference drew participants from all over Central and Eastern Europe, with the exception of Romania and Albania. The Western countries were mainly represented by the United States of America because the initiator and sponsor of the conference was the Hastings Center. The Center has continued to play a key role in helping to bring together Central and Eastern European medical ethicists and their Western counterparts. It has provided books, journals, forums, and scholarships to a number of medical ethicists in the region. The Centre for the Study of Philosophy and Health Care of Swansea, Wales, joined the Hastings Center's Eastern European Program. The Welch Centre obtained support from the Nuffield Foundation, which has been quite generous in giving scholarships, libraries, and journals to many, then still Communist countries. Excellent opportunities opened up for Central and East Europeans who were interested in medical ethics. The resulting journals, libraries, scholarships, invitations to conferences, and (to) face-to-face meetings have been milestones in many respects for medical ethics and medical ethicists in the region.

One of the results of this collaboration was the creation of the Central and East European Association of Bioethics with the generous help of the Open Society Foundation of New York. This association has initiated cooperation, prompted free exchanges of ideas, and advanced the ideal of human rights in the eighteen countries that have so far joined the Association. Members seem to agree that medical ethics is an important tool to rehumanize and democratize medicine in post-Communist Europe, and at the same time, to elevate the general moral level of their societies. In many of these countries, progressive health laws have been enacted recently that codify many patient rights. In Hungary, for example, a whole chapter of such legislation is dedicated to these rights (Magyar 1997).

Medical ethicists in the region have played significant roles in bringing about these welcome policy changes. If progress is to continue, medical ethics has but one alternative: to take advantage of the slow blossoming of democracy in Eastern Europe and to work to achieve respect and prominence for medical ethics among students, health professionals, policy makers, and citizens.

VIII. Conclusion

More than four decades of Communism have had their effect on the minds of those living today in the post-Communist world. As the Pole, Szawarski, has stated:

> Though all these countries speak different languages, and have different cultural and historical heritage, they have shared a common political fate: for more than 40 years they were all under the political control of the Soviet Union, and their whole social life was permeated by the ideology of Marxism-Leninism. Although the communist

dictatorship belongs to the past it would be unwise to ignore its immense impact on the life and behavior of common people. (Szawarski 1992, 13)

The earlier-quoted Russian authors expressed their skepticism about a quick change:

> A long period of time will be needed for people to believe that physicians have a right not to inform state authorities against their clients, and that there is a strong legal protection for that kind of right. But such a belief could develop only on the ground of respect for the power and authority of law. In Russia there has never been strong legal tradition . . . It will need a lot of time to overturn the vertical relationship of servile "brotherness" of patients and physicians under supervision of the state authority, into a horizontal relationship of civil "otherness" under protection of the law. (Tichtchenko and Yudin 1992, 32–33)

It is quite obvious to many living in post-totalitarian countries that the disappearance of Communism does not mean that its mentality, after many decades of brainwashing, hypocrisy, personality cult, and dynastic rule, has also disappeared. Unfortunately, it is still present. Medical ethics in service to an ideology had and still can have very detrimental consequences. In connection with the ideological influence, for example, in Poland, a prominent medical ethicist made the following comment:

> Recent political changes are increasing the power of vested ecclesiastical interests to impose an authoritarian "ethical" regime on the universities and the population in general. Very conservative laws are being processed in areas such as abortion and contraception, for example. (Evans 1991, 20)

When a government puts all its power and bureaucratic mechanisms in the service of a particular ideology, people suffer. Some are stigmatized, discredited, and even persecuted. Ideologies – sooner or later – are fueled by thirst for power. They generate hatred and permanent conflicts, especially in those countries – like those of Eastern Europe – that had no traditions of democracy. Thus societies could not and cannot protect themselves from ideologies that are forced on them from above by those in power. Morally weak people can easily take advantage of a current ideology to advance themselves. No wonder that some of the hard-line Communists have become impassioned Christians immediately after the demise of the Communist system. One of the lasting effects of Communist ideology is the long and difficult learning process of democracy and the general acceptance of freedom of thought and expression as a primary value, as opposed to identification with an ideology.

NOTE

1. "Tipping" is a particular and unique social phenomenon in the health care systems of the former "Socialist" countries (see also Chapter 41). It is a product of that society, where – mainly due to all kinds of shortages – goods and services could only be obtained by tips that in many circumstances they were nothing else but bribes. After the Communist take over, tipping has spread into all aspects of patient-physician relationship. In the 1990s, ironically tips (usually envelopes padded with money) were taxed by law, so even today, at least theoretically, physicians must pay tax after their tips. There are only guesses about the annual amount of this extra money received by health professionals. Generally, it is estimated to be around 50 billion Forint (approx. $1 = 250$ Forint). This figure, however, does not seem to be reliable, for one thing: because in many cases not even the physician's spouse knows about the exact amount of this 'secret' income. Another reason is that tipping can take many forms: all kind of goods: food, drinks, antique items, books, compact disks; all kinds of favors, for instance, political (promotion), police connection (fixing traffic tickets); better grades to children, easier admittance to schools; free labor with expertise or without it. The practice of tipping – which is still present today – threatens the whole mechanism of the health care system, and it blocks, or at least hinders every reform attempt. It discriminates between rich and poor (in a nominally free health care system!) and divides physicians beyond the possibility of reconciliation.

CHAPTER 57

THE ETHICS OF MILITARY MEDICAL RESEARCH IN THE UNITED STATES DURING THE COLD WAR

Jonathan D. Moreno

I. INTRODUCTION: PROBLEMS AND ISSUES

The role of military establishments in human medical research is one of the least understood aspects of the history of medical ethics. Yet, experimentation involving persons in military service, whether as subjects or as officials authorizing these activities, not only carries with it vexing legal and political but ethical issues as well. The U.S. military also has made important and largely unappreciated contributions to the evolution of regulations concerning medical experiments. One of the ironies of this history is that the deliberate avoidance of the use of soldiers as experimental subjects has often led to abuses of vulnerable persons in their place (Moreno 2001). This chapter sketches this complex story, focusing mainly on certain critical events and incidents immediately preceding and during the Cold War. Medical experimentation during World War II in Germany and Japan is considered for its influence, in the case of Germany, and relative lack of influence, in the case of Japan, on the United States' military policies and guidelines that developed during the Cold War period. These policies and guidelines often anticipated advances in medical ethics in the civilian world. In spite of a number of shocking and unacceptable abuses, much of the conversation and conceptual apparatus that later characterized the bioethics movement that

began in the 1960s took shape in the context of military medicine.

II. THE UNIQUE STANDING OF MILITARY PERSONNEL

Military personnel are generally required to accept medical care that will enable them to return to their post or to accept medical care that will protect their ability to execute their duties. Thus, following the Uniform Code of Military Justice (UCMJ), U.S. Army Command Policy (AR 600–20) states that: "A soldier on active duty or active duty for training will usually be required to submit to medical care considered necessary to preserve his or her life, alleviate undue suffering, or protect or maintain the health of others" (U.S. Department of the Army 1999). A salient issue is whether participation in research can be considered "medical care" and therefore required. Military personnel are protected from coercion or threat of UCMJ punishment by AR 70–25, which states:

> Moral, ethical and legal concepts on the use of human subjects will be followed as outlined in this regulation. Voluntary consent of the human subject is essential. Military personnel are not subject to punishment under the Uniform Code of

Military Justice for choosing not to take part as human subjects. Further, no administrative sanctions will be taken against military or civilian personnel for choosing not to participate as human subjects. (U.S. Department of the Army 1990)

The Department of Defense is also governed by the Common Rule, a standard regulatory regime for seventeen federal agencies that conduct or sponsor research involving human subjects. Current U.S. policy on the use of human subjects is the result of a lengthy and complex debate within the military establishment, a debate that has taken place both in the United States and elsewhere. Although this debate focused particularly on the research participation of military personnel, it applied as well to the funding of medical research for national security purposes that involves civilians as study subjects. This chapter examines the evolving policies and practices in the area of military medical research.

One area that is not covered in this chapter (with the partial exception of the Japanese experiments in China in the 1930s and 1940s) is field tests of chemical and biological weapons. These activities would take us outside the field of medical research proper. Similarly, the role of secrecy in national security research, although mentioned, is not discussed in detail. Nonetheless, one can hardly do justice to the ethics of military medical research involving human subjects without taking into account the security environment within which such studies have often been conducted.

III. Policies and Practices before World War II

Soldiers have long seemed natural candidates for experimentation. After all, the essence of their duties includes exposure to significant risks, including risks proper to innovations that might gain some strategic or tactical advantage over an adversary. Sometimes these innovations are pharmaceutical in nature. Prior to the twentieth century, some deliberate (albeit uncontrolled) drug experiments for military purposes were conducted using soldiers as subjects. In 1883, Bavarian soldiers were given cocaine without their knowledge to see if it would help stave off fatigue. Not all of these activities were nonvoluntary. During the Boer War at the turn of the century, British soldiers were offered typhoid vaccine; few took it in spite of many deaths from the disease (Altman 1998).

No incident in the history of the ethics of military medical experiments is more significant than Walter Reed's turn-of-the-century yellow fever experiment in Havana, Cuba. Before and during World War II, Reed's work was often cited in the United States as a model of ethical military medical human experiments. By 1900, the yellow fever epidemic in Cuba had killed thousands more American soldiers than had the Spanish army in the recent war. Captain Reed and his colleagues on the Yellow Fever Commission were aware of Giuseppe Sanarelli's theory that a mosquito was the responsible vector, although his results were clouded by ethical protests that his subjects had not given permission for the experiment and three had died. The epidemiology of the disease, often affecting all the inhabitants of one house and then skipping several dwellings seemed to support the mosquito theory (Altman 1998).

Several members of the Yellow Fever Commission, although not Reed himself, were among the first to volunteer to "take the bite." One of this first group died, as did a nurse who volunteered later on. To provide decisive confirmation with larger numbers, American soldiers and Spanish workers were recruited. Those who agreed to participate signed an innovative contract designed by Reed that warned them that they might die in the experiment. The workers were also offered 100 dollars in gold to sign up and an additional 100 dollars if they contracted the disease. Their families were to receive the money if they died.

In the decades following the Reed experience, the American military had rules on record that only "volunteers" are to be used in research. At least as early as 1925 the U.S. Army had regulations on "The Prevention of Communicable Diseases in Man – General." By the early 1930s the Navy created a policy for sailors who were working on a new submarine escape device at the Navy Yard in Washington D.C. In 1932, the Secretary of the Navy was given a protocol for the planned experiments. "SecNav approved the request for the work," according to an internal Navy history, "with the understanding that all subjects should be informed volunteers; that the detailed protocol be approved in advance, and that every precaution be taken to prevent accidents." During World War II, the Navy secretary sent a memo "to all ships and stations" requiring that all human experiments involving service personnel receive his approval before they can begin (Moreno 2001, 22). These requirements were not always followed, and in fact they masked a deep ambivalence about how far military personnel could be required to go in serving their country as part of an experiment. In a 1993 report the National Academy of Sciences (NAS) estimated that during World War II more than 60,000 servicemen were used in chemical research, 4,000 with mustard gas or lewisite, its chemical relative. This was a far larger number than had been suspected before the NAS study. Remarkably, virtually all of the subjects kept their promise of silence for decades, partly out of patriotism and partly out of fear of reprisals. Only in the 1980s did their stories come out, when they sought compensation for long-term medical problems they attributed to their gas exposures (NAS 1993).

IV. THE NUREMBERG TRIALS AND THE CONTROVERSY ABOUT MEDICAL ETHICS

Public concern about military medical experiments was largely muted in the first half of the twentieth century; however, human experiments in the military context came under extraordinary scrutiny during the trials of Nazi doctors and bureaucrats at Nuremberg in 1946 and 1947 (see Chapters 34, 50, and 54). It is not generally appreciated that many of the Nazi medical experiments were undertaken for military purposes. The Nazi experiments involved the exploitation of defenseless concentration camp inmates rather than German military personnel. They are relevant to our story precisely because Jews, Gypsies, political prisoners, and others were regarded as preferable to the sacrifice of the flower of German youth. Those labeled as criminals because of their ethnic group or political activity would also have to serve the war effort, in this instance as human subjects (Moreno 2001, 59).

There were four indictments against the twenty-three defendants at the "doctors' trial": conspiracy, war crimes, crimes against humanity, and membership in criminal organizations. The distinction between crimes against humanity and war crimes is important. Crimes against humanity were undertaken in the reckless pursuit of scientific knowledge or from sheer sadism, but war crimes were acts intended to aid the Nazi military. In this indictment, one can perceive the close relationship between the Third Reich's military aims and concentration camp medical experiments (Moreno 2001, 59–62). Many different medical experiments aimed at battlefield medical problems: typhus, phosphorous burns, bone and muscle grafts, the use of new drugs to treat infections, sterilization techniques, and others. Rarely amnesty was granted to those who survived; usually victims were exterminated to eliminate witnesses. Several of the experiments in the war crimes indictment were directed at the air–sea rescue needs of the Luftwaffe: high-altitude rescue experiments, experiments with sustained low temperatures (hypothermia), and experiments in making sea water potable (Moreno 2001, 60–2).

Although the Nazi's defense argued that they were either not personally culpable for the experiments or in some cases not even aware of them, there were two other important themes specific to medical ethics: that there was no international consensus in the medical profession on the rules of human use and that in any case in war medical ethics could justifiably be suspended. On the first point, the judges seem to have been persuaded because they constructed their ten-point Nuremberg Code (actually a third

section of their decision in the case) to address the need for guidance.

On the second point, the Nazi defense also made headway, focusing on human research practices in the United States and elsewhere. Among the most spectacular examples they entered into evidence was the role of 800 American prisoners in a malaria experiment sponsored by the president's Committee on Medical Research. The experiment had been the subject of a several-page photo-spread in *Life Magazine* for June 1945. The subjects were imprisoned at several federal penitentiaries. The defense lawyers also noted poison experiments conducted on eleven condemned prisoners in Manila, cholera and plague experiments on children, and other questionable research with human beings (Moreno 2001, 66–7). In response, the prosecution mainly returned to its contention that the case was not about medical ethics but about homicide: "the use of involuntary subjects in a medical experiment is a crime and, if it results in death, it is the crime of murder" (Moreno 2001, 73–4). The doctor is responsible for ensuring that the subject is a volunteer who understands the nature and hazards of the experiment. No allowance or exception was permissible, according to the prosecution, for reasons of national security. As for the defense doctrine of "superior orders," they could mitigate a soldier's guilt in the heat of battle but not in the case of medical experiments far from combat.

Regardless of the medical ethics controversy, in the end the Nuremberg judges accepted the prosecution's contention that the essential issue before the court was murder. Seven of the defendants were found guilty and hanged, eight were given lengthy prison sentences, and the rest were acquitted, in at least some instances for lack of evidence (Moreno 2001, 81).

V. THE JAPANESE CHEMICAL AND BIOLOGICAL WARFARE PROGRAM

The Germans were not the only Axis military establishment to exploit innocent civilians in experiments that might advance the war effort. From the mid-1930s to 1945 the Japanese military conducted extensive biological and chemical warfare experiments in occupied China (see Chapter 53). The most famous of the individuals in charge of these projects was Dr. Ishii Shiro, whose Unit 731 first operated in and around Harbin, Manchuria, at a prison and laboratory complex of 100 brick buildings. As many as 1,000 prisoners were inoculated with various diseases, in the early years mainly anthrax, glanders (a disease found mostly in horses that can be fatal in humans), and plague, but also cholera. When the subjects became too weak to be of further value they were killed by a poison injection. There were also experiments with cyanide, phosgene gas, and deadly electrical shocks. A much larger facility was built on hundreds of acres in Ping Fan, including 150 buildings with administrative offices, laboratories, worker dormitories, barracks, barns, stables, a farm, greenhouses, a power plant, furnaces to incinerate human and animal remains, a prison for human guinea pigs, and recreational facilities for the Japanese personnel, numbering several thousand. High security was maintained, including constant aerial surveillance above the site. Officially, this was the local Water Purification Bureau installation (Harris 1994, 105). In addition to the experiments on individuals, activity on an immense scale was devoted to the manufacture of pathogens for field testing. Equipment included four one-ton capacity boilers and fourteen autoclaves, each of which held thirty cultivators that Ishii designed. At its peak production the Ping Fan complex apparatus could produce enough cells to provide forty billion pathogenic bacteria over several days. Among the agents produced were plague, typhoid, parathyroid A and B, typhus, smallpox, tularemia, infectious jaundice, gas gangrene, tetanus, cholera, dysentery, glanders, scarlet fever, undulant fever, tick encephalitis, and hemorrhagic fever (Harris 1994, 106).

Various delivery systems were tested, including using several kinds of bombs in the creation of bacterial clouds. From 1939 to 1942, Unit 731 personnel tested their weapons on Soviet soldiers and local populations by using a vast array of methods. More than 1,000 wells were poisoned with typhoid bacilli, for example, and Ishii created a cholera epidemic by "vaccinating" locals in Changchun. He dumped thyroid and parathyroid bacteria into wells and marshes in Nanking and left sweet cakes laced with the stuff where they would be found by poor inhabitants. Rats were released carrying plague-infested fleas, and in Ning Bo the reservoir was stocked with pathogens of cholera, typhus, and plague while they were being sprayed on wheat fields from the air. There were also chemical warfare experiments on Chinese prisoners with mustard gas, altitude experiments in low-pressure chambers, and even frostbite studies. Various means of delivering biological agents with bombs were explored (Harris 1994, 106).

There were no war crimes trials of Dr. Ishii and his colleagues, in spite of several rounds of investigation by American experts. It appears that a decision was made by U.S. occupational forces to exploit whatever information the Japanese military had acquired for their own purposes and to deny it to other powers. The Soviet Union did try a number of lower-ranking Japanese participants in the experiments in 1949, but the defendants were pronounced guilty and given light sentences (Moreno 2001, 114). There has been a longstanding but inconclusive scholarly debate about allegations that the United States used information gained from the Japanese during the Korean War to conduct field experiments against North Korean and Communist Chinese forces. The absence of war crimes trials of Japanese physicians after World War II may explain

the relative lack of influence of the Japanese chemical and biological warfare program on the subsequent development of American military policy and practice in research ethics during the Cold War.

VI. THE EARLY ATOMIC ENERGY COMMISSION AND THE AFTERMATH OF THE FIRST SEVENTEEN PLUTONIUM INJECTIONS

U.S. national security agencies other than the armed forces played a crucial role after World War II, when government officials attempted to develop rules concerning the use of human subjects in unclassified medical experiments. In the course of these post-war deliberations, concepts that would prove critical to the later bioethics movement emerged, but they were soon forgotten and lay dormant for decades.

During the war, Manhattan Project officials had secretly sponsored the first seventeen of eighteen plutonium injections in hospitalized patients. The purposes of these experiments were primarily to assess and improve radiation worker safety conditions, and secondarily to evaluate the potential for the use of radioisotopes in the treatment of cancer (Advisory Committee on Human Radiation Experiments 1996, 135–71). In December 1946, just before the Atomic Energy Commission's (AEC) assumption of control over the nation's atomic establishment, the Manhattan Project suspended human studies until the AEC had the opportunity to set standards and approve the proposed research (Nichols 1946).

In January 1947, the AEC's Interim Medical Advisory Board recommended resumption of the human experiments program that had been suspended with the end of the Manhattan Project. The AEC's general counsel approved an interim authorization for a program of "clinical testing" with radioisotopes, pending full commission approval. The interim authorization included the condition that "It be susceptible of proof that any individual patient, prior to treatment, was in an understanding state of mind and that the nature of the treatment and possible risk involved be explained very clearly and that the patient express his willingness to receive treatment" (Warren 1947).

The AEC general counsel's office at first suggested a written patient "release" for each subject, but modified this position in the face of the objections of the chairman of the Interim Medical Advisory Board, Dr. Stafford Warren. As a compromise, it was agreed that at least two doctors would "certify in writing" that the patient had received an explanation and had agreed to the experimental "treatment" (Advisory Committee on Human Radiation Experiments 1996, 47). The consent issue was much on the minds of AEC officials at this time, partly due to what they had learned about the Manhattan Project's plutonium injection experiments.

The chief of the AEC's Medical Division argued that the plutonium injections should remain classified, citing the "medical legal aspects in the use of plutonium in human beings" (Brundage 1947). It was in this context that the AEC General Manager, Carroll Wilson, wrote to Warren in April 1947 indicating the Commission's formal approval of a continued research program with radioisotopes and describing the standards to be used in clinical research with human subjects. Wilson first stated, "treatment (which may involve clinical testing) will be administered to a patient only when there is expectation that it may have therapeutic effect." Second, consistent with the compromise worked out by the General Counsel's office, Wilson stated:

> It should be susceptible of proof from official records, that, prior to treatment, each individual patient, being in an understanding state of mind, was clearly informed of the nature of the treatment and its possible effects, and expressed his willingness to receive the treatment. (Wilson 1947a)

The letter went on, "in every case two doctors should certify in writing (made part of an official record) to the patient's understanding state of mind, to the explanation furnished him, and to his willingness to accept the treatment" (Wilson 1947a). These three elements – understanding, explanation, and voluntariness – are still considered crucial to the informed consent process. They also appear in the first article of the Nuremberg Code, which was being drafted around the same time as the AEC was developing its statements. In neither case is the historical record complete enough to assess fully the arguments or considerations underlying the selection of these elements. It appears that the AEC's requirement was in fact applied to the eighteenth plutonium injection, the only one conducted under AEC sponsorship. The medical records of the patient at the University of California in June 1947 include a notation stating that the patient, who was "fully oriented and in sane mind," agreed to the procedure after its experimental nature was "explained" to him. This notation met the consent condition set forth in the April compromise, although apparently not the requirement for "therapeutic effect" (Advisory Committee on Human Radiation Experiments 1996, 155).

In addition to the deliberations and negotiations in conjunction with the Interim Medical Advisory Board, a parallel process was taking place within the AEC throughout much of 1947. In June of that year an independent, blue ribbon Medical Board of Review was convened, composed of distinguished physicians and scientists. Their charge was to help set the new agency's biomedical research mission. During its 3-day meeting the Board also considered the conditions under which human experiments could proceed.

These conditions were communicated by Carroll Wilson in response to the inquiry of an AEC-sponsored researcher, Robert Stone of the University of California, who had been associated with three plutonium injections at the University of Chicago. Stone asked to have reports of his research declassified for publication. Wilson denied this request. In a November 1947 letter, he also advised Stone of the policy drafted by the Medical Board of Review in June 1947, which was subsequently endorsed by the Advisory Committee on Biology and Medicine that fall.

In his letter to Stone, Wilson noted that the Medical Board of Review, in approving "the position taken by the medical staff of the AEC," indicated without further qualification that no "substance known to be, or suspected of being, poisonous or harmful" should be used in human subjects unless all of the following conditions were met:

> (a) that a reasonable hope exists that the administration of such a substance will improve the condition of the patient, (b) that the patient give his complete and *informed consent* in writing, and (c) that the responsible next of kin give in writing a similarly complete and informed consent, revocable at any time during the course of such treatment. (Wilson 1947b, emphasis added)

Wilson's November 5 letter to Stone reiterated the dual requirements for a prospect of therapeutic effect and consent (put even more strongly and originally as *"informed consent in writing"*) that were expressed in his April 30 letter to Stafford Warren. The November letter adds a further condition for written informed consent for the next of kin.

Why did the rules that emerged from the Medical Board of Review process, and which resulted in the November letter to Stone, exceed in rigor those worked out by the AEC administrators in consultation with their regular physician advisors, represented in the April letter to Stafford Warren? An answer can be gleaned from the Medical Board of Review's statement of the standards for human research:

> Were it not for the extreme value and pressure for securing reliable information on the limits of human tolerance of radioactive substances there would be no need for explicit reference to this subject [human testing] ... we believe that since secrecy must of necessity mark much of the medical research supported by the federally-sponsored AEC, particular care must be taken in all matters that under other circumstances would be open to investigation and publicity. (Wilson 1947b)

It is not known what the meaning of "particular care" is in this statement. A benign interpretation would be that, considering the burdens of secrecy under which the

AEC operated, the special review board evidently decided that even higher human research standards should apply than those that had already been adopted by the AEC. If this were the case, however, then the subjects themselves would have to be cleared for security purposes, so they could be fully informed. Yet, the review board made no statement on this matter.

VII. THE PENTAGON ADOPTS THE NUREMBERG CODE

During the post–World War II era the AEC was not the only agency within the national security establishment to develop consent rules for human experiments. The Department of Defense went through a lengthy and historic policy-making process of its own in the early 1950s. A 1975 Army Inspector General Report on "Use of Volunteers in Chemical Agent Research" points out that two major events had occurred that influenced discussions in this period. First, the 1947 Nuremberg Code articulated ten rules to govern medical experiments with human subjects. Second, the 1950 Army Reorganization Act vested authority to approve research and development in the Secretary.

The documentary history bears out the Army Inspector General's conclusion. At its September 8, 1952 meeting the Armed Forces Medical Policy Council (AFMPC) heard a presentation from the Chief of Preventive Medicine of the Army Surgeon General's Office concerning the medical services' role in the development of defensive measures and devices.

> It was pointed out that the research had reached a point beyond which essential data could not be obtained unless human volunteers were utilize for such experimentation . . . Following detailed discussion, it was unanimously agreed that the use of human volunteers in this type of research be approved.

The chair of the AFMPC subsequently reported:

> The Armed Forces Medical Policy Council again considered the subject [of human experimentation] at their meeting on 13 October 1952, in view of certain changes in the conditions under which experiments were to be conducted. It was resolved that the ten rules promulgated at the Nuremberg Trials be adopted as the guiding principles to be followed. (Casberg 1952)

Why were the Nuremberg rules proposed as the basis for the Pentagon's policy on human experiments? The answer comes in a letter written by the Administrator of the Armed Forces Epidemiological Board on March 2, 1953.

> It was on Mr. Jackson's insistence that the "Nuremberg Principles" were used in toto in the document [the proposed Pentagon policy], since he stated, *these already had international juridical sanction*, and to modify them would open us to severe criticism along the line – "see they use only that which suits them." (Rapalski 1953, emphasis added)

Stephen Jackson was the assistant general counsel assigned to the AFMPC. It is interesting that a Pentagon attorney in 1953 cited the 1947 ruling by the judges at the Nuremberg Medical Trial as setting international legal precedent to which American researchers should be held. Jackson was joined in his support for this measure by Anna M. Rosenberg, the Assistant Secretary for Manpower and Personnel. Rosenberg was a nationally recognized authority on labor relations. On October 22, 1952, 9 days after the AFMPC passed their Nuremberg Code recommendation, Jackson wrote Casberg the following memorandum:

> I discussed the attached with Mrs. Rosenberg on Saturday. She concurred in the conditions except that she recommended that a provision be added 1. Requiring that the consent be expressed in writing before at least one witness.
>
> I have added such language in the appropriate place under number 1. The new matter is underlined. Mrs. Rosenberg has approved this language.
>
> Mr. Kent the General Counsel, has approved this addition from the legal standpoint.
>
> I recommend that the conditions be so amended. (Jackson 1952)

Thus, not only was the Nuremberg Code and its consent requirement adopted, but also an even stronger written and witnessed consent provision was added. On January 13, 1953 the AFMPC's memo to the Secretary of Defense "strongly recommended that a policy be established for the use of human volunteers (military and civilian employees) in experimental research at Armed Forces facilities," and that such use "shall be subject to the principles and conditions laid down as a result of the Nuremberg Trials" (Casberg 1953).

Finally, on February 26, 1953, the new Defense Secretary signed off on the Council's proposed policy. The memorandum was given the number TS-01188. Paragraph 1 states:

> Based upon a recommendation of the Armed Force Medical Policy Council, that human subjects be employed, under recognized safeguards, as the only feasible means for realistic evaluation and/or development of effective preventive measures of defense against atomic, biological or chemical agents, the policy set forth below will govern the use of human

volunteers by the Department of Defense in experimental research in the fields of atomic, biological and/or chemical warfare. (Wilson 1953)

The use of the term volunteers is common in documents in both the worlds of civilian and military medicine during the period in question. Prior to the 1960s, the term does not appear to have been subjected to close analysis. Rather, it was generally presumed that one was a volunteer if one expressed willingness to cooperate. Short of physical coercion, it was not obvious what the disqualifying conditions would be. The word subject was often used as well, apparently without any systematic intent to use one term or the other.

The second paragraph of the Pentagon policy states:

By reason of the basic medical responsibility in connection with the development of defenses of all types against atomic, biological and/or chemical warfare agents, Armed Services personnel and/or civilians on duty at installations engaged in such research shall be permitted to actively participate in all phases of the program, such participation shall be subject to the following conditions. (Wilson 1953)

The rest of the document mainly recites the Nuremberg Code verbatim, but without acknowledging the origination of the policy in the trials, or that it repeats the Code. One addition is paragraph 2.a. (2). Written in language distinctly more legalistic in tone than that of the Code, it states, "The consent of the human subject shall be in writing, his signature shall be affixed to a written instrument setting forth substantially the aforementioned requirements and shall be signed in the presence of at least one witness who shall attest to such signature in writing." This is the section inserted at the direction of Assistant Secretary Rosenberg.

Routine efforts to pass the defense secretary's top-secret order down the chain of command, and to declassify its content, started almost immediately. Unfortunately, the process was not always successful. According to a report published by the Army Inspector General in 1975, one operation called Top Hat took place at the Chemical Corps School at Fort McClellan, Alabama, between September 15 and September 19, 1953. As described in the 1975 Army Inspector General's report:

This research project, which was termed a 'local field exercise' involved the use of Chemical Corps troops in testing methods of decontaminating biological warfare agents, mustard gas, and nerve gas. A review of the scant literature available on the exercise indicated that it was conducted in contravention of the intent of the Department of Defense and Department of the Army policies. (United States Department of the Army 1975)

The 1975 Army report concluded that Operation Top Hat was probably thought to fall within the "line of duty" of a Chemical Corps exercise and was not regarded as an experiment. Other Army experiments, including especially lysergic acid diethylamide (LSD) testing involving thousands of soldiers during the 1960s without adequate consent, were clearly incompatible with the Pentagon policy.

In another well-known case, a 42-year-old patient at the New York State Psychiatric Institute died in 1953 following an apparently involuntary experiment with a mescaline derivative. The classified research was being conducted through a contract with the Army Chemical Corps, and the circumstances of the death were covered up by the Army and the State of New York (Moreno 2001, 194–9). On the whole, the Army Inspector General reported in 1975 that there had been a "startling . . . lack of consistency in the interpretations" of the Department of Defense policy, citing several examples (United States Department of the Army 1975). The army thus concluded that it had failed to implement its own human experimentation requirements.

VIII. CONCLUSION

The record discussed in this chapter is a mixed one. On one hand, military and national security officials deliberated seriously about the human subjects and conditions most appropriate for human experimentation, and did so with an intensity greater than civilian discussions of medical ethics at the time. On the other hand, the deeper meaning and applications of the policies that were articulated were poorly understood and inadequately communicated to those with authority over human subjects. Soldiers were variously regarded as suitable for exposure to hazardous conditions due to their inherently risky pursuits, or as precious resources not to be "wasted" as human guinea pigs.

As noted above, today the Department of Defense is a signatory of the federal Common Rule, which requires both prior review of research protocols and the informed consent of the subject. By executive memorandum from the president, following the recommendations of the Advisory Committee on Human Radiation Experiments in 1995, classified research must also be reviewed by a suitably cleared internal review board and informed consent is required from human subjects with appropriate security clearances. A permanent rule to this effect is expected to be adopted as part of the Common Rule.

Normal volunteer programs are operated at medical research facilities, for example, at the United States Army Medical Research Institute for Infectious Diseases (USAMRIID) at Fort Detrick in Frederick, Maryland. By treaty only defensive research on biological and chemical weapons is permitted. Volunteers at USAMRIID are drawn from a pool of medics called Medical Research

Volunteer Subjects (MRVS) on assignment at Fort Detrick. A unique aspect of the MRVS program is their representation on the institute's Human Use Committee (Moreno 2001, 276–81)

In general, medical research conducted by the military is today as carefully regulated as any in the nation. There are fully fleshed out rules and procedures, approval takes place at multiple levels, and there is close review and monitoring. Today's military research system is a product of earlier lessons learned. By contrast, civilian medical research involving academic and corporate sponsorship lacks the care and accountability the U.S. military has finally achieved. Other nations' reluctance to allow access to information concerning their medical military activities, including the Western allies, limits the opportunities for similar judgments abroad.

CHAPTER 58

MEDICAL ETHICS AND THE MILITARY IN SOUTH AFRICA DURING APARTHEID: JUDGING HISTORY

Wendy Orr

I. INTRODUCTION

It is well recognized that physicians in the military confront ethical challenges emerging from the dual loyalties of the role of physician, to protect and promote the health-related interests of the patient, and that of the military officer, to protect and promote the legitimate interests of the state through the application of organized violence (or threat of same). The justification for military physicians using medical knowledge for purposes of state interests other than healing patients becomes an ethical challenge, especially when the health or even lives of patients or others are put at risk when physicians pursue such purposes (see Chapters 53 and 57). The role of military medicine in South Africa during apartheid provides a crucial case study of military medical ethics during the post-World War II period. The purpose of this chapter is to explore the ethical issues raised by the conduct of physicians in the service of the South African state and its policies of apartheid.

This chapter examines critically the "just war" justification of using medical knowledge and skill for purposes of the state other than healing patients. This justification is found wanting in the context of international statements on medical ethics that make the role of physician and its moral obligations primary. For example, the

Declaration of Geneva commits a physician to not using "medical knowledge contrary to the laws of humanity" (WMA 1948, 1). The World Medical Association (WMA) Regulations in Time of Armed Conflict state, "Any procedure detrimental to the health, physical or mental integrity of a human being is forbidden unless therapeutically justifiable" (WMA 1956, 1). These statements create a burden of proof that the just war defense cannot meet.

II. THE "JUST WAR" JUSTIFICATION OF THE USE OF MEDICAL KNOWLEDGE FOR PURPOSES OTHER THAN HEALING

No discussion of medical ethics and the military would be complete without a consideration of the just war debate. Many military health personnel invoke just war theory to justify what might otherwise be deemed to be unethical conduct, if judged only on the basis of accepted, international ethical norms for health professionals. In particular, military medical personnel in South Africa who participated in torture, administration of psychotropic drugs for purposes of interrogation, and other human rights violations have justified their conduct with the "just war" argument. In other words, when the safety and security of the state are threatened, the state is justified in taking whatever steps may be necessary to protect itself and its citizens.

As an agent and employee and citizen of that threatened state, the military doctor thus participates in actions that are necessary to preserve the state and are therefore ethically justifiable. This argument is deeply flawed, both in its misuse of the "just war" theory (which, even used correctly, is questioned by many political theorists and ethicists) (Holmes 1989; Howard 1979) and in the complete disregard for the need for ethical medical conduct that takes context, circumstances, and all interests into account.

Just war proponents assume that war is justified "and ask only under what conditions it is justified and how it is to be conducted justly" (Holmes 1992, 212). Various writers have postulated conditions that would fulfill the requirements for the justice of going to war (*jus ad bellum*) and the just conduct of war (*jus in bello*) (Johnson 1984; Osgood and Tucker 1967; Walzer 1977). Numerous international conventions, such as those quoted previously, address the same issue. In summary, for one to be justified in resorting to war, the conditions to be met include: (1) just cause, (2) competent authority, (3) comparative justice, (4) right intention, (5) last resort, (6) probability of success, and (7) proportionality (United States Catholic Bishops' Conference 1983, 30). The principles governing the conduct of war may be summarized as (1) proportionality and (2) discrimination (i.e., the lives of innocent people and noncombatants may not be taken directly) (United States Catholic Bishops' Conference 1983, 30).

If a medical professional working for the military is satisfied that the above conditions for the justice of resorting to war and the just conduct of war have been met (and it would be interesting to determine how many such professionals do indeed take the time to consider this), is he or she then justified in using his or her medical knowledge for purposes other than healing? Is this a situation in which the interests of the patient may "give way to the principle 'The interests of third parties come first'" (Beauchamp and McCullough 1984, 164)? Human rights advocates would argue that individual rights always take precedence and that where medical ethics are subjugated to the just war theory or ethics of war, human rights are inevitably abused.

III. DOCTORS WITH DUAL OBLIGATIONS

1. The Problem of Divided Loyalties

The problem of dual or divided loyalties – simultaneous obligations, express or implied, to the patient and to a third party, especially the state – remains a continuing challenge for health professionals. Health professionals who are also military personnel probably exemplify more than any others the conflict between serving the interests of an employer, the state or institution, and upholding the rights of patients. On the one hand, such physicians are subject to the ethics governing their conduct as health care professionals. On the other hand, they have obligations to protect the safety and security of the state by which they are employed. It is inevitable that these dual obligations will at times seem to be, or actually will be, opposed to each other. The duty of undivided loyalty to one's patient has become a central feature of bioethics. Physicians, nurses, and other health professionals, however, are increasingly called upon by the state or other entities to use medical skills to interact with individuals for purposes other than diagnosis and treatment (Physicians for Human Rights 2000, 1).

Recent experiences of health professionals in Chile, Kosovo, Turkey, and the United States and many other countries demonstrate that the problem of dual loyalty and upholding the human rights of patients is a worldwide problem (Physicians for Human Rights 2000, 1; British Medical Association 1992, 33–63; Stover and Nightingale 1985, 31–5; Chapman and Rubenstein 1998). International codes and statements on medical ethics provide a framework within which dual loyalties can be addressed. The problem of the physician's dual loyalties becomes especially acute in the context of armed conflict. How dual loyalties should be addressed in this context depends vitally on whether the conflict in question meets accepted criteria for being a just war, both *jus ad bellum* and *jus in bello*.

In some situations, subordination of patient interests to the requirements of the state undeniably serves legitimate purposes. For example, reporting evidence of child abuse to authorities may violate confidentiality, but would, hopefully, prevent abuse from recurring. More frequently, however, elevating the interests of the state over those of the patient leads to violations of that patient's rights. For example, in Chile, physicians participated in torture under orders from the military (Stover 1987, 21–34). In South Africa, doctors in the employ of the military injected detainees with lethal substances like Tubarine.[1] Indeed, the information revealed by the South African Truth and Reconciliation Commission (TRC) and the subsequent trial of Dr. Wouter Basson (see later) have demonstrated that medical personnel working for the South African Defence Force (SADF) demonstrated a staggering disregard for human life, medical ethics, and patient rights, which they justified on the basis that they were "fighting a war."

2. Dual Loyalties and International Statements of Medical Ethics

International declarations on medical ethics and research ethics, as well as codes of conduct, have been developed to guide and govern the ethical conduct and practice of the medical profession (see Chapters 50 and 51). Most of these declarations have been developed by the WMA, but some emanate from the United Nations (UN). All member countries of these organizations have ratified the declarations and medical doctors practicing in those countries are expected to adhere to the codes of conduct embodied in the declarations.

It is crucial for the case study undertaken here that these declarations are unequivocal about a physician's primary loyalty. The WMA's *International Code of Medical Ethics* states the following:

> A physician shall... act only in the patient's interest; owe his patients complete loyalty and all the resources of his science; not permit motives of profit to influence the free and independent exercise of professional judgment on behalf of patients. (WMA 1946, 2)

The *Declaration of Geneva* makes a similar, unequivocal claim:

> The health of my patient will be my first consideration; I will maintain the utmost respect for human life; I will not permit consideration of age, disease or disability, creed, ethnic origin, gender, nationality, political affiliation, race, sexual orientation, or social standing to intervene between my duty and my patient. (WMA 1949, 1)

The WMA's *Declaration on Physician Independence and Professional Freedom* continues along the same lines:

> Physicians must recognize and support the rights of
>   their patients.
> Physicians must have the professional freedom
>   to care for their patients without interference.
>   (WMA 1986a, 1)

Many authors have, however, questioned whether the principle, reiterated in these declarations and codes, that "the best interests of the patient come first" is indeed absolute.

> It is a rebuttable presumption that must sometimes give way to the principle 'The interests of third parties come first'... any adequate account of the physician's moral responsibilities must accommodate interests of (other) parties... Some forms of conflict are best resolved in favor of the patient, others present genuine dilemmas, and still others are best resolved in favor of the third party. (Beauchamp and McCullough 1984, 164)

The international declarations quoted above, however, clearly emphasize the primacy of the physician's obligation to protect and promote the patient's health-related interests and the physician's autonomy in determining the nature and limits of this obligation.

Joseph M. Jacob, rather disparagingly, describes professional codes of medical ethics as "a formal, but crude, mixture of morality and etiquette" (Jacob 1988, 7). As shown in many other chapters of this volume, however, it is a serious mistake to read such codes and statements as concerned with only intraprofessional matters or (mere) etiquette (see Chapter 1).

Health professionals working for the military are undoubtedly subject to the same ethical principles, guidelines, and conflicts as any other health care professional. It would thus appear as if, depending on context and circumstances, health professionals working for the military could, at times, justifiably place the interests of the state and/or their employer, above those of the patient. The lack of an absolute principle only aggravates the military doctor's dilemma. What should govern the decision as to whose interests should prevail? Self-interest, and indeed self-preservation, also become considerations, in that the health professional himself or herself may be under threat if he or she does not prioritize the needs of the state. The above international statements would demand that the interests of patients are primary and that physicians should be willing, if necessary, to risk self-interest in order to fulfill the primary and overriding obligations of their role as physicians.

3. Military Doctors and Civilians in South Africa

Military doctors have, historically, played an important role in providing health care services to civilian populations in times of peace. In South Africa, doctors doing compulsory military service were frequently sent to rural hospitals in isolated areas, where few doctors would voluntarily go (South African Medical Services 1997, 6). In addition, doctors in the military services of many nations have provided invaluable services during times of natural disasters and epidemics. For example, South African and British military doctors performed lifesaving relief work during the floods in Mozambique in February 2000.

Even this beneficent role is not without ethical dilemmas. When South Africa invaded Angola and set up bases in northern South West Africa (as it was then called), the doctors and nurses assigned to these bases provided medical care to the local population at times when they were not needed to attend to military personnel. It was common knowledge, however, that this service was part of the propaganda strategy of "winning (the) hearts and minds" of the local population to ensure that they cooperated with the military by passing on information about rebel force movements and by refusing to harbor members of the opposition forces in their villages. When SADF forces (and doctors) were withdrawn from these areas, the local population was abandoned without any sustainable access to health care (TRC of South Africa 1998, 4:121). In such a situation, it is doubtful whether health care workers can truly act with "professional independence" and "without interference" (WMA 1986a, 1).

In times of conflict, military bases are very often the best-equipped and resourced facilities offering medical care. Military doctors are obliged to care first for members of their own armed services however. Physicians and other health professionals employed by the military may be expected or requested to participate in the interrogation and torture of prisoners of war. More frequently, they are expected to provide medical care to such prisoners after the torture episodes, without asking questions or taking any steps to prevent further abuses (TRC of South Africa Report 1998, 4:123, 125; British Medical Association 1992, 40–2).

Regulations adopted by the WMA, state, for example, that:

> Medical ethics in time of armed conflict is identical to medical ethics in time of peace... The primary task of the medical profession is to preserve health and save life... Human experimentation... is strictly forbidden on all persons deprived of their liberty, especially civilian and military prisoners and the population of occupied countries... In emergencies, the physician must always give the required care impartially. (WMA 1956, 1–2)

These guidelines are of minimal assistance in a situation in which a military doctor is under pressure, and indeed desires, to serve the medical needs of his or her injured comrades or believes sincerely that it is necessary to acquire certain information from prisoners of war to prevent further death and destruction.

IV. Chemical and Biological Warfare

1. General Issues

After World War I, which saw the use on an unprecedented scale of chemical agents as weapons of war, the UN General Assembly addressed the issue of the "Use in War of Asphyxiating, Poisonous or other Gases, and of Bacteriological Methods of Warfare" in the Geneva Protocol (UN Organization, UN General Assembly 1952). The provisions of this protocol were elaborated on and refined in the Conventions on the "Prohibition of the Development, Production and Stockpiling of Bacteriological (Biological) and Toxin Weapons and on their Destruction" (UN General Assembly 1972) and the "Prohibition of the Development, Production, Stockpiling and Use of Chemical

Weapons and on their Destruction" (UN Organization, UN General Assembly 1993).

These two latter UN treaties state that, in regard to chemical and biological weapons, signatories to the conventions

> shall never under any circumstances... develop, produce, otherwise acquire, stockpile or retain (such) weapons; use (such) weapons; or engage in any military preparations to use (such) weapons.

In addition, each state that is a signatory to the Conventions shall "undertake to destroy all (such) weapons it owns or possesses."

Subsequent declarations by the World Health Organization (WHO) and the WMA make it clear that it is ethically and morally unacceptable for medical personnel to be involved in the development and/or use of chemical and biological weapons. The WMA Declaration states:

> Therefore, the World Medical Association considers that it would be unethical for the physician, whose mission it is to provide health care, to participate in the research and development of chemical and biological weapons, and to use his or her personal and scientific knowledge in the conception and manufacture of such weapons. (WMA 1990, 1)

The WHO "calls upon all medical associations and medical workers to consider it their moral and professional duty to give every possible assistance to the international movement directed towards the complete prohibition of chemical and bacteriological (biological) means of waging war" (WHO 1970, 1).

2. Offensive and Defensive Chemical and Biological Capacity in South Africa

Doctors and other scientists working for the military may well find themselves in a position in which they are asked to assist in the development of chemical and biological weapon (CBW) or warfare capacity. In such cases, the justification is very often that such capacity is necessary to prepare a defense against a possible CBW attack from an enemy. The argument runs along the lines of: If one is not completely familiar with the agents that an enemy might use, or indeed even one step ahead, one cannot defend one's country against such an attack.

The UN *Convention on Chemical Weapons* declares that

> Purposes not prohibited under this convention means:
>
> a) Industrial, agricultural, research, medical, pharmaceutical or other peaceful purposes;
> b) Protective purposes, namely those purposes directly related to protection against toxic

chemicals and to protection against chemical weapons;

c) Military purposes not connected with the use of chemical weapons and not dependent on the use of toxic properties of chemicals as a method of warfare;

d) Law enforcement including domestic riot control purposes.[2] (UN Organization, UN General Assembly 1993, Article II:9)

The UN Convention on Biological Weapons also allows for research into and exchange of scientific information about bacteriological agents and toxins "for prevention of disease, or for other peaceful purposes" (UN Organization, UN General Assembly 1972, Article X:1).

These clauses leave huge gaps in the so-called prohibition of the development and use of CBW. The interpretation of "peaceful" or "defensive" purposes can be (and has been) perverted to mean whatever the power concerned wants it to mean. In the TRC hearing into the South African Chemical and Biological Warfare Program, Dr. Schalk van Rensburg, a scientist involved in the research and development aspects of a supposedly defensive CBW capacity, held up a piece of paper and said "The difference between defensive and offensive is this thin – depending on what side of the paper is uppermost, your program can be defensive one day and offensive the next" (TRC of South Africa hearings transcripts 1998b).

Once again medicine in the military finds itself subject to two different sets of rules – UN Conventions that allow for the development of chemical and biological agents under certain conditions, WHO and WMA "guidelines" that prohibit the involvement of doctors in CBW under any circumstances. Moreover, interpreting and applying these rules is the very state or the military, to whom the doctor owes allegiance and loyalty as an employee.

3. Project Coast in South Africa

Project Coast, South Africa's chemical and biological warfare program, was conceptualized by the SADF in the late 1970s and initiated in the early 1980s. It was implemented supposedly as a response to the threat of chemical attack from "Communist" (Cuban) forces in the Angolan war arena. Evidence of alleged chemical weapon usage and its effect on civilians in Angola was presented as a justification for the development of a defensive CBW capacity by the SADF.

The program was placed under the auspices of the Surgeon-General of the SADF (who was the Project Manager) and a high-powered "beheerkommittee" (Coordinating Management Committee), but day-to-day control and decision making were in the hands of the Project Officer, Dr. Wouter Basson, a medical doctor. The

Surgeon-General and Dr. Basson both belonged to the medical arm of the SADF, the South African Medical Services (SAMS). The project was thus very clearly located as being formally under the control of military health professionals, although scientists other than medical doctors were also involved in the research and development of chemical and biological agents. It also became evident in the TRC hearing that, although Dr. Basson supposedly reported to the project manager, he also at times reported independently (and without the knowledge of the project manager) to the Head of Special Forces, the Minister of Defence, chief of the SADF, the chief of staff intelligence, and the commissioner of police.

Dr. Basson and other members of Project Coast traveled extensively and established wide-ranging international networks and connections. Travels in the early 1980s, while the program was being set up, included contact with China, the United States, Israel, and West Germany. Once the program was established, further contact was made with the United Kingdom, Belgium, Libya, Croatia and, Switzerland. Although the formal role of foreign governments in supporting Project Coast has not been clarified, it is evident that, without some level of foreign assistance, this project would not have been possible.

Throughout the TRC investigation into Project Coast and the subsequent trial of Dr. Wouter Basson, the Surgeon-General has maintained that the aims and objectives of the program were to develop a defensive capacity only. The exception to this was the intention of the military to develop new crowd control agents, for use in internal riot situations (as permitted by the UN Convention). The evidence produced thus far has revealed gross aberrations of intent, discipline, actions, command structures, financial dealings, and professional relationships. It has also revealed allegations of widespread human rights abuses perpetrated by, under the orders, or with the assistance of doctors working for SAMS or Special Forces.

In addition to the manufacture and stockpiling of large numbers of toxins and bacteriological agents, such as cholera and anthrax, scientists engaged in the project also conducted work, at the behest of Dr. Basson, into anti-fertility agents that would selectively affect black women, produced massive amounts of street drugs such as mandrax and ecstasy (supposedly for use as crowd control agents), and designed and made murder weapons from screwdrivers that could inject poison and umbrellas that could shoot tiny poisoned ball bearings. Perhaps one of the most sinister pieces of evidence to emerge at the TRC hearings was the "verkope lys" (shopping list). This was a list of items supposedly ordered by Dr. Basson from scientists working at Roodeplaat Research Laboratories – a Project Coast front company. The items on the list include cigarettes laced with anthrax,[3] poisoned chocolates, botulinum[4] in milk, paraoxon[5] in whisky, and shampoo mixed with parathion.[6] Not one witness at the hearing was able to explain adequately how such items could be part of a defensive CBW program. In the Commission's view these were clearly murder weapons. This impression was supported by the fact that members of the Civil Cooperation Bureau (a secret government hit squad) revealed in interviews with TRC investigators that it was common knowledge that SADF doctors could provide them with toxins to be used in assassinations.

Evidence has been given at the trial of Dr. Wouter Basson (who has been charged with, among other things, fraud, conspiracy to commit murder, murder, and manufacturing and dealing in illegal drugs) that Basson and other SADF doctors and operatives had been involved in "testing" various toxic agents on detainees. A specific focus of Project Coast seems to have been the development of highly toxic agents, which could be easily and surreptitiously administered, would cause death, and then be undetectable on postmortem.

One individual who gave such evidence was Dr. Kobus Bothma, a doctor with SAMS in the 1980s, who left South Africa in 1993 to practice medicine in Canada. At some stage in the mid-1980s, Dr. Bothma had been given a gel-like substance by Dr. Basson and told to rub it on the skin of a number of detainees to see whether it would have a lethal effect. Dr. Bothma traveled by helicopter with the detainees to a remote part of Kwazulu-Natal, where the experiment was conducted. The gel appeared to have no adverse effects. Dr. Bothma's instructions from Basson were allegedly that, once the experiment was completed, he should inject the detainees with Tubarine, have their bodies loaded into the helicopter and dump the bodies over the Indian Ocean. Dr. Bothma could not bring himself to carry out the instructions, but gave the prisoners a ketamine[7] injection (to relieve their suffering, he reported), then left them with a member of Special Forces, who administered the Tubarine. The bodies were then thrown into the sea from the helicopter. Other operatives gave similar and supporting evidence.

The picture that has emerged from the TRC hearings and investigation and the trial proceedings against Dr. Basson are of science and medicine perverted by the military. The image of scientists in white coats, professors, doctors, veterinarians, biochemists, and engineers, propping up apartheid with the support of an extensive international network and with the might of the South African military machinery behind them is a particularly chilling one. Here was evidence of science being subverted to cause disease, to produce murder weapons, agents of mass destruction, and massive amounts of street drugs –

the latter apparently purely for the personal financial gain of some project members.

V. Conclusion

Of most concern, however, is that almost every doctor or scientist challenged to explain how he or she could have been involved in such unethical research and development work, or even in blatantly gross violations of human rights, resorted to the "just war" argument, to "the challenge of science" justification, or to the "I did not know" refuge.

The "just war" argument has been discussed previously. The "challenge of science" justification rationalizes that a scientific task, undertaken in isolation in a laboratory, can become so absorbing that the end result or ultimate purpose of the experiment or research becomes subsumed by the excitement of solving the scientific challenge and achieving technological breakthroughs.[8] The "I did not know" refuge is an all too familiar one – I did not know that I was working for an SADF front-company, I did not know that my research would be used to develop murder weapons, I did not know what my research would be used for, I did not know that the apartheid government was killing its opponents in cold-blood, I did not know why I was asked to culture millions of cholera organisms, I did not know.

These arguments echo the voices of many of the Nazi doctors at the Nuremberg Trials. It seems that little has changed and that years of war have not taught the medical profession anything about ethics in war or the ethics of war. Hours of deliberations and pages of guidelines and declarations have not brought about any greater protection against abuses. The growth of bioethics as a discipline has done little to guide the day-to-day conduct of medical professionals along more ethical paths. It is immensely difficult for doctors honestly and ethically to fulfill dual obligations. Specifically, the forms of conflict presented to the military doctor seldom present anything other than "a genuine dilemma" (Beauchamp and McCullough 1984, 164) and the basic ethical principles of respect for autonomy, nonmaleficence, beneficence, and justice can seldom be upheld in a situation in which those principles are constantly being challenged.

There are authors who argue that "in principle physicians and psychotherapists can function in the military and can render valuable service to wounded soldiers, even in an unjust war, without violating moral principles. They render service to the soldier as a human being rather than to the soldier as a soldier" (Beauchamp and Childress 1989, 346). At the same time these authors also acknowledge, however, that "Some actions grossly violate canons of medical ethics and thereby warrant disobedience to orders rather than conformity to them. An example is an order for a physician to help torture a prisoner in order to gain information."

History has shown that all too often the needs of the military master supersede those of the patient. Undoubtedly, the services of health professionals are needed in the military, both for the good of civilians and military personnel. Whether those professionals should be employed by and beholden to the military master and subject to military discipline for disobeying an order that conflicts with or "grossly violates" medical ethics is an issue that deserves ongoing consideration and debate.

NOTES

1. Tubarine is an agent used to induce muscle paralysis. Without respiratory support, death from suffocation will result.

2. It is remarkable that this convention prohibits the use of chemical riot control agents as a method of warfare, but allows them to be used internally (against a state's own citizens) for riot control purposes.

3. Anthrax is a highly infectious bacterium, which is usually lethal if acquired via the respiratory tract.

4. Botulinum is a potentially lethal toxin produced by the *Clostridium botulinum* bacterium.

5. Paraoxon is a breakdown product of parathion, which is a pesticide poison.

6. Parathion is a pesticide poison.

7. Ketamine is an anesthetic drug used to induce unconsciousness and amnesia.

8. This specific rationale was offered in the TRC Hearings by Dr. Jan Lourens, a bioengineer who was responsible for developing the euphemistically named "applicators" or murder weapons like the screwdrivers and umbrellas mentioned in the previous section.

C. Medical Ethics and Health Policy

Chapter 59

Making Distinctions "Natural": The Science of Social Categorization in the United States in the Twentieth Century

Dorothy Nelkin and David Rosner

I. Introduction

Biological explanations do political work, writes anthropologist Margaret Lock, "creating the rules for belonging and exclusion" (Lock 1999, 83–113). Scientific criteria have long served as a means to create and justify social categories on the basis of "natural" distinctions. The biological sciences have been used to differentiate "good citizens" (those who, in a prevailing social context, will contribute to work, economic growth, and prosperity) from "bad citizens" (those who are criminally inclined, dependent, unhealthy, or likely to be costly risks). They have been used to identify membership in particular racial and ethnic groups for purposes of entitlements, and they have been used to explain inequalities by casting the differential treatment and status of particular groups as a natural consequence of essential, immutable traits.

The power of science as a means of categorizing people expanded in the late nineteenth century when clinicians and public health officials began to explore the etiology of disease in the distinctive features and susceptibilities of individual patients and their social milieu. Historian Matthew Jacobson describes how the increased focus on the individual had significant implications for many areas of social policy (Jacobson 1998, 113). Scientific fields such as craniometry and phrenology were

developed to evaluate and categorize people according to their behavioral characteristics, susceptibility to disease, and ability to do particular types of work. They became tools in criminal investigations and provided guidelines for employment practices. Immigration authorities also welcomed these scientifically sanctioned techniques as a way to shape the contours of the American citizenry and to weed out those who were likely to become public charges (Jacobson 1998).

These nineteenth-century sciences shared the assumption that outer physical characteristics – body contours, brain size, and skin color – were markers of immutable and heritable traits. Later, eugenicists shifted scientific attention from gross to hidden body systems: they believed that the germplasm determined individual health, character, and personality – and was the basis of group distinctions.

Scientists today use genetic tests to draw distinctions among citizens on the basis of physical, although often nonevident, differences. Identifying "genetic predispositions" through genetic tests is a way to differentiate among individuals. Also, looking for genetic mutations – that is, for the variants that account for the diseases characteristic of certain populations – is a way to identify traits and predispositions that are associated with particular race and ethnic groups. Just as science in the past supported policies based on population stereotypes, science today continues to create social categories, resulting in the exclusion of individuals – from work or immigration – on the basis of the anticipated health risks and the purported behavioral predispositions of particular groups.

This chapter addresses patterns in the use of science-based technologies in creating and reifying social distinctions on the basis of biological categories. Clearly, poverty, social class, and other socio-economic factors are important explanations of disease and behavior. Selective attention, however, has often focused on biological rather than social sources of social problems, and biological explanations, supported by the presumed neutrality of science, have had significant political clout. The contemporary use of biological categories follows directly from the tendency to focus on individual susceptibilities and predispositions in nineteenth- and early twentieth-century medicine. We show how the idea of individual susceptibility underlying the germ theory of disease laid the groundwork for defining suspect groups. The medical community at that time sought to distinguish between and among populations based on heredity, class, or supposed genetic differences. Their scientific assumptions reflected prevailing economic demands and social stereotypes.

Historian Robert Young has noted that: it is often "impossible to distinguish biological science from its economic and political context and from the generalizations which serve both as the motives for the research and which are fed back into social and political debate" (Young 1971, 177–206). We will suggest how both the early sciences of classification and later research on genetic diversity have integrated political ideologies and social agendas into their methods and constructs. Today, scientists argue that race is not a meaningful biological category. Yet, the concept of genetic predisposition has become a way to once again create social categories on the basis of race distinctions. We provide examples of how biology has entered social debate and influenced policies and institutional practices.

II. The Concept of Individual Susceptibility

Our modern notions of science developed in the context of the rapidly growing economy and changing social environment of the late nineteenth century. The constraints, possibilities, and problems of that changing society shaped the sciences of the time in ways that were to significantly affect future social policies. The field of bacteriology, perhaps the most important of the modern medical and public health sciences, is a case in point. This field emerged in the United States in the midst of massive immigration of peoples from Southern and Eastern Europe. In little over four decades, millions of Eastern European Jews, Slavs, Greeks, and Italian Catholics fundamentally altered the demographics of the nation. So too, immigration fundamentally altered the assumptions underlying public health and medical practice. Whereas older sanitarians had sought ways to alter the environmental circumstances of the poor to stop the transmission of disease, the new public health and medical practitioners increasingly defined disease in terms of a particular entity – the germ. Before the bacteriological revolution, wrote historian Charles Rosenberg, "the body was seen, metaphorically, as a system of dynamic interactions with its environment. Health or disease resulted from a cumulative interaction between constitutional endowment and environmental circumstance" (Vogel and Rosenberg 1979, 5). Hibbert Hill described the changes at the end of the nineteenth century, "The old public health was concerned with the environment; the new is concerned with the individual. The old sought the sources of infectious disease in the surroundings of man; the new finds them in man himself" (Hill 1916, 8).

Before the 1880s, clinicians and public health workers held significantly different conceptions of health. Whereas physicians saw sick patients and sought to identify the cause of disease and treat its symptoms, public health workers addressed the problem of environmental control, stressing the importance of personal and public hygiene. Sanitation, the inspection of meats, sewage, housing, immigration control, and the provision of clean water and air were critical to the mandate of the public health professional.

The discoveries of Pasteur, Lister, and Koch created a new faith in laboratory science not only among physicians but also among public health workers. "Bacteriology became an ideological marker, sharply differentiating the 'old' public health, the province of untrained amateurs, from the 'new' public health, which belonged to scientifically trained professionals," points out Elizabeth Fee (Fee 1987, 19; Rosenkrantz 1972, Chapters 3 and 4). Despite their different professional mandates, public health workers and physicians began to share a common faith in the significance of the disease-specific germ entity.

These changing ideas about communicable diseases were especially important to the understanding of tuberculosis, commonly called phthisis or consumption. For much of the nineteenth century, consumption was assumed to be a disease peculiar to an individual's social position as well as personal qualities. A coal miner, for example, might contract a special form of consumption known as "miners' con," whereas glass blowers, rock cutters, grinders and others were considered particularly susceptible to industry-specific forms of the disease. According to Ludwig Teleky, a noted industrial physician and author of the first history of industrial hygiene, by 1881, the year of Koch's discovery, there was "a vast knowledge of [the importance of] dust on the lungs" and its relationship to consumption (Teleky 1948, 199). Suddenly, the study of its industrial etiology and the effect of dust in the workplace ceased: "All cases [of phthisis] were [now] diagnosed as tuberculosis," a bacterial disease caused by a germ, not one's social class circumstances (Vogt 1948).

American public health and medical professionals sought to reconcile the many symptoms of phthisis and consumption with the new "scientific" germ model of disease. If they were to mount an effective campaign to eliminate the sources of the disease, the modes of transmission of the bacteria had to be isolated and the most vulnerable populations identified. Questions turned to the differential susceptibility of various groups. Why was it that the poor were so likely to be struck by disease? It was because the germ propagated and spread among a population weakened by innate susceptibilities rooted in both their inherited as well as environmental circumstance. Why was it that children appeared to be a high-risk group? It was because tainted milk from tubercular cows poisoned children from particular social classes or ethnic groups. How was it that individuals outside of particular risk groups came down with the disease? Because they had a hereditary predisposition that left them vulnerable to infection.

Although all those suffering from the common symptoms of coughing, wheezing, and spitting blood had phthisis, the disease seemed to take on different meanings for different social classes. For middle class sufferers, the disease appeared in an almost romantic light. The translucent flush of Victorian ladies suffering from this disease became a standard image in the nineteenth-century novel. For the working class, huddled together in the slum dwellings of large cities such as London, Paris, New York, the disease was far more sinister (Dubos and Dubos [1952] 1987, 69).

The apparent idiosyncrasy of the symptoms that marked phthisis among different individuals and social classes during most of the nineteenth century reinforced prevailing ideas about the nature, cause, and treatment of disease. Phthisis could be linked to the on-going, long-term moral and social environment that predisposed a victim to a disease process. It could be rooted in personal behavior such as drinking, social position, poor living quarters, malaise of urban life style, or unhealthful work. "Treatment was to be sensitively gauged not to a disease entity but to such distinctive features of the patient as age, gender, ethnicity, socioeconomic position, and moral status, and to attributes of place like climate, topography and population density" (Warner 1986, 158). The nineteenth-century practitioner needed to have a complete knowledge of the life history of the patient to make an accurate diagnosis and plan of treatment.

As phthisis was redefined as a bacterial crisis of susceptible individuals, the very victims of disease were presented as its propagators: "A careless or ignorant expectorating consumptive can eliminate and distribute seven billions of bacilli in twenty-four hours," warned S. A. Knopf in

the journal *Charities* in 1901. "You know that the expectoration . . . when allowed to dry and pulverize, may, when inhaled with the dust of the atmosphere, give tuberculosis" (Knopf 1901, 76). A focus on the victims was also the solution to threatened epidemics. Journals declared that responsible tuberculars could stem the disease. They were encouraged to carry and use flasks to dispose of their spittle so that "it cannot dry and be blown about to be inhaled by others." The leaders in public health practice believed that "to control tuberculosis, it was not necessary to improve the living conditions of the 100 million people in the United States, only to prevent the 200,000 active tuberculosis cases from infecting others" (Fee 1987, 20–1).

If the specificity of the bacterial agent and the assumed biological characteristics of the target group were most important, the earlier emphasis on cleaning up the general environment seemed misdirected. This shift in emphasis had a profound impact on the practice and organization of environmental control and on social policies in the early years of the century. After all, if the victims' bodies were the source of disease, public authorities would be relieved from the burdensome responsibility of controlling the forces of production, industrialization, and housing.

III. From Individual Susceptibility to Suspect Groups

The attention placed on the characteristics and vulnerability of individuals had particular salience in the United States in the decades between 1880 and 1920 when nearly 20 million poor Southern and Eastern Europeans arrived. These immigrants faced a mixed reception. The industrial revolution and the labor needs of the changing factory in the nineteenth century called for an increased supply of cheap labor, so the seemingly endless flow of immigrants was convenient. The demand of the new industrial workplace shaped assumptions about the physical, cultural, and intellectual characteristics of a "healthy" and productive citizen. Independence, creativity, and skill were often less valued than the ability to adapt to the industrial assembly line and the scientifically managed factory. At the same time, the desire to create a cheap and obedient labor force drawn from the ranks of immigrants conflicted with the interests of domestic workers who wanted to avoid competition from cheap immigrant labor. The need for cheap labor often conflicted with government concerns about draining public health and social service resources and the desire to exclude those likely to carry disease or to become public charges. Debates ensued concerning the relative importance of moral quality, high IQ, or robust physical health in shaping the new American citizenry

The eugenics movement guided social policies during this period. Driving the eugenics movement was the belief that biological improvement was a critical national need. American competitiveness, economic stability, and social order seemed to rest on the differential reproduction of certain classes and races, and on selective immigration policies. The assumptions of eugenics incorporated a complex set of beliefs based on the idea that hereditary material (the "germplasm") was the determiner of disease susceptibility, character, behavior, and personality traits.

Eugenics was not a single coherent idea but a fragmented public discussion that served many agendas. According to eugenicists, intelligence and feeblemindedness, special talents and criminal tendencies, industriousness, alcoholism, laziness, poverty, loquacity, harlotry, and vagrancy were all hereditary traits that distinguished certain families and groups. Scientists and public health workers searched for pathological families. The Race Betterment Society offered awards for fitter families and "better babies."

Leading authorities in the fields of medicine, public health, and other scientific fields formed an implicit alliance to focus on individual heredity as the basis of social reform. "That the marriage of those carrying hereditary taint should not be permitted is the general opinion and the same is sustained by the science of eugenics," wrote Dr. J. N. Hurty, President of the American Public Health Association and Commissioner of Health for the State of Indiana in 1912: "[C]ertain persons should not be permitted parenthood" (Hurty 1912, 315–20). Hurty, speaking for a good portion of the public health community, was seeking to develop a uniform system for the regulation of marriage throughout the country.

From Hurty's public health perspective, the passing of heritable traits from one generation to the next promised to weaken and destroy the character as well as the health of Americans. He reminded his readers of the Jukes family, ostensibly a family of "imbeciles," that proved the heritability of intelligence. Hurty noted that various states had prohibited the young, siblings, parents and children, syphilitics, and whites and blacks from marrying. Why not establish uniform codes that extended local laws to include imbeciles? Indiana, he proudly noted, already banned the marriage of imbeciles, epileptics, along with "any male person who is or has been within five years an inmate of any county asylum or home for indigent persons" (Hurty 1912).

Immigration was also troubling to many Americans bent on perpetuating "good American stock." Nativists were convinced of the biological inferiority of specific groups, their feeblemindedness, propensity for degeneracy and crime, and congenitally poor health. Stereotypes – of the neurasthenic Jews, the criminally inclined and tubercular Italians, and the parasite-infected Asians – proliferated (Markel 1997). The dumping of "heterogeneous masses" wrote Thurman Rice, a eugenicist from Indiana in a book called *Racial Hygiene*, defied the laws of biology, "the laws of nature" (Rice 1929).

Consumption, particularly, became viewed as a "foreign" disease, one that resided among the immigrant and the poor. The poor were "carriers," spreading disease to the unsuspecting and the defenseless Americans. The poor themselves and the communities in which they lived, were often considered "seedbeds" of tuberculosis in the early 1900s, remembered Frances Perkins, the Secretary of Labor under Franklin D. Roosevelt. "It was our happy practice to console ourselves with the thought that the residents of [the Lower East Side of New York] were almost entirely of Irish extraction," Perkins wrote, "and the Irish, we thought, were the 'seedbed' of tuberculosis" (Perkins 1940, 7–0–4(3)).

Nativists also assumed that the physical and ethnic differences of immigrant groups were markers of their moral and intellectual qualities. They sought to restrict immigration to "those who looked like Americans" (Jacobson 1998, 78). To Harry Laughlin, a prominent eugenicist, immigration was an "investment in hereditary traits." Backed by eugenic studies sponsored by the Carnegie Foundation, he petitioned Congress for race quotas – meaning at that time limiting Mediterranean peoples and encouraging Nordics who would become "useful citizens."

The United States Marine Hospital Service, to become the Public Health Service in 1912, was given the dubious task of inspecting in-coming immigrants for physical and mental disabilities that would disqualify them for entrance. At Ellis Island and at other ports throughout the country, medical officers, in their forbidding military uniforms, were among the first officials faced by new immigrants as they were inspected and screened for communicable diseases or mental limitations. The murky boundaries between science and social prejudice often informed the reason for exclusion or quarantine (Fairchild 1997).

To justify exclusionary practices, officials sought out scientific tools of evaluation. They needed "objective" criteria – ways to measure "natural" human differences, detect health risks, and help decide who should be admitted or excluded. The tools and concepts of science were viewed as neutral ways to refine immigration polices and workplace practices, but scientific measurements themselves were influenced by prevailing stereotypes about natural distinctions.

IV. EVALUATING PEOPLE THROUGH SCIENTIFIC MEASUREMENTS

Eugenicists assumed that social, moral, and intellectual differences had physical manifestations (Cooter 1984). The bodies of criminals, wrote anthropologist Henry M. Boies, "Diverge in some essential respect from the normal type of mankind" (Rafter 1997). So, they employed the nineteenth-century sciences of craniometry and phrenology to identify these distinctions. Scientists measured the heads of prisoners to study the relationship of skull contours to behavior. They disinterred Native American bones to study the physical manifestations of behavioral differences between races and they used the remains to support theories that nonwhites were intellectually and morally inferior.

Brain collections, documenting and demonstrating human differences, proliferated. Burt Green Wilder, a professor of animal husbandry at Cornell University created at Cornell the first brain collection in the United States, intending to show the relationship between brain structure and race, and intelligence and personal idiosyncrasies. He collected nearly 200 brains, including those of criminals, common people, college professors, and women.

The new discipline of psychology emerged in the early twentieth century as a further means to evaluate and categorize people on the basis of natural distinctions. Tracing the historical development of psychology as a credible scientific discourse, sociologist Nikolas Rose, documents how the discipline was driven by the needs of schools, reformatories, the army, and the factory. These institutions, faced with rapid social change, tried to identify individual differences and to predict future pathologies to meet their evolving demands. The field of psychology developed "as the science of individual differences, of their conceptualization and their measurement . . . and of the prognoses of future conduct in terms of them" (Rose 1985, 5).

The psychometric instruments developed by psychologists were widely used to evaluate new immigrants. These tests, evaluating intelligence, generally ignored the effect of cultural and language differences. Yet psychologist Henry Goddard claimed they demonstrated that two of five immigrants could be classified as feebleminded and that the Mediterranean races were intellectually inferior to the Nordic race (Kevles 1985).

Ideas about "natural distinctions" also shaped the development of scientific measures to evaluate production workers and to create a more efficient workplace. The human body has long been conceived of as the basic production unit that has created wealth and capital. From the early debates over workers' compensation legislation, insurance industry death benefits, and compulsory health insurance to the recent litigation over asbestosis and silicosis and other occupational diseases, the workers body has been valued, monetarized, and commodified and effectively regarded as a machine. This mechanistic and monetary view of the workers body encouraged placing differential value on human beings. The very language used to describe workers' bodies has reflected such evaluations. The "counting" of the industrial dead; the death "toll" of industry; the "costs" of industrial expansion were constant metaphors in the legal, popular, and professional literature describing industrial accidents and disease. Degrading human life by measuring its worth in dollars and cents had the practical impact of controlling and amortizing the costs of production as industries sought to rationalize their own accounting, as well as production processes (Rosner and Markowitz 1987).

Reducing biological complexity to the physical interactions of springs, levers, molecules or, most recently, to molecular and genetic components is fundamental to certain traditions in biological thought (La Mettrie [1748] 1994, 93). The metaphor of the body as machine also became a tool in broader social debates about who should work, where, and under what conditions.

In the years between the Civil War and World War I, the United States emerged as a dominant industrial power. Substantially agricultural in the years before the Civil War, the United States quickly emerged as the leading producer of coal, steel, railroad tracks, outstripping England, Germany, and France in virtually every index of industrial production. A chronic shortage of labor led to historically high wages among the artisans – and a significant degree of labor militancy – among skilled workers who, for most of the nineteenth century, controlled production.

This chronic problem of high wages, labor shortages, union militancy, and unparalleled abundance of untapped resources led many to grudgingly accept the rapid influx of immigrants into America's cities in the late nineteenth and early twentieth centuries. Immigration promised relief from the chronic labor unrest, high wages, and unity that had led to paralyzing strikes in the 1870s and 1880s. This need for the efficient use of relatively scarce labor also created an unparalleled attention to efficiency in production. In place of a system of factory work where skilled artisans controlled the entire production of an object from beginning to end, theorists began to develop systems of "scientific management" that sought to replace the empowered worker with replaceable, interchangeable, and powerless cogs. The assembly line transformed the lives of the labor classes.

In 1911, Frederick Winslow Taylor, in his famous manifesto on *The Principles of Scientific Management*, posited that work could be broken down into discrete, interchangeable tasks and that workers could be taught to perform specific discrete tasks efficiently. Taylor's followers maintained that, if work were organized properly, workers' bodies were effectively interchangeable parts that could be replaced when they became too demanding, too inefficient, or broken. Challenging the prevailing system of production in which skilled labor controlled the speed and methods of production, Taylor, and the industrialists who adopted his scheme, sought, according to historian David Montgomery, to take the brain [read: control] of the worker and put it under the manager's cap (Taylor [1911] 1985, 114–15).

Workers, once skilled and largely in control of the speed of work and hence the levels of production, were now preconceived as units of value, and categorized by their supposed biological limitations and potentials. A language of accounting slowly assumed a centrality in the new field of "scientific management," that saw the common laborer as a mechanical part of the production process that could be replaced at the behest of management. This popular image of workers as little more than an interchangeable part played an important role in management's war with labor. The creation of a workers' compensation system that required the evaluation of lost limbs, lost eyes, or hearing, provided further evidence of the commodification of the body. The adjustments of compensation in court cases according to age and potential earning capacity of the injured worker linked the value of the human body to the work place.

If the changing methods of production redefined the workers body, they also influenced the definition of disease. Just as epidemic diseases, borne by water, air, or human contact were paradigmatic of nineteenth-century urban life, so short-term industrial poisonings and long-term industrially related illnesses characterized twentieth-century industrialization. Devastating lung conditions such as silicosis increased among working class populations as high-speed pneumatic drills and jackhammers, sand blasting equipment, and dynamite replaced the pick and shovel. Similarly, angiosarcoma of the liver, as well as bladder and brain cancers increased among workers in the growing plastics and petrochemical industries. The rigors of the new work environment called for the selection of workers whose bodies could withstand the pressures and poisons of the workplace.

The reductionist and mechanical images of the body underlying the tools of Taylorism and the practices of scientific management were to influence the reception and applications of the "new biology" that began to emerge in the 1970s. For advances in genetics offered new possibilities of evaluation and selection on the basis of scientific predictions about future health and behavior.

V. The New Biology after World War II

After World War II, the much-publicized payoffs for medicine – the Salk vaccine, antibiotics, transplantation – brought considerable prestige to the medical sciences. The new biology, following Watson and Crick's discovery of the double helix, was expected to produce the next medical miracle, and biotechnology was expected to generate unprecedented economic progress. As a reporter put it: "After years of being a dowdy old lady, biology has become belle of the ball" (Nelkin 1995).

The diagnostic possibilities arising from the new biology were welcomed for their economic as well as clinical implications. Just as eugenics had once appealed as a tool of evaluation and classification, so the predictive power of genetics appealed as a way to anticipate who was fit to survive in an increasingly competitive world. Genetic testing could provide predictive tools for institutions hoping to make actuarial calculations about their workers on the basis of science (Nelkin and Tancredi 1995).

The explanatory powers of genetics also had ideological utility. The rapid growth of cities during the 1970s had generated controversies over how to deal with the social problems of urbanization – the urban violence, drug use, the disruption of the nuclear family. Who was to blame? Just as planting the blame for infectious disease on individual vulnerabilities appealed to nineteenth-century public health officials, so too, the idea that some people are genetically predisposed to "bad" behavior appealed in a way to relieve the state and society from collective responsibility for social problems. For some, it offered an antidote to the liberal egalitarian theories of the 1960s and its expression in the controversial Great Society Programs (Murray 1984). Distinctions among individuals could be attributed not to social conditions but to the genes, and differences among groups could be interpreted as biologically ordained.

In 1969, Arthur Jensen published his well-known essay: "How Much can we boost IQ and Scholastic Achievement." Jensen argued that there was a significant average difference in IQ between blacks and whites and attributed this difference in part to genes. The pubic discussion of Jensen's work opened the floodgates to others opposing the Great Society Programs. Richard Herrnstein wrote, in a 1971 *Atlantic Monthly* article, that intelligence was 80% genetic and that the genetic inferiority of blacks accounted for their lower social position. The Pioneer Fund, a eugenic organization formed in 1937 by the eugenicist Harry Laughlin, supported many scientific studies purporting to show the biological bases of race stereotypes. The Fund both supported and publicized this work and directed it to influential policy makers.

By focusing on biology as a determining factor, these studies tried to undermine the optimistic visionary Great Society advocates whose claim for social policy resources assumed the mutability and improvability of human beings. Ideas about biological distinctions appealed in the context of growing concerns about domestic problems. The increasing cost of welfare programs and the changing ethnic composition of cities, encouraged speculation about the role of racial characteristics in perpetuating poverty and violence. Terms such as "welfare mothers" and "urban underclass" became euphemisms for race, and the biological arguments had policy influence.

In a speech describing primate studies, Dr. Frederick Goodwin, Director of the National Institute of Mental Health under the G. H. W. Bush administration suggested that "the loss of social structure in this society and particularly within the high impact inner city areas has removed some of the civilizing evolutionary things that we have built up, and maybe it isn't just the careless use of the word when people call certain areas of certain cities, 'jungles'" (Goodwin 1992). He later created the Violence Initiative at National Institute of Mental Health that included research efforts to identify people who may be biologically prone to violent behavior.

A number of popular books appeared in the early 1990s offering genetic and evolutionary explanations for race distinctions. Among the most inflammatory writers was J. Philippe Rushton who argued that blacks have larger penises and smaller brains than whites, explaining differences in educational and reproductive performance. Racial variations, he contends, are a consequence of evolutionary pressures. As humans entered the colder climates of Europe, the environment favored those who had genes for organizational skills and sexual and personal restraints. There was, he claims, a tradeoff between brain size and reproductive potency (Rushton 1994). Rushton's ideas were a modern variant of the old hypothesis that bodily differences between race groups account for differences in social, political, and economic status. He was not the only person disseminating these ideas. Race theorists were increasingly willing to express their views about the biological basis of race differences and suggest the implications for social policy. Then, Richard Herrnstein and Charles Murray, in *The Bell Curve*, moved the debate over genetic differences to center stage (Herrnstein and Murray 1994).

These social categorizations are beginning to take on a more "scientific" tone as fields such as behavioral psychology, evolutionary biology, and sociobiology draw authority from "harder" scientific developments in molecular biology and genetics. The writing in these fields, directed to a broad readership is providing a language through which group differences can be interpreted as biologically ordained. These sciences play a strategic role in continued debates over race and ethnic differences, reinforcing old ideas about human distinctions and the role of individual susceptibility in the understanding of human behavior and disease.

VI. Genetics and Natural Distinctions

The Human Genome Project has justified its budgetary demands by promising to resolve the problems of diseased bodies and deviant minds through an understanding of the genetic basis of behavior and disease. The work of geneticists involves the study of the gene variants that correlate with predisposition to disease. Genetic textbooks and research proposals begin with a common narrative: health and behavioral problems lie in "genetic predispositions."

Since 1994, improvements in automatic sequencing and information processing have enhanced the ability to analyze DNA proteins and other gene products, and to isolate the alleles that are disruptive of normal functioning. These changes have accelerated the development of tests that can detect ever-more subtle biological differences and predict disease before the manifestation of symptoms. A 1996 survey by the National Institutes of Health Task Force on Genetic Testing found that more than 450 research programs were developing genetic tests for hundreds of genetic conditions, allowing the prediction of the health status of asymptomatic individuals (NIH/DOE Task Force 1997). The research includes efforts to detect predisposition to behavioral and personality characteristics as well as disease.

The concept of predisposition – of genetic risk – is open to broad interpretation. Technically, a predisposition is a biological condition signaling that an individual may suffer a future disease or behavioral aberration: predisposition is a statistical risk calculation, not a prediction. In its clinical meaning, to be predisposed is to be at risk for a disease or condition that may or may not be expressed in the future.

In its social meaning, however, DNA – like the germplasm of the eugenics movement – is a "blueprint of destiny." Those who carry the traits for certain disorders can be reconceptualized as "persons at risk" whose potential condition differentiates them from "the normal," and labels them unsuited for normal opportunities (Lippman 1991). People diagnosed as predisposed to a behavior or disease are treated as if it were certain to be expressed, even when the relationship between genetic mutations and their phenotypic expression is conditional, poorly understood, and subject to interpretive fallacies (Billings et al. 1992, 476–82).

Uncertainties in the interpretation of genetic information are especially problematic when tests are used to screen populations – for example, in screening workers for genetic susceptibility to toxic substances. The purpose of screening (unlike clinical testing) is not to discover the cause of manifest symptoms in an individual, but to deduce statistical levels of disease in a population. Population susceptibilities – for example, the prevalence of sickle cell anemia among African Americans or breast cancer among women of Ashkenazi descent – are based on statistical assumptions and say little about the health status of a given individual. Yet, risk predictions on the basis of genetic information about a population can have consequences for individuals identified with that population regardless of their individual state. In effect, such predictions become a measure of natural distinctions.

The association of genetic predispositions with different populations is an old story, reflected in the early immigration debates; however their revival is especially ironic in light of current scientific understanding. One of the insights of genetic research is the profound similarities at the level of DNA among human beings. The lesson of molecular genetics could be that we are all very much alike. Moreover, modern geneticists seek to set themselves apart from early eugenicists by focusing on individual predispositions. Yet, genetics is still appropriated to support arguments about distinctions among populations, and the research in this field is itself based on tracing these population distinctions (Duster 2001).

Geneticists acquire information about predispositions by finding the markers that co-segregate with genes for illness among members of families or groups with a significant prevalence of a particular hereditary disease. So far, genes have been located for disorders such as Huntington's and Tay Sachs that are caused by mutation in a single gene. Scientists are now seeking to decipher the genetic basis of more complex diseases, and they are also trying to isolate the genetic basis of behavioral traits and disorders – from manic depression to Alzheimer's disease, from shyness to aggression.

Research on predispositions has led to quests for the sources of genetic diversity and for particularly "interesting" and, therefore, potentially valuable genes in various populations. Scientists are searching for the genetic variants that leave some people more susceptible than others to the effect of environmental chemicals. The Centers for Disease Control and Prevention is developing a program on genetics and public health. The purpose is to assess the population distribution of selected genotypes and the public health impact of interactions between genetic variation and environmental risk factors.

Studies of the social and ethical implications of the Human Genome Project have proliferated, often supported by the ethical, legal, and social (ELSI) implications of the project. They mainly focus on the implications for individuals as predictive information about their health becomes increasingly available. They raise questions about the privacy of genetic information, the potential for abuse, and the dilemmas of individual choice when there are few therapeutic options. A distinct set of implications has to do with collective risks – the way information about genetic predisposition can affect race and ethnic groups through the association of genetic diseases with particular populations. As institutions use predictive information from genetic tests to create distinctions on the basis of anticipated health risks and behavioral predispositions, they may categorize individuals, not because of their personal condition, but the predispositions attributed to their group or race (Juengst 1999, 61–82).

VII. RACE DIFFERENCES AND THE METHODS OF SCIENCE

The virtual continuum of genetic variation suggests that, scientifically, race is a meaningless category. Yet underlying the search for disease genes is an assumption that genetic diversity is an important clue to differential

predispositions. Geneticists thus rely on and search out distinctions to do their research. Populations known to be susceptible to a particular disease are valuable resources for studies of genetic risk. With a stunning blindness to historical sensitivities, geneticists have employed recruitment strategies (e.g., advertising for Jewish genes) that emphasize the correlations between race and specific diseases. Ideally, scientists hope to find "genetically pure" populations, assuming their genes will reveal information about genetic variation. This assumption underlies the Human Genome Diversity Project (HGDP), planned in 1992, and the "gene hunting" by biotechnology companies seeking disease genes from isolated populations throughout the world.

Many genetic diseases and conditions are indeed statistically associated with particular ethnic populations. Tay Sachs disease and certain forms of breast and colon cancer are prevalent among Jews of Ashkenazi descent; Thalassemia among Mediterranean people; and sickle cell, hypertension, and diabetes among people of African descent. Some genes predispose certain groups to particular diseases – asthma susceptibility genes are found among the isolated people of Tristan da Cunha, Easter Island, and the Brazilian Highlands. Huntington's disease is prevalent on an island in Venezuela, high blood pressure among many American Indians, diabetes in Ghana and Nigeria, and deafness among the Bedouins.

Geneticists also collect genes that seem to protect certain peoples against particular diseases – including resistance to human immunodeficiency virus infection among some Ugandans, leukemia in Papua, New Guinea, and Alzheimer's among the Cherokee in Oklahoma. The Icelandic people, isolated for centuries and thus relatively "pure" in a country that has kept excellent medical and genealogical records, have become a valuable resource for the study of genetic mutations linked to disease.

In 1998, a National Academy of Sciences review of the HGDP reported that "studies of human genetic variation have the potential to be particularly effective. . . . The incidence of disease can depend strongly on the biologic origins of a human population" (National Research Council 1997, 19–20). The report was encouraging to the gene hunters targeting "pure" populations to assess their genetic differences. Yet, the search for the disease genes that are characteristic of particular groups has embroiled the HGDP in controversy. Some scientists are strongly critical of the effort. Biological anthropologist Jonathan Marks questions whether genes are in fact the most important cause of variation in the risk of disease. He argues that much of this variation is due not to fundamental genetic differences but to historical-cultural factors. "Between-group variations is largely accounted by four variables – dietary salt intake, body fat, physical activity level, and stress – while in-group variation appears to have a significant genetic component" (Marks 1995, 212).

Contemporary research, he says, is not designed to collect adequate information about environmental factors and other information that is essential to understanding the complexities of disease.

Anthropologist Margaret Lock questions whether there are, in fact, any "genetically pure" populations to study. The premise of this research on genetic mutations, she says, may reflect unprovable assumptions (Lock 1999). Bioethicist Eric Juengst notes that the very process of reifying certain groups as "pure types" reinforces the old idea that humans can be classified according to biological categories. This, he fears, adds fuel to popular notions about the biology of race and their implementation in social policy (Juengst 1999).

Molecular biologist Herbert Nickens, concerned about the implications of genetic research for African Americans, calls genetics a "science of inequality" that "entwines society's racial, ethnic and economic biases with genetic differences that can be detected, particularly if any of these differences are differentially distributed by race, ethnicity or class." In a society that tends to stigmatize specific populations, he writes, the Human Genome Project offers opportunities for further stigmatization on the basis of potential risk for disease.

Genetics is not necessarily a science of inequality, as Nickens suggests; however, the concept of predisposition, like earlier ideas about susceptibility, is malleable – easily appropriated and readily exported from science to social policy (Tribe 1971, 1329). Observations associating ethnicity and disease are often useful in identifying risk factors in individuals for purposes of medical care, and genetic information, buttressed by scientific expertise, is useful well beyond the clinical arena. Such information is becoming a convenient and accepted way of creating social categories, preserving existing social arrangements, and enhancing the control of certain groups over others.

VIII. Implications: The Social Meaning of Genetic Prediction

There are significant economic and policy interests in risk information (Nelkin and Tancredi 1994). Pressured to maintain economic viability, efficiency, and accountability, institutions need to anticipate future contingencies and to avoid future risks. Genetics appears to be one means to differentiate individuals on the basis of ostensibly natural categories. Associating genetic predisposition with particular groups seems an efficient way to resolve ambiguities while limiting the role of arbitrary interpretation. As Nickens noted, however, genetics, like the earlier sciences described by Matthew Jacobson, is often a racialized science, influenced by social stereotypes and biases. Ideologies and expectations frame the interpretation, use, and management of genetic information. Just as social stereotypes amplify the meaning of genetic

predisposition, so identification of the genetic predisposition of specific ethic groups can reify social stereotypes.

Several examples illustrate how identification of differential predispositions, and explanations of these differences are entering decisions and debates in the contexts of work, criminal justice, and immigration policy – how they are creating rules for belonging and exclusion.

1. In the Workplace

Employers in the early part of the century had used gross physical markers to define the worker's body and its fitness for particular types of work. Today, the markers are hidden, but can be disclosed through DNA tests. The consequences, however, may be similar. Take the lawsuit filed by seven African-American employees against the Lawrence Berkeley Laboratory at the University of California. During mandatory physical examinations, the company doctor drew their blood supposedly for a cholesterol test. In 1995, they discovered that – without their knowledge or consent – they had been tested for the sickle cell genetic mutation. They were so incensed about the genetic tests that they filed suit against the laboratory and the U.S. Department of Energy that runs it, for invading their privacy and violating their civil rights.

The laboratory employs approximately 3,400 people – all had blood taken during physical examinations. Only the blood of African Americans and Latino employees was tested for risk of genetic disease. The laboratory provided no explanation of why genetic information was necessary, other than a vague assertion that the testing was done for the employees benefit. The plaintiffs, however, believed the selective testing reflected assumptions about their genetic inferiority. The Federal District Court sided with the employer, saying that the practice was not an invasion of privacy because the employees had agreed to the physical examinations, but the 9th Circuit Court of Appeals reversed the lower court decision, confirming the need for consent (Lehrman 1997).

Related to sickle cell anemia is a condition called glucose-6-phosphate dehydrogenase deficiency (G6PD), suspected to enhance the susceptibility of individuals to illness from toxic substances. Genetic screening techniques have been used in the workplace to identify and exclude workers with this deficiency (Rothstein 1983; Draper 1991). Justified in the first instance as a way to protect employee health, tests that identify vulnerable individuals can also be used to control compensation claims and avoid costly changes in the workplace environment, reducing a company's burden of responsibility to provide safe working conditions. It is the worker, viewed as a replaceable commodity, who is excluded from the workplace. Given the association of G6PD with sickle cell anemia, African American employees – even those without the allele – have been especially vulnerable to exclusion

(Duster 1989). The population susceptibilities that are associated with a genetic predisposition can be readily applied to individuals who assume the burden and blame (United States Congress, Office of Technology Assessment 1990).

Vulnerability to occupational hazards led to the creation, in 1998, of a National Institute of Environmental Health Sciences. This Institute systematically seeks out genes that are important predictors of environmentally related diseases. This would allow the identification of those who are at risk. The plan is to test Americans representing the ethnic diversity of the country, on the assumption that susceptibility will vary among different ethnic groups – that there are natural distinctions (Kaiser 1997, 569–70).

2. In the Criminal Justice System

The shape of the skull is no longer considered a meaningful indicator of a person's character. Similar impulses, to use the body and brain as a means to categorize and differentiate people, however, are shaping contemporary science. Experimental imaging technologies such as positron emission tomography and magnetic resonance imaging allow scientists to visualize and assess how various parts of the brain function under specific stimuli and to study the relationship between brain functioning and particular behavior among different people. Positron emission tomography scans of violent patients have linked their deviant behavior to specific brain abnormalities. Imaging techniques can be used to detect the actual presence of brain abnormalities but also to predict who may be violent in the future.

DNA analysis was developed in a medical context as a technique to identify the markers that indicate familial disorders. In 1983, a British geneticist used the technology to identify a rapist. Subsequently, DNA testing spread out of the medical sphere into the sphere of public surveillance. It is a convenient technology. A wad of spit, a spot of blood, a semen stain, or a single hair is all that is necessary to create a DNA profile, and the sample can be stored and later used to detect a person's genetic predispositions.

In light of prevailing stereotypes associating race and crime, Hispanics and African Americans have been likely targets for DNA surveillance. In 1995, for example, the police in Ann Arbor, Michigan ran a DNA dragnet operation. Hoping to find a serial rapist on the basis of a vague description, police officers questioned more than 700 African American men and took blood samples for DNA testing from 160 of them. One man was stopped eight times, and each time was required to show a receipt proving that his blood had already been tested. The receipt, in effect, became his "passport" to avoid further questioning. It "proved" his genetic innocence.

Similarly, in 1998, police in Florida asked 50 African American hospital employees to provide saliva samples in a DNA dragnet search for the strangler of a nursing home administrator. According to police chief, John S. Farrell: "It is a way to focus the investigation efficiently ... It would save time and money ... It is an extremely cost-effective tool." The African Americans tested felt they were targets of discriminatory suspicion – that they were suspect because of stereotypes associating blacks with crime (Andrews and Nelkin 2001).

The techniques used in forensic science can reinforce stereotypes. Scientists use reference groups to assess the evidentiary value of DNA matches between crime samples and suspect samples. They use population polymorphism frequency statistics drawn from FBI and police databases. These samples differentially represent African Americans who comprise the majority of the prison population. There are many social reasons for this situation, but DNA analysis encourages biological explanations and generalizations.

Specific markers are available to identify some ethnic groups from a DNA sample. This allows forensic teams to predict the racial origins of suspects before anyone is arrested. Apparently efficient, such predictions are also problematic; the notion of homogeneous, well-defined racial types is illusory, for race reflects social categorization. Yet, the probabilistic predictions from a DNA sample, can bolster popular beliefs about race differences. "Genetic data seems more real, more definitive than the old cultural classifications" – and more useful as a political tool (Vines 1995).

Dissenting in a Virginia lawsuit challenging the state's program to collect blood samples for genetic testing from nonviolent offenders, Judge Murnagnan worried that arguments for administrative efficiency could justify "the testing of other discrete populations, e.g., racial minorities or residents of underprivileged areas" (*Jones v. Murray* 1992). The state could simply go into the inner city and demand blood samples as a way to manage risk. Ronald Walters, a political scientist at Howard University, speculates: "Let's just assume we find a genetic link (to violence) ... The question I have always raised is how will this finding be used? There is a good case, on the basis of history, that it could be used in a racially oppressive way, which is to say you could mount drug programs in inner-city communities based upon this identification of so-called genetic markers" (Stolberg 1995).

Research on the biological basis of behavior is likely to increase abuses. If behavioral geneticists identify genes associated with aggressive behavior, it would be easy to envision the creation of risk management measures to prevent crime more efficiently by circumscribing the rights of people thought to have criminal genes. This, as sociologist Nikolas Rose observes, is consistent with recent trends toward employing preventive models in the efforts to control crime. These models call for calculating risk probabilities based not on individual dangerousness implied by a person's actions, but on population predictions that might indicate potential risk (Rose 1998, 177–95). Preventive measures could include identifying those supposedly "predisposed" to antisocial behavior and keeping certain groups under surveillance.

3. In Immigration Debates

During the early part of the century, eugenic ideas had framed debates about immigration (Kraut 1994). Anti-immigration groups saw potential immigrants as economic and health risks – a drain on public services. They were categorized as intrinsically unhealthy and biologically inferior. The biology-based theories of the eugenics movement led to the 1924 Immigration Act with its restrictions on immigration from Central, Southern, and Eastern Europe.

After World War II, eugenic arguments virtually disappeared from public discourse. Today, reflecting the public visibility of genetics along with renewed concern about immigration, similar arguments are reappearing in the rhetoric of nativist groups (Nelkin and Michaels 1998, 33–59). This rhetoric builds on assumptions about the biological differences among ethnic and race groups, and their differential health, reproductive patterns, and behavioral predispositions. Nativists contend that genetically determined physical and behavioral traits are characteristic of specific racial groups, and that cultures themselves are an expression of biological characteristics.

The language of genetics and especially arguments about genetic diversity, appeal to nativist groups as a way to define their agenda not as racist, but as rational and scientific. The National Alliance, for example, opposes immigration because of "the natural laws of heredity," and a conviction that the inferiority of some races is a "biological fact" based on evolutionary history (Cotten 1993). Coming from extremists, such views are hardly new, but they also appear in mainstream media as race theorists promote their views about genetic differences. Peter Brimelow, in a best selling anti-immigration book called *Alien Nation* (1995), notes that America's core population comes from "European stock" (picking up the early eugenics language of animal breeding). In *The Bell Curve* (1995), Herrnstein and Murray argue that economic inequities are a ratification of "genetic justice" and insist that immigration policy must consider that Latino and Black immigrants "are putting downward pressure on the distribution of intelligence. The cognitive capacity of the country is at stake." Such claims are built on ideas about natural distinctions.

The leap from science to social policy, which is sometimes encouraged by scientists, has helped to foster such arguments. Daniel Koshland, molecular biologist and former editor of *Science*, has argued that genetics is important in selecting people with "superior skills" for "as society gets more complex, perhaps it must select for individuals more capable of coping with its complex problems (Koshland 1988–89, 10–13).

Concepts of genetic diversity and differential predispositions are easily translated into social policy. By defining what is "natural," science has long been appropriated to create and justify social categories, that is, to do the political work that serves policy agendas. Critics, however, question the deterministic assumptions underlying genetic predictions. Steven Rose, a British neuroscientist, writes that such predictions are based on "a faulty reductive sequence whose steps include: reification, arbitrary agglomeration, improper quantification . . . misplaced causality and dichotomous partitioning between genetic and environmental causes" (Rose 1995, 380–2).

The search for differences in genetic predispositions among diverse populations recasts old and pervasive beliefs about the importance of "blood" in powerful scientific terms. The rich and healthy are what they are because of their genetic endowments. So too, the deviant or dysfunctional – and those "at risk" – are fated by their genes. As genetics becomes the basis of classifying and categorizing people, of creating "natural" distinctions, this science is as easily appropriated and readily politicized today as craniometry, phrenology, and eugenics were a century ago.

IX. CONCLUSION

The significance of scientific information rests, of course, on how it is used. Beyond employers, law enforcement officials, and immigration authorities, there are many other institutions – motor vehicle bureaus, schools, creditors, adoption agencies, organ transplant registries, professional sports teams, sexual partners, the military, mortgage lenders, even university tenure committees – with reasons for wanting access to information about the future health status of people in their domain. As in the Lawrence Livermore case, their use of such information is likely to be influenced by expectations and assumptions concerning population susceptibilities to particular conditions.

Research in molecular biology is yielding new information about latent predispositions and future risks. This research has high status today, perceived as the basis of future medicine and science, institutions are understandably attracted to the predictions promised by a genetic "map" and to the apparent certainties implied by genetic testing. The idea of genetic predisposition is a useful and convenient construct. As scientists increasingly associate risk with specific populations, however, it is also a dangerous construct. Looking back at the efforts to classify and categorize people during the earlier days of industrialization and mass immigration, it is easy to see the fallacies in past scientific formulations. Similar beliefs have reemerged in the persistent preoccupation with what makes people different. Amplified by ideological agendas, the growing appeal of genetic predictions can ultimately serve to reify biological explanations of human differences and to reinforce social stereotypes.

ACKNOWLEDGMENTS

We would like to acknowledge material provided by Troy Duster, and comments from the members of the New York University Law Faculty at a "bag lunch" presentation.

CHAPTER 60

HISTORY OF PUBLIC HEALTH ETHICS IN THE UNITED STATES

Barron H. Lerner and Ronald Bayer

I. INTRODUCTION

Although "public health ethics" as a concept has existed for less than two decades, political leaders and medical officials have long made moral and value-laden decisions designed to protect the health of the community. History, by revealing the social and cultural forces that inform scientific policies, is an ideal approach for understanding the controversies that have arisen in public health – both before and after they were termed "ethical" in nature (Fee 1993). This chapter will focus on public health ethics in the United States since 1900, drawing, where appropriate, on events that occurred prior to the twentieth century and in other countries. It will highlight a series of controversies that have characterized public health ethics, explicitly noting the relevance of these issues for modern ethicists, health officials, clinicians, and the general public.

In contrast to medical practice, which emphasizes the care of specific patients, and bioethics, which stresses patients' rights, public health is concerned with health and disease among populations. Although public health interventions are justified in terms of their potential benefit to the populace, they may do so by restricting the liberties of other citizens. Thus, a central theme of public health ethics is the tension between protecting the overall health of such populations and the rights of specific individuals who live in these communities. How have public health officials pursued this duty to the greater good with restrictive – and at times coercive – measures? Given that infectious diseases and other public health threats disproportionately affect disadvantaged persons, how equitably have public health policies been implemented?

The types of interventions proposed by health officials have evolved with the changing prevalence of disease and the growing knowledge of how diseases spread. During the second half of the nineteenth century, officials focused on sanitary measures, such as purification of sewage systems and improvement of trash collection, as methods for lowering the rates of disease in the community. With the development of the germ theory, however, the concern shifted to sick individuals apt to infect the healthy. As a result, certain infected persons became subject to restrictions, including forcible confinement in institutions that were routinely deemed appropriate by governmental officials and legal authorities. Attempts to challenge public health powers were typically either ignored or dismissed by the courts.

The conflicts engendered by public health interventions assumed center stage in the 1980s and 1990s with the appearance of the acquired immunodeficiency syndrome (AIDS), an infection primarily spread through sexual contact, the sharing of drug-injection equipment, and during childbirth, and the resurgence of tuberculosis (TB), a communicable disease spread through respiratory secretions. Confronted with alarming mortality rates, some public health officials considered reviving many of the older, more restrictive policies of the past. Yet, these dual epidemics had arisen in an era that had come to recognize the preeminence of individual rights and an era in which bioethics had done so much to advance the rights of patients. AIDS activists, in particular, refused to accept the restrictive and at times paternalistic features that accompanied traditional public health measures.

Out of these late twentieth-century controversies emerged the discipline of "public health ethics." Indeed, public health ethicists would play a major role in devising solutions to public health controversies in which civil liberties were given much broader birth than at the turn of the twentieth century. Yet, as outright coercion became a less acceptable strategy for protecting the public health, elements of paternalism reemerged, masked in terms of the protection of third parties. One notable example of this process has occurred in the campaign to lower smoking rates. Over the next decades, those involved in shaping the new public health ethics will need to confront the question of whether such efforts are essential to public health or represent an unacceptable intrusion on liberty.

II. EARLY PUBLIC HEALTH POWERS

Evidence of restricted liberties in the name of public health dates back thousands of years. For example, the Bible discusses the segregation of those with leprosy, a disfiguring disease believed to be contagious: "All the days wherein the plague shall be in him he shall be defiled; he is unclean: he shall dwell alone; without the camp shall his habitation be" (Leviticus 13:46). One of the first official state-imposed systems of mandatory segregation was the quarantining of ships in Venice and other European cities in the fourteenth century. These efforts, which entailed the isolation of passengers for 40 days (hence the term "quarantine"), sought to prevent the entry of the bubonic plague, a dreaded epidemic disease that killed up to one-third of the population of Europe during the Middle Ages and the Renaissance. Although the mechanism of transmission was unknown, officials knew that the plague flared after the arrival of foreign ships from cities undergoing outbreaks of the disease.

The most comprehensive use of governmental authority to protect the public's health in the early modern era was the system of "medical police" established in Germany by Johann Peter Frank (1745–1811) in the late eighteenth century. Frank encouraged local officials to monitor and intervene in all aspects of the public's health, including marriage, childbirth, housing, nutrition, accident prevention, and the management of diseases presumed to be communicable (Rosen 1993, 140). The association of Frank's

efforts with authoritarian political regimes led some historians to criticize the medical police as an intrusive intervention primarily designed to serve the state. It is worth noting, however, that Frank cautioned against excessive intrusions into the lives of private citizens (Sigerist 1956, 59). In addition, many of his strategies subsequently became routine components of public health practice in democratic societies.

Most historians situate the origins of modern public health not in Frank's Germany but in the "Great Sanitary Awakening" of the mid-nineteenth century. The growing interest in sanitation, in turn, had arisen from the French Enlightenment, which emphasized the state's role in bettering the human condition (Rosen 1993, 109), and utilitarianism, which urged civil legislation designed to achieve the greatest happiness for the largest number of people" (Porter 1999, 116). Sanitarianism first gained favor in England, thanks to the efforts of the reformer Edwin Chadwick (1800–1890), a disciple of the utilitarian Jeremy Bentham (1748–1832). Chadwick had helped to draft a new Poor Law Amendment in 1834, which had promoted the migration of workers to rapidly industrializing English cities. A major repercussion of this population shift was the deteriorating health of laborers, which Chadwick believed was due to the overcrowded and filthy urban dwellings into which they had settled.

Chadwick confirmed his hypothesis in his famous 1842 publication, *Report on the Sanitary Condition of the Labouring Population of Great Britain*. In this report, Chadwick documented higher rates of disease among poorer populations and proposed a series of reforms, including better drainage of sewage, improved water supplies and prompt removal of all refuse (Chadwick 1842). In its proposal of bureaucratic interventions that could improve the lives of poor laborers, bolster Britain's free market economy, and potentially protect the upper classes from communicable diseases, Chadwick's report received considerable praise. By 1848, the government had passed the First British Public Health Act, which instituted some of the proposed reforms. Chadwick's work was even supported by John Stuart Mill, the author of "On Liberty," the famous 1859 essay delineating the limits of state intervention into the lives of citizens (Porter 1999, 145).

Reformers outside of England, such as the German physician Rudolph Virchow (1821–1900), echoed Chadwick's conclusions about the duty of government and medicine to improve the health and lives of the poor (Porter 1999, 107). Only with better housing, diet and education, argued the German hygienist Max von Pettenkofer, British statistician William Farr, and others, could the poor hope to defend themselves against disease (Porter 1999, 108; Hamlin 1990).

Chadwick had not only justified governmental intervention based on its ability to improve the population's health, he also saw better sanitation as a way to improve the morals of the poor, whom he described as "short-lived, improvident, reckless, and intemperate, and with habitual avidity for sensual gratifications" (Rothman, Marcus, and Kiceluk 1995, 238). As would continue to be the case, such characterizations tended to conflate moralistic judgments about the poor with the actual public health threat that they represented.

As Great Britain further developed its public health apparatus, objections began to occur that at times resembled those confronted by Johann Frank. For example, some contemporary critics charged the government with "despotic interference" into both individual lives and the free market" (Porter 1999, 120). Later measures, such as the institution of mandatory smallpox vaccination in 1853 and the compulsory examination and possible detention of women with venereal diseases, drew additional charges of "medical despotism" (Porter 1999, 130).

In the United States, no centralized public health apparatus emerged. Although commentators acknowledged the growing presence of overcrowded, disease-ridden slums in industrializing American cities, efforts to prevent disease remained localized and based on voluntarism. These characteristics reflected the antistatist tradition of American federalism. Many of the earliest reformers were neither politicians nor physicians but religious figures who blamed sin for outbreaks of cholera and other epidemic diseases that periodically attacked American cities. Preaching the "gospel of hygiene" (Porter 1999, 152), these reformers argued that sanitary interventions strongly supplemented the ability of prayer to improve the health of the poor. Gradually, local governments, such as New York City and the state of Massachusetts, began to implement the types of sanitary reforms proposed by Chadwick (Rosenkrantz 1972; Duffy 1990).

III. BACTERIOLOGY AND THE NEW PUBLIC HEALTH

The underlying rationale for sanitary intervention was about to undergo a major challenge. Like most (but not all) of his contemporaries, Chadwick believed that the majority of infectious diseases – such as cholera, typhus, and consumption – were not contagious. Rather, they spread through miasmas, invisible clouds of matter produced by decaying garbage and waste. This theory led naturally to Chadwick's assumption that environmental purification would lower rates of disease. "[F]or Chadwick," the historian Dorothy Porter has written, "disease was smell" (Porter 1999, 119). The elucidation of the germ theory of disease repudiated the miasmatic hypothesis. Through an elegant series of experiments conducted in the 1870s and 1880s, Louis Pasteur, Robert Koch, and other scientists demonstrated that many infectious diseases were caused by specific bacteria that could be passed from diseased to healthy individuals. For example, cholera was spread

when a healthy individual accidentally ingested bacteria expelled in the diarrhea of a sick person. Consumption, later known as TB, developed due to the inhalation of aerosolized respiratory droplets coughed up by individuals with active disease.

Armed with the precise scientific knowledge so valued in the Progressive era, public health officials in the United States revisited earlier assumptions. Among the most prominent innovators was Providence, Rhode Island, health officer Charles V. Chapin (Cassedy 1962). Although Chapin and his compatriots thought that purifying water and removing sewage were likely of some value in preventing water-borne infections, they believed that monitoring the behavior of the sick was of much greater importance. Thus, persons with infectious diarrhea needed to defecate apart from other family members and wash their hands fastidiously. Individuals sick with TB needed to cough into handkerchiefs, dispose of their sputum properly and, at times, leave their apartments for hospitalization in sanatoria. Children with diphtheria or scarlet fever had to stay home from school until health officials deemed them noninfectious (Chapin 1910; Hill 1916, 158–72).

One ardent champion of the so-called new public health was Minnesota health official and Chapin disciple Hibbert W. Hill. "The old public health was concerned with the environment," he wrote in 1916. "The new is concerned with the individual" (Hill 1916, 8). Control of infectious diseases, therefore, needed to focus on preventing the transit of specific bacteria between individuals. Developing programs to combat individual infections fit well with the Progressive emphasis on efficient bureaucratic interventions. Hill's allegiance to disease specificity is revealed in his own words. Within a single sentence he would repeat the word four times: "[S]pecific troubles must be met by specific measures directed specifically against the real specific cause of that trouble" (Hill 1916, 3).

Although some health officials who accepted the germ theory also continued to call for better housing, nutrition, and jobs for the urban poor (Chadwick 1842; Galdston 1941), Hill and most of his colleagues had lost interest in the old sanitarian strategies for preventing disease. "A bullet," he wrote, "will travel equally as far through the soldier who is physically perfect as through him who is a physical wreck" (Hill 1916, 1). To be sure, Hill based his recommendations on the prevailing understanding of medical evidence. The growing emphasis on promoting healthier behaviors also represented a political decision to distance public health strategies from broader welfare programs designed to benefit the poor. Hill's emphasis on the prevention of specific diseases would become a centerpiece of public health practice in the twentieth century (Lerner 1998, 170–5).

Linked to this perspective, and the health officer's "sociological supervision" of the infected (Hill 1916, 93), was the inevitable question about the rights of the individual in the context of public health. Building on the prestige of the new science of bacteriology, United States health officials attained their most far-reaching authority in the early twentieth century. In combating both epidemic and endemic infections, they were able to compel citizens to perform whatever behaviors were deemed necessary to protect the community's health. In the rare instances when there were legal challenges, the courts sided with the state. In the celebrated 1905 case, *Jacobson v. Massachusetts*, the United States Supreme Court ruled that Massachusetts' mandatory smallpox vaccination statute was constitutional. Noting the existence of other "restraints and burdens in order to secure the general comfort, health, and prosperity of the State," the court termed the regulation "necessary for the public health or the public safety" (*Jacobson v. Massachusetts* 1905). This decision well exemplified the Roman dictum *"Salus publica suprema lex"* (Public health is the highest law).

Quarantine was a central feature of the new focus on the dangers posed by infected individuals and the risks they posed to others. With the authority to isolate came an inevitable abuse of power. Public health officers frequently used quarantine in an arbitrary manner, imposing restrictions on the poor and disadvantaged – "those who were least able to protest" (Porter and Porter 1988). Although acknowledging that infectious diseases did predominate among such individuals, historians of public health have nevertheless argued that impositions were often unreasonable, extending beyond any criteria that contemporary science could have justified.

One victimized group was immigrants, who were at times forcibly evicted from their dwellings or subject to strict home quarantine simply because they belonged to the same ethnic groups as persons suffering from cholera, the bubonic plague, or other epidemic diseases (Markel 1997; Kraut 1994; Musto 1986). In February 1892, for example, New York City health officers quarantined roughly 1,200 Russian Jews at Riverside Hospital, located on North Brother Island in the East River. Although some of these persons had recently acquired typhus fever after arriving on the *S. S. Massilia*, the vast majority were healthy individuals who had the misfortune of living near those who had become ill. While on the island, as many as 49 of this latter group themselves became diseased, presumably having been infected during the quarantine (Markel 1997, 67). Meanwhile, as Howard Markel has detailed, the city declined to quarantine non-Jewish New York residents concurrently discovered to have typhus. Serving as a convenient scapegoat for the epidemic, the fate of the Russian immigrants "was that of quarantine, physically, spiritually, and emotionally" (Markel 1997, 55).

Public health quarantine served as a precedent for anti-immigrant legislation that emerged as a result of growing eugenic sentiments in the 1910s and 1920s (Pernick 1996). Having singled out poor immigrants as one of several populations in American society that were threats to the biological and racial purity of the nation, eugenicists helped convince the U.S. Congress to pass the 1924 Johnson Act that selectively restricted immigration from Eastern Europe. The eugenics movement also supported other restrictive public health measures aimed at protecting the "purity" of the White Anglo-Saxon population. One particularly egregious example was the forced eugenic sterilization of the mentally retarded, criminals and so-called defective populations (see Chapter 54).

Historians studying endemic diseases, such as TB, have documented similar overuse of public health powers. In 1903, for example, New York City made a portion of Riverside Hospital into a detention facility for uncooperative TB patients. It is no surprise that New York was home to this effort. The city's famous public health officer, Hermann Biggs (1859–1923), was among the country's most vocal proponents of aggressive public health regulations, terming disease "a removable evil" (Rosen 1993, 440). "We are prepared, when necessary," he wrote, "to introduce and enforce measures which might seem radical and arbitrary, if they were not plainly designed for the public good" (Garrett 2000, 112). Yet institutions such as Riverside, Sheila Rothman has argued, served less as public health facilities than repositories for homeless vagrants (Rothman 1994). The adjectives used to describe such patients, for example, "ignorant," "vicious" and "wanton," suggest that they were isolated as a form of punishment (Lerner 1998, 117–18, 137).

Efforts to control the spread of venereal diseases during World War I also led to the questionable use of detention. Fearing the debilitating effects of syphilis and gonorrhea on U.S. soldiers, the federal government quarantined more than 30,000 prostitutes who supposedly harbored one or both of these diseases. Barbed wire surrounded many of the institutions used for detention. Pointing out that infected men were not quarantined and that some of the women may not have even had active infection, Allan Brandt has criticized this episode as "the most concerted attack on civil liberties in the name of public health in American history" (Brandt 1985).

Perhaps the best-known example of aggressive public health detention was the case of Mary Mallon, also known as "Typhoid Mary." When the New York City Department of Health first identified Mallon as spreading typhoid fever in 1907, it represented a great triumph of the new public health. Scientists had just learned that seemingly healthy persons could silently harbor – and then transmit to others – the bacterium that caused the disease. Mallon, an Irish immigrant who worked as a cook, had inadvertently spread typhoid fever to several families when preparing food. Yet when confronted with a Department of Health edict forbidding her from continuing her chosen profession, Mallon refused to comply. Ultimately, health officials took her into custody again, but not before she had caused at least 47 cases of the disease and three deaths (Kraut 1994, 102; Leavitt 1996). Mallon was ultimately quarantined on North Brother Island for 23 years. Noting that Mallon, a laborer, an immigrant and a woman, was confined, while other typhoid carriers were allowed to remain free, historians have characterized her as a victim of discrimination by overzealous public health officials.

But as Judith Leavitt has shown, the Typhoid Mary story is more complicated. Mallon was not only a victim but stubbornly rejected a series of compromises proposed by health officials (Leavitt 1996). A similarly complex story occurred when health departments revived Biggs' strategy of forcible detention for noncompliant TB patients after World War II. For example, at Firland, a TB sanatorium in Seattle, Washington, health officials went well beyond what was warranted by the public health standards of the era. Having established a locked ward to detain patients who represented a true threat to the community's health, these officials ultimately used the ward as a way to control unruly tuberculous Skid Row alcoholics who disrupted sanatorium routine. Yet, Seattle officials believed that their use of coercion – while excessive – represented the only feasible mechanism for curing TB in Skid Row alcoholics, and thus enabling such men to resume relatively healthy and independent lives (Lerner 1998). With the rise of bioethics and the patients' rights movement after 1970, such paternalistic justifications for restrictive public health measures would become increasingly unacceptable.

IV. EARLY VOICES OF PROTEST

The first protests against public health mandates, however, had occurred much earlier. For example, in response to the September 1892 quarantining of Eastern European Jews feared to be harboring cholera, Yiddish language journalist Abraham Cahan charged New York officials with subjecting the immigrants to "murderous injustice and inequalities" (Markel 1997, 113). When Jacobson unsuccessfully objected to Massachusetts' mandatory smallpox vaccination a decade later, he had argued that the statute violated "the inherent right of every free man to care for his own body and health in such way as to him seems best" (*Jacobson v. Massachusetts* 1905). Mary Mallon had described herself as "an innocent human being" who had "committed no crime" but was being "treated like an outcast – a criminal" (Kraut 1994, 100).

At times, those criticizing public health excesses were not individually aggrieved citizens but the medical profession. For example, New York physicians in the 1890s had objected to Biggs' insistence that they report all cases of TB to the health department. Such a regulation, they believed, interfered with the confidential doctor–patient relationship (Fox 1975). In other instances, doctors opposed public health measures that they saw as medically misguided or as promoting "socialized medicine." A critic of one such intervention, the fluoridation of the water supply after World War II, termed it a "hoax" that encouraged public health "dictatorship" (Lerner 1998, 50).

Episodic protests also accompanied the growing use of detention for TB patients in the 1950s. Not surprisingly, some of the most vocal objections occurred in Seattle, with its aggressive policy of confining Skid Row alcoholics. In 1956 and 1957, a series of patients at Firland Sanatorium began a letter-writing campaign that accused the hospital staff and local health officials of abusing public health powers. Among the charges leveled were that "people who have had negative [noninfectious] sputum for months may be placed under quarantine" and that a detained patient "is not allowed to defend himself in any manner, as he could in a court of law" (Lerner 1998, 140–1). "Free-born people," importuned two of the most vocal critics, "are not accustomed to dictatorship that forces indignaties [sic] on them while they are helpless" (Lerner 1998, 140).

The Firland patients sent their missives widely, attempting to interest newspapers and politicians at both the local and national level; however, they received a positive response from only one group: the Washington state chapter of the American Civil Liberties Union (ACLU) (Lerner 1998, 142). In 1957, the ACLU sent a subcommittee of its civil liberties committee to investigate the patients' complaints. In a subsequent report, the group "independently confirmed and enlarged upon" the charges, documenting the following "abuses" at Firland: "mis-use of quarantine, opening of patients' mail, the assignment of patients to maximum security wards, and the use of solitary confinement" (Lerner 1998 142). Yet reflecting the typical dominance of public health claims in this era, subcommittee members basically let the issue drop. Not until 7 years later did the ACLU return, helping to implement a unique system in which a local judge traveled to Firland to conduct informal detention hearings.

The willingness of a judge to consider the previously ignored objections of a group of Skid Row alcoholics spoke to emerging concerns about institutionalization and other civil liberties violations in the United States. Beginning in the early 1960s, a small group of lawyers and psychiatrists, notably Thomas Szasz of the State University of New York at Syracuse, had begun to object to the frequent civil commitment of the mentally ill (Szasz 1963, 40–1). Although some of Szasz's critique stemmed from his radical notion that mental illness was a "myth," he convincingly argued that many psychiatric patients were being inappropriately committed to institutions and, once there, deprived of basic rights such as bodily privacy and legal counsel. By the 1970s, numerous rulings by the Supreme

Court and state courts had invoked the due process clause of the Fourteenth Amendment to ensure the civil liberties of both the mentally ill and persons charged with criminal wrongdoing (Lerner 1998, 147). These cases, plus an occasional ruling opposing the detention of a TB patient, served to discourage the continued expansive reliance on coercion in the face of perceived epidemics of contagious disease. The relatively small number of cases specific to TB in all likelihood stemmed from the continued decline of the disease during the 1960s and 1970s.

V. PUBLIC HEALTH ETHICS: EARLY DISCUSSIONS

The seeds for a fundamental conceptual shift were sewn in these years, when advocates for the weak and disempowered framed their claims for redress in the language of rights. It was in this context that the contemporary bioethics movement took shape. The fundamental thrust of the new medical ethics was to revisit the balance of power between doctors and patients and between researchers and their subjects. In so doing, the architects of bioethics – physicians, philosophers, theologians, lawyers, and social scientists – could draw on the legacy of efforts to impose ethical constraints on research involving human subjects and the history of legal norms that required that competent adults give their consent to medical interventions. The new efforts were also indelibly marked by the upsurge in the broad struggle for rights that characterized the 1960s and 1970s. In this context, medical paternalism was the target; patient autonomy became the linchpin of the attempt to frame a new ethics of medicine.

As bioethics took shape, its central focus was on the clinical encounter. This emphasis on the rights of patients and research subjects drew upon prevailing conceptions of American individualism. Even when those involved in the first generation of bioethics strayed beyond the doctor–patient dyad, the emphasis was on autonomy: the antagonism to paternalism was manifest. This was true of efforts to examine genetic counseling, screening programs for sickle cell trait and disease, and the uses of psychiatry in promoting behavior control. A different set of moral claims arose in only one instance – when there were questions about access, whether to scarce resources such as hemodialysis or to medical care in general. Here the issue of justice was paramount.

What is most striking about the bioethics that took hold in the United States was that it paid virtually no attention to matters of public health. The rare exceptions to the dominant concerns with clinical medicine and research only serve to highlight this point. For example, in the 1970s it had become clear that the patterns of morbidity and mortality in the United States and other advanced industrialized nations were being dramatically affected by exposure to environmental toxins and by personal

behaviors, such as poor diet, smoking, and lack of exercise. Marc Lalonde's 1978 analysis, *A New Perspective on the Health of Canadians*, provided an official imprimatur: "Self-imposed risks and the environment are the principal or important underlying factors in each of the five major causes of death between age one and age seventy, and we can only conclude, that unless the environment is changed and the self-imposed risks are reduced, the death rates will not be significantly improved" (Lalonde 1974, 15). Lalonde was clear about the moral implications of this new perspective. "The ultimate issue . . . is whether and to what extent government can get into the business of modifying human behaviors, even if it does so to improve health" (Lalonde 1974, 36).

In his introduction to the American analogue of the Lalonde report, *Healthy People*, published 1 year later, U.S. Secretary of Health, Education and Welfare Joseph Califano was blunt as well.

> You the individual can do more for your own health and well being than any doctor, any hospital, any drug, any exotic medical device . . . If we are to mount a successful public health revolution in the next generation [the changes required] go far beyond the traditional health care community. (U.S. Department of Health, Education, and Welfare, 1957, viii–ix)

Califano virtually called for an open debate of the ethical implications of his claims.

> There will be controversy – and there should be – about what role the government should play, if any, in urging citizens to give up these pleasurable but damaging habits. But there can be no denying the public consequences of those private habits. (U.S. Department of Health, Education, and Welfare 1957, 12)

John Knowles, president of the Rockefeller Foundation, summarized the emerging mood when he declared in a widely read and influential statement, "I believe the idea of a 'right' to health should be replaced by the idea of an individual moral obligation to preserve one's own health – a public duty if you will" (Knowles 1979). From a very different ideological perspective, Ivan Illich, in his *Medical Nemesis*, underscored the limits, indeed the damaging impact, of medicine on public health and made clear that communal well-being could not result from professional interventions (Illich 1976a, 1976b).

That the health of populations was centrally a function of broad social conditions and that medicine itself played a small role in secular trends in morbidity and mortality was not a new thesis. It had been the claim of British Professor of Social Medicine Thomas McKeown since the 1950s (McKeown 1976). What was remarkable was that commentators across the political spectrum had now seized upon this perspective. There were worries, however, some of which had been signaled by Marc Lalonde and Joseph Califano, others by commentators who viewed the new turn as a form of victim blaming.

It was in this setting that New York's Hastings Center, then the country's preeminent bioethics research institute, convened a working group to examine the ethical challenges posed by the focus on behavior and health. In the course of its work, the group addressed meanings of personal responsibility, the extent to which social factors imposed morally relevant limits on the capacity of individuals to choose behaviors that might enhance health, and the dangers of the perspective that justified behavioral modification based on the social costs of unregulated activities (Moreno and Bayer 1985). More radically, consideration was given to the possibility of jettisoning the central formulations of a liberalism focused on individuals in favor of a communitarian approach (Beauchamp 1985).

Very different was the effort on the part of the Hastings Center to examine the ethical challenges posed by threats to the health of workers. Here the Center sought to examine not only matters of professional ethics – that is, the duties of scientists, engineers, and occupational health physicians – but more importantly, the ethics of setting standards in occupational health. In the course of this undertaking, Center members had to confront several complex questions. What did justice require when workplace exposure had to be established in the face of limited or uncertain data? Should standards reflect the needs and vulnerabilities of those at special risk? (Bingham 1985). Should women be subject to unique restrictions because of the possible threat of toxicity to unborn fetuses? In the end, it was necessary to address the question of whether the constraints of the market created burdens on workers that rendered free choice a meaningless concept (Daniels 1985).

Little sustained effort to examine the ethics of occupational health or the relationship between behavior and public health followed these undertakings. When the efforts ended, discussion of the ethics of public health faded. It would take an event of extreme severity and extended duration – the AIDS epidemic – for issues of public health ethics to finally take center stage.

VI. The Emergence of AIDS

The first report of what would come to be known as AIDS, issued in June 1981, shattered the assumption that infectious threats no longer posed a challenge to advanced industrial societies. That recognition and the emerging dread about the magnitude of the epidemic led to the realization that a host of new ethical questions needed to be addressed. Not surprisingly, the first encounter between ethics and AIDS involved an issue at the heart of bioethics, that of confidentiality and research. A working group

constituted by the Hastings Center and involving public health officials, researchers, clinicians, lawyers, ethicists, and the first generation of AIDS activists addressed the question of how to facilitate critically important epidemiological research into a disease borne by stigmatized and fearful populations (Bayer, Levine, and Murray 1984).

What resulted from this Hastings Center undertaking was, in a way, far more important than the set of research guidelines generated by the group. An understanding emerged that there was a set of critical public health matters that would challenge ethical perspectives first developed in the clinical setting. Based on this understanding, the Hastings Center undertook innovative work in the epidemic's formative period, paving the way for many ethicists who would study AIDS during the next decade. Among the ethical questions these scholars would address were the following:

- Should public settings, like gay bathhouses, that facilitated multiple sexual contacts, be closed?
- What restrictions should be placed on blood donation by those at risk of HIV infection?
- How aggressively should HIV antibody testing, under conditions of confidentiality, be encouraged?
- Was anonymity in testing preferable to confidentiality? And, if so, under what circumstances?
- Should the results of antibody tests be reportable – with full identification – to public health officials?
- Should contact notification programs, so central to the history of TB and venereal disease control, be applied to AIDS?
- Were there circumstances when the duty to warn unsuspecting sexual partners should take priority over the duty to protect physician–patient confidentiality?
- Should intravenous drug users be provided with sterile needles even if such moves would be perceived as fostering the use of illicit and dangerous drugs?
- Should public health officials have the power to quarantine human immunodeficiency virus (HIV)-infected individuals who willfully or recklessly exposed others to risk?

Not surprisingly, the most important early contribution of ethicists to the policy debates surrounding AIDS involved HIV testing – an issue relevant to both public health and clinical practice. From the outset, the test developed to detect antibodies to the AIDS virus – and first used on a broad scale in blood banking – was mired in controversy. Uncertainty about the significance of the test's findings and about its quality and accuracy led to disputes over privacy, communal health, social and economic discrimination, coercion, and liberty. For those who feared that public anxiety about AIDS would turn individuals infected with the AIDS virus into targets of destructive social policy and practice, the antibody test generated enormous concern. Vigorous encouragement of testing, critics feared, would ineluctably lead to mandatory approaches given the authoritarian history of public health. Because confidentiality would not be preserved, the infected would suffer stigmatization and deprivation of the right to work, go to school, and obtain insurance. Most ominously, the identification of HIV-positive persons could threaten freedom itself. No marginal advance of the public health, opponents of wide-scale testing asserted, could warrant such a catastrophic array of personal burdens.

Conversely, those who believed that the identification of the infected or potentially infected provided an opportunity for modifying risky behavior saw in the test a great opportunity. Some advocates of testing were attentive to matters of privacy so forcefully articulated by gay groups, civil libertarians and ethicists. They opposed the use of coercion and stressed the importance of protecting the confidentiality of test results, preserving the right of each individual to choose or decline testing, and guaranteeing the social and economic rights of those who tested positive for HIV. This strategy sought to combine an aggressive defense of the public health with a commitment to the privacy and social interests of the infected.

The Hastings Center published its pioneering and collaborative work on HIV testing in the *Journal of the American Medical Association* in 1986 (Bayer, Levine, and Wolf 1986). Reflecting both an antipathy to coercion and a commitment to liberal values characteristic of bioethics, the center's guidelines concluded,

> We believe that the greatest hope for stopping the spread of HIV infection lies in the voluntary cooperation of those at higher risk – their willingness to undergo testing and to alter their personal behavior and goals in the interests of the community. But we can expect this voluntary cooperation – in some cases, sacrifice – only if the legitimate interests of these groups and individuals in being protected from discrimination are heeded by legislators, professionals, and the public. (Bayer, Levine, and Wolf 1986, 1774)

A group working out of the Johns Hopkins School of Public Health struck a similar posture when addressing the ethical issue of mandatory screening of pregnant women for HIV infection. The group concluded that the implementation of counseling and screening policies that interfered with women's reproductive freedom, or that resulted in the unfair stigmatization of vulnerable social groups was unacceptable (Faden, Geller, and Powers 1991).

Both the Hopkins and Hastings Center statements reflected a much broader development in AIDS policy during the epidemic's first decade. Thanks in large part to those concerned with issues of ethics a determination had been made to treat AIDS differently from other sexually transmitted and infectious diseases. This AIDS "exceptionalism" signaled a commitment to HIV prevention measures that were noncoercive – that is, those that respected the privacy and social rights of those at risk for HIV infection. In diverging from the tradition of public health practice forged by Hermann Biggs and others at the turn of the century, this perspective eschewed threats and quarantine in favor of mass education and voluntary testing and counseling. At the core of this voluntarist approach was a belief that recourse to traditional public health measures would drive the epidemic underground. Thus, gay leaders concerned about privacy, civil libertarians concerned about limiting unwarranted state intrusions, public health officials concerned about effective disease control, and ethicists opposed to the overbearing application of medical authority found common ground (Bayer 1989).

But as the first decade of the epidemic drew to a close in the early 1990s, the factors that had made possible a broad-based commitment to exceptionalism began to change (Bayer 1991). For example, the epidemiology of the epidemic began to shift, with increasing numbers of cases occurring among injection drug users. Meanwhile, public health officials increasingly came to believe that some of their traditional strategies were applicable to AIDS. Most important were the advances in therapeutics. The ability to prevent HIV-related opportunistic infections and assumptions about the ability to slow the course of HIV progression itself suggested the importance of early identification of those infected. To achieve this, mass screening, the "return of HIV testing to the medical mainstream," and familiar public health interventions – such as name-based reporting and mandatory partner notification – became increasingly attractive.

With the "normalization" of AIDS in the late 1990s, the innovative ethical formulations that had prevailed at the epidemic's outset began to wane. For some, this development represented the triumph of tradition over principle. Others disagreed, arguing that AIDS had established an important precedent in public health ethics. Respect for individual autonomy and privacy had become critical components of epidemic control, even if communal well-being necessitated a perspective derived from a focus on populations rather than an exclusive preoccupation with individual rights. Most significantly, this perspective took on international dimensions in the effort to forge a link between health and human rights (Mann et al. 1994).

VII. TUBERCULOSIS RESURGENT

As AIDS exceptionalism waned, a new challenge to public health surfaced. Beginning in 1985, there was a resurgence of TB in the United States, fueled, in part, by the epidemic of HIV infection. In New York City, the rate of new cases of TB, which had reached a nadir in 1979, had tripled by 1992. This increase translated into 3,811 new cases of the disease in the city. Health officials estimated that there were 52,100 "excess" TB cases across the United States. Of special concern was the high percentage of TB cases that were resistant to one or more of the standard antibiotics. Multidrug-resistant cases often proved fatal, especially to those with immune systems already compromised by HIV infection (Frieden et al. 1993).

This epidemiological challenge drew the attention of a number of ethicists who had helped develop the notion of AIDS exceptionalism (Dubler et al. 1992). TB, however, was not AIDS. First, it was an airborne disease that could be transmitted to contacts who were unaware that they were being placed at risk. Second, the availability of treatments that could render those with TB noninfectious provided a public health justification for the aggressive use of antibiotic therapy. Nevertheless, drawing on the rights-based focus of bioethics and evolving constitutional principles regarding the burden borne by the state when it sought to deprive individuals of liberty, ethicists came to see the legal regime surrounding TB as "antiquated," involving measures that "predate[d] modern concepts of constitutional law and the need for a flexible range of public health powers" (Gostin 1993).

As the ethical issues posed by TB came into focus, there was remarkably little controversy over whether infectious individuals should be required to undergo therapy in the name of public health. John Stuart Mill's harm principle provided a sufficient basis for such restrictions on autonomy, as did the constitutional principles enumerated by the Supreme Court in the 1905 *Jacobson* decision (*Jacobson v. Massachusetts*). Given the developments in mental health law and the experiences with AIDS, there was a recognition that, however justified the imposition of constraints, due process protections needed to be recognized. Individuals with TB who might be deprived of their liberty in the name of public health were entitled to a hearing before an impartial tribunal, representation by counsel, and the opportunity to cross-examine witnesses.

The situation was more complicated. Most of the drug-resistant cases of TB that so fueled anxiety in the late 1980s and early 1990s had resulted from erratic compliance of patients with medical therapy. Thus, the problem of public health officials was not only to ensure the treatment for infectious individuals but also to assume the completion of therapy once such persons were no longer contagious. This conceptual shift from the immediate threat of the infectious TB patient to the noninfectious patient who could pose a *future* threat to the community required a broadening of the ethical and legal warrant for the imposition of treatment. The emphasis on treatment completion had one further implication: the need to create mechanisms to monitor patients to ensure that they, in fact, took their medications. It was here that controversy did surface.

An approach that had increasingly gained favor since the 1970s was directly observed therapy (DOT), in which tuberculous patients took their medications in the presence of a health care provider. So effective was DOT that a number of TB experts had begun to argue that all patients be deemed at risk for noncompletion of therapy and hence be required to participate in DOT (Iseman, Cohn, and Sbarbaro 1993). Yet this strategy could be viewed as overly broad, imposing burdens on those who might be adherent without DOT as well as those who would fail to take their medications. Because the vast majority of TB cases involved minorities, drug users, psychiatrically impaired persons and the HIV-infected, universal DOT would potentially revisit the unjust impositions inflicted on past TB patients.

Indeed, when a working group on the ethics of TB control met in New York in the early 1990s, it could not reach consensus on the matter of universal mandatory DOT. Civil libertarians and AIDS activists insisted that DOT be imposed only on those who had demonstrated noncompliance. Others, including some ethicists, had asserted that the threat of drug-resistant TB justified an approach that jettisoned individualized assessments for a population-based conception of risk (Dubler et al. 1992). Ultimately, although DOT was encouraged by health officials throughout the country in the 1990s, mandatory DOT typically remained limited to those who had failed one or more trials of voluntary compliance with medications. Those who remained noncompliant despite DOT – more than 500 persons nationwide between 1984 and 2000 – were subject to forcible detention. Because such individuals were overwhelmingly from disadvantaged populations, some argued that public health officials continued to use their powers unjustly, despite the increased attention to due process protections (Lerner 1999).

By 1999, the TB crisis in the United States had abated; the number of new cases was at the lowest point in recorded American history. Commentators credited this achievement to the widespread use of DOT and enhanced public health efforts. Whether detention of persistently nonadherent patients, including those who were noninfectious, had also made much of a contribution remained a matter of dispute. It was at this time that the Centers for Disease Control and Prevention asked the Institute of Medicine to undertake a study of the prospects of TB elimination in the United States. Its report, *Ending Neglect* (Institute of Medicine (IOM)), proposed a new conceptual shift that would entail the aggressive 6-month prophylactic "treatment" of those with latent infection – those who harbored the TB bacillus but were not sick with the disease (and who were therefore incapable of transmitting infection to others).

As such treatment was to be voluntary in nature for most individuals, it raised no critical ethical challenges. It was, however, the IOM's endorsement of *mandatory* treatment of latent infection among immigrants that represented a major policy departure, with important ethical implications. Epidemiological data had revealed that upward of half of all new cases of TB in the United States occurred in the foreign born. Starting with this finding, the committee that authored *Ending Neglect* ultimately concluded that all immigrants from nations with high TB prevalence be required to undergo screening for both active and latent infection. Those who were infected, the committee continued, should be obliged to undergo prophylactic therapy as a condition for the regularization of their immigration status. In addressing the question of whether mandatory identification and treatment of latent infection represented an unacceptable intrusion on the rights of immigrants, the committee concluded, "The issues of screening and treatment for latent infection compel society to address the question of when, if ever, it is appropriate to use compulsory health powers and how to balance the collective well-being against the rights of the individual to be free of intrusions when the threat he or she poses to other is only statistical (IOM 2000, 48) . . . The committee can see no fundamental reason why the logic of current TB screening should not be extended to those with latent infection" (IOM 2000, 95).

Among those who endorsed the committee's position were constitutional lawyers, experts on immigration law, and advocates for the foreign-born. Nevertheless, given the long record of civil liberties abuses against immigrants and other disadvantaged populations, it is remarkable that so significant an extension of the public health powers of the state should have elicited no significant discussion among ethicists.

VIII. ANTISMOKING EFFORTS: PATERNALISM REDUX?

Both AIDS and TB raised questions about the appropriate use of restrictive public health powers on diseased individuals who might pose risk to others. As the public health campaign against smoking in the United States intensified in the 1990s, it became necessary to address different questions – those first raised by the publication of the *Lalonde Report* (Lalonde 1974) and *Healthy People* (United States Department of Health, Education and Welfare 1957) two decades earlier. Here the central antagonism of bioethics to paternalism would need to be confronted.

When, as was the case with cigarette smoking, individuals engaged in behaviors that threatened their health and lives, what was the appropriate role of the state? Was it to inform, to warn, and to cajole through health education, or could it go further? In the name of the public health, could the state act more forcefully, imposing

burdens, restrictions or prohibitions that reflected a tutelary, even paternalistic role?

It is the mark of the hegemony of the Millian perspective on the limits of state power that the central justifications for antismoking policies adopted by the U.S. government in the years since the Surgeon General's 1964 report have sedulously sought to avoid the appearance of paternalism. Perhaps more striking, the arguments put forth by antismoking activists have typically avoided such assertions as well. These antitobacco strategies were threefold, focusing on the restriction on advertising and other educational initiatives, the limitation of smoking in public settings, and the imposition of taxes (Feldman and Bayer 2004).

Initially, health announcements weakly sought to warn smokers about the risks to which they were exposing themselves. Such efforts posed few challenges to civil libertarians. Of greater concern were early attempts to prohibit advertising. Although most public health officials and ultimately the American Medical Association advocated such restrictions, they had to confront the opposition not only of the tobacco industry but of those who favored strict First Amendment protections for commercial speech (Bayer et al. 2003).

Confronted with forceful opposition based on freedom of expression, public health officials and their allies began to emphasize how advertising lured vulnerable young people into a lifelong addiction to smoking. It was but a small step, subsequently, to assert that the protection of children represented a justifiable form of paternalism, even if such restrictions inevitably interfered with the ability of adults to make unfettered choices. In its 1994 report, *Growing Up Tobacco Free*, the IOM declared:

> Portraying a deadly addiction as a healthful and sensual experience tugs against the nation's efforts to promote a tobacco-free norm and to discourage tobacco use by children and youths. This warrants legislation restricting the features of advertising and promotion that make tobacco use attractive to youths. (IOM 2000, 131)

When the Food and Drug Administration later sought, ultimately ineffectively, to impose severe restrictions on all public displays of tobacco, it justified such limits almost entirely on the need to protect children from smoking, now defined as a "pediatric illness" (Bayer 2002).

The second element of the antismoking strategy involved increasingly burdensome restrictions on smoking in public settings. Here, too, the justification centered on the protection of vulnerable third parties placed at risk by smoke and smokers. As the executive director of Americans for Nonsmokers Rights stated in 1986, "We're just telling smokers to step outside, not how to save their lives" (Bayer and Colgrove 2002). In addressing himself to other activists, he underscored the strategic importance of focusing on the protection of innocents. "Activists," he advised, "should state that they are not 'antismoker' but rather environmentalists concerned with clean air for everyone. The issue should be framed in the rhetoric of the environment, toxic chemicals, and public health rather than the rhetoric of saving smokers from themselves or the cigarette companies" (Bayer and Colgrove 2002, 952). That such restrictions would have a dramatic impact on smokers' ability to smoke, and hence on cigarette consumption, was portrayed as a salutary secondary benefit from instituting necessary protections against second-hand smoke.

The third and final dimension of anti-tobacco efforts involved raising taxes on cigarettes. Although it was readily understood that such taxes were regressive, falling disproportionately on those least able to afford them, it was also appreciated that increases in prices would have a depressive effect on consumption. As with the benefits of restrictions on smoking in public settings, health officials would increasingly argue that higher taxes simply internalized the social costs of smoking. Because smokers got sick, and required medical care, they imposed economic burdens on nonsmokers. Fairness dictated that smokers themselves shoulder the costs. As one antitobacco activist stated, "Tobacco users [need to] start to pay their fair share for their use of tobacco products. It's a user fee, just like with other recreational activities. We're saying, 'If you want to ski the slope, you've got to buy the lift ticket.' It's only fair" (McNamara 1994). When it became increasingly clear that the early deaths of smokers mitigated these supposed economic burdens, proponents of higher taxes were compelled to emphasize the extent to which higher taxes and higher prices protected children and adolescents from smoking because they had less disposable income (Centers for Disease Control 1998). Once again, it was innocents who were to be protected.

A striking indication of the extent to which the growing field of bioethics had largely ignored issues within public health was its almost complete absence from the decades-long debate over how best to confront cigarette smoking, with its attendant human suffering. Only in 1989, a quarter of a century after the *Surgeon General's Report* was issued, did a philosopher publish an extended analysis of the ethics of tobacco control. In *No Smoking*, Robert Goodin sought to lay an ethical groundwork for severe restrictions on tobacco, and although he attended to the conventional arguments about how smoking represented a public health threat to others, he was most innovative in justifying state interference based on the harm that smokers imposed on themselves. Goodin was able to make this argument because he rejected the injunctions of John Stuart Mill. "To a very large extent ... the justification of public health measures in general must

be baldly paternalistic," he claimed. "Their fundamental point is to promote the wellbeing of people who might otherwise be inclined cavalierly to court certain sorts of diseases" (Goodin 1989, 31). Remarkably, this analysis sought to provide a foundation for a public health ethics utterly incompatible with the fundamental elements of bioethics.

IX. Conclusion: Public Health Ethics

During the 20 years that followed the onset of the AIDS epidemic, a number of ethicists were drawn to questions posed by threats to the public health; however, their efforts have been episodic rather than sustained. Particular challenges posed by AIDS, such as privacy, consent, and the limits of confidentiality, generated lively debate. The short-lived resurgence of TB in the early 1990s refocused attention on the uses and limits of coercion in the name of public health. With the sense of crisis surrounding AIDS having receded and with TB once again on the decline, interest in public health ethics has lost some of its vigor. The only exception has been the work of those ethicists involved in the global epidemics of AIDS and TB. On turning to these massive challenges, they have been compelled to address the vast inequalities between wealthy and Third World countries, the extent to which those in the Third World have moral claims to expensive therapeutic interventions, and the degree to which the wealthy have a moral duty to provide rescue.

Despite the striking contributions of those who ventured to address AIDS and TB, it is clear that public health ethics is still at a very formative stage. If conference halls could now be filled with individuals who see the work of medical ethics as central, it would be no exaggeration to state that those concerned with public health ethics could but fill a seminar room. This may be partially explained by the fact that those involved in public health policy making or practice still rarely characterize their work as having an ethical dimension.

Furthermore, it is clear that the absence of sustained effort on the part of those drawn to the moral challenges of public health has left a conceptual void. Given bioethics' commitment to the protection of patients and research subjects from the abuse of medical authority, and its inherent opposition to paternalism, it is not surprising that those who have sought to address public health ethics have found themselves in a conceptual bind. Forging an ethics of public health will necessitate fresh approaches to the protection and enhancement of the well-being of populations – as opposed to specific patients or subjects. Such an effort will inevitably generate conflicts between individual interests and rights and collective needs. How to resolve these conflicts remains the challenge. What is clear is that recourse to Mill's harm principle will be insufficient. Although constitutional principles and values will inevitably influence the development of public health ethics in the United States, such principles should not replace ethical norms in this process.

An ethics of public health that can address environmental and occupational threats to health, that considers the enduring challenge of infectious diseases, that addresses the relationship between individual and social behavior and chronic illness, and that is attuned to the relationship between morbidity and mortality and the social structure, should be enough to keep legions busy. Whatever the limited attainments of the past two decades, it is clear that the task has just begun.

CHAPTER 61

ETHICS AND HEALTH POLICY IN THE UNITED KINGDOM AND THE UNITED STATES: LEGISLATION AND REGULATION

Daniel M. Fox and Rudolf Klein

I. INTRODUCTION

A chapter by authors whose expertise is politics and policy making is appropriately an underinformed and perhaps overly cynical contribution to a history of medical ethics, which we take to mean disciplined statements about what is proper in relationships between health professionals and patients and between persons responsible for public health and populations. Whatever the achievements of ethicists in other arenas (Jonsen 1998), their influence on the development of legislation and regulation in the United Kingdom and the United States has been at best mixed.

Ethical doctrines have sometimes influenced the development of public policy, such as regulations in the United States for the protection of human subjects of research (see Chapters 50, 51, and 57). Ethical doctrines have also influenced how policy is implemented. That is, ethicists have helped to implement policies made for other reasons than the persuasiveness of their reasoning. Moreover, ethicists have helped to shape public opinion and, perhaps, the views of some of the elected and appointed officials who make policy, sometimes through commissions appointed by public bodies. Unfortunately, we do not know how to isolate the influence of ethical doctrines

from that of the vast amount of other information available to policy makers. In particular, it is impossible to distinguish the contribution of ethical doctrines to the minestrone of ideas – often inconsistent and always evolving – that shape the public philosophy or public morality that guides, and constrains, the conduct of policy makers in any country at any one time and that makes certain policy options unacceptable (for example, euthanasia of, or experiments on, the mentally handicapped).

In this chapter, we define policy as accountable action by legislative bodies and appointed heads of executive agencies. We avoid the difficult subject, on which we are not expert, of the implications of court decisions for policy and the ways in which judges use the discourse of ethicists. We will discuss general characteristics of the politics of policy making and then closely examine some examples of the modest role of medical ethics in the development and implementation of policy in the United Kingdom and the United States. We do so as a counterpoint to self-congratulatory accounts of influence. In doing so, we hope to persuade readers of two points. The first is that to survive and succeed, policy makers frequently pay more attention to what is prudent than to what others, and sometimes even they themselves, think is proper. Our second point is that on occasion statements about what is proper, and even ethicists themselves, have helped policy makers to reduce public turmoil as well as to dodge direct responsibility for actions that could increase the number of their enemies.

Our aim has been to analyze the role of ethics and ethicists in the policy process and to explain why it turns out to be so limited in practice. Others might want to adopt a more prescriptive approach, arguing the case for a more extended role. (For the alternative view, see Chapter 18.)

II. THE POLITICS OF POLICY MAKING

Health policy is a subset of general public policy. By health policy we mean deliberate efforts within particular jurisdictions to prevent, postpone, treat, or accommodate illness or injury for significant groups of people. These efforts are usually expressed in legislation, regulation, or policy guidance from executive agencies and legislative oversight committees. For convenience, we divide health policies in the public sector into two groups, using terms borrowed from economics: those that affect the supply of health services (e.g., policies for research, professional education, building facilities, and purchasing drugs and equipment) and those that affect the demand for services (especially policy for financing care and for removing barriers to access).

General policy frames health policy. Health policy is deeply affected by whom a government taxes (and the tax burden on different groups) and by how it prioritizes health services and improvements in health status in comparison to, for example, economic growth and employment, infrastructure, and national security. The same people who make general policy are responsible for the most important decisions about health policy: executives, legislative leaders, and persons accountable for budget and finance (Fox 1995; Klein 2000).

Many people who are active in the health affairs of each country focus their attention entirely on the health sector and on the interests they cherish within it. They accord scant attention to the relationship between health and general policy. Because the health sector is such a large percentage of the economy, especially in the United States, many health professionals, managers, and even health officials in public service can easily spend their entire careers ignoring how closely health and general policy are linked.

Many health professionals, again including persons on public payrolls, complain about the ignorance and intrusiveness of persons who make general public policy. Senior policy makers are familiar with these complaints, which they attribute to disloyalty, ideology, or professional self-interest. As a result, many senior policy makers in general

government (notably persons who run for office or manage executive departments responsible for budget and finance) reflexively distrust anyone who advocates for health policies that involve new costs or new risks of public controversy.

Persons in general government usually discount claims by health professionals, public health officials, and even by pharmaceutical manufacturers and by ethicists, that they are morally superior to the general run of advocates. They hear such claims every day from groups pressing for action on every issue about which government makes policy.

Persons in general government also know, however, that illness and its attendant suffering matter deeply to the public. A politician can pay dearly for media coverage that suggests that he or she is not properly sensitive to public anxiety about the spread of disease or lack of access to health services. On more than a few occasions, policy makers in each country have given proponents of particular health policies an easier time than other interest groups.

They or their successors have had reason to regret such indulgence. Because of their insularity and self-righteousness, health professionals – especially members of the medical profession – are a famously ungrateful interest group. Similarly, advocates for persons suffering from particular diseases typically interpret any success in obtaining more public funds for research or treatment as an invitation to demand more. During the second half of the twentieth century, health care interest groups were second only to Cold Warriors in successfully manipulating the politics of creating and resolving impending crises.

Leaders in general government also differ from many specialists in health politics and policy in having a deeper appreciation of how political institutions shape what policy is made, when, how, and by whom. By political institutions we mean both constitutional arrangements, whether written as in the United States or unwritten as in the United Kingdom, and the formal and informal rules that govern relationships among levels of government and within particular legislative and judicial bodies, executive departments, and political parties.

Some political institutions are not governmental in a formal sense, for example, the media, business and professional associations, labor unions, advocacy organizations, and often charities and foundations. Each of these institutions has a history, often going back a century or more. Ignorance of that history has frequently been fatal to persons who aspire to initiate or to change policy.

In summary, as a result of the politics of policy making, precepts and discourse of medical ethics that are deduced from theories are fundamentally incompatible with the conduct of public affairs. Ethicists who base their advice on the analysis of cases, as various presidential commissions in the United States have done, are more likely to inform the judgments of policy makers. Even inductive ethicists, however, have on occasion crossed the boundary between analysis and advocacy.

Although we know less about what ethicists think and do than we know about the work of policy makers, we venture five generalizations about the grounds for this incompatibility:

- Ethicists, whether deductive or inductive, usually value clarity and precision, as do most people who earn their livings as intellectuals. Policy makers are often required to prefer ambiguity, inconsistency, and at times obfuscation.
- Ethicists who reason from well-defined principles to practical conclusions have different habits of mind than do policy makers, who have to deal with situations in which principles conflict or in which their translation into policy is problematic. With general goals in mind, policy makers assess the interests and behavior of competing groups and negotiate with persons within and outside public bodies to achieve a result that can be implemented.
- Ethicists who accord the highest value to principles and the precepts they deduce from them have different priorities than do leaders of government. Public policy makers usually value loyalty to allies and party over loyalty to convictions – and they value political survival above all else.
- Ethicists, both inductive and deductive, accord high value to solving problems. Policy makers often prefer to postpone problems rather than imposing solutions that have intolerable political costs.
- Medical ethicists, by occupational definition, accord priority to the proper conduct of health professionals and health affairs in general. Policy makers often sacrifice improvements in health services and health status to the exigencies of other areas of policy.

In what follows, we test these propositions by examining selected issues on which medical ethicists have been active, or where they might have been expected to make a significant contribution to the policy process. These are debates first about rationing and second about policy for regulating physician behavior. In both cases, we compare the United States and the United Kingdom experiences to see whether our propositions are robust enough to justify general conclusions about the role of medical ethics in the policy process, that is, whether they hold irrespective of the particular institutions and political culture of individual liberal democracies.

We do not claim that our conclusions apply to totalitarian, or even to kleptocratic regimes, although in these cases one would expect the role of ethical doctrine to be even more limited. Examples include the practice of euthanasia and experiments on the mentally handicapped in Nazi Germany (see Chapter 54), the use of psychiatric diagnoses to incarcerate dissidents in the Soviet Union (see Chapter 55), as well as bribery and the international narcotics trade in contemporary Africa, Asia, and South America.

The other two cases, regulation of research in the United States and acquired immunodeficiency syndrome/human immunodeficiency virus policy in the United Kingdom focus on a single country because, having made our comparative point, we chose not to repeat ourselves. Instead we offer evidence from two additional areas in which ethics served but did not drive policy makers in carrying out their responsibilities.

Both the United States and the United Kingdom can, very broadly, be described as liberal democracies, subscribing to such notions as the rule of law, decision making by elected representatives, and so on. Nevertheless, in many other respects, crucial for an understanding of the policy process, they differ. The United States has a pluralistic system, offering a multiplicity of "veto points" (Immergut 1992). The division of responsibility between the President and Congress and among federal, state, and local governments means that policy is the product of coalition building and bargaining. In contrast, the United Kingdom system of government, sometimes described as an elective dictatorship, means that the administration of the day tends to have an automatic majority in Parliament, giving it the ability to drive through its policy proposals even in the face of strong public (and professional) opposition. The role of local government is limited to the delivery of services within parameters determined by the central administration.

Whereas the United States can be characterized as an example of diffused decision making, the United Kingdom can be categorized as an example of concentrated decision making. The opportunities for interest groups to influence policy are accordingly much greater in the former than in the latter: only contrast the fate of President Clinton's health plan with Mrs. Thatcher's ability to drive through her 1991 reform of the National Health Service (NHS) in the face of strenuous opposition. Add to these factors that the law plays a much larger part in the American political culture than in the British case – where the notion of legally enforceable rights is alien, where the courts are rarely called upon to decide health policy issues and even more rarely call on medical ethicists to give evidence – and we are clearly dealing with very different policy-making environments. We shall indeed find significant differences in both policy processes and outcomes in the examples that follow – but, we would claim, that they have one common element: that, in line with our propositions, there is in some cases little evidence that medical ethics have either directly shaped or made a persisting contribution to the implementation of public policy.

III. RATIONING AND ALLOCATION

1. The United States

During the past half-century, medical ethicists and their allies in the United States have frequently urged policy makers to address systematically the allocation of scarce resources. In general, advocacy for reallocation has had two purposes. One was to increase access to health care for the poor and the underserved, mainly by establishing a universal entitlement to health insurance. The other purpose was the just distribution of new, high-technology clinical interventions that promised to extend or to save lives (Ubel 2000). Ethicists' allies in promoting both purposes included advocates for the poor and for persons suffering from particular life-threatening diseases. Policy makers in the federal government and the states rejected most advice from ethicists and their allies about how they could achieve either purpose.

Most policy makers believed that their rejection of this advocacy was principled. They reasoned that they were elected or appointed to office to act on behalf of a public that was unwilling to be taxed to pay for universal coverage and that abhorred the word rationing.

Most Americans consistently told pollsters and the persons they elected to public office that they preferred to believe that access and allocation were separate issues. They supported policies for access that created direct insurance subsidies for the elderly, for persons with severe disabilities, and for children who had the misfortune of living in households where income fell below the poverty line. They also endorsed policies that subsidized health insurance through the tax system when employers chose to offer it to employees and later extended this subsidy to self-employed persons. They agreed that poor adults ought to have a regular source of health care and that everyone ought to have emergency care (Jacobs 1993).

These policies created uneven – many would say inequitable – access to health services. Millions of people had no insurance for all or part of each year. Public safety net services for both emergencies and preventive services were unevenly available across the country.

This result has been politically acceptable. Disappointed advocates of universal coverage sometimes accused the majority of Americans of being mean-spirited or ethically challenged. Others complained about the conspiratorial power of interest groups to mobilize opposition to reform among policy makers and the public. Yet opponents of universal coverage were too prominent to be conspiratorial. They have included, for example, most private employers and labor union locals, the insurance industry, and many health professionals.

It is more likely that American policy for health coverage is politically acceptable for three other reasons. One reason is that a vast number of Americans – like people in every leading industrial country except Britain, according to a recent survey – prefer more disposable income to higher taxes (Editorial 2000). The second reason is that most Americans do not accord health coverage the same priority that advocates do. The third reason is that Americans express their empathy with sick people by opposing any explicit rationing of health services.

Americans have expressed their abhorrence of rationing by making it clear to public officials that health policy should rescue persons in dire situations and that the newest promising interventions ought to be available to all persons who need them. The only Americans who have endorsed explicit rationing have done so in hypothetical situations: for example, in responses to questions asked by social scientists or in formal meetings in which they debated variants of the general question, "Who shall live and who shall die" (Ubel 2000)?

Policy makers have received countless complaints from their constituents about services denied them by government programs, health maintenance organizations, and insurance companies. They have understood quite well the difference between political behavior and what respondents in scientifically selected samples told social scientists or what people who wanted to be regarded as earnest and thoughtful by their neighbors said at community meetings.

From an orderly and principled – an ethical – point of view it may seem nonsensical that the same public that demands access to any potentially beneficial service also supports rigorous cost containment and rejects proposals for universal access to health care. Politicians prefer to be orderly and principled; their responsibilities make such behavior difficult and sometimes impossible.

Policy makers, whether elected or appointed, are required to accord close attention to the complexity of human behavior in political communities. As a result, they know that some members of the public do not carefully examine their opinions about who ought to be covered for what services by health insurance until they are confronted personally with pain and suffering, their own or that of a person close to them. Policy makers also understand that many people express generous instincts – and Americans are famously generous people – without computing the cost of acting on those instincts to themselves, their health plan, or government. Moreover, many Americans have been persuaded by generations of medical and media propaganda claiming that investment in the supply side of health care, that is in hospital construction, advanced training for medical specialists, and biomedical research, would improve everyone's health ever more efficiently. In addition, as philosopher-ethicist Daniel Callahan wrote, "Americans are in general just not certain what role to give to the pursuit of health and the avoidance of disease in their lives" (Callahan 2000).

There are numerous examples in point. The first health care rationing issue to receive wide national attention was the limited availability of kidney dialysis when that intervention ceased to be experimental in the early 1960s. Beginning with concern about whether the so-called God Committee at the University of Washington should judge the personal worth of candidates for dialysis, the media, ethicists and policy makers debated alternative ways to allocate this new resource (Jonsen 1998; see also Chapter 38).

To truncate a very long story, after a decade of public debate, the United States Congress solved the problem in 1972 by passing legislation to finance dialysis for persons of all ages suffering from end-stage renal disease as an entitlement under the Medicare program. Because members of Congress were sensitive to the political culture in which they lived, they chose to avoid the issue of rationing facilities for dialysis.

The most widely publicized rationing debate of the 1990s was about the list of medical interventions, ranked in priority order, devised by a public commission in Oregon to guide the allocation of resources among persons with low incomes who were or would be enrolled in the federal/state Medicaid program. Oregon policy makers wanted guidance about allocating resources fairly as part of a new policy that would double the size of the population covered by Medicaid (Fox and Leichter 1991).

Ethicists and policy analysts from many countries pronounced about the Oregon process. Considerable publicity attended community meetings around the state about allocation preferences. Professional ethicists staffed some of these meetings, which appealed to their colleagues in other jurisdictions; however, the majority of persons attending the meetings worked in health care or lived in the same household as people who did. Even greater publicity greeted the first report of a commission appointed by state government to rank particular interventions by using methods of cost effectiveness analysis that incorporated decisions about values.

To truncate a long story again: The policy makers who eventually implemented the Oregon Health Plan used their professional and political judgment, as well as analytical tools, to decide what would or would not be covered at different levels of aggregate funding. Most of these political judgments occurred within the state; others were negotiated between Oregon officials and officials of the federal government under two administrations. Some ethicists claim that their intervention made it possible for state officials to replace "simple utilitarian cost effectiveness" with a more politically acceptable "rule of rescue" principle as the basis of policy. This claim confuses the work of a commission that advised policy makers with the opportunities and constraints of Oregon and federal politics.

By 2000, persons who still paid attention (very few of whom now lived outside the state) agreed that the expansion of Oregon's Medicaid program during the 1990s had been a considerable success. More Oregonians received decent health coverage and as a result their health status and access to educational and economic opportunity had improved. The unusual public debate about the ethics of rationing was an interlude in the normal politics of policy making (Leichter 1999).

2. The United Kingdom

Britain's NHS is often held up as an example – and a reproach – to the United States. Indeed it presents a very different picture from that drawn in the previous section. Whereas the United States enters the new millennium with an incomplete, chaotic yet exorbitantly expensive system of health care, Britain in 1948 succeeded at a stroke in achieving what successive generations of American politicians have failed to bring about: universal health coverage. Moreover, the principle that resources should be allocated according to need, as distinct from the ability to pay, was enshrined in the founding constitution of the NHS. Here would seem to be an example of an institution deliberately created to enshrine an ethical imperative. Despite changes in the internal structure and organization of the NHS over the decades, there has not been any weakening in the commitment to either universalism or equity in the allocation of resources. Funded out of general taxation the NHS is a powerful instrument of redistribution – to the poor and the old, both of whom make disproportionately large demands on services – but nevertheless has continued to enjoy overwhelming public support even while criticism of its actual performance has grown over the years. Successive governments, Conservative as well as Labor, have competed in proclaiming their commitment to the principles of the NHS. The achievement of equity in both access to health care and the treatment offered has remained a dominant policy goal, endorsed if not necessarily actively pursued by governments irrespective of political ideology. Over the decades, great efforts have been invested in devising formulae for distributing the central budget equitably to the component geographical units of the NHS, that is, according to various measures of need.

All in all, therefore, the United Kingdom would appear to provide an example of ethical considerations driving policy. Equity as the guiding principle of the NHS has become institutionalized. Further the United Kingdom experience would also seem to suggest that there is an inverse relationship between the professional strength of medical ethicists and their influence on public policy. In the United Kingdom, in strong contrast to the United States, medical ethicists are a rare species without a strong base either in academia or the health care system.

The picture of the NHS as an example of ethics triumphing over political expediency – contrary to our propositions – must, however, be modified in important respects. The first point to note is that the image of the NHS as equity institutionalized represents a gross historical oversimplification. In its origins the NHS is the child of a marriage between technocratic paternalism (Fox 1986) and Labor Party ideology. The former wanted to create an institution in which the wonders of modern medicine could be organized rationally and efficiently: a system in which the state would allow (and fund) the professionals to deliver the best care as defined by them and to distribute it according to their criteria of need. The latter wanted to create an institution that would remove all financial barriers to access and, in the words of the NHS's political architect, Aneurin "Nye" Bevan (1897–1960), devise a system that would "generalise the best." If the NHS embodies the Good Samaritan principle – as Richard Titmuss (1970) put it – in this particular instance the Good Samaritan is wearing a white coat. Interestingly the Beveridge Report (Beveridge 1942) which is often – although wrongly – seen as leading to the creation of the NHS was extremely parsimonious in its appeal to ethical principles as distinct from administrative rationality. In the very short section of the report devoted to health care, Beveridge simply noted, "restoration of a sick person to health is a duty of the State and the sick person." Equity did not feature in his arguments.

In its conception, the NHS therefore reflects an unacknowledged stress between two ethical principles. On the one hand, openly celebrated, is the equity principle. On the other hand, seldom even mentioned, is the autonomy principle. The case for providing free health care to all is (externalities apart) precisely the argument that health care is, in Rawlsian terms, a requirement for achieving fair equality of opportunity: maximizing people's ability to function, within the limits set by their personal inheritance of genes, is seen as a necessary condition for the autonomous framing and pursuit of individual life plans. Egalitarianism is, in short, justified in terms of autonomy. The NHS offends, in crucial respects, against the autonomy principle. It is, as noted above, a monument to technocratic paternalism: a system geared to meeting need as defined by the professional providers, not to respond to the wants of users. Despite the semantic transformation of the patient (an essentially passive concept) into the consumer (an active concept) in recent years, it is professional practices, not public preferences, that dictate the pattern of health care provision. The ability to choose between different doctors or hospitals – a necessary if not sufficient condition, surely, for autonomy – is conspicuous by its absence in the NHS.

In the 1990s, successive governments have sought to change the balance, exhorting the NHS to be more responsive and introducing a kind of top-down consumerism by command. So, for example, the conservative administration introduced the principle of "patient rights" – something of a misnomer because the rights, as set out in the Patient's Charter, were not legally enforceable. The New Labor government elected in 1997 has since developed this strategy further. It is important, however, to be clear as to why this change has taken place. There has been no great debate about the ethical underpinnings of the NHS and the tension between equity and autonomy. Even though there has been much discussion of the ethics of the doctor–patient relationship, and the need to put this on a more equal footing, this has not been translated into a wider discussion of how this is to be achieved within the constraints of the NHS.

If governments have acted, it is for very different reasons. There was mounting public dissatisfaction with the services provided by the NHS: the political costs of maintaining the NHS were beginning to outweigh the economic advantages of a system that provided universal coverage at half the cost (in terms of the proportion of gross domestic product spent on health care) of the United States. There was further a growing awareness, not least among Labor Ministers, that a provider-dominated health service was something of an anomaly in the emergent supermarket society. Political expediency thus went hand in hand with sociological analysis (Giddens 1998) in bringing about a new emphasis in policies toward the NHS. Whether the attempt to transform technocratic paternalism into consumer responsiveness within the existing framework of the NHS is a feasible long-term policy is, of course, another question. For the purposes of this chapter, it suffices to demonstrate that the new direction of health policy owes nothing to ethical principles.

One piece of evidence, suggesting that the NHS's concentration on equity at the expense of autonomy is at odds with citizen preferences, is the growth of the private sector of health care. Something like 11 percent of the population are now covered by private health care insurance; others use the private sector on a pay as you go basis. Too much should not be made of this. The rise in private health care insurance, and use, has flattened out in recent years. The private sector remains specialized, concentrating on elective surgery. Most users do not exit from the NHS – they continue to use it, both for general practitioner services and for life-threatening conditions – and remain loyal to it. The incentive is to use the private sector selectively: to jump NHS waiting lists, to ensure choice of a consultant and to have better hotel services while hospitalized.

The real significance of the private sector, from the perspective of our analysis, is the dog that has not barked for 50 years. Without question, the private sector is an offense against the equity principle of the NHS. It allows money to talk. The original decision to allow NHS consultants to engage in private practice – the foundation of the private sector – was a quite conscious concession to political expediency: the price Bevan was prepared to pay to win the support of the prestigious Royal Colleges for his scheme. Yet, no government since 1948 has even questioned whether the continued existence of the private sector is compatible with the ethical imperative that led to the creation of the NHS. In the 1970s, Harold Wilson's Labor government sought to reduce the scope of the private sector, with a famous lack of success. Mrs. Thatcher's Conservative governments sought to encourage private health care insurance by offering limited tax breaks. The New Labor government is seeking to restrict the private practice activities of NHS consultants without, however, challenging the principle.

Although analyzing the extent to which there is equity in access to the NHS has become something of an academic industry, the wider effects on equity of the private sector have virtually been ignored in public debate. For Labor the private sector is a beast best left undisturbed. For hospital consultants private practice fees can double or even triple their NHS salaries: any move to restrict the sector therefore risks a major confrontation with the medical profession (as it did in the 1970s). For the Conservatives, the private sector appears to offer a way of diminishing the demands on, and the financial appetite of, the NHS. In neither case do ethical considerations shape party policies, although ideological biases undoubtedly color them. No attempt has been made to balance explicitly the rival ethical claims of equity and autonomy: in political debate (in contrast to academic discussion) there are no prizes for clarity on this issue. As in the case of schooling – where Britain notoriously has a two-tier system – liberalism appears to set a limit to egalitarianism. It is political expediency, however, that ensures that this limit remains a fuzzy frontier.

The attractions and advantages of fuzziness in policy making are further illustrated by the case of rationing in the United Kingdom. The NHS has, since its inception, been an example of rationing in health care. Operating within fixed budgets, it has had to allocate limited resources among competing demands. It has rationed by denial: imposing restrictive conditions for access to particular types of treatment (e.g., by age – as in the case of renal dialysis) or refusing to prescribe certain expensive drugs. It has rationed by delay: witness the notorious waiting lists. It has rationed by dilution: poor standards of care on chronic wards are an example. It has rationed by deflection: the long-term care of the elderly has largely been diverted to the social services sector. (See also Chapter 7.)

The distinguishing characteristic of most of these rationing strategies is that they do not reflect explicit decisions by policy makers in central government. Central decisions about allocating envelopes of resources – to particular services or to health authorities responsi-

ble for providing health care to given populations – have been transmuted into clinical decisions about who should be treated, how, and to what level of intensity. Politicians have, in effect, sheltered behind the doctrine of clinical autonomy. For most of the history of the NHS, this arrangement suited both partners in the enterprise. Politicians benefited because the consequences of their decisions about resources were not directly attributable to them: essentially, it was a blame-diffusion strategy. The medical profession benefited because its members enjoyed a degree of autonomy and immunity from scrutiny that would be unimaginable in the United States.

The position has begun to change in recent years. There has been an increasing degree of scrutiny of medical practice; in turn, the medical profession has become increasingly unhappy about accepting responsibility for delivering less than acceptable standards of care (as it saw it). Further, one consequence of the 1991 reforms of the NHS was to give greater visibility to the activities of the NHS by separating the roles of purchasers and providers and generating more information about what was on offer to the public. The media seized upon instances of what came to be known as "postcode rationing" – that is, geographical variations in access to, and the availability of, different forms of treatment. The practice of rationing appeared to be not only arbitrary but also incompatible with the NHS's equity principle.

The first reaction of policy makers in the United Kingdom was, like their counterparts in the United States, to expunge the word rationing from their vocabulary. To the argument that equity required explicit central decisions about what should or should not be provided by the NHS – that access and availability should not be determined by the lottery of geography – they responded by pointing out that it would be wrong to dictate what clinicians should or should not do when faced with the particular circumstances of individual patients. More recently, the New Labor government has taken a somewhat different tack. It has invoked technical expertise as an alternative to political decision making. It has created a National Institute for Clinical Excellence to provide best-practice guidance to clinicians. In effect, Bevan's hyperbolic policy ambition of "generalising the best" has been revived.

If the instruments of policy are changing, the underlying goal has not. Policy makers are still seeking to side-step the challenge of taking direct responsibility for the criteria to be used in allocating resources. To put it crudely, they are engaged in an exercise in ethical evasion in the absence of ethical consensus. Should resources be used to maximize the health of the population or to minimize social class inequalities in health care status? Should utilitarianism rule supreme or is there a role for the rule of rescue? What if the effectiveness criterion – the main tool of the experts – does not offer an unambiguous recipe for resource allocation? The questions are all familiar to those concerned with the ethics of rationing. They are, however, also questions that policy makers prefer not to address: a response that, given the lack of agreement among ethicists themselves, may be proper as well as prudent public policy.

IV. REGULATING THE BEHAVIOR OF DOCTORS

1. The United States

Medical ethics has been integral to policy for regulating the behavior of doctors (called physicians in the United States and hence throughout this section) because government, for centuries, has delegated considerable authority to the medical profession to police itself (Fox 1993; see also Chapter 47). During the nineteenth century, each state established a board of medicine. Although technically public bodies they engaged in professional self-regulation. The members of the board were, in fact or effect, chosen by the leaders of state and county medical societies.

The boards made and implemented public policy, especially policy that protected the economic interests of the profession. For example, they established requirements for licensure and the scope of medical practice as well as defining and penalizing unethical behavior – with particular emphasis on referral practices that could divert patients' fees to healers who did not accept the discipline of organized medicine. The boards adjudicated complaints about individual physicians and had the authority to suspend or remove the license of any member of the profession who violated the ethical and economic doctrines expressed in the diction of ethics that had been the basis of policy (Ameringer 1999).

The scope of the boards' informal authority increased in the twentieth century. Boards in most states had considerable influence on the establishment or closure of medical schools and the size of their entering classes. Moreover, as a result of the power of organized medicine, medical boards often made policy, formally and informally, about the scope of practice of other professions, for example, optometry and nursing.

In the last quarter of the twentieth century, the boards acquired new formal authority but as accountable agents of government rather than as self-regulators who prioritized the interests of their profession. Boards now managed therapeutic interventions for impaired physicians and those who exploited their patients sexually as an extension of their role in licensure. In many states, boards of medicine regulated persons who practiced such alternative therapies as acupuncture and naturopathy. Perhaps most important, the boards regulated the prescribing of drugs that were also controlled substances; a role in which they were often in tension or even conflict with federal and state officials responsible for narcotics control and criminal justice.

General government had encouraged the boards to use the precepts and codes of medical ethics to make policy. The medical profession, in turn, used "codes of ethics and disciplinary rules . . . to reclaim political power" that its members were losing to collective purchasers in government and business and to the insurance industry under managed care (Ameringer 1999, 113). Governors and state legislators were usually delighted to devolve difficult decisions to the boards. These decisions were particularly difficult because someone always loses when a complaint against a physician is resolved; either a complaining patient or the physician complained against, or a patient's family members, or physicians who testified against a colleague.

The delegation of quasi-judicial authority to the boards to implement policy based on principles of medical ethics enabled policy makers to take credit for justice being done without incurring blame from any of their constituents. As the number of health professions seeking recognition and insurance reimbursement proliferated in the last third of the century, wary legislators augmented the responsibilities of medical boards or created new boards to regulate emerging professions. Boards became participants in the politics of policy making for health professionals' access to the public and its money.

The boards' links to the leaders of organized medicine diminished as medical care became an increasingly complicated and expensive enterprise. Legislators and governors could no longer risk being accused of ceding regulatory authority to members of a profession who made the most significant decisions about individuals in a sector of the economy that received approximately 60 percent of its income from government spending (Fox and Fronstin 2000).

As the complexity of the issues the boards addressed increased, they became more dependent on professional staff, that is, on managers and lawyers on the public payroll. The boards came to resemble other regulatory bodies, for example those that set and implemented standards for education and public utilities. Procedures and decisions were now determined by statutes and case law, just as they were for other regulated groups and industries, not by explicit ethical doctrines. Ethics remained part of the discourse of policy making, influencing but not determining law and regulation.

During the 1990s, policy makers in general government in a growing number of states encouraged medical boards to change their priority from regulating (and often, still protecting) the profession to advocacy and representation on behalf of consumers. General policy makers eagerly deflected to the boards the rising political heat they felt from aggrieved consumers and alternative healers. Many boards now appointed consumers to membership (Milbank Memorial Fund 1998). Legislation and, in some states, ballot initiatives augmented the boards' authority to regulate the prescribing of narcotics to control pain; especially in situations in which the prescription could have the "double effect" of relieving pain and hastening death. This expansion of their duties made the boards even more dependent on professional staff and on legal procedures than on codes of ethics. The medical profession, far from holding the boards captive, now pleaded with the boards, as they did with other regulatory agencies, to help them negotiate with consumers and health plans.

Unfortunately for the boards, however, their role is being eroded by changes in the organization of medical practice and the consequent introduction of techniques of quality improvement that are grounded in statistical analysis and management science rather than in ethical principles. As more physicians practiced in corporate environments – investor-owned or nonprofit health maintenance organizations and physician-owned multispecialty practices – more of them are required to be accountable within an institutional (more precisely, an industrial) rather than, as in the past, a professional framework. Continuous Quality Improvement (CQI) and its successor methodologies promise to make obsolete regulatory structures, like medical boards, that punish physicians who transgress against principles (Ameringer 1999; Robinson 1999).

2. United Kingdom

The General Medical Council (GMC), set up by an Act of Parliament in 1858, is a paradigm example of professional self-regulation. Its creation represented a victory for the medical profession. To quote the words of the GMC itself (cited in Stacey 1992, 20), the Act "was passed largely as a result of initiative within the profession, and the establishment of the Council was desired as much for the protection of the duly qualified medical practitioner from the competition of unqualified practitioners as for the protection of the public." Its subsequent history consolidated that victory: the medical profession maintained its grip over the GMC, autonomously deciding how doctors should be educated, who should be admitted to the register of medical practitioners and what criteria (and processes) should be used to strike off those deemed to have offended against the profession's standards of conduct and code of ethics. Although the proportion of lay members nominated by the government has, over the past three decades crept up to 25 percent, the GMC remains very much dominated by the medical profession – in part elected by the profession, in part representing academic institutions. (See also Chapter 36.)

This picture of a medical monolith has begun to change over the past decade and a half. The important point, from the perspective of this analysis, is that very few of the changes have been prompted by explicit public policy interventions. They represent the adaptive strategy of a medical profession under threat first from a changing social environment in which deferential respect for the authority of doctors could no longer be taken for granted – in which legitimacy and trust have to be earned – and under pressure, in the past few years, from a Labor government with a radical strategy for improving quality in the NHS. The result has been a degree of change unprecedented in terms of both direction and pace. So far at least, it is change initiated by the GMC itself: control of the agenda of reform still remains – if somewhat precariously – in the hands of the institution itself.

In 1975, a government-appointed Committee of Inquiry reported on the regulation of the medical profession: the Merrison report (Merrison 1975). Significantly this committee was appointed not because of dissatisfaction among policy makers or the public about the way in which the GMC performed its role but because of pressure from the medical profession itself. There had been a long-simmering dispute not about ethics but about money: doctors were angry about the introduction of an annual fee (instead of a once and for all payment) for having their names retained on the medical register. The details of the report's recommendations are of no concern here: they included changes in the composition of the GMC's governing body (more members elected by the profession and more lay people). Two points, however, need to be noted. The medical profession itself largely dominated the process of translating the report's recommendations into legislation: so, for example, the recommendation that the GMC should have its own investigative unit for inquiring into complaints was ignored (Stacey 1992). Second, was the report's illuminating characterization of the GMC's role:

> An instructive way of looking at regulation is to see it as a contract between public and profession, by which the public go to the profession for medical treatment because the profession has made sure that it will provide satisfactory treatment.

Was the GMC keeping to its side of the contract? In the 1980s, and even more in the 1990s, the question was asked with increasing urgency. As deferential patients began to be transformed into demanding consumers, as Mrs. Thatcher started to swing her handbag at the professions, criticism of the GMC began to mount. In particular, there was much criticism of the way in which the GMC dealt with complaints about doctors – rejecting the vast majority without explanation – and the grindingly slow pace of its disciplinary proceedings. In turn, the leadership of the GMC began to realize that a changing social culture demanded a changing medical culture. The GMC accordingly began to move from the ethics of medical self-protection to the ethics of consumer protection.

Two booklets setting out the GMC's code of practice for doctors illustrate the change. The 1977 booklet, *Professional Conduct and Discipline*, concentrates on conduct by doctors that might bring the profession into disrepute. It is essentially about character, behavior, and relations with other doctors. Thus doctors risked disciplinary censure (or being struck off the register) if convicted of taking drugs, driving under the influence of drink, fraud, and indecent behavior or found guilty of sleeping with their patients, attacking the professional skills of a colleague, or advertising. Two paragraphs deal with neglect or disregard of personal responsibilities to patients for their care and treatment; two pages are devoted to "signposts or notice-boards relating to health centres or medical centres."

More than 20 years on the GMC's *Good Medical Practice* – defining the duties of a doctor – marks a transformation. Here the emphasis is squarely on the responsibilities of doctors to deliver good-quality care. These include keeping knowledge and skills up to date, working within the limits of their competence, taking part in medical audit, respecting the views and dignity of patients and accepting responsibility for working collegially in teams. Whereas the 1977 document stressed that doctors should not criticize their colleagues, the 1998 document imposed a duty on doctors to take action if they believed that "a doctor's or other colleague's health, conduct, or performance "was a threat to patients. Traditional concerns – improper personal relationship, fiscal integrity, and so on – still feature, but very much in a minor key.

Changes in the focus of the GMC were accompanied by changes in its machinery. New procedures for examining the performance (as distinct from the conduct of doctors) came into operation in 1997. These are designed to deal with doctors who, while chaste and honest, have failed to maintain their professional skills adequately. It remains to be seen how this new procedure will work. More important, the GMC's ability to set its own course – to redefine professional ethics and responsibilities autonomously – was threatened by external events.

First, there was the election in 1997 of a New Labor government committed to a quality agenda in the NHS. Second, the same year the GMC began hearings in the notorious Bristol case in which two pediatric cardiac surgeons (and the medically qualified chief executive of the trust) were found guilty of misconduct following the deaths of a series of young children. The Bristol case was followed by a number of other examples of medical failures or misdeeds. The procession of erring doctors culminated in the case of Dr. Shipman – a GP found guilty of murdering fifteen of his patients – found guilty of drug abuse by the GMC decades earlier but subsequently reinstated (thus fueling the suspicion that doctors tended to be overly lenient toward their colleagues). The issue of medical standards, and the role of the GMC in safeguarding them, thus became a subject of intense media and political concern for the first time in the history of the NHS. Although external pressure strengthened the hand of the GMC's President – Sir Donald Irvine, elected on a reform ticket in 1995 – in persuading an often-reluctant profession to change, it also threatened the ability of the medical profession to determine the agenda. So, for example, Sir Donald was able to persuade the medical profession to accept – in the wake of the Bristol case – the principle of revalidation of professional qualifications. The switch of emphasis from inputs (medical education) to outputs (medical performance) seemed complete – propriety redefined as competence.

In the meantime, however, the government was pursuing its own agenda. It was not an agenda driven by an interest in medical ethics but rather by a determination to ensure that the medical profession was meeting its side of the implicit contract with the public, as defined in the Merrison report, by providing "satisfactory treatment." A variety of measures were introduced. A statutory responsibility for quality was imposed on the chief executives and boards of NHS trusts; a Commission for Health Improvement, in effect an NHS inspectorate, was created to ensure that providers were meeting quality standards. In short, a proactive was replacing a reactive system of maintaining medical standards. Whereas previously the GMC had to wait for cases to be brought to it, now there is a machinery (in theory at least) for systematically generating work for it: the number of doctors charged with serious disciplinary offenses by the GMC more than doubled between 1998 and 1999, rising from 80 to 181 (Laurence 2000).

If so, the change will be symbolic. The glass wall between a self-regulating medical profession and policy making is cracking: interestingly in the Bristol case, the Secretary of State for Health publicly criticized the GMC for striking only two of the doctors off the register and pronouncing a more lenient sentence on the third. In a sense, the GMC is becoming an instrument of government policy, just as boards of medicine have in the United States. It is a trend that has already produced a backlash in the profession. Caught between government pressure and professional reluctance, the future of the GMC is therefore in some doubt: Professional regulation is, to an extent at least, becoming publicly regulated. At the time of writing the GMC is, under government pressure, proposing to reform its structure and procedures radically: among other changes, it is planning to increase sharply the proportion of lay members (GMC 2001).

V. CONCLUSION

We have described how policy makers, driven by considerations of political and administrative feasibility, routinely, and without great anguish, make trade-offs between competing ethical principles in a process that rarely (if ever) involves addressing or invoking those principles directly. Moreover, subordinating ethics to politics may also be a sensible way to avoid inflicting harm on vulnerable people: for instance the consideration accorded persons with severe disabilities under implicit and explicit rationing policies in both countries. Prudence, that is, may reinforce propriety.

Policy makers have good reasons to farm out tricky ethical issues to others. The cases of both rationing and regulation illustrate how official and semi-official groups of peers can alleviate protracted controversies over irreconcilable differences and also insulate general government from criticism.

Many ethicists in the United States take pride in having helped policy makers resolve profound differences among religious groups about the definition of death. Ethicists took a major role in proposing a Uniform Definition of Death Act for adoption by the states and in promoting its passage during the 1980s (Gray 1995; see Chapter 63). The Uniform Act, along with such related measures as statutes requiring consent to physicians' Do Not Resuscitate (DNR) orders, however, have failed in practice in most jurisdictions (Light and McGee 1998; Zuckerman 1999). As a practitioner of general government, the majority leader of a state legislative chamber, complained about the Uniform Act (not for attribution), "There is no chance of implementing this policy successfully when the same physiological situation creates a dead Catholic and a living Jew."

In practice, the implicit value systems of policy makers are more important than explicit ethical debate. These value systems often become institutionalized – as in the commitment to equity as symbolized by Britain's NHS and the commitment to liberty as symbolized by the high value that most Americans place on having choices about physicians, hospitals and health plans.

The importance of these value systems in shaping policy appears to be more important in the United Kingdom than in the United States – partly because of differences in political institutions and partly because (at least until recently) there was a more cohesive elite in the United Kingdom. Nevertheless appearance is misleading in this instance. Policy debates in the United States, especially in

state politics, about when life begins and how it is permissible for it to end have been about values. This is emphatically not to say, however, that policy for these matters has been made in deference to any consistent set of ethical principles; indeed ethical principles conflict. American politics and policy are also characterized by both generosity toward persons in need of rescue and unwillingness to compromise liberty by creating a compulsory insurance system.

We began this chapter by arguing that ethicists and their doctrines have been more influential in the implementation than in the development of policy, at least in the United Kingdom and the United States. We explained why and how the practice of policy making by persons in general government is inconsistent with the preferences and intellectual habits of professional ethicists. Then we demonstrated our point by telling stories about policy issues in the two countries. We concluded that values matter, that ethics matter, but that neither alone are sufficient grounds for policy making in liberal democracies.

We do not intend to denigrate ethics and ethicists. Our theme is the complexity of the politics of policy making. We share the view of one historian that the "history of ethics ... has less to do with great thinkers and their teachings than with collective shifts of moral sensibility that occur over a period of decades or centuries" (Haskell 1998). Similarly, we are sympathetic to the complaint of a noted American jurist that "academic moralists pick and choose from an a la carte menu the moral principles that coincide with their social set" (Ryerson 2000), and note that a leading ethicist concludes that the policy prescriptions he and his colleagues advocate are usually "personal rather than political" (Wikler 1991). Of course, some jurists and persons in many other professions also confuse the personal and the political.

Here, then, is our personal message, grounded in the preceding analysis. We offer any aspiring Philosopher Kings (and Queens in an equal-opportunity world) – and we know that many, perhaps most, ethicists do not have such aspirations – the same caution each of us has offered on other occasions to aspiring Economist Kings: aspirants to such thrones will always be disappointed by the politics of policy making in any countries that are fit to live in.

CHAPTER 62

ETHICAL ISSUES IN ORGAN TRANSPLANTATION IN THE UNITED STATES

Judith P. Swazey and Renée C. Fox

I. INTRODUCTION

The modern era of human solid organ transplantation began in the 1950s, when the first successful outcomes began to be achieved with live donor kidney transplants. During these early years of clinical transplants, however, successful results were rare and usually ephemeral, given the many unknown and uncontrolled factors involved in moving from the animal laboratory to humans and the drastic illnesses of the patients. Pioneering transplant surgeon Francis D. Moore has called the decade from 1952–1962 the "black years" between the introduction of whole body radiation and the discovery of immunosuppressive chemotherapy to forestall the inexorable rejection of an organ from anyone but an identical twin (Moore 1968, 384). By 1963, 194 kidney transplants had been reported in the literature; of the 103 non-twin transplants in this total, fewer than 10 percent survived for 3 months (Goodwin and Martin 1963).

Kidneys also began to be obtained from the "newly dead" – from cadaveric donors. Beyond the limited supply of live donors, there were other reasons, both explicit and latent, why transplant surgeons showed a growing preference for cadaveric organs. Foremost among these reasons has been the deep concern, bordering on dread, about the fact that live organ transplantation engages them in an act that deliberately inflicts surgical damage on a healthy person, albeit for the good of someone else. As such, it constitutes a hands-on violation of one of the most fundamental moral principles of the profession of medicine – the injunction to "do no harm" – and incurs the daunting ultimate risk that it could even result in the death of a live, healthy donor (see Chapter 38).

Transplant teams also felt a great deal of uneasiness and, beyond that, suspicion about the motivations of living donors for volunteering to give a part of themselves in the hope of saving the life of a family member or even a "stranger." Two other sources of disquiet involved, first, defining who was eligible to be a live donor other than someone who is biologically related to a recipient, such as a sibling or birth parent. Should a person who is "related" by other forms of kinship, such as a spouse or adopted child, be allowed to be a donor? Second, transplant teams found that there could be a range of complex social and psychiatric dynamics involved in live donor-recipient-family interactions, both before and after an organ graft (Abram 1972; Bevan 1971; Fellner and Schwartz 1971).

Many of these types of medical, ethical, and psychosocial uncertainties and complexities that physicians and their teams, donors, recipients, and their families have persistently encountered are grounded in the gatekeeping and gift-exchange dimensions of organ transplantation (Fox and Swazey 1978; Fox and Swazey 1992). From the outset, in the United States the use of a kidney from both live and cadaveric donors was defined and portrayed as a "gift of life" by those engaged in obtaining and transplanting organs. At first, the notion of organs as gifts was used metaphorically, with little awareness of the implications of this conceptualization. Gradually, through clinical experience and interpretive analyses by psychiatrists, social workers, and social scientists, the meaning and effects of the gift-exchange aspects of transplantation became better recognized.

What became more apparent is that psychologically, socially, and culturally, giving and receiving an organ is neither an absolute nor a random freedom. These freedoms are mediated and governed, on the one hand, by the at-once biomedical, psychological, and sociological screening processes exercised by transplant professionals in their role as gatekeepers, vested with the authority to decide who may give and who may receive an organ, and by the norms of gift-exchange on the other. In his classic anthropological work, *The Gift*, as we wrote in our first book on transplantation, Marcel Mauss pointed out that "although gift exchange is an expressive set of acts through which something symbolic and interpersonal as well as material is transmitted, it is not totally spontaneous. Rather, it is structured by a triple set of norms: the obligations to give, to receive, and repay," which Mauss defined as "symmetrical and reciprocal." By this, he meant that under certain socioculturally defined circumstances, an individual or a group is supposed to offer a gift to a particular person. In turn, the person or persons to whom a gift is proffered is expected to accept it. The recipient is then under social and moral pressure to eventually balance out the exchange by giving the donor a thing of equivalent worth. "Failure to live up to any of these entwined expectations produces disequilibrium and social stress that affects the donor, the recipient, and those closely associated with them" (Fox and Swazey 1978, 5–6; Mauss 1954). If one thinks about our common, everyday experiences with the ways in which gift exchange can be conscripting and obligating as well as fulfilling, one begins to appreciate the ways in which organ exchange can be inordinately more complicated: the pressures to offer a potentially life-saving gift, to accept such a gift if it is offered, the strains for all parties in the transaction if the recipient's body rejects the gift, and the dilemmas of how one can repay an essentially unrepayable gift of life.

Using only cadaveric kidneys could free transplant teams to some extent from the issues involved in live donor transplants and the gift-exchange framework in which they are embedded. Transplant teams learned, however, that obtaining kidneys from deceased rather than living donors, as well as other vital organs, such as livers and hearts, when these began to be transplanted in 1963

and 1967, respectively, still involved inner and outer gift-giving pressures. Those engaged in the transplantation endeavor discovered that complex psychosocial issues were associated with the use of cadaveric organs. Notable among these were the emotional reactions of recipients to receiving organs from an unknown "stranger," who had had to die for them to live, and their tendency to imbue these organs with what they imagined might be the donors' personal attributes, as they grappled with the implications of incorporating them into their bodies and lives.

Two of the more macrosocietal issues that developed around cadaveric transplantation were those surrounding the so-called definition of death, and efforts to increase the supply of organs for the growing numbers of patients on transplant waiting lists. We will focus on how these issues have crystallized and been responded to in the United States.

II. Getting Organs: What and When is Death?

The evolving concept of death in the second half of the twentieth century, which has been shaped by scientific, medical, social, and cultural factors, is integrally entwined with the history of organ transplantation and its uses of the dead by the living. There is a powerful imagery and symbolism in the term "harvesting," which until recently, was commonly used by transplant surgeons to describe procuring cadaveric organs. How do we define death and "know" that a person is "really" dead before physicians harvest their organs? There is a medical need to procure organs in as "living" a state as possible while making sure the donor is medically, legally, and ethically "dead" (see Chapter 63).

During the 1960s, both the medical and legal communities were uncertain about the status of people from whom organs were being procured. These donors were variously described in the medical literature, for example, as "irreversibly dying," "imminently dead," "virtually dead," or simply "dead." The growing capabilities and use of respirators and other resuscitative and life support technologies also contributed to unease and uncertainty among anesthesiologists and neurologists about the use of the traditional criteria – cessation of heartbeat and respiration – for determining when death occurs (Wolstenholme and O'Connor 1966). Cadaveric donors and life support systems thus brought in their wake complex and persisting problems of determining when a mechanically supported patient is dead, when it is morally as well as technically acceptable to stop life-sustaining treatment, and how the organs of a potential cadaver donor can be kept viable for transplantation without violating the so-called dead donor rule that prohibits causing death by removing vital organs before a donor's demise.

The formulation and institutionalization of the concept of "brain death" – the determination and declaration of a person's death based on irreversible cessation of all functions of the entire brain, including the brain stem – emerged in part as a response to these uncertainties. In August 1968, an ad hoc committee at Harvard Medical School, convened and chaired by anesthesiologist Henry K. Beecher, published a report in the *Journal of the American Medical Association* that defined "irreversible coma as a new criterion for death" (Ad Hoc Committee of the Harvard Medical School 1968). Despite its weaknesses – such as the confusion between "irreversible coma" and "brain death" evident in the paper's title – the Harvard committee's proposed new criterion gained rapid medical and legal acceptance. By the end of the 1970s, twenty-seven states had passed legislation recognizing the new criterion, model statutes had been proposed by the American Bar Association and the American Medical Association, and various European and international bodies had issued statements on brain death.

The Harvard report and related developments, however, also generated both medical and legal confusion about the roles of traditional cardiopulmonary criteria and the new neurologically based brain death definition: what do these two sets of standards mean for deciding exactly what "death" is, and when it can be deemed to have occurred? These and related questions were deliberated and debated by various individuals and groups, such as The Hastings Center's Task Force on Death and Dying (Kass 1971; Morison 1971; Task Force on Death and Dying 1972). More importantly, from an ethical and moral perspective, the brain death definition also fostered profound disquietude and criticisms about what some saw as its overly utilitarian linkage with the desire to procure more organs, and the implications of the new formulation for our understanding of human life and personhood. These deep philosophically and religiously grounded concerns were articulated by several of the seminal figures in the emerging field of bioethics, most prominently by philosopher Hans Jonas (1903–1993) and theologian Paul Ramsey (1913–1988) (Jonas 1970, 1974; Ramsey 1970b). Speaking from both his metaphysical and religious perspectives on scientific and technological progress and on human mortality, Jonas' "emphatic verdict" was that brain death was acceptable only "[a]s long as it is merely a question of when it is permitted to cease the artificial prolongation of certain functions (like heartbeat) traditionally regarded as signs of life . . . to break off a sustaining intervention and let things take their course." What he found not only "disquieting" but even "ominous" was combining "the quest for a new definition of death" with organ procurement. "The patient must be absolutely sure that his doctor does not become his executioner," Jonas affirmed, and the dying patient's "expiring moments should be

watched over with piety and be safe from exploitation" (Jonas 1970:26–28).

The importance of such persisting concerns about what and when is death were recognized in the 1978 legislation establishing the President's Commission for the Study of Ethical Problems in Medicine and Biomedical and Behavioral Research. The Commission's first charge was to study "the ethical and legal implications of the matter of defining death, including the advisability of developing a uniform definition of death." In 1981, the Commission issued its landmark report, *Defining Death*, with an accompanying appendix, *Guidelines for the Determination of Death*. The Commission held that "death is a unitary phenomenon that can be accurately demonstrated either on the traditional grounds of irreversible cessation of heart and lung functions or on the basis of irreversible functions of the entire brain," and on that basis concluded that there was a need to "[restate] the standards traditionally recognized for determining that death has occurred." Given the variability that existed among state laws, the Commission further recommended, "such a restatement ought preferably to be a matter of [uniform] statutory law." With respect to the two catalysts for the 1968 Harvard report and the subsequent events leading to the Commission's work, its *Defining Death* report further recommended, "any statutory 'definition' should be kept separate and distinct from provisions governing the donation of cadaver organs and from any legal rules on decisions to terminate life-sustaining treatment" (President's Commission [1981] 1998a, 15). Drawing on a model statute developed by lawyer Alexander Capron (who became Executive Director of the Commission) and physician–scientist Leon Kass as part of the Hasting Center Task Force's work (Capron and Kass 1972), the Commission proposed the language of a Uniform Determination of Death Act that soon was enacted nationwide.

Although there has seemed to be a widespread medical, legal, and ethical consensus about brain death, it has remained an uncertain and imperfect one. There is still a deep underlying disquietude and lack of consensus about what death is, why brain death is death and how it is related to cardiopulmonary death, and about the timing of when death occurs in the trajectory of a person's dying. These basic issues have resurfaced in the debates about various attempts to increase the supply of cadaveric organs. There have been, for example, proposals to "relax" the dead donor rule, providing exceptions to it or interpreting it more broadly to allow the removal of vital organs without brain death. These strategies, which raise profound questions about what it means to be "fully human" or a "person," include removing organs from anencephalic newborns before brain stem activity has stopped, and – an extension of using anencephalic infants as donors – adopting "neocortical death" rather than whole brain death as the criterion for pronouncing a person dead and harvesting their organs (American Medical Association 1995; Robertson 1999; Truog and Fletcher 1989; Veatch 1975).

The most recent effort to increase the supply of organs by changing criteria for pronouncing death, initiated in the early 1990s, has been the use of what are termed planned or controlled "non-heart-beating donors." In such cases, a family agrees to have a life-sustaining treatment withdrawn from a close relative who is terminally ill but not brain dead. In effect, this is a return to the way that early donors of cadaveric organ were declared dead on the basis of cardiopulmonary criteria, before brain dead "heart-beating cadaver" donors became the norm. The use of non-heart-beating donors has fomented considerable medical and ethical debate about matters such as how irreversible the loss of pulmonary and cardiac function is; how long the interval should be after the complete cessation of circulatory function before death is declared; whether giving drugs to these donors to sustain organ viability before they are pronounced dead could hasten or cause their death; and whether these dying persons and their families are treated humanely and respectfully during the prospective donor's planned "terminal management" (Fox 1993; Institute of Medicine 1997; Non-heart-beating donor protocols 1993; Youngner, Arnold, and DeVita 1999)?

III. Other Efforts to Increase the Supply of Cadaveric Organs

In addition to redefining death, numerous other efforts have been made to meet the constantly growing demand for organs in the decades since the 1960s. The "supply–demand problem" has escalated because the number of available organs has increased at a much lower percentage than the numbers of candidates for the increasing array of organs being transplanted, singly or in combinations, for various diseases and medical conditions. The demand also has been fueled by growth in the number of centers doing transplants, and by expanding eligibility criteria for transplant recipients that has created larger waiting lists and exacerbated ethical and social policy questions about how to most fairly and equitably allocate these scarce resources.

Since the 1950s, as discussed previously, organ donation has been conceptualized and promoted as a "gift of life." Concomitant with the introduction of brain death criteria, the gift-exchange framework for cadaveric donation began to be codified in 1968 with the drafting of a model law, the Uniform Anatomical Gift Act, by the National Conference of Commissioners on Uniform State Laws. By the end of the 1970s, all states had adopted the Act, which legally permits competent adults to declare their intent to donate their organs or other bodily parts

after death, or, without such a declaration, permits family members to authorize donation unless the deceased has specifically indicated he or she does not want to be a donor (Sadler, Sadler, and Stason 1968).

In the 1980s, a further, largely unsuccessful effort to increase the rate of cadaveric donations was made in the form of a "required request" concept, subsequently enacted in federal legislation, requiring hospital personnel to seek permission from a newly dead person's next of kin to harvest organs (Caplan 1988; Martyn, Wright, and Clark 1988). Two other proposed strategies to procure more cadaveric organs have not, thus far, been implemented or attracted much support in the United States, largely because they fall outside of, and would negate, the profound social, moral, and spiritual meaning of the at-once literal and transcendent gift-of-self to a known or unknown other that underlies the gift-exchange framework. These are, first, "presumed consent" legislation, which is operative in several other countries, that permits the routine harvesting of organs unless the decedent, prior to death, has registered a specific objection to being a donor. Secondly, there have been a number of proposals to provide financial compensation to prospective donors premortem or to their families postmortem. None of these entail the outright buying and selling of organs, which was forbidden in the United States in the National Organ Transplantation Act, enacted in 1984 (Public Law 98–507). Rather, they involve various types of what is called "regulated compensation" or "rewarded gifting," none of which has yet been implemented. The most commercially based of these ideas has been the proposal to establish a "futures market" in cadaveric organs that would allow healthy persons to contract for the sale of their organs, to be retrieved, delivered, and transplanted after their death (Cohen 1989; Hansmann 1989). Other suggested strategies have sought to maintain a boundary between "direct payments and individual incentives" by providing such things as "coverage for a donor's medical expenses" or "payment for the burial expenses of a deceased donor" (Childress 1989). To various degrees, all of the compensation-for-donation proposals have elicited opposition about what their critics view as the dangerous step toward placing organs in a market framework, commodifying them, and undermining the "altruistic gift" basis of organ donation that it might constitute.

As long as the organ shortage has existed, there have been cycles of moving toward and away from the use of market and compensation mechanisms to augment the number of donated organs. What has remained more constant has been the condemnatory stand that medical and human rights organizations have taken against the organized buying, selling, and brokering of human organs, primarily, but not only, kidneys from living "donors," that extensively occur in a number of developing countries, most notably in India (Chengappa 1990; Trucco 1989).

Given the moral objections to organ markets in developing countries, it is both socially and ethically ironic that some 85 percent of the fifty-nine nonprofit organ procurement agencies in the United States have established lucrative sources of income by selling body parts "directly to for-profit biomedical firms or to tissue banks with corporate connections" (Heisel and Katches 2000). According to a June 2000 investigative report and an accompanying survey, a majority of the agencies are harvesting far more tissues – such as bone, skin, heart valves, veins, and tendons – than organs from cadaveric donors. In contrast to the consent requirements for organ donation, the agencies have acknowledged that, unless asked, they do not tell the families of deceased donors about retrieving tissues, seek their permission to do so, or disclose to whom and for how much these "gifts" will be sold. At present, laws in the United States against selling human tissue, which are "treated as commodities," are "vague and untested." In the wake of the media disclosure, the Secretary of Health and Human Services (HHS) ordered a probe of the "tissue trade," and the Board of Directors of the United Network for Organ Sharing issued a statement "urging state and federal regulators to give the tissue business more scrutiny" (Heisel and Katches 2000).

Biomedical criteria for what are judged to be "acceptable" cadaveric organs also have been liberalized and expanded in the drive to obtain more organs. The more expansive criteria "include, importantly, increasing age (up to 80 years) in some programs, but also donors with diabetes, hypertension, some infections, high-risk social history but negative HIV test, some hemodynamic instability, some chemical imbalances, increased organ preservation time . . . or increased time after death in the body" (Institute of Medicine 1997, 10). Transplant experts predict that these expanded criteria could increase the cadaver donor supply by 25 to 39 percent; however, they also admit that using donors "of greater age and in less satisfactory medical conditions . . . exact a price in increased procurement costs; increased cost of transplantation; and lower graft and recipient survival." These financial and human costs, an Institute of Medicine task force pointed out, "must be weighed against the morbidity, death, and economic and other costs in patients on the waiting list" (Institute of Medicine 1997, 11).

The drive to procure more solid organs also has fueled a resurgence and increase in the use of live donors. In addition to live donor kidneys, which account for approximately half of the renal transplants performed today at many centers, living donors increasingly provide segments of livers and lungs, and, in smaller numbers, portions of the small intestine and distal segment of the pancreas. These developments, the members of a "live organ donor consensus group" wrote in a December 2000 statement, "have necessitated a reexamination of the med-

ical and ethical issues involving live organ donors" (Live Organ Donor Consensus Group 2000). The conclusion of the 100-plus member group, which included "physicians, nurses, ethicists, psychologists, lawyers, scientists, social workers, transplant recipients, and living donors," attested to the continuing medical, ethical, and psychosocial concerns about the use of live donors, nearly half a century after the first successful identical twin graft was performed:

> The person who gives consent to be a live organ donor should be competent, willing to donate, free from coercion, medically and psychosocially suitable, fully informed of the risks and benefits as a donor, and fully informed of the risks, benefits, and alternative treatment available to the recipient. The benefits to both donor and recipient must outweigh the risks associated with the donation and transplantation of the living donor organ. (Live Organ Donor Consensus Group 2000, 2919)

IV. ORGAN REPLACEMENT AND ISSUES OF EQUITY

Since their inception, kidney and other types of cadaveric transplants, as well as maintenance dialysis, have raised, in paradigmatic form, "life boat ethics" questions about how we can most justly or equitably allocate scarce, potentially lifesaving resources (Childress 1970; Fox and Swazey 1996). One set of equity issues has been raised by studies that "have shown convincingly that minorities, women, and persons with low income have reduced access to kidney transplantation" in terms of referral to a transplant center for evaluation, placement on a waiting list, or receiving a kidney (Levinsky 1999, 1692).

Other questions of fairness involve the national system for procuring and distributing donor organs within and across the geographical regions of the Organ Procurement and Transplantation Network, established under the National Organ Donor Transplant Act of 1984. The system, run by the nonprofit United Network for Organ Sharing (UNOS) under contract with the federal government, generally distributes organs within local areas first, even if there are sicker patients, more urgently in need of transplants listed in another geographical region. In response to the contention that this policy causes significant disparities in waiting time across the Network's sixty-two geographical regions, the U.S. Department of HHS proposed a Final Rule in 1998 to "assure that allocation of scarce organs will be based on common medical criteria, not accidents of geography" (United States Department of HHS 1998). The Rule generated so much controversy and opposition within segments of the transplantation community that, as of fall 2000, it had not been enacted. One of the strongest objections concerned the greater federal oversight of the distribution system that it would establish through new policy-making authority given to the Secretary of HSS. Spokespersons for UNOS and transplant surgeons vehemently argued that organ allocation is rightfully a medical decision – one that should be entrusted to medical experts and not vested in or shared with the government.

Another persistent allocation issue, which emanates primarily from within the professional transplant culture, is whether the common practice of retransplanting organs in patients whose graft has failed is a "justifiable use of scarce cadaveric donor organs." Patients view transplantation "as a 'second chance' for healthy and productive life after end-stage organ failure," a transplant surgeon has written, but "[u]nfortunately, many first transplants are not successful" (Kahan 1997, 2). Transplant physicians are deeply reluctant to confine themselves to performing only one transplant on a patient, or to restrict the number of times they will retransplant an organ in a patient. If an organ graft is unsuccessful, for whatever reason, transplant surgeons are strongly disposed to perform another graft on that patient, even though they acknowledge that heart and liver recipients do not do as well as first-time recipients with respect to organ survival or patient mortality, and that although first and second kidney transplants may sometimes be equivalent in outcome, graft survival is poorer in third transplants. Transplant professionals realize that serious questions of equity are posed by their propensity toward retransplantation, given the insufficient number of organs available for all those awaiting a transplant, and the fact that patients on the waiting list who have never received a transplant have a greater probability of doing well with a first graft than candidates for retransplant. By and large, these physicians subscribe to the principles that the optimum allocation of organs should be based on relative efficacy of outcome and the probability of benefit and that to ensure the best use of donor organs "only patients with a reasonable chance of survival after retransplantation should be regrafted" (Tokat 1995). Nevertheless, their emotional and moral commitment to prolonging the lives

of patients whom they have already "salvaged" from end-stage illness make them feel, to use their own language, that they are "abandoning" these patients if they do not pursue retransplant following graft failure (Fox 1997, 6). In addition, a sense of responsibility for what they term "iatrogenic organ failure" due to the increasing number of "marginal" organs they are using inclines transplant surgeon toward regrafting a recipient of such an organ. There is pathos in these physicianly sentiments, that are institutionally supported by the UNOS policy of according retransplant candidates the same access to available organs as those awaiting first transplants.

V. Conclusion

In 1968, recalling the wartime act of recreating a new car with spare parts obtained from two useless vehicles, two physician pioneers of human organ transplantation, with a mixture of awe and dread, raised the following question: "Does the surgeon have the right to remove a liver, a heart, or a kidney from a cadaver in order to practice what [has been termed] 'cannibalizing?'" Although they had "committed themselves to the adventure of . . . transplantation in man," they wrote, they were among "the first to admit how difficult it [was] to be certain that one is following the proper road in this regard" (Hamburger and Crosnier 1968, 37). Today, more than 30 years later, moral uncertainty about this "cannibalizing" use of the dead to perpetuate the lives of the living still has not been entirely dispelled.

Acknowledgments

Preparation of this chapter was supported by grants for The Acadia Institute Project on Bioethics in American Society from the Greenwall Foundation, the National Library of Medicine 1RO1-LM06893, and the National Science Foundation SBR-9710579.

CHAPTER 63

DEFINING AND REDEFINING LIFE AND DEATH

Robert M. Veatch

I. INTRODUCTION

Debates about the definitions of life and death have played important roles in the history of biomedical ethics (see Chapter 38). After exploring some of those meanings, this chapter examines the positions taken prior to the time of the transplantation of human organs (see Chapter 62). This is followed by a more extensive discussion of the definition of death in the transplant era and controversies that can be expected over that definition in the coming century.

II. CONCEPTUAL ISSUES

The terms, "life" and "death," each have a number of different meanings. They are terms playing important roles in biology, sociocultural communication, and in moral, legal, and public policy debates.

1. The Meaning of Life

To know what it means for a human to be dead, one must first reflect on what it means to be alive. The *Webster's Third New International Dictionary of the English Language Unabridged* (Gove 1971, 3333) contains no fewer than twenty-one definitions of the term, "life," many of which include multiple subcategories. The first group of definitions view life as a biological phenomenon; the second group view it more metaphorically as the existence of anything such as a culture. A third group of definitions use the term to assign moral or legal or public policy status to an entity.

A. Biological Uses

The first definition is that life means "an animate being; the quality that distinguishes a vital and functional being from a dead body or purely chemical matter." Often certain functions are identified as essential such as metabolism, growth, reproduction, or responsiveness. Based on the presence of these functions, a living entity of any species can be differentiated from the dead body (mortal remains) of one of that species. This biological use does not imply moral or legal or public policy status.

B. Social and Cultural Uses

Metaphorically the language also permits people to speak of entities as having a life in a social or cultural sense. With this usage, people sometimes speak of a language or culture or a state of being alive or dead. The speaker is merely distinguishing between those that continue to function with their essential characteristics in tact and those that have ceased to maintain their essential features. A "dead" culture is one that no longer exists. Of course, in this metaphorical use of the term, life, it can be very difficult to identify the essential defining features so it is hard to tell the exact point at which the Mayan civilization ended and the Aztecs began or that Latin ended and Italian began. In general terms, however, we understand what is meant by speaking of a culture as living or dead.

C. Moral, Legal, and Public Policy Uses

In medical ethics, the term, life, is sometimes used to convey some normative judgment: which beings have "moral standing," to whom certain legal or moral rights apply, and to whom public policies are addressed. For example, the United Nations Declaration of Human Rights is said to affirm rights of all living human beings. Prohibition of homicide governs the legal and moral status of all living individuals. It does not apply once an individual is "dead." In the debates over the morality of abortion, even though embryos and early fetuses obviously are made up of living human tissue, some attempt to claim that they are not yet living beings as a way of claiming that they do not bear the moral and legal protections that are attributed to the living. Others insist that life begins at conception because they wish to convey that the conceptus bears certain rights including the right not to be killed.

Not everyone uses the word, "life," as if anyone who is alive must bear such rights. Hence, liberals on abortion may claim that even though an embryo is a living human being, it does not bear full moral standing and conservatives might acknowledge that to establish that living fetuses bear moral or legal standing requires more than proving that they are biologically living. In biomedical ethics, the claim that a being is alive is often meant to be a moral claim rather than a biological or ontological one.

2. The Meaning of Death

The word, "death," can be used in these same three ways. Some insist that death, when applied to a biological organism, is strictly a biological concept (Becker 1975; Lamb 1985). Others use the term metaphorically to refer to the death of a language or a culture. In recent biomedical ethics, the term, "death," has been assigned important moral, legal, and public policy meaning. To say that a human is "dead" is to say that, for public policy purposes, there has been an important change in legal and moral status. Certain legal rights, including the right not to be killed and other rights in constitutional and common law, no longer apply. Morally, if one claims an individual has died, one is claiming that a radical change in

moral status has occurred. Many things that could not be tolerated morally while one was considered alive, including conduct of dissection and invasive research as well as procuring of organs for transplant, become tolerable when death has occurred. In fact, a wide range of behavioral social changes are signaled when death occurs: relatives go into mourning, an individual's assets are dispersed, life insurance pays off, health insurance ceases, the marital status of the spouse changes, and, in some cases, medical treatments that were previously considered appropriate are no longer deemed necessary. Death, then, is the radical change in the moral and legal status of a being when it loses the essential characteristics of its being. The philosophical question through the ages has been what constitutes those essential characteristics.

III. PRIOR TO THE TRANSPLANT ERA

1. In Ancient Culture

Prehistorical cultures have been divided into the *primitive*, such as the aboriginal Australian and the *archaic* cultures of tribes of Africa, Polynesia, and the New World (Bellah 1965). We have little information about the exact beliefs of the most primitive cultures in terms of the meaning of life and death. We know that by the time of tribal culture, life was associated with "spirit" and that such spirits had a way of departing from bodies, thus causing death. Ancestral spirits might find their way back into the bodies of future descendants, thus leading to a view that the life of one generation was literally a coming again of the deceased.

By the time of the *historical* cultures, that is the cultures with sufficient literacy to leave a written record of their beliefs, there is a much more complex belief system that includes a transcendental supernatural world and an identifiable deity or deities. Death becomes conceptualized as a transition to a new life in another realm. The concept of the soul emerges as a defining characteristic of life and its departure from the body marks the end of life in its present bodily form. In the *Phaedo* Plato recounts Socrates conversation with Cebes in which Socrates asks:

> Then, tell me, what must be present in a body to
> make it alive?
> Soul.
> Is this always so?
> Of course.
> So, whenever soul takes possession of a body, it
> always brings life with it?
> Yes, it does.
> Is there an opposite to life, or not?
> Yes, there is.
> What?

Death.

Does it follow, then from our earlier agreement, that soul will never admit the opposite of that which accompanies it?

Most definitely, said Cebes.

Very good. And what do we call that which does not admit death?

Immortal.

And soul does not admit death?

No.

So soul is immortal.

Yes, it is immortal.

Well, said Socrates, can we say that that has been proved? What do you think?

Most completely, Socrates. (*Phaedo* 105A–105E)

Thus for Socrates, the soul is the life principle and it is immortal. Something similar can be said of Aristotle:

What is ensouled is distinguished from what is unensouled by living. But living is spoken of in many ways, and if even one of these belong to something, we say that it is alive, that is: thought; perception; motion and rest with respect to place; and further motion with respect to nourishment, decay and growth. (*De Anima* 413ᵃ 20–6; Shields 1999)

Whereas for the Greeks, death is often seen as an escape from the body, Jews and Christians have a very different understanding. In earliest Judaism, life is associated with breath: its absence with death. There is no doctrine of the immortality of the soul; rather there is a belief in a resurrection in bodily form, a matter that will be of concern when society develops the capacity to transplant human organs (Stendahl 1965).

2. Modern Western Culture

Modern western culture continues to be influenced by both Greek and Judeo-Christian beliefs about the meaning of life and death. The secularization of society, however, has led to a more mundane set of beliefs about the meaning of life and death. The traditional association of life with breath developed to the point that life was increasingly associated with the body's capacity for circulation and respiration. The tests for death were measures of loss of circulatory and respiratory function, the feeling for a pulse or the mirror to the nostrils to detect respiration. The absence of these functions was taken to be the end of life, the end of the society's commitment to treat the human the way living people were treated. It was clearly recognized that these tests had to be applied in such a manner that *irreversible* loss could be established. Temporary stoppage of the heart or of breathing was never properly understood to be death. Although the first breath as the fetus emerges from the birth canal has continued to

be taken by some Jews as the beginning of human life with full moral standing, most members of western society understood that capacity for respiration and circulation emerges during fetal development so they attributed the full moral standing associated with this normative meaning of the word, life, to prenatal life as well. Those who associate full moral standing with the unique, genetically determined potential for these capacities saw life with full moral significance as present from conception; those who associated it with the emergence of the actual capacities for these functions tended to take a more incrementalist view, seeing life, in this normative sense, emerging as circulatory and respiratory functions developed prenatally.

IV. The Era of Transplants

This presumption that life was associated with circulatory and respiratory function and that death was the irreversible loss of these functions persisted throughout the modern period. The medical capacity to intervene during the decline and irreversible loss of these functions was so limited that once the process of loss of these functions began (what can be called *dying*), the entire process progressed so rapidly that there was no need to be more precise about exactly which functions of the body were critical in deciding whether someone was alive or dead. Death would occur very rapidly so that loss of heart and lung function, circulation and respiration, as well as the associated neurological functions did not need to be analyzed any more precisely. A major concern in the nineteenth century was that someone would mistakenly be taken for dead when the loss of these functions proved not to be irreversible. Elaborate devices were created so that one buried prematurely could pull an alarm that would raise a flag or sound an alarm and open the coffin. Still, no one seriously questioned precisely what bodily functions needed to be measured to determine whether death had occurred.

1. Pre-1970: The Discovery of Important Uses of the Dead Body

A. Death, Autopsy, and the Anatomy Laboratory

Gradually, medical scientists and others began to discover that there were potential uses of the dead body, including dissection for medical education, autopsy to determine the cause of death, and research for the advancement of medical knowledge. Although there was nearly unanimous agreement that the living person could not be used for these purposes, such uses of the dead were gradually seen as acceptable. Some, including many Orthodox Jews, placed stringent limits on medical uses of the dead body, but even they supported autopsy if identifiable human life could be saved from such invasion.

B. The Birth of Organ Transplantation and the Importance of the Concept of Death

By the middle of the twentieth century, medical scientists and others began to realize that there were other more exciting and more controversial uses of the dead body. Organ transplants from animal species had been part of mythology since ancient times. Human-to-human kidney transplants were attempted as early as the 1930s. The first successful human organ transplant occurred in 1954 when a kidney was transplanted to an identical twin at the Peter Bent Brigham Hospital in Boston. During this same period advances in medical technology led to the development of the artificial ventilator so that bodily functions of persons without central nervous system control of respiration could be maintained for increasingly long periods of time. For the first time, it could make a critical, lifesaving difference to clarify exactly what functions were essential to the presence of life (see Chapter 62).

C. The French and Coma Dépassé

In 1959, a group of French neurophysiologists reported their findings based on research dealing with patients in extremely deep coma. These patients were ventilator dependent and lacked reflexes and electrophysiological activity. They referred to the condition as *"coma dépassé"* (Mollaret and Coulon 1959). They had, in effect, identified a group of patients who would later be described as having completely dead brains. Postmortem examination would reveal necrosis and autolysis.

D. The Harvard Ad Hoc Committee

The stakes were to escalate still further in December of 1967 when South African surgeon, Christiaan Bernard, cut out the heart of Louis Washkansky and transplanted it into a patient in heart failure. Although kidneys and other organs could, in principle, be procured from persons who had died based on irreversible loss of cardiac functions, by definition, hearts could not be. An irreversibly destroyed heart could never beat again. Concurrent with the explosion of heart transplants a committee at Harvard Medical School was convened by physician Henry K. Beecher. The group, known as the Ad Hoc Committee of the Harvard Medical School to examine the Definition of Brain Death, published its report in May of 1968 (Ad Hoc Committee of Harvard Medical School 1968). That report is credited with establishing the concept of "brain death." In fact, all it did was set out criteria for measuring what it called "irreversible coma." A person was considered to be in irreversible coma if hypothermia and drug

overdose were excluded and four criteria were met: unreceptivity and unresponsitivity, no movements or breathing, no reflexes, and a flat electroencephalogram (which, the committee emphasized, was "of great confirmatory value" but not an essential requirement for measuring the death of the brain). The committee members believed that, if the first three criteria were met, the fourth had to be as well. It assumed, as did everyone else at the time, that irreversible coma was synonymous with the death of the brain, an assumption later found to be erroneous. It is now clear that people can be irreversibly unconscious, in fact comatose, without having all tissues of the entire brain completely dead.

Even more critically, it assumed, without any argument, that the death of the brain should be taken as the death of the person as a whole. The tremendous prestige of the committee and its sponsor apparently convinced a public that if the committee claims that people with dead brains should be treated as dead people, then it must be so. The view has a certain plausibility to it. As we have seen, from ancient times both Greek and Christian cultures sometimes associated being "alive" (in the sense of having full moral and legal standing) with functions we now associate with the brain. No one seriously questioned why a committee of medical scientists would have the authority to advocate converting the longstanding commitment to a cardiac- and respiratory-oriented understanding of death to one based on neurological function. Likewise, no one seriously questioned why a committee setting out to develop empirical neurological measures of a particular brain pathology would add a few nonscientists – a theologian, a historian of science and a lawyer, for example. These nonscientists were never permitted to offer any philosophical, theological, legal, or historical arguments in favor of considering people with dead brains as people who should be treated the way we treat dead people.

2. The 1970s: The Emergence of the Brain-based Concept of Death

Soon after the appearance of the Harvard Report, there was widespread excitement about the adoption of a brain-oriented concept of death. The clinicians saw it as an opportunity to procure organs as well as obtain bodies and body parts for others uses including teaching, research, and therapy.

A. Early United States Legislative Efforts

In 1970 the State of Kansas passed a new law defining death (*Kan. Stat. Ann.* 77–202 (Supp. 1971)). Its statute provided two alternative definitions of death, a feature soon to be criticized. A person was considered dead if there is the absence of spontaneous respiratory and cardiac function and attempts at resuscitation are considered hopeless; however, a person was also considered dead if there is an absence of spontaneous brain function and restoration was considered hopeless. The State of Maryland soon passed a similar law (*Maryland Session Laws* 1972 Ch. 693) and other states of the United States followed so that by the end of the century all states had laws in one form or another calling for death pronouncement based on irreversible loss of brain function.

B. Early European Developments

Interest in brain-based definitions of death appeared in several European countries as well. Swedish physician Gunner Biorck had called for examination of the definition of death (Biorck 1968). In the Netherlands, Baronness Adrienne van Till-d'Aulnis de Bourouill encouraged support of brain-based death pronouncement, supporting what she called the Austro-German criteria in which angiography was performed to measure the absence of intracranial blood circulation (Van Till-d'Aulnis de Bourouill 1975). The Law Reform Commission of Canada formally endorsed death based on brain criteria in 1981. These developments led to a widespread European and North American consensus supporting a brain-based alternative to the traditional cardiac-oriented death definition.

C. The Institute of Society, Ethics and the Life Sciences (The Hastings Center) Task Force of Death and Dying: The Beginnings of the Intellectual Refinement

Although a pragmatic consensus was emerging, there was increasing discomfort in the intellectual community. This discomfort was expressed in the most sustained way by the Task Force on Death and Dying of the Institute of Society, Ethics and the Life Sciences (Task Force on Death and Dying 1972). Its report identified confusion over whether death is a process or a single event, concern that death should not be redefined merely for purposes of procuring organs for transplant, troubles that can result if two alternative definitions of death are endorsed (such as in the Kansas law), and insistence that the definition of death must be kept distinct from the moral question of when it is acceptable to stop treatment on a still-living person. That group also was clearly aware that a definition of death could be further updated so that someone might be considered dead even though some brain functions remained, a development that would dominate the discussion in the decades to come. Another product of that Task Force was the so-called Capron/Kass model statute (Capron and Kass 1972).

D. Voices Dissenting from the Consensus

Although there existed, in the 1970s, a substantial consensus sympathetic to the use of brain criteria for death pronouncement, the commentators were not unanimous. First, some in the philosophical, religious, legal, and medical community continued to support more traditional heart and lung criteria (Bleich 1973; Byrne, O'Reilly, and Quay 1979; Jonas 1974; Nilges 1984). The Danish Council of Ethics, a body established by Danish law to assist the Danish Parliament in regulating biomedical activities, insisted that heart, circulatory, respiratory, and brain function must all "totally and irreversibly have ceased" for a person to be dead, a position contrary to the thinking in virtually all Western countries (The Danish Council of Ethics 1989). These critics made clear that the question of when people should be treated as dead was not a scientific question. No medical evidence could be brought forward to establish that these critics were mistaken, even if the dominant view was that, philosophically and theologically, they had made an unwise choice.

Dissent also emerged in Great Britain where, under the influence of outspoken London neurologist Chris Pallis, support emerged for what he called "brain stem" death (Pallis 1982a, 1982b). His claim was that death occurred when there was irreversible loss of capacity for both consciousness and respiration and that the destruction of the brain stem, which is the path necessary for mediating conscious activity as well as the site responsible for respiration, necessarily meant one was dead (regardless of the state of the other brain centers including the cerebrum).

In this support of the brain stem as the critical site for diagnosing death, almost no one other than the British have concurred. Pallis's critics point out that, while the destruction of the brain stem necessarily means that, given the present state of neurological science, we cannot be conscious of the outside world, as long as cerebral activity remains, there is no logical reason why one could not remain conscious. In fact, they claim that, were someone some day able to invent input and outputs to the cerebrum that mimicked the brain stem's ability to arouse activity in the cerebrum, it would be possible to envision a conscious, communicating human without a brain stem. This hypothetical, the critics of brain stem death say, makes clear that death requires destruction of the whole brain, not merely the brain stem.

E. Formal Proposals to Change the Definition of Death

This emerging consensus in favor of a brain-oriented definition of death has led many public and professional organizations to endorse the use of brain criteria to pronounce death for public policy purposes. Some have nevertheless advocated that these changes occur informally through the development of a professional consensus. Others, however, have endorsed statutes that would formally and legally change the definition of death.

Following the dissatisfaction with the Kansas and Maryland proposals, a number of groups have followed the lead of Capron and Kass to endorse statutory language that would make death pronouncement based on irreversible loss of brain function the law. Often these proposals state or assume that there may be various tests or criteria for measuring the loss of brain function, including the use of traditional heart and lung criteria in those cases in which anoxia has existed for a sufficiently long time that brain function could not possibly survive.

By 1980, the American Bar Association, the American Medical Association (AMA), and the National Conference of Commissioners of Uniform State Laws had each adopted model language in addition to the Capron/Kass proposal. There was a need for uniformity. This was accomplished in the United States through the work of the President's Commission for the Study of Ethical Problems in Medicine and Biomedical and Behavioral Research. Its report, *Defining Death*, synthesized these proposals into the Uniform Determination of Death Act (President's Commission for the Study of Ethical Problems in Medicine and Biomedical and Behavioral Research [1981] 1998a, 2). The text of that brief proposal reads:

> An individual who has sustained either (1) irreversible cessation of circulatory and respiratory functions, or (2) irreversible cessation of all functions of the entire brain, including the brain stem, is dead. A determination of death must be made in accordance with accepted medical standards.

The British continue to dissent from both the policy of adopting a formal statute and the insistence that the entire brain's functions must be destroyed. Other countries including Australia and Canada have, however, adopted statutes endorsing death based on loss of all brain functions. Only Asian countries have continued to resist definitions of death based on brain-oriented criteria. In 1997 Japan endorsed a very limited use of brain-criteria for death pronouncement provided organs were to be procured for transplant and both the individual while alive and the family have consented to the use of brain criteria.

3. The Whole-Brain/Higher-Brain Conflict

During this period of the 1970s, philosophical doubt emerged not only from supporters of cardiac-oriented and brain-stem-oriented definitions of death, but also from those who became convinced that humans could be treated as dead even though lower-brain (brain stem) functions remained. In 1971, J. B. Brierley and colleagues published a provocative article describing two patients who seemed clearly to have permanently lost cerebral function (their cerebrums were shown on autopsy to have lost cellular structure), yet, because of intact brain stems, they could breathe on their own (Brierley et al. 1971). The patient survived breathing on their own for five months

each. Clearly, they could not be considered dead, based on irreversible loss of all functions of the entire brain; their brain stems had to be functional to control respiration. Nevertheless, they were not ever going to be capable of consciousness. They were in what was informally called a "coma" or, more precisely, a persistent vegetative state.

A. The Emerging Philosophical Doubt

The cases were debated heatedly at the meetings of the Task Force on Death and Dying of the Institute of Society, Ethics and the Life Sciences. It became obvious that the Harvard criteria that equated "coma" with the death of the entire brain had conflated mere irreversible coma with destruction of all brain tissues. The question was now open for debate: Should a person who retains brain stem function, but has irreversibly lost cerebral function and with it the capacity for consciousness, be considered dead or alive? All the brain-oriented definitions proposed to this time would treat such patients as alive. They had brain-based respiratory control and perhaps also some brain stem reflexes. Nevertheless, some began to ask whether a permanently unconscious person – one with no future capacity for any mental functioning – could really be considered alive any more than one with a dead brain could be (Engelhardt 1975, 587–90; Veatch 1975). What emerged was a proposal for further revision of the definition of death, one that came to be called the "higher-brain-oriented" definition because it considered people dead if there was irreversible loss of all "higher" brain functions. Sometimes this has been referred to as a cerebral, a cortical, or a neocortical definition, on the assumption that the cortex, specifically the neocortex of the cerebrum, is the locus of consciousness. Others prefer the purposely vague term "higher" because they realize that, in theory one might have lost these higher functions, such as consciousness, even though some cerebral cortex (for example, motor cortex) remained alive. By choosing the vague term "higher" they force a discussion of exactly which functions are the most important. Usually, the answer has to do with any capacity for consciousness.

B. The Rejection of Higher-Brain Formulations by the United States President's Commission

By the time the United States President's Commission took up the topic of the definition of death, the choice between a "higher-brain-oriented" definition and a "whole-brain-oriented" one was apparent. Both the consultants to the Commission on the subject had publicly endorsed the higher-brain view (Green and Wikler 1980; Veatch 1975). Nevertheless, the Commission, whose executive director was Alex Capron, the coauthor of the whole-brain-oriented Capron/Kass proposal, endorsed the whole-brain position.

C. *Remaining Support of the Higher-Brain Formulations*

By the end of the twentieth century no government had adopted the higher-brain view although a significant number of the philosophers and theologians considering the topic, perhaps a majority of them, had done so. Additional controversy on the subject emerged from the debate over the procurement of organs from anencephalic infants. Although many fetuses with anencephaly are born dead and others die almost immediately at birth, some have sufficient neurological development that, in principle, organs could be procured from them after birth. Anencephalic infants, in spite of the term, which means "without encephalon" or "without brain," actually have considerable brain tissue. Some can respire on their own although true anencephalic infants cannot be conscious because they do not have the cerebral tissue to sustain consciousness. Thus, these infants are not dead by whole-brain criteria.

Nevertheless some clinicians and some parents of these infants realize that their organs, which are thought to be of no value to these infants, could bring life-sustaining benefits to others. In Germany, some proposed that these infants be classified as "brain absent" (Beller and Reeve 1989). This turns out to be a mistake, however, because the anencephalic infant, actually has a brain, in some cases one capable of carrying out functions for a prolonged period. The functions, however, are those of the brain stem.

Recognizing the important value of the organs of these infants, the AMA's Council on Ethical and Judicial Affairs proposed that an exception be made to the dead donor rule so that organs could be taken from living humans who were anencephalics (AMA 1995). The reaction was swift and hostile. Within 24 hours, the Ethics Committee of the United Network for Organ Sharing had condemned the proposal. Some critics pointed out that if organs could be taken from anencephalic infants while alive, there was no reason given why they could not also be taken from those in a persistent vegetative state. They had a similar irreversible loss of consciousness. These critics wanted to hold the line at the whole-brain standard whereby all functions of the *entire* brain had to be gone for a person to be dead and a person had to be dead before organs could be procured.

Others were critical of the AMA position even though they did not object to organ procurement. Holding to the higher-brain definition of death, they believed that anencephalics (and the persistently vegetative) were, in fact, already dead. They hold that organs could thus be procured without violating the dead donor rule. Anencephalics should not be made an exception whereby organs could

be taken form the living, but should be reclassified as deceased (or more accurately, never having been alive).

V. CONCLUSION: CONTROVERSIES FOR THE TWENTY-FIRST CENTURY

At the beginning of the twenty-first century there is little more agreement on the definition of life and death than there was a half century earlier. A minority in the West (and perhaps a majority in the East) still clings to the cardiac-oriented definition of death. Most have adopted some version of a brain-oriented definition, but now the dispute has shifted to one between higher-brain and whole-brain views. Newer controversies remain (Youngner et al. 1999).

The newest dimension to the debate is the realization that there are not merely two brain-oriented views, but countless variations. Although most prefer a definition based on critical bodily functions, some insist that the underlying structure must be destroyed for death to occur. Whereas most consider individual cellular functions irrelevant, some insist that a function is a function and that, if the law says *all* functions of the entire brain must be destroyed, then cellular functions must all be dead before death is diagnosed. Many find it harder and harder to believe that every single supercellular function of the brain must be destroyed for death to occur. They cannot see that the presence of a single gag reflex mediated through the brain stem should count as a sign of life of the person as a whole. One neurologist paradoxically insists that whole "nests of cells" in the brain might continue to perform their functions without counting as a sign of life while he simultaneously insists that he has not abandoned the whole-brain view, that is, the view that holds that every function of the entire brain must be gone before death is pronounced (Bernat 1992). Anyone who adopts this view must be prepared to articulate criteria upon which the functions of nests of living cells should be classified as significant or insignificant and, even then, it seems hard to call the resulting position a "whole-brain" view. Recent research has revealed that not only are electrical functions retained in some brains classified as dead, but neurohormonal functions may remain as well (Halevy and Brody 1993).

There is increasing awareness that insisting on loss of every function is implausible. Some differentiation between significant and insignificant brain functions seems essential. The critical question is just which functions are insignificant. Does the integrating of bodily functions count as life even if no mental function is possible? That would be the view of those who take a more organic bodily function view. Does mental function have to be present? That would be the position of those who take views more closely associated with the classical Greek thought. Do both mental functions and some integrating organic functions have to be present? That would be the view closer to classical Christian theology. If there are countless possible answers to these questions and no scientific basis upon which they can be answered, we may have to resign ourselves to the possibility that there will not at any time soon be agreement on a societal definition of life and death.

Two recent proposals to respond to this dilemma may have to be considered. First, we may recognize that as science can stretch out the process of dying, there will be no one point at which all death-related behaviors are all appropriate. We may be forced to abandon the quest for a single, univocal point that we call death at which society approves of stopping treatment, going into mourning, establishing the role of the widow, reading a will, instituting succession in public office, and taking organs. Each of these activities may find its own appropriate time in the dying process and death, itself, will cease to have meaning.

The second possibility is that society will continue to seek a single point at which most if not all of these behaviors seem appropriate, the point we have traditionally labeled death. In a complex pluralistic world, however, we may have to acknowledge that people from different religions and cultures cannot agree on exactly what that point is. Some have proposed that society adopt a "default definition" that will be used unless an individual while competent has executed an advance directive choosing some other definition of death for use in his or her own case (Veatch 1976). If the individual has not spoken while competent, that task might be left to the next of kin or other valid surrogate. This proposal for a conscience clause has generated considerable debate. The President's Commission considered and rejected it as creating chaos in the public policy arena. Certainly, if an unlimited range of choice were permitted that would be the case. Some could insist that they were dead even though heart, brain stem, and cerebral function all remained in tact. Others might insist that they be considered alive even though all of these had ceased and the body had begun to putrefy. For public health reasons, if no other, some limits would have to be placed on the discretion among plausible definitions of death. Recognizing those limits, however, some are finding a policy of a default definition with conscientious choice among a limited range of options a policy worth further consideration (Veatch 1999). The State of New Jersey adopted a definition of death law with a conscience clause in 1991 (New Jersey Declaration of Death Act 1991). In 1997 Japan adopted a limited version of a conscience clause to be used only if organ procurement is contemplated (Japan 1997; see Chapter 43).

APPENDIX

BIOGRAPHIES: WHO WAS WHO IN THE HISTORY OF MEDICAL ETHICS

ALEXANDER, LEOPOLD (LEO) (Vienna, Austria 1905–Boston, Massachusetts 1985)

Austrian-American neurologist, and war crimes investigator, Leo Alexander was born into an assimilated Viennese Jewish family. After completing his training in neurology in 1933 Alexander visited China as a Lecturer. Unable to return to Germany because of Nazi policies excluding Jews from employment in medicine and science, he immigrated to the U.S. in 1934. In 1943, Alexander enlisted in the U.S. army, joining the 7th Army War Crimes Group in 1945, ultimately serving as a consultant to the U.S. prosecution team at the Nuremberg War Crimes Trials (1946–1947).

Inspired by a proposal from another prosecution expert, Andrew Ivy (1893–1978), and concerned that a proposed medical oath (the World Medical Association's [WMA's] 1948 Physician's Oath) (WMA [1948] 1995a) would not suffice to prevent the recurrence of unethical experimentation on human subjects, Alexander penned three memoranda for the prosecution between December 1946 and April 1947. In these memoranda, Alexander proposed that a code of ethics be included in the Tribunal's final judgment to state standards of ethical research on human subjects. The Tribunal adopted Alexander's proposal and the

code, which came to be known as the Nuremberg Code, and ultimately set the standard for research ethics for the second half of the twentieth century (*United States v. Karl Brandt et al.* 1947). According to a leading historian of the Code, Paul Weindling, eight of the Code's ten provisions were formulated in Alexander's memoranda and the Code often replicates lines from Alexander's memoranda word-for-word. (The two provisions in the Code that were absent from Alexander's memos are the subject's right to end an experiment at will and the scientist's duty to end any experiment that might result if the subject's injury or death appears likely.)

Returning to civilian life in 1948–1949, Alexander published eight papers on war crimes and human experimentation. The most influential was Science under Dictatorship, which appeared in the *New England Journal of Medicine* (Alexander, 1949b). Alexander was also a critic of unrepentant "de-Nazified" researchers. When Dutch delegates protested inviting Julius Hallervorden (1882–1965) to the Fifth International Conference of Neurologists (Lisbon 1953), Alexander became a central figure in a controversy. Documents assembled by Alexander in his role as war crimes investigator showed that Hallervorden had done research on more than 600 brains from victims of the Nazi eugenic-euthanasia program and was present at the killing of more than sixty children and adolescents. Alexander had also documented Hallervorden's statement, "Look here now, boys, if you are going to kill all those people, at least take the brains out so that the material could be utilized." "I accepted the brains, of course." Hallervorden had told Alexander, "where [the brains] came from and how they came to me was really none of my business."

In the immediate postwar environment of reconciliation, Nazi war crimes and the Nuremberg Code were obliterated from short-term memory. Neurologists felt that Alexander was "overreacting," some even argued that Alexander owed Hallervorden an apology. The neurological community would later point to Hallervorden with pride as one of its founders (Richardson 1990). Alexander's biographer, Ulf Schmidt, remarks that the Hallervorden "affair left Alexander as a lonely and controversial voice in a sea of experts who longed for a return to normality" (Schmidt 2004, 273).

Robert B. Baker

Arnald of Villanova (c. 1260–1311 Montpellier, France)

Professor of Medicine in Montpellier; personal physician of two kings of Spain (Peter III, James II); author of numerous philosophical, theological, and medical works; alchemist; Arnald was one of the most significant and influential intellectuals of his time. Medically speaking, Arnald was a devoted supporter of Galen, but his scripts also contain repeated calls on the scholastic-Arabic theory to be more practice-orientated. As well as commentaries on Hippocrates and Galen, he also composed *Speculum medicinae* (Medical Reflections), the *Parabolae medicationis* (Medical Aphorisms); a new version of Avicenna's script, *De viribus cordis* (On the Forces of the Heart); and *Regimen sanitatis* (Sanitary Regimen) for Peter of Aragon. His knowledge of Arabic enabled him to produce many important translations. Magic, astrology, and alchemy are all dealt with in his works. Through the nineteenth century, many works were wrongly attributed to Arnald.

Arnald studied the "artes liberals," theology, medicine, and the Arabic language in Montpellier and Naples. At the start of his career, he was the personal physician of Peter III and James II of Aragon. From 1291 onward, he held the Chair of Medicine in Montpellier. Around 1300, he took the side of the spirituals in the Franciscan "poverty conflict" and shared their eschatological expectations. He later became the personal physician of Boniface VIII in Rome, whose successor, Benedict XI, imprisoned him in Perugia. Arnald, a central character of this period, was later an advisor to Fredrick III of Aragon (King of Sicily) and to Clement V, whom he encouraged to carry out a reform

of the Church. He was an important mediator between politics, medicine, and theology.

Klaus Bergdolt

Bacon, Francis (January 22, 1561, London–April 9, 1626, London)

Francis Bacon's philosophy of science and medicine had considerable impact on the history of medical ethics, especially in the eighteenth century in the work of John Gregory (1724–1773) and Thomas Percival (1740–1804). Bacon insisted that medicine be based on "experience," that is, carefully observed results of natural and designed experiments, anticipating by almost four centuries the emergence of evidence-based medicine. He also set out an ethics for medicine, especially concerning end-of-life care that was widely influential.

Bacon was the son of Sir Nicholas Bacon, Keeper of the Seal, and Lady Anne Cooke, a learned woman from the nobility. After being educated at home, Bacon entered Trinity University at the age of 12, after which he read law at Gray's Inn. He was elected to serve in the Parliament in 1584 and served his constituency for 36 years. Bacon's political career had its ups and downs, taking a strong upturn with James I's succession of Queen Elizabeth in 1603. His career culminated in his appointment as Lord Chancellor in 1618, a position he held for 3 years, when he was convicted of bribery. He devoted his remaining years to intellectual work. During this period he produced the first of his two books of *Magna Instauratio, the Dignity and Advancement of Learning* and the *New Organon*.

In these works, Bacon set out his philosophy of science and medicine. Both should aim at the relief of "man's estate," that is, the reduction of mortality and morbidity. To achieve this goal, science and medicine needed to be reformed, by putting them on reliable empirical foundations. Such foundations were to be found in observation and experiment, conducted according to a rigorous method designed to minimize bias. Bacon attacked scientific and medical claims that lacked a basis in experience, especially those based in metaphysical systems that, because they lacked any empirical foundations, he labeled speculative. Bacon should be understood to have set out the components of scientific method that still shape scientific and clinical investigation. For example, he faults physicians for not following a regular use of medications, so that their hypothesized effects can be reliably identified and investigation undertaken to determine whether the medication does indeed cause the hypothesized effect.

Bacon argued that the "offices" or capacities of medicine should be the preservation of health, the cure of diseases (when "cure" meant any improvement in symptoms, not arresting or removing pathology), and the prolongation of life. By the last, Bacon meant that the then-frightful rates of mortality (60 percent or more by the age of 16) should be reduced, with the aim of having more people live longer. He also meant that the diseases and infirmities of old age should become a main focus of medical care, thus anticipating the creation of the specialty of geriatrics by almost four centuries. Bacon was also concerned about the quality of care for dying patients and called for medicine to develop the capacity to provide for *"outward Euthanasia, or the easy dying of the body."*

Bacon's experience-based method for science and medicine had a deep, shaping influence on the English and Scottish Enlightenments. Gregory and Percival appeal explicitly to Bacon in their attempts to reform medicine into a scientifically disciplined profession worthy of the intellectual trust of the sick. Gregory also appeals to Bacon's concept of "outward euthanasia" in calling for physician's not to abandon gravely ill patients and to "smooth the avenues of death."

Laurence B. McCullough

BACON, ROGER (c. 1219 [traditionally 1214], Ilchester–1292, Paris)

Scholastic philosopher, Franciscan Roman Catholic theologian, mathematician, philologist, and scientist, Roger Bacon was one of the most important intellectuals of the Middle Ages. Bacon's theological goal was the reconciliation of science and theology. In the prefaces of his main works, the *Opus maius*, the *Opus minus*, and the *Opus tertium* Bacon called for a reform of biological science and medicine. Being *"scientiae experimentales"* (experimental sciences) these were characterized by *"experimentum"* (experimentation) rather than mathematics, which was regarded as a model for the other natural sciences.

Bacon was considered a "magus" because he described the process of making gunpowder and proposed flying machines and motorized ships and carriages. His geographical tracts were still considered relevant in the time of Columbus. Bacon joined the Franciscans in 1250, taught in Oxford and Paris, and was a supporter of the Millenarian ideas of Joachim de Fiore (c. 1135–1204). In 1260, a conflict arose with his superiors in the order, possibly because he did not respect the internal censure rules of the order of Bonaventura. Forbidden to travel, Bacon sent the *Opus Maius* to Clement IV (1265). Bacon was temporarily imprisoned, probably because of a ban on Aristotle (1277). Girolamo d'Ascoli, later Pope Nicholas IV, claimed that Bacon's work contained *"suspectas novitates"* (suspicious novelties).

In his *Opus Maius*, Bacon chastised the shortcomings of scholastic medicine, accusing physicians of possessing no more than superficial knowledge (Bacon 1964; Brewer 1959). Their knowledge of medicinal herbs was especially lacking. Old herbs were applied instead of fresh ones, and false drugs were sold as genuine. Bacon identified thirty-six weak points (*errores*) of medicaments (*composita*). He also analyzed the contradictions between the medical doctrines and claimed that there were no norms or rules for pharmaceutical formulae. "This is why death, physical decline and other illnesses often occur. Cursed (*maledicta*) drugs are more frequent that blessed ones (*benedicta*)." Bacon accused physicians of not striving to increase their knowledge and of passing their responsibility on to others.

Klaus Bergdolt

BALLARD, MARTHA MOORE (1735, Oxford, Massachusetts–1812, Hallowell, Maine)

Ballard was a lay midwife and an outstanding example of an observant, caring woman whose diary (1787–1812) reveals extensive work as a midwife and lay healer. She possessed a deep religious faith and became quite skillful in preparing herbal remedies for parturient women and other patients. Although formally unschooled, she was fully aware of university education and the medical profession. Her uncle was a Yale graduate and a physician, and two brothers-in-law were physicians. Her brother, Jonathan, was a Harvard graduate and a Congregationalist pastor. In 1754, Martha Moore married Ephraim Ballard in Oxford, Massachusetts. In 1777, she and five children joined her husband, a miller, in Hallowell, Maine. Their ninth child was born in 1779; three had died in a diphtheria epidemic in 1769. Between 1785 and 1812, she assisted 816 women in childbirth. She prescribed herbs internally as teas and syrups, and externally as poultices and ointments. She used anise, balm, burdock, camomile, coriander, and other local plants and seeds. She purchased aloes, camphor, licorice, myrrh, Dragon's blood, and other medicinal ingredients. She was a devout Congregationalist.

Chester R. Burns

BARD, SAMUEL (1742, Philadelphia, Pennsylvania–1821, Hyde Park, New York)

Samuel Bard studied medicine with his father, John Bard, and attended King's College. He then matriculated at the University of Edinburgh and received a medical degree in 1765. After returning to New York City, he and several colleagues began a medical school at King's College in 1767, the second to be established in British North America. Bard taught at this school for more than 40 years. In 1769, Bard gave a commencement address about the duties of physicians to the first graduating class at King's College Medical School (now Columbia College of Physicians and Surgeons). It was published in the same year and is considered the first publication on this subject by a colonial physician in British North America. In this address, Bard appeals to the concepts of benevolence, tenderness, honor, and humanity as the basis for the physician's obligations to the sick. "In your behavior to the sick" he admonished the graduating class at Kings, "remember always that your patient is the object of the tenderest affection; it is therefore your duty not only to preserve his life but avoid wounding the sensibility of a tender parent, a distressed wife, or an affectionate child. Let your carriage be humane and attentive, be interested in his welfare, and show your apprehension of his danger rather by your assiduity to relieve, than by any harsh or brutal expressions of it." He also makes an appeal for the support of the New York Hospital, which was a hospital for the sick poor modeled on the infirmaries in Britain.

Chester R. Burns

had toyed with the notion of grounding medical morality in the law. This tradition was embraced by such Anglo-American writers as Michael Ryan (1800–1841), Alfred S. Taylor (1806–1880), and Beck. Beck envisioned law and medicine as interlocked and believed that a working knowledge of medical jurisprudence was indispensable to ordinary medical practitioners (Crowther 1993; Mohr 1992; Ryan 1831, 1832; Taylor, 1844, 1944).

Beck's two-volume work revolutionized the field by focusing on the scientific basis of what we would today call "forensic medicine." Volume One covered feigned diseases, impotence, sterility, intersex, rape, pregnancy, delivery, abortion and infanticide, the identification of corpses, and insanity. Volume Two covered persons found dead, wounds, and poisons. Knowledge of medical jurisprudence was considered indispensable to competent practitioners and the subject was taught at all major medical schools, using Beck's book. By the end of the century, however, medical educators lost faith in the value of medical jurisprudence. The subject lost its place in the medical curriculum, and the concept of medical jurisprudence rapidly obsolesced (Mohr 1993).

Robert B. Baker

BECK, THEODORIC ROMEYN (April 11, 1791, Schenectady, New York–November 19, 1855, Utica, New York)

Author of a seminal textbook on forensic medicine, Theodoric Beck was a graduate of Union College, Schenectady (1807), and of the (Columbia) College of Physicians and Surgeons (1811). After an unsuccessful stint at private medical practice, he became principal of the Albany Academy (1817–1848) and professor of medical jurisprudence and *materia medica* at various medical colleges. In 1823, he founded the Albany Lyceum of Natural History, which ultimately became the Albany Institute of History and Art and the New York State Museum. In 1829, he was elected president of the Medical Society of the State of New York and a manager of the New York state lunatic asylum (becoming president of the board of managers in 1854). From 1849 to 1853, Beck edited the *American Journal of Insanity* (Hamilton 1856; Mohr 1992).

Beck's most lasting contribution was *Elements of Medical Jurisprudence* (Beck 1823, various editions through 1842, reprinted 1997). Written with his brother, John Brodhead Beck (1794–1851), the book was intended to establish medical jurisprudence in a role that encompassed both forensic medicine and medical ethics. Like "medical ethics," the concept of "medical jurisprudence" was introduced to English by Thomas Percival (1740–1804), who

BEECHER, HENRY KNOWLES (nee Harry Unangst, 1904 Peck, Kansas–1976 Boston, Massachusetts)

Henry Knowles Beecher was Chief of Anesthesia at the Massachusetts General Hospital (1936–1969), a member of the Harvard Medical School Faculty (1936–1969, and, after 1941, Henry Isaiah Dorr Professor of Anesthesia Research at Harvard – the first endowed chair in anesthesiology in the U.S. He pioneered the epidemiological assessment of medical interventions in anesthesiology (Beecher and Todd 1954), did ground-breaking research on the placebo effect (Beecher 1946, 1955), and was an early champion of the prospective, double-blind, placebo-controlled clinical trial (Beecher 1959, 1963). Beecher favored a utilitarian theory of triage (Beecher 1970) and chaired the Ad Hoc Committee of the Harvard Medical School to Examine the Definition of Brain Death, whose 1968 report provided the catalyst prompting a worldwide substitution of neurological for cardiopulmonary criteria of death.

Although initially resistant to imposing the Nuremberg Code's requirement of "informed voluntary consent" on "therapeutic research" (Beecher 1963), after discovering dozens of cases of abusive research conducted by well-known researchers, Beecher publicized their activities in an internationally famous "whistle-blowing" article, "Ethics and Clinical Research" published in the *New England*

Journal of Medicine (Beecher 1966). The article detailed twenty-two cases of abusive research including such infamous cases as the Jewish Chronic Disease–Sloan Kettering cancer implant studies, and the U.S. Public Health Service's Tuskegee syphilis study. The article alerted the medical world to these experiments and, by informing the public at large (Beecher 1970), laid the groundwork for investigations by the U.S. Congress. These investigations culminated in the National Research Act (1974), which established Institutional Review Boards (IRBs) to monitor the activities of researchers; it also led to the appointment of a National Commission for the Protection of Human Subjects of Biomedical and Behavioral Research (1974–1978). The Commission's Belmont Report (1979) stated basic principles for research on human subjects, and facilitated the negotiation of "the Common Rule," that is, research ethics regulations shared by U.S. government agencies and funding bodies. This trio – IRBs guided by the principles in the Belmont Report and the regulations detailed in the Common Rule – would govern human subjects research in the United States through the end of the twentieth century.

Robert B. Baker

BINDING, KARL (April 6, 1841, Frankfurt/Main–April 7, 1920, Freiburg (Breslau, Germany)

Binding was a German lawyer, and professor of criminal and constitutional jurisprudence at the universities of Basel, Freiburg im Breslau, Strassburg, and Leipzig, where he was twice elected rector of the University. Binding's *Die Normen und ihre Übertretung* (1872–1919) (*Norms and their Transgression*) earned him a reputation as a leading German theoretician of the "classical" school of penal law, which adhered to a conception of justice as retaliation.

In 1920, Binding and psychiatrist Alfred E. Hoche (1865–1943) published a two-part tract *Die Freigabe der Vernichtung lebensunwerten Lebens* (Permission for the Destruction of Life Unworthy of Life) (Hafner and Winau 1974), the most influential work on "euthanasia" in interwar Germany. The tract, which might have been written as an ethical rationalization of the starvation of the mentally ill and disabled that had happened during World War I, triggered heated discussion within the legal, medical, and theological worlds. It combined an analysis of legal norms with medical ethical arguments to critique the traditional moral belief system, which advocated care and compassion for the disabled. Binding and Hoche saw the disabled as "life unworthy of life," "ballast existences," and "useless eaters" overburdening a financially bankrupt welfare system.

Most of the medical community denounced the involuntary "euthanasia" of the handicapped as murder. Many feared that it would undermine existing humanitarian and ethical values of care and cure. Others were anxious that the debate on "euthanasia" could poison fragile postwar doctor–patient relationships and tarnish the image of medical institutions. Although some favored eugenic sterilization of the mentally disabled, almost all opposed killing them. In 1921, the German medical profession rejected a proposal to legitimize the "destruction of life unworthy of life."

Debate over the tract adumbrated the "euthanasia" policy of the National Socialists. Some of the defendants in the Nuremberg Doctors' Trial, for example, Hitler's escort physician Karl Brandt (1904–1948), referred to the book to justify their role in the Nazi "euthanasia" program. Social Darwinist thought had been influential in Germany from the 1880s onward. The shock of the loss of World War and the cultural and economical crises of the postwar period brought about a radicalization of these ideas, which received further legitimation from the tract and the status of its authors. Binding and Hoche's tract prepared the way ideologically for the "euthanasia" program of the National Socialists who would later appeal to it as an academic "authority." (See also: Hoche, Alfred.)

Andreas-Holger Maehle and Ulf Schmidt

BRANDT, KARL (January 8, 1904, Mühlkhausen, Alsace–June 2, 1948, Landsberg am Lech, Germany)

Brandt was Hitler's personal escort physician, medical professor at the University of Berlin, Hitler's commissioner for the "euthanasia" program, head of the "Action Brandt," Reich Commissioner for Health and Sanitation, Special Plenipotentiary for Chemical Warfare, Major General in the SS, and Major General in the *Waffen-SS*. He was also defendant No. 1 in the Nuremberg Doctors' Trial.

Brandt studied medicine at the Universities of Jena, Freiburg im Breslau, Munich and Berlin. He became a member of the NSDAP (Nazi party) in 1932 (No. 1,009,617) and joined the SA in 1933. He married Anni Rehborn on March 17, 1934 (NSDAP membership No. 1264305). He was appointed Hitler's escort physician in June 1934. Throughout the late 1930s, Brandt, constantly in Hitler's vicinity, enjoyed the "ear of the Führer," and was given special assignments by Hitler to circumvent established administrative structures.

From the beginning, Brandt was involved in the planning of the Nazi euthanasia program, the murder of handicapped children and adults. In the autumn of 1939, Brandt was appointed to oversee the introduction of the program.

Following the formal cessation of the centrally organized euthanasia program in 1941, the killings continued on a more decentralized level under the code name, "Aktion Brandt," to free hospital bed-space for war-wounded German soldiers and civilians. The euthanasia program was the Nazi's first systematic murder of tens of thousand of people. It provided the Nazi leadership with expertise and personnel for the systematic mass murder of a large number of people in the Holocaust. On August 20, 1942, Hitler appointed Brandt to General Commissioner for Health and Sanitation to coordinate the military and civilian sectors of the health system. Brandt's position allowed him to become the dominating personality in the German health service. He was only answerable to Hitler directly.

Brandt was also a member of the Reich Research Council, in charge of German medical research and Special Plenipotentiary for Chemical Warfare. In this capacity, he became implicated in numerous medical experiments that German doctors conducted on concentration camp inmates, especially those concerned with epidemic jaundice and chemical warfare agents. From September 12, 1946 to August 20, 1947, Brandt was tried as part of a group of twenty-three defendants in the Nuremberg War Crimes Tribunal's Doctors' Trial. He was charged with, and found guilty of, war crimes, crimes against humanity, and membership in an organization declared criminal by the judgement of the International Military Tribunal. Brandt was sentenced to death on August 20, 1947 and hanged on August 2, 1948, at Landsberg prison.

Ulf Schmidt

Burns, Chester (December 5, 1937, Nashville, Tennessee–December 27, 2006, New York, New York)

Pioneer historian of medical ethics, medical humanist, and medical educator, Chester Burns was awarded a bachelors degree with a major in philosophy and a medical doctorate from Vanderbilt University in Nashville (1959 and 1963, respectively). He became a Fellow at the Johns Hopkins University Institute of Medicine (1964–1969) and in June 1969 was the first American-born physician to receive a Ph.D. in the history of medicine from Hopkins. His thesis was "Medical Ethics in the United States before the Civil War" (Burns 1969b). With his newly minted M.D. and Ph.D. in hand, Burns joined the University of Texas Medical Branch (1969) where he founded the Institute for the Medical Humanities, from which he retired as James Wade Rockwell Professor of the History of Medicine in 2006. From 1975–1976, he served as president of the Society for Health and Human Values, a predecessor to the American Society of Bioethics and Humanities (ASBH).

He was the official ASBH historian from the organization's founding in 1998. In 2005, he received the ASBH's distinguished service award.

Superlatively equipped to explore the history of medical ethics by his training in history, medicine, and philosophy, in 1977, Burns edited a ground-breaking volume, *Legacies in Ethics and Medicine* that reprinted significant publications on the history of medical ethics by historians of medicine (Burns 1977a). Among the essays reprinted was one by Burns himself that firmly asserted the ethical nature of Percival's *Medical Ethics* (Percival 1803b), challenging the then received view that *Medical Ethics* dealt with medical etiquette not medical ethics (Leake 1927; Berlant 1975; Waddington 1975). Burns also wrote an authoritative history of American medical ethics for the various editions of the *Encyclopedia of Bioethics* (Reich 1978, 1995; Post 2004), and was an enthusiastic contributor to this volume and its biography section.

Robert B. Baker

Cannon, Walter Bradford (October 18, 1871, Prairie du Chien, Wisconsin–October 1, 1945, Franklin, New Hampshire)

Walter B. Cannon, Professor of Physiology at Harvard (1906–1942), President of the American Physiological Society (1914–1916) was an inventor of two major physiological concepts (homeostasis and traumatic shock) a pioneer in the use of X-rays to study physiological processes, and a founder of the two fields: psychosomatic medicine and psychophysiology. He received his B.A., M.A., and M.D. from Harvard University in 1896, 1897, and 1900, respectively. There he became a student of Henry Pickering Bowditch (1840–1911), whom he succeeded as George Higginson Professor of Physiology in 1906. Cannon was the first American physician to lobby for ethics standards that would protect the rights of animal and human research subjects.

Born and raised a Calvinist, as a high school student, Cannon struggled over the conflict between his faith and his belief in the theory of evolution, turning from Calvinism to Unitarianism. Motivated by his Unitarian beliefs Cannon had a lifelong commitment to social justice, supporting the Loyalist struggle against Fascism in Spain, Chinese resistance to the Japanese invasion, and the Soviet–American alliance during World War II. He became President of the American–Soviet Medical Society in 1943, despite rising United States–Soviet tensions.

As founding Chair of the American Medical Association's Council for the Defense of Medical Research (1908–1926), Cannon was a militant opponent of antivivisectionist initiatives prohibiting all experimentation on animals.

Seeking a less radical alternative that would still provide for the humane treatment of animals in scientific experimentation, in 1909–1910 Cannon negotiated an arrangement under which American medical laboratories would voluntarily adopt standards for the humane treatment of animals used in research. In 1915–1916, he attempted to negotiate a similar solution to the treatment of the human subjects of scientific research by getting journal editors to voluntarily embrace a policy prohibiting publications that reported research on humans conducted without the informed consent of the subject. He also proposed that the American Medical Association (AMA) adopt an ethical principle prohibiting such research. To this end, in 1916, Cannon wrote an editorial in the *Journal of the American Medical Association* in which he declared that experiments conducted "without the consent of the person on whom it is tried" violated the "fundamental right which any individual possesses … of controlling the uses to which his own body is put."

These efforts established Cannon as the first American physician to propose formally the integration of research subjects protections into the AMA's Principles of Medical Ethics and the first to propose that, as a matter of policy, journals refuse to publish unethical experiments. Both initiatives were stymied. Pathologist Simon Flexner (1863–1946), founding Director of the Rockefeller Institute for Medical Research (1906–1935) and the public voice of the research establishment, had been Cannon's close ally in the fight to protect research science against militant antivivisectionism. When the issue turned to protecting human subjects, however, Flexner, who in 1914 became the President of the Association of American Physicians – an organization committed to medical science free from the disputes surrounding the AMA's code of ethics – was reluctant to support Cannon's efforts, and may have subverted them. In the end, Flexner's *Journal of Experimental Medicine* challenged the proposed prohibition on publishing unconsented research by publishing precisely such an article. The AMA never voted on Cannon's proposal for principles of research ethics and Cannon's initiative foundered.

Robert B. Baker

DE CASTRO, RODRIGO (c. 1546 Lisbon–Hamburg, 20 January 1627)

Professor of Medicine in Hamburg, author of various different medical works, and personal physician of the King of Denmark, Rodrigo came from a Jewish Portuguese family. Following his medical studies in Portugal and Spain, he moved, for political reasons (possibly to avoid religious persecution), to the harbor city of Hamburg – an important center of trade and commerce. Here he took up an important position as a physician, his patients including the King of Denmark and many princes from North Germany. His son, Benedict (Baruch Nehemias) de Castro, was also a leading physician and scholar. Benedict's paper "Flagellum calumniantium, in quo anonymi cuiusdam libelli adversus medicos hebraeolusitanos calumniae refutantur" shows that both father and son, who in their publications self-identify as "Lusitani," a term indicating Jewish origins, had many adversaries and enemies.

Rodrigo was an important physician in Hamburg where he also worked during the plague. At this time, he wrote the "Tractatus brevis de natura et causis pestis quae hoc anno 1596 Hamburgensem civitatem affigit … " (Hamburg 1596) and the script "De universa muliebrum morborum medicina, novo et antehac a nemine tentato ordine opus absolutissimum … " (Hamburg 1603, 1604, 1617, Cologne 1628, Hamburg 1662). In 1614, the "Medicus politicus" was also published in Hamburg. The book, a classic treatise on the politic physician that employs a casuistic approach to issues that later eras will identify with "medical ethics," is also considered a classic of medical humanism. One of its themes is that "whoever is requesting individual medical care, the physician should take that person up and attempt to cure that person with all diligence, whether Christian, Jew, Turk or heathen; for all are linked by the law of *humanitas* (humanity, humanism), and *humanitas* requires that they all be treated equally by the physician."

Klaus Bergdolt and Robert B. Baker

CELSUS, AULUS CORNELIUS (C. 25 BCE–C. 50)

Celsus was an encyclopedist and perhaps a physician. Little is known about his life. His *De Medicina* (Celsus 1915) divided medicine into diet, pharmacy, and surgery, and provided early accounts of inflammation, the pharmacological management of diseases and injuries, the use of opioids (a mixture of opium poppy and wine), and a variety of surgical procedures. Celsus compared medicine to agriculture: just as the latter produces nourishment for the body, medicine should aim at producing health. Medicine seeks to explain disease in terms of natural causes and should seek a rational form of medical practice. Celsus emphasized compassion as a virtue of physicians, although he believed that compassion should not interfere with surgical procedures. "Now a surgeon should be youthful or at any rate nearer youth than age; with a strong and steady hand which never trembles, and ready to use the left hand as well as the right; with vision sharp and clear, and spirit undaunted; filled with pity, so that he wishes to cure his patient, yet is not moved by his cries, to go too fast, or cut less than is necessary; but he does everything just as if the cries of pain cause him no emotion" (Celsus 1935–1938, Book 7, §4). Celsus opposed human vivisection but not dissection: "But to lay open the bodies of men whilst still alive is as cruel as it is needless; that of the dead is a necessity for the learner, who should know positions and relations, which the dead body exhibits better than does a living and wounded man" (Celsus 1935–1938, Proem, §74).

Laurence B. McCullough

COTTA, JOHN (1575?–1650?)

In *A Short Discoverie of the Unobserved Dangers of Severall Sorts of Ignorant and Unconsiderate Practisers of Physicke in England* (1612), Cotta, a physician, argued that only university-educated physicians should practice medicine. In defending learned medicine, Cotta attacked other types of practitioners. He equated learning with medical ability and the lack of it with dangerous and hence unethical medicine. Cotta argued that only the physician learned in Greek medicine could safely prescribe medicines, matching treatment to the individual state of a patient. Cotta attacked empirics, unlearned surgeons, apothecaries, and women who practiced as physicians; he also criticized astrologers, uroscopists, and travelers who bring back exotic medicines from the far corners of the world without knowing how to use them. Cotta saw patients as often deluded, as misled by bystanders at the bedside, and deceived by the rhetoric of rival practitioners. He condemned the medicine of empirics, Paracelsians, and others as dangerous. His ethical stance was that Galenic medicine is the safest and hence most ethical form of medicine.

The failings of patients were attributed to their lack of knowledge about what made a proper physician. To address this problem, Cotta set out the characteristics of the "true artist" or physician. These consisted of long study, the use of reason, knowledge of the constant laws of nature set in the world by God, and the ability to observe nature in detail and to aid her. Although the virtue of the physician is mentioned, knowledge is more important. Christian ethical values are signally absent from Cotta's treatise. The need for charity in a physician is explicitly denied. Classical Galenic medicine is presented as safe and good whereas all other types of medicine are dangerous and morally suspect. Cotta's ethics center on the right type of knowledge and are underpinned by the need to create a monopoly of practice for like-minded physicians.

Andrew Wear

EKIKEN, KAIBARA (December 17, 1630–October 15, 1714)

Confucian botanist and philosopher Ekiken's work on medical ethics belongs to a genre of Japanese writings concerned with the "care of life" or Yojo. He was the author of more than 100 philosophical works, including moral instruction for women (*The Great Learning for Women*) and for children that was based on Confucianism and was influential for many centuries. Originally trained as a physician, in 1657, while still in his twenties, Ekiken left medicine for the study of Confucianism.

Ekiken's major work in medical ethics, *Yojokun* (Teaching for the Care of Life), appeared in 1713 (Kaibara [1713a] 1961). The proper care of life in oneself requires mastery of a lifelong discipline of thought and behavior by ritual and other activities. Ekiken taught that the practice of medicine should be a "humanitarian art." Physicians should be motivated mainly by a concern to protect the interests of their patients rather than by the pursuit of self-interest, so that medicine becomes a life of service defined by fulfilling obligations to the sick. To achieve this life of service the physician must immerse himself in Confucian ethics, which is modeled on filial piety or obligation, the moral relationship of obedience of a dutiful son to his father. This paradigmatic moral relationship was generalized into the life of service or obligation to the sick. Ekiken's medical ethics writings continue to influence contemporary Japanese medical ethics.

Laurence B. McCullough

FLETCHER, JOSEPH (April 10, 1905–October 28, 1991)

An ordained minister of the Episcopal Church, Joseph Fletcher taught ethics for many years in the Episcopal Divinity School in Cambridge, Massachusetts. Initially interested in problems of social justice, he turned to medical ethics in 1949. At that time, the field was bereft of philosophical analysis and Fletcher took up several important questions, such as the patients' right to know the truth about their condition and the moral permissibility of euthanasia. He lectured on these questions at Harvard and subsequently published these lectures, *Medicine and Morals*, which took unconventional positions but nonetheless had a wide and generally favorable reception (Fletcher 1954).

Written before bioethics emerged as a discipline, *Medicine and Morals* might be designated as transitional work conserving the preoccupations of the old medical ethics while heralding the appearance of a new style. Fletcher took up traditional questions of medical ethics but criticized traditional answers by affirming the patient's right to know the truth and to receive desired services, even euthanasia. He thus anticipated the powerful role that the ethical principle of respect for autonomy would play in bioethics. Fletcher continued to write on problems of medical ethics, particularly those associated with advances in genetics and reproductive science. His explicit account of his ethical system, *Situation Ethics: The New Morality* (Fletcher 1966) attracted attention for its departure from an ethics of rules and principles in favor of a judgment of what love demands in the situation. Fletcher became Visiting Professor of Medical Ethics in the School of Medicine, University of Virginia. Freed from ecclesiastical constraints, he elaborated a humanistic ethic and applied it to many issues in bioethics. His other principal books are *Ethics of Genetic Control: Ending Reproductive Roulette* (Fletcher 1974) and *Humanhood: Essays in Biomedical Ethics* (Fletcher 1974). Fletcher's stress on responsible human freedom had a significant effect on the development of bioethics.

Albert R. Jonsen

FOREEST, PIETER VAN [FORESTUS, PETRUS] (1522, Alkmaar, Netherlands–1597, Delft, Netherlands)

Known as the "Hippocrates of Holland," van Foreest was town physician for Delft. His *Observationes et Curationes Medicinales* (Medicinal Observations and Cures) (1588, enlarged edition 1591) was famous for its descriptions of the plague in Delft and of a large number of clinical cases.

Van Foreest was a critic of uroscopists and other rivals of learned physicians in the medical marketplace (van Foreest 1589). In the Middle Ages, uroscopy relied on the examination of urine as the sole method of diagnosis and prognosis and had been used by the newly emerging cadre of Galenic physicians as a diagnostic tool to impress clients. Sixteenth-century physicians, in contrast, favored Galen's method of healing, which held that the individual circumstances of the patient were the key to safe and true healing. Van Foreest accepted the value of uroscopy, but only if seen as one among many indications that could be used to assess a patient's condition. He presented Galenic medicine as the only valid form of medicine. In his vitriolic attacks upon uroscopists, mountebanks, and ignorant patients, van Foreest implicitly created a medical ethics in which the learning of the Galenic physicians was the guarantee of good medical practice, implicitly linking a proper knowledge of medicine with moral worth. From this perspective, patient choice of treatment and of practitioner was only allowable if directed toward Galenic medicine.

Andrew Wear

GALEN (Claudius Gelenus of Pergamum) (c. 129, Pergamum [modern day Bergama, Turkey]–c. 200, Rome)

Galen was a Greek philosopher-physician practicing in the Roman period. He spent 4 years of his youth as an attendant in a temple dedicated to Asclepius, the god of healing. Thereafter, he became a gladiator, which gave him direct experience with wounds. He moved to Rome in 162 where he lectured and wrote on anatomy, became a successful medical practitioner and court physician to the Emperor Marcus Aurelius.

Galen preserved and transmitted the humoral theory of medicine, influencing the subsequent history of medicine for more than 1,000 years. His ethics revolve around three principles: love of the truth/knowledge, love of the creator, and love of humanity or *philanthropia*. Galen called for physicians to seek knowledge and truth through empirical research on living animals and human cadavers, to be truthful in their communications to their patients, and to resist their self-interested temptation to avoid being the bearer of bad news. Exceptions to truthfulness are permissible, but only if they benefit the patient.

Galen's conception of *philanthropia* entailed that a physician's behavior was a crucial component of good patient care. Physicians should not be motivated by material gain or greed in their practice, but by love of humanity. They should also be dedicated to hard work in service of the sick. Galen treats Hippocrates as an exemplar of the virtues of the philanthropic physician, even though this concept does not appear in the Hippocratic texts. Galen called for medicine and philosophy to be closely connected. He is well known for holding *quod optimus medicus sit quoque philosophus*, "That the best doctor is also a philosopher," the title of one of his works.

Laurence B. McCullough

GALTON, SIR FRANCIS (February 16, 1822, Birmingham, England–January 17, 1911, London)

Galton was a Victorian polymath, natural scientist, writer, doctor, geographer, meteorologist, tropical explorer, statistician, anthropologist – and, not least, a cousin of Charles Darwin. He coined the term "eugenics," by which he meant the science of improving human hereditary characteristics.

Galton was taught in Boulogne, in Kenilworth, and at the King Edwards's School in Birmingham. He studied medicine at the General Hospital in Birmingham and at King's College, London. He also studied mathematics at Cambridge University. In the 1840s and 1850s, he undertook extensive travels to Egypt, Khartoum, Syria, and tropical Africa. Following Charles Darwin's publication on the *Origin of Species* (1859), Galton began research into heredity and in 1865 published his first results. In 1869, he published his book, *Hereditary Genius: An Inquiry into its Laws and Consequences*. Galton wanted to demonstrate the inheritance of physical and psychological characteristics in humans by means of biostatistical research and twin studies. By the mid-1860s, he developed the outlines of a new theory to improve the inherited conditions of a race to the highest ideal, a concept for which he coined the term, "national eugenics," in 1883. The theory of eugenics applied evolutionary biology and cell theory to modern society and state government. Eugenics established key elements of Social Darwinism in which the social problems of society were transformed into perceived illnesses of society. Galton's eugenics was relatively vague in making concrete policy proposals for the improvement of the human race. He made some negative eugenic proposals including the idea of removing habitual criminals from society and prohibiting the procreation of the mentally ill. Further biometrical studies on plants and animals and work on heredity turned Galton into a widely known proponent of the eugenics movement (Galton 1889).

Ulf Schmidt

GISBORNE, THOMAS (October 31, 1758, Bridge Gate, Derby, England Derbyshire England–March 24, 1846. Yoxall Lodge, Derbyshire, England: buried Barton-under-Needwood, Straffordshire, England)

The Reverend Thomas Gisborne was an Evangelical Anglican minister, an essayist, a poet, a political philosopher, and a social reformer. A Harrow-educated alumnus of St. John's College, Cambridge, he became a curate in 1783. Along with parliamentarian William Wilberforce (1759–1833) and the writer and playwright, Hannah More (1745–1835), Gisborne was a leading member of the Clapham sect (fl. 1790–1830), a group of social reformers dedicated to the reform of the penal system and the abolition of slavery.

Like most abolitionists seeking secular philosophical reasons to justify their position, Gisborne drew inspiration from John Locke (1632–1704), whose theory of god-given natural rights shared equally by all humanity, and whose contention that governmental authority derives from a social contract with the governed, directly challenged the propriety of slavery (Locke 1690). As it happened, however, the leading political philosophy textbook of Gisborne's day, *The Principles of Moral and Political Philosophy*, dismissed Locke's social contract as "founded upon a supposition false in fact, and leading to dangerous

conclusions" (Paley 1785, 292). The textbook's author was another Cambridge theologian, William Paley (1743–1805), who is best remembered today for his teleological arguments for the intelligent design of the universe (Paley 1802). In two quite different works, Gisborne attempted to rebut Paley's critique of Locke. *The Principles of Moral Philosophy Investigated and Briefly Applied To the Constitution of Civil Society* (Gisborne 1789) contends that the Lockean social contract was tacit and thus not subject to Paley's criticisms. *An Enquiry into the Duties of Men in the Higher and Middle Classes of Society in Great Britain Resulting from Their Respective Stations, Professions and Employment* (Gisborne 1794) unpacks the social contract tacitly accepted by gentlemen by dint of their professions and social status: magistrate, minister, lawyer – and physician. Gisborne also wrote a similar book about the tacitly accepted social responsibilities of ladies (Gisborne 1797). Both works transform a traditional genre, the gentleman or gentlewoman's guide to proper conduct, into works of "applied moral philosophy."

While drafting the chapter on the responsibilities of physicians, Gisborne entered into correspondence with an eminent older reformer, the physician, Thomas Percival (1740–1804). Gisborne drew from this correspondence an experienced practitioner's sense of the physician's responsibilities; in turn, he inspired Percival to reformulate rules for the Manchester Infirmary into a formal code of professional medical ethics (Baker 1993; Percival 1803). Percival acknowledged his debt, praising Gisborne's *Enquiry* as "the most complete system, extant, of Practical Ethics" (Percival 1803, 5). The system was complete enough to address such emerging problems as the abuse of sick poor patients in infirmaries (i.e., charity hospitals) as involuntary human guinea pigs, "strongly reprobat[ing] every experiment rashly or hastily adopted; or carried out by the selfish, the ignorant, the careless or the obstinate. Proceedings of this nature are highly criminal, partly because they involve the health and life of sufferers in needless hazards" (Gisborne 1794, 408–9).

Nineteenth-century British medicine accepted ideals of a tacit medical ethics based on gentlemanly honor, much like that championed by Gisborne. At mid-century, a physician at Trinity College, Oxford, William Alexander Greenhill (1814–1894), reprinted classic works in medical ethics, beginning with the most important. He reprinted Gisborne before Percival. In the twentieth century, however, Gisborne fell out of print. His work on medical ethics only began to receive attention at the end of the century, as medical historians began the challenging project of reconstructing the history of British medical ethics – a daunting enterprise because the ethics of tacit understandings championed by Gisborne is difficult to document (Baker 1993; Haakonssen 1997; Porter 1993; Veatch 2005, 53–6).

Robert B. Baker

Gregory of Tours (538 or 539, Averni [modern Clermont]–November 17, 593 or 594, probably Tours)

Bishop of Tours, historian, and author of theological and historic works, Gregory is famous for the *Decem Libri Historiarum: Historia Francorum* (Ten Historical Books, The History of the Franks). The work begins with a retrospective look at the history of the world from Adam to St. Martin, the patron saint of Tours (deceased 397), and includes an in-depth history of the kingdom of the Franks. It ends with a history of the bishops of Tours and a calculation of the age of the world. Gregory held that history was influenced by causal occurrences in worldly events as well as by divine influence.

Gregory considered the success of medical treatment to be entirely dependent on the will of God. Thus, prayers and intercessions were more effective than ointments and surgical instruments. Gregory rejected medicine as a "worldly" science, whose pagan origin was no coincidence. He saw it a moral problem that the "cataract couchers" and healers only reasoned in a "causal" way, while illnesses were in reality divine punishments or trials. Ethics in medicine required both the patient and the healer to demonstrate piety and acceptance of the divine will.

Klaus Bergdolt

Gregory, John (June 23, 1724, Aberdeen, Scotland–February 9, 1773, Edinburgh, Scotland)

Born into an academically distinguished family of mathematicians, astronomers, and physicians, John Gregory wrote the first modern, philosophical medical ethics in the English language. After studying at Kings College in Aberdeen, Gregory attended the University of Edinburgh (1742–1745) and the University of Leiden (1745–1746) for his medical studies. He was awarded an unearned medical degree from the University of Aberdeen in 1746. From 1746 to 1754, Gregory served as Professor of Philosophy at King's College in Aberdeen. He relocated to London in 1754, to start his own medical practice, returning to Aberdeen as Professor of Physic at King's in 1755. In 1764, he moved to Edinburgh, and was made a fellow of the Royal College of Physicians of Edinburgh in 1765. In 1766, he was appointed Professor of the Practice of Medicine by the Edinburgh Town Council. That same year saw him appointed First Physician to His Majesty for Scotland and granted the high honor of Freedom of the City of Edinburgh. He died in his sleep of hereditary gout at the age of only 49.

At Edinburgh, Gregory expanded considerably upon the tradition of giving lectures on medical ethics before students undertook their clinical experiences at the Royal Infirmary (McCullough 1998a). Student note sets of his lectures exist from as early as 1767 (Gregory 1767, 1767–1768, 1769, 1772). In 1770, these lectures appeared as *Observations on the Duties and Qualifications of a Physician, and on the Method of Prosecuting Enquiries in Philosophy*. The book was well received and Gregory revised it in 1772 as *Lectures on the Duties and Qualifications of a Physician*.

Gregory's medical ethics rests on the twin sources of Francis Bacon's (1561–1626) philosophy of science and medicine, which insisted that science be based on the results of careful observation and experimentation, and Scottish moral sense theory, which grounds morality in sympathy, the natural capacity of fellow-feeling. Inspired by these sources Gregory extols the intellectual virtue of candor, being open to evidence from any source, and the moral virtues of tenderness and steadiness. Gregory deploys this virtue-based approach to address such topics as confidentiality, honestly informing seriously ill patients ("one of the most disagreeable duties in the profession"), the adoption of new remedies, and the obligation not to abandon the dying but to "smooth the avenues of death," and the relationship between medicine and religion. Gregory also set out an ethics for clinical research with human subjects, appealing to a version of the Golden Rule.

Laurence B. McCullough

Haeckel, Ernst Heinrich (February 16, 1834, Potsdam–August 8, 1919, Jena)

Haeckel was a zoologist, biologist, philosopher, anthropologist, psychologist, cosmologist, and a leading proponent of monism. Haeckel is known for his statement that "ontogeny recapitulates phylogeny." His evolutionary and monist philosophy helped to establish and justify Social Darwinism and German racial hygiene. Haeckel's views about "artificial selection" in man's struggle for survival served as argument in favor of negative eugenic measures in German racial policy. Nazi propagandists used his phrase that "politics is applied biology." Ernst Haeckel was the son of a Prussian government official, Carl Haeckel, and Charlotte, née Sethe. From early on, Heackel was fascinated by plant and animal science. He studied medicine at the Universities of Berlin, Würzburg, and Vienna, and, in 1856, he became the assistant of Rudolf Virchow at the University of Würzburg. Prompted by a number of study trips to Italy in the 1850s, he became increasingly interested in comparative anatomy and zoology. In Sicily, he discovered 144 new species of radiolarians (amoeboid protozoa). Other research focused on poriferans (sponges) and annelids (segmented worms). In 1862, Haeckel was appointed to extraordinary professor at the University of Jena and, in 1866, published his *Generelle Morphologie der Organismen* (General Morphology of Organisms).

An advocate of Darwin's evolutionary theory, Haeckel developed the concept of monism, which rejected the idea of an all powerful, controlling God, but which saw God as the sum of all forces and matter. He campaigned for the abolition of religious teaching in schools, which he wanted to have replaced with the teaching of natural sciences. Research into evolutionary biology and developmental theory shaped the formulation of Haeckel's "law of recapitulation," that the "ontogeny recapitulates phylogeny," namely, that the history of the species is recapitulated in embryological development. In 1874, he published *Anthropogenie oder Entwicklungsgeschichte des Menschen* (Anthropogeny or Evolution of Man) that linked the development of human society with evolutionary theory. Haeckel projected Darwin's "struggle for existence" onto society and argued that two kinds of selective processes existed in nature. Whereas man's struggle for survival determined "natural selection," there was also "artificial selection," the active process of "weeding out" the weak and burdensome members of society. To give his argument greater legitimacy, Haeckel referred to the society of the Spartans, who apparently had killed their weak, ill, or handicapped offspring. In 1894 the University of Jena appointed him to professor of geology and palaeontology. Five years later he published his major work on *Die Welträtsel. Gemeinverständliche Studien über biologische Philosophie* (Worlds' Mysteries: General Studies on Biological Philosophy) (1899) in which he expanded on materialism, the role of the natural sciences and monism. The book was translated into twenty-five languages. In 1904, Haeckel participated at the international peace congress in Rome and, in 1906, he founded the "German Monist Association" in Jena.

Ulf Schmidt

HAYS, ISAAC (July 5, 1796, Philadelphia, Pennsylvania–April 12, 1879, Philadelphia, Pennsylvania)

Isaac Hays, "the most gifted medical journalist of the nineteenth century" (Gross 1879), received his medical degree from the University of Pennsylvania in 1820. He would ultimately become a member of the American Philosophical Society, of the College of Physicians of Philadelphia, and President of the Philadelphia Academy of Natural Science (1865–1869). Philadelphians admired the socially gracious Hays for his skill as an editor and for his personal qualities – including his public adherence to Judaism.

Public tolerance of Judaism, however, was limited in the rest of nineteenth-century America. Hays's colleague, Richard Arnold (1808–1876), had to apologize to his daughter for the behavior of a "Lady" who had come calling but refused to enter their house when she realized that Arnold's daughter was entertaining a Jewess. "Among" this lady's "other religious aversions" Arnold wrote apologetically, was "a peculiar one for Israelites" (Shyrock [1929] 1970, 86). Not surprisingly, given the prejudices of the age, when Hays became founding editor of the *American Journal of the Medical Science* (1827), originally the *Philadelphia Journal of the Medical Physical Science*, 1820–1827) he had to do so anonymously. His name did not appear on the masthead for 14 years (1841). Memorial notes on Hays's remark the role of anti-Semitism in shaping his life. "By birth a Hebrew . . . [Hays] through long life adhered to the ancient faith . . . often quoting Pope's lines: 'For modes of faith let graceless zealots fight: His can't be wrong whose life is in the right'" (Stillé 1880, 35).

In 1846, Hays attended a national conference on reforming medical education organized at the behest of Nathan Smith Davis (1817–1904). Unfortunately, the conference was unable to reach a consensus. Rather than see it end in failure, Hays proposed the creation of a national medical association that could deal with ongoing problems facing American medicine – including reforming education and developing a code of ethics for American physicians. When this resolution passed, Hays was charged with organizing the founding convention for what would become the AMA and was appointed to a committee to draft its code of ethics.

Hays and the committee chair, John Bell (1796–1872), decided to base the new AMA code on an edition of Percival's *Medical Ethics* that they had edited for the Kappa Lambda society of Philadelphia two decades earlier (Kappa Lambda 1827). Hays took charge of the editorial process, and Bell took charge of introducing the new code to the AMA's founding convention. During the actual presentation of the code, Hays remained off-stage as Bell read to convention notes from him stating, "this code . . . carefully preserved the words of Percival" (Hays [1847] 1999, 315). Evoking the name of the eminent, eminently Christian, and safely deceased British physician, Thomas Percival (1740–1804), deflected potential anti-Semitic murmurings and effectively valorized the many radically new ideas in the proposed code, which the AMA voted unanimously to adopt (AMA [1847] 1999). After the convention, Hays continued to play an off-stage role at the AMA chairing its publication committee (1847–1853) and serving as treasurer (1848–1852). He attended his last national meeting at the age of 64 in 1858 (Brinton 1879; Gross 1879; Stillé 1880).

Survivors write history. In 1897, when the AMA met to celebrate its semicentennial Nathan Smith Davis, the sole founding member attending, seized the laurel of "father of the AMA." Davis's preemption effectively eclipsed Hays's role, obscuring the fact that it was Hays, rather than Davis, who had actually proposed the establishment of the AMA, who had organized its founding meeting, and who had edited its code of ethics.

By the twentieth century, Hays was dimly remembered as the AMA's first treasurer (Fishbein 1947; Moore 1947) but his role in founding the AMA and crafting its code of ethics was forgotten. The only history of American medical ethics published in the twentieth century ignored Hays entirely (Konold 1962). A half-century after Hays's death, however, American ophthalmologists began to claim him as a founder of their field (Flaxman 1936; Albert, Schele 1965; Morgenstern 2002) and Jewish physicians began to embrace him as a forbearer (Kagan 1939a; 1939b, 19–21; Kagan 1941, 11). In the 1990s, historians preparing for the celebration of the AMA's sesquicentennial discovered the proposal to establish the AMA among Hays's papers, written in his hand. Comparisons of the AMA's code with Percival's code also made clear that Bell and Hays had edited Percival's language to introduce their own radically new conception of professional ethics. A more tolerant age could readily acknowledge what an earlier era had found awkward to accept: a Sephardic Jew played a leading role in founding the AMA, crafting its code of ethics, and creating a new conception of professional ethics (Baker 1995, 1999; Jonsen 2000, 69–70; Veatch 2005, 115–19).

Robert B. Baker

Hellegers, André Eugène Désiré Joseph (June 5, 1926, Venlo, The Netherlands–May, 18, 1979, Amsterdam, the Netherlands)

"The Pope's Biologist," founder and founding director of the Kennedy Institute of Ethics, André Hellegers was educated at the Jesuit preparatory school, Stonyhurst, at Oxford, at the University of Edinburgh (medical degree 1951) and at the Sorbonne (1952–1956), where he studied space medicine. After a residency in obstetrics and gynecology at Johns Hopkins (1953–1956), Hellegers spent 11 years (1956–1967) dividing his time between Hopkins and Yale. In 1967, he moved to Georgetown University as a physiologist; in 1971, he became the founding Director of the Kennedy Institute of Ethics.

A bibliographic review of Hellegers' work compiled by The Kennedy Institute of Ethics' Library (Goldstein 1999) lists 231 publications. From his first scientific article on vitamins and pregnancy to his last posthumous publication on maternal–fetal physiological interactions, pregnancy and maternal–fetal interactions were the focal point of Hellegers' scientific oeuvre. In 1963, this preoccupation led to his appointment as scientific advisor to the Pontifical Commission for the Study of Population, the Family, and Birth (1963–1965) – popularly known as the "Papal Birth Control Commission." The commission was to assist Pope John XXIII (1881–1963, pontiff from 1958 to 1963) in rethinking the Roman Catholic church's position on birth control. With the majority of the Commission, Hellegers recommended that the Church abandon its view that contraception was intrinsically sinful. When the Commission's report was sent to John XXIII's successor, Pope Paul VI (1897–1978, pontiff from 1963 to 1978), Pope Paul rejected its recommendation, reaffirming traditional Catholic teachings condemning all forms of birth control, except for the rhythm system. Hellegers believed that the Church "would someday repudiate [Pope Paul VI's 1968 encyclical, *Humane Vitae*] just as it had ... official pronouncements condemning religious liberty and freedom of conscience" (McClory 1995, 141).

Hellegers returned to Georgetown preoccupied with questions about the moral status of the fetus, the ethics of contraception, medically induced death, and research ethics – lifelong concerns. Seeking to explore these issues further, he applied to the Joseph P. Kennedy, Jr. Foundation for funds to bring to Georgetown, the Princeton-based Protestant theologian Paul Ramsey (1913–1988). Ramsey spent the 1968–1969 academic year at Georgetown. The experience of having an "ethicist" in residence proved so successful that Hellegers applied to the Kennedy Foundation to fund a Georgetown ethics institute. In 1971, the new institute opened its doors as "The Joseph and Rose Kennedy Center for the Study of Human Reproduction and Bioethics." Its name was eventually shortened to "The Kennedy Institute of Ethics."

The Institute began with two resident ethicists: LeRoy Walters, a Yale-educated Mennonite theologian and Warren Reich, a dissident Catholic theologian, formerly of Catholic University. Hellegers was ultimately to bring to the Institute such seminal figures in the fledgling field of bioethics as Tom Beauchamp, James Childress, John Connery, Charles Curran, H. Tristram Engelhardt, Jr., Richard McCormick (1922–2000), William May, Gene Outka, Edmund Pellegrino, Terry Pinkard, and Robert Veatch. He also raised funds for the projects that created the infrastructure of the new field of bioethics: the *Bibliography of Bioethics* (1975–), the *Encyclopedia of Bioethics* (Reich 1978, 1995a) and the National Reference Center for Bioethics Literature (1975–). Although Hellegers had envisioned the new interdisciplinary field, he never lived to see the enterprise become a household word, "bioethics."

Hellegers was recognized as an important figure in Roman Catholic moral theology in his lifetime (Anonymous no date, 1971; Kaiser 1985; McClory 1995) and was affectionately memorialized after his death (Anonymous 1979, 1983; Beller 1979; Bruns 1979; de Wachter 1979; Healey 1979; McCormick 1979a, 1979b, 1983; Queenan 1996; Schifferli 1979; Shriver 1979; Tauber 1979). His role in founding bioethics and the Kennedy Institute is less widely known but has been well documented (Anonymous 1993; Harvey 2004; Jonsen 1998; McCarthy 1979; Reich 1994, 1995, 1996, 1999; Walters 1985, 2003).

Robert B. Baker

HELMONT, JOHANNES BAPTISTA VAN (January 12, 1579, Brussels–December 30, 1644, Brussels, Belgium)

Helmont was a Flemish nobleman, mystic, chemist, and doctor of medicine. Some of van Helmont's writings were published in his life and his collected works were published posthumously as *Ortus Medicinae* (The Origin of Medicine) (1648) with the *Opuscula* appended. The *Ortus* was translated into English (1662), German (1683), and French in selections (1671). In these works, van Helmont set out a new medicine that was influenced by Paracelsus (see Paracelsus) yet also strongly independent of him. He developed through experiment and quantification the theories that each type of material had a "gas" that was its spiritual essence and that water was the basic material of the world. He saw digestion as produced by acid. Rejecting the classical notion of disease as an imbalance of the humors or as putrefaction, van Helmont conceived disease in ontological terms, as an *ens* or being, that could be produced by an external agent. By an almost mysterious process, the idea or picture of the disease created illness.

Running through van Helmont's writings was not only a strong mystical Neo-Platonic thread but also a deeply held belief in the idea of the Christian physician motivated by the values of charity and of not harming the patient. Like Paracelsus, van Helmont believed that God endowed the chemical physician with the gift of healing and with chemical insight.

Van Helmont studied at Louvain where he received his M.D. in 1599. He visited Switzerland, Italy, France, and England between 1600 and 1605. In 1609, he married Margerite van Ranst and became lord of Merode and other estates and began a program of private study and research. Van Helmont came under prolonged ecclesiastical inves-

tigation and was placed under house arrest from 1634 to 1636 for his treatise on the magical properties of the weapon salve *De Magneticae Vulnerum Curatione* (On the Magnetic Cure of Wounds). He was finally cleared in 1642. Van Helmont's son, Fraciseus Mercurius, published an edition of his father's writings in 1648 and publicized them through Europe (Pagel 1944, 1982).

Andrew Wear

HENRY OF MONDEVILLE (c. 1260, Emondeville–after 1325, probably Paris)

Professor of surgery and anatomy at Montpellier and Paris, personal physician of the King of France, and a diplomat, Henry of Mondeville's fame in the history of medicine is mainly due to his comprehensive work *Chirurgia* (Surgery), which was begun in 1304, and which remained uncompleted at his death. As early as 1314 parts of the text were translated by the author himself into French. Parts of the original Latin text were published in 1889; the entire text was published in 1892.

Henry probably came from Hermondaville in the present-day French department of La Manche. He was *Chirurgien du Roi* (Surgeon to the King) under Philip IV and Louis X and participated in their campaigns. He taught medicine, anatomy, and surgery in Montpellier and from 1306 in Paris. Of the planned five sections of the *Chirurgia*, he was only able to complete the ones about anatomy and the treatment of wounds. The work is remarkable for its anatomical illustrations. In keeping with the methodology and didactic style of the university medicine circa 1300, *Chirurgia* was constructed in a scholastic manner. Henry propagated rules on how physicians should behave to address common complaints about surgeons' conduct, and to improve the reputation of surgery as a subject in the universities. Cheats were condemned. Anyone who had not entered surgery through the "right door," that is, through a study of medicine, was dismissed as an unscrupulous, greedy, and irresponsible quack, "an intruder or thief, traitor and cheat." Unlike the barber-surgeon, a medical surgeon must have an all-encompassing understanding of medicine. There was thus only one correct type of medicine, which was taught at university. All other forms were judged to be illegitimate, because "through the mistakes of these people, especially fortune-tellers, religious people, monks and hermits . . . which the people have such great faith in, illnesses which were originally curable become incurable or worse than before." Such "healers" kill people!

Henry believed that God was a healer who was assisted in his work by physicians and surgeons. Henry denounced the greed of the scholastic "physicians" who sometimes performed useless treatments or delayed necessary surgical operations for their own financial gain. Surgeons and physicians should each recognize the limits of their training. The former were responsible for illnesses with pains that could be localized and for external injuries, the latter for internal illnesses.

Klaus Bergdolt

Hippocrates (c. 460 BCE, Kos, Greece– c. 375–351 BCE, Larissa, Thessaly, Greece)

Lauded in his own lifetime by Plato and Aristotle as the world's greatest physician, Hippocrates and his sons, Thessalus and Dracon, founded a school of medicine. Their school abandoned magico-religious models of sickness, replacing them with a model that sought to explain health and illness in terms of natural physical processes and that diagnosed illness by observing physical signs and symptoms. Associated with the Hippocratic School is a collection of more than sixty-three medical treatises known as the *Corpus Hippocratum* (Jones 1923–1931; Jouanna 1999, 373–416; Littré 1839–1861). Although the entire corpus was originally attributed to Hippocrates, the works were actually written by different authors over a period spanning several centuries. Many of the treatises appear to have been written by physicians associated with the Hippocratic School, others do not.

Scholars continue to debate which of these treatises, if any, is attributable to Hippocrates himself. It is not clear that the most famous document in the in corpus, the Hippocratic Oath, is attributable to Hippocrates. According to a manuscript attributed to the Greco-Roman physician, Galen (Claudius Galenus of Pergamum, 129–c. 199 to 216), the Oath was drafted when the Hippocratic family opened their school of medicine to nonfamily members. Unfortunately, the date of this event is as uncertain as the authorship of the document. What is clear is that the Oath formalizes the moral ideals of the Hippocratic family and commits those who swear it to practice according to these ideals – and to protect the family's trade secrets (Jounana 1999, 46–8).

Successive generations of physicians and scholars have drawn on the corpus to construct accounts of Hippocrates's life, Hippocratic medicine, and Hippocratic medical ethics. When virtues ethics was fashionable, Hippocrates became a paragon of medical virtue. In eras in which moral taste ran to the deontological (i.e., toward an ethics of duty), attention tended to focus on the Hippocratic Oath. Over the course of two and one-half millennia, era after era has remodeled Hippocrates and Hippocratic ethics to suit its taste (Cantor 2003; Coulter 1975; Edelstein 1943; Galvão-Sobrinho 1996;

Goldberg 1963; Heidel 1941; Jones 1923–1931; Levine 1971; Littré 1839–1861; Miles 2004; Phillips 1973; Rutten and Reppert-Bismarch 1996; Sargent 1982; Smith 1996; von Staden 1996). It is beyond the scope of this short "biography" to attempt to inventory either the texts out of which various eras have constructed their Hippocratic model or the various interpretations offered – and it is certainly beyond its scope to attempt to assess which is the most historically "accurate." It is possible, however, to offer an example of the reinvention process by examining two competing interpretations of the nature of the Hippocratic physician, both derive from a line in a letter attributed to Hippocrates.

The line has Hippocrates stating, "It is not proper that I should . . . save Persians from disease, since they are the enemies of the Greeks" (Jouanna 1999, 23). In 1801, when the eminent American physician Benjamin Rush presented a lecture, "On the Vices and Virtues of Physicians" to his students at the University of Pennsylvania, he drew on this line to extol the virtues of physicians as patriots, soldiers, and defenders of their country (Rush 1811, 134–137). The Roman statesmen, Cato the Elder (234–139 BCE), read this line in the same way. He concluded that because Greeks would not heal their enemies, Romans should not put themselves in the hands of Greek physicians. "Beware of them all" he warned his countrymen (Temkin 1991, 60). Defending his own integrity and that of other Greek physicians practicing in Rome, Scribonious Largus (fl. 14–54) searched the corpus and found that the Hippocratic physician has a heart full of mercy and humanity (Hamilton 1986, 213–214), hence:

> A man lawfully bound to medicine by [the Hippocratic] oath will not give a bad drug even to enemies (though as a soldier and a good citizen he will pursue them by any means when the state [se] demands). For medicine does not evaluate people by [their] fortune or character but promises to bring help to all equally and vows never to harm them. (Temkin 1991, 61)

Rush, a signer of the American Declaration of Independence and physician to George Washington's army at Valley Forge, looked into the *Corpus Hippocratum* and found Hippocrates the patriot, so did Cato the Elder. Scribonius searched the corpus and found Hippocrates the humanist whose heart was full of mercy and who never harmed anyone while playing the role of physician, not even an enemy. The corpus has proved an enduring treasure trove of plausible interpretations that allows each generation of physicians and scholars to reinvent their own Hippocrates and their own conception of Hippocratic medical ethics (Cantor 2002).

Robert B. Baker

HOCHE, ALFRED E. (August 1, 1865, Wildenheim, Germany–May 16, 1943, Wildenheim, Germany)

Hoche was a psychiatrist, neuropathologist, professor of neuropathology at the university of Freiburg im Breslau, and coauthor with Karl Binding of the two-part tract *Die Freigabe der Vernichtung lebensunwerten Lebens* (Permission for the Destruction of Life Unworthy of Life) (1920). (For more on this book, see the biography of Karl Binding; see also Chapters 18, 34, and 54.) In 1891, Hoche completed his habilitation (second doctorate) at the University of Strasbourg and was appointed assistant professor in 1899. From 1902, Hoche was professor of neuropathology at the University of Freiburg im Breslau. Later in his career Hoche became one of the most prominent advocates of the state-sanctioned killing of mentally and physically handicapped patients whom he saw as "ballast existences" and "useless eaters." His writings were strongly influenced by the death of his only son at the battle of Langemark during World War I. For Hoche, handicapped children and adults apparently placed a financial and emotional burden on relatives, the community, and the state. According to Hoche, no financial resources should be spent on "inferior elements" and "half-, quarter-, or eighth-forces." He called for the elimination of "life unworthy of life." Both Binding and Hoche brushed aside the possibility of error in implementing their radical measures. Whereas Binding argued that mankind would lose so many on account of error that "one more or less hardly counts in the balance," Hoche claimed that there was "one hundred per cent certainty in selection." Binding and Hoche's arguments were of great significance for those trying to justify the killing of the handicapped, particularly during the Nazi "euthanasia" program.

Ulf Schmidt

HOFFMANN, FRIEDRICH (February 19, 1660, Halle, Germany–November 12, 1742, Halle, Germany)

Friedrich Hoffmann was a German physician who wrote a highly influential text on medical ethics, *Medicus Politicus*, or the politic doctor. By this expression, Hoffmann meant that the physician should base the ethics of clinical practice on the moral virtue of prudential self-interest. Hoffmann insisted that in doing so the physician was not simply to look at his own interests in isolation from the interests of others but instead take the interests of others into account to achieve enlightened self-interest.

Hoffmann taught medicine at the medical school at Halle starting in 1693. He is credited with introducing ether into clinical practice under the name, "Anodyne." He is also credited with helping to originate pediatrics and he is thought to be the first to clinically describe appendicitis and German measles.

Adopting Francis Bacon's (1561–1626) scientific method and philosophy of medicine, Hoffmann's research led him to articulate a corpuscular theory, which held that the first principles or causes in nature were matter and motion. He rejected explanations based on substantial forms, that is, unchanging essences that defined the species to which an individual should be assigned. As static entities, substantial forms could not explain the motion or change that which was essential to life. Hoffmann held that human life comprises a complex of mind and body. Motion or change in the human body was to be explained by appeal to a soul or vital principle, a real, constitutive causal component of things in which their function or physiology originates. This vital principle, in turn, explains the observed, regular order of change or function in the human body, as well as purposeful movement. Hoffmann's work had considerable influence on the subsequent develop of the science of physiology.

Hoffmann's account of prudence emphasized the mutual love or natural connectedness among human beings, which emulates God's relationship to man and man's to God. The physician becomes a physician by undertaking a life of service to the sick, based on enlightened self-interest. On this basis, Hoffmann instructed physicians to be chaste and to be cautious in reaching clinical judgment. Physicians should not be evasive in communicating their clinical circumstances to those who are gravely ill "but always . . . admit that danger is near." The physician should not fear challenging the more optimistic views of other physicians or even of the patient when the circumstances warrant doing so. When the physician has reached the judgment that the patient's condition is incurable, however, a prudential regard to protect his reputation supports the obligation to withdraw in such cases. Prudence instructs the physician to avoid becoming known as a physician whose patients die as a result of his ministrations.

Laurence B. McCullough

HOOKER, WORTHINGTON (March 3, 1806, Springfield, Massachusetts–November 6, 1867, New Haven, Connecticut)

A lineal descendant of the Puritan, Reverend Thomas Hooker (1586–1641), the spiritual leader whose band of pioneers founded Hartford and the Connecticut colony, Worthington Hooker was one of America's first science educators. After receiving his baccalaureate from Yale (1825) and his medical doctorate from Harvard (1829), he practiced medicine in Connecticut (1829–1852), becoming professor of medicine at Yale (1852–1867). An ardent champion of the AMA and its Code of Ethics (AMA Vice President, 1864), Hooker believed that the AMA was the sole force in American life supporting scientific medicine against the politically powerful and popular tide of homeopathy and kindred "medical delusions."

Hooker is sometimes credited with introducing the Latin precept, *primum non nocere* (first do no harm), into English language medical ethics (Herranz 2002) but his major contribution to medical ethics lay in his articulation of a comprehensive conception of the physician–patient relationship based on professionalism, honesty, sympathy, and science. Hooker presented an overview of his position in *Physician and Patient* (Hooker 1849), the only American monograph on medical ethics published in the nineteenth century. Details of his conception of the physician–patient relationship were worked out in a series of books and lectures published over the decade and one-half from 1844 to 1857 (Hooker 1844, 1849, 1852a, 1852b, 1857).

Vexed by the popularity and political clout of medical theories that he believed unscientific – homeopathy, hydropathy, Thomsonianism, and so forth – Hooker was fearful that these "medical delusions" would gain hegemony in popular mind (Hooker 1850, 1852a). Later in his life, he devoted himself to writing science textbooks and to educating the public and their children about the nature of science and scientific evidence (Hooker, 1862, 1867, 1871, 1884). He also tried to develop a science-based "rational therapeutics" that could be deployed by practitioners to distinguish scientific from unscientific therapies (Hooker 1857).

Like Samuel Bard (1742–1821) and John Gregory (1724–1773) before him, Hooker believed that sympathy lay at the foundation of the physician–patient relationship, and, like them, he was challenged by the problem of revealing terminal prognoses to patients. In Hooker's view (as in Bard's and Gregory's), a professional physician–patient relationship should be based on honesty and mutual respect. Yet, Hooker feared that to tell patients of impending death might deprive them of hope and even of some slim chance of life. Prudence and sympathy thus seemed to demand a degree of deception incompatible with the honesty that Hooker believed essential to the physician–patient relationship. Seeking to reconcile these positions, Hooker held that although physicians should never utter falsehoods, they have

> a right... to withhold his opinion from [the patient] if he can do it without falsehood or equivocation. He might say... something like this: "You are very sick... I hope the remedies will do so and so (pointing out somewhat the effects ordinarily to be expected) but I cannot tell." Something of this kind... is perfectly consistent with the truth and good faith... and very often when more is

> said... the physician goes beyond the limits which infinite wisdom has thought best to set to his knowledge. (Hooker 1849, 384)

Hooker was a well-known figure in his own time. In the second half of the twentieth century, he was remembered as a pioneering science educator, a writer of science books for children (Musto 1984), a Yale worthy (Burns 1976; Young 1980) and, later, as a medical ethicist whose views anticipated those propounded by the bioethics movement of the 1970s (Beauchamp 1995; Burns 1995, 1999; Halpern 2001; Hooker 1972). The Worthington Hooker School in New Haven Connecticut is named in his honor.

Robert B. Baker and Chester R. Burns

Hufeland, Christoph Wilhelm (August 12, 1762, Langensalza/Thüringen, Germany– August 25, 1836, Berlin, Germany)

Hufeland was a German court physician, professor of medicine (Universities of Jena and Berlin), and Prussian State Councillor. Hufeland became Personal Physician to the Duke of Sachsen-Weimar and taught at the University of Jena. In 1801 he moved to Berlin as Physician-in-Ordinary to the Prussian King. There he became director of the Charité, the training hospital for military doctors. In 1810, he was among the founders of the University of Berlin and its first Medical Dean. Promoted to Prussian State Councillor for Health, he directed health care for the indigent, introducing Berlin's first free policlinic. Hufeland thought and acted according to scientific and social principles of the Enlightenment. Linking health, disease, mortality, and social conditions, he developed an interventionist and prototechnical understanding of medicine in his *Makrobiotik oder die Kunst, das Menschliche Leben zu Verlängern* (The Art of Prolonging Life), (1796 – still in print). He initiated medical discussion circles, one being the "Journal für praktische Heilkunde und Wundarzneykunst" (1795–1836). Hufeland's manual of medical practice *Enchiridion Medicum, oder Anleitung zur Medizinischen Praxis* (Code of Medical Practice), appeared in more than ten editions. Hufeland was in many ways one of the most influential German doctors of his time.

Ulf Schmidt

Ibn Baz, ʿAbd Al-ʾAziz B. ʿAbd Allah (1912, Riadh, Saudi Arabia–1999, al-Taʾif buried in Mecca)

He was the head of the supreme religious Council of the Land of Saudi Arabia. From the age of approximately

16, he was blind, but he continued his education until he was ordained as *qadi* at approximately age 25. Since that time he held several leading positions in religious universities in Saudi Arabia, as well as heading various bodies issuing *fatwas* within the Kingdom and outside. He is considered a relative moderate, and, in 1991, he issued an appeal to King Fahd to reform the nondemocratic regime in the kingdom and eliminate corruption. His fatwas have been gathered in the collection *Fatawa Islamiyya* (1988–1995). He also authored books on such topics as prayer, dogmatics, almsgiving, and women's dress code.

Vardit Rispler-Chaim

IVY, ANDREW CONWAY (February 25, 1893, Farmington, Missouri–February 7, 1978, Oak Park, Illinois)

American physiologist and physician, Andrew C. Ivy, earned his doctorate in physiology from the University of Chicago (1918) and his medical doctorate from Rush Medical School (1922). President of the American Physiological Society (1939–1941) and Executive Director of the National Advisory Cancer Council (1947–1951), Ivy served on the faculties of the University of Chicago (1917–1919, 1923–1925), Loyola University School of Medicine (1919–1923), Northwestern University (1923–1946), and the University of Illinois (1946–1962).

Although a pacifist, in the 1940s, Ivy became founding Scientific Director of the Naval Medical Research Institute. Following in the tradition of U.S. Army physician Walter Reed (1851–1902), Ivy's Naval research laboratories required all human subjects to be consenting volunteers and restricted life-threatening experiments to those in which members of the research team themselves served as subjects. In 1946, on the recommendation of the AMA, Ivy served as the U.S. Government's Scientific Expert at the Nuremberg War Crimes Tribunal (*United States v. Karl Brandt et al.* 1947).

In a report to the AMA about the Nazi war crimes, Ivy proposed that it adopt a formal statement of research ethics to underline the differences between American and Nazi research practices (Ivy 1946, 1949). Ivy included in this memorandum a statement of research ethics based on the practices that his laboratories had followed. The AMA adopted a truncated version of Ivy's recommended principles as its Principles of Research Ethics (AMA 1946) – the first principles of research ethics formally adopted by any American medical society.

Returning to the Nuremberg war crimes trial, Ivy represented the AMA's principles, not as the practices of the Naval Medical Research Institute, but as standard practice in the United States and throughout the civilized world. As evidence, he noted similarities between the AMA's principles and the pre-Nazi German research regulations. The Tribunal drew on his testimony to condemn the Nazi experiments as a violation of basic ethical standards accepted throughout the civilized world. In retrospect, some scholars have described Ivy's characterization of the state of research ethics, in 1946, as "mythic," others have suggested that Ivy came perilously close to committing perjury (Baker 1998; Marrus 1999). Yet, in combination with a set of principles proposed by another American expert witness, Colonel Leopold (Leo) Alexander (1905–1985), Ivy's principles were adopted by the Tribunal as the Nuremberg Code – the basis for all modern research ethics. Ironically, by insisting on the truth of mythic universal principles, Ivy made his myth become truly universal (Baker 1998; Marrus 1999; Pross 1992; Schmidt 2004; Shuster 1998; Temme 2003; Vaux and Schade 1988; Weindling 2001, 2004).

Ivy was a medical luminary in his lifetime. Between 1919 and 1955, he and his coworkers published more than 1,500 papers: an average of more than forty papers per year for more than 35 years. The Science Citation Index shows that, from 1964 to 1971, Ivy's articles were cited more often than any other scientist in the world. Unfortunately, after 1953 Ivy zealously championed an alternative cancer treatment, Kreibiozen. Introduced to Kreibiozen by its inventor, Dr. Stevan Durovic of the Instituto Biologica Duga (Buenos Aires, Argentina), Ivy established that the substance was safe by injecting it into himself and some of his colleagues. He then tested Kreibiozen on a small number of cancer patients with positive results. After establishing to his own satisfaction that his small study confirmed Dr. Durovic's impressive reports on Kreibiozen's efficacy, in 1951, Ivy called a press conference to announce a new cure for cancer. When multi-institutional studies failed to confirm Ivy's preliminary findings, Ivy and Durovic responded by alleging a conspiracy on the part of the American Cancer Society and the American pharmaceutical industry to suppress a cancer cure (Ivy 1952, 1953a, 1953b; Ivy et al. 1956). Ivy is remembered today for his seminal work in physiology, for his role in the creating the Nuremberg Code – and for the Kreibozen fiasco (Boyle 1968; Dill 1979; Dragstedt 1944; Fenn 1963; Harkness 1999; Snell 1952; Ward 1984).

Robert B. Baker

JAD AL-HAQQ, ALI JAD AL-HAQQ (1917, Batra, Egypt–1997, Cairo, Egypt)

After receiving a diploma in *Shar'i* law in 1945, he was appointed *qadi* in 1954. He was appointed *Mufti Al-Diyar*

Al-Misriyya (prime *mufti* of Egypt) in 1978, Minister of Religious Endowments in 1983, and was Sheikh Al-Azhar from 1982 until his death. His *fatwas* were published in *Al-Fatawa Al-Islamiyya* volumes 8, 9, 10. There is also a collection of his works titled *Buhuth waFatawa Islamiyya fi Qadaya Mu'asira* (Islamic researches and fatwas on contemporary issues) 1995. Cairo: Al-Azhar al-Sharif, al-Amana al-'Amma lillajna al-Ulya lilDa'wa al-Islamiyya. In this collection, medical dilemmas are discussed aside other social and scientific topics

Vardit Rispler-Chaim

JAKOBOVITS, IMMANUEL, BARON JAKOBOVITS (February 8, 1921, Königsberg, East Prussia–October 31, 1999, London, UK)

Drawing on his knowledge of the ethical discourse of Judaism, known as the *halakkah* (see Chapter 16) Rabbi Jakobovits created the field of Jewish medical ethics (Rosner 2001). Son of a rabbi who left Germany before the Nazi persecutions of Jews, Jakobovits was educated in Germany and in London. In 1949, he became the Chief Rabbi of Ireland; in 1958, he served as rabbi of the Fifth Avenue Synagogue in New York City. He subsequently became Chief Rabbi of the United Hebrew Congregations of the British Commonwealth, retiring in 1991. Jakobovits was knighted in 1981 and made a life peer in 1988. In 1991, he was awarded the prestigious Templeton Prize for Progress in Religion.

Rabbi Jakobovits once referred to himself as the "grandfather" of Jewish medical ethics (Rosner 2001, 306). He addressed medical ethics systematically in *Jewish Medical Ethics* (Jakobovits 1959, 1975). The book's subtitle, *A Comparative and Historical Study of the Jewish Religious Attitude to Medicine and its Practice*, reveals its scope. Jakobovits frames his book as the "first attempt at a comprehensive presentation of the Jewish medical legislation," guiding the activities of physicians and scientists (Rosner 2001). He addressed topics that have become staples of bioethics, including artificial insemination, birth control, abortion, eugenics, sterilization, euthanasia, and autopsies.

In other works, Jakobovits addressed the ethics of human experimentation ([1966] 1979). Research on human subjects is ethically permissible in both healthy and sick subjects, Jakobovits held; however, there is no ethical obligation for any person, sick or well, to subject themselves to research. Moreover, clinical research is permissible only if it has therapeutic intent.

Laurence B. McCullough

MAHMUD, ABD AL-HALIM (1910, Abu Ahmad, province al-Sharqiyya, Egypt–1978, Cairo, Egypt)

He served as Sheikh Al-Azhar between 1973 and 1978, the successor of Shaltut. He was a sincere Sufi (follower of mystical Islam), an Al-Azhar graduate, and he also obtained a doctoral degree from the Sorbonne, France in 1940. He taught philosophy in the Islamic Religion Department at al-Azhar, and also at universities in Tunisia, Libya, Iraq, and Sudan. He believed in the need to apply the *Shari'a* law in all areas of life in Egypt. His *fatwa* collection is titled *Fatawa 'Abd al-Halim Mahmud* (1986).

Vardit Rispler-Chaim

MAIMONIDES, MOSES (March 30, 1135, Cordoba, Spain–December 12, 1204, Fostat, Egypt)

Moshe ben Maimon, better known in the West as Maimonides and in the Islamic world as Abu Imran Mussa bin Maimun ibn Abdallah al-Qurtubi al-Israili, was a renowned Jewish rabbi, physician, and philosopher. He studied Torah under his father, who, to escape the forced conversion of Jews to Islam, relocated the family to Morocco. Maimonides subsequently lived in what is now modern Israel and settled in Egypt, where he became the Grand Vizier Alfadhil. Maimonides' many writings influenced both Jewish and non-Jewish thinkers. Scholars differ on whether Maimonides should be read as having attempted a synthesis between Jewish thought and Aristotelianism or primarily as a philosopher who took Aristotelianism to be true and Judaism to be allegorical. His major contribution to Judaism is the *Mishneh Torah*, or code of Jewish law.

The relationship between theological and philosophical ideas and discourses in Maimonides's works is complex. He held that preservation of one's life was a religious obligation. Developing and strengthening the capacity of medicine to heal thus becomes a matter of obligation and medical care could be pursued without violating one's religious obligations.

The so-called Oath of Maimonides and the Daily Prayer of a Physician have been attributed to Maimonides; however, it was probably written in the 1790s by Marcus Herz (1747–1803), a German physician-philosopher, one of Immanuel Kant's (1724–1804) students. The "Prayer" states: "Thou hast endowed man with the wisdom to relieve the sufferings of his brother, to recognize his disorders, to extract the healing substances, to discover their powers and to prepare and to apply them to suit every ill."

The "Prayer" sets out a general medical ethics, emphasizing the life of service to the sick and the physician's ethical obligation to keep self-interest in a systematically secondary place. It admonishes: "Do not allow thirst for profit, ambition for renown and admiration, to interfere with my profession, for these are the enemies of truth and of love for mankind and they can lead astray in the great task of attending to the welfare of thy creatures." The "Prayer" also warns against intellectual and clinical complacency.

Laurence B. McCullough

MAKHLUF, HASANAYN MUHAMMAD (1890, Bani ʿAdiyy, Egypt–1990, Cairo, Egypt)

Known as the *"Mufti of the Egyptian Lands,"* he graduated from Al-Azhar University in Egypt in 1914, and was appointed *mufti* of Egypt in 1945. In 1948, he was appointed member of *Hay'at Kibar Ulama' Al-Azhar* (the Council of Great *Muftis* attached to Al-Azhar). There is a collection of *fatwas* that he issued, *Fatawa Shar'iyya waBuhuth Islamiyya* (1965), and he wrote books on Islamic law and the Qurʾan.

Vardit Rispler-Chaim

MARX, KARL FRIEDRICH HEINRICH (1796, Karlsruhe, Germany–1877, Göttingen, Germany)

Marx was a German physician, medical historian, and Professor of Medicine, University of Göttingen. Marx read medicine and philosophy in Heidelberg, Vienna, and Jena and was appointed to a position at the university library of Göttingen, where he became a reader in 1822, and a full professor of medicine in 1831. Marx taught and published on all theoretical and clinical fields of medicine but became best known by his writings on the ethics of physicians. These included his inaugural lecture *"De euthanasia medica"* (Medical Euthanasia) (1826), *"Über die Abnahme der Krankheiten durch die Zunahme der Civilisation"* (On the decrease of diseases because of the increase of civilization)" (1844) and *"Ueber das Verdienst der Aerzte um das Verschwinden der dämonischen Krankheiten"* (On the merit of doctors with the disappearance of daemonic diseases)" (1859). Marx challenged the view that medicine was strictly based on natural science and called for high moral standards in the practice of the healing art. He held that ethical behavior at the bedside would have beneficial effects. His works were controversial. Although some saw in Marx the founder of "ethical" medicine, others viewed him as an outsider, whose ideas faded away without major resonance.

Andreas-Holger Maehle

MATHER, COTTON (February 12, 1663, Boston, Massachusetts–February 13, 1728, Boston Massachusetts)

Mather was a Puritan cleric who delineated specific duties for physicians in his widely read book, *Bonifacius, or Essays to Do Good* (1710). He designated combined roles of cleric and physician as an "angelic conjunction," thereby encouraging colonials to adopt these dual roles. In opposition to local doctors, he advocated smallpox variolation in 1721 as a way to reduce mortality during epidemics in Boston. Cotton Mather's paternal grandfather had studied at Oxford and his maternal grandfather had graduated from Cambridge. Both ministers migrated to Massachusetts and six of their sons became Puritan divines. Fifteen-year-old Cotton earned his B.A. from Harvard College in 1678, his M.A. in 1681 – with the latter diploma presented by his grandfather, Increase Mather, who had recently become president of Harvard. Ordained in May 1685, Cotton Mather devoted more than 40 years to the Puritan cause, preaching a final sermon in December 1727, about 6 weeks before his death. Mather was an ardent scholar and scientific observer. Between 1711 and 1723, he sent eighty-two scientific manuscripts to the Royal Society in London. Mather was a prolific author with 388 published works, hundreds of unpublished pages, and several thousand letters. Two books are pertinent to the history of medical ethics: *Bonifacius* published in 1710 and *The Angel of Bethesda* completed in 1724, but not published until 1972. The Puritans of New England wanted each individual and community group firmly connected by a theistic system of beliefs, arguments, rules, and policies. To demonstrate these connections and provide guidelines for daily living, Mather wrote *Bonifacius, or Essays to Do Good*. Published in 1710, this widely read book was issued in more than fifteen editions. *Bonifacius* provided specific imperatives for ministers, schoolteachers, magistrates, lawyers, physicians, and others. Cotton Mather devoted many hours to the preparation of a self-help medical guide for Puritans that he titled *The Angel of Bethesda*. It is divided into sixty-six chapters that deal with such topics as cures by charms, medicinal waters, tobacco, hiccoughs, scabies, hemorrhoids, jaundice, asthma, nosebleeds, apoplexy, bladder stones, gout, headaches, madness, nightmares, exercise and other nonnaturals, and "Nishmath-Chajim." Almost every chapter included recommendations about remedies and ways to stay healthy.

Chester R. Burns

MOLL, ALBERT (1862, Lissa, Posen, Prussia–1939, Berlin, Germany)

Albert Moll was a German neurologist and psychotherapist, who had a private practice in Berlin

(1887–1933). His 650-page handbook of medical ethics, *Ärztliche Ethik* (Doctors' Ethics) (1902), discussed in unprecedented detail both the professional duties of the physician and ethical problems in contemporary medicine. Built on the concept of a tacit contract between doctor and patient, his ethics responded to the challenges of medical professionalization and scientific research in medicine.

Moll studied medicine in Breslau, Freiburg (Breisgau), Jena, and Berlin. Having completed a M.D. thesis under the Berlin orthopedic surgeon Julius Wolff in 1885, he embarked on a grand tour through the clinics of Vienna, Budapest, London, Paris, and Nancy. He experimented with therapy by hypnosis in his Berlin practice from 1887, and began to specialize in psychotherapy and sexology, becoming an adversary of Sigmund Freud's psychoanalysis. Moll's publications include *Der Hypnotismus* (Hypnotism, 1889, 5th ed. 1924, English 1890), *Die konträre Sexualempfindung* ([Homosexuality] 1891, 4th ed. 1914, French 1893, English 1931), *Das Sexualleben des Kindes* (The Sexual Life of the Child, 1908, English 1912), and *Handbuch der Sexualwissenschaften* ([Handbook of Sexology], 1912, 3rd ed. 1926). Moll was an active member of the Berlin Chamber of Physicians, serving as chairman of its panel for contracts with health insurers in the district of Great Berlin and as a member of its committee against quackery. Although Moll converted from the Jewish to the Christian (Protestant) faith in 1896 and had been a member of the nationalist Deutsche Vaterlandspartei since 1917, the Nazi regime treated Moll as a Jew and withdrew his license to practice medicine in 1933, as it did with Jewish doctors generally. Still Moll managed to publish his autobiography, *Ein Leben als Arzt der Seele* (A Life as a Doctor of the Mind), in 1936.

Moll's *Ärztliche Ethik. Die Pflichten des Arztes in allen Beziehungen seiner Thätigkeit* (Doctors' Ethics. The Duties of the Doctor with regard to all his Activities) was influential on both German and Russian medical ethics. Moll applied the concept of a tacit contract between doctor and patient to the manifold issues of professional ethics and medical morality in late nineteenth-century Germany. His ethics displayed both features of medical paternalism and respect for the self-determination of the patient.

Moll rejected such systems of moral philosophy as utilitarianism and evolutionary ethics as a basis for medical ethics because, in his view, they challenged the foundational nature of the physician–patient relationship. In the context of contemporary public debates on abuses of human subjects in German hospitals, Moll's text dedicates a great deal of space to discussions of ethical requirements in clinical research. He also discusses in great detail the relationship between doctor and client (patient), including issues such as medical confidentiality and euthanasia; the different roles various categories of physicians (e.g., the panel doctor, the specialist, the hospital doctor) play with respect to their clients (e.g., mental patients);

morally problematic medical activities, such as deceiving patients, risky treatments, and abortion; the economic aspects of medical practice; professional ethics and private life of the physician; the doctor's role in public health; medical certificates; animal experimentation; pathological autopsy; and medical education.

Andreas-Holger Maehle

NICHOLAS OF POLAND (Second Half of the Thirteenth Century, Kraków)

Dominican priest, medical teacher, Nicholas had an important role in the history of "alternative medicine." Focusing on the God-given forces of nature, Nicholas opposed scholastic, or Galenistic, medicine and propagated a treatment based on the "vilia," the simplest of substances, and on trust in God. Although we know that Nicholas was a member of the Dominican order of Kraków, there are many gaps in his biography. He is thought to have studied and worked for 20 years in Montpellier, possibly in the "studium generale" founded there by the Dominicans in 1248. His main work, the *Antihippocras* (Antipocras) appeared around 1270. It was published by Karl Sudhoff in 1916 (see K. Sudhoff, Antipocras). The *Antihippocras* is a pamphlet directed at a readership of religious and educated lay people that is viciously critical of school medicine. Nicholas also castigates the conduct of overly intellectual physicians trained at the universities who were too removed from the people. He criticizes Hippocrates and Galen, while praising Hermes Trismegistos and (his own contemporary) Albertus Magnus. Nicholas argued that the most effective treatments consisted of powders or preserved pieces of snakes, frogs, and insects. Amulets were considered very important, as well as astrology and "occult" sciences. Nicholas demanded that the doctors return to humility and the acceptance of the God-given "via caelestis" (the way of heaven) that is present in the simplest plants.

Klaus Bergdolt

PAGEL, JULIUS LEOPOLD (May 29, 1851, Pollnow/Pommern–January 31, 1912, Berlin, Germany)

Julius Pagel was a German medical historian and practicing physician. In 1898, he was appointed titular professor, and in 1901 Associate Professor of the History of Medicine at the University of Berlin. Pagel's primary scholarly contributions lie predominantly in the field of History of Medicine; however, his booklet, *Medicinische Deontologie* (Medical Deontology 1897), deserves attention as a contribution to the *"savoir faire* literature – a precursor to modern medical ethics. Written in response to problems of competition among medical practitioners in the period following the introduction of compulsory health insurance for workers in the German Reich in 1883, the book is noteworthy for its conservative views on the appropriate conduct of doctors.

Pagel studied medicine in Berlin from 1871. After completing a thesis on the Göttingen medical school of the eighteenth century, supervised by the Berlin medical historian and pathologist August Hirsch (1817–1894), Pagel was promoted M.D. in 1875. Having collaborated with Hirsch on the latter's bio-bibliography of prominent doctors, *Biographisches Lexikon hervorragender Aerzte aller Zeiten und Völker* (Biographical Dictionary of Eminent Doctors of all Times and Nations) (6 vols., 1884–1888), he was granted a teaching license (Habilitation) for History of Medicine in 1891. Pagel argued for the usefulness of medico-historical knowledge for doctors. Specializing in medieval medicine he became one of the most prominent representatives of the emerging academic discipline of History of Medicine. His publications include *Die Chirurgie des Heinrich von Mondeville* (The Surgery of Henri de Mondeville) (1892), *Einführung in die Geschichte der Medizin* (Introduction to the History of Medicine) (1898), *Einführung in das Studium der Medizin* (Introduction to the Study of Medicine) (1899), *Biographisches Lexikon hervorragender Aerzte des 19. Jahrhunderts* (Biographical Dictionary of Eminent Doctors of the 19th Century) (1901), and, with Max Neuburger, *Handbuch der Geschichte der Medizin* (Handbook of the History of Medicine) (3 vols., 1902–1905). As a Jew, he was prevented from obtaining a full professorship and earned his living as a panel doctor and poor law physician.

Pagel's *Medicinische Deontologie. Ein kleiner Katechismus für angehende Praktiker* (Medical Deontology: A Brief Catechism for Future Practitioners) was in the tradition of medical *savoir faire* literature. This text advised the young practitioner on proper and prudent behavior toward colleagues and patients. Originally published as a series of thirteen articles in the *Allgemeine Medicinische Central-Zeitung* (General Medical Central Newspaper) in 1896, Pagel's *Deontologie* addressed questions of medical etiquette and professional ethics that had been raised by fierce competition among practitioners. It dealt in detail with the duties of "collegiality," especially during consultations. Pagel appealed to the "threefold honor" of the doctor: as a man, an academic, and a member of the medical profession. His advice covered the setting up and running of a medical practice; relations with pharmacists, midwives, and other health care providers; the different duties of doctors practicing in town and in the countryside; and the specific demands on doctors practicing under health insurance contracts, communal poor relief schemes, or as officers of health. Pagel's discussion of the doctor's relationship to patients was guided by overt medical paternalism, demanding that

the doctor must be, or at least appear to be "sovereign" in the interest of the welfare of the sick. Consent seeking was only deemed necessary for major surgical interventions. *Deontologie* also included a historical chapter on the of medical deontological literature, which devoted much space to Friedrich Hoffmann's *Medicus Politicus* (The Political Doctor) (1738, German 1752), which Pagel valorized as a paradigmatic work of this genre.

Andreas-Holger Maehle

PAPPWORTH, MAURICE HENRY, M.B., CH.B. (nee Maurice Papperovitch, January 9, 1910, Liverpool, United Kingdom – Vale Lodge, Vale of Health, Hampstead, London, October 12, 1994)

Pappworth was an internationally recognized advocate of patients' rights in medical research. He is best known for his *Human Guinea Pigs. Experimentation on Man* (1967). In the book, Pappworth described more than 200 ethically questionable medical experiments, conducted on human subjects in British hospitals, institutions, and prisons. Although the British medical establishment's initial response of was overwhelmingly hostile, Pappworth's book was highly influential and assisted the establishment of ethics committees to supervise clinical research in Britain.

Pappworth was a medical outsider. He was denied a consultancy because "no Jew could ever be a gentleman" (Booth 1994) and made a living tutoring others for positions denied to him. Pappworth's other main contribution to British medicine was as a clinical teacher, who successfully coached hundreds of young doctors in their attempts to achieve Membership of the Royal College of Physicians. His interest in the ethics of research arose in part from the ethical doubts some of his tutees had about the experimental work they had to take part in for career reasons. In addition to *Human Guinea Pigs*, Pappworth was the author of primers on passing medical examinations.

Kenneth Boyd

PARACELSUS, THEOPHRASTUS PHILIPPUS AUREOLUS BOMBASTUS VON HOHENHEIM (November 11 or December 17, 1493, Einsiedeln, Switzerland–September 24, 1541, Salzburg, Austria)

A Swiss-German chemist, physician, and vitalist-mystic, Paracelsus was the creator of a new medical system based on chemical principles, which was opposed to the university-based Galenic medicine. He placed a strong emphasis on Christian ethical values in contrast to the "heathenish" medicine of Galen.

Paracelsus came from a humble background. His early "educational" experiences included mining, religion, and magic as well as of botany and medicine. This practical and occult mix was joined with a free-thinking approach to religion and a radical social stance (Paracelsus supported the German's peasant revolt) that characterized much of his work.

Paracelsus attacked Greek and Arabic medicine and the humoral theory taught in the universities. He believed that the body worked according to spiritual quasimagical chemical principles. Disease could be caused by an outside agent disturbing the workings of the body's *archeus* or internal chemist. His ontological view of disease as a specific entity looks very modern; however, it was integrated into a vitalistic, animate view underpinned by Paracelsus's belief that there were correspondences and links between the macrocosm (the universe) and the microcosm (the body). Stars could send emanations of disease or a plant could cure a part of the body that looked similar to it (the doctrine of signatures), so that a walnut could cure the brain. Despite foul-mouthed sections in his writings, Paracelsus brought a strong Christian ethic to his medicine. He believed that God granted the physician the gift of healing and thus that physicians did not become physician by studying in the universities. The godly physician displayed the Christian virtue of charity to the poor in his practice, while producing an ethically safe and effective series of chemical medicines that, because they were the products of a laboratory inspired by God, bore God's imprimatur. This ethical–religious approach is diffused through Paracelsus's works.

Paracelsus's only official post was town physician of Basel from 1527 to 1528. He then led a wandering existence traveling through Germany, Switzerland, and Austria. Few of Paracelsus' writings were published in his lifetime; most were published in the second half of the sixteenth century. (For a modern collected edition of Paracelsus's works see Sudhoff, 1922–1933; Pagel, 1958; Webster, 1982; Grell, Ole Peter 1998.)

Andrew Wear

Percival, Thomas (September 29, 1740, Warrington, Lancashire–August 30, 1804, Manchester, England)

Inventor of the expressions "medical ethics" and "professional ethics'" and author of the first modern code of professional medical ethics, Thomas Percival elected to become a Unitarian at the age of 17. The decision was principled and momentous because British law denied civil rights to Unitarians and other dissenters. In 1757, Percival became the first student at Warrington (1757–1786), a dissenting academy, where he studied under the classicist, John Aiken (1713–1780), the theologian, John Taylor (1694–1761), and the chemist Joseph Priestly (1733–1804), discoverer of oxygen and cofounder of the American Unitarian Church. As a Unitarian, Percival was denied access to Cambridge and Oxford, so he continued his education at Edinburgh (1761–1764) and Leiden (1765), where he earned his doctorate in medicine.

In 1765, Percival, then a newly graduated 25-year-old physician, became a member of the Royal Society of London (1765). Within 2 years, he married the daughter of a wealthy merchant and moved to Manchester. From this point onwards, Percival's life centered on five interlinked themes: family and community; education; religion; public health; and moral-political reform (Percival 1807). His writings mirror his life. Puzzled about inoculating his children against small pox, Percival wrote on the subject (Percival 1768) and proposed a reform of small pox data collection (Percival 1773). As his children matured, he wrote *A Father's Instructions to his Children* (Percival 1775, 1777, 1803) – a "best selling" children's book. From the mid-1770s onward, Percival regularly published collections of his literary-philosophical (Percival 1781, 1784, 1789) and medical-scientific essays (Percival 1769, 1772, 1773, 1788–1789).

In the 1780s, Percival became a leading figure at the Manchester Infirmary (1752–present), and founded the Manchester Literary and Philosophical Society (1781–present). Life became precarious for Percival and other dissenters during the 1790s, when, in the run up to war with revolutionary France, the British began to treat dissenters as traitors. On July 11, 1791, a mob burned the Unitarian meeting house and the private home and the laboratory of Percival's friend and mentor, Joseph Priestly – who fled to America.

Percival's magnum opus, *Medical Ethics*, was begun in 1793, in response to a dispute roiling the Manchester Infirmary. In 1794, Percival circulated a draft of the work (Percival 1794) dedicated to a son bound for medical school. When that son died, Percival lost interest in the project. Eight years later, when another dispute roiled the Manchester Infirmary and when another son was headed to medical school, Percival returned to the project – perhaps as an assertion of Enlightenment idealism in the face of the continued political repression (Pickstone 1993).

Percival introduced *Medical Ethics* as a system of "professional ethics," a neologism that he coined to encapsulate his novel conception of medicine as a self-regulating occupation dedicated to the service of the sick, whose "prerogatives are public trusts" (Percival 1803b, 52, Chap. II, Art. XXXII). In eighty-nine numbered articles, Percival offers a formal code of professional conduct for physicians and surgeons. The code obligates medical professionals to be mindful of their duty to "minister to the sick" with "skill, attention and fidelity" because "the ease, the health, and the lives" of their patients is "committed to their charge." It also enjoins confidentiality, tenderness, steadiness, humaneness, consensual treatment, peer review of research proposals, and treating the sick poor in hospitals comparably to paying private patients. Finally, because it was created to resolve disputes, it formulates elaborate rules for preventing and adjudicating intraprofessional conflict.

The British medical establishment never accepted Percival's concept of formal professional ethics – although his work was occasionally reprinted in Britain (Anonymous 1827, Percival 1849, Brown 1850). Americans were more receptive. In 1847, the newly formed AMA adopted a code of ethics based on an Americanized edition of Percival's *Medical Ethics* (Baker 1999) and Americans have kept *Medical Ethics* continuously in print (Percival 1927, 1975, 1985) and have a rich history of debating and reinterpreting the text and its significance (Baker 1993a, 1999; Baker et al. 1999, xiv–xx; Beecher 1970, 218; Belkin 1998; Berlant 1975; Burns 1977; Haakonssen 1997; Katz 1969, 486–7; 1972, 321; 1984; 2002, 17; Pellegrino 1985a, 1985b, 1986; Pickstone 1993; Pickstone and Butler 1984; Veatch 2005, 56–72; Waddington 1975, 1984).

Robert B. Baker

PLOETZ, ALFRED (1860, Swinemünde, Breslau–1940, Herrsching am Ammersee)

Founder and leading proponent of the German racial hygiene movement. In 1895, Ploetz coined the term, "racial hygiene," for the science of the improvement of hereditary characteristics of human races. Ploetz's writings were of significant importance in legitimizing Nazi racial hygiene. He briefly studied economics at the Universities of Breslau and Zurich, where he became familiar with socialist and social-democratic conceptions of society, ideas that later influenced his racial utopian writings. In Zurich he became acquainted with the psychiatrists Auguste Forel (1848–1931) and Ernst Rüdin (1874–1952) as well as with the gynecologist Agnes Bluhm (1862–1943). He was also a friend of the Hauptmann brothers, and of Frank Wedekind (1864–1918). Bismarck's anti-socialist legislation (1878–1890) prompted Ploetz to spend time abroad, especially in the United States, Switzerland, and France. In 1885, he visited a number of utopian "colonies" in the United States, for example, the "Ikarier"-community in Corning, Iowa, whose members attempted to turn their socialist and utopian vision into reality. In 1888, Ploetz was naturalized as a Swiss citizen in

Witikon. In May 1890, he married Rüdin's sister Pauline in St. Gallen. They first moved to Paris where Ploetz wanted to pursue his medical studies. Later they moved to Springfield, Illinois, to establish a medical practice. He divorced her in 1898. Ploetz was an ardent advocate of nonsmoking and antialcoholism. In 1895, he published his book, *Die Tüchtigkeit unsrer Rasse und der Schutz der Schwachen* (The Competence of Our Race and the Protection of the Weak). The subtitle of the book was *Ein Versuch über Rassenhygiene und ihr Verhältnis zu den humanen Idealen, besonders zum Socialismus* (An Attempt about Race Hygiene and Its Relationship to the Ideals of Man, Especially to Socialism). Ploetz's (see Ploetz 1895a, 1895b) racial utopia stressed artificial "selection" by strengthening the best in society, but also called for Spartan methods of infanticide to improve the human race: "If it transpires however that the new-born is a weakling or a degenerate, then a group of doctors . . . will produce a mild death, let's say by a small dose of morphine. The parents, educated in strict honour of the well-being of the race, don't leave themselves to rebellious feelings, but try it a second time, fresh and cheerfully, if their certificate on the ability to procreate grants them permission." Ploetz's main concept was to move the artificial selection from those already born to those not yet born. His aim was to combine a social policy with artificial selection, and diffuse the Darwinian "struggle for existence" by prenatal selection. It was an attempt to provide a basis for reconciling socialism with Darwinism. In his original conception, Ploetz did not intend that racial hygiene would necessarily be anti-Semitic. He saw the Jews, together with the Aryans, as one of the most "cultured races" and anti-Semitism as a "useless ploy" that would disappear with the advances of the natural sciences. Yet, the increasing popularity and influence of the racial hygiene movement brought Ploetz closer to right-wing ideologies. In 1918, Ploetz founded the *Widarbund*, a conglomeration of ultraconservative, elitist, and sometimes anti-Semitic racial hygienists. Ploetz wanted to promote his racial utopia in countries such as the United States, which he saw as a "bold leader in the realm of eugenics." After the Nazi assumption of power, Ploetz and Rüdin remarked that "through his deeds Hitler would advance to the ranks of one of our greatest leaders of all times," thus providing the Nazi leadership with scientific and professional legitimacy.

Ulf Schmidt

RAMSEY, PAUL (Mendenhall, Mississippi, December 10, 1913–February 29, 1988, Princeton, New Jersey)

Ramsey Paul, a graduate of Milsaps College in Mississippi and Yale Divinity School and Professor of Christian Religion at Princeton University, in 1969, Paul Ramsey was invited to lecture at Yale Divinity School on the emerging problems in medical ethics. A book, based on those lectures, *The Patient as Person. Explorations in Medical Ethics* (Ramsey 1970) situated medical ethics in a theological doctrine of the sanctity of life and the covenant of fidelity, and used philosophically acute analyses to formulate articulate moral positions on major bioethical questions.

This was the first major book in the new field of bioethics. Ramsey begins by positing a moral foundation for his review of particular ethical issues involved in the patient–physician relationship: that relationship is a sacred covenant of trust in which physicians promise loyalty to those who entrust their lives to them. Pushing beyond the physician–patient relationship Ramsey also analyses human experimentation, the determination of death, and organ transplantation. In exploring these issues, Ramsey repudiates utilitarian reasoning about medical-moral issues because such reasoning often violates the canon of loyalty on which medicine and medical research must rest. He continued to study these and other issues, particularly those concerned with care of the dying patient and with genetics. Other books are *Fabricated Man: the Ethics of Genetic Control* (Ramsey 1970), and *Ethics at the Edges of Life* (Ramsey 1978).

Albert R. Jonsen

RIDA, MUHAMMAD RASHID (1865, Qalmun (near Trippoli), Syria–1935, Cairo, Egypt)

Born in Syria, then moving to Egypt, he was a student of Muhammad Abduh (d. 1905), he was the founder of the *Salafiyya* movement and fundamentalist Islam, and Sheikh Al-Azhar (the highest Islamic institution of Islamic scholarship) until his death. He is the author of many religious books, a commentary to the Qurʾan, a *fatwa* collection, and *Al-Manar*, the journal published by the fundamentalist movement in Egypt in thirty-four volumes. His fatwa collection is titled *Fatawa al-Imam Muhammad Rashid Rida*, 6 vols., 1970.

Vardit Rispler-Chaim

RUSH, BENJAMIN (December 24, 1745, Byberry, Pennsylvania–April 19, 1813, Philadelphia, Pennsylvania)

As a student at the College of New Jersey (now Princeton) from which he graduated in 1760, Rush became familiar with the new moral philosophy espoused by several English and Scottish professors. After apprenticing himself to a prominent Philadelphia doctor for 5 years, Rush studied medicine at the University of Edinburgh, receiving a medical degree in 1768. He returned to Philadelphia in 1769 and became one of America's most distinguished practitioners and medical educators. He signed the Declaration of Independence, helped to organize the Pennsylvania Society for Promoting the Abolition of Slavery, was a founding trustee of Dickinson College, advocated prison reform, condemned capital punishment, helped to organize the College of Physicians of Philadelphia, and wrote the first American book about the medical care of the mentally ill.

After practicing and teaching for two decades, 44-year-old Benjamin Rush gave his first lecture on the duties of physicians in February 1789. He subsequent years, he gave other lectures on medical ethics. A brief review of six lectures is helpful in understanding the ways in which their topics were connected in Rush's mind. Several duties were announced in 1789 (Rush 1818, 254–264). Doctors should honor Christian ideals, be patient and cheerful with sick persons, show special regard for the poor, and discover ways to improve medical knowledge (see also Rush 1811, 141–65). Rush reformulated these duties as virtues and vices in an 1801 lecture (Rush 1811, 120–40). Fulfilling one's duties resulted in behaviors that exemplify the virtues of piety, humanity, and patriotism. The "pleasures and pains" of a physician's life were causally connected to the virtues and vices, connections explored in a lecture given in 1803 (Rush 1811, 210–31). A truly virtuous doctor would be happy: a vicious one miserable.

In a lecture given in 1807, Rush identified a causal connection among virtues, duties, happiness, and business success (Rush 1811, 232–55). A virtuous doctor used honorable means to attract patients and establish a reputation: respect for public worship, decent clothes and polite manners, sympathy and respect for patients, and special attention to the sick poor. In these lectures, Rush usually exemplified logical opposites. Failures to discharge one's duties confirmed vices, created pains, resulted in loss of business, and retarded medical progress. Vices include a fondness for public amusements and clubs and theaters, careless examinations of patients and harsh answers to their questions, an unwillingness to attend patients at night, desertion of patients during an epidemic, and extravagant fees. Rush extended his analysis of patriotism in a lecture given in 1810 (Rush 1811, 363–95). He urged doctors to honor their special civic duties, such as testifying in courts about matters of forensic medicine and providing assistance to public authorities in developing sanitary policies for local communities. A patriotic doctor shared medical expertise needed by courts and governing officials.

Chester R. Burns

RYAN, MICHAEL (Burrisoleigh, Tipperary, Ireland 1794 or 1800–London, December 11, 1840)

The first person to ever denominate himself a "Professor of Medical Ethics," Michael Ryan, man-midwife, surgeon, lecturer on medical jurisprudence, and editor of the *London Medical and Surgical Journal* (1829–1837), received his medical training in Dublin and Edinburgh. He was awarded a medical doctorate from Edinburgh in 1821, after which he began to practice in Kilkenny and later in Tipperary. He moved to London around 1827 where he began offering lectures on midwifery, medical jurisprudence and medical ethics in 1828 (Brody et al. 2008). In these lectures, Ryan appears to have been the sole nineteenth-century British proponent of the concept of medical ethics introduced by Thomas Percival (1740–1804) and the only nineteenth-century British medical educator to have expressly lectured to his students about the substantive content of the writings of Percival and John Gregory (1724–1773) (Burns 1977b).

The lectures first appeared as part of a series on medical ethics and medical jurisprudence published in Ryan's *London Medical Surgical Journal* (1829–1831), and later in the two editions of Ryan's *Manual of Medical Jurisprudence* (Ryan 1831b, 1832). They are something of a hodge-podge consisting of more or less historically ordered précis of the writings of others, stitched together by segues, comments and observations. Ryan is not always clear about where his renditions of the views of others end, and his own commentaries begin. Nonetheless, these lectures contrast strikingly with those of his contemporaries, if for no other reason than they focus on subjects that virtually all of his British contemporaries neglected – medical ethics and medical jurisprudence.

Ryan's most original contribution was in the field of research ethics. He argued that a duty stipulated in the medical oath of Edinburgh University (which was signed by all matriculates since at least 1762), the duty of caution, means that physicians must take "care not to expose the sick to any unnecessary danger." Ryan interpreted this to mean that a physician must not "administer a dangerous medicine to gratify . . . zeal for science [or] to ascertain the comparative advantage or disadvantage of some new remedy." Ryan further condemns all dangerous experiments on human subjects as "a breach of ethics . . . and a great breach of trust towards his patient . . . [that] the profession . . . has always reprobated" (Ryan 1831b, 37). Ryan concludes that, "in this age . . . all experiments are made upon inferior animals" (Ryan 1831b, 37).

Ryan's view that experimentation on human subjects must be constrained by medical ethics, and must be preceded by experiments on animals, was so out of keeping with the spirit of unregulated experimentation common in the nineteenth century that a reviewer in the *Lancet* publicly lampooned it. "Will it be believed that Dr. Ryan can be so ignorant, as to be unaware that to the experiments he repudiates we are indebted for the discovery of . . . the therapeutic effects of all our remedial agents? . . . As to the performance of *therapeutic* experiments on *inferior* animals – such a thing is scarcely heard of" (Anonymous 1831c, 141).

Ryan replied "that dangerous experiments should not be made on the sick without their consent." "Perhaps in his zeal for science" the reviewer "would allow a few experiments to be made on himself. . . . Or would he prefer the application of these things on the poor?" (Ryan 1831a, 224). Neither Gregory, nor Percival, nor anyone else cited by Ryan as major figures in the history of medical ethics, had stated that the informed consent of the research subject was an essential prerequisite for ethical experimentation on humans. Ryan would thus appear to have been the first medical ethicist to champion this ideal.

It is unclear how Ryan's theories of medical ethics and research ethics would have evolved had he the opportunity to develop them further. Sadly, like many medical reformers of the period, he became entangled in a series of flytes and lawsuits and he was ultimately forced into bankruptcy because of them. When he died in 1840 at the comparatively young age of 40 or 46 a collection was taken up to support his widow.

Robert B. Baker

SHALTUT, MAHMUD (1893, Minyat Bani Mansur, Egypt–1963, Cairo, Egypt)

Born to a peasant family in Egypt, Shaltut was educated at Al-Azhar. After graduating in 1918, he worked as a lawyer at the Shari'a courts and in journalism, and held several positions at Al-Azhar until he was declared Sheikh Al-Azhar, in 1958, at the age of 65. During his rectorship he received visitors from all over the world. He saw the importance of independent thought and is considered a reformist among the religious scholars. His *Al-Fatawa* collection (an edited volume of *fatwas* published in daily newspapers and over the radio) is widely read and often quoted (*Al-Fatawa* 1974).

Vardit Rispler-Chaim

SHA'RAWI, MUHAMMAD MUTAWALLI AL- (1911, Daqadus, Egypt–1998, Daqadus, Eygpt)

He was educated at Al-Azhar, appointed Minister of Religious Affairs in Al-Sadat's cabinet 1976–1978, and several *fatwa* collections (relatively short *fatwas*) have been compiled from his numerous *fatwas*. He wrote a commentary on the Qur'an and many other books. His fatwa collection is *Al-Fatawa, kull ma yahimm al-Muslim fi Hayatihi wayawmihi waghaddihi* (1981–1982).

Vardit Rispler-Chaim

al-Qasim, Saudi Arabia and served as a member of the Supreme Council of Ulama in Saudi Arabia. He wrote books on Islamic law and theology and commentaries to the Qur'an.

Vardit Rispler-Chaim

SIMON, MAXMILIEN ISIDORE AMAND (1807, fl. 1845–1865)

Little is known about the life of Simon. In addition to his work on medical ethics, he published books on epidemics and on the hygiene of the body and soul. He also introduced the concept of deontology into modern French medical ethics, borrowing the concept from the work of the English philosopher, Jeremy Bentham (1748–1832), for whom it meant a "science of obligation," – a broader understanding of "deontology" than that current in Anglo-American philosophical ethics. The term "medical deontology'" continues to be used in this broad sense in French and continental European medical ethics.

Simon's *Déontologie Médicale* (Medical Deontology) appeared in 1835 (Spanish translation 1852). Citing Bacon's scientific method (*"méthode baconniene"* (Simon 1845, 98) and its rigorous application to the improvement of medicine, Simon advocated clinical research. To protect human subjects, however, he wanted such research to be conducted only in large hospitals under the direction of experienced academic physicians. Simon's clinical ethics emphasized the responsible management of clinical uncertainty, an enduring ethical consideration; he called upon physicians to develop therapeutic prudence (*"la prudence thérapeutique;"* Simon 1845, 102). Simon invoked Jesus Christ as a moral exemplar for physicians to model themselves upon in their professional practice. He called for physicians to be self-sacrificing and never to refuse their beneficent art (*"art bienfaisant;"* Simon 1845, 209) to the sick. The life of a physician is one of complete study and self-sacrifice (*"La vie du médicin . . . est une vie toute d'étude et de dévoument;"* Simon 1835, 212). This includes the duty to care for the sick during epidemics, a commitment that influenced the 1847 Code of Ethics of the AMA (Bell [1847] 1999, 317).

Laurence B. McCullough

UTHAYMIN, MUHAMMAD B. SALIH AL- (1926, Unayzah, Saudi Arabia–2001, Jedda, Saudi Arabia)

One of the great *muftis* of Saudi Arabia, a disciple of Sheikh Ibn Baz. He was the director of the school of Islamic law at the Imam Muhammad b. Saud Islamic University in

ZARQA', MUSTAFA AL- (1904, Aleppo, Syria–1998, Riyad, Saudi Arabia)

He studied at the Shar'i school, which his father had founded. He studied at the Faculty of law at Damascus University and graduated in 1933. Later, he was appointed professor there of Civil Law and Islamic Law. He wrote many books, among them his well-known collection of *fatwas, Fatawa al-Shaykh Mustafa al-Zarqa'.*

Vardit Rispler-Chaim

ZERBI, GABRIELE (also Zerbis) (1445, Verona, Italy–1505, Dalmatia, Croatia)

Professor of Medicine in Padua, Zerbi was very successful as a medical author. Among his books are: *Gerontocomica, scilicet de senum cura, atque victu* (On the care of the aged) (Rome 1489); *Anatomiae corporis humani et singulorum illius membrorum liber* (Anatomy of the human body) (Venice 1502, 1533); and, *De cautelis medicorum liber* (Advice to medical men) (Venice 1495, 1503, Pavia 1508, 1517, Lyon 1524, 1582, Pavia 1528). Zerbi studied medicine in Pavia and practiced in Verona. He was a Professor of Medicine in Padua for many years, where he also taught the "artes liberales" (liberal arts). He later became the personal physician of prominent contemporaries in Bologna, Venice, Rome, and at the Court of the Bosnian Sultan. In *Gerontocomica* (1489), he described an individual life force, which came from nature and which, with the correct dietary conditions, could optimize the quality of life. In *De Cautelis Medicorum*, he developed rules of conduct for physicians, which also included philosophical and religious aspects. *De cautelis medicorum* is one of the first comprehensive books on medical deontology of the Renaissance. The physician must commit himself to practice and to expanding his knowledge, his behavior thus consisting of a "duplex actus" (*Medicus non potest esse perfectus nisi exercitatus;* the physician cannot be perfect without having exerted himself). Academic study and practice complement each other.

In this emphasis on practice, we can identify a moving away from the university schools' blind trust in the antique and Arabic authorities. Zerbi based his theories on Hippocrates, Galen, Haly Abbas, Avicenna, Mesue,

Alkindi, and also on the scriptures. He made special mention of the Hippocratic Oath. A physician must have knowledge of philosophy and of the artes liberales (liberal arts). He should be modest and taciturn and inspire confidence,while also accepting the advice of colleagues.

He should not consider fame and money to be of primary importance. Zerbi is believed to have been murdered in Turkey for not having been able to cure a Pascha.

Klaus Bergdolt

BIBLIOGRAPHY

Aaron, Henry, and William Schwartz. 1984. *The Painful Prescription: Rationing Hospital Care*. Washington DC: Brookings Institution.

Abbott, Walter M., ed. 1966. *The Documents of Vatican II*. London: Geoffrey Chapman.

Abdul-Rauf, Muhammad. 1977. *The Islamic View of Women and the Family*. New York: Robert Speller & Sons.

Abellán, José Luis. 1972. *La idea de América: Origen y evolución*. Madrid: Istmo.

Abellán, José Luis. 1981. *Historia Crítica del Pensamiento Español, Tomo III: Del Barroco a la Ilustración (Siglos XVII y XVIII)*. Madrid: Espasa-Calpe.

Abellán, José Luis. 1984. *Historia Crítica del Pensamiento Español, Tomo IV: Liberalismo y Romanticismo (1808–1874)*. Madrid: Espasa-Calpe.

ʿAbd al-Hamid, Muhammad Muhyi al-Din. 1966. *Al-Ahwal al-Shakhsiyya fi al-Shariʾa al-Islamiyya (Personal Status in the Islamic Shariʾa)*. Cairo: Maktabat al-Sabih waAwladuhu.

Abram, Harry S. 1972. "Psychological Dilemmas of Medical Progress." *Psychiatry in Medicine*. 3: 51–8.

Abū Dāwūd, Sulaimān b. al-Ašʾat al-Siğistānī. 1994. *Sunan Abī Dāwūd*. 4 vols., edited by Ṣidqī Muḥammad Ğamīl. Bairūt: Dār al-Fikr.

Abū l-Qāsim, al-Zahrāwī. 1973. *Abulcasis On Surgery and Instruments: A Definitive Edition of the Arabic Text with English Translation*, translated by Martin S. Spink and George L. Lewis. London: Wellcome Institute of the History of Medicine.

Acosta, Joseph de. [1590] 1962. *Historia natural y moral de las Indias*. México: Fondo de Cultura Económica.

Acuña, Sebastian de. 1746. *Dissertaciones sobre el orden, que los medicos deben observar en las juntas para evitar discordias y conservar la autorida, y prerrogativa, de que goza cada uno; en defensa de las Universidades de España, del Real Protho-Medicato, de los Medicos de Camara de su Magestad y de los de su Real Familia; dedicase a la ilustrissima y Novilissima Universidad de Alcalá*. Madrid: Luis Correa.

Ádám, György. 1978. *Tipping in Hungary*. Budapest: Magvető Kiadó.

Ádám, György. 1984a. "Az orvosi hálapénz körüli vitához (On the Controversy of Tipping Physicians)." *Társadalmi Szemle (Social Review)*. (October): 135–44.

Ádám, György. 1984b. "Az orvosi hálapénz hatályos jogunkban (Physicians' Tipping in Our Contemporary Laws)." *Jogtudományi Közlöny (Juridical Gazette)*. (November): 642–50.

Ádám, György. 1985a. "Az orvosi hálapénz története Magyarországon (History of Physicians' Tipping in Hungary, first part)." *Mozgó Világ (Moving World)*. (February): 56–69.

Ádám, György. 1985b. "Az orvosi hálapénz története Magyarországon (History of Physicians' Tipping in Hungary, second part)." *Mozgó Világ (Moving World).* (March): 49–61.

Ádám, György. 1986a. *Az orvosi hálapénz Magyarországon (Tipping Physicians in Hungary).* Budapest: Magvető Kiadó.

Ádám, György. 1986b. "The Legal Judgment of the Gratuity for Doctors in Hungary." *Acta Juridica Academiae Scientiarum Hungaricae.* 28: 57–78.

Ádám, György. 1989a. *Adóztatás után (After Tax Tipping).* Budapest: Magvető Kiadó.

Ádám, György. 1989b. "Gratuity for Doctors and Medical Ethics." *Journal of Medicine and Philosophy.* 14: 315–22.

Adams, Mark B., ed. 1990. *The Wellborn Science: Eugenics in Germany, France, Brazil, and Russia.* New York/Oxford: Oxford University Press.

Ademuwagun, Z. A., et al., eds. 1979. *African Therapeutic Systems.* Los Angeles: Crossroads Press.

Adeva y Pacheco, Juan de. 1753. *Verdadera medicina y desengaños de la adulacion medica, para la conservacion de la salud del cuerpo humano.* Madrid: Joaquin Ibarra.

Adhikari, Ramesh K. 1999. "Medical Ethics in the Nepalese Context." In *Health Ethics in Six SEAR Countries,* edited by Nimal Kasturiaratchi, Reidar Lie, and Jens Seeberg, 64–75. New Delhi: WHO-SEARO, World Health Organization, Regional Office for South-East Asia.

Ad Hoc Committee of the Harvard Medical School to Examine the Definition of Brain Death. 1968. "A Definition of Irreversible Coma: A Report of the Ad Hoc Committee of the Harvard Medical School to Examine the Definition of Brain Death. *Journal of the American Medical Association.* 205: 337–40.

Advisory Committee on Human Radiation Experiments (ACHRE, Ruth R. Faden, Chair). 1996. *The Human Radiation Experiments: Final Report of the President's Advisory Committee on Human Radiation Experiments.* New York: Oxford University Press.

Advisory Committee to the Director, National Institutes of Health. 1988. *Report of the Human Fetal Tissue Transplantation Research Panel.* Washington DC: National Institutes of Health. In *Source Book in Bioethics: A Documentary History,* edited by Albert R. Jonsen, Robert M. Veatch, and LeRoy Walters, 103–110. Washington DC: Georgetown University Press.

Agulhon, Maurice. 1977. *Le Cercle dans la France Bourgeoise, 1810–1848: Etude d'une mutation de Sociabilité.* Paris: Colin.

Aikema, Bernard, and Dulcia Meijers. 1989. *Nel Regno dei Poveri: Arte e Storia dei Grandi Ospedali Veneziani in Età Moderna.* Venice: Arsenale.

Aird, John S. 1990. *Slaughter of the Innocents: Coercive Birth Control in China.* Washington DC: The American Enterprise Institute.

Airedale NHS Trust v. Bland. 1 All ER 821. (1993).

Al-Ahram Weekly. 11 July 1991. "Islamic Ulema against Genetic Determination."

Al-Ahram Weekly. 7 November 1991, 12.

Al-ʾAlam Al-Islami. 5–11 Aug. 1996, 14.

Al-ʾAlam Al-Islami. 16–22 Dec. 1996, 13.

Al-ʾAlam Al-Islami. 20–26 Jan. 1997, 6.

Albert, D. M., and H. G. Schele. 1965. *A History of Ophthalmology at the University of Pennsylvania,* 107–20. Springfield IL: Charles C Thomas.

Alexander, Leo. 1945. "The Treatment of Shock from Prolonged Exposure to Cold, Especially in Water." *CIOS Target No. 24, Medical, Combined Intelligence Objectives Sub-Committee,* G-2 Division, SHAEF (Rear), APO 413, 10 July 1945.

Alexander, Leo. [1947] 1977. "Ethical and Non-Ethical Experimentation on Human Beings, April 15, 1947." Reprinted in "Ethics of Human Experimentation." *Psychiatric Journal of the University of Ottawa.* 1: 40–6.

Alexander, Leo. 1948a. "Sociopsychologic Structures of the SS." *Archives of Neurology and Psychiatry.* 59: 622–34.

Alexander, Leo. 1948b. "War Crimes and Their Motivation, the Socio-Psychological Structure of the SS and the Criminalization of a Society." *Journal of Criminal Law and Criminology.* 39: 298–326.

Alexander, Leo. 1948c. "War Crimes: Their Social-Psychological Aspects." *American Journal of Psychiatry.* 105: 170–7.

Alexander, Leo. 1949a. "Introductory Statement." In *Doctors of Infamy: The Story of the Nazi Medical Crimes,* edited by Alexander Mitscherlich and Fred Mielke, translated by Heinz Norden, xxix–xxxiv. New York: Henry Schuman.

Alexander Leo. 1949b. "Medical Science Under Dictatorship." *New England Journal of Medicine.* 241: 39–47.

Alexander, Leo. 1949c. "The Molding of Personality Under Dictatorship: The Importance of Destructive Drives in the Socio-Psychological Structure of Nazism." *Journal of Criminal Law and Criminology.* 40: 3–27.

Alexander, Leo. 1949d. "Science Under Dictatorship." *March of Medicine.* 14: 51–106.

Alexander, Leo. 1950. "Science under Dictatorship: The One Hundred and Fiftieth Anniversary Discourse of the New York Academy of Medicine," 51–56. New York: New York Academy of Medicine.

Alexander, Leo. 1954. "Why I Became a Doctor and Why I Became the Sort of Doctor I Am." In *Why We Became Doctors,* edited by Noah Daniel Fabricant, 75–9. New York: Grune & Stratton.

Alexander, Leo. 1966a. "Limitations in Experimental Research on Human Beings with Special Reference to Psychiatric Patients." *Diseases of the Nervous System.* 27: 61–5.

Alexander, Leo. 1966b. "Limitations in Experimental Research on Human Beings." *Lex et Scientia: International Journal of Law and Science*. 3: 8–24.

Alexander, Leo. 1967. "Protections of Privacy in Behavioral Research." *Lex et Scientia, International Journal of Law and Science*. 4: 34–8.

Alexander, Leo. 1973. "Temporal Laws and Medical Ethics in Conflict: Letter to the Editor." *New England Journal of Medicine*. 289: 324–5.

Alexander, Leo. 1975a. "How Euthanasia Worked." *Our Family*. 28: 12–13.

Alexander, Leo. 1975b. "Medical Science under Dictatorship." *The Catholic Digest*. 38: 45–7.

Alexander, Leo. 1975c. "Medicine Under the Nazis." *Private Practice*. 7: 36–9

Alexander, Leo. 1977. "Ethics of Human Experimentation." *Psychiatric Journal of the University of Ottawa*. 1 (1–2): 40–6.

Alexander, Shana. 1962. "They Decide Who Lives, Who Dies." *Life*. 53: 102–25.

Alexandrinus, Iulius. 1557. *De medicina et medico dialogus libris quinque distinctus*. Basel: Andreas Gesnerus.

ʿAlī ibn Riḍwān, b. ʿAlī b. Ǧaʾfar. [1409] 1982. *Maqālat ʿAlī b. Riḍwān fī t-taṭarruq biṭ-ṭibb ilā s-saʾāda*, translated and commentary by Albert Dietrich. Göttingen: Vandenhoeck and Ruprecht.

Ali Riza Bey, Balikhane Nazırı. 2001. *Eski zamanlarda İstanbul Hayatı*. Istanbul: Kitabevi.

Almeras, Jean-Pierre, and Henri Pequignot. 1996. *La Déontologie Médicale*. Paris: Litec.

Alonso Muñoyerro, Luis. 1934. *Código de Deontología Médica*. Madrid: Ediciones Fax.

Alonso Muñoyerro, Luis. 1940. *Moral Médica en los Sacramentos de la Iglesia*. Madrid: Ediciones Fax.

Alonso Muñoyerro, Luis. 1950. *Código de Deontología Farmacéutica*. Madrid: Ediciones Fax.

Alter, D., et al. 2002. "Biology or Bias: Practice Patterns and Long-Term Outcomes for Men and Women with Acute Myocardial Infarction." *Journal of the American College of Cardiology*. 39 (12): 1909–16.

Altman, Lawrence K. 1998. *Who Goes First? The Story of Self-Experimentation in Medicine*. Berkeley CA: University of California Press.

Álvarez Millán, Cristina. 1999. "Graeco-Roman Case Histories and their Influence on Medieval Islamic Clinical Accounts." *Social History of Medicine*. 12: 19–43.

Álvarez Millán, Cristina. 2000. "Practice versus Theory: Tenth-Century Case Histories from the Islamic Middle East." *Social History of Medicine*. 13: 293–306.

Álvarez-Sierra, José. 1963. *Diccionario de Autoridades Médicas*. Madrid: Editora Nacional.

Aly, Götz, ed. 1989. *Aktion T4, 1939–1945: Die "Euthanasie" – Zentrale in der Tiergartenstraße 4*. Berlin: Edition Hentrich.

Aly, Götz, et al. 1985. *Reform und Gewissen: "Euthanasie" im Dienst des Fortschritts*. Berlin: Rotbuch.

Aly, Götz, Peter Chroust, and Christian Pross. 1994. *Cleansing the Fatherland: Nazi Medicine and Racial Hygiene*, translated by Belinda Cooper. Baltimore: Johns Hopkins University Press.

Ambroselli, Claire. 1988. *L'Éthique Médicale*. Paris: Presses Universitaires de France.

American Hospital Association. 1973. "Statement on a Patient's Bill of Rights." *Hospitals*. 47: 41.

American Hospital Association. [1973] 1992. *The Patient's Bill of Rights*. Chicago: American Hospital Association.

American Institute of Homeopathy; American Medical Association; National Eclectic Medical Association. 1888. *The Three Ethical Codes: The Code of Ethics of the American Medical Association, its Constitution and By-Laws; The Code of Ethics of the American Institute of Homeopathy; The Code of Ethics of the National Eclectic Medical Association*. Detroit MI: The Illustrated Medical Journal Co.

American Medical Association. [1847] 1999a. *Code of Ethics*. In *The American Medical Ethics Revolution: How the AMA's Code of Ethics Has Transformed Physicians' Relationships to Patients, Professionals, and Society*, edited by Robert Baker et al., 324–34. Baltimore: Johns Hopkins University Press.

American Medical Association. 1868, 1869. *Transactions of the American Medical Association*. Chicago: American Medical Association.

American Medical Association. [1903] 1999b. *Principles of Medical Ethics*. In *The American Medical Ethics Revolution: How the AMA's Code of Ethics Has Transformed Physicians' Relationships to Patients, Professionals, and Society*, edited by Robert Baker et al., 335–45. Baltimore: Johns Hopkins University Press.

American Medical Association. [1912] 1999c. *Principles of Medical Ethics*. In *The American Medical Ethics Revolution: How the AMA's Code of Ethics Has Transformed Physicians' Relationships to Patients, Professionals, and Society*, edited by Robert Baker et al., 346–54. Baltimore: Johns Hopkins University Press.

American Medical Association. [1957] 1999d. *Principles of Medical Ethics*. In *The American Medical Ethics Revolution: How the AMA's Code of Ethics Has Transformed Physicians' Relationships to Patients, Professionals, and Society*, edited by Robert Baker et al., 355–7. Baltimore: Johns Hopkins University Press.

American Medical Association. [1980] 1999e. *Principles of Medical Ethics*. In *The American Medical Ethics Revolution: How the AMA's Code of Ethics Has Transformed Physicians' Relationships to Patients, Professionals, and Society*, edited by Robert Baker et al., 358–9. Baltimore: Johns Hopkins University Press.

American Medical Association. [1990, 1994a] 1999f. *Fundamental Elements of the Patient-Physician Relationship*. In *The American Medical Ethics Revolution: How the AMA's Code of Ethics Has Transformed Physicians' Relationships to Patients, Professionals, and Society*, edited by Robert Baker et al., 360–1. Baltimore: Johns Hopkins University Press.

American Medical Association. [1994b] 1999g. "Withholding or Withdrawing Life-Sustaining Medical Treatment." *Code of Medical Ethics: Current Opinions with Annotations, 1998–1999*. 2.20: 45–6. Chicago: American Medical Association.

American Medical Association. 1999h. *Code of Medical Ethics: Current Opinions with Annotations, 1998–1999*. Chicago: American Medical Association.

American Medical Association. n.d. *Proceedings of the House of Delegates [PHD]*. Chicago: American Medical Association.

American Medical Association Committee on the Protection of Medical Research. 1914. "Report of the Committee on the Protection of Medical Research." *Journal of the American Medical Association*. 63: 94.

American Medical Association Council of Ethical and Judicial Affairs. 1986. *CEJA Report B – I-86: Statement on AIDS*. Chicago: American Medical Association.

American Medical Association Council of Ethical and Judicial Affairs. 1987. *Report of the Council on Ethical and Judicial Affairs A – I-87, Ethical Issues Involved in the Growing AIDS Crisis*. Chicago: American Medical Association.

American Medical Association Council on Ethical and Judicial Affairs. 1995. "The Use of Anencephalic Neonates as Organ Donors." *Journal of the American Medical Association*. 273: 1614–8.

American Medical Association Council on Ethical and Judicial Affairs. 1998. *Code of Medical Ethics: Current Opinions and Annotations 1998–1999*. Chicago: American Medical Association.

American Medical Association, House of Delegates. 1946. "Principles of Research Ethics." *Journal of the American Medical Association*. 133: 35.

American Medical Association Judicial Council. 1958. "Principles of Medical Ethics; Opinions and Reports of the Judicial Council; Abstracted and Annotated." *Journal of the American Medical Association*. Special Edition. June 7, 1958.

American Medical Association Judicial Council. 1977. *Opinions and Reports of the Judicial Council: Including the Principles of Medical Ethics and Rules of the Judicial Council*. Chicago: American Medical Association.

Ameringer, Carl F. 1999. *State Medical Boards and the Politics of Public Protection*. Baltimore: Johns Hopkins University Press.

Ampofu, O., and F. D. Johnson-Romauld. 1987. "Traditional Medicine and its Role in the Development of Health Services in Africa." Background paper for the technical discussions of the 26th, 26th, and 27th sessions of the Regional Committee for Africa. Brazzaville: World Health Organization.

Amundsen, Darrel W. 1977. "Medical Deontology and Pestilential Disease in the Late Middle Ages." *Journal of the History of Medicine and Allied Sciences*. 32: 403–21.

Amundsen, Darrel W. 1978a. "History of Medical Ethics. IV: Europe and the Americas: A. Ancient and Medieval Periods: 2. Medieval Europe: Fourth to Sixteenth Century." In *The Encyclopedia of Bioethics*, edited by Warren T. Reich, 938–51. New York: Macmillan.

Amundsen, Darrel W. 1978b. "Medieval Canon Law on Medical and Surgical Practice by the Clergy." *Bulletin of the History of Medicine*. 52: 22–44.

Amundsen, Darrel W. 1982. "Medicine and Faith in Early Christianity." *Bulletin of the History of Medicine*. 56: 326–50.

Amundsen, Darrel W. 1995a. "History of Medical Ethics: IV. Europe: A. Ancient and Medieval: 2. Early Christianity." In *Encyclopedia of Bioethics*, edited by Warren Reich, 1516–22. New York: Simon & Schuster Macmillan.

Amundsen, Darrel W. 1995b. "History of Medical Ethics: IV. Europe: A. Ancient and Medieval: 3. Medieval Christian Europe." In *Encyclopedia of Bioethics*, edited by Warren T. Reich, 1522–36. New York: Simon & Schuster Macmillan.

Amundsen, Darrel W. 1996. *Medicine, Society, and Faith in the Ancient and Medieval Worlds*. Baltimore: Johns Hopkins University Press.

Amundsen, Darrel W. 2001. "History." In *Methods in Medical Ethics*, edited by Jeremy Sugerman and Daniel P. Sulmasy, 126–45. Washington DC: Georgetown University Press.

Amundsen, Darrel W., and Gary B. Ferngren. 1982. "Philanthropy in Medicine: Some Historical Perspectives." In *Beneficence and Health Care*, edited by Earl E. Shelp, 1–31. Dordrecht: D. Reidel.

Amundsen, Darrel W., and Gary B. Ferngren. [1986] 1998. "The Early Christian Tradition." In *Caring and Curing: Health and Medicine in the Western Religious Traditions*, edited by Ronald L. Numbers and Darrel W. Amundsen, 40–64. [New York: Macmillan]. Reprint. Baltimore: Johns Hopkins University Press.

Amundsen, Darrel W., and Gary B. Ferngren. 1996. "The Perception of Disease and Disease Causality in the New Testament." In *Aufstieg und Niedergang der Römischen Welt II*. 37. 3, edited by Wolfgang Haase, 2934–56. Berlin/New York: Walter de Gruyter.

Andreae, Johann Valentin. 1975. *Christianopolis. Aus dem Lateinischen übersetzt von W. Biesterfeld*. Stuttgart: Reclam Universalbibliothek 9786.

Andrews, Lori B., and Dorothy Nelkin. 2001. *Body Bazaar: The Market for Human Tissue in the Biotechnology Age*. New York: Crown Publishers.

Anees, Munawar A. 1989. *Islam and Biological Futures: Ethics, Gender, and Technology*. London: Mansell.

Angell, Marcia. 1992. "Editorial Responsibility: Protecting Human Rights by Restricting Publication of Unethical Research." In *The Nazi Doctors and the Nuremberg Code: Human Rights in Human Experimentation*, edited by George J. Annas and Michael A. Grodin, 276–85. New York/Oxford: Oxford University Press.

Angell, Marcia. 2000. "Is Academic Medicine for Sale?" *New England Journal of Medicine*. 342: 1516–18.

Annas, George J., and Michale A. Grodin, eds. 1992. *The Nazi Doctors and the Nuremberg Code: Human Rights in Human Experimentation*. New York/Oxford: Oxford University Press.

Annas, George J., and Michael A. Grodin. 1999. "Medicine and Human Rights: Reflections on the Fiftieth Anniversary of the Doctors' Trial." In *Health and Human Rights*, edited by Jonathan M. Mann et al., 301–11. New York/London: Routledge.

Anonymous. n.d. "Bibliography of Andre E. Hellegers, M.D." Unpublished document, National Reference Center for Bioethics Literature. Copied from the Georgetown University Archives at Lauinger Library.

Anonymous. 1693. *The Statutes of the College of Physicians London*. London: n.p.

Anonymous. [1723] 1986. *Onania, or, The Heinous sin of self-pollution. A supplement to the Onania*. New York: Garland Publishing.

Anonymous. 1730. *Breviarium Italicae Historiae a temporibus Frederici Secondi Augusti usque ad annum MCCCLIV ab anonimo Italo. . . .* In *Rerum Italicarum Scriptores*. 16, edited by Ludovico Antonio Muratori, col. 285f. Milano: n. p.

Anonymous. 1823. *Extracts from the Medical Ethics of Dr. Percival*. Philadelphia: Kappa Lambda.

Anonymous. 1825. "Editorial." *New York Monthly Chronicle of Medicine and Surgery*.

Anonymous. 1827a. *Medical Ethics; or, a Code of Institutes and Precepts, Adapted to the Professional Conduct of Physicians and Surgeons. by the Late Thomas Percival with Additions, Illustrative of the Past and Present State of the Profession and its Collegiate Institutions, in Great Britain*. London: Jackson, Borough.

Anonymous. 1827b. "Review of Medical Ethics, or a Code of Institutes and Precepts adopted to the Professional Conduct of Physicians and Surgeons: by the later Dr. THOMAS PERCIVAL, M.D., F.R.S, & c. With Additions illustrative of the past and present state of the Profession, and its Collegiate Institutions in Britain." Small 8 vol. pp. 360; London,

1827; Jackson, Borough." *The Lancet*. (1826–1827) 12 (series 2): 696–7.

Anonymous. 1831a. "Editor's Reply to Dr. Ryan." *The Lancet*. 1831–1832, 1 (November 5, 1831): 221–22; 224–27.

Anonymous. 1831b. "Prosecution of Dr. Ryan by the Old Ladies of Rhubarb Hall." *The Lancet*. 1831–1832, 1 (April 2, 1831): 18–20.

Anonymous. 1831c. "Review of A Manual of Medical Jurisprudence, compiled from the best Medical and Legal Works &c, &c, being an Analysis of a Course of Lectures on Forensic Medicine &c" by Michael Ryan, M.D. &c. &c. London: Renshaw and Rush. 8 vol. pp. 309." *The Lancet*. 1831–1832, 1 (October 29, 1831): 137–43.

Anonymous. 1870. "Essays of the Birmingham Speculative Club." *The Saturday Review*. 30: 632–4.

Anonymous. 1878. *A FEW RULES OF MEDICAL ETIQUETTE by A LICENTATE OF THE ROYAL COLLEGE OF PHYSICIANS*. London: Bailliere, Tindall and Cox.

Anonymous. 1904. "A Review of 'The Confessions of a Physician' by V. Veresaeff," translated from Russian by S. Linden. *British Medical Journal*. 1: 1020–2.

Anonymous. 1928. "Novoe vo vrachebnoi etike." *Voprosy Zdravookhranenija Sredne-Volzhskoi Oblasti*. 1: 19–20.

Anonymous. 1945. *Walter Bradford Cannon, 1871–1945: a memorial exercise: held at the Harvard Medical School, Monday, November 5, 1945*. Boston MA.

Anonymous. 1955. "De more medicorum: Ein parodistisch-satirisches Gedicht des 13. Jahrhunderts." *Sudhoffs Archiv*, edited by Franz Brunhölzl. 39: 289–315.

Anonymous. 1963. "Walter Bradford Cannon." *Physiologist*. 6: 4–5.

Anonymous. 1971. "An Interview (with André Hellegers)." *Georgetown Medical Bulletin*. 24 (3): 4–10. February.

Anonymous. 1978. *De Decem Quaestionibus de Medicorum Statu. Ein spaetmittelalterlicher Dialog zur aerztlichen Standeskunde*, edited by Rudolf Peitz. Wuerzburger Medizinhistorische Forschungen 11. Pattensen: Horst Wellm.

Anonymous. 1979. "Dr. André Eugène Désiré Joseph Hellegers, M.D." *Stonyhurst Magazine*. 41 (468): 160–4.

Anonymous. 1983. "André Hellegers." *European Journal of Obstetrics, Gynecology, and Reproductive Biology*. 14 (5): 279–81.

Anonymous. 1993. "How Bioethics Got Its Name." *Hastings Center Report*. 23 (6, Supplement): S6–S7.

Anonymous Salernitanus. 1853. "De adventu medici ad aegrotum libellus." In *Collectio Salernitana II*, edited by Salvatore de Renzi, 74–80. Napoli: Filiatre Sebezio.

Anonymous Salernitanus. 1856. "De secretis mulierum." In *Collectio Salernitana IV,1*, edited by Salvatore de Renzi, 2–176. Napoli: Filiatre-Sebezio.

Antes, Peter. 1982. *Ethik und Politik im Islam*. Stuttgart: Kohlhammer.

Antiochian Orthodox Christian Archdiocese. 1989. *The Liturgikon*. Englewood NJ: Antiochian Orthodox Christian Archdiocese.

Antoninus of Florence, Saint. [1454, 1740] 1959. *Summa Moralis (or Summa Theologica)*. Reprint of the 1740 edition. Graz: Akademische Druck- und Verlagsanstalt.

Anyinam, Charles A. 1987. "Persistence with Change: A Rural-Urban Study of Ethno-Medical Practices in Contemporary Ghana." Ph.D. diss., Queens University, Kingston.

Aquinas, Thomas. 1964. *Summa Theologiae*. Cambridge UK: Blackfriars.

Arbesmann, Rudolph. 1954. "The Concept of 'Christus Medicus' in St. Augustine." *Traditio*. 10: 1–28.

Argentina. Comisión Nacional sobre la Desaparición de Personas (CONADEP). 1984. *Nunca Más*. Buenos Aires: Eudeba.

Ariès, Philippe. 1962. *Centuries of Childhood: A Social History of Childhood*, translated by Robert Baldick. New York: Random House.

Ariès, Philippe. 1983. *The Hour of Our Death*. Hammondsworth: Penguin Books.

Aristoteles. [1911] 1985. *Nikomachische Ethik*, translated by Eugen Rolfes. Hamburg: Felix Meiner Verlag.

Arluke, Arnold, and Clinton R. Sanders. 1996. *Regarding Animals*. Philadelphia: Temple University Press.

Arndt, William F., and F. Wilbur Gingrich. 1957. *A Greek-English Lexicon of the New Testament and Other Early Christian Literature; A Translation and Adaptation of Walter Bauer's Griechisch-Deutsches Wörterbuch zu den Schriften des Neuen Testaments und der übrigen urchristlichen Literatur*. 4th ed. Chicago: University of Chicago Press.

Arnold, Pascal, and Dominique Sprumont. 1997. "Der Nürnberger Kodex: Regeln des Völkerrechts." In *Ethik und Medizin: 1947–1997*, edited by Ulrich Tröhler and Stella Reiter-Theil, 115–30. Göttingen: Wallstein.

Arnold, Pascal, and Dominique Sprumont. 1998. "The 'Nuremberg Code': Rules of Public International Law." In *Ethics Codes in Medicine: Foundations and Achievements of Codification since 1947*, edited by Ulrich Tröhler and Stella Reiter-Theil, 84–96. Aldershot/Brookfield/Singapore/Sydney: Ashgate.

Aronowitz, Robert A. 1998. *Making Sense of Illness: Studies in Twentieth-Century Medical Thought*. New York: Cambridge University Press.

Ärztetag. 1889. "Grundsätze einer ärztlichen Standesordnung." *Aerztliches Vereinsblatt für Deutschland*. 18: 273.

Ärztlicher, Bezirksverein München. 1875. *Der aerztliche Stand und das Publikum: Eine Darlegung der beiderseitigen und gegenseitigen Pflichten*. Munich: Verlag von J. A. Finsterlin.

Ärztlicher, Kreisverein Karlsruhe. [1876] 1900. "Standesordnung." Reprinted in *Aerztliche Ehrengerichte und ärztliche Standesorganisation in Preußen*, edited by F. Altmann, 179–83. Berlin: Verlag von H. W. Müller.

Ärztlicher, Kreisverein Karlsruhe. [1897] 1907. "Vollzugs-Verordnung zu § 22 der ärztlichen Standesordnung für den Kreisverein Karlsruhe, Schiedsgericht Betreffend." Reprinted in *Die Entwickelung des ärztlichen Standes seit den ersten Dezennien des 19. Jahrhunderts*, edited by Christoph Marx, 152–3. Berlin: Verlag von Struppe & Winckler.

Asad, Muhammad, trans. 1980. *The Message of the Qurʾān*. Gibraltar: Dar Al-Andalus.

Aschheim, Steven E. 1992. *The Nietzsche Legacy in Germany, 1890–1990*. Berkeley CA: University of California Press.

Ash, Mitchell G., and Alfons Söllner, eds. 1996. *Forced Migration and Scientific Change: Emigré German-Speaking Scientists and Scholars after 1933*. Cambridge/New York: Cambridge University Press.

Ashcroft, R., et al. 1998. "Teaching Medical Ethics and Law within Medical Education: A Model for the UK Core Curriculum." *Journal of Medical Ethics*. 24: 188–92.

Association of Boston Physicians. [1808] 1995. "The Boston Medical Police." In *The Codification of Medical Morality: Historical and Philosophical Studies of the Formalization of Western Medical Morality in the Eighteenth and Nineteenth Centuries: Volume Two: Anglo-American Medical Ethics and Medical Jurisprudence in the Nineteenth Century*, edited by Robert Baker, 41–6. Boston: Kluwer Academic Publishers.

Asti, Astesanus de. [1317] 1478. *Summa de Casibus Conscientia*. Venice (no imprint).

Athanasius. 1950. *The Life of St. Anthony*, translated by R. T. Meyer. Ancient Christian Writers 10. Westminster: Newman Press.

Atwater, Edward. 1978. "'Squeezing Mother Nature': Experimental Physiology in the United States before 1870." *Bulletin of the History of Medicine*. 52: 313–35.

Augustine, Saint. 1957–72. *City of God against the Pagans*. 7 vols., LOEB CLASSICAL LIBRARY, 411–7. Cambridge MA: Harvard University Press.

Augustinus. n.d. *Sancti Aurelii Augustini Sermones I–CCCXVI*. Patrologia Latina (Migne), 38–39. Brepol.

Azor, Juan. 1603. *Institutionum Moralium: In quibus universae quaestiones ad conscientiam recte... Tomus primus*. Lugduni: Horatij Cardon.

Azor, Juan. 1607. *Institutionum Moralium: In quibus universae quaestiones ad conscientiam recte... Tomus secundus*. Lugduni: Horatij Cardon.

Baader, Gerhard, and Ullrich Schultz, eds. 1989. *Medizin und Nationalsozialismus: Tabuisierte Vergangenheit—Ungebrochene Tradition?* Frankfurt: Mabuse.

Bachmann, Peter. 1965. "Galens Abhandlung darüber, dass der vorzügliche Arzt Philosoph sein muss." *Nachrichten der Akademie der Wissenschaften in Göttingen.* Phil.-Hist. Klasse.

Bacon, Francis. [1620] 2000. *The New Organon,* edited by Lisa Jardine and Michael Silverthorne. Cambridge: Cambridge University Press. Reprinted in *The Works of Francis Bacon,* vol. 4, edited by J. Spedding, R. L. Ellis, and D. D. Heath, 39–248. London: Longmans, Cumpers, and Co.

Bacon, Francis. [1623] 1868. *De Augmentis Scientiarum (Of The Dignity and Advancement of Learning).* In *The Works of Francis Bacon, Baron of Verulam, Viscount St. Alban and Lord High Chancellor of England,* vol. 4, edited and translated by J. Spedding, R. L. Ellis, and D. D. Heath. London: Longman and Co.

Bacon, Francis. [1630] 1969. *Elements of the Common Lawes of England.* New York: Da Capo Press.

Bacon, Francis. 1854. *Preface to Novum Organum.* In *Bacon: The Works,* edited and translated by Basil Montague, 343–71. Philadelphia: Parry and MacMillan (available at http://history.hanover.edu/texts/Bacon/novorg.html).

Bacon, Francis. 1858. "De dignitate et augmentis scientiarum." In *The Works of Francis Bacon,* vol. 1, edited by J. Spedding, R. L. Ellis, and D. D. Heath, 423–837. London: Longmans.

Bacon, Francis. 1875. "On the Dignity and Advancement of Learning." In *The Works of Francis Bacon,* edited by J. Spedding, R. L. Ellis, and D. D. Heath, 273–498. London: Longmans, Cumpers, and Co.

Bacon, Francis. 1974. *The Advancement of Learning and New Atlantis,* edited by Arthur Johnston. Oxford: Clarendon Press.

Bacon, Roger. [1897–1900] 1964. *The 'Opus majus' of Roger Bacon,* edited, with introduction, and analytical table by John Henry Bridges. Reprint. Frankfurt/Main: Minerva.

Bailey, William H. 1881. "Anniversary Address." In *Transactions of the Medical Society of New York,* 107–12. New York: Medical Society of the State of New York.

Bainbridge, Margaret. 1982. "Life-Cycle Rituals of the Turks of Turkey." In *Research Papers: Muslims in Europe.* 16: 1–11.

Bakar, Osman. 1999. *The History and Philosophy of Islamic Science.* Cambridge UK: Islamic Text Society.

Baker, Ian. 1997. *The Tibetan Art of Healing.* San Francisco CA: Chronicle Books.

Baker, Robert. 1989. "The Evolution of DNR Policy." In *Rationing of Medical Care for the Critically Ill,* edited by Martin A. Strosberg and I. Alan Fein, 52–63. Washington DC: Brookings Institution.

Baker, Robert. 1993a. "Deciphering Percival's Code." In *The Codification of Medical Morality: Historical and Philosophical Studies of the Formalization of Western Medical Morality in the Eighteenth and Nineteenth Centuries: Volume One: Medical Ethics and Etiquette in the Eighteenth Century,* edited by Robert Baker, Dorothy Porter, and Roy Porter, 179–211. Dordrecht: Kluwer Academic Publishers.

Baker, Robert. 1993b. "Medical Propriety and Impropriety in the English-Speaking World Prior to the Formalization of Medical Ethics: Introduction." In *The Codification of Medical Morality: Historical and Philosophical Studies of the Formalization of Western Medical Morality in the Eighteenth and Nineteenth Centuries: Volume One: Medical Ethics and Etiquette in the Eighteenth Century,* edited by Robert Baker, Dorothy Porter, and Roy Porter, 15–17. Dordrecht: Kluwer Academic Publishers.

Baker, Robert. 1993c. "Professional Integrity and Global Budgeting: A Study of Physician Gatekeeping in the British National Health Service." *Professional Ethics.* 2: 3–34.

Baker, Robert. 1993d. "Visibility and the Just Allocation of Health Care: A Study of Age-Rationing in the British National Health Service." *Health Care Analysis.* 1.2: 139–50.

Baker, Robert, ed. 1995a. *The Codification of Medical Morality: Historical and Philosophical Studies of the Formalization of Western Medical Morality in the Eighteenth and Nineteenth Centuries: Volume Two: Anglo American Medical Ethics and Medical Jurisprudence in the Nineteenth Century.* Boston: Kluwer Academic Publishers.

Baker, Robert. 1995b. "An Introduction to the Boston Medical Police of 1808." In *The Codification of Medical Morality: Historical and Philosophical Studies of the Formalization of Western Medical Morality in the Eighteenth and Nineteenth Centuries: Volume Two: Anglo-American Medical Ethics and Medical Jurisprudence in the Nineteenth Century,* edited by Robert Baker, 25–40. Boston: Kluwer Academic Publishers.

Baker, Robert. 1995c. "The Historical Context of the American Medical Association's 1847 *Code of Ethics.*" In *The Codification of Medical Morality: Historical and Philosophical Studies of the Formalization of Western Medical Morality in the Eighteenth and Nineteenth Centuries: Volume Two: Anglo-American Medical Ethics and Medical Jurisprudence in the Nineteenth Century,* edited by Robert Baker, 47–64. Boston: Kluwer Academic Publishers.

Baker, Robert. 1996. "Resistance To Medical Ethics Reform In The Nineteenth Century." *Malloch Room Newsletter of The New York Academy of Medicine.* 13: Spring.

Baker, Robert. 1998a. "Multiculturalism, Postmodernism And The Bankruptcy Of Fundamentalism." *Kennedy Institute of Ethics Journal.* 8 (3): 210–31.

Baker, Robert. 1998b. "A Theory of International Bioethics: The Negotiable and the

Non-Negotiable." *Kennedy Institute of Ethics Journal.* 8: 233–73.

Baker, Robert. 1998c. "Transcultural Medical Ethics and Human Rights." In *Ethics Codes in Medicine: Foundations and Achievements of Codification since 1947,* edited by Ulrich Tröhler and Stella Reiter-Theil, 312–31. Aldershot/Brookfield/Singapore/Sydney: Ashgate.

Baker, Robert. 1999. "The American Medical Ethics Revolution." In *The American Medical Ethics Revolution: How the AMA's Code of Ethics Has Transformed Physicians' Relationships to Patients, Professionals, and Society,* edited by Robert Baker et al., 17–51. Baltimore: Johns Hopkins University Press.

Baker, Robert. 2001. "Bioethics and Human Rights: A Historical Perspective." *Cambridge Quarterly of Healthcare Ethics.* 10: 241–52.

Baker Robert. 2002a "Bioethics and History." *Journal of Medicine and Philosophy.* 27: 447–74.

Baker, Robert. 2002b. "From Metaethicist to Bioethicist." *CQ: Cambridge Quarterly of Healthcare Ethics.* 11.4: 369–79.

Baker, Robert, et al., eds. 1999. *The American Medical Ethics Revolution.* Baltimore: Johns Hopkins University Press.

Baker, Robert, and Linda Emanuel. 2000. "The Efficacy of Professional Ethics: The AMA Code of Ethics in Historical and Current Perspective." *Hastings Center Report.* 30: S13–17.

Baker, Robert, and Victoria Hargreaves. 2001. "Transplantation: A Historical Perspective." In *Advances in Bioethics: Volume 7: The Ethics of Organ Transplantation,* edited by Wayne Shelton, 1–42. New York: Elsevier Science Publications.

Baker, Robert, Dorothy Porter, and Roy Porter, eds. 1993. *The Codification of Medical Morality: Historical and Philosophical Studies of the Formalization of Western Medical Morality in the Eighteenth and Nineteenth Centuries: Volume One: Medical Ethics and Etiquette in the Eighteenth Century.* Dordrecht: Kluwer Academic Publishers.

Baker, Robert, and Martin Strosberg. 1995. *Legislating Medical Ethics: A Study of New York State's Do Not Resuscitate Law.* Dordrecht: Kluwer Academic Publications.

Bakstanovszkij, V. I., et al. 1978. *Marxist Ethics.* Budapest: Kossuth Publisher.

Balasubramanium, K. 2001. "Lanka Must Protect Its Access to Affordable Medicines." *The Daily Mirror Online* (Colombo). www.dailymirror.lk/inside/health/021115.html (visited January 17, 2003): 1–2.

Bald, R. C. 1970. *John Donne: A Life.* New York/Oxford: Oxford University Press.

Baltimore Medico-Chirurgical Society. 1832. *A System of Medical Ethics, Adopted by the Medico-Chirurgical Society of Baltimore; Being the Report of the Committee on Ethics, and Published by Order of the Society.* Baltimore: James Lucas and E. K. Deaver.

Banco, Mundial. 1993. *Informe sobre el Desarrollo Mundial 1993.* Washington DC: The World Bank.

Banks, Abraham. 1839. *Medical Etiquette; or An Essay upon the Laws and Regulations Which Ought Properly to Govern the Conduct of Members of the Medical Profession in Their Relation to Each Other.* London: Charles Fox.

Bar, Muhammad Ali al-. 1981. *Khalq al-Insan bayna al-Tibb wal-Qur'an (The Creation of Man between Medicine and the Qur'an).* Saudi Arabia: n.p.

Bard, Samuel. 1769. *A Discourse upon the Duties of a Physician, with Some Sentiments, on the Usefulness and Necessity of a Public Hospital, Delivered before the President and the Governors of King's College, at the Commencement, Held on the 16th of May, 1769. As Advice to Those Gentlemen Who Then Received the First Medical Degrees Conferred by That University.* New York: A & J Robertson.

Bardi, Girolamo. 1644. *Medicus politico catholicus.* Genoa: Maria Farroni.

Barger, A. C. 1981. "New technology for a new century: Walter B. Cannon and the invisible rays." *Physiologist.* 24 (5): 6–14.

Barker-Benfield, G. J. 1976. *The Horrors of the Half-Known Life: Male Attitudes toward Women and Sexuality in Nineteenth-Century America.* New York: Harper & Row Publishers.

Barnes, Jonathan. 1991. "Galen on Logic and Therapy." In *Galen's Method of Healing,* edited by Fridolf Kudlien and Richard J. Durling, 50–102. Leiden: E. J. Brill.

Barry, Jonathan. 1985. "Piety and the Patient: Medicine and Religion in Eighteenth-Century Bristol." In *Patients and Practitioners: Lay Perceptions of Medicine in Pre-Industrial Society,* edited by Roy Porter, 145–76. Cambridge UK: Cambridge University Press.

Bar Sela, Ariel, and Hebbel E. Hoff. 1962. "Isaac Israeli's Fifty Admonitions to the Physicians." *Journal for the History of Medicine.* 17: 245–57.

Barstein, E. A. 1936. *Kakim Dolzhen Byt' Vrach-stakhanovets?* Ural'sk: Zapadno-Kazakhstanskoe oblastnoe otdelenie Medsantrud, Gostipografija.

Bartrip, Peter. 1995a. "An Introduction to Jukes Styrap's *A Code of Medical Ethics* (1878)." In *The Codification of Medical Morality: Historical and Philosophical Studies of the Formalization of Western Medical Morality in the Eighteenth and Nineteenth Centuries: Volume Two: Anglo-American Medical Ethics and Medical Jurisprudence in the Nineteenth Century,* edited by Robert Baker, 145–8. Boston: Kluwer Academic Publishers.

Bartrip, Peter. 1995b. "Secret Remedies, Medical Ethics, and the Finances of the *British Medical Journal.*" In *The Codification of Medical Morality: Historical and Philosophical Studies of the Formalization of Western Medical Morality in the Eighteenth and Nineteenth Centuries: Volume Two: Anglo-American Medical Ethics and Medical Jurisprudence in the Nineteenth Century*, edited by Robert Baker, 191–204. Boston: Kluwer Academic Publishers.

Basha, Hassan Shamsi. 1996. "Al-Siyam wal-Amrad al-ʾAsabiyya wal-Nafsiyya (The Fasts and Neuropsychological Diseases)." In *Majallat al-Hajj*. 3: 23–4.

Basham, A. L. 1976. "The Practice of Medicine in Ancient and Medieval India." In *Asian Medical Systems: A Comparative Study*, edited by Charles Leslie, 18–43. Berkeley CA: University of California Press.

Basil, Saint. 1962. *The Long Rules*, translated by Sister Monica Wagner. Washington DC: Catholic University of America Press.

Basil, Saint. 1983. "The Ninety-Two Canons of our Father among Saints Basil the Great." In *The Rudder of the Orthodox Catholic Church*, edited by Sts. Nicodemus and Agapius, translated by D. Cummings, 772–863. New York: Luna Printing.

Basil, Saint. 1994. "The Hexaemeron." In *Nicene and Post-Nicene Fathers*. 2nd series, vol. 8, edited by Philip Schaff and Henry Wace, 52–107. Peabody MA: Hendrickson Publishers.

Bassiouni, M. C., T. G. Baffers, and J. T. Evard. 1981. "An Appraisal of Human Experimentation in International Law and Practice: The Need for International Regulation of Human Experimentation." *International Journal of Criminal Law and Criminology*. 72: 1597–666.

Bauer, Axel. 2001. "Streitfall Anatomie und Öffentlichkeit." In *Schöne Neue Körperwelten: Der Streit um die Ausstellung*, edited by Franz Josef Wetz and Brigitte Tag, 171–203. Stuttgart: Klett-Cotta.

Bayer, Ronald. 1988. "Scientists, Engineers, and the Burdens of Occupational Exposure: The Case of the Lead Standard." In *The Health and Safety of Workers: Case Studies in the Politics of Professional Responsibility*, edited by Ronald Bayer. New York: Oxford University Press.

Bayer, Ronald. 1989. *Private Acts, Social Consequences: AIDS and the Politics of Public Health*. New York: Free Press.

Bayer, Ronald. 1991. "Public Health Policy and the AIDS Epidemic: An End to HIV Exceptionalism?" *New England Journal of Medicine*. 324: 1500–4.

Bayer, Ronald. 2002. "Tobacco, Commercial Speech, and Libertarian Values: The End of the Line for Restrictions on Advertising?" *American Journal of Public Health*. 92: 356–9.

Bayer, Ronald, et al. 2003. "Tobacco Advertising in the United States: A Proposal for a Constitutionally Acceptable Form of Regulation." *Journal of the American Medical Association*. 287: 2990–5.

Bayer, Ronald, and James Colgrove. 2002. "Science, Politics and Ideology in the Campaign Against Environmental Tobacco Smoke." *American Journal of Public Health*. 92: 949–54.

Bayer, Ronald, Carol Levine, and Thomas H. Murray. 1984. "Guidelines for Confidentiality in Research on AIDS." *IRB*. 6.6: 1–7.

Bayer, Ronald, Carol Levine, and S. M. Wolf. 1986. "HIV Antibody Screening: An Ethical Framework for Evaluating Proposed Programs." *Journal of the American Medical Association*. 256: 1768–74.

Bayertz, Kurt. 1994. *The Concept of Moral Consensus: The Case of Technological Interventions into Human Reproduction*. Dordrecht/Boston: Kluwer Academic Press.

Bayle, Françoise. 1950. *Croix Gammée Contre Caducée: Les Expériences Humaines en Allemagne pendant la Deuxième Guerre Mondiale*. Berlin/Neustadt: Palatinat.

Beauchamp, Dan. 1985. "Community: The Neglected Tradition of Public Health." *Hastings Center Report*. 15: 28–36.

Beauchamp, Tom L. 1995. "Worthington Hooker on Ethics in Clinical Medicine." In *The Codification of Medical Morality: Historical and Philosophical Studies of the Formalization of Western Medical Morality in the Eighteenth and Nineteenth Centuries: Volume Two: Anglo American Medical Ethics and Medical Jurisprudence in the Nineteenth Century*, edited by Robert Baker, 105–19. Boston: Kluwer Academic Publishers.

Beauchamp, Tom. 2003. "The Origins, Goals, and Core Commitments of The Belmont Report and Principles of Biomedical Ethics." In *The Story of Bioethics: From Seminal Works to Contemporary Explorations*, edited by Jennifer K. Walter and Eran P. Klein, 17–46. Washington DC: Georgetown University Press.

Beauchamp, Tom L. 2007. "History and Theory in 'Applied Ethics'." *Kennedy Institute of Ethics Journal*. 17: 55–64.

Beauchamp, Tom L., and James F. Childress. 1979. *Principles of Biomedical Ethics*. New York: Oxford University Press.

Beauchamp, Tom L., and James F. Childress. 1983. *Principles of Biomedical Ethics*. 2nd ed. New York: Oxford University Press.

Beauchamp, Tom L., and James F. Childress. 1989. *Principles of Biomedical Ethics*. 3rd ed. New York: Oxford University Press.

Beauchamp, Tom L., and James F. Childress. 1994. *Principles of Biomedical Ethics*. 4th ed. New York: Oxford University Press.

Beauchamp, Tom L., and James F. Childress. 2001. *Principles of Biomedical Ethics*. 6th ed. New York: Oxford University Press.

Beauchamp, Tom L., and Laurence B. McCullough. 1984. *Medical Ethics: The Moral Responsibilities of Physicians*. Englewood Cliffs NJ: Prentice Hall.

Beck, Theodric Romeyn. 1823. *Elements of Medical Jurisprudence*. Albany NY: Webster and Skinner.

Beck, Theodric Romeyn. 1836. "Original Reports of the Revisers." In *The Revised Statutes of New-York . . . 1828 to 1835 Inclusive*, appendix to vol. III, 829–30. Albany NY: State of New York.

Beck, Theodric Romeyn. 1997. *Elements of Medical Jurisprudence*. Reprinted by The Lawbook Exchange, Ltd. Albany NY: Websters and Skinners.

Becker, Lawrence C. 1975. "Human Being: The Boundaries of the Concept." *Philosophy and Public Affairs*. 4: 334–59.

Becker, Peter E. 1988. *Zur Geschichte der Rassenhygiene: Wege ins Dritte Reich*. Stuttgart/New York: G. Thieme.

Beddoes, Thomas, ed. 1799. *Contributions to Physical and Medical Knowledge, Principally from the West of England*. London: T. N. Longman and O. Rees.

Beddoes, Thomas. 1802. *Hygeia: or Essays Moral and Medical, on the Causes Affecting the Personal State of our Middling and Affluent Classes*. Bristol: J. Mills.

Beddoes, Thomas. 1806. *Manual of Health: or, the Invalid Conducted Safely Through the Seasons*. London: Johnson.

Beecher, Henry K. 1946. "Pain in Men Wounded in Battle." *Annals of Surgery*. 123: 96–105.

Beecher, Henry K. 1955. "The Powerful Placebo." *Journal of the American Medical Association*. 159: 1602–6.

Beecher, Henry K. 1959. *Measurements of Subjective Responses: Quantitative Effects of Drugs*. New York: Oxford University Press.

Beecher, Henry K. 1963. "Ethics and Experimental Therapy." *Journal of the American Medical Association*. 186: 858–9.

Beecher, Henry K. 1966. "Ethics and Clinical Research." *New England Journal of Medicine*. 274: 1354–60.

Beecher, Henry K. 1970. *Research and the Individual: Human Studies*. Boston: Little Brown.

Beecher, Henry K., and D. P. Todd. 1954. "A Study of Deaths Associated with Anesthesia and Surgery." *Annals of Surgery*. 149: 2–34.

Beese, Wolfgang. 1991. "Points." *Bulletin of Medical Ethics*. 66: 24.

Beier, Lucinda. 1985. "In Sickness and in Health: A Seventeenth-Century Family's Experience." In *Patients and Practitioners: Lay Perceptions of Medicine in Pre-Industrial Society*, edited by Roy Porter, 101–28. Cambridge UK: Cambridge University Press.

Belkin, Gary S. 1998. "History and Bioethics: The Uses of Thomas Percival." *Medical Humanities Review*. 12: 39–59.

Belkin, Samuel. 1960. *In His Image: The Jewish Philosophy of Man as Expressed in Rabbinic Tradition*. London/New York/Toronto: Abelard-Schuman.

Bell, John. [1847] 1999. "Introduction to the 1847 Code of Ethics." In *The American Medical Ethics Revolution: How the AMA's Code of Ethics Has Transformed Physicians' Relationships to Patients, Professionals, and Society*, edited by Robert Baker et al., 317–23. Baltimore: Johns Hopkins University Press.

Bell, John, and Isaac Hays, eds. 1823. *Extracts from the Medical Ethics of Dr. Percival*. Philadelphia: Kappa Lambda Society of Hippocrates.

Bell, Richard, trans. 1939. *The Qurʾān*. 2 vols. Edinburgh: T. & T. Clark.

Bell, Whitfield J., Jr. 1975. *The Colonial Physician & Other Essays*. New York: Science History Publications.

Bellah, Robert N. 1965. "Religious Evolution." In *Reader in Comparative Religion: An Anthropological Approach*, edited by William A. Lessa and Evon T. Vogt, 73–87. New York: Harper & Row.

Beller, F. K. 1983. "André E. Hellegers as a Philosopher Portrayed by His Thinking. In Memoriam of an Admired Friend." *European Journal of Obstetrics, Gynecology and Reproductive Biology*. 14 (5): 289–97.

Beller, Fritz K., and Julia Reeve. 1989. "Brain Life and Brain Death – The Anencephalic as an Explanatory Example: A Contribution to Transplantation." *Journal of Medicine and Philosophy*. 14: 5–23.

Belloni, Luigi. 1958. "La medicina a Milano fino al Seicento." *La storia di Milano*. 11: 595–696. Milano: Fondazione Treccani degli Alfieri.

Benedict XV. 1914. *Ad Beatissimi Apostolorum*. www.papalencyclicals.net.

Benedict, Saint. 1992. *Regula Benedicti – Die Benediktsregel. Lateinisch-Deutsch*, hrsg. von der Salzburger Äbtekonferenz. Beuron: Beuroner Kunstverlag.

Benison, S., and A. C. Barger. 1978. "Walter Bradford Cannon." In *Dictionary of Scientific Biography*. 15: 71–7. New York: Scribner.

Benison, Saul, A. Clifford Barger, and Elin L. Wolfe. 1987. *Walter B. Cannon: The Life and Times of a Young Scientist*. Cambridge MA: Belknap Press.

Bennet, F. J., and J. Maneno, eds. 1986. *National Guidelines for the Implementation of Primary Health Care in Kenya*. Nairobi: Ministry of Health, NGO's of Kenya, WHO and UNICEF.

Benoit, E. 1966. "Status, Status Types, and Status Interrelations." In *Role Theory: Concepts and Research*, edited by Bruce Biddle and Edwin Thomas, 77–80. New York: Wiley.

Bentham, Jeremy. [1789] 1970. *An Introduction to the Principles of Morals and Legislation*, edited by J. H. Burns and H. L. A. Hart. London: Athlone Press.

Bentham, Jeremy. 2004. *The Auto-Icon*. http://www.ucl.ac.uk/Bentham-Project/info/auto-iconhtm.htm (visited November 16, 2007).

Benzenhoefer, Udo. 1999. *Der gute Tod: Euthanasie und Sterbehilfe in Geschichte und Gegenwart*. München: C. H. Beck.

Berg, J. H. van den. 1969. *Medische Macht en Medische Ethiek*. Nijkerk: Callenbach.

Berg, J. W., et al. 2001. *Informed Consent: Legal Theory and Clinical Practice*. Oxford: Oxford University Press.

Bergdolt, Klaus, ed. 1989. *Die Pest 1348 in Italien: 50 zeitgenössische Quellen*. Heidelberg: Manutius.

Bergdolt, Klaus. 1991. "Zur antischolastischen Arztkritik des 13. Jahrhunderts." *Medizin-Historisches Journal.* 26: 264–82.

Bergdolt, Klaus. 1992. *Arzt, Krankheit und Therapie bei Petrarca: Die Kritik an Arzt und Naturwissenschaft im italienischen Frühhumanismus.* Weinheim: VCH.

Bergdolt, Klaus. 1994. *Der Schwarze Tod: Die Grosse Pest und das Ende des Mittelalters.* München: C. H. Beck.

Bergdolt, Klaus. 1998. "Medizinische Ethik (Historisch)." In *Lexikon der Bioethik*, vol. 2, edited by Wilhelm Korff, Lutwin Beck, and Paul Mikat, 647–52. Gütersloh: Gütersloher Verlagshaus.

Berger, Robert L. 1992. "Nazi Science: Comments on the Validation of the Dachau Human Hypothermia Experiments." In *When Medicine Went Mad: Bioethics and the Holocaust*, edited by Arthur L. Caplan, 109–33. Totowa NJ: Humana Press.

Berlant, Jeffrey L. 1975. *Profession and Monopoly: A Study of Medicine in the United States and Great Britain.* Berkeley CA: University of California Press.

Bernard, Claude. 1865. *Introduction à l'étude de la médecine expérimentale.* Paris: J.B. Baillière.

Bernard, Claude. [1865a] 1949. *Introduction à l'Etude de la Médecine Expérimentale.* Reprinted as *An Introduction to the Study of Experimental Medicine*, translated by H. C. Greene. New York: Schuman.

Bernard, Claude. [1865b, 1927] 1957a. *An Introduction to the Study of Experimental Medicine*, edited by I. Bernard Cohen, translated by Henry Copley Greene. New York: Dover Publications.

Bernard, Claude. 1957b. *Introduction to the Study of Experimental Medicine*, translated by Henry Copley Greene. New York: Dover.

Bernard, Jean. 1994. *Médecin dans le Siècle.* Paris: Robert Laffont.

Bernhard of Clairvaux. 1994. *Sermones super Cantica Canticorum.* In *Sämtliche Werke.* 5. Innsbruck: Tyrolia.

Bernat, James L. 1992. "How Much of the Brain Must Die on Brain Death?" *Journal of Clinical Ethics.* 3: 21–26.

Bevan, William. 1971. "On Stimulating the Gift of Blood." *Science.* 173: 583.

Beveridge, William. 1942. *Social Insurance and Allied Services.* London: Her Majesty's Stationary Office Cmd. 6404.

Bhardwaj, Minakshi. 2001. "Biotechnology, Bioethics, and the Poor." *Electronic Journal of Biotechnology.* 4.3. http://ejbiotechnology.ucv.cl/content/vol4/issue3/issues/04/ (visited January 30, 2008).

Bhardwaj, Minakshi and Jayapaul Azariah (1999). "Cloning: Paradox, Paradigm and Ethics in Indian Society." *Eubios Journal of Asian and International Bioethics* 9(3): 71–3.

Bhishagratna, K. K., ed. and trans. 1963. *An English Translation of the Suśruta Saṃhitā: Based on Original Sanskrit Text.* Chowkhamba Sanskrit Studies. Varanasi: Chowkhamba Sanskrit Series Office.

Bhishagratna, Kunjalal K., trans. and ed. [1918] 1963. *An English Translation of the Suśruta Saṃhitā: Based on Original Sanskrit Text.* 2nd ed., 3 vols. Chowkhamba Sanskrit Studies. Varanasi: Chowkhamba Sanskrit Series Office.

Biagini, Hugo. 1989. *Filosofía americana e identidad.* Buenos Aires: Eudeba.

Bickel, Marcel H. 2000. *Die Entwicklung zur experimentellen Pharmakologie, 1790–1850: Wegbereiter von Rudolf Buchheim.* Basle: Schwabe.

Biesterfeldt, Hans Hinrich. 1984. "Some Opinions on the Physician's Remuneration in Medieval Islam." *Bulletin of the History of Medicine.* 58: 16–27.

Bihl, Geoffrey. 2001. "Drugs and Donors: Limiting Factors to Transplantation in South Africa." *Medscape Transplantation.* 2. 2. Conference report presented at the 19th South African Transplantation Society Congress, Bloemfontein, South Africa, September 16–19, 2001.

Bilimoria, Purushottama, and Renuka Sharma. 1998. "Issues in Health Ethics in Modern India." In *The Other Revolution: NGO and Feminist Perspectives from South and East Asia*, edited by Renuka Sharma, 252–70. Delhi: Indian Books Centre in Association with Open Wisdom Publications.

Billings, P. R., et al. 1992. "Discrimination as a Consequence of Genetic Testing." *American Journal of Human Genetics.* 50.3: 476–82.

Bilmen, Ömer N. 1986. *Büyük İslâm İlmihali.* Istanbul: Bilmen Yayinevi.

Binder, Jochen. 2000. *Zwischen Standesrecht und Marktwirtschaft: Ärztliche Werbung zu Beginn des 20. Jahrhunderts im deutsch-englischen Vergleich.* Frankfurt/Main: P. Lang.

Binding, Karl, and Alfred E. Hoche. 1920. *Die Freigabe der Vernichtung lebensunwerten Lebens: Ihr Mass und ihre Form.* Leipzig: Verlag von Felix Meiner.

Binding, Karl, and Alfred E. Hoche. [1920] 1975. *The Release and Destruction of Life Devoid of Value: Its Measure and its Form*, translated by Robert Sassone. Santa Ana CA: Robert Sassone.

Bingham, Eula. 1985. "Hypersusceptibility to Occupational Hazards." In *Hazards: Technology and Fairness*, National Academy of Engineering, ed., 79–88. Washington DC: National Academy Press.

Biorck, Gunnar. 1968. "Thoughts on Life and Death." *Perspectives in Biology and Medicine.* 11: 527–43.

Birch, Thomas. 1756–1757. *The History of the Royal Society of London for Improving of Natural Knowledge, from Its First Rise. In Which the Most Considerable of Those Papers Communicated to the Society, Which Have Hitherto Not Been Published, Are Inserted in Their Proper Order, as a Supplement to the Philosophical Transactions.* London: A. Millar.

Birnbaum, Raoul. 1989. "Chinese Buddhist Traditions of Healing and the Life-Cycle." In *Healing and Restoring: Health and Medicine in the World's Religious Traditions*, edited by Lawrence E. Sullivan, 33–57. New York: Macmillan.

Blackstone, Sir William. 1768. *Commentaries on the Laws of England*, vol. 3. Oxford: Clarendon Press.

Blanton, Wyndham B. 1930. *Medicine in Seventeenth-Century Virginia*. Richmond VA: William Byrd Press.

Blaschke, Andreas. 1998. *Beschneidung: Zeugnisse der Bibel und verwandter Texte*. Tübingen: Francke.

Blasius, Dirk. 1980. *Der verwaltete Wahnsinn: Eine Sozialgeschichte des Irrenhauses*. Frankfurt: S. Fischer Taschenbuch.

Blasszauer, Béla. 1984a. *A jó halál (Good Death: Euthanasia – Pro & Con)*. Budapest: Gondolat Publishing.

Blasszauer, Béla. 1984b. "Az orvosi hálapénzről – etikai alapon (On the Tipping of Physicians – On Ethical Basis)." *Valóság (Reality)*. 2: 98–9.

Blasszauer, Béla. 1995a. *Orvosi etika (Medical Ethics)*. Budapest: Medicina Publishing.

Blasszauer, Béla. 1995b. "History of Medical Ethics: IV. Europe: D. Contemporary Period: 8. Central and Eastern Europe." In *Encyclopedia of Bioethics*. 2nd ed., edited by Warren T. Reich, 1595–1601. New York: Simon & Schuster Macmillan.

Blasszauer, Béla. 1997a. *Eutanázia (Euthanasia)*. Budapest: Medicina Publishing.

Blasszauer, Béla. 1997b. "Guest Editorial: Petty Corruption in Health Care." *Journal of Medical Ethics*. 23: 133–4.

Blasszauer, Béla, and E. Kismodi. 2001. "Ethics Committees in Hungary." In *Ethics Committees in Central and Eastern Europe*, edited by Jozef Glasa, 191–6. Bratislava: Charis-IMEB FDN.

Bleich, J. David. 1973. "Establishing Criteria of Death." *Tradition*. 13: 90–113.

Bleich, J. David. 1977–1995. *Contemporary Halakhic Problems*. 4 vols. New York: Ktav.

Bleich, J. David. 1981. *Judaism and Healing: Halakhic Perspectives*. New York: Ktav.

Bleich, J. David. 1998. *Bioethical Dilemmas: a Jewish Perspective*. Hoboken NJ: Ktav.

Bleich, J. David, and Fred Rosner. 1979. *Jewish Bioethics*. New York: Hebrew Publishing Co.

Bleker, Johanna, and Norbert Jachertz. 1993. *Medizin im Dritten Reich*. Cologne: Deutscher Ärzte-Verlag.

Blijham, G. H., and L. Tjabbes-Meijer. 2002. "Euthanasia and Assisted Suicide – Respecting the Patient's Will." In *Health and Health Care in the Netherlands: A Critical Self-Assessment of Dutch Experts in Medical and Health Sciences*, edited by A. J. P. Schrijvers and Liliane Droyan Kodner, 285–91. Maarssen: Elsevier Gezondheitszorg.

Bliss, Michael. 1999. *William Osler: A Life in Medicine*. Oxford: Oxford University Press.

Blokhin, Nikolai N. 1977. *Deontologija v Onkologii*. Moscow: Meditsyna.

Bóc, Imre. 1984. "Ingyenesség mellett szabad orvosválasztást (Let's have free choice of physicians, besides our free health care system!)." *Valóság (Reality)*. 2: 100–1.

Böcher, Otto. 1970. *Dämonenfurcht und Dämonenabwehr: Ein Beitrag zur Vorgeschichte der chrsitlichen Taufe*. Stuttgart: Kohlhammer.

Böcher, Otto. 1972a. *Christus Exorcista: Dämonismus und Taufe im Neuen Testament*. Stuttgart: Kohlhammer.

Böcher, Otto. 1972b. *Das neue Testament und die dämonischen Mächte*. Stuttgart: Kohlhammer.

Bock, Gisela. 1986. *Zwangssterilisation im Nationalsozialismus: Studien zur Rassenpolitik und Frauenpolitik*. Opladen: Westdeutscher Verlag.

Bock, Hieronymus. 1543. *Kreutterbuch....* Strassburg: Josiam Rihel.

Bodmer, Walter, Sir. 1992. "Animal Experimentation and Cancer Research." In *Animal Experimentation and the Future of Medical Research*, edited by Jack H. Botting, 75–89. London: Portland Press.

Bohn, Johann. 1704. *De officio medici duplici, clinici nimirum ac forensis,....* Leipzig: Friedrich Gleditsch.

Boisvert, Mathieu. 2000. "Conception and Intrauterine Life in the Pali Canon." *Studies in Religion*. 29: 301–11.

Bolam v. Friern. HMC. 2 All ER 118. (1957).

Boleda, Cristóbal de. n.d. *Question medico-moral en qve resolvtiva y solidamente se disputa que tiempo sea el oportuno para administrar la extrema-vncion y se defiende ser en el que el medico ordena el viatico al enfermo*. Sevilla: Lucas martín de Hermosilla.

Bonah, Christian. 2002. "Experimental Rage: the Development of Medical Ethics and the Genesis of Scientific Facts." *Social History of Medicine*. 15: 187–207.

Bonah, Christian. 2003. "Le drame de Lübeck; la vaccination BCG, le 'procès Calmette' et les Richtlinien de 1931." In *La Médecine Expérimentale au Tribunal: Implications Éthiques de quelques Procès Médicaux du Xxe siècle Européen*, edited by Christian Bonah, Etienne Lepicard, and Volker Roelcke, 65–94. Paris: Editions des Archives Contemporaines.

Bonati, Maurizio Rippa. 1994. "L'anatomia "teatrale" nelle descrizioni e nell'iconografia." In *Il Teatro Anatomico: Storia e restauri*, edited by Camillo Semenzato, 55–81. Limena/Padua: Offset Invicta.

Bonnar, Alphonsus. 1939. *The Catholic Doctor*. 2nd ed. London: Burns, Oates, and Washbourne.

Bonner, Thomas Neville. 1992. *To the Ends of the Earth: Women's Search for Education in Medicine*. Cambridge MA: Harvard University Press.

Boorse, Christopher. 1975. "On the Distinction Between Disease and Illness." *Philosophy and Public Affairs*. 5: 49–68.

Booth, Christopher. 1994. "Obituary." *British Medical Journal*. 309: 1577–8.

Borisov, Peter Ya. 1902a. "Obzor deayatel'nosti tovarisheskikh besed chlenov S-Peterburgskogo Vrachebnogo obshestva vzaimnoi pomoshi." *Vestnik Sankt-Peterburgskogo Vrachebnogo Obshestva Vzaimnoi Pomoshi*. 1: 28–38.

Borisov, Peter Ya. 1902b. "Retsenzija na knigu Albert Moll Aertzliche Ethik." *Russkii Vrach*. 17: 669–70.

Boston Medical Association. 1852. *The Medical Police and Rules and Regulations of the Boston Medical Association*. Boston: Boston Medical Association.

Botting, Jack H., ed. 1992. *Animal Experimentation and the Future of Medical Research*. London: Portland Press.

Boudewyns, Michiel. 1666. *Ventilabrum Medico-Theologicum*. Antwerp: Cornelius Woons.

Bouillon-Jensen, Cindy. 1995. "Infants: II. History of Infanticide." *Encyclopedia Of Bioethics*. 2nd ed., edited by Warren T. Reich, 1200–6. New York: Simon and Schuster Macmillan.

Bouillon-Jensen, Cindy, and David Larson. 2004. "Infanticide." *Encyclopedia Of Bioethics*. 3rd ed., edited by Stephen Post, 1236–44. New York: Thomson-Gale.

Bowen, Donna L. 1997. "Abortion, Islam, and the 1994 Cairo Population Conference." *International Journal of Middle East Studies*. 29: 161–84.

Boyd, Ann, Pinit Ratanakul, and Attajenda Deepudong. 1998. "Compassion as Common Ground." *Eubios Journal of Asian and International Bioethics*. 8: 34–7.

Boyd, Kenneth M., ed. 1979. *The Ethics of Resource Allocation in Health Care*. Edinburgh: Edinburgh University Press.

Boyd, Kennth M., ed. 1987. *The Pond Report on the Teaching of Medical Ethics*. London: IME Publications.

Boyd, Kenneth M. 1995. "What Can Medical Ethics Learn from History?" *Journal of Medical Ethics*. 21: 197–8.

Boyle, James David (Interviewer). 1968. "Andrew Conway Ivy: transcript of an oral history, interviewed by James David Boyle, Nov. 4, 1968." Bethesda MD: National Library of Medicine, Unique ID: 2935142R.

Boyle, John P. 1979. "The Ordinary Magisterium: Towards a History of the Concept." *Heythrop Journal*. 20: 380–98.

Boyle, Robert. 1744. *The Works of the Honourable Robert Boyle*. 5 vols. London: A. Millar.

Brain, Peter. 1977. "Galen on the Ideal of the Physician." *South African Medical Journal*. 52: 936–8.

Brand, Ulrich. 1977. *Ärztliche Ethik im 19. Jahrhundert: Der Wandel ethischer Inhalte im medizinischen Schrifttum. Ein Beitrag zum Verständnis der Arzt-Patient-Beziehung*. Freiburg: H. F. Schulz Verlag.

Brandt, Allan M. 1985. *No Magic Bullet: A Social History of Venereal Disease in the United States since 1880*. New York: Oxford University Press.

Brandt, Richard B. [1972] 1974. "The Morality of Abortion." *The Monist*. 56: 504–26. Reprinted in *Abortion: Pro and Con*, edited by Robert L. Perkins, 151–69. Cambridge MA: Schenkman.

Braun, Lucien. 1988. *Paracelsus, Alchimist, Chemiker, Erneuerer der Heilkunde: Eine Bildbiographie*. Zürich: SV International/Schweizer Verlagshaus.

Bray, Francesca. 1997. *Technology and Gender: Fabric of Power in Late Imperial China*. Berkeley CA: University of California Press.

Breck, John. 1998. *The Sacred Gift of Life*. Crestwood NY: St. Vladimir's Seminary Press.

Breen, Louise A. 1991. "Cotton Mather, the 'Angelical Ministry,' and Inoculation." *Journal of the History of Medicine and Allied Sciences*. 46: 333–57.

Brennan, Troyan A. 1999. "Proposed Revisions to the Declaration of Helsinki – Will They Weaken the Ethical Principles Underlying Human Research?" *New England Journal of Medicine*. 341: 527–31.

Brennan, Troyen A., and Donald Berwick. 1996. *New Rules: Regulation, Markets and the Quality of American Health Care*. San Francisco CA: Jossey Bass.

Brewer, John Sherren. 1859. *Fratris Rogeri Bacon Opera quaedam hactenus inedita*. London: Longman, Green, Roberts.

Brierley, J. B., et al. 1971. "Neocortical Death after Cardiac Arrest: A Clinical, Neurophysiological, and Neuropathological Report of Two Cases." *The Lancet*. 2: 560–5.

Brimelow, Peter. 1995. *Alien Nation: Common Sense about America's Immigration Disaster*. New York: Random House.

Brinker, Wendy. 2000. "J. Marion Sims: One Among Many Monumental Mistakes: A Biographical Sketch." *Chicken Bones: A Journal for Literary and Artistic African-American Themes*. http://www.nathanielturner.com/jmarionsims.htm/ (visited January 30, 2008).

Brinton, D. G. 1879. "Memorial: Isaac Hays." *Proceedings of the American Philosophical Society*. 18: 259–60.

British Foreign Office. 1949. *Scientific Results of German Medical War Crimes*. London: HMSO.

British Medical Association, Working Party. 1992. *Medicine Betrayed: The Participation of Doctors in Human Rights Abuses*. London: Zed Books Ltd.

Brock, Thomas D. 1999. *Robert Koch: A Life in Medicine and Bacteriology*. Washington DC: ASM Press.

Brockliss, Laurence, and Colin Jones. 1997. *The Medical World of Early Modern France*. Oxford: Clarendon Press.

Brodie, Sir Benjamin C. 1843. *Introductory Discourse on the Duty and Conduct of Medical Students and Practitioners: Addressed to the Students of the Medical School of St. Georges*

Hosptial, October 2, 1843. London: Longman, Brown, Green, and Longmans.

Brody, Baruch A. 1975. *Abortion and the Sanctity of Human Life*. Cambridge MA: MIT Press.

Brody, Baruch A. 1983. "The Use of Halakhic Material in Discussions of Medical Ethics." *Journal of Medicine and Philosophy*. 8: 317–28.

Brody, Baruch A. 1998. *The Ethics of Biomedical Research: An International Perspective*. Oxford/New York: Oxford University Press.

Brody, Baruch A. 2002. "Ethical Issues in Clinical Trials in Developing Countries." *Statistics in Medicine*. 21: 2853–88.

Brody, Howard. 1976. *Ethical Decisions in Medicine*. New York: Little Brown.

Brody, Howard, Zahara Meghani, and Kimberly Ann Greenwald, eds. 2009. *Michael Ryan's Writings on Medical Ethics*. Dordrecht: Kluwer Academic Publishers.

Bron, T. 1928. "Vrachebnaya etika." In *Bolshaya Meditsynskaya Entsyclopedija*. 1st ed., vol. 5, edited by N. A. Semashko, 584–6. Moscow: Sovetskaya Entsyclopedija.

Brouardel, Paul. 1893a. *La Profession Médicale au Commencement du XXe Siècle*. Paris: Baillière.

Brouardel, Paul. 1893b. *Le Secret Médical*. 2nd ed. Paris: Baillière.

Brown, John. 1850. *Review of Works On Medical Ethics by Thomas Percival and Others*. Edinburgh: Murray & Gibb.

Browne, Edward G. 1921. *Arabian Medicine*. London: Cambridge University Press.

Browne, Oswald. 1894. *On the Care of the Dying: A Lecture to Nurses*. London: George Allen.

Brundage, B. M. 1947. United States Army Medical Division. Memorandum to Declassification Section, 19 March.

Brunfels, Otto. 1532. *Contrafact Kreuterbuch*. Strassburg: Hans Schotten.

Bruns, Paul. 1979. "The Man André." *Kennedy Institute Quarterly Report*. 5 (1).

Buchan, William. 1769. *Domestic Medicine, or the Family Physician*. Edinburgh: Balfour, Auld and Smellie.

Buchanan, Allen E. 1996. "Is There a Medical Profession in the House?" In *Conflicts of Interest in Clinical Practice and Research*, edited by Robert G. Speece, D. S. Shimm, and Allen E. Buchanan, 105–36. New York: Oxford University Press.

Buchanan, Allen E., et al. 2000. *From Chance to Choice: Genetics and Justice*. New York: Cambridge University Press.

Büchner, Franz. [1941] 1985. "Der Eid des Hippokrates: Wortlaut des am 18. November 1941 in der Aula der Universität Freiburg gehaltenen öffentlichen Vortages." In Franz Büchner *Der Mensch in der Sicht moderner Medizin*, 131–51. Freiburg/Basel/Wien: Herder.

Buck v. Bell. 274 U.S. 200. (1927).

Buess, Heinrich. 1946. *Die historischen Grundlagen der intravenösen Injektion*. Aarau: Sauerländer.

Buḫārī, Muḥammad b. Ismāʿīl Ibrāhīm b. al-Muġīra. 1985. *Ṣaḥīḥ al-Buḫārī*. 9 vols., translated by Muhammad M. Khan (Arabic to English). Bairūt: Dar al-Arabia.

Bürgel, Johann Christoph. 1966. "Die 'Bildung des Arztes': Eine arabische Schrift zum ärztlichen Leben aus dem 9. Jahrhundert." *Sudhoffs Archiv*. 50: 337–60.

Bürgel, Johann Christoph. 1967a. "Adab und ictidāl in ar-Ruhāwīs Adab aṭ-Ṭabīb." *Zeitschrift der Deutschen Morgenländischen Gesellschaft*. 117: 90–102.

Bürgel, Johann Christoph. 1967b. "Die wissenschaftliche Medizin im Kräftefeld der islamischen Kultur." In *Bustan: Österreichische Zeitschrift für Kultur, Politik und Wirtschaft der islamischen Länder*, no.1: 9–19.

Bürgel, Johann Christoph. 1970. "Untersuchungen zum ärztlichen Leben und Denken im arabischen Mittelalter." Habil. diss., University of Göttingen.

Bürgel, Johann Christoph. 1973. "Psychosomatic Methods of Cures in the Islamic Middle Ages." *Humaniora Islamica*. 1: 157–72.

Bürgel, Johann Christoph. 1991. *Allmacht und Mächtigkeit, Religion und Welt im Islam*. München: C. H. Beck.

Burguiere, Paul, Danielle Gourevitch, and Yves Malinas, eds. and trans. 1988–1994. *Soranos d'Ephese: Maladies des Femmes*. 3 vols. Paris: Les Belles Lettres.

Burke, M. E. 1977. *The Royal College of San Carlos: Surgery and Spanish Medical Reform in the Late Eighteenth Century*. Durham NC: Duke University Press.

Burleigh, Michael. 1994. *Death and Deliverance: "Euthanasia" in Germany, 1900–1945*. Cambridge/New York: Cambridge University Press.

Burleigh, Michael, ed. 1996a. *Confronting the Nazi Past: New Debates on Modern German History*. London: Collins & Brown.

Burleigh, Michael. 1996b. "Saving Money, Spending Lives: Psychiatry, Society, and the "Euthanasia" Programme." In *Confronting the Nazi Past: New Debates on Modern German History*, edited by Michael Burleigh, 98–111. London: Collins & Brown.

Burleigh, Michael. 1997. *Ethics and Extermination: Reflections on Nazi Genocide*. Cambridge/New York: Cambridge University Press.

Burleigh, Michael, and Wolfgang Wippermann. 1991. *The Racial State: Germany 1933–1945*. Cambridge/New York: Cambridge University Press.

Burnham, John C. 1998. *How the Concept of Profession Changed the Writing of Medical History*. London: Wellcome Institute for the History of Medicine.

Burnham, John C. 1999. "A Brief History of Medical Practitioners and Professional Historians as Writers of Medical History." *Health & History*. 1: 250–73.

Burns, Chester R. 1967. "Worthington Hooker: Physician, Teacher, Reformer." *Yale Medicine*. 2 (2): 17–8.

Burns, Chester R. 1969a. "Malpractice Suits in American Medicine before the Civil War." *Bulletin of the History of Medicine.* 43: 41–56.

Burns, Chester R. 1969b. "Medical Ethics in the United States before the Civil War." Ph.D. diss., Johns Hopkins University, Maryland.

Burns, Chester R., ed. 1977a. *Legacies in Ethics and Medicine.* New York: Science History Publications.

Burns, Chester R. 1977b. "Reciprocity in the development of Anglo-American medical ethics, 1765–1865." In *Legacies in Ethics and Medicine,* edited by Chester R. Burns, 300–6. New York: Science History Publications.

Burns, Chester R. 1995a. "History of Medical Ethics: V. The Americas: A. Colonial North America and Nineteenth-Century United States." In *Encyclopedia of Bioethics.* 2nd ed., edited by Warren Reich, 1610–6. New York: Simon & Schuster Macmillan.

Burns, Chester R. 1995b. "Reciprocity in the development of Anglo-American medical ethics, 1765–1865." In *The Codification of Medical Morality: Historical and Philosophical Studies of the Formalization of Western Medical Morality in the Eighteenth and Nineteenth Centuries: Volume Two: Anglo-American Medical Ethics and Medical Jurisprudence in the Nineteenth Century,* edited by Robert Baker, 135–43. Boston: Kluwer Academic Publishers.

Burns, Chester R. 1999a. "Setting the Stage: Moral Philosophy, Benjamin Rush, and Medical Ethics in the United States before 1846." In *The American Medical Ethics Revolution: How the AMA's Code of Ethics Has Transformed Physicians' Relationships to Patients, Professionals, and Society,* edited by Robert Baker et al., 3–16. Baltimore: Johns Hopkins University Press.

Burns, Chester R. 1999b. "Worthington Hooker." *American National Biography,* edited by John A. Garraty and Mark C. Carnes, vol. 11, 139–40. New York: Oxford University Press.

Burns, Chester R. 2000. "Writing the History of Medical Ethics: A New Era for the New Millenium." *Medical Humanities Review.* 14: 35–41.

Burrell, David B. 1993. *Freedom and Creation in Three Traditions.* Notre Dame IN: University of Notre Dame Press.

Bussche, Hendrik van den. 1989a. *Im Dienste der "Volksgemeinschaft." Studienreform im Nationalsozialismus am Beispiel der ärztlichen Ausbildung.* Berlin: Dietrich Reimer.

Bussche, Hendrik van den, ed. 1989b. *Medizinische Wissenschaft im "Dritten Reich." Kontinuität, Anpassung und Opposition an der Hamburger Medizinischen Fakultät.* Berlin: Dietrich Reimer.

Butterfield, Herbert. 1931. *The Whig Interpretation of History.* London: G. Bell and Sons.

Bylebyl, Jerome. 1991. "Teaching Methodus Medendi in the Renaissance." In *Galen's Method of Teaching,* edited by F. Kudlien and R. J. Durling, 157–89. Leiden: E. J. Brill.

Bynum, William F. 1980. "Health, Disease and Medical Care." In *The Ferment of Knowledge: Studies in the Historiography of Eighteenth-Century Science,* edited by G. S. Rousseau and Roy Porter, 211–54. Cambridge UK: Cambridge University Press.

Bynum, William F. 1994. *Science and the Practice of Medicine in the Nineteenth Century.* Cambridge UK: Cambridge University Press.

Bynum, William F., E. J. Browne, and Roy Porter, eds. 1981. *Dictionary of the History of Science.* Princeton NJ: Princeton University Press.

Bynum, William F., and Roy Porter, eds. 1987. *Medical Fringe & Medical Orthodoxy 1750–1850.* London: Croon Helm.

Byrne, Paul A., Sean O'Reilly, and Paul M. Quay. 1979. "Brain Death – An Opposing Viewpoint." *Journal of the American Medical Association.* 242: 1985–90.

Cabanis, Pierre-Jean-Georges. 1802. *Rapports du physique et du moral de l'homme.* Paris: Crapart, Caille et Ravier libraries.

Cabanis, Pierre-Jean-Georges. 1816. *El grado de certidumbre en medicina: memoria escrita en francés por Mr. Cabanis; traducida al castellano de la última edición publicada en agosto de 1803 por Luis Guarnerio y Allavenia.* Madrid: Imprenta de Repullés.

Cahill, Lisa Sowle. 1995. "Abortion: III. Religious Traditions: B. Roman Catholic Perspectives." In *Encyclopedia of Bioethics.* 2nd ed., edited by Warren T. Reich, 30–4. New York: Simon & Schuster Macmillan.

Callahan, Daniel. 1970. *Abortion: Law, Choice, and Morality.* New York: Macmillan.

Callahan, Daniel. 1973. "Bioethics as a Discipline." *Hastings Center Studies.* 1: 66–73.

Callahan, Daniel. 1987. *Setting Limits: Medical Goals in an Aging Society.* New York: Simon and Shuster.

Callahan, Daniel. 1990. *What Kind of Life: The Limits of Medical Progress.* New York: Simon and Shuster.

Callahan, Daniel. 2000. "Freedom, Healthism, and Health Promotion: Finding the Right Balance." In *Promoting Healthy Behavior: How Much Freedom? Whose Responsibility?,* edited by Daniel Callahan, 138–52. Washington DC: Georgetown University Press.

Callahan, Daniel. 2003. *What Price Better Health? Hazards of the Research Imperative.* Berkeley CA: University of California Press.

Campbell, Alastair V. 1972. *Moral Dilemmas in Medicine: A Coursebook in Ethics for Doctors and Nurses.* Edinburgh: Churchill Livingstone.

Campbell, Alastair V. 2000. "My Country tis of Thee'– The Myopia of American Bioethics." *Medicine, Health Care and Philosophy.* 3: 195–8.

Campbell, Courtney S. 2000. "Religious Views on Biotechnology: Protestant." In *Encyclopedia of Ethical, Legal, and Policy Issues in Biotechnology,* edited by

Thomas J. Murray and Maxwell J. Mehlman, 938–47. New York: John Wiley & Sons.

Canan, İbrahim. 1988. *Kütüb-i Sitte Muhtasarı Tercüme ve Şerhi*. 18 vols. Ankara: Akçağ.

Cangiamila, Francesco. 1774. *Embriología Sagrada o Tratado de la obligación que tienen los curas, confesores, médicos, comadres, y otras personas, de cooperar á la salvación de los niños que aun no han nacido, de los que nacen al parecer muertos, de los abortivos, de los monstruos, &c; reducida á compendio, y puesta en francés con varias adiciones por Mr. El Abate Dinouart; y traducida del frances al castellano por Joaquin Castellot*. Vol. 2. Madrid: Imprenta de Pedro Marin.

Cannon, Bradford. 1994. "Walter Bradford Cannon: Reflections on the Man and His Contributions." *International Journal of Stress Management*. 1 (2).

Cannon, Walter Bradford. 1909. "The Responsibility of the General for Freedom of Medical Research." *Boston Medical Surgical Journal*. 161: 430.

Cannon, Walter Bradford. 1911. *The Mechanical Factors of Digestion*. New York: Longmans, Green & Co.

Cannon, Walter Bradford. 1915, 1920, 1929. *Bodily Changes in Pain, Hunger, Fear, and Rage: an account of recent researches into the function of emotional excitement*. New York: D. Appleton and Co.

Cannon, Walter Bradford. 1916. "The Right and Wrong of Making Experiments on Human Beings." *Journal of the American Medical Association*. 67: 1372–3.

Cannon, Walter Bradford. 1923. *Traumatic Shock*. New York: Appleton.

Cannon, Walter Bradford. 1932, 1939. *The Wisdom of the Body*. New York: W. W. Norton.

Cannon, Walter Bradford. 1945. *The Way of an Investigator: A Scientist's Experiences in Medical Research*. New York: W. W. Norton.

Cannon, Walter Bradford, and William Beaumont. 1933. *Experiments and Observations on the Gastric Juice and the Physiology of Digestion: Some modern extensions of Beaumont's studies on Alexis St. Martin*. The Beaumont Foundation lectures [no. 12].

Cannon, Walter Bradford, and Arturo Rosenblueth. 1949. *The Supersensitivity of Denervated Structures; a Law of Denervation*. New York: Macmillan.

Cantor, David, ed. 2002. *Reinventing Hippocrates*. Aldershot: Ashgate.

Capellmann, Carl. 1879. *Pastoral Medicine*. New York: Fr. Pustet.

Caplan, Arthur L. 1988. "Professional Arrogance and Public Misunderstanding." *Hastings Center Report*. 18: 34–37.

Caplan, Arthur L., ed. 1992. *When Medicine Went Mad: Bioethics and the Holocaust*. Totowa NJ: Humana Press.

Capron, Alexander, and Leon Kass. 1972. "A Statutory Definition of the Standards for Determining Human Death: An Appraisal and a Proposal." *University of Pennsylvania Law Review*. 121: 87–118.

Caraka Saṃhitā: Text with English Translation and Critical Exposition Based on Cakrapāṇi Datta's Āyurveda Dīpikā. 1976–1977. Vol. 1–2. First Edition. Varanasi, Chowkhamba Sanskrit Series Office.

Caramuel, Juan. 1645. *Theologia Moralis: Ad prima eaque clarissima principia reducta*. Lovanii: Petri Zangrii.

Cariage, J. L. 1959. *L' Exercice de la Médecine en France à la fin du XIXe Siècle*. Besançon: Priv. Printed.

Carlos II (of Spain). 1680. *Recopilación de las leyes de los reinos de Indias*. Madrid: n. p.

Carrell, Alexis. [1936] 1988. *Man the Unknown*. New York: Harper & Brothers.

Carrick, Paul. 1985. *Medical Ethics in Antiquity: Philosophical Perspectives on Abortion and Euthanasia*. Dordrecht: Reidel.

Carter, Jennifer J., and Joan H. Pittock, eds. *Aberdeen and the Enlightenment: Proceedings of a Conference Held at the University of Aberdeen*. Aberdeen: Aberdeen University Press.

Carvais, Robert. 1986. "Le Microbe et la Résponsabilité Médicale." In *Pasteur et la Révolution Pastorienne*, edited by Claire Salomon-Bayet, 217–75. Paris: Payot.

Casberg, Melvin A. 1952. United States Department of Defense Armed Forces Medical Policy Council. Memorandum to the Secretary of Defense, 24 December.

Casberg, Melvin A. 1953. United States Department of Defense Armed Forces Medical Policy Council. Memorandum to the Secretary of Defense, 13 January.

Cassedy, James H. 1962. *Charles V. Chapin and the Public Health Movement*. Cambridge MA: Harvard University Press.

Cassedy, James H. 1991. *Medicine in America: A Short History*. Baltimore: Johns Hopkins University Press.

Cassine, Léon. n.d. *Le Médecin dans la Société Actuelle*. Saint-Quintin: Baudry-Baudry.

Cassiodor. 1894. "Cassiodori Senatoris Variae." *Monumenta Germaniae Historica*. 12, 191f, edited by Theodor Mommsen. Berlin: Weidmann.

Cassiodor. 1937. *Cassiodoris Senatoris Institutiones*, edited by R. A. B. Mynors. Oxford: Clarendon Press.

Castro, Rodnezia. 1614. *Roderici à Castro Lusitani Philosophorum et Medicorum Doctoris per Europam Notissimi Medicus politicus sive De Officiis Medico-Politicis Tractatus, Quatuor distinctus Libris*. Hamburg: Zacharias Hertel.

Castro, Rodrigo de. 1614. *Medicus-politicus; sive, De officiis medico-politicis tractatus, quatuor distinctus libris*. Hamburg: Frobenianus.

Catechism of the Catholic Church. 2000. 2nd ed. Vatican City: Liberia Editrice Vaticana.

Cathell, D. W. 1898. *Book on the Physician Himself and Things that Concern His Reputation and Success.* 10th ed. Philadelphia: F. A. Davis Co.

Celsus, Aulus Cornelius. 1915. *De Medicina,* edited by Friedrich Marx. Lipsiae: Tuebner.

Celsus, Aulus Cornelius. 1935–1938. *De Medicina, with an English Translation by W. G. Spencer.* Cambridge MA: Harvard University Press, Loeb Classical Library.

Centers for Disease Control. 1998. "Response to Increases in Cigarette Prices by Race-Ethnicity, Income, and Age Groups – United States, 1976–1993." *Morbidity and Mortality Weekly Report.* 47: 605–9.

Centre for Conflict Resolution, South Africa. *Weekly Reports on the Trial of Dr. Wouter Basson.* http://ccrweb.ccr.uct.ac.za/cbw (visited June 3, 2000).

Chaadaev, Peter Ya. 1906. *Philosophicheskie Pis'ma.* Perevod s frantsuzskogo M. O. Gershenzona. Moscow: I. N. Kushnerev I Ko.

Chaadaev, Peter Ya. 1969. "The Philosophical Letters Addressed to a Lady: Letter 1." In *The Major Works of Peter Chaadaev,* translation and commentary by Raymond T. McNally, 38–39. Notre Dame IN/London: University of Notre Dame Press.

Chadwick, Edwin. 1842. *Report on the Sanitary Condition of the Labouring Population of Great Britain.* London: Clowes.

Chaicharoen, Pitak, and Pinit Ratanakul. 1998. "Letting-Go or Killing: Thai Buddhist Perspectives on Euthanasia." *Eubios Journal of Asian and International Bioethics.* 8: 37–40.

Chalmers, Iain, et al., eds. 2003. *The James Lind Library: Documenting the Evolution of Fair Trials.* www.jameslindlibrary.org (visited November 16, 2007).

Chamber of Physicians of West Germany. [1947] 1949. "Proceedings: June 14, 1947; October 18, 1947; November 29, 1947." *World Medical Association Bulletin.* 1: 9.

Chambers, Tod. 1998. "Retrodiction and the Histories of Bioethics." *Medical Humanities Review.* 12: 9–22.

Chan, J. 1998. "From Chinese Bioethics to Human Cloning: A Methodological Reflection." *Chinese and International Philosophy of Medicine.* 1: 49–71. [Chinese].

Chan, Wing-Tsit. 1963. *A Source Book in Chinese Philosophy.* Princeton NJ: Princeton University Press.

Chandler, Brooks, Koizumi, Kiyomi, and James O. Pinkston. 1975. *The Life and Contributions of Walter Bradford Cannon, 1871–1945: His Influence on the Development of Physiology in the Twentieth Century.* Albany NY: State University of New York Press.

Chapin, Charles V. 1910. *The Sources and Modes of Infection.* New York: John Wiley.

Chapman, Audrey R., and Leonard S. Rubenstein, eds. 1998. *Human Rights and Health: The Legacy of Apartheid.* Washington DC: American Association for the Advancement of Science.

Chapman, Carleton B. 1984. *Physicians, Law and Ethics.* New York: New York University Press.

Charatan, Fred B. 1996. "Anatomy Textbook has Nazi Origins." *British Medical Journal.* 313: 1422.

Charcot, J. M. 1867. *Leçons Cliniques sur Les Maladies des Vieillards et Les Maladies Chroniques.* Paris: Delahaye.

Chebotareva, E. P. 1970. *Vrachebnaya Etika.* Moscow: Meditsyna.

Chekhov, Anton P. 1987. "Zapisnaya knizhka I." *Sobranie Sochinenii i Pisem v 30 Tomakh.* T. 17, 8. Moscow: Nauka.

Chen, Menglei. [1723] 1962. *Gujin Tushu Jicheng Yibu Quanlu (Collection of Ancient and Modern Books, The Part of Medicine), Book 12: General Discussions, (Volumes 501–520 in original).* Beijing: People's Health Press.

Chen, Rongxia. 2001. "Why Bring Up the Past Tragedy Again?" *Eubios Journal of Asian and International Bioethics.* 11: 107.

Chen, Shou (Jin). 1995. *San Guo Zhi (Annals of the Three Kingdoms).* Beining: Chinese Book House.

Chen, Yuan-Fang. 1997. "Japanese Death Factories and the American Cover-Up." *Cambridge Quarterly of Healthcare Ethics.* 6: 240–2.

Chengappa, R. 1990. "The Organs Bazaar." *India Today,* July 31, 30–7.

Childress, James F. 1970. "Who Shall Live When Not All Can Live?" *Soundings.* 53: 339–55.

Childress, James F. 1989. "Ethical Criteria for Procuring and Distributing Organs for Transplantation." In *Organ Transplantation Policy: Issues and Prospects,* edited by James F. Blumenstein and Frank A. Sloan, 87–113. Durham NC: Duke University Press.

Childress, James F. 2003. "Principles of Biomedical Ethics: Reflections on A Work in Progress." In *The Story of Bioethics: From Seminal Works to Contemporary Explorations,* edited by Jennifer K. Walter and Eran P. Klein, 47–66. Washington DC: Georgetown University Press.

Chinese Central Archive, et al., eds. 1989 [1991–1992]. *(Japanese) Bacteriological and Chemical Warfare.* Beijing: Chinese Bookstore [Translated into Japanese. Tokyo: Dobunkan].

Christianson, Eric H. 1980. "The Medical Practitioners of Massachusetts, 1630–1800: Patterns of Change and Continuity." In *Medicine in Colonial Massachusetts, 1620–1820,* edited by Philip Cash, Eric H. Christianson, and J. Worth Estes, 49–67. Boston: The Colonial Society of Massachusetts.

Christianson, Eric H. 1987. "Medicine in New England." In *Medicine in the New World: New Spain, New France, and New England,* edited by Ronald L. Numbers, 101–53. Knoxville TN: University of Tennessee Press.

Chrysostom, Saint John, 1986. *On Marriage and Family Life*, translated by Catherine Roth and David Anderson. Crestwood NY: St. Vladimir's Seminary Press.

Church Information Office. 1975. *On Dying Well*. London: Church Information Office.

Cicero, Marcus Tullius. 1921. *De Officiis*, translated by Walter Miller. Cambridge MA/New York: Loeb Classical Library, Macmillan.

Clark, Sir George N. 1964–1966. *A History of the Royal College of Physicians of London*. 2 vols. Oxford: Clarendon Press.

Clavijero, Francisco Javier. [1781] 1976. *Historia Antigua de México*. 6th ed. México: Porrúa.

Clement of Alexandria. 1994. "The Stromata." In *Ante-Nicene Fathers*, vol. 2, edited by Alexander Roberts and James Donaldson, 523–67. Peabody MA: Hendrickson Publishers.

Clifford, Terry. 1984. *Tibetan Buddhist Medicine and Psychiatry: The Diamond Healing*. York Beach ME: S. Weiser.

Clinton, William Jefferson. 1997. "Remarks by the President in Apology for Study Done in Tuskegee." Washington DC: The White House. http://clinton4.nara.gov/textonly/New/Remarks/Fri/19970516/898.html (visited January 30, 2008).

Cocks, Geoffrey. 1985. *Psychotherapy in the Third Reich: The Göring Institute*. New York: Oxford University Press.

Codronchi, Giovan Battista. 1591. *De Christiana, ac tuta medendi ratione, ...* Ferrara: Mammarell.

Cohen, I. Bernard. 1985. *Revolution in Science*. Cambridge MA: Belknap Press of Harvard University Press.

Cohen, L. R. 1989. "Increasing the Supply of Transplant Organs: The Virtues of a Futures Market." *George Washington Law Review*. 58: 1–51.

Coleman, William, and Frederic L. Holmes, eds. 1988. *The Investigative Enterprise: Experimental Physiology in Nineteenth-Century Medicine*. Berkeley CA: University of California Press.

Cole-Turner, Ronald. 1993. *The New Genesis: Theology and the Genetic Revolution*. Louisville KY: Westminster/John Knox Press.

Cole-Turner, Ronald. 1997. *Human Cloning: Religious Responses*. Philadelphia: Westminster/John Knox Press.

College of Physicians of London. n.d. *Annals of the College of Physicians of London*, typescript transcription and translation by the Royal College of Physicians.

Colombo, Realdo. [1559] 1983. *De re anatomica libri XV*. Reprint. Brussels: Culture et Civilisation.

Colón, Cristóbal. [1492–1506] 1982. *Textos y documentos completes*, edited by Consuelo Varela. Madrid: Alianza Editorial.

Committee on Tipping. 2000. *Jelentés az orvosi hálapénzről: Helyzetelemzés és következtetések (Report on Medical Tipping: Situation Analysis and Conclusions)*. Budapest: Springer Orvosi Kiadó Kft (Springer Medical Publisher Limited).

Comte Rendu de la Première Session de Congrès International de Médicine Professional. 1900. Paris: Masson.

Condrochius, Baptista. 1591. *De Christiana, ac Tuta Medendi Ratione*. Ferrara: Mammarellus.

Cong, Y. 1998. "Ethical Challenges in Critical Care Medicine: A Chinese Perspective." *Journal of Medicine and Philosophy*. 23: 581–600.

Congar, Yves. 1982a. "A Brief History of the Forms of the Magisterium and Its Relations with Scholars." In *Readings in Moral Theology No. 3: The Magisterium and Morality*, edited by Charles E. Curran and Richard A. McCormick, 314–31. New York: Paulist Press.

Congar, Yves. 1982b. "A Semantic History of the Term 'Magisterium'." In *Readings in Moral Theology No. 3: The Magisterium and Morality*, edited by Charles E. Curran and Richard A. McCormick, 297–313. New York: Paulist Press.

Congregation for the Doctrine of the Faith. 1987. *Donum Vitae*. www.seminarianlifelink.org.

Connery, John R. 1978. "Abortion III: Roman Catholic Perspectives." In *Encyclopedia of Bioethics*, edited by Warren T. Reich, 9–13. New York: Macmillan.

Conrad, Lawrence I. 1985. "The Social Structure of Medicine in Medieval Islam." *The Society for the Social History of Medicine Bulletin*. 37: 11–15.

Constantelos, Demetrios J. 1991. *Byzantine Philanthropy and Social Welfare*. 2nd ed. New Rochelle NY: Aristide Caratzas.

"Constitution of Sri Lanka." *Official Website of the Government of Sri Lanka*. http://www.priu.gov.lk/Cons/1978Constitution/Introduction.htm (visited January 30, 2008).

Cook, Harold J. 1986. *The Decline of the Old Medical Regime in Stuart London*. Ithaca NY: Cornell University Press.

Cook, Harold J. 1990. "The Rose Case Reconsidered: Physicians, Apothecaries, and the Law in Augustan England." *Journal of the History of Medicine and Allied Sciences*. 45: 527–55.

Cook, Harold J. 1995. "History of Medical Ethics: IV. Europe: B. Renaissance and Enlightenment." In *Encyclopedia of Bioethics*. 2nd ed., edited by Warren T. Reich, 1537–43. New York: Simon & Schuster Macmillan.

Cook-Deegan, Robert. 1994. *The Gene Wars: Science, Politics, and the Human Genome*. New York: W. W. Norton.

Cooper, David E. 2002. "The 'Frankensteinian' Nature of Biotechnology." In *Historical and Philosophical Perspectives on Biomedical Ethics: From Paternalism to Autonomy?*, edited by Andreas-Holger Maehle and Johanna Geyer-Kordesch, 139–49. Aldershot: Ashgate.

Cooter, Roger. 1984. *Cultural Meaning of Modern Science: Phrenology and the Organization of Consent in 19th Century Britain*. Cambridge UK: Cambridge University Press.

Cooter, Roger. 1995. "The Resistible Rise of Medical Ethics." *Social History of Medicine.* 8: 257–70.

Cooter, Roger. 2000. "The Ethical Body." In *Medicine in the Twentieth Century,* edited by Roger Cooter and John Pickstone, 451–68. Amsterdam: Harwood Academic Publishers.

Coppens, Charles. 1897. *Moral Principles and Medical Practice: The Basis of Medical Jurisprudence.* New York: Benziger Brothers.

Cornarius, Janus. 1545. *Hippocratis Coi medicorum omnium longe principis opera . . . per Ianum Cornarium medicum physicum lingua Latina conscripta.* Basel Froben.

Cortés, Hernán. [1522] 1976. *Cartas de Relación.* 9th ed. México: Porrúa.

Cotta, John. 1612. *A Short Discoverie of the Unobserved Dangers of Several Sorts of Ignorant and Unconsiderate Practisers of Physicke in England.* London: Imprinted for William Iones, and Richard Boyle dwelling in the Blacke-Friars.

Cotten, Richard. 1993. "American Dissident Voices." *Minuteman Bulletin Board.* (September 11).

Coulter, Harris L. 1975. *Divided Legacy: A history of the Schism in Medical Thought. Vol. 1, The Patterns Emerge: Hippocrates to Paracelsus.* Washington DC: Wehawken Book Co.

Council in Ancyra. 1983. "The Twenty-Five Canons of the Holy Regional Council Held in Ancyra." In *The Rudder of the Orthodox Catholic Church,* edited by Sts. Nicodemus and Agapius, translated by D. Cummings, 489–505. New York: Luna Printing.

Council of Europe. 1996. "Convention for Protection of Human Rights and Dignity of the Human Being with Regard to the Application of Biology and Biomedicine: Convention on Human Rights and Biomedicine." *Kennedy Institute of Ethics Journal.* 7: 277–90.

Council of Europe. 1997a. *Convention for the Protection of Human Rights and Dignity of the Human Being with Regard to the Application of Biology and Medicine: Convention on Human Rights and Biomedicine.* www.conventions. coe.int/treaty/en/treaties/html/164.htm (visited November 16, 2007).

Council of Europe. 1997b. "Convention for the Protection of Human Rights and Dignity of the Human Being with Regard to the Application of Biology and Medicine." *Convention on Human Rights and Biomedicine,* (Orviedo, U. IV, 1997). European Treaty Series, No. 164.

Council of Europe. 2000. *Convention on Human Rights and Biomedicine.* http://conventions.coe.int (visited November 16, 2007).

Council of Europe Steering Committee on Bioethics. 1997. *Convention on Human Rights and Biomedicine.* Oviedo. www.coe.int/T/E/Legal_affairs/Legal_co-operation/Bioethics/ (visited November 16, 2007).

Council of Europe Steering Committee on Bioethics. 2002. *Chart of signatures and ratifications of the Convention on Human Rights and Biomedicine, the Protocol on the Prohibition of Cloning Human Beings, and the Protocol concerning Transplantation of Organs and Tissues of Human Origin.* www.coe.int/T/E/Legal_affairs/Legal_co-operation/Bioethics/ (visited November 16, 2007).

Council of International Organizations of Medical Sciences. 1993. *International Ethical Guidelines for Biomedical Research involving Human Subjects.* www.cioms.ch. (visited November 16, 2007).

Council for International Organizations of Medical Sciences and the World Health Organization. 1993. *International Ethical Guidelines for Biomedical Research Involving Human Subjects.* Geneva: CIOMS, WHO.

Crawford, Catherine. 1993. "Medicine and the Law." In *Companion Encyclopedia of the History of Medicine,* edited by William F. Bynum and Roy Porter, 1619–40. London/New York: Routledge.

Crawford, Catherine. 1994. "Legalizing Medicine: Early Modern Legal Systems and the Growth of Medico-Legal Knowledge." In *Legal Medicine in History,* edited by Michael Clark and Catherine Crawford, 89–116. Cambridge UK: Cambridge University Press.

Crawford, Catherine. 2000. "Patients' Rights and the Law of Contract in Eighteenth-Century England." *Social History of Medicine.* 13: 381–410.

Cressy, David. 1997. *Birth, Marriage and Death: Ritual, Religion and the Life Cycle in Tudor and Stuart England.* Oxford: Oxford University Press.

Crocker, Lester. 1991. "Introduction." In *The Blackwell Companion to the Enlightenment,* edited by John W. Yolton, et. al., 1–10. London: Blackwell Publishers.

Cronin, Archibald Joseph. [1937] 1965. *The Citadel.* Boston: Little Brown.

Crowther, M. Anne. 1995. "Forensic Medicine and Medical Ethics in Nineteenth-Century Britain." In *The Codification of Medical Morality: Historical and Philosophical Studies of the Formalization of Western Medical Morality in the Eighteenth and Nineteenth Centuries: Volume Two: Anglo American Medical Ethics and Medical Jurisprudence in the Nineteenth Century,* edited by Robert Baker, 173–90. Boston: Kluwer Academic Publishers.

Cruzan v. Director, Missouri Department of Health. 111 Led2d 225, SCT 2841. (1990).

Cui, H. 1999. "Patients' Determination vs. Physicians' Beneficence." *Chinese and International Philosophy of Medicine.* 2: 83–93 [Chinese].

Cullen, Christopher. 1993. "Patients and Healers in Late Imperial China: Evidence from the Jinpingmei." *History of Science.* 31: 99–150.

Cullen, William. 1768. *Clinical Lectures of Doct' W'' Cullen . . . delivered in the Royal Infirmary of Edinburgh 1768 & 1769.* Student notes, author unknown. MS 1/9/7. Glasgow: Royal College of Physicians and Surgeons of Glasgow.

Cullen, William. n.d. *Clinical Lectures by William Cullen.* Notes by Dr. Rhodes. Cage 10a-247, Lecture 6, Section 1. Philadelphia: College of Physicians of Philadelphia.

Culpeper, Nicholas. 1649. *A Physical Directory or a Translation of the London Dispensary Made by the College of Physicians of London.* London: P. Cole.

Cunningham, Andrew, and Perry Williams, eds. 1992. *The Laboratory Revolution in Medicine.* Cambridge UK: Cambridge University Press.

Cunningham, Lawrence S., et al. 1993. "Veritatis Splendor." *Commonweal.* 12. 18 (October 22): 11–18.

Curran, Charles E. 1975. *Ongoing Revision: Studies in Moral Theology.* Notre Dame IN: Fides.

Curran, Charles E. 1977. "Utilitarianism and Contemporary Moral Theology." *Louvain Studies* 6: 239–55.

Curran, Charles E. 1985. *Directions in Fundamental Moral Theology.* Notre Dame IN: University of Notre Dame Press.

Curran, Charles E. 1986. *Faithful Dissent.* Kansas City MO: Sheed and Ward.

Curran, Charles E. 1995. "Roman Catholicism." In *Encyclopedia of Bioethics.* 2nd ed., edited by Warren T. Reich, 2321–31. New York: Simon & Schuster Macmillan.

Curran, Charles E. 2003. "The Catholic Moral Tradition in Bioethics." In *The Story of Bioethics: From Seminal Works to Contemporary Explorations,* edited by Jennifer K. Walter and Eran P. Klein, 113–30. Washington DC: Georgetown University Press.

Curran, Charles E. 2005. "A Place for Dissent: My Argument with Joseph Ratziner." *Commonweal.* 132.9 (May 6): 18–20.

Curran, Charles E., and Richard A. McCormick, eds. 1988. *Dissent in the Church.* New York: Paulist Press.

Currie, James. 1804. *Medical Reports on the Effects of Water, Cold and Warm as a Remedy in ever and Febrile Diseases,* vol. 2. Liverpool/London: McCreery and Cadell.

Dahl, Matthias. 1998. *Endstation Spiegelgrund: Die Tötung behinderter Kinder während des Nationalsozialismus am Beispiel einer Kinderfachabteilung in Wien 1940 bis 1945.* Vienna: Erasmus.

Daiches, W. S. 1986. *The Scottish Enlightenment: An Introduction.* Edinburgh: The Saltire Society.

Daniels, Norman. 1985. *Just Health Care.* New York: Cambridge University Press.

Daniels, Norman. 1988. *Am I My Parents Keeper? An Essay on Justice Between the Young and Old.* Oxford: Oxford University Press.

Danilevsky, Vladimir Ya. 1921. *Vrach, Ego Prizvanie i Obrazovanie.* Khar'kov.

Danish Council of Ethics, The. 1989. *Death Criteria: A Report.* Copenhagen: The Danish Council of Ethics.

Dante Alighieri. 1956. *Die Göttliche Komödie (Divina Commedia), Italienisch und Deutsch,* edited by August Vezin. Freiburg/Rom: Herder.

Daqr, Nada Muhammad Na'im al-. 1997. *Mawt al-Dimagh bayna al-Tibb wal-Islam (Brain Death between Medicine and Islam).* Damascus: Dar al-Fikr.

Darwin, Francis. 1995. *The Life of Charles Darwin.* London: Studio Editions Ltd.

Darwin, Robert. 1789. *Appeal to the Faculty Concerning the Case of Mrs. Houlston.* Shrewsbury: P. Sandford.

Dastidar, Koyeli Ghosh. 1987. "Individual Autonomy in Traditional Indian Thought." *Journal of Indian Philosophy.* 15: 99–107.

Daube, David. 1965. *Collaboration with Tyranny in Rabbinic Law.* London: Oxford University Press.

Daum, Monika, and Hans-Ulrich Deppe, eds. 1991. *Zwangssterilisation in Frankfurt am Main, 1933–1945.* Frankfurt/New York: Campus.

d'Avenel, Vicomte. 1907. "Les Riches Depuis Septs Cents Ans. Honoraires des Professions Libérales: Médecins et Chirurgiens." *Revue des Deux Mondes.* 37: 117–48.

Davies, G. 1991. *The Scottish Enlightenment and Other Essays.* Edinburgh: Polygon.

Davis, Dena, S. 1991. "Beyond Rabbi Hiyya's Wife: Women's Voices in Jewish Bioethics." *Second Opinion.* 16: 10–30.

Davis, Michael. 2003. "What Can We Learn by Looking for the First Code of Professional Ethics?" *Theoretical Medicine and Bioethics.* 24: 433–54.

Davis, Natalie Zemon. 1975. "Poor Relief, Humanism, and Heresy." In *Society and Culture in Early Modern France,* edited by Natalie Zemon Davis, 17–64. Stanford CA: Stanford University Press.

Davis, Nathan Smith. [1903] 1907. *History of Medicine with The Code of Medical Ethics.* Chicago: Cleveland Press.

Dechambre, Amédée. 1882. "Déontologie." *Dictionnaire Encyclopédique des Sciences Médicales,* première série. Paris: Masson.

DeGrazia, David. 1999. "The Ethics of Animal Research: What are the Prospects for Agreement?" *Cambridge Quarterly of Healthcare Ethics.* 8: 23–34.

Deichgräber, Karl. 1950. *Professio medici, Zum Vorwort des Scribonius Largus.* Mainz: Akademie der Wissenschaften.

Deichgräber, Karl. 1955. *Der Hippokratische Eid.* Stuttgart: Hippokrates-Verlag.

Deichgräber, Karl. 1970. *Medicus Gratiosus: Untersuchungen zu einem griechischen Arztbild. Mit einem Anhang: Testamentum Hippocratis und Rhazes' De indulgentia medici.* Mainz: Akademie der Wissenschaften und der Literatur.

Deichgräber, Karl. 1983. *Der Hippokratische Eid.* 4th ed. Stuttgart: Hippokrates-Verlag.

Deichmann, Ute. 1996. *Biologists Under Hitler,* translated by Thomas Dunlap. Cambridge MA: Harvard University Press.

Delafield, Francis. 1886. "President's Address: Proceedings of the Association of American Physicians." *Journal of the American Medical Association.* 7: 16.

Dembo, Gregory I. 1930. "Vrachebnoe pravo i vrachebnaya etika." In *Vrachebnaya Taina I Vrachebnaya Etika. Rechi i Stat'i*, edited by V. I. Voyachek and V. P. Osipov, 26–40. Leningrad: Krasnaya Gazeta.

Demiéville, Paul. 1985. *Buddhism and Healing: Demiéville's Article "Byō" from Hōbogirin.* Trans. Mark Tatz. Lanham: University Press of America.

Denzinger, Henricus, and Adolfus Schonmetzer. 1973. *Enchiridion Symbolorum Definitionum et Declarationum de Rebus Fidei et Morum.* 35th ed. Freiburg: Herder.

Denzinger, Heinrich, and Peter Hünermann. 1991. *Enchiridion Symbolorum Definitionum et Declarationum de Rebus Fidei et Morum.* Friburgo de Brisgovia: Herder.

Deontologicheskii Kodex Vostochno-Galitsiiskoi Vrachebnoi Palaty. 1908. *Zhurnal Obshestva Russkikh Vrachei v Pamyat' N. I. Pirogova.* 6: 646–51; 7: 769–72.

Department of Health and Social Security, United Kingdom. 1984. *Report of the Committee of Inquiry into Human Fertilisation and Embryology.* London: Her Majesty's Stationery Office.

Department of Health, United Kingdom. 2000. *Stem Cell Research: Medical Progress with Responsibility: A Report from the Chief Medical Officer's Expert Group Reviewing the Potential of Developments in Stem Cell Research and Cell Nuclear Replacement to Benefit Human Health.* London: Department of Health. http://www.liebertonline.com/doi/abs/10.1089/152045500436113?cookieSet=1&journalCode=clo.1 (visited January 30, 2008).

Derbyshire, Robert C. 1969. *Medical Licensure and Discipline in the United States.* Baltimore: Johns Hopkins University Press.

De Renzi, Salvatore. 1865. *Collectio Salernitana*, vol. 2. Naples: Filatre-Sebezio.

Desai, Prakash N. 1989. *Health and Medicine in the Hindu Tradition: Continuity and Cohesion.* New York: Crossroads.

Descartes, René. 1960. *Discours de la méthode*, edited by Lüder Gäbe. Hamburg: Meiner.

Dessing, Nathal M. 2001. *Rituals of Birth: Circumcision, Marriage, and Death among Muslims in the Netherlands.* Leuven: Peeters.

Deutsch, Erwin. 1998. "The Nuremberg Code: The Proceedings in the Medical Case, the Ten Principles of Nuremberg, and the Lasting Effect of the Nuremberg Code." In *Ethics Codes in Medicine: Foundations and Achievements of Codification since 1947*, edited by Ulrich Tröhler and Stella Reiter-Theil, 71–83. Aldershot/Brookfield/Singapore/Sydney: Ashgate.

Developing World Bioethics. 2001. Oxford/Boston: Blackwell Publishers.

DeVille, Kenneth A. 1990. *Medical Malpractice in Nineteenth-Century America: Origins and Legacy.* New York: New York University Press.

DeVries, Raymond, and Janardan Subedi, eds. 1998. *Bioethics and Society: Constructing the Ethical Enterprise.* Upper Saddle River NJ: Prentice Hall.

Dhand, Arti. 2000. "Poison, Snake, the Sharp Edge of a Razor: Yet the Highest of Gurus: Defining Female Sexuality in the Mahàbhàrata." Ph.D. diss., McGill University, Montreal.

Dharmasiri, Gunapala. 1989. *Fundamentals of Buddhist Ethics.* Antioch CA: Golden Leaves.

Díaz del Castillo, Bernal. [1632] 1976. *Historia de la Conquista de Nueva España.* 11th ed. México: Porrúa.

Dienel, Christiane. 1993. "Das 20. Jahrhundert (I): Frauenbewegung, Klassenjustiz und das Recht auf Selbstbestimmung der Frau." In *Geschichte der Abtreibung: Von der Antike bis zur Gegenwart*, edited by Robert Jütte, 140–68. Munich: Verlag C. H. Beck.

Dietrich, Albert. 1984. "ʿAlī ibn Riḍwān über den Wert medizinischer Lehrbücher (Kanānīsh)." In *Studi in onore di Francesco Gabrieli nel suo ottanesimo compleanno*, a cura di Renato Traini, 269–77. Roma: Università di Roma "La Sapienza," Dipartimento di studi orientali.

Dietrich, Albert. 1991. "ʿAlī ibn Riḍwān: Über den Wert medizinischer Kommentare (tafāsīr)." In *Yād-Nāma in memoria di Alessandro Bausani.* 2, a cura di Biancamaria Scarcia Amoretti e Lucia Rostagno, 59–74. Roma: Bardi.

Dikotter, Frank. 1998. *Imperfect Conception: Medical Knowledge, Birth Defects, and Eugenics in China.* New York: Columbia University Press.

Dill, David B. 1979. "A. C. Ivy – Reminiscences." *Physiologist.* 22(5): 21–2.

Diller, H., ed. 1962. *Hippokrates: Schriften.* Reinbeck bei Hamburg: Rowholt.

d'Irsay, Stephen. 1927. "Patristic Medicine." *Annals of Medical History.* 9: 364–78.

Dixon, Suzanne. 1988. *The Roman Mother.* Norman OK: University of Oklahoma Press.

Diyanet, İşleri Başkanlığı. 1995. *Fetvalar.* Ankara: Diyanet İşleri Başkanlığı Yayınları.

Dolbin, Anatoly G. 2003. Interview with author. Moscow, January.

Dols, Michael W. 1984. *Medieval Islamic Medicine: Ibn Ridwān's Treatise "On the Prevention of Bodily Ills in Egypt"*, translated with an introduction. Arabic text edited by Adil S. Gamal. Berkeley CA: University of California Press.

Dong, P., and X. Wang. 1998. "Caring for Terminally Patients: The Daoist Perspective." *Chinese and International Philosophy of Medicine.* 1: 107–20 [Chinese].

Donne, John. 1982. *Biathanatos*, edited by M. Ruddick and M. P. Battin. New York: Garland.

Doppelfeld, Elmar. 2000a. *Paper read at international symposium, "Das Menschenrechtsübereinkommen des*

Europarates – taugliches Vorbild für eine weltweit geltende Regelung?" Heidelberg, Akademie der Wissenschaften, 19 September, 2000, and personal communication.

Doppelfeld, Elmar. 2000b. "Weltärztebund – Probe für die Glaubwürdigkeit." *Deutsches Ärzteblatt.* 97, A-1587–A-1592.

Doppelfeld, Elmar. 2002. "Das Menschenrechtsübereinkommen zur Biomedizin: Entstehungsgeschichte und Regelungsgehalt." In *Das Menschenrechtsübereinkommen zur Biomedizin des Europarates: taugliches Vorbild für eine weltweit geltende Regelung?* Jochen Taupitz (Hrsg), 15–27. Berlin: Springer.

Dorff, Elliot N. 1998. *Matters of Life and Death: A Jewish Approach to Modern Medical Ethics.* Philadelphia: Jewish Publication Society.

Döring, Ole, ed. 1999. *Chinese Scientists and Responsibility: Ethical Issues of Human Genetics in Chinese and International Contexts.* Hamburg: Institute for Asian Studies.

Döring, Ole. 2001. "Comments on Inhumanity in the Name of Medicine: Old Cases and New Voices for Responsible Medical Ethics from Japan and China." *Eubios Journal of Asian and International Bioethics.* 11: 44–7.

Döring, Ole. 2003. "China's Struggle for Practical Regulations in Medical Ethics." *Nature Reviews Genetics.* 4: 233–9.

Döring, Ole, and Chen Renbiao, eds. 2002. *Advances in Chinese Medical Ethics: Chinese and International Perspectives.* Hamburg: Institute for Asian Studies.

Dörner, Klaus. 2000. "Nationalsozialismus und Medizin – Wurden die Lehren Gezogen?" In *NS-Euthanasie in Wien,* edited by Eberhard Gabriel and Wolfgang Neugebauer, 131–6. Vienna/Cologne/Weimar: Böhlau.

Dörner, Klaus, et al. 1980. *Der Krieg gegen die psychisch Kranken.* Rehburg-Loccum: Psychiatrie Verlag.

Dörner, Klaus, and Angelika Ebbinghaus, eds. 1999. *The Nuremberg Doctors' Trial, 1946–47.* Munich: K. G. Saur. Mikrofiche.

Dörner, Klaus, and Angelika Ebbinghaus, eds. 2000. *Vernichten und Heilen: Der Nürnberger Ärzteprozeß und seine Folgen.* Berlin: Aufbau.

Dorotheos of Gaza. 1977. *Discourses and Sayings,* translated by Eric Wheeler. Kalamazoo MI: Cistercian Publications.

Dover, K. J. 1989. *Greek Homosexuality.* Cambridge MA: Harvard University Press.

Doyal, Len, and Jeffery S. Tobias. 2001. *Informed Consent in Medical Research.* London: BMJ Books.

D. P. M. P. M. [Prudencio María Pascual]. 1820. *Arte de pensar y de obrar bien, o filosofía racional y moral.* Madrid: Imprenta de la Viuda de Aznar.

Dragstedt, Carl A. 1944. "Andrew Conway Ivy." *Quarterly Bulletin of the Northwestern University Medical School.* 18: 139–40.

Drane, James F. 1988. "Universal Medical Ethics." *Quirón.* 29: 53–64.

Drane, James F. 1996. "Bioethical Perspectives from Ibero-America." *Journal of Medicine and Philosophy.* 21: 557–69.

Drane, James F. 1999. "Complejo Bioético: Pigmalión, Narciso y Knock." *Acta psiquiátrica y psicológica de América latina.* 45: 109–21. Commentary to José A. Mainetti.

Drane, James F., and Hernán Fuenzalida. 1991. "Medical Ethics in Latin America: A New Interest and Commitment." *Kennedy Institute of Ethics Journal.* 1: 325–38.

Draper, Elaine. 1991. *Risky Business.* New York: Cambridge University Press.

Drinan, Robert F. 1992. "The Nuremberg Principles in International Law." In *The Nazi Doctors and the Nuremberg Code: Human Rights in Human Experimentation,* edited by George J. Annas and Michael A. Grodin, 174–82. New York/Oxford: Oxford University Press.

Du, Z. 1999. "Health Care Reform: Practical and Reasonable Choices." *Chinese and International Philosophy of Medicine.* 2: 5–25 [Chinese].

Dubé, Paul. 1669. *Le Medecin des Pauvres.* Paris: E Couterot.

Dubler, Nancy N., et al. 1992. "Tuberculosis in the 1990s: Ethical, Legal and Public Policy Issues in Screening, Treatment and the Protection of those in Congregate Facilities: A Report from the Working Group on TB and HIV." In *The Tuberculosis Revival: Individual Rights and Societal Obligations in a Time of AIDS.* New York: United Hospital Fund.

Dubois, Abbe J. A., and Henry K. Beauchamp. [1906] 1959. *Hindu Manners, Customs and Ceremonies.* 3rd ed. Oxford: Claredon Press.

Dubos, René, and Jean Dubos. [1952] 1987. *The White Plague: Tuberculosis, Man, and Society.* [Boston: Little, Brown]. Reprint. New Brunswick NJ: Rutgers University Press.

Duden, Barbara. 1987. *Geschichte unter der Haut: Ein Eisenacher Arzt und seine Patientinnen um 1730.* Stuttgart: Klett-Cotta.

Duden, Barbara. 1991. *The Woman Beneath the Skin.* Cambridge MA: Harvard University Press.

Duff, R. S., and A. G. M. Campbell. 1973. "Moral and Ethical Dilemmas in the Special-Care Nursery." *New England Journal of Medicine.* 289: 980–4.

Duffy, John. 1964. "Anglo-American Reaction to Obstetrical Anesthesia." *Bulletin of the History of Medicine.* 38: 32–44.

Duffy, John. 1990. *The Sanitarians: A History of American Public Health.* Chicago: University of Illinois Press.

Dulieu, Louis. 1988a. *La Médecine à Montpellier*, tome IV. Paris: Presses Universelles.

Dulieu, Louis. 1988b. *La Médecine à Montpellier*, Vol. 4. Paris: Les Presses Universitaires.

Duncan, A. S., G. R. Dunstan, and R. B. Welbourn, eds. 1981. *Dictionary of Medical Ethics*. London: Darton, Longman and Todd.

Dunlop, D. M., and Bedi N. Şehsuvaroğlu. 1960. "Bīmāristān." In *The Encyclopaedia of Islam*. 1: 1222–6. Leiden: E. J. Brill.

Dunn, Fred L. 1976. "Traditional Asian Medicine and Cosmopolitan Medicine as Adaptive Systems." In *Asian Medical Systems: A Comparative Study*, edited by Charles Leslie, 133–58. Berkeley CA: University of California Press.

Dunstan, G. R., et al. 1972. *The Problem of Euthanasia*. Edinburgh: Contact (Pastoral) Ltd.

Dupré, Louis. 1964. *Contraception and Catholics: A New Appraisal*. Baltimore: Helicon.

Duster, Troy. 1989. *Backdoor to Eugenics*. New York: Routledge.

Duster, Troy. 2001. "The Premature and Ill Conceived Burial of Race in Science." In *Anthopology in the Age of Genetics*, edited by Alan Goodman, Deborah Heath, and Susan Lindee. Berkeley CA: University of California Press.

du Toit, Brian, and Ismail H. Abdalla. 1985. *African Healing Strategies*. Owerri, Nigeria/New York: Trado-Medic Books.

Dwivedi, Ramanath. 1974. "Paramedicine in the Classical Indian Medical Literature (Ayurveda)." In *Religion and Medicine*, edited by K. N. Udupa and Gurmohan Singh, 85–94. Varanasi: Institute of Medical Sciences.

Dwork, Debórah. 1993. "Childhood." In *Companion Encyclopedia of the History of Medicine*, edited by William F. Bynum and Roy Porter, 1072–91. London/New York: Routledge.

Dyer, Frederick N. 1999. *Champion of Women and the Unborn: Horatio Robinson Storer, M.D.* Canton MA: Science History Publications.

Eamon, William, and Gundolf Keil. 1986. "Plebs amat Empirica: Nicolas of Poland and his Critique of the Medieval Medical Establishment." In *Sudhoffs Archiv*. 70: 180–96.

Eben, Antonia K. 1998. *Medizinische Ethik im weltanschaulich-religiösen Kontext: Albert Moll und Albert Niedermeyer im Vergleich*. Munich: Uni-Druck.

Eberstein, Winfried C. J. 1999. *Das Tierschutzrecht in Deutschland bis zum Erlass des Reichs-Tierschutzgesetzes vom 24. November 1933. Unter Berücksichtigung der Entwicklung in England*. Frankfurt/Main: P. Lang.

Ebisawa, Arimichi. 1944. *Kirishitan no Syakaikatsudo oyobi Nanbanigaku (The Japanese Kirishitan's Social Activities and Nanban Medicine)*. Tokyo: Fuzanbo.

Ebrahim, Abul Fadl Mohsin. 1989. *Abortion, Birth Control, and Surrogate Parenting: An Islamic Perspective*. Indianapolis IN: American Trust Publication.

Ebrahim, Abul Fadl Mohsin. 1991. *Islamic Ethics and the Implications of Modern Biomedical Technology*. Ann Arbor MI: University Microfilms International.

Ebrahim, Abul Fadl Mohsin. 1992. *Islamic Guidelines on Animal Experimentation*. Islamic Medical Association of South Africa: Qualbert S.A.

Ebrahim, Abul Fadl Mohsin. 1993. *Biomedical Issues: Islamic Perspective*. Kuala Lumpur: A. S. Nordeen.

Eckart, Wolfgang U. 1984. "'Medicus Politicus' oder 'Machiavellus medicus'? Wechselwirkungen von Ideal und Realität des Arzttypus im 17. Jahrhundert." *Medizinhistorisches Journal*. 19: 210–24.

Eckart, Wolfgang U. 2001. "Moll, Albert." In *Ärzte Lexikon. Von der Antike bis zur Gegenwart*. 2nd ed., edited by Wolfgang U. Eckart and Christoph Gradmann, 222–3. Berlin: Springer.

Edelson, Paul. 2001. "Henry K. Beecher and Maurice Pappworth: Informed Consent in Human Experimentation and the Physician's Response." In *Informed Consent in Medical Research*, edited by Len Doyal and Jeffrey S. Tobias, 20–7. London: BMJ Books.

Edelstein, Ludwig. 1943. *The Hippocratic Oath: Text, Translation, and Interpretation*. Baltimore: Johns Hopkins University Press.

Edelstein, Ludwig. 1967. *Ancient Medicine: Selected Papers of Ludwig Edelstein*, edited by Owsei Temkin and C. Lilian Temkin. Baltimore: Johns Hopkins University Press.

Editorial. 1899. *Charities*. 3: 3. State of Connecticut. 1908. *Report of the Special Commission Appointed to Investigate Tuberculosis*. Hartford.

Editorial. 1967. "Johann Peter Frank (1745–1821): Public Health by Decree." *Journal of the American Medical Association*. 202: 228–9.

Editorial. 1979. "The Straw and the Camel." *Philosophy*. 54: 277–8.

Editorial. 1994. "World Medical Association Is Reanimated." *Bulletin of Medical Ethics*. 101 (September): 3–5.

Editorial. 2000. "Taxation: Spend, Spend Spend." *The Economist*, March 16.

Editorial. 2001. "What are the Effects of the Fifth Revision of the Declaration of Helsinki?" *British Medical Journal*. 323: 1417–23.

Editorial. 2001. "Many Doctors in South Africa Favor Mercy Killing." *The Daily Dispatch*, May. www.dispatch.co.za/2001/05/17/southafrica/CADOCTOR.HTM (visited November 15, 2007).

Editorial. 2002. "Patient-Centred Healthcare." *The Sunday Times: The Daily Mirror Online*. www.dailymirror.lk/2002/11/13/editorial.html (visited November 15, 2007): 1–2.

Editors of Lingua Franca, eds. 2000. *The Sokal Hoax: The Sham that Shook the Academy.* Lincoln: University of Nebraska Press.

Egwang, Thomas E. 2001. "Biotechnology Issues in Africa." *EJB Electronic Journal of Biotechnology.* 4.3. http://www.scielo.cl/scielo.php?pid=S0717–34582001000300005&script=sci_arttext (visited January 30, 2008).

Eimontova, R. G. 1998. *Idei Prosveshenija v Obnovljayusheisja Rossii: 50–60-e Gody XIX Veka.* Moscow: Institut rossiskoi istorii RAN.

Elaut, L. 1958. "Le 'Medicus Politicus' de Friedrich Hoffman." *Janus.* 47: 166–79.

Elgood, Cyril. 1962. "Tibb-ul Nabbi or Medicine of the Prophet." *Osiris.* 14: 33–192.

Elkadi, Ahmed. 1976. "Professional Ethics: Ethics in the Medical Profession." In *The Journal of the Islamic Medical Association.* (September): 27–30.

Elkeles, Barbara. 1985. "Medizinische Menschenversuche gegen Ende des 19. Jahrhunderts und der Fall Neisser. Rechtfertigung und Kritik einer wissenschaftlichen Methode." *Medizinhistorisches Journal.* 20: 135–48.

Elkeles, Barbara. 1996. *Der moralische Diskurs über das medizinische Menschenexperiment im 19. Jahrhundert.* Stuttgart: Gustav Fischer.

Elon, Menachem. 1969. "Jewish Law and Modern Medicine." *Israel Law Review.* 4: 467–78.

Elon, Menachem. 1994. *Jewish Law: History, Sources, Principles,* translated by B. Auerbach and M. J. Sykes. Philadelphia: Jewish Publication Society.

El'shtein, Natan V. 1986. "Etika meditsynskaya." In *Bol'shaya Meditsynskaya Entsiclopedija.* 3rd ed., 28: 368–71. Moscow: Sovietskaya Entsiclopedija.

Elston, Mary Ann. 1990. "Women and Anti-Vivisection in Victorian England, 1870–1900." In *Vivisection in Historical Perspective.* 2nd ed., edited by Nicolaas A. Rupke, 259–94. London: Routledge.

Elwan, Omaia. 1967. "Empfängnisregelung und Abtreibung im Islam." In *Rechtsvergleichung und Rechtsvereinheitlichung,* edited by Eduard Wahl et al., 439–70. Heidelberg: Winter.

Elwan, Omaia. 1968. "Das Problem der Empfängnisregelung und Abtreibung. Die herrschende Auffassung des Staates und der religiösen Kreise in islamischen Ländern." *Zeitschrift für vergleichende Rechtswissenschaft.* 70: 25–80.

Elwell, John J. 1860. *A Medico-Legal Treatise on Malpractice and Medical Evidence.* New York: J. S. Voorhies.

Emanuel, Ezekiel J. 1994. "The History of Euthanasia Debates in the United States and Britain." *Annals of Internal Medicine.* 121.10: 793–802.

Emanuel, Linda, and Stephen Latham. 1999. "Who Needs Physicians' Professional Ethics?" In *The American Medical Ethics Revolution: How the AMA's Code of Ethics Has Transformed Physicians' Relationships to Patients, Professionals, and Society,* edited by Robert Baker et al., 192–203. Baltimore: Johns Hopkins University Press.

Engelhardt, H. Tristram, Jr. 1974. "The Disease of Masturbation: Values and the Concept of Disease." *Bulletin of the History of Medicine.* 48: 234–48.

Engelhardt, H. Tristram, Jr. [1974] 1981. "The Disease of Masturbation: Values and the Concept of Disease." In *Concepts of Health and Disease: Interdisciplinary Perspectives,* edited by Arthur L. Caplan, H. Tristram Engelhardt Jr., and James J. McCartney; foreword by Denton Cooley, 267–80. Reprint. Reading MA: Addison-Wesley, Advanced Book Program (World Science Division).

Engelhardt, H. Tristram, Jr. 1975. "Defining Death: A Philosophical Problem for Medicine and Law." *The American Review of Respiratory Disease.* 112: 587–90.

Engelhardt, H. Tristram, Jr. 1986a. *The Foundations of Bioethics.* New York: Oxford University Press.

Engelhardt, H. Tristram, Jr. 1986b. "The Languages of Medicalization." In H. Tristram Engelhardt, *The Foundations of Bioethics,* 157–201. New York: Oxford University Press.

Engelhardt, H. Tristram, Jr. 1996. *The Foundations of Bioethics.* 2nd ed. New York: Oxford University Press.

Engelhardt, H. Tristram, Jr. 2000. *The Foundations of Christian Bioethics.* Lisse: Swets & Zeitlinger.

Engelhardt, H. Tristram, Jr. 2002. "The Ordination of Bioethicists as Secular Moral Experts." *Social Philosophy & Policy.* 19.2: 59–82.

Engelhardt, H. Tristram, Jr., and Daniel Callahan, eds. 1980. *Knowing and Valuing: The Search for Common Roots.* Hastings-on-Hudson NY: The Hastings Center.

Erikson, Erik H. 1959. "Growth and Crises of the Healthy Personality." In Erik Erikson, *Identity and the Life Cycle: Selected Papers; with a historical introduction by David Rapaport.* Psychological Issues Series, Monograph 1, 50–100. New York: International Universities Press.

Erikson, Erik, H. 1968. *Ghandi's Truth: On the Origins of Militant Non-Violence.* New York: W. W. Norton.

Escobar, Antonio. 1652–1663. *Universae theologiae moralis: receptiores absque lite sententiae nec non problematicae disquisitiones. Volumen primum: Generalia principa. Volumen secundum: Sacramenta. Tomi tertii pars prima: Adhuc sacramenta. Tomi tertii pars alatera: Matrimonii sacramenti. Volumen quartum: Decalogi praecepta. Tomus quintus. Tomus sextus. Tomus septimus et ultimus: Triplex status: ecclesiasticus, religiosus & saecularis.* Lugduni: Philippi Borde, Laurentii Arnaud & Claudii Rigaud.

Escobar, Triana Javier. 1996. "Humanistic and Social Education for Physicians: The Experience of the Colombian School of Medicine." *Journal of Medicine and Philosophy.* 21: 651–7.

Ess, Josef van. 1980. "Islam." In *Die fünf großen Weltreligionen*, edited by Emma Brunner-Traut, 67–87. Freiburg: Herder.

Essex, M. 1994. "The Etiology of AIDS." In *AIDS in Africa*, edited by M. Essex, 1–20. New York: Raven Press.

Europa. 2001. *Official Journal of the European Communities*. (May 1): L 121, vol. 44: 34.

Eusebius. [1926, 1932] 1992, 1994. *The Ecclesiastical History*. [2 vols.] Reprint. Loeb Classical Library 153/265. Cambridge MA/London: Harvard University Press.

Evagrios the Solitary. 1988. "On Prayer." In *The Philokalia*, edited and translated by G. E. H. Palmer, Philip Sherrard, and Kallistos Ware, 1:55–71. Boston: Faber and Faber.

Evans, Donald. 1991. "Building Libraries in Eastern Europe." *Bulletin of Medical Ethics*. 66: 20–2.

Evans, John Grimley. 1997. "Geriatric Medicine: A Brief History." *British Medical Journal*. 315: 1075–7.

Evans, John H. 2002. *Playing God? Human Genetic Engineering and the Rationalization of Public Bioethical Debate*. Chicago: University of Chicago Press.

Evans-Pritchard, E. E. 1937. *Witchcraft, Oracles and Magic among the Azande*. Oxford: Clarendon Press.

Eve, A., and I. J. Higginson. 2000. "Minimum Dataset Activity for Hospice and Hospital Palliative Care Services in the UK 1997/98." *Palliative Medicine*. 14. 5: 395–404.

Evenden, Doreen. 2000. *The Midwives of Seventeenth-Century London*. Cambridge UK: Cambridge University Press.

Evidence-Based Medicine Working Group. 1992. "Evidence-Based Medicine: A New Approach to Teaching the Practice of Medicine." *Journal of the American Medical Association*. 268: 2420–5.

Evleth, Donna. 1995. "Vichy France and the Continuity of Medical Nationalism." *Social History of Medicine*. 8.1: 95–116.

Faden, Ruth R., and Tom Beauchamp. 1986. *A History and Theory of Informed Consent*. Oxford: Oxford University Press.

Faden, Ruth R., G. Geller, and M. B. Powers. 1991. *AIDS, Women, and the Next Generation: Towards a Morally Acceptable Public Policy for HIV Testing of Pregnant Women and Newborns*. New York: Oxford University Press.

Faden, Ruth R., Susan E. Lederer, and Jonathan D. Moreno. 1996. "U.S. Medical Researchers, the Nuremberg Doctors' Trial, and the Nuremberg Code." *Journal of the American Medical Association*. 276: 1667–71.

Fadiman, Anne. 1997. *The Spirit Catches You and You Fall Down: A Hmong Child, Her American Doctors, and the Collision of Two Cultures*. New York: Farrar, Straus and Giroux.

Fainshtein. 1904. "Zasedanie Pravlenija Obshestva 13 Janvarja 1904 g." *Vestnik Sankt-Peterburgskogo Obshestva Vzaimnoi Pomoshi*. 9–10: 58–67.

Fairchild, Amy L. 1997. "Science at the Borders: Immigrant Medical Inspection in Defense of the Nation, 1891–1930." Ph.D. diss., Columbia University, New York.

Fairchild, Amy L., and Ronald Bayer. 1999. "The Uses and Abuses of Tuskegee." *Science*. 284: 919–21.

Fan, Minsheng. 1999. "Who Should Sign the Consent Form? Family Members' View in Medical Practice." *Chinese and International Philosophy of Medicine*. 2: 87–110 [Chinese].

Fan, Ruiping. 1997. "Self-determination vs. Family-Determination: Two Incommensurable Principles of Autonomy." *Bioethics*. 11: 309–22.

Fan, Ruiping. 1998. "Human Cloning and Human Dignity: Pluralist Society and the Confucian Moral Community." *Chinese and International Philosophy of Medicine*. 1: 73–93 [Chinese].

Faradj, Abdalmalik. [1935] 1996. *Relations médicales hispano-maghrébines au XIIe siècle*. [Thèse de médecine, Paris. Paris: Les Éditions Véga]. Reprinted in *Abu 'l-Alā' ibn Zuhr (d. 525/1130) and his Son Abū Marwān Ibn Zuhr (d. 557/1161): Texts and Studies*, edited by Fuat Sezgin, 323–84. Frankfurt am Main: Institute for the History of Arabic-Islamic Science.

Farkas, Endre. 1978. *The Basis of Marxist Ethics*. Budapest: Textbook, Co.

Faulstich, Heinz. 1998. *Hungersterben in der Psychiatrie 1914–1949: Mit einer Topographie der NS-Psychiatrie*. Freiburg im Breisgau: Lambertus.

Faure, Olivier. 1993. *Les Français et Leur Médecine au XIXe Siècle*. Paris: Belin.

Faust, Bernhard Christoph. 1794. *Gesundheits-Katechismus für Aeltern und Lehrern in zusammenhängende Rede gebracht*. Bückeburg: Althaus.

Fee, Elizabeth. 1987. *Disease and Discovery: A History of The Johns Hopkins School of Hygiene and Public Health, 1916–1939*. Baltimore: Johns Hopkins University Press.

Fee, Elizabeth. 1993. "Public Health, Past and Present: A Shared Social Vision." In *A History of Public Health*, expanded edition, edited by George Rosen, ix–xl. Baltimore: Johns Hopkins University Press.

Feijoo, Benito Jerónimo. 1726–1740. *Teatro crítico universal*. 9 vols. Madrid: Herederos de Francisco del Hierro.

Feijoo, Benito Jerónimo. 1742–1760. *Cartas eruditas y curiosas*. 5 vols. Madrid: Herederos de Francisco del Hierro.

Feinberg, Joel, ed. 1973. *The Problem of Abortion*. Belmont CA: Wadsworth.

Feinberg, John S. 1979. *Theologies and Evil*. Lanham MD: University Press of America.

Feinberg, Nikolai G. 1903. "Retsenzija na Knigu Albert Moll 'Aertzliche Ethik.'" *Vestnik Sankt-Peterburgskogo Vrachebnogo Obshestva Vzaimnoi Pomoschi*. 4: 304–13.

Feingold, Aaron J. 1996. *Three Jewish Physicians of the Renaissance*. Tel Aviv: American Friends of Beth Hatefutsoth.

Feldman, Eric A., and Ronald Bayer, eds. 2004. *Unfiltered: Conflicts Over Tobacco Policy and Public Health*. Cambridge MA: Harvard University Press.

Felipe IV (of Spain). 1640. *Recopilación de las leyes destos Reynos*. Madrid: n. p.

Fellner, C. H., and S. H. Schwartz. 1971. "Altruism in Disrepute: Medical vs. Public Attitudes Toward the Living Organ Donor." *New England Journal of Medicine*. 284: 582–5.

Fenn, W. O. 1963. *History of the American Physiological Society: The Third Quarter Century, 1937–1962*, 5–7. Washington DC: American Physiological Society.

Ferguson, Everett, ed. 1990. *An Encyclopedia of Early Christianity*. New York: Garland Publishing.

Ferngren, Gary B. 1987. "The Imago Dei and the Sanctity of Life: The Origins of an Idea." In *Euthanasia and the Newborn: Conflicts Regarding Saving Lives*, edited by R. C. McMillan, H. Tristram Engelhardt Jr., and S. F. Spicker, 23–45. Dordrecht/Boston: D. Reidel.

Ferngren, Gary B. 1988. "The Organisation of the Care of the Sick in Early Christianity." In *Actes/Proceedings of the XXX International Congress of the History of Medicine*, edited by H. Schadewaldt and K.-H. Leven, 192–8. Düsseldorf: Vicom KG.

Ferngren, Gary. 1989. "The Ethics of Suicide in the Renaissance and Reformation." In *Suicide and Euthanasia: Historical and Contemporary Themes*, edited by Baruch A. Brody, 155–81. Dordrecht/Boston: Kluwer Academic Publishers.

Ferngren, Gary. 1992. "Early Christianity as a Religion of Healing." *Bulletin of the History of Medicine*. 66: 1–15.

Ferngren, Gary B. 2000. "Early Christian Views of the Demonic Etiology of Disease." In *From Athens to Jerusalem: Medicine in Hellenized Jewish Lore and in Early Christian Literature*, edited by Samuel Kottek, et al. 183–201. Rotterdam: Erasmus Publishing.

Ferngren, Gary B., and Darrel W. Amundsen. 1996. "Medicine and Christianity in the Roman Empire: Compatibilities and Tensions." In *Aufstieg und Niedergang der Römischen Welt II. 37. 3*, edited by Wolfgang Haase, 2957–80. Berlin: Walter de Gruyter.

Figueroa, Patricio R., and Hernán Fuenzalida. 1996. "Bioethics in Ibero-America and the Caribbean." *Journal of Medicine and Philosophy*. 21: 611–27.

Filippi, Gian Giuseppe. 1996. *Mṛtyu: Concept of Death in Indian Traditions*, translated by Antonio Rigopoulos. New Delhi: D. K. Printworld.

Finch, Charles. 1990. *The African Background to Medical Science: Essays on African History, Science and Civilization*. London: Karnak House.

First-and-Second Council. 1983. "The Seventeen Canons of the so-called First-and-Second Council." In *The Rudder of the Orthodox Catholic Church*, edited by Sts. Nicodemus and Agapius, translated by D. Cummings, 455–74. New York: Luna Printing.

First International Conference on Islamic Medicine. 1981. *Islamic Code of Medical Ethics*. (January). Kuwiet.

Fischer, Alfons. 1933. *Geschichte des deutschen Gesundheitswesens. Vol. 2: Von den Anfängen der hygienischen Ortsbeschreibungen bis zur Gründung des Reichsgesundheitsamtes (Das 18. und 19. Jahrhundert)*. Berlin: Kommissionsverlag F. A. Herbig.

Fischer, Christian Ernst. 1799. *Versuch einer Anleitung zur medizinischen Armenpraxis*. Göttingen: Dieterich.

Fischer, David Hackett. 1970. *Historians' Fallacies: Toward a Logic of Historical Thought*. New York: Harper & Row.

Fischer, Joseph. A. ed. 1956. *Die Apostolischen Väter*. 2 vols. Darmstadt: Wissenschaftliche Buchgemeinschaft.

Fischer-Homburger, Esther. 1989. *Medizin vor Gericht: Zur Sozialgeschichte der Gerichtsmedizin*. Darmstadt: Luchterhand.

Fischer-Kamel, Doris S. 1987. "The Midwife in History with Special Emphasis on Practice in Medieval Europe and the Islamic World." M.A. diss., University of Arizona, Ann Arbor: UMI 1991. 1330519.

Fishbein, Morris. 1947. *A History of the American Medical Association 1847 to 1947*. Philadelphia: W. B. Saunders.

Fissell, Mary E. 1991. *Patients, Power, and the Poor in Eighteenth-Century Bristol*. Cambridge UK: Cambridge University Press.

Fissell, Mary E. 1993. "Innocent and Honorable Bribes: Medical Manners in Eighteenth- Century Britain." In *The Codification of Medical Morality: Historical and Philosophical Studies of the Formalization of Western Medical Morality in the Eighteenth and Nineteenth Centuries: Volume One: Medical Ethics and Etiquette in the Eighteenth Century*, edited by Robert Baker, Dorothy Porter, and Roy Porter, 19–45. Dordrecht: Kluwer Academic Publishers.

Fitz, Reginald H. 1895. "The Legislative Control of Medical Practice." *Medical Correspondence of the Massachusetts Medical Society*. 16: 275–360.

Flashar, Hellmut, and Jacques Jouanna. 1996. *Médecine et Morale dans l'Antiquité*. Vandoeuvres, Geneva: Fondation Hardt.

Flaxman, N. 1936. "Isaac Hays: Pioneer American Ophthalmologist." *Archives of Ophthalmology*. 16: 78–90.

Fleming, D. 1973. "Walter Bradford Cannon." In *Dictionary of American Biography*, suppl. 3: 133–7. New York: Scribner.

Fletcher, Joseph. 1954. *Morals and Medicine: The Moral Problems of the Patient's Right to Know the Truth, Contraception, Artificial Insemination, Sterilization, and Euthanasia*. Princeton NJ: Princeton University Press.

Fletcher, Joseph. 1966. *Situation Ethics: The New Morality*. Philadelphia: Westminster Press.

Fletcher, Joseph. 1974a. *Ethics of Genetic Control: Ending Reproductive Roulette*. Garden City NJ: Anchor Press.

Fletcher, Joseph. 1974b. *Humanhood: Essays in Biomedical Ethics*. Buffalo NY: Prometheus Books.

Flexner, Abraham. [1910] 1973. *Medical Education in the United States and Canada: A Report to the Carnegie Foundation for the Advancement of Teaching*. Buffalo NY: Heritage Press.

Florida, Robert E. 1991. "Buddhist Approaches to Abortion." *Asian Philosophy*. 1: 39–50.

Florida, Robert E. 1994. "Buddhism and the Four Principles." In *Principles of Health Care Ethics*, edited by R. Gillon and A. Lloyd, 105–16. Chichester: John Wiley and Sons.

Florida, Robert E. 1999. "Abortion in Buddhist Thailand." In *Buddhism and Abortion*, edited by Damien Keown, 11–29. Honolulu HI: University of Hawaii Press.

Flower, Elizabeth, and Murray G. Murphey. 1977. *A History of Philosophy in America*. New York: Capricorn Books.

Fluss, Sev S. 1999. "International Guidelines on Bioethics." *EFGCP News*. (December): Supplement.

Foesius, Anutius. 1595. *Hippocratis Opera Omnia*. Frankfurt: Wechel.

Foltz, Bruce V. 2001. "Hidden Patency: On the Iconic Character of Human Life." *Christian Bioethics*. 7: 317–31.

Fontaine, Nicolas. 1738. *Mémoires pour servir a l'histoire du Port-Royal*. 2 vols. Cologne: Aux dépens de la Compagnie.

Ford, John C., and Gerald Kelly. 1982. "Doctrinal Value and Interpretation of Papal Teaching." In *Readings in Moral Theology No. 3: The Magisterium and Morality*, edited by Charles E. Curran and Richard A. McCormick, 1–13. New York: Paulist Press.

Forestus, Petrus. 1589. *De Incerto Fallaci, Urinarum Iudicio quo Uromantes, ad Perniciem Multorum Aegrotantium Utuntur*. Leiden: Plantin for Franciscus Raphelengius.

Forestus, Petrus. 1653. *Domini Petri Foresti Alcmariani medicinae doctoris . . . opera omnia*. 2 vols. Frankfurt: Berthelin.

Forssmann, Werner. 1974. *Experiments on Myself: Memoirs of a Surgeon in Germany*. New York: St. Martin's Press.

Forster, Heidi, Ezekiel Emanuel, and Christine Grady. 2001. "The 2000 Revision of the Declaration of Helsinki: A Step Forward or More Confusion?" *The Lancet*. 358: 1449–53.

Foucault, Michel. [1963] 1973. *Naissance de la clinique: Une archéologie du regard médical*, translated as *The Birth of the Clinic: An Archaeology of Medical Perception* by A. M. Sheridan Smith. New York: Pantheon.

Fox, Claire G., Gordon L. Miller, and Jacquelyn C. Miller. 1996. *Benjamin Rush, MD: A Bibliographic Guide*. Westport CT: Greenwood Press.

Fox, Daniel M. 1975. "Social Policy and City Politics: Tuberculosis Reporting in New York, 1889–1900." *Bulletin of the History of Medicine*. 49: 169–75.

Fox, Daniel M. 1979. "The Segregation of Medical Ethics: A Problem in Modern Intellectual History." *Journal of Medicine and Philosophy*. 4: 81–97.

Fox, Daniel M. 1986. *Health Policies, Health Politics: The British and American Experience, 1911–1965*. Princeton NJ: Princeton University Press.

Fox, Daniel M. 1993. "The Medical Institutions and the State." In *Companion Encyclopedia of the History of Medicine*, edited by William F. Bynum and Roy Porter, 1204–30. London/New York: Routledge.

Fox, Daniel M. 1995. *Power and Illness: The Failure and Future of American Health Policy*. Berkeley/Los Angeles/London: University of California Press.

Fox, Daniel M., and Paul Fronstin. 2000. "Public Spending for Health Care Approaches 60 Percent." *Health Affairs*. 19: 271–4.

Fox, Daniel M., and Howard Leichter. 1991. "Rationing Care in Oregon: The New Accountability." *Health Affairs*. 10: 7–27.

Fox, Renée C. 1993. "An Ignoble Form of Cannibalism: Reflections on the Pittsburgh Protocol for Procuring Organs from Non-Heart-Beating Cadavers." *Kennedy Institute of Ethics Journal*. 3: 231–9.

Fox, Renée C. 1997. "Ethics of Retransplantation." *Transplantation & Immunology Letter*. XIII: 3, 6.

Fox, Renée C., and Judith P. Swazey. 1974. *The Courage to Fail: A Social View of Organ Transplants and Dialysis*. Chicago: University of Chicago Press.

Fox, Renée C., and Judith P. Swazey. 1978. *The Courage To Fail: A Social View of Organ Transplants and Dialysis*. 2nd revised ed. Chicago: University of Chicago Press.

Fox, Renée C., and Judith P. Swazey. 1984. "Medical Morality is not Bioethics: Medical Ethics in China and the United States." *Perspectives in Biology and Medicine*. 27: 336–60.

Fox, Renée C., and Judith P. Swazey. 1992. *Spare Parts: Organ Replacement in American Society*. New York: Oxford University Press.

Fox, Renée C., and Judith P. Swazey. 1996. "Transplantation and the Medical Commons." In *Perspectives in Medical Sociology*. 2nd ed., edited by Peter Brown, 399–415. Prospect Heights IL: Waveland Press.

Frank, Johann Peter. 1779–1827. *System einer vollständigen medicinischen Polizei*. 9 vols. Mannheim: C. F. Schwann.

Frede, Michael. 1987. *Essays in Ancient Philosophy*. Oxford: Clarendon Press.

Freedman, Benjamin. 1999. *Duty and Healing: Foundations of a Jewish Bioethic*. New York: Routledge.

Freidson, Eliot. 1961. *Patients' Views of Medical Practice*. New York: Russell Sage Foundation.

Freidson, Eliot. 1999. "Professionalism and Institutional Ethics." In *The American Medical Ethics Revolution: How the AMA's Code of Ethics Has Transformed Physicians' Relationships to Patients, Professionals, and Society*, edited by Robert Baker et al., 124–43. Baltimore: Johns Hopkins University Press.

French, Richard. 1975. *Antivivisection and Medical Science in Victorian Society*. Princeton NJ: Princeton University Press.

French, Roger. 1993. "The Medical Ethics of Gabriele de Zerbi." In *Doctors and Ethics: The Earlier Historical Setting of Professional Ethics*, edited by Andrew Wear, Johanna Geyer-Kordesch, and Roger French, 72–97. Amsterdam: Rodopi.

French, Roger. 1999. *Dissection and Vivisection in the European Renaissance*. Aldershot: Ashgate.

Freud, Sigmund. 1971. *Heredity and the Aetiology of the Neuroses*. In *The Standard Edition of the Complete Psychological Works of Sigmund Freud*. London: Hogarth Press.

Freund, Richard A. 1990. *Understanding Jewish Ethics*. San Francisco CA: EM Text.

Frewer, Andreas. 2000. *Medizin und Moral in Weimarer Republik und Nationalsozialismus: Die Zeitschrift "Ethik" unter Emil Abderhalden*. Frankfurt/New York: Campus.

Frewer, Andreas, and Clemens Eickhoff, eds. 2000. *Euthanasie und die Aktualität der historischen Diskussion – Zur Interaktion von Geschichte und Ethik in der Medizin*. Göttingen: Campus.

Frewer, Andreas, and Josef N. Neumann, eds. 2001. *Medizingeschichte ind Medizinethik 1990–1950*. Göttingen: Campus.

Frewer, Andreas, and Claudia Wiesemann, eds. 1999. *Medizinverbrechen vor Gericht. Das Urteil im Nürnberger Ärzteprozeß gegen Karl Brandt und andere sowie aus dem Prozeß gegen Generalfeldmarschall Milch*. Erlangen/Jena: Palm & Enke.

Frewer, Andreas, and Rolf Winau, eds. 1997. *Geschichte und Theorie der Ethik in der Medizin*. Erlangen/Jena: Palm & Enke.

Friedberg, E., ed. [1879] 1959. *Corpus Iuris Canonici*. Reprint. Graz: Akademische Druck- und Verlagsanstalt.

Frieden, T., et al. 1993. "The Emergence of Drug-Resistant Tuberculosis in New York City." *New England Journal of Medicine*. 328: 521–6.

Friedenwald, Harry. 1944. *The Jews and Medicine*. Baltimore: Johns Hopkins University Press.

Friedlander, Henry. 1995. *The Origins of Nazi Genocide: From Euthanasia to the Final Solution*. Chapel Hill NC/London: University of North Carolina Press.

Frings, Hermann-Josef. 1959. *Medizin und Arzt bei den griechischen Kirchenvätern bis Chrysostomos*. Ph.D. diss., University of Bonn, Bonn.

Frois, Luis. [1585] 1983. *Furoisu no Nippon Oboegaki (Memorandum on Japan)*, translated by Kiichi Matsuda and Engelbert Jorissen. Tokyo: Chuo Koron Sha.

Fu, Charles Wei-hsun. 1991. "From Paramartha-satya to Samvrti-satya: An Attempt at Constructive Modernization of (Mahayana) Buddhist Ethics." In *Buddhist Ethics and Modern Society: An International Symposium*, edited by Charles Wei-Hsun Fu and Sandra A. Wawrytko, 313–29. New York: Greenwood Press.

Fuchs, Leonhart. 1543. *New Kreuterbuch*. Basel: Michael Isingrin.

Fuenzalida-Puelma, Hernán, and Susan Scholle Connor, eds. 1989. *The Right to Health in the Americas: A Comparative Constitutional Study*. Washington DC: Panamerican Health Organization.

Fujiii, Shizue. 1997. *Unit 731*. Taipei: Wenyintang.

Fujikawa, Yu. [1904] 1941. *Nippon Igakushi (The Japanese Medical History)*. Tokyo: Nisshin Shoin.

Fujikawa, Yu. [1934] 1978. *Japanese Medicine*. New York: AMS Press.

Fukasawa, Shichiro. 1981. *Narayamabushi Ko, Shincho Gendai Bungaku (Thoughts on The Narayama Ballade, Contemporary Literature)*, vol. 47. Tokyo: Shincho Sha.

Fukuyama, Francis. 2003. *Our Posthuman Future: Consequences of the Biotechnology Revolution*. New York: Picador.

Fumus, Bartholomaeus. [1538] 1627. *Summa Armilla*. Cologne (no imprint).

Furth, Charlotte. 1999. *A Flourishing Yin: Gender in China's Medical History, 960–1665*. Berkeley CA: University of California Press.

Fye, Bruce. 1978. "Active Euthanasia: An Historical Survey of its Conceptual Origins and Introduction to Medical Thought." *Bulletin of the History of Medicine*. 52.4: 492–502.

Gabriel, Eberhard, and Wolfgang Neugebauer, eds. 2000. *NS-Euthanasie in Wien*. Vienna/Cologne/Weimar: Böhlau.

Gadamer, Hans-Georg. 1996. *The Enigma of Health: The Art of Healing in a Scientific Age*. Stanford CA: Stanford University Press.

Galdston, Iago. 1941. "Humanism and Public Health." *Annals of Medical History*. 3rd series. 3: 513–23.

Galeano, Eduardo. [1971] 1981. *Las venas abiertas de América Latina*. 3rd ed. Madrid: Siglo XXI de España Editores.

Galen. [1830] 1965. "Claudii Galeni De libris propriis." In *Claudii Galeni Opera Omnia XIX*, edited by C. G. Kühn, 8–48. Hildesheim: Georg Olms.

Galen. 1976. *On the Affected Parts*, translated by R. E. Siegel. Basle, Switzerland: Karger Publishers.

Galen. 1988. *On Examinations by Which the Best Physicians are Recognized*, edition of the Arabic version with English translation and commentary by Albert Z. Iskandar. Berlin: Akademie Verlag.

Galérant, Germain. 1990. *Médecine de Campagne: De La Révolution à La Belle Époque*. Paris: Christian de Boutiller.

Gallinger, Senator Jacob H. [1900] 1995. "A Bill for the Regulation of Scientific Experiments upon Human Beings in the District of Columbia. S.3424, 56th Congress, 1st Session, March 1900." In Susan E. Lederer, *Subjected to Science: Human Experimentation in*

American before the Second World War, 142–6. Baltimore: Johns Hopkins University Press.

Galton, Francis. 1865. "Hereditary Talent and Character." *Macmillian's Magazine*. no. 12: 157–66, 318–27.

Galton, Francis. 1869. *Hereditary Genius: An Inquiry into its Laws and Consequences*. London: Macmillan.

Galton, Francis. 1883. *Inquiries into Human Faculty and its Development*. London/New York: Macmillan.

Galton, Francis. 1889. *Natural Inheritance*. London/New York: Macmillan.

Gálvao-Sobrinho, Carlos R. 1996. "Hippocratic Ideals, Medical Ethics, and the Practice of Medicine in the Early Middle Ages." *Journal of the History of Medicine and Allied Sciences*. 51: 438–55.

Gan, Zhuwang. 1995. *Sun Simiao Pingzhuan (Review of Sun Simiao)*. Nanjing: Nanjing University Press.

Ganssmüller, Christian. 1987. *Die Erbgesundheitspolitik des Dritten Reiches: Planung, Durchführung und Durchsetzung*. Cologne: Böhlau.

Gante, Michael. 1993. "Das 20. Jahrhundert (II): Rechtspolitik und Rechtswirklichkeit, 1927–1976." In *Geschichte der Abtreibung. Von der Antike bis zur Gegenwart*, edited by Robert Jütte, 169–206. Munich: Verlag C. H. Beck.

Ganzini, Linda, et al. 2000. "Physicians' Experiences with the Oregon Death with Dignity Act." *New England Journal of Medicine*. 342: 557–63.

Garcia, Juan César. 1972. *La educación médica en la América Latina*. Washington DC: Organización Panamericana de la Salud.

Garcia-Ballester, Luis. 1993. "Medical Ethics in Transition in the Latin Medicine of the Thirteenth and Fourteenth Centuries: New Perspectives on the Physician-Patient Relationship and the Doctor's Fee." In *Doctors and Ethics: The Earlier Historical Setting of Professional Ethics*, edited by Andrew Wear, Johanna Geyer-Kordesch, and Roger French, 38–71. Amsterdam: Rodopi.

Garcia-Ballester, Luis. 1996. "Ethical Problems in the Relationship Between Doctors and Patients in Fourteenth-Century Spain: On Christian and Jewish Practitioners." In *Medicine and Medical Ethics in Medieval and Early Modern Spain: An Intercultural Approach*, edited by Samuel S. Kottek and Luis Garcia-Ballester, 11–32. Jerusalem: Magnes Press.

Garçon, Émile. 1956. *Code Pénal Annoté*. Nouv. Ed. Paris: Sirey.

Garner, Robert. 1998. *Political Animals: Animal Protection Policies in Britain and the United States*. New York: St. Martin's Press.

Garofalo, Ivan, ed. 1988. *Erasistrati fragmenta*. Pisa: Giardini.

Garrafa, Volnei. 2000. "A Bioethical Radiography of Brazil." *Acta Bioética*. VI: 177–82.

Garrett, Laurie. 2000. *Betrayal of Trust: The Collapse of Global Public Health*. New York: Hyperion.

Garzya, Antonio. 1996. "Science et Conscience dans la Pratique Médicale de l'Antiquité Tardive et Byzantine." In *Médecine et Morale dans l'Antiquité*, edited by Hellmut Flashar and Jacques Jouanna, 337–64. Vandoeuvres, Geneva: Fondation Hardt.

Gaup, R. 1915. "Hysterie und Kriegsdienst." *Münchener Medizinische Wochenschrift*. 62: 361–3.

Gaup, R. 1916. "Kriegsneurosen." *Zeitschrift für die Gesamte Neurologie und Psychiatrie*. 34: 357–90.

Gefenas, E. 2001a. "Is 'Failure to Thrive' Syndrom Relevant to Lithuanian Healthcare Ethics Committees?" *HEC Forum*. 4: 381–92.

Gefenas, E. 2001b. "Social Justice and Solidarity." In *Bioethics in a European Perspective*, edited by Henk A. M. J. ten Have and B. Gordjin, 119–229. Dordrecht: Kluwer Academic Publishers.

Geison, Gerald L. 1995. *The Private Science of Louis Pasteur*. Princeton NJ: Princeton University Press.

Gekker, M. 1928. "Materal'noe polozhenie vrachei na Ukraine." *Acta Medica*. 19: 18–26.

General Medical Council. 1971. "General Medical Council: Disciplinary Committee." *British Medical Journal Supplement*. 3542: 79–80.

General Medical Council. 2001. *Protecting Patients: A Summary Consultative Document*. London: General Medical Council.

Gens, A. B. 1927. "K probleme legalizatsii aborta V RSFSR." *Aborty v 1925 Godu*, 21–8. Moscow: TsSu SSSR.

Gens, A. B. 1929. *Problema Aborta*. Moscow: Gosmedizdat.

Gentilcore, David. 1994. "'All that Pertains to Medicine': Protomedici and Protomedicate in Early Modern Italy." *Medical History*. 38: 121–42.

Gentilcore, David. 1995. "'Charlatans, Mountebanks and Other Similar People': The Regulation and Role of Itinerant Practitioners in Early Modern Italy." *Social History*. 20: 297–314.

Gentilcore, David. 1998. *Healers and Healing in Early Modern Italy*. Manchester: Manchester University Press.

Geraghty, Karen. 2001. "Guarding the Art: Edmund D. Pellegrino, MD." *Virtual Mentor: Journal of the American Medical Association*. (October). www.ama-assn.org/ama/pub/category/6572.html (visited February 22, 2004).

Gernet, Jacques. 1996. *A History of Chinese Civilization*. 2nd ed., translated by J. R. Foster and Charles Hartman. Cambridge UK: Cambridge University Press.

Gernet, M. I. 1927. "Abort v zakone i statistika abortov." In *Aborty v 1925 Godu*, 3–20. Moscow: TsSU SSSR.

Gershenzon, Mikhail O., ed. 1911. *Epokha Nikolaja I*. Moscow: Obrazovanie.

Getchell, J. P., et al. 1987. "Human Immunodeficiency Virus Isolated from a Serum Sample Collected in 1976 in Central Africa." *Journal of Infectious Diseases*. 156.5: 833–87.

Geuter, Ulfried. 1992. *The Professionalisation of Psychology in Nazi Germany*, translated by Richard J. Holmes. Cambridge/New York: Cambridge University Press.

Geyer-Kordesch, Johanna. 1993. "Natural Law and Medical Ethics in the Eighteenth Century." In *The Codification of Medical Morality: Historical and Philosophical Studies of the Formalization of Western Medical Morality in the Eighteenth and Nineteenth Centuries: Volume One: Medical Ethics and Etiquette in the Eighteenth Century*, edited by Robert Baker, Dorothy Porter, and Roy Porter, 123–39. Dordrecht: Kluwer Academic Publishers.

Ghāfiqī, Muḥammad ibn Qassūm ibn Aslam al-. [1933] 1986. *Kitāb al-Murshid fī l-kuḥl (Al-Morchid fi'l-Kohhl), ou Le Guide d'oculistique*, traduction des parties ophtalmologiques d'après le manuscrit conservé à la Bibliothèque de L'Escurial par Max Meyerhof. [Masnou, Barcelona: Laboratoires du Nord de l'Espagne]. Reprint in *Augenheilkunde im Islam: Texte, Studien und Übersetzungen*, herausgegeben von Fuat Sezgin. 4 vols, 2: 519–743. Frankfurt am Main: Institut für Geschichte der Arabisch-Islamischen Wissenschaften.

Ghanem, Isam. 1982. *Islamic Medical Jurisprudence*. London: Arthur Probsthain.

Ghanem, Isam. 1989. "The Response of Islamic Jurisprudence to Ectopic Pregnancies, Frozen Embryo Implantation, and Euthanasia." In *Arab Law Quarterly*. 4: 345–9.

al-Ghazālī, Abū-Ḥāmid Muḥammad Ibn-Muḥammad. [1352] 1933. *Iḥyāʾ ʿulūm ad-dīn*. 4 vols. Kairo: Matbaʾa al-ʾUtmānīya.

al-Ghazzālī, Abū-Ḥāmid Muḥammad Ibn-Muḥammad. 1958. *Tahāfut al-Falāsifa*. Sulaimān Dunyā (red). Al-Qāhira: Dar al-Maʾarif.

al-Ghazzālī, Abū-Ḥāmid Muḥammad Ibn-Muḥammad. 1962. *Iḥyāʾ ʿulūm ad-dīn, Kitāb al-ʾilm*, translated by Nabih Amin Faris. Lahore: Ashraf Press.

al-Ghazzālī, Abū-Ḥāmid Muḥammad Ibn-Muḥammad. 1992. *The Ninety-Nine Beautiful Names of God (Al-Maqṣad al-asnā fī sharḥ asmāʾ al-ḥusnā)*, translated by David B. Burrell and Nazih Daher. Cambridge UK: The Islamic Text Society.

al-Ghazzālī, Abū-Ḥāmid Muḥammad Ibn-Muḥammad. 1998. *Kīmiyāʾ as-Saʾāda. Das Elixier der Glückseligkeit*, translated by Hellmut Ritter. München: Diderichs.

Giddens, Anthony. 1998. *The Third Way*. Cambridge UK: Polity Press.

Gil'adi, Avner. 1992. *Children of Islam: Concepts of Childhood in Medieval Muslim Society*. London: Macmillan.

Gil'adi, Avner. 1999. *Infants, Parents, and Wet Nurses: Medieval Islamic views on Breastfeeding and their Social Implications*. Leiden: E. J. Brill.

Gilles de Corbeil. 1826. *Aegidii Corboliensis carmina medic*, edited by Ludwig Choulant. Leipzig: Voss.

Gillon, Ranaan. 1986. *Philosophical Medical Ethics*. Chichester: John Wiley & Sons.

Gillon, Ranaan, and A. Lloyd. 1994. *Principles of Health Care Ethics*. Chichester: John Wiley & Sons.

Giordano, Ralf. 1987. *Die zweite Schuld oder von der Last Deutscher zu sein*. Hamburg: Rasch und Röhring.

Girgolav, S. 1930. "Eksperimenty na lyudjakh." In *Vrachebnaya Taina i Vrachebnaya Etika. Rechi i Stat'i*, edited by V. I. Voyachek and V. P. Osipov, 21–5. Leningrad: Krasnaya Gazeta.

Girolamo, Mercuriale, and Michele Colombo. 1588. *Hippocratis Coi Opera quae exstant Graece et Latine veterum codicum collatione restituta . . . .* Venice: Giunta.

Gisborne, Thomas. 1789. *The Principles of Moral Philosophy Investigated and briefly Applied to the Constitution of Civil Society*. London: B. & J. White.

Gisborne, Thomas. 1794. *An Enquiry into the Duties of Men in the Higher and Middle Classes of Society in Great Britain Resulting from their Respective Stations, Professions and Employment*. London: B. & J. White.

Gisborne, Thomas. [1794] 1847. W. A. Greenhill editor, *On the Duties of Physicians: Resulting from their Profession*. Oxford: J. H. Parker; London: J. Churchill.

Gisborne, Thomas. 1797. *An Enquiry into the Duties of the Female Sex*. London: B. & J. White.

Glasa, Jozef, ed. 1992. *Contemporary Problems of Medical Ethics in Central Europe*. Bratislave, Yugoslavia: Institute Medical Ethics and Bioethics.

Glasa, Jozef, et al. 2000. "Ethics Committees in the Slovak Republic." In *Ethics Committees in Central and Eastern Europe*, edited by Jozef Glasa, 229–38. Bratislava: Charis-IMEB FDN.

Glover, Jonathan. 1999. *Humanity: A Moral History of the Twentieth Century*. London: Jonathan Cape.

Goerke, Heinz. 1984. *Berliner Ärzte*. 2nd ed. Berlin: Berlin Verlag.

Goerke, Heinz. 1994. "Moll, Albert." In *Neue Deutsche Biographie*, edited by Historische Kommission bei der Bayerischen Akademie der Wissenschaften, vol. 17, 733. Berlin: Duncker & Humblot.

Goerke, Heinz. 1999. "Pagel, Julius Leopold." In *Neue Deutsche Biographie*, edited by Historische Kommission bei der Bayerischen Akademie der Wissenschaften, vol. 19, 759. Berlin: Duncker & Humblot.

Goitein, Shelomo Dov. 1967–1993. *A Mediterranean Society: The Jewish Communities of the Arab World as Portrayed in the Documents of the Cairo Geniza*. 6 vols. Berkeley CA: University of California Press.

Gold, Hal. 1996. *Unit 731 Testimony*. Tokyo: Charles E Tuttle Co.

Goldberg, Herbert S. 1963. *Hippocrates, Father of Medicine*. New York: Franklin Watts.

Goldstein, Doris Mueller. 1999. "Bibliography of Resources by and about André E. Hellegers." *Kennedy Institute of Ethics Journal*. 9(1): 89–107.

Goldstein, S. 1989. *Suicide in Rabbinic Literature*. Hoboken NJ: Ktav.

Gomez, Pedro León. 1744. *Dissertaciones morales, y medicas: en que se expressan los casos, en que pueden declarar los medicos no obliga el comer de viernes, guardar la forma del fasting, decir, ó oir missa, el rezo, ó la assitencia al choro*. Madrid: Manuel Fernández.

Gomez, Pedro León. 1768. *Disertación de pulsos: en que se da a entender lo mucho que hay que saber sobre su conocimiento y pronosticos. Y un breve apéndice de las disertaciones morales y medicas*. Madrid: Viuda de Manuel Fernández.

González, Ceferino. 1873. *Filosofía elemental*. 2 vols. Madrid: Imprenta de Policarpo López.

Good, Charles M. 1987. *Ethnomedical Systems in Africa: Patterns of Traditional Medicine in Rural and Urban Kenya*. New York: Guilford Press.

Goodin, Robert E. 1989. *No Smoking: The Ethical Issues*. Chicago: University of Chicago Press.

Goodman, Nathan G. 1934. *Benjamin Rush: Physician and Citizen, 1746–1813*. Philadelphia: University of Pennsylvania Press.

Goodwin, W. E., and D. C. Martin. 1963. "Transplantation of the Kidney." *Urological Survey*. 13: 229–48.

Gorski, A. J., and Z. Zalewski. 2000. "Recent Developments in Bioethics in Polish Science and Medicine." In *Ethics Committees in Central and Eastern Europe*, edited by Jozef Glasa, 209–16. Bratislava: Charis-IMEB FDN.

Goslar, H., ed. 1930. *Hygiene und Judentum*. Dresden: Sternlicht.

Gostin, Lawrence O. 1993. "Controlling the Resurgent Tuberculosis Epidemic: A 50-State Survey of TB Statutes and Proposals for Reform." *Journal of the American Medical Association*. 269: 255–61.

Gotthard, Joseph Friedrich. 1793. *Leitfaden für angehende Aerzte Kranke zu prüfen und Krankheiten zu erforschen mit einer Kranken- und Witterungsbeobachtungstabelle*. Erlangen: Palm.

Gourevitch, Danielle. 1984. *Le triangle hippocratique dans le monde greco-romain: Le malade, sa maladie, et son medecin (Bibliotheque des Ecoles francaises d'Athenes et de Rome, 251)*. Rome: Ecole francaise de Rome.

Gove, Philip Babcock, ed. 1971. *Webster's Third New International Dictionary of the English Language Unabridged*. Springfield MA: G. & C. Merriam Co.

Government of Japan. 1997. *The Long Term Care Insurance Law (Kaigo Hoken Ho)*.

Government of Japan, Ministry of Health, Labor and Welfare (MHLW). 2003. *White Paper on Health, Labor, and Welfare*. Tokyo: Gyosei.

Govinda, Lama Angarika. 1974. *The Psychological Attitude of Early Buddhist Philosophy*. New York: Samuel Weiser.

Gracia, Diego. 1980. "Ideología y ciencia clínica en la España de la primera mitad del siglo XIX." *Estudios de Historia Social*. 12–13: 229–43.

Gracia, Diego. 1987. "Spain: From the Decree to the Proposal." *Hastings Center Report*. 17: S29–S31.

Gracia, Diego. 1988. "Spain: New Problems, New Books." *Hastings Center Report*. 18: S29–S30.

Gracia, Diego. 1995. "Hard Times, Hard Choices: Founding Bioethics Today." *Bioethics*. 9: 192–206.

Gracia, Diego. 1996. "Bioethics in the Spanish-Speaking World." In *History of Bioethics: International Perspectives*, edited by Roberto dell'Oro and Corrado Viafora, 169–97. San Francisco CA: International Scholars Publications.

Gracia, Diego, and Teresa Gracia. 1995. "History of Medical Ethics: IV. Europe: D. Contemporary Period: 2. Southern Europe." In *Encyclopedia of Bioethics*. 2nd ed., edited by Warren T. Reich, 1556–63. New York: Simon & Schuster Macmillan.

Gradmann, Christoph. 2001. "Robert Koch and the Pressures of Scientific Research: Tuberculosis and Tuberculin." *Medical History*. 45: 1–32.

Gräf, Erwin. 1967. "Die Stellungnahme des islamischen Rechts zu Geburtenregelung (tanāīm al-nasl) und Geburtenbeschränkung (taḥdīd al-nasl)." In *Der Orient in der Forschung*, edited by Wilhelm Hoenerbach, 209–32. Wiesbaden: Otto Harrosowitz.

Gräf, Erwin. 1976. "Auffassungen vom Tod im Rahmen islamischer Anthropologie." In *Der Mensch und sein Tod*, edited by Johannes Schwartländer, 126–45. Göttingen: Vandenhoeck Ruprecht.

Graham, Stephen. 1935. *Tsar of Freedom: The Life and Reign of Alexander II*. New Haven CT: Yale University Press.

Granjel, Luis S. 1979. *La Medicina española del siglo XVIII*. Salamanca: Ediciones Universidad de Salamanca.

Granjel, Luis S. 1986. *La Medicina española contemporánea*. Salamanca: Ediciones Universidad de Salamanca.

Grasset, Joseph. 1900a. *Principes Fondamentaux de la Déontologie Médicale*. Paris: Masson.

Grasset, Joseph. 1900b. "Rapport: Sur les principes fondamentaux de la déontologie médicale." In *Congrès international de médecine professionelle et de déontologie médicale, 1er., Paris, 1900. Compte Rendu*, edited by Jules Glover, 293–371. Paris: Masson & Cie.

Gray, Bradford H. 1995. "Bioethics Commissions: What Can We Learn from Past Successes and Failures?" In *Society's Choices: Social and Ethical Decision Making in Biomedicine*, edited by R. E. Bulger, E. M. Bobby, and H. V. Fineberg, 261–306. Washington DC: National Academy Press.

Green, Michael B., and Daniel Wikler. 1980. "Brain Death and Personal Identity." *Philosophy and Public Affairs*. 9: 105–33.

Green, R. M. 1985. "Contemporary Jewish Bioethics: A Critical Assessment." In *Theology and Bioethics*, edited by Earl E. Shelp, 245–66. Dordrecht: D. Reidel.

Greenberg, Moshe. 1960. "Some Postulates of Biblical Criminal Law." In *Yehezkel Kaufmann Jubilee Volume*, edited by M. Haran, 5–28. Jerusalem: Magness Press.

Greene, N. M. 1976. "Henry Knowles Beecher, 1904–1976 (obituary)." *Anesthesiology*. 45: 377–8.

Greene, Velvl W. 1992. "Can Scientists Use Information Derived from the Concentration Camps?" In *When Medicine Went Mad: Bioethics and the Holocaust*, edited by Arthur L. Caplan, 155–70. Totowa NJ: Humana Press.

Gregory XVI. 1832. *Mirari Vos Arbitramur*. www.papalencyclicals.net.

Gregory, James. 1800. *Memorial to the Managers of Royal Infirmary*. Edinburgh: Murray and Cochrane.

Gregory, John. 1759. *An Inquiry into Those Faculties which Distinguish Man from the Rest of Animal Creation*. Aberdeen University Library, MS 3107/1/4.

Gregory, John. 1765. *A Comparative View of the State and Faculties of Man with those of the Animal World*. London: J. Dodsley.

Gregory, John. 1770. *Observations on the Duties and Offices of a Physician, and on the Method of Prosecuting Enquiries in Philosophy*. London: W. Strahan and T. Cadell.

Gregory, John. [1770] 1998a. *Observations on the Duties and Offices of a Physician, and on the Method of Prosecuting Enquiries in Philosophy*. [London: W. Strahan and T. Cadell]. Reprinted in *John Gregory's Writings on Medical Ethics and Philosophy of Medicine*, edited by Laurence B. McCullough, 93–159. Dordrecht: Kluwer Academic Publishers.

Gregory, John. 1771. "Clinical Lectures by Dr. Gregory 1771 & Dr. Cullen 1772." Student notes, author unknown. Royal College of Surgeons of Edinburgh MS 36.

Gregory, John. [1772a] 1817. *Lectures on the Duties and Qualifications of a Physician*. Philadelphia: M. Carey & Son.

Gregory, John. [1772b] 1998b. *Lectures on the Duties and Qualifications of a Physician*. [London: W. Strahan and T. Cadell]. Reprinted in *John Gregory's Writings on Medical Ethics and Philosophy of Medicine*, edited by Laurence B. McCullough, 161–245. Dordrecht: Kluwer Academic Publishers.

Gregory, John. 1774. *A Father's Legacy to his Daughters*. London: W. Strahan and T. Cadell.

Gregory, John. 1778. *Vorlesungen über die Pflichten und Eigenschaften eines Artzes: Aus dem Englischen nach der neuen und verbesserten Ausgabe*, translator unknown. Leipzig: Caspar Fritsch.

Gregory, John. 1787. *Discours sur les devoirs, les qualities et les connaissances du médicin, avec un cour d'études*, translated by B. Verlac. Paris: Crapart & Briands.

Gregory, John. 1789. *Lexioni Sopra I Doveri e la Qualita di un Medico*, translated by F. F. Padovano. Florence: Gaetano Cambiagi.

Gregory, Juan. 1803. *Discurso sobre los deberes, qualidades y conocimientos del medico, con el método de sus estudios*. Madrid: Imprenta Real.

Gregory of Nazianzus. n.d. *Funebra in laudem Caesarii fratris*. Patrologia Graeca 36: 755–88.

Gregory of Nazianzus. 1908. *St. Grégoire de Nazianze: Discours funèbres en l'honneur de son frère Césaire et de Basile de Césarée (Oratio 8; 43)*, edited by F. Boulanger, 2–56. Paris: Picard.

Gregory of Tours. 1988. *Fränkische Geschichte I–X. Nach der Übersetzung von Wilhelm von Giesebrecht. Neu bearbeitet von Manfred Gebauer*. 3 vols. Essen/Stuttgart: Phaidon.

Grell, Ole Peter. 1993a. "Caspar Bartholin and the Education of the Pious Physician." In *Medicine and the Reformation*, edited by Ole Peter Grell and Andrew Cunningham, 78–100. London: Routledge.

Grell, Ole Peter. 1993b. "Conflicting Duties: Plague and the Obligations of Early Modern Physicians Towards Patients and Commonwealth in England and the Netherlands." In *Doctors and Ethics: The Earlier Historical Setting of Professional Ethics*, edited by Andrew Wear, Johanna Geyer-Kordesch, and Roger French, 131–52. Amsterdam: Rodopi.

Grelletry, J. Lucien. 1900. *L'Héroisme Médical*. Macon: Protat Frères.

Grin, I. V. 1914. *Abort – prestuplenie ili operatsija?* Moscow.

Grisez, Germain. 1993. "Revelation versus Dissent." *The Tablet*. 247: 1329–31.

Grodin, Michael A. 1992. "Historical Origins of the Nuremberg Code." In *The Nazi Doctors and the Nuremberg Code*, edited by George J. Annas and Michael A. Grodin, 121–44. New York: Oxford University Press.

Gromer, Johann. 1985. *Julius Leopold Pagel (1851–1912). Medizinhistoriker und Arzt*. Cologne: Kohlhauer.

Gross, Samuel. 1879. "Memorial: Isaac Hays." *American Journal of the Medical Sciences*. NS. 78: 281–92.

Gruman, Gerald. 1966. "A History of Ideas About the Prolongation of Life: The Evolution of the Prolongevity Hypothesis to 1800." *Transactions of the American Philosophical Society*. 56.9: 1–102.

Grysanowski, Ernst. 1897. *Gesammelte antivivisectionistische Schriften*. Münster: Basch.

Guarnieri, Patrizia. 1990. "Moritz Schiff (1823–1896): Experimental Physiology and Noble Sentiment in Florence." In *Vivisection in Historical Perspective*. 2nd ed., edited by Nicolaas A. Rupke, 105–24. London: Routledge.

Guerra, Francisco. 1972. "Medicina colonial en Hispanoamérica." In *Historia Universal de la Medicina*. IV, edited by Pedro Laín Entralgo, 346–55. Barcelona: Salvat.

Guerrini, Anita. 1989. "The Ethics of Animal Experimentation in Seventeenth-Century England." *Journal of the History of Ideas*. 50: 391–407.

Guido d'Arezzo. 1984. *Guido d'Arezzo der Jüngere und sein, Liber mitis*, edited by Konrad Goehl. Würzburger Medizinhistorische Forschungen 32. Pattensen: Horst Wellm.

Guillaume, Pierre. 1996. *Le Rôle Social du Médecin Depuis Deux Siècles, 1800–1945*. Paris: Association Pour l'Etude de L'Histoire de la Secutité Sociale.

Gulyaev, A. V. 1970. "Voprosy deontologii v khirurgii." In *Pervaya Vsesoyuznaya Konferentsija po Problemam Meditsynskoi Deontologii: Moskva, 28–29 janvarja 1969g*, edited by A. F. Bilibin et al., 71–81. Moscow: Meditsyna.

Guo, Chengzhou, ed. 1997. *Records of Japanese Bacteriological Warfare in China*. Beijing: Yanshan Press.

Guo, X., et al. 1998. "Chinese Values Regarding Euthanasia." *Chinese and International Philosophy of Medicine*. 1.1: 137–49 [Chinese].

Gurlt, Ernst. 1931. Christoph Wilhelm Hufeland. In: *Biographisches Lexikon der hervorragenden Ärzte aller Zeiten und Völker*. 2nd ed., edited by August Hirsch, Vol. 3, 329–32. Berlin: Urban & Schwarzenberg.

Guroian, Vigen. 1996. *Life's Living toward Dying*. Grand Rapids MI: Wm. Eerdmans.

Gustafson, James M. 1978. *Protestant and Roman Catholic Ethics: Prospects for Rapprochement*. Chicago: University of Chicago Press.

Guthrie, George James. 1815. *On Gun-Shot Wounds of the Extremities*. London: Longman.

Haakonssen, Lisbeth. 1997. *Medicine and Morals in the Enlightenment: John Gregory, Thomas Percival, and Benjamin Rush*. Amsterdam: Rodopi.

Haber, Samuel. 1991. *The Quest for Authority and Honor in the American Professions 1750–1900*. Chicago: University of Chicago Press.

Hachmeister, Sylke. 1992. *Kinopropaganda gegen Kranke: Die Instrumentalisierung des Spielfilms "Ich klage an" für das nationalsozialistische "Euthanasieprogramm."* Baden Baden: Nomos.

Hacking, Ian. 1975. *The Emergence of Probability*. Cambridge UK: Cambridge University Press.

Haddad, Farid S. 1982. "Arabic Medical Ethics." *Studies in History of Medicine*. 6: 122–36.

Haeckel, Ernst. 1866. *Generelle Morphologie der Organismen: Allgemeine Grundzüge der organischen Formenwissenschaft, mechanisch begründet durch die von Charles Darwin reformirte Descendenz-Theorie*. Berlin: G. Reimer.

Haeckel, Ernst. 1874. *Anthropogenie oder Entwicklungsgeschichte des Menschen*. Leipzig: W. Engelmann.

Haeckel, Ernst. 1899. *Die Welträtsel. Gemeinverständliche Studien über biologische Philosophie*. Bonn: E. Strauss.

Hafner, Karl Heinz, and Rolf Winau. 1974. "'Die Freigabe der Vernichtung lebensunwerten Lebens.' Eine Untersuchung zu der Schrift von Karl Binding und Alfred Hoche." *Medizinhistorisches Journal*. 9: 227–54.

Hagemann, Ludwig. 1985. "Eschatologie im Islam." In *Weiterleben nach dem Tode?*, edited by Adel Th. Khoury and Peter Hünermann, 103–20. Freiburg i. Br.: Herder.

Hahn, Susanne. 1984. "Die ärztliche Ethik im Leben eines Arztes der Seele – Überlegungen zur medizinisch-ethischen Konzeption Albert Molls (1862–1936)." *Zeitschrift für die gesamte innere Medizin*. 39: 558–61.

Hahn, Susanne. 1995. "'Der Lübecker Totentanz': Zur rechtlichen und ethischen Problematik der Katastrophe bei der Erprobung der Tuberkuloseimpfung 1930 in Deutschland." *Medizinhistorisches Journal*. 30: 61–79.

Halbfass, Wilhelm. 1988. *India and Europe: An Essay in Understanding*. Albany NY: State University of New York Press.

Haldar, Jnanranjan R. 1977. *Medical Science in Pali Literature*. Calcutta: Indian Museum.

Haldar, Jnanranjan R. 1992. *Development of Public Health in Buddhism*. Varanasi: Indological Book House.

Halevy, Amir, and Baruch Brody. 1993. "Brain Death: Reconciling Definitions, Criteria, and Tests." *Annals of Internal Medicine*. 119: 519–25.

Hall, Marshall. 1831. *A Critical and Experimental Essay on the Circulation of the Blood*. London: Seeley and Burnside.

Haller, Albrecht von. 1756–60. *Mémoires sur la nature sensible et irritable, des parties du corps animal*. 4 vols. Lausanne: Bousquet and d'Arnay.

Haller, John S. 1981. *American Medicine in Transition 1840–1910*. Urbana IL: University of Illinois Press.

Halper, Thomas. 1989. *The Misfortunes of Others: End-Stage Renal Disease in the United Kingdom*. Cambridge UK: Cambridge University Press.

Halpern, Jodi. 2001. *From Detached Concern to Empathy: Humanizing Medical Practice*. New York: Oxford University Press.

Hamarneh, Sami K. 1964. "Origin and Functions of the Hisbah System in Islam and its Impact on the Health Professions." *Sudhoffs Archiv*. 48: 157–73.

Hamarneh, Sami K. 1997. *Background of Yunani (Unani), Arabic and Islamic Medicine and Pharmacy*. Karachi: Hamdard Foundation.

Hamburger, Jean, and Jean Crosnier. 1968. "Moral and Ethical Problems in Transplantation." In *Human Transplantation*, edited by Felix T. Rappaport and Jean Dausset. New York: Grune and Stratton.

Hamilton, Frank H. 1856. *Eulogy on the Life and Character of Theodric Romeyn Beck, M. D., LL. D., delivered before the Medical Society of the state of New-York*. Albany NY: Medical Society of the State of New York.

Hamilton, J. S. 1986. "Scribonius Largus on the Medical Profession." *Bulletin of the History of Medicine.* 60: 209–16.

Hamlin, Christopher. 1990. *Public Health and Social Justice in the Age of Chadwick.* Cambridge UK: Cambridge University Press.

Hampson, Judith. 1990. "Legislation: A Practical Solution to the Vivisection Dilemma?" In *Vivisection in Historical Perspective.* 2nd ed., edited by Nicolaas A. Rupke, 314–39. London: Routledge.

Hankinson, R. J. 1992. "Galen's Philosophical Eclecticism." In *Aufstieg und Niedergang der romischen Welt.* II, 36.5, edited by Wofgang Haase and Hildegard Temporini, 3505–22. Berlin/New York: Walter De Gruyter.

Hankinson, R. J. 1994. "Galen's Concept of Scientific Progress." In *Aufstieg und Niedergang der romischen Welt.* II, 37.2, edited by Wofgang Haase and Hildegard Temporini, 1775- 89. Berlin/New York: Walter De Gruyter.

Hankinson, R. J., ed. 1998. *Galen On Antecedent Causes,* edited with an introduction, translation, and commentary by R. J. Hankinson. Cambridge UK: Cambridge University Press.

Hansmann, H. 1989. "The Economics and Ethics of Markets for Human Organs." In *Organ Transplantation Policy: Issues and Prospects,* edited by James F. Blumenstein and Frank A. Sloan, 57–85. Durham NC: Duke University Press.

Harakas, Stanley. 1990. *Health and Medicine in the Eastern Orthodox Tradition.* New York: Crossroad.

Harandi, Sheikh Mustafa al-. 1997. *Al-Istinsakh al-Bashari waHuquq al-Shari'a al-Islamiyya. (Human Cloning and the Rights of the Islamic Shari'a).* Kuwait: Maktabat al-Alfayn.

Harbison, E. Harris. 1964. "The Protestant Reformation." In E. Harris Harbison, *Christianity and History: Essays,* 141–56. Princeton NJ: Princeton University Press.

Hardacre, Helen. 1994. "Response of Buddhism and Shinto to the Issue of Brain Death and Organ Transplant." *Cambridge Quarterly of Healthcare Ethics.* 3: 585–601.

Häring, Bernard. 1968. "The Encyclical Crisis." *Commonweal.* 88: 588–94.

Häring, Bernard. 1973. *Medical Ethics,* edited by Gabrielle L. Jean. Notre Dame IN: Fides.

Häring, Bernard. 1993. "A Distrust That Wounds." *The Tablet.* 247: 1378–9.

Harkness, Jon M. 1996a. "Nuremberg and the Issue of Wartime Experiments on U.S. Prisoners: The Green Committee." *Journal of the American Medical Association.* 276: 1672–75.

Harkness, Jon M. 1996b. "Research Behind Bars: A History of Medical Experimentation on American Prisoners." Ph.D. diss., University of Wisconsin, Wisconsin.

Harkness, Jon M. 1998. "The Significance of the Nuremberg Code." *New England Journal of Medicine.* 338: 995–6.

Harkness, Jon M. 1999. "Beecher, Henry Knowles." In *American National Biography,* edited by John A. Garraty and Mark C. Carnes, vol. 2, 456–67. New York: Oxford University Press.

Harkness, Jon M. 1999b. "Ivy, Andrew C." In *American National Biography,* edited by John A. Garraty and Mark C. Carnes, Vol. 11, 726–28. New York: Oxford University Press.

Harley, David. 1990. "Honour and Property: The Structure of Professional Disputes in Eighteenth-Century English Medicine." In *The Medical Enlightenment of the Eighteenth Century,* edited by Andrew Cunningham and Roger French, 138–64. Cambridge UK: Cambridge University Press.

Harley, David. 1993a. "Ethics and Dispute Behavior in the Career of Henry Bracken of Lancaster: Surgeon, Physician and Manmidwife." In *The Codification of Medical Morality: Historical and Philosophical Studies of the Formalization of Western Medical Morality in the Eighteenth and Nineteenth Centuries: Volume One: Medical Ethics and Etiquette in the Eighteenth Century,* edited by Robert Baker, Dorothy Porter, and Roy Porter, 47–71. Dordrecht: Kluwer Academic Publishers.

Harley, David. 1993b. "Medical Metaphors in English Moral Theology, 1560–1660." *Journal of the History of Medicine.* 48: 396–435.

Harley, David. 1994. "The Scope of Legal Medicine in Lancashire and Cheshire, 1660–1760." In *Legal Medicine in History,* edited by Michael Clark and Catherine Crawford, 45–63. Cambridge UK: Cambridge University Press.

Harnack, Adolf. 1892. "Medicinisches aus der ältesten Kirchengeschichte." *Texte und Untersuchungen zur Geschichte der altchristlichen Literatur.* 8.4: 37–152.

Harrell, David Edwin, Jr. 1975. *All Things Are Possible: The Healing and Charismatic Revivals in Modern America.* Bloomington IN: Indiana University Press.

Harris, John. 1985. *The Value of Life.* London: Routledge & Kegan Paul.

Harris, John. 2004. "Immortal Ethics." In *Strategies for Engineered Negligible Senescence: Why Genuine Control of Aging May Be Foreseeable,* edited by Aubrey D. N. J. de Grey, 527–34. New York: Annals of the New York Academy of Sciences.

Harris, John. 2005. "The Age Indifference Principle and Equality." *Cambridge Quarterly of Healthcare Ethics.* 14: 93–9.

Harris, Sheldon R. 1994. *Factories of Death: Japanese Biological Warfare, 1932–1945, and the American Cover-Up.* London/New York: Routledge.

Harris, Sheldon R. 2000. "Japanese Medical Atrocities in World War II: Unit 731 was not an Isolated Aberration." Presented at the International Citizens Forum on War Crimes and Redress, Tokyo. December 11, 1999; updated February 25, 2000. www.vcn.bc.ca/alpha/speech/Harris.htm (visited October 28, 2007).

Harrison, Carol E. 1999. *The Bourgeois Citizen in Nineteenth-Century France: Gender, Sociability, and the Uses of Emulation.* Oxford: Oxford University Press.

Harsin, Jill. 1989. "Syphilis, Wives, and Physicians: Medical Ethics and the Family in Nineteenth-Century French Medicine." *French Historical Studies.* 16.1 (Spring): 72–95.

Hart, James. 1623. *The Arraignment of Urines Wherein Are Set Downe the Manifold Errors and Abuses of Ignorant Urinemongering Empirickes, Cozening Quacksalvers, Women-physitians . . . Written First by Peter Forrest . . . Newly Epitomized and Translated . . . by James Hart.* London: G. Eld for Robert Mylbourne.

Harvey, John Collins. 2004. "André Hellegers and Carroll House: Architect and Blueprint for the Kennedy Institute of Ethics." *Kennedy Institute of Ethics Journal.* 14 (2): 199–206.

Harvey, Peter. 2000. *An Introduction to Buddhist Ethics.* Cambridge UK: Cambridge University Press.

Harvey, Susan Ashbrook. 1985. "Physicians and Ascetics in John of Ephesus: An Expedient Alliance." In *Symposium on Byzantine Medicine,* edited by John Scarborough, 87–93. Washington DC: Dumbarton Oaks Library and Collection.

Harvey, William. [1628] 1928. *Exercitatio anatomica de motu cordis et sanguinis in animalibus.* Reprint. Florence: R. Lier.

Haskell, Thomas L. 1998. *Objectivity is not Neutrality: Explanatory Schemes in History.* Baltimore/London: Johns Hopkins University Press.

Hastedt, Heiner. 1998. *Der Wert des Einzelnen: Eine Verteidigung des Individualismus.* Frankfurt: Suhrkamp.

Hathout, Hassan. 1990. "The Ethics of Genetic Engineering: An Islamic Viewpoint." *Journal of the Islamic Medical Association of North America.* 22: 99–101.

Hathout, Hassan. 1992. "Islamic Basis for Biomedical Ethics." In *Transcultural Dimensions in Medical Ethics,* edited by Edmund Pellegrino et al., 57–72. Frederick MD: University Publishing Group.

Hathout, Hassan, and B. Andrew Lustig. 1993. "Bioethical Developments in Islam." In *Theological Developments in Bioethics: 1990–92,* edited by B. Andrew Lustig, 133–47. Dordrecht: Kluwer Academic Publishers.

Hauerwas, Stanley. 1986. *Suffering Presence: Theological Reflections on Medicine, the Mentally Handicapped, and the Church.* Notre Dame IN: University of Notre Dame Press.

Hayʾat, Kibar al-Ulamaa. 1994. *Abhath Hayʾat Kibar al-Ulamaa bilMamlaka al-Arabiyya Al-Suʾudiyya (Research of the Supreme Council of Scholars).* Cairo: Maktabat al-Sunna.

Hays, Isaac. 1834–1836. *The American Cyclopedia of Practical Medicine and Surgery; a Digest of Medical Literature.* Philadelphia: Carey, Lea, and Blanchard.

Hays, Isaac. [1847] 1999. "Note to the 1847 Convention." In *The American Medical Ethics Revolution: How the AMA's Code of Ethics Has Transformed Physicians' Relationships to Patients, Professionals, and Society,* edited by Robert Baker et al., 315. Baltimore: Johns Hopkins University Press.

Hazelgrove, Jenny. 2002. "The Old Faith and the New Science: The Nuremberg Code and Human Experimentation Ethics in Britain, 1946–73." *Social History of Medicine.* 15: 109–35.

He, Lun, and Shi Weixing. 1988. *Modern Medical Ethics.* Zhejiang Education Press.

He, Zhaoxong, ed. 1988. *A History of Medical Morality in China.* Shanghai: Shanghai Medical University Press.

Health Education Library for People. [November 17, 1999, In *Times of India*]. 1999. "Rally for Ban on Sex Selection Tests, Female Foeticide." *Health Education Library for People.* http://www.healthlibrary.com/news/15-21nov99/rally.htm (visited July 5, 2002).

Healy, Edwin F. 1956. *Medical Ethics.* Chicago: Loyola University Press.

Healy, Timothy. 1979. "The Renaissance Man." *Kennedy Institute Quarterly Report.* 5 (1).

Heidel, William Arthur. 1941. *Hippocratic Medicine: Its Spirit and Method.* New York: Columbia University Press.

Heilmann, Karl Eugen. 1973. *Kräuterbücher in Bild und Geschichte.* München: Kölbl.

Heinisch, Klaus J. 1968. *Kaiser Friedrich II. in Briefen und Berichten seiner Zeit,* edited by Klaus J. Heinisch. Darmstadt: Wissenschaftliche Buchgesellschaft.

Heisel, William, and Mark Katches. 2000. "Organ Agencies: Aid For-Profit Supplier." *Orange County (CA) Register.* www.ocregister.com/health/body/organ.

Heister, Lorenz. 1728. *De anatomes subtilioris utilitate.* Helmstedt: Schnorr.

Hellegers, André. 1966. "Contraception and Motivation." *Bulletin of the Guild of Catholic Psychiatrists.* 13: 237.

Hellegers, André. 1967. "Abortion, the Law and the Common Good." *Medical Opinion and Review.* 3: 76. Reprinted as: "Law and the Common Good." *Commonweal.* 86 (15): 418–23.

Hellegers, André. 1969a. "Critique of an Encyclical." *Medical Opinion and Review.* 5: 71.

Hellegers, André. 1969b. "A Scientist's Analysis." In *Contraception, Authority and Dissent,* edited by Charles E. Curran, 216–39. New York: Herder and Herder.

Hellegers, André. 1973a. "Hopkins Case Raises Issue: How Long to Maintain Life?" *Internal Medicine News.* 6 (16): 34–5.

Hellegers, André. 1973b. "The Abortion Ruling: Analysis and Prognosis; Commentary: Dr. Hellegers." *Hospital Progress.* 54 (3): 86–7.

Hellegers, André. 1973c. "Amazing Historical and Biological Errors in Abortion Decision." *Hospital Progress.* 54 (5): 16–7.

Hellegers, André. 1973d. "Government Planning and the Principle of Subsidiarity." In *The Population Crisis and Moral Responsibility,* edited by J. Philip Wogaman, 137–44. Washington DC: Public Affairs Press.

Hellegers, André. 1973e. "The Beginnings of Personhood: Medical Considerations." *Perkins Journal.* 27 (1): 11–5.

Hellegers, André. 1973f. "What Is 'Extraordinary' in Maintaining Life?" *Obstetrics and Gynecology News.* 8 (14): 14. Also in *Family Practice News.* 3 (14): 16; *Internal Medicine News.* 6 (16): 34–5.

Hellegers, André. 1973g. "Population, Rhythm, Contraception and Abortion Policy Questions." *Linacre Quarterly.* 40 (2): 91–6.

Hellegers, André. 1973h. "The Johns Hopkins Case." *Obstetrics and Gynecology News.* 8 (12): 40–1. Also in *Pediatric News.* 7 (6): 36–7; *Family Practice News.* 3 (12): 20–1; *Internal Medicine News.* 6 (14): 16–7.

Hellegers, André. 1973i. "*Wade* and *Bolton:* Medical Critique." *Catholic Lawyer.* 19 (4): 251–8.

Hellegers, André. 1974a. "Ethical Problems in Human Reproduction." In *Obstetrics & Gynecology Annual,* edited by Ralph M. Wynn, Vol. 3, 1–5. New York: Appleton-Century-Crofts.

Hellegers, André. 1974b. "Ethics of Drug Introductions." *Internal Medicine News.* 7 (22): 20.

Hellegers, André. 1975a. "Bioethical Debates in Gynecology and Obstetrics." In *Gynecology and Obstetrics: The Health Care of Women,* edited by Seymour L. Romney, et al., 33–44. New York: McGraw-Hill.

Hellegers, André. 1975b. "The Ethics of the Edelin Case." *Obstetrics and Gynecology News.* 10 (10): 14. Also in *Family Practice News.* 5 (8): 44–5; *Pediatric News.* 9 (4): 22–3.

Hellegers, André. 1975c. "Abortion: Another Form of Birth Control?" *Human Life Review.* 1 (1): 21–5.

Hellegers, André. 1975d. "'I Would Have Pulled the Plug, If....'" *Obstetrics and Gynecology News.* 10 (22): 24–5. Also in *Family Practice News.* 5 (22): 46–7; *Internal Medicine News.* 18 (21): 10.

Hellegers, André. 1975e. "The Etiology of Bioethics." *Obstetrics and Gynecology News.* 10 (20): 14. Also in *Family Practice News.* 5 (14): 18.

Hellegers, André. 1976a, 1977. "Research Money for Death." *Family Practice News.* 6 (22). Also in *Obstetrics and Gynecology News.* 12 (3): 16–7.

Hellegers, André. 1976b. "Interest in Bioethics Grows." *Obstetrics and Gynecology News.* 11 (14): 32. Also in *Internal Medicine News.* 9 (21): 41; *Family Practice News.* 6 (12): 43.

Hellegers, André. 1976c. "Rising Vogue of Bioethics." *Family Practice News.* 6 (12): 43.

Hellegers, André. 1976d. "Le Problème des Choix en Politique Médicale." *Concilium: Revue Internationale de Théologie.* 110: 73–80.

Hellegers, André. 1976e. "2nd Round on Fetal Research." *Obstetrics and Gynecology News.* 11 (10): 14–5. Also in *Family Practice News.* 6 (8): 30.

Hellegers, André. 1976f. "Ethical Aspects of Research." *Obstetrics and Gynecology News.* 11 (6): 26–7. Also in *Family Practice News.* 6 (2): 36.

Hellegers, André. 1976g. "Formal Education in Ethics." *Internal Medicine News.* 9 (21): 41.

Hellegers, André. 1976h. "Funds for Spiritual Research?" *Family Practice News.* 6 (2): 36.

Hellegers, André. 1976i. "Medische en ethische problemen in de adolescentie." *Nederlands Artsenverbond Informatiebulletin.* 3 (2): 3–18.

Hellegers, André. 1976j. "New Commission, New Focus." *Obstetrics and Gynecology News.* 11 (8): 54–5.

Hellegers, André. 1976k. "Quinlan: No Sweeping Precedent." *Obstetrics and Gynecology News* 11 (15): 16, 1.

Hellegers, André. 1976l. "Right to Work in Pregnancy?" *Family Practice News.* 6 (16): 28.

Hellegers, André. 1976m. "Should Pregnant Women Work?" *Obstetrics and Gynecology News.* 11 (17): 29. Also in *Family Practice News.* 6 (16): 28.

Hellegers, André. 1977a. "Biostatistische Grundlagen der Bevölkerungsentwicklung." In *Geburtshilfliche-gynäkologische Praxis,* edited by Fritz K. Beller and Heinz-D. Bottcher, 87–101. Stuttgart: Georg Thieme Verlag.

Hellegers, André. 1977b. "It's OK with Me, Doc. Why Do You Object?" *Contemporary Ob/Gyn.* 10 (5): 86–90.

Hellegers, André. 1977c. "Round Table Discussion: The Physician as Moral Agent." In *Philosophical Medical Ethics: Its Nature and Significance,* edited by Stuart F. Spicker and H. Tristram Engelhardt, 225–30. Boston: D. Reidel.

Hellegers, André. 1977d "A Lottery for Lives?" *Obstetrics and Gynecology News.* 12 (7): 20–1. Also in *Family Practice News.* 6 (24): 34; *Internal Medicine News.* 10 (21): 18.

Hellegers, André. 1977e. "Biologic Origins of Bioethical Problems." In *Obstetrics and Gynecology Annual,* vol. 6, edited by Ralph M. Wynn, 1–9. New York: Appleton-Century-Crofts.

Hellegers, André. 1977f. "Children and Consent." *Pediatric News.* 11 (1): 41.

Hellegers, André. 1977g. "Consent for Those Who Cannot." *Family Practice News.* 7 (10): 35.

Hellegers, André. 1977h. "Legal and Ethical Implications for Health Policy." In *Death and Dying: An Examination of Legislative and Policy Issues*, edited by Janet L. Dinsmore, 49–57. Washington DC: Health Policy Center, Georgetown University.

Hellegers, André. 1977i. "Making the Difficult Choices." *Internal Medicine News*. 10 (21): 18.

Hellegers, André. 1977j. "The Field of Bioethics." In *CRS Bioethics Workshop for Congress*, edited by Vikki Z. Zegel and Donna Parratt, 17–21. Washington DC: Congressional Research Service, Library of Congress.

Hellegers, André. 1978a. "Abortion." In *The Encyclopedia of Bioethics*, edited by Warren T. Reich, 1–5. New York: Macmillan.

Hellegers, André. 1978b. "Fetal Research." In *The Encyclopedia of Bioethics*, edited by Warren T. Reich, 489–93. New York: Macmillan.

Hellegers, André. 1978c. "Moral Education and Development. Part VI: Bioethics." *Today's Catholic Teacher*. 11 (6): 62–3.

Hellegers, André. 1979a. "Reflections on Health Care and Its Possible Future." *Kennedy Institute Quarterly Report*. 5 (1): Summer.

Hellegers, André. 1979b. "A Tyranny of Facts in Medicine." *New Physician*. 28 (6): 37–8.

Hellegers, André. 1979c. "The Ethical Dilemmas of Medical Research." In *Regulation of Scientific Inquiry: Societal Concerns with Research*, edited by Keith M. Wulff. Boulder CO: Westview Press.

Hellegers, André. 1979d "Artifice in Procreation." *Obstetrics and Gynecology News*. 14 (6): 20–1.

Hellegers, André, et al. 1968. *The Terrible Choice: The Abortion Dilemma*. New York: Bantam Books.

Hellegers, André, et al. 1979. *Biology, Ethics and Society: Questions and Issues*. New York: Prospective International.

Hellegers, André, et al. 1983. "Effect of Fetal Hypercapnia on Maternal and Fetal Cardiovascular and Respiratory Function." *European Journal of Obstetrics, Gynecology and Reproductive Biology*. 14 (5): 311–5.

Hellegers, André, and Albert R. Jonsen. 1976. "Conceptual Foundations for an Ethics of Medical Care." In *Ethics and Health Policy*, edited by Robert M. Veatch and Roy Branson, 17–33. Cambridge MA: Ballinger.

Hellegers, André, and Richard A. McCormick. 1977. "Legislation and the Living Will." *America*. 136 (10): 210–3.

Hellegers, André, and Richard A. McCormick. 1978a. "The Specter of Joseph Saikewicz: Mental Incompetence and the Law." *America*. 138 (12): 257–60.

Hellegers, André, and Richard A. McCormick. 1978b. "Unanswered Questions on Test Tube Life." *America*. 139 (4): 74–8.

Hellegers, André, Albert R., Jonsen and Paul Ramsey. 1974, 1976. "Conceptual Foundations for an Ethics of Medical Care." In *Ethics of Health Care: Papers of the Conference on Health Care and Changing Values, 27–29 November 1973*, edited by Laurence R. Tancredi, 3–20. Washington DC: National Academy of Sciences. Reprinted in Robert M. Veatch and Roy Branson, eds. 1976. *Ethics and Health Policy*, 17–33. Cambridge MA: Ballinger.

Helmchen, Hanfried, and Rolf Winau, eds. 1986. *Versuche mit Menschen in Medizin, Humanwissenschaft und Politik*. Berlin and New York: De Gruyter.

Helmont, Johannes Baptista van. 1621. *De Mageneticae Vulnerum Curatione*. Paris: Victorem le Roy.

Helmont, Johannes Baptista van. 1642. *Febrium Doctrina Inaudita*. Antwerp: Widow of Cnobbarus.

Helmont, Johannes Baptista van. 1644. *Opuscula Medica Inaudita*. Amsterdam: L. Elzevier.

Helmont, Johannes Baptista van. 1648. *Ortus Medicinae . . . Opuscula Medica Inaudita*. Amsterdam: L. Elzevier.

Helpage International. 2000. *Aging Issues in Africa: A Summary*. http://www.helpage.org/Resources/Policyreports (visited January 30, 2008).

Hendin, H. 2002. "The Dutch Experience." *Issues in Law and Medicine*. 17.3: 223–46.

Hendrick, George. 1977. *Henry Salt, Humanitarian Reformer and Man of Letters*. Urbana IL: University of Illinois Press.

Henry, Jean. (c. 1482). *Livre de vie active des Religieuses de l'Hoteldieu*. H. D. L.1425 fol.11v. Musée de l'assistance publique. Paris.

Herranz, Gonzalo. 1992. *Comentarios al Código de Etica y Deontologia Médica*. Pamplona: Eunsa.

Herranz, Gonzalo. 1998. "The Inclusion of the Ten Principles of Nuremberg in Professional Codes of Ethics: An International Comparison." In *Ethics Codes in Medicine: Foundations and Achievements of Codification since 1947*, edited by Ulrich Tröhler and Stella Reiter-Theil, 127–39. Aldershot/Brookfield/Singapore/Sydney: Ashgate.

Herranz, Gonzalo. 2002. "The Origin of Primum Non Nocere." *British Medical Journal*, electronic responses and commentary. (September 1).

Herrnstein, Richard, and Charles Murray. 1994. *The Bell Curve*. New York: Free Press.

Hertzen, Alexander I. 1956. *Sobranie Sochinenii v 30 Tomakh*, tom 7. Moscow: Izdatel'stvo Akademii Nauk SSSR.

Hibbard, James F. 1879. "The Relations of the Code of Ethics to State and Municipal Sanitary Organizations." *Transactions of the American Medical Association*. 30: 383–7.

Hick, John. 1985. *Evil and the God of Love*. 2nd ed. Basinstoke UK: Macmillan.

Higgs, R. 1997. "As, rule of." In *The New Dictionary of Medical Ethics*, edited by K. Boyd, R. Higgs, and J. Pinching, 1. London: BMJ Publishing Group.

Hildegard von Bingen. 1998. *Hildegard von Bingen, 1098– 1179*, edited by Hans-Juergen Kotzur. Mainz: Philipp von Zabern.

Hildreth, Charles T. 1834. "Case of Notencephale, with Engravings." Boston: Published privately for the author, not paginated.

Hildreth, Martha. 1987. *Doctors, Bureaucrats, and Public Health in France, 1888–1902*. New York: Garland.

Hill, Christopher. 1964. *Society and Puritanism in Pre-Revolutionary England*. London: Secker & Warburg.

Hill, Hibbert Winslow. 1916. *The New Public Health*. New York: Macmillan.

Hippocrates. 1923a. *Hippocrates, Volume I*, translated by W. H. S. Jones. Cambridge MA: Harvard University Press.

Hippocrates. 1923b. *Hippocrates, Volume II*, translated by W. H. S. Jones. Cambridge MA: Harvard University Press.

Hippocrates. 1928. *Hippocrates, Volume III*, translated by E. T. Withington. Cambridge MA: Harvard University Press.

Hippocrates. 1931. *Hippocrates, Volume IV*, translated by W. H. S. Jones. Cambridge MA: Harvard University Press.

Hippocrates. 1959a. *Decorum*. Hippocrates Works II, 269–301. Loeb Classical Library. London/Cambridge MA: William Heinemann, Harvard University Press.

Hippocrates. 1959b. *Humours*. Hippocrates Works IV, 62–95. Loeb Classical Library. London/Cambridge MA: William Heinemann, Harvard University Press.

Hippocrates. 1962a. *Oath*. Hippocrates Works I, 291–7. Loeb Classical Library. London/Cambridge MA: William Heinemann, Harvard University Press.

Hippocrates. 1962b. *Precepts*. Hippocrates Works I, 312–23. Loeb Classical Library. London/Cambridge MA: William Heinemann, Harvard University Press.

Hippocrates. [1962] 1994. *Epidemics*. Hippocrates Works I, 139–287 (Epidemics 1–3), VII, 18–415 (Epidemics 2; 4–7). Loeb Classical Library. London/Cambridge MA: Harvard University Press.

Hippocrates. 1988a. *Hippocrates, Volume V*, translated by Paul Potter. Cambridge MA: Harvard University Press.

Hippocrates. 1988b. *Hippocrates, Volume VI*, translated by Paul Potter. Cambridge MA: Harvard University Press.

Hippocrates. 1991. *Hippocrates, Volume VII*, translated by Wesley D. Smith. Cambridge MA: Harvard University Press.

Hippocrates. 1995. *Hippocrates, Volume VIII*, translated by Paul Potter. Cambridge MA: Harvard University Press.

Hiroi, Yoshinori. 1996. *Genetic Technologies, Genetic Thoughts*. Tokyo: Chuou Kouronsha Publishers [Japanese].

Hitchcock, Richard. 1990. "Arabic Medicine: The Andalusi Context." In *The Human Embryo: Aristotle and the Arabic and European Traditions*, edited by G. R. Dunstan, 70–8. Exeter: University of Exeter Press.

Hitler, Adolf. [1926] 1939. *Mein Kampf*. New York: Stackpole Sons.

Hitler, Adolf. 1936. *Mein Kampf*. Munich: Zentralverlag der NSDAP.

Ho, P. Y., and F. P. Lisowski. 1997. *A Brief History of Chinese Medicine*. 2nd ed. Singapore: World Scientific.

Hodge, Hugh L. [1839a] 1854. *On Criminal Abortion; A Lecture Introductory to the Course on Obstetrics, and Diseases of Women and Childern. University of Pennsylvania, Sesion 1854–5*. Philadelphia: T. K. and P. G. Colling.

Hodge, Hugh L. [1839b] 1872. *On Criminal Abortion; A Lecture Introductory to the Course on Obstetrics, and Diseases of Women and Childern. University of Pennsylvania, Sesion 1854–5*. Philadelphia: Lindsay and Blakiston.

Hodge, Hugh L. 1864. *The Principles and Practice of Obstetrcs*. Philadelphia: Blanchard and Lea.

Hoedeman, Paul. 1991. *Hitler or Hippocrates: Medical Experiments and Euthanasia in the Third Reich*, translated by Ralph de Rijke. Sussex: Book Guild.

Hoffer, Peter C., and N. E. H. Hull. 1981. *Murdering Mothers: Infanticide In England And New England, 1558–1803*. New York: New York University Press.

Hoffman, Yoel. 1986. *Japanese Death Poems*. Tokyo: Charles E. Tuttles.

Hoffmann, Friedrich. 1738. *Medicus Politicus; sive, Regulae Prudentiae secundum quas Medicus Juvenis Studia sua & Vitae Rationem Dirigere Debet*. Leiden: Philip Bonk.

Hoffmann, Friedrich. 1749. *Medicus Politicus, sive Regulae Prudentiae secundum quas Medicus Juvenis Studia sua et Vitae Rationem Dirigere Debet*. In Friedrich Hoffmann, *Operum Omnium Physico-Medicorum Supplementum in Dias Partes Distributum*. Genevae: Fratres de Tournes.

Holmes, Oliver Wendell. [1882, 1891] 2001. *The Professor at the Breakfast Table*, edited by David Widger. Project Gutenberg E-text. www.gutenberg.net/ etext01/prabt11.txt (visited October 28, 2007).

Holmes, Oliver Wendell. 1891. *Medical Essays, 1842–1882*. Boston: Houghton Mifflin.

Holmes, Oliver Wendell. 1942. "The Contagiousness of Puerperal Fever." In *Sourcebook of Medical History*, edited by Logan Clendening, 605–6. New York: Dover Books.

Holmes, Robert L. 1989. *On War and Morality*. Princeton NJ: Princeton University Press.

Holmes, Robert L. 1992. "Can War be Morally Justified? The Just War Theory." In *Just War Theory*, edited by

Jean B. Elshtain, 197–233. Oxford: Basil Blackwell Ltd.

Hooker, Worthington. 1844. *Dissertation on the respect due to the medical profession, and the reasons why it is not awarded by the community.* Norwich CT: J. G. Cooley.

Hooker, Worthington. 1849. *Physician and Patient, or, A practical view of the mutual duties, relations and interests of the medical profession and the community.* New York: Baker and Scribner.

Hooker, Worthington. 1850. *Lessons from the history of medical delusions.* Fiske Fund prize dissertation of the Rhode Island Medical Society, no. 13. New York: Baker and Scribner.

Hooker, Worthington. 1852a. *Homoeopathy: an examination of its doctrines and evidences.* Fiske Fund prize dissertation of the Rhode Island Medical Society, no. 14. New York: Scribner.

Hooker, Worthington. 1852b. *Inaugural Address.* New Haven, Connecticut.

Hooker, Worthington. 1857. *Prize essay. Rational therapeutics; or, the comparative value of different curative means, and the principles of their application.* Boston: J. Wilson & Son.

Hooker, Worthington. 1862. *Human physiology, designed for colleges and the higher classes in schools, and for general reading.* New York: Sheldon.

Hooker, Worthington. 1867. *The Child's Book of Nature. Three Parts in One. Part I. Plants. Part II. Animals. Part III. Air, Water, Heat, Light, &C.* New York: Harper & Brothers.

Hooker, Worthington. 1871. *Science for the School and Family. Part III. Mineralogy And Geology.* New York: Harper & Brothers.

Hooker, Worthington. 1884. *Natural History. For the Use of Schools and Families.* New York: Harper & Brothers.

Hooker, Worthington. 1972. *Physician and Patient: Or, A Practical View of the Mutual Duties, Relations and Interests of the Medical Profession and the Community.* New York: Arno Press & The New York Times.

Hopkins, Donald. 1983. *Princes and Peasants: Smallpox in History.* Chicago: University of Chicago Press.

Hopkins, Keith. 1965–1966. "Contraception in the Roman Empire." *Comparative Studies in Society and History.* 8: 124–51.

Hornblum, Allen M. 1998. *Acres of Skin: Human Experimentation at Holmesburg Prison.* New York/London: Routledge.

Horner, I. B., trans. and ed. 1949. *The Book of Discipline (Vinaya-Pitaka). Vol. 1.* London: Luzac & Company for the Pāli Text Society.

Horner, I. B., trans. and ed. 1959. "Discourse on an Exhortation to Channa (Channovādda-sutta)," In *The Middle Length Sayings (Majjhima-nikāya), Vol. 3,* 315–19 London: Luzac & Company for the Pāli Text Society.

Horner, I. B., trans. [1963–1964] 1969–1990. *Milindapañha* London: Luzac.

Horst, W. D. 2001. "Biotechnology and Human Development in Developing Countries." *EJB Electronic Journal of Biotechnology.* ISSN:0717–3458. http://www.scielo.cl/scielo.php?pid = S0717-34582001000300002&script = sci_arttext (visited January 30, 2008).

Houlbrooke, Ralph A. 1998. *Death, Religion, and the Family in England, 1480–1750.* Oxford: Clarendon Press.

House of Lords, United Kingdom. 1994. *Report of Select Committee on Medical Ethics.* London: HMSO.

Houtzager, H. L., ed. 1989. *Pieter van Foreest. Een Hollands Medicus in de Zestiende Eeuw.* Amsterdam: Rodopi.

Hoven, Friedrich Wilhelm von. [1840] 1984. *Lebenserinnerungen, with an introduction and notes by Hans-Günther Thalheim and Evelyn Laufer.* Berlin: Rütten & Loening.

Howard, Michael, ed. 1979. *Restraints on War: Studies in the Limitation of Armed Conflict.* Oxford: Oxford University Press.

Howard-Jones, N. 1982. "Human Experimentation in Historical and Ethical Perspectives." *Social Science and Medicine.* 16: 1429–48.

Howell, Trevor Henry. 1975. *Old Age: Some Practical Points in Geriatrics.* 3rd ed. London: Lewis.

Howell, W. H., and C. W. Greene. 1938. *History of the American Physiological Society Semicentennial, 1887–1937,* 94–6. Baltimore: American Physiological Society.

Huang Di Nei Jing Su Wen (The Yellow Emperor's Internal Medicine). 1995. (For a recent English translation, see *The Yellow Emperor's Classic of Medicine,* translated by Ni Maoshing. Boston: Shambhala).

Hubenstorf, Michael. 1984. "Österreichische Ärzteemigration 1934–1945 – Zwischen neuem Tätigkeitsgebiet und organisierten Rückkehrplänen." *Berichte zur Wissenschaftsgeschichte.* 7: 85–107.

Hubenstorf, Michael. 1987. "Österreichische Ärzteemigration." In *Vertriebene Vernunft I: Emigration und Exil österreichischer Wissenschaft, 1930–1940,* edited by Friedrich Stadler, 359–415. Vienna/Munich: Jugend und Volk.

Huber, Samuel J., and Matthew K. Wynia. 2004. "When Pestilence Prevails . . . Physician Responsibilities in Epidemics." *American Journal of Bioethics.* 4: W5–W11.

Huerkamp, Claudia. 1985. *Der Aufstieg der Ärzte im 19. Jahrhundert: Vom gelehrten Stand zum professionellen Experten: Das Beispiel Preußens.* Göttingen: Vandenhoeck & Ruprecht.

Hufeland, Christoph Wilhelm. 1797. *Die Kunst das menschliche Leben zu verlängern, von D. Christoph Wilhelm Hufeland.* Wien, Prag: Bey Franz Haas, Buchhandler.

Hufeland, Christoph Wilhelm. 1806. "Die Verhältnisse des Arztes." *Journal der practischen Arzneykunde und Wundarzneykunst.* 23: 5–36.

Hufeland, Christoph Wilhelm. 1836. *Enchiridion medicum oder Anleitung zur medizinischen Praxis: Vermächtnis einer funfzigjährigen Erfahrung*. 2nd ed. Berlin: Jonas Verlagsbuchhandlung.

Hufeland, Christoph Wilhelm. [1836] 1844. *Manual of the Practice of Medicine: The Results of Fifty Years Experience*, translated by C. Bruchhausen and R. Nelson. London/Paris: Hippolyte Baillière.

Hughes, James. 1999. "Buddhism and Abortion: A Western Approach." In *Buddhism and Abortion*, edited by Damien Keown, 183–98. Honolulu HI: University of Hawaii Press.

Huisman, Frank. 1992. *Stadsbelang en standsbesef: Gezondheidszorg en medisch beroep in Groningen, 1500–1730*. Rotterda: Erasmus Publishing.

Hulot-Pietri, E. 1989. *La Médecine Malgré Elle: Témoignage sur l'idéologie médicale francaise*. Paris: L'Harmattan.

Human Body Shop, The. 1998. *Indian Culture*. http://indianculture.about.com/culture/indianculture/library/weekly/aa021698.htm.

Humboldt, Alejandro de. [1808] 1978. *Ensayo político sobre el Reino de la Nueva España*. 3rd ed. México: Porrúa.

Hume, David. [1739] 2000. *A Treatise of Human Nature*, edited by David Fate Norton and Mary J. Norton. Oxford: Oxford University Press.

Hume, David. [1777] 1987. "Of National Characters." In *David Hume: Essays Moral, Political, and Literary*, edited by E. F. Miller, 197–215. Indianapolis IN: Liberty Classics.

Hurty, John Newell. 1912. "Regulation of Marriage." *American Journal of Public Health*. 2: 315–20.

Husemann, Theodor. 1932. "Karl Friedrich Heinrich Marx." In *Biographisches Lexikon der hervorragenden Ärzte aller Zeiten und Völker*. 2nd ed., edited by August Hirsch, vol. 4, 105–7. Berlin: Urban & Schwarzenberg.

Ianni, Octavio. 1976. *Esclavitud y capitalismo*. México: Siglo XXI Editores.

Ibn ʿAbdūn. 1947. *Séville musulmane au début du XIIᵉ siècle. Le traité d'Ibn ʿAbdūn sur la vie urbaine et les corps de metiers*, traduit avec une introduction et des notes [par] Évariste Lévi-Provençal. Paris: Librairie orientale et américaine G. P. Maisonneuve.

Ibn ʿAbdūn. 1955. "Risāla fī l-Qaḍāʾ wa-l-ḥisba (On the Offices of the Judge and the Market Inspector)." In *Documents arabes inédits sur la vie sociale et économique en occident musulman au moyen âge, publiés avec une introduction et un glossaire par Évariste Lévi-Provençal. Première série: Trois traités hispaniques de ḥisba (Texte arabe)*, 1–65. Le Caire: Institut Français d'Archéologie Orientale du Caire.

Ibn Abī Uṣayba. 1884. *ʿUyūn al-anbāʾ fī ṭabaqāt al-aṭibbāʾ*, edited by August Müller. Königsberg: Selbstverlag.

Ibn Abī Uṣaybiʿa, Muwaffaq al-Dīn Abū l-ʿAbbās Aḥmad ibn al-Qāsim. [1882–1884] 1972. *ʿUyūn al-anbāʾ fī ṭabaqāt al-aṭibbāʾ (Gems of Information on the Classes of Physicians)*. Herausgegeben von August Müller. 2 vols. Kairo, Königsberg. Reprint (2 vols, in 1). Westmead, Farnborough: Gregg International Publishers.

Ibn al-Ukhuwwa. 1938. *The Maʿālim al-qurba fī aḥkām al-ḥbba of Ḍiyāʾ al-Dīn Muḥammad ibn Muḥammad al-Qurashī al-Shāfiʿī Known as Ibn al-Ukhuwwa*, edited with abstract of contents, glossary and indices by Reuben Levy. Cambridge UK: Cambridge University Press, and London: Luzac.

Ibn Baz, ʿAbd al-Aziz. 1988. *Fatawa Islamiyya li ʿAbd al-ʾAziz b. Baz, Muhammad b. al-ʾUthaymin, ʿAbdAllah b. Jibrin (Islamic fatwas by ʿAbd al-ʾAziz b. Baz, Muhammad b. al-ʾUthaymin, ʿAbdAllah b. Jibrin)*. Beirut: Dar al-Qalam.

Ibn Buṭlān. 1984. *Das Ärztebankett. Aus arabischen Handschriften übersetzt und mit einer Einleitung sowie Anmerkungen versehen von Felix Klein-Franke*. Stuttgart: Hippokrates Verlag.

Ibn Buṭlān. 1985. *The Physicians' Dinner Party*, edited from Arabic Manuscripts and with an Introduction by Felix Klein-Franke. Wiesbaden: Otto Harrassowitz.

Ibn Buṭlān, Abu l-Ḥasan al-Muḫtār ibn ʿAbdūn. [1054] 1984. *Daʾwat al-aṭibbāʾ ʿala Maḏhab Kalīla wa Dimna*, translated by Felix Klein-Franke. Stuttgart: Hippokrates Verlag.

Ibn Hindū, Abū l-Faraj ʿAlī ibn al-Ḥusayn. 1989. *Miftāḥ al-Ṭibb wa-Minhāj al-Ṭullāb (The Key to the Science of Medicine and the Students' Guide)*, edited by M. Mohaghegh and M. T. Daneshpazuh. Tehran: Tehran University Press.

Ibn Idris, Sharif b. Adwal. 1997. *Kitman al-Sirr waIfshaʾuhu (Concealing Secrets and Revealing Them)*. Amman: Dar al-Nafaʾis.

Ibn Jumayʿ, Hibatallāh ibn Yūsuf al-Isrāʾīlī. 1983. *Treatise to Ṣalāḥ ad-Dīn on the Revival of the Art of Medicine*, edited and translated by Hartmut Fähndrich. Wiesbaden: Kommission Franz Steiner.

Ibn Khaldûn. 1967. *The Muqaddimah: An Introduction to History*. 3 vols., translated by Franz Rosenthal. New York: Princeton University Press.

Ibn Qayyim al-Ǧauzīya, Abū ʿAbd-Allāh Muḥammad b. Abī Bakr. 1994. *Aṭ-Ṭibb an-Nabawī*, edited by Bašīr Muḥammad ʿUyūn. Damaskus: Dār al-Bayān.

Ibn Riḍ ān, ʿAlī. 1982. *Über den Weg zur Glückseligkeit durch den ärztlichen Beruf. Arabischer Text nebst kommentierter deutscher Übersetzung, herausgegeben von Albert Dietrich*. Göttingen: Vandenhoeck & Ruprecht.

Iborra, Pascual. 1987. *Historia del Protomedicato en España, 1477–1822*. Valladolid: Secretariado de Publicaciones de la Universidad de Valladolid.

ICH. 1996. *Guideline for Good Clinical Practice.* www.ich.org.

Ikegami, Naoki, and J. C. Cambell. 1996. *The Art of Balance in Health Policy: Maintaining Japan's Low-Cost, Egalitarian System.* Cambridge UK: Cambridge University Press.

Ilkilic, Ilhan. 2001. "The Autonomy of the Patient and the Muslim Patient in a Society with Pluralist Values." *Concilium: an International Review of Theology.* 4: 135–46.

Ilkilic, Ilhan. 2002. *Der muslimische Patient: Medizinethische Aspekte des muslimischen Krankheitsverständnisses in einer wertpluralen Gesellschaft.* Münster: Lit.

Ilkilic, Ilhan. 2003a. *Begegnung und Umgang mit muslimischen Patienten.* 3rd ed. Tübingen: IZEW.

Ilkilic, Ilhan. 2003b. "Das kranke Kind muslimischer Eltern in Deutschland – zum Fall des Mukarim Emil." In *Das Kind als Patient. Ethische Konflikte zwischen Kindeswohl und Kindeswille,* edited by Claudia Wieseman et al., 203–16. Frankfurt: Campus.

Ilkilic, Ilhan, and Raphaela Veit. 2004. *Gesundheitsmündigkeit und Patientenethik in der islamischen Tradition.* Bochum: Zentrum für Medizinische Ethik.

Illich, Ivan. 1976a. *Limits to Medicine: Medical Nemesis, the Expropriation of Health.* London: Marion Boyars Publishers Ltd.

Illich, Ivan. 1976b. *Medical Nemesis: The Expropriation of Health.* New York: Pantheon Books.

Imam Malik ibn Anas. 1989. *Al-Muwatta of Imam Malik ibn Anas,* translated by Aisha A. Bewley. London: Keagan Paul International.

Immergut, Ellen M. 1992. *Health Politics.* Cambridge UK: Cambridge University Press.

In re Quinlan. 70 NJ 10, 355 A.2d 647 (1976).

Institute of Medicine. 1994. *Growing Up Tobacco Free: Preventing Nicotine Addiction in Children and Youth.* Washington DC: National Academy Press.

Institute of Medicine. 1997. *Non-Heart-Beating Organ Transplantation: Medical and Ethical Issues in Procurement.* Washington DC: National Academy Press.

Institute of Medicine. 1999. *Organ Procurement and Transplantation: Assessing Current Policies and the Potential Impact of the DHHS Final Rule.* Washington DC: National Academy Press.

Institute of Medicine. 2000. *Ending Neglect: The Elimination of Tuberculosis in the United States.* Washington DC: National Academy Press.

Isaacs, Haskell D. 1994. *Medical and Para-Medical Manuscripts in the Cambridge Genizah Collections,* with the assistance of Colin F. Baker. Cambridge UK: Cambridge University Press.

Iseman, M. D., D. L. Cohn, and J. A. Sbarbaro. 1993. "Directly Observed Treatment of Tuberculosis: We Can't Afford Not to Try It." *New England Journal of Medicine.* 328: 576–8.

Ishida, Ichiro. 1963. *Nippon Shisoshi Gairon (The Outline of Japanese History of Thoughts).* Tokyo: Yoshikawa Kobunkan.

Ishida, Yasuo. 1997. "A Book Review of *Factories of Death* by Seldon H. Harris, published by Routledge (first edition)." *Metro Medicine.* (April): 36–7.

Iskandar, Albert Z. 1960. "Al-Rāzī wa-miḥnat al-ṭabīb (Al-Rāzī and the Examination of the Physician)." *Al-Machriq.* 54: 471–522.

Iskandar, Albert Z. 1962. "Galen and Rhazes on Examining Physicians." *Bulletin of the History of Medicine.* 36: 362–5.

Iskandar, Albert Z. 1976. "An Attempted Reconstruction of the Late Alexandrian Medical Curriculum." *Medical History.* 20: 235–58.

Ivaniushkin, A. 1983. "Conception of Marxist Ethics and Professional Medical Ethics." In *Medical Ethics and Deontology,* edited by G. B. Morozov and G. I. Caregorodcev, 51–65. Moscow: Medicina [Russian].

Ivanyuskin, A. Ya. 1998. "Vrachebnaya etika v Rossii (XIX-nachalo XX veka)." In *Bioetika: Printsypy, Pravila, Problemy,* edited by Boris Yudin, 93–110. Moscow: Editorial URSS.

Ivy, Andrew C. 1946. "Report on War Crimes of a Medical Nature Committed in Germany and Elsewhere On German Nationals and the Nationals of Occupied Countries by the Nazi Regime during World War II." Chicago: American Medical Association Archives.

Ivy, Andrew C. 1948. "The History and Ethics of the Use of Human Subjects in Medical Experiments." *Science.* 108: 1–5.

Ivy, Andrew C. 1949. "Statement." In *Doctors of Infamy: The Story of the Nazi Medical Crimes,* edited by Alexander Mitscherlich and Fred Mielke, translated by Heinz Norden. New York: Henry Schuman.

Ivy, Andrew C. 1952. *Observations on Krebiozen; Preliminary Study to Determine if Krebiozen is Biologically Active in the Management of the Cancer Patient, a Report.* Chicago: self-published.

Ivy, Andrew C. 1953a. *Is Krebiozen of Value in the Treatment of Cancer?* Chicago: Gunthrop-Warren.

Ivy, Andrew C. 1953b. *Statement Prepared for Presentation to the Committee of Fourteen on House Joint Resolution No. 10, for the Purpose of Ascertaining the Facts of the Controversy That has Arisen at the University of Illinois Concerning Research on Krebiozen.* Chicago: Gunthrop-Warren.

Ivy, Andrew C., Pick, John F., and W. F. P. Phillips. 1956. *Observations on Krebiozen in the Management of Cancer.* Chicago: H. Regnery Co.

Izvestija. 2003. No. 12. Jan. 24, IV.

Izutsu, Toshihiko. 1980. *The Concept of Belief in Islamic Theology: A Semantic Analysis of Îmân and Islâm.* New York: Arno Press.

Jackson, Mark. 2002. *Infanticide: Historical Perspectives on Child Murder and Concealment, 1550–2000.* Aldershot: Ashgate.

Jackson, Stephen M. 1952. Office of the Secretary of Defense. Memorandum to M. Casberg, 22 October.

Jacob, Joseph M. 1988. *Doctors and Rules.* London: Routledge.

Jacobi, Abraham. 1909. "The Modern Hippokrates." *The New York State Journal of Medicine.* 9: 81–90.

Jacobs, Lawrence R. 1993. *The Health of Nations: Public Opinion and the Making of American and British Health Policy.* Ithaca NY: Cornell University Press.

Jacobson v. Massachusetts. 197 U.S. 11. (1905).

Jacobson, Matthew F. 1998. *Whiteness of A Different Color.* Cambridge MA: Harvard University Press.

Jacquart, Danielle. 1998. *La Médecine médiévale dans le cadre Parisien: XIVe-XVe siècle.* Paris: Fayard.

Jad al-Haqq, Ali Jad al-Haqq. 29. 12. 1980. In *Al-Fatawa al-Islamiyya.* 9: 3110–5; 9: 3087–92 (11. 2. 1979); 9: 3213–28 (23. 3. 1980).

Jakobovits, Immanuel. 1959. *Jewish Medical Ethics: A Comparative and Historical Study of the Jewish Religious Attitude to Medicine and its Practice.* New York: Bloch Publishing Company.

Jakobovits, Immanuel. 1975. *Jewish Medical Ethics: A Comparative and Historical Study of the Jewish Religious Attitude to Medicine and its Practice.* 2nd ed. New York: Bloch Publishing Company.

Jakobovits, Immanuel. [1977] 1979. "Medical Experimentation on Humans in Jewish Law." *Proceedings of the Association of Orthodox Jewish Scientists,* Vol. 1. New York NY. Reprinted in Fred Rosner and David J. Bleich, eds. 1979. *Jewish Bioethics,* 377–83. New York: Sanhedrin Press.

Jalland, Pat. 1996. *Death in the Victorian Family.* Oxford: Oxford University Press.

James, William. 1967. "The Moral Philosopher and the Moral Life." In *The Writings of William James,* edited by John J. McDermott, 610–28. Chicago: University of Chicago Press.

Jamili, Al-Sayyid al-. 1987. *Al-Iʾjaz al-Tibbi fi al-Qurʾan (Divine Medicine in the Qurʾan).* Beirut: Dar Maktabat ak-Hilal.

Janer, Félix. 1831. *Elementos de moral médica ó Tratado de las obligaciones del médico y del cirujano, en que se exponen las reglas de su conducta moral y política en el ejercicio de su profesión.* Barcelona: Joachin Verdaguer.

Janer, Félix. 1835. *Preliminares clínicos o introducción a la práctica de la Medicina.* Barcelona: Imp. De F. Garriga.

Janer, Félix. 1847. *Tratado elemental completo de moral médica o Exposición de las obligaciones del médico y del cirujano: en que se establecen las reglas de su conducta moral y política en el ejercicio de su profesión.* Madrid: Librería de los señores viuda e hijos de Calleja.

Jankrift, Kai-Peter. 1995. *Leprose als Streiter Gottes: Institutionalisierung und Organisation des Ordens vom Heiligen Lazarus zu Jerusalem von seinen Anfängen bis zum Jahre 1350.* Münster: Lit.

Janssens, R. J., and Henk A. M. J. ten Have. 1999. "Hospice and Euthanasia in The Netherlands: An Ethical Point of View." *Journal of Medical Ethics.* 25: 408–12.

Japan. 1997. *The Law Concerning Human Organ Transplants (Law No. 104).*

Japanese Medical Association. 2000. "Physician's Code of Ethics with Annotations." *Journal of the Japan Medical Association.* 124.

Javashvili, Givi, and G. Kiknadze. 2000. "Ethics Committees in Georgia." In *Ethics Committees in Central and Eastern Europe,* edited by Jozef Glasa, 179–86. Bratislava: Charis-IMEB FDN.

Jayakody, Lal, and Nimal Kasturiaratchi. 1999. "Status of the Teaching and Practice of Medical Ethics in Sri Lanka." In *Health Ethics in Six SEAR Countries,* edited by Nimal Kasturiaratchi, Reidar Lie, and Jens Seeberg, 76–84. New Delhi: WHO-SEAR, World Health Organization, Regional Office of South-East Asia.

Jayatilleke, Kulatissa Nanda. 1972. *Ethics in Buddhist Perspective.* Kandy: Buddhist Publication Society.

Jenyns, Soame. 1790. *The Works of Soame Jenyns, Esq.* 4 vols., edited by Charles Nalson Cole. London: Cadell.

Jerome, Saint. 1991. *Select Letters of St. Jerome.* 262. Loeb Classical Library. Cambridge MA: Harvard University Press.

Jerouschek, Günther. 1988. *Lebensschutz und Lebensbeginn: Kulturgeschichte des Abtreibungsverbots. Medizin in Recht und Ethik 17.* Stuttgart: Enke.

Jerouschek, Günther. 1993. "Mittelalter: Antikes Erbe, weltliche Gesetzgebung und Kanonisches Recht." In *Geschichte der Abtreibung: Von der Antike bis zur Gegenwart,* edited by Robert Jütte, 44–67. München: C. H. Beck.

Jetter, Dieter. 1986. *Das europäische Hospital: Von der Spätantike bis 1800.* Köln: Dumont.

Jewson, N. D. 1974. "Medical Knowledge and the Patronage System in Eighteenth-Century England." *Sociology.* 8: 369–85.

Jewson, N. D. 1976. "The Disappearance of the Sick Man from Medical Cosmology, 1770–1870." *Sociology.* 10: 225–44.

Jie, Xueshi, et al. 1998. *War and Plague: A Historical Study of the Crimes of Unit 731.* Beijing: People's Press.

John the Faster, Saint. 1983. "The 35 Canons of John the Faster." In *The Rudder of the Orthodox Catholic Church,* edited by Sts. Nicodemus and Agapius, translated by D. Cummings, 931–52. New York: Luna Printing.

John Paul II. 1981. *Familiaris Consortio.* www. papalencyclicals.net.

John Paul II. 1987a. *Donum Vitae (Instruction on Respect for Human Life)*. www.vatican.va/roman_curia/congregations/cfaith/documents/rc_con_cfaith_doc_19870222_respect-for-human-life_en.html.

John Paul II. 1987b. *Spiritus Domini*. www.papal-library.saint-mike.org.

John Paul II. 1992. *Fidei Depositum*. www.papalencyclicals.net.

John Paul II. 1993. *Veritatis Splendor*. www.papalencyclicals.net.

John Paul II. 1995a. *Evangelium Vitae*. www.papalencyclicals.net.

John Paul II. 1995b. *Evangelium Vitae (The Gospel of Life)*. www.ewtn.com/library/ENCYC/JP2EVANG.HTM.

John Paul II. 1997. *Laetamur Magnopere*. www.papallibrary.saint-mike.org.

John of Salisbury. 1855. "Metalogicon." In *Johannes Saresberiensis Opera Omnia*. Patrologia Latina (Migne), 199, col. 824–946: Paris.

Johnson, James T. 1984. *Can Modern War Be Just?* New Haven CT: Yale University Press.

Johnson, Samuel. [1755] 1979. *A Dictionary of the English Language*. [London: W. Strahan]. Reprint. R. W. Burchfield, ed. New York: Arno Press.

Jonas, Hans. 1969. "Philosophical Reflections on Human Experimentation." *Daedalus*. 98: 219–47.

Jonas, Hans. 1970. "Philosophical Reflections on Experimenting with Human Subjects." In *Experimentation with Human Subjects*, edited by Paul A. Freund, 1–31. New York: George Braziller.

Jonas, Hans. 1974. "Against the Stream: Comments on the Definition and Redefinition of Death." In Hans Jonas, *Philosophical Essays: From Ancient Creed to Technological Man*, 132–40. Englewood Cliffs NJ: Prentice Hall.

Jones v. Murray. 962 F.2d 302 at 313. (Judge Murnaghan dissent, 1992).

Jones, James H. 1981. *Bad Blood: The Tuskegee Syphilis Experiment*. New York: Free Press.

Jones, James H. 1993. *Bad Blood: The Tuskegee Syphilis Experiment*, revised edition. New York: The Free Press.

Jones, W. H. S., ed. 1923. *Hippocrates*. Cambridge MA: Harvard University Press.

Jones, W. H. S. 1923–1931. *Hippocrates*. 4 vols. London: Heinemann.

Jones, W. H. S. 1924. *The Doctor's Oath: An Essay in the History of Medicine*. Cambridge UK: Cambridge University Press.

Jones, W. H. S., et al., eds. 1923–1995. *Hippocrates, with an English translation by W. H. S. Jones*. 8 vols. Loeb Classical Library. Cambridge/London: Harvard University Press.

Jonsen, Albert R., ed. 1993. "The Birth of Bioethics." *Hastings Center Report*. 23: S1–S16.

Jonsen, Albert R. 1998. *The Birth of Bioethics*. New York/Oxford: Oxford University Press.

Jonsen, Albert R. 2000. *A Short History of Medical Ethics*. New York: Oxford University Press.

Jonsen, Albert R., Mark Siegler, and William Winslade. 1986. *Clinical Ethics*. 4th ed. New York: McGraw-Hill.

Jonsen, Albert R., and Stephen Toulmin. 1988. *The Abuse of Casuistry: A History of Moral Reasoning*. Berkeley CA: University of California Press.

Jonsen, Albert R., Robert M. Veatch, and LeRoy Walters, eds. 1998. *Source Book in Bioethics: A Documentary History*. Washington DC: Georgetown University Press.

Jost, Adolf. 1895. *Das Recht Auf den Tod: Social Studie*. Göttingen: Dieterich'sche Verlangbuchhandlung.

Jouanna, Jacques. 1992. *Hippocrate*. Paris: Fayard.

Jouanna, Jacques. 1996. "Un Témoin Méconnu de la Tradition Hippocratique: l'Ambrosianus gr. 134 (B 113 sup.), fol. 1–2 (avec une Nouvelle Édition du Serment et de la Loi)." In *Storia e Ecdotica dei Testi Medici Greci*, edited by Antonio Garzya, 253–72. Naples: M. D'Auria.

Jouanna, Jacques. 1997. "La lecture de l'ethique hippocratique chez Galien." In *Médecine et morale dans l'Antiquité: Dix exposés suivis de discussions*, edited by Hellmut Flashar and Jacques Jouanna, 211–53. Vandoeuvres, Geneva: Fondation Hardt.

Jouanna, Jacques. 1998. *Hippocrate: Les Vents*. Paris: Les Belles Lettres.

Jouanna, Jacques. 1999. *Hippocrates*. Baltimore MD and London: Johns Hopkins University Press.

Joubert, Laurent. 1578. *Erreurs populaires au fait de la Medicine au Régime de Santé*. Avignon: Bertrand.

Joubert, Laurent. [1578] 1989. *Popular Errors*, translated by Gregory David de Rocher. Tuscaloosa AL: University of Alabama Press.

Journal of Medical Ethics, vols. 1–28, 1975–2002. London: BMJ Publishing Group.

Juengst, Eric. 1999. "I-DNA-Fiction: Personal Privacy and Genetic Justice." *Chicago-Kent Law Review*. 74: 61–82.

Juhel-Rénoy, Edouard. 1892. *Vie Professionelle et Devoirs du Médecin*. Paris: Doin.

Jütte, Robert. 1994. *Poverty and Deviance in Early Modern Europe*. Cambridge UK: Cambridge University Press.

Juynboll, W. Th. 1960. "Adhān." In *The Encyclopaedia of Islam*. 1: 187–88. Leiden: E. J. Brill.

Juynboll, W. Th., and J. Pedersen. 1960. "ʿAkīka." In *The Encyclopaedia of Islam*. 1: 337. Leiden: E. J. Brill.

Kagan, Solmon R. 1939a. "Two Great American Physicians." *Medical Leaves*. 2: 65–8.

Kagan, Solmon R. 1939b. *Jewish Contributions to Medicine in America, from Colonial Times to the Present*. Boston: Boston Medical Publishing Company.

Kagan, Solomon R. 1942. *American Jewish Physicians of Note.* Boston: The Boston Medical Publishing Company.

Kahan, Barry D. 1997. "A Third Chance?" *Transplantation & Immunology Letter*, XIII: 2.

Kahn, Richard J., and Patricia G. Kahn. 1997. "The Medical Repository: The First U.S. Medical Journal (1797–1824)." *New England Journal of Medicine.* 337: 1926–30.

Kaibara, Ekiken. [1711a] 1961a. *Wazoku Dojikun (The Japanese Popular Teachings for Children).* Iwanami Bunko, 33–010–1. Tokyo: Iwanami Shoten.

Kaibara, Ekiken. [1711b] 1970. *Gojokun (Five Constant Teachings).* Nippon Shiso Taikei, no. 34. Tokyo: Iwanami Shoten.

Kaibara, Ekiken. [1713a] 1961b. *Yojokun (The Teaching for the Care of Life).* Tokyo: Iwanami Shoten.

Kaibara, Ekiken. [1713b] 1974. *Yojokun (Japanese Secret of Good Health),* translated by Masao Kunihiro. Tokyo: Tokuma Shoten Publishing Co. Ltd.

Kaiser, Jocelyn. 1997. "Environmental Institute Lays Plans for Gene Hunt." *Science.* 278: 569–70.

Kaiser, Robert Blair. 1985. *The Politics of Sex and Religion: A Case History in the Development of Doctrine, 1962–1984.* Kansas City MO: Leven Press.

Kamisar, Yale, and Leo Alexander. [1971] 1987. *The Slide Toward "Mercy Killing".* Oak Park IL.: National Commission on Human Life, Reproduction and Rhythm.

Kanovitch, Bernhard. 1998. "The Medical Experiments in Nazi Concentration Camps." In *Ethics Codes in Medicine: Foundations and Achievements of Codification since 1947,* edited by Ulrich Tröhler and Stella Reiter-Theil, 60–70. Aldershot: Ashgate.

Kan. Stat. Ann. 77–202 (Supp. 1971).

Kane, Pandurang Vaman. 1930 [1968]. *History of Dharmaśāstra.* Vol. 1. Second. Poona, Bhandarkar Oriental Research Institute.

Kane, Pandurang Vaman. [1941] 1974. *History of Dharmaśāstra.* Vol. 2. [1st ed., 2 parts] 2nd ed., 2 parts. Poona, India: Bhandarkar Oriental Research Institute.

Kane, Pandurang Vaman. [1946] 1973. *History of Dharmaśāstra.* Vol. 3. Third Edition. Poona, Bhandarkar Oriental Research Institute.

Kangle, R. P., trans. and ed. [1969] 1988. *The Kauṭilīya Arthasàstra.* Vol. 1. Delhi: Motilal Banarsidass.

Kant, Immanuel. [1797] 1907. "Die Metaphysik der Sitten." In *Kant's gesammelte Schriften. 1 Abt.: Werke.* 9 vols., edited by Königlich Preußische Akademie der Wissenschaften, 1902–23. Vol. 6: 203–494. Berlin: Reimer.

Kappa Lambda. 1821. *Extracts from the Medical Ethics or A Code of Institutes and Precepts, Adapted to the Professional Conduct of Physicians & Surgeons in Private or General Practice, by Thomas Percival, MD.* Lexington KY: T. Smith at the Reporter Office.

Kappa Lambda. 1823. *Extracts from the Medical Ethics of Dr. Percival.* Philadelphia: Kappa Lambda.

Karambelkar, Vinayak Waman. 1961. *The Athavaveda and the Ayur-Veda.* Nagpur: Nagpur India (City) University.

Karmi, Ghada. 1981. "State Control of the Physicians in the Middle Ages: An Islamic Model." In *The Town and State Physician in Europe from the Middle Ages to the Enlightenment,* edited by Andrew W. Russell, 63–84. Wolfenbüttel: Herzog August Bibliothek.

Kass, Leon. 1971. "Death as an Event: A Commentary on Robert Morison." *Science.* 173: 698–702.

Kasturiaratchi, Nimal, Lie Reidar, and Jens Seeberg, eds. 1999. *Health Ethics in Six SEAR Countries.* New Delhi: WHO-SEARO, World Health Organization, Regional Office for South-East Asia.

Kasule, O. Hassan. 1998. *Euthanasia: An Islamic Perspective.* http://iiu.edu.my/medic/islmed/Lecmed/euthanasia98.nov.html (visited July 23, 2002).

Kater, Michael H. 1985. "Medizinsche Fakultäten und Medizinstudenten: Eine Skizze." In *Ärzte im Nationalsozialismus,* edited by Fridolf Kudlien, 82–104. Cologne: Kiepenheuer und Witsch.

Kater, Michael H. 1989. *Doctors Under Hitler.* Chapel Hill NC/London: University of North Carolina Press.

Katsube, Mitake. 1978. *Nippon Shiso no Bunsuirei (The Watershed of Japanese Thoughts).* Tokyo: Keiso Shobo.

Katz, Jay. 1966. *Experimentation with Human Beings: Materials & Cases.* New Haven CT: Yale University Press.

Katz, Jay. 1969. "The Education of the Physician Investigator." *Daedalus.* (Spring): 480–501.

Katz, Jay. 1972. *Experimentation with Human Beings: The Authority of the Investigator, Subject, Profession, and State in the Human Experimentation Process.* New York: Russell Saga Foundation.

Katz, Jay. 1984. *The Silent World of Doctor and Patient.* New York: Free Press.

Katz, Jay. 1992. "The Consent Principle of the Nuremberg Code: Its Significance Then and Now." In *The Nazi Doctors and the Nuremberg Code: Human Rights in Human Experimentation,* edited by George J. Annas and Michael A. Grodin, 227–39. New York/Oxford: Oxford University Press.

Katz, Jay. 1996. "The Nuremberg Code and the Nuremberg Trial: A Reappraisal." *Journal of the American Medical Association.* 276: 1662–6.

Katz, Jay. 1997. "Human Sacrifice and Human Experimentation: Reflections at Nuremberg." *Yale Journal of International Law.* 22: 401–18.

Katz, Jay. 2002. *The Silent World of Doctor and Patient,* with a new foreword by Alexander Morgan Caplan. Baltimore: Johns Hopkins University Press.

Kaufmann, Doris, ed. 2000. *Geschichte der Kaiser-Wilhelm-Gesellschaft im Nationalsozialismus: Bestandsaufnahme und Perspektiven der Forschung.* 2 vol. Göttingen: Wallstein.

Kaufmann, Doris, and Hans-Walter Schmuhl, eds. 2001. *Rassenforschung im Nationalsozialismus: Konzepte und wissenschaftliche Praxis unter dem Dach der Kaiser-Wilhelm-Gesellschaft.* Göttingen: Wallstein.

Kaupen-Haas, Heidrun.1969. *Heidrun, Stabilitat und Wandel arztlicher Autoritat: Eine Anwendung soziologischer Theorie auf Aspekte der Arzt-Patient-Beziehung.* Stuttgart: Enke.

Kaupen-Haas, Heidrun, ed. 1986. *Der Griff nach der Bevölkerung: Aktualität und Kontinuität nazistischer Bevölkerungspolitik.* Nördlingen: Greno.

Kean, Hilda. 1998. *Animal Rights: Political and Social Change in Britain since 1800.* London: Reaktion Books.

Keenan, James F., and Thomas A. Shannon, eds. 1995. *The Context of Casuistry.* Washington DC: Georgetown University Press.

Keenan, Mary Emily. 1941. "St. Gregory of Nazianzus and Early Byzantine Medicine." *Bulletin of the History of Medicine.* 9: 8–30.

Keenan, Mary Emily. 1944. "St. Gregory of Nyssa and the Medical Profession." *Bulletin of the History of Medicine.* 15: 150–61.

Kelly, David F. 1979. *The Emergence of Roman Catholic Medical Ethics in North America: A Historical-Methodological-Bibliographical Study.* New York/Toronto: The Edwin Mellen Press.

Kelly, Gerald A. 1956. "The Morality of Mutilation: Towards a Revision of the Treatise." *Theological Studies.* 17: 322–44.

Kelly, Gerald A. 1958. *Medico-Moral Problems.* St. Louis MO: Catholic Hospital Association.

Kelsey, M. T. 1976. *Healing and Christianity in Ancient Thought and Modern Times.* New York: Harper and Row.

Kemeny, M. Margaret, et al. 2003. "Barriers to Clinical Trial Participation by Older Women with Breast Cancer." *Journal of Clinical Oncology.* 21.12; June 15: 2268–75.

Kemp, N. D. A. 2002. *'Merciful Release': The History of the British Euthanasia Movement.* Manchester: Manchester University Press.

Kennedy, Ian. 1981. *The Unmasking of Medicine.* London: George Allen & Unwin.

Keown, Damien. 1992. *The Nature of Buddhist Ethics.* Basingstoke: Macmillan.

Keown, Damien. 1995. *Buddhism and Bioethics.* London: St. Martin's Press.

Keown, Damien, ed. 1999a. *Buddhism and Abortion.* Honolulu: University of Hawaii Press.

Keown, Damien. 1999b. "Buddhism and Abortion: Is There a Middle Way?" In *Buddhism and Abortion,* edited by Damien Keown, 199–218. Honolulu HI: University of Hawaii Press.

Kershaw, Ian. 1994. *Der NS-Staat, Geschichtsinterpretation und Kontroversen im Überblick.* Reinbek bei Hamburg: Rohwohlt.

Kersting, Franz-Werner. 1996. *Anstaltsärzte zwischen Kaiserreich und Bundesrepublik: Das Beispiel Westfalen.* Paderborn: Ferdinand Schöningh.

Kersting, Franz-Werner, Karl Teppe, and Bernd Walter, eds. 1993. *Nach Hadamar: Zum Verhältnis von Psychiatrie und Gesellschaft im 20. Jahrhundert.* Paderborn: Ferdinand Schöningh.

Kett, Joseph. 1968. *The Formation of the American Medical Profession: The Role of Institutions, 1780–1860.* New Haven CT: Yale University Press.

Kevles, Daniel J. 1985. *In the Name of Eugenics.* New York: Knopf.

Kevles, Daniel J. 1993. "Is the Past Prologue? Eugenics and the Human Genome Project." *Contention: Debates in Society, Culture, and Science.* 2: 21–37.

Khabarovsk Trial Materials, The. 1950. *Materials Relating to the Trial of Former Servicemen of the Japanese Army Charged with Manufacturing and Employing Bacteriological Weapons.* Moscow: Foreign Languages Publishing House.

Khoury, Adel T. 1981. "Abtreibung im Islam." In *CIBEDO-Dokumentation,* no. 11: 1–29.

Kibre, Pearl. 1985. *Hippocrates Latinus.* New York: Fordham University Press.

Kiev, Ari., ed. 1964. *Magic, Faith, and Healing: Studies in Primitive Psychiatry Today.* New York: Free Press of Glencoe.

Kimani, Violet Nyambura. 1981. "The Unsystematic Alternative: Towards Plural Health Care Among the Kikuyu of Central Kenya." *Social Science & Medicine.* 15B: 333–40.

Kimsma, Gerrit, and B. J. van Duin. 1998. "Teaching Euthanasia: The Integration of the Practice of Euthanasia into Grief, Death and Dying Curriculum of Post-Graduate Family Medicine Training." In *Asking to Die: Inside the Dutch Debate about Euthanasia,* edited by David C. Thomasma, et al., 107–112. Dordrecht: Kluwer Academic Publishers.

Kimsma, Gerrit, and Evert van Leeuwen. 1998. "Euthanasia and Assisted Suicide in the Netherlands and the USA: Comparing Practices, Justifications and Key Concepts in Bioethics and Law." In *Asking to Die: Inside the Dutch Debate about Euthanasia,* edited by David C. Thomasma et al., 35–70. Dordrecht: Kluwer Academic Publishers.

Kimura, Rihito. 1987a. *Inochi o Kangaeru (Thinking of Life).* Tokyo: Nippon Hyoron Sha.

Kimura, Rihito. 1987b. "Bioethics as a Prescription for Civic Action: The Japanese Interpretation." *Journal of Medicine and Philosophy.* 12: 267–77.

Kimura, Rihito. 1991. "Fiduciary Relationships and the Medical Profession: A Japanese Point of View." In *Ethics, Trust, and the Professions: Philosophical and Cultural Aspects,* edited by Edmund D. Pellegrino, Robert M. Veatch, and John P. Langan, 235–45. Washington DC: Georgetown University Press.

Kimura, Rihito. 1994. "Bioethics and Japanese Health Care." *Washington-Japan Journal*, 3 (1, Winter): 2–4.

Kimura, Rihito. 1995. "History of Medical Ethics: III. South and East Asia: D. Japan: 2. Contemporary Japan." In *Encyclopedia of Bioethics*. 2nd ed., edited by Warren T. Reich, 1496–1505. New York: Simon & Schuster Macmillan.

Kimura, Rihito. 1997. "The Need for New Images." *World Health Forum*. 18. Geneva: World Health Organization.

Kimura, Rihito. 1998a. "Death, Dying, and Advance Directives in Japan: Sociocultural and Legal Points of View." In *Advance Directives and Surrogate Decision Making in Health Care – United States, Germany, and Japan*, edited by Hans-Martin Sass, Robert M. Veatch, and Rihito Kimura, 187–208. Baltimore MD and London: Johns Hopkins University Press.

Kimura, Rihito. 1998b. "Organ Transplantation and Brain-Death in Japan: Cultural, Legal, and Bioethical Background." *Annals of Transplantation*. 3: 55–8.

Kimura, Rihito. 2000. *Jibun no Inochi wa Jibunde Kimeru-Sho, Ro, Byo, Shi no Baioeshikkusu (Make Your Own Decision for Your Own Life – Bioethics of Birth, Sickness, Aging and Death)*. Tokyo: Shueisha.

Kimura, Rihito. 2003. *Baieshikkusu Hanndobukku (Bioethics Handbook)*. Tokyo: Hoken.

Kimura, Rihito. 2004. "IV. Japan: B. Contemporary Japan" In *Encyclopedia of Bioethics*. 3rd ed., edited by Stephen Post, 1706. New York: Macmillan.

King, Lester S. 1958. *The Medical World of the Eighteenth Century*. Chicago: University of Chicago Press.

King, Lester S. 1983. "The AMA Sets A New Code of Ethics." *Journal of the American Medical Association*. 249: 1338–42.

King, Steven, and Alan Weaver. 2000. "Lives in Many Hands: The Medical Landscape in Lancashire, 1700–1820." *Medical History*. 44: 173–200.

Kinsey, Alfred. 1948. *Sexual Behavior in the Human Male*. Philadelphia: W. B. Saunders.

Kinsey, Alfred. 1953. *Sexual Behavior in the Human Female*. Philadelphia: W. B. Saunders.

Kinsley, David. 1996. *Health, Healing, and Religion: A Cross-Cultural Perspective*. Upper Saddle River NJ: Prentice Hall.

Kırbaşoğlu, M. Hayri. 1993. *İslam Düşüncesinde Sünnet*. Istanbul: Fecr.

Kircher, Bettine. 1986. "Alfred Hoche (1865–1943): Versuch einer Analyse seiner Psychiatrischen Krankheitslehre." Med. diss., Albert-Ludwigs-Universität Freiburg.

Kirchner, E. 1927. "Anfänge rassenhygienischen Denkens in Morus 'Utopia' und Campanellas 'Sonnenstadt'." *Archiv für Rassen- und Gesellschaftsbiologie*. 21.

Kirk, Beate. 1999. *Der Contergan-Fall: Eine unvermeidbare Arzneimittelkatastrophe?*. Stuttgart: Wissenschaftliche Verlagsgesellschaft.

Kitagawa, Joseph Mitsuo. 1989. "Buddhist Medical History." In *Healing and Restoring: Health and Medicine in the World's Religious Traditions*, edited by Lawrence E. Sullivan, 9–32. New York: Macmillan.

Klee, Ernst. 1983. *'Euthanasie' im NS-Staat: Die Vernichtung lebensunwerten Lebens*. Frankfurt: S. Fischer.

Klee, Ernst, ed. 1985. *Dokumente zur 'Euthanasie'*. Frankfurt: S. Fischer.

Klee, Ernst. 1997. *Auschwitz: Die NS-Medizin und Ihre Opfer*. Frankfurt: S. Fischer.

Klee, Ernst. 2001. *Deutsche Medizin im Dritten Reich. Karrieren vor und nach 1945*. Frankfurt: S. Fischer.

Klein, Rudolf. 2000. *The New Politics of the National Health Service*. 4th ed. Harlow Essex: Prentice Hall.

Klein-Franke, Felix. 1982. *Vorlesungen über die Medizin im Islam*. Wiesbaden: Franz Steiner Verlag.

Klinkhammer, Gisela. 2000. "Medizinische Forschung am Menschen: Abkehr von einheitlichen Standards." *Deutsches Ärzteblatt*. 97: A-2205–A-6.

Knauer, Peter. 1967. "The Hermeneutic Function of the Principle of Double Effect." *Natural Law Forum*. 12: 132–62.

Knipe, David M. 1989. "Hinduism and the Tradition of Āyurveda." In *Healing and Restoring: Health and Medicine in the World's Religious Traditions*, edited by Lawrence E. Sullivan, 89–110. New York: MacMillan Publishing Company.

Knopf, S. A. 1901. "Our Duties Toward the Consumptive Poor." *Charities*. 6: 76.

Knowles, John. 1979. "The Responsibility of the Individual." *Daedalus*. 106: 57–80.

Knowles, L. P. 2001. "The Lingua Franca of Human Rights and the Rise of a Global Bioethic." *Cambridge Quarterly of Healthcare Ethics*. 10: 253–63.

Kocher, Paul H. 1950. "The Idea of God in Elizabethan Medicine." *Journal of the History of Ideas*. 11: 3–29.

Kogon, Eugen. 1995. *Ideologie und Praxis der Unmenschlichkeit: Erfahrungen mit dem Nationalsozialismus*. Berlin: Quadriga.

Kogon, Eugen, Hermann Langbein, and Adalbert Rückerl. 1983. *Nationalsozialistische Massentötungen durch Giftgas*. Frankfurt: S. Fischer.

Kolakowski, Leszek. 1978. *Main Current of Marxism – Its Origin, Growth and Dissolution*, translated by P. S. Falla. New York: Palladio Press.

Kolb, Stephan, and Horst Seithe, eds. 1998. *Medizin und Gewissen: 50 Jahre nach dem Nürnberger Ärzteprozeß*. Frankfurt: Mabuse.

Koni, Anatoly F. 1901. "Vrachebnaya taina." *Entziclopedichesky Slovar' Brokgauza i Efrona*. T. 64: 494–5.

Koni, Anatoly F. 1914. *Feodor Petrovich Gaaz: Biografich-eskii Ocherk*. 6th ed. Moscow: Tipografija T-va I. D.Sytina.

Koni, Anatoly F. 1928. "K materialam o vrachebnoi etike." *Acta Medica*. 19: 10–17.

Konold, Donald E. 1962. *A History of American Medical Ethics, 1847–1912*. Madison WI: The State Historical Society of Wisconsin.

Kopp, Vincent J. 1999. "Henry K. Beecher, M.D.: Contrarian (1904–1976)." *ASA Newsletter*. 63.

Korotkikh, Raisa V. 1989. "Teoreticheskoe Obosno-vanie Razvitija Vrachebnoi Etiki i Meditsynskoi Deontologii v Sovetskom Zdravookhranenii." Diss. Doct. Med. Nauk. Gosudarstvennaya Tsentral'naya Nauchnaya Meditsinskaya Biblioteka. Moscow.

Koshland, Daniel E., Jr. 1988–1989. "The Future of Biological Research." *MBL Science*. 3: 10–13.

Kottek, Samuel S. 1967. "Le symbole du lion dans la medicine de l'antiquite." *Revue Histoire de Medicine Hebrait*. 78: 161–8.

Kottek, Samuel S. 1996. "Medical Practice and Jewish Law: Nahmanides' *Sefer Torat Haadam*." In *Medicine and Medical Ethics in Medieval and Early Modern Spain: An Intercultural Approach*, edited by Samuel S. Kottek and Luis Garcia-Ballester, 163–72. Jerusalem: Magnes Press.

Kovács, József. 1991. "Bribery and Medical Ethics in Hungary." *Bulletin of Medical Ethics*. 66: 13–8.

Kovács, József. 1997. *A modern orvosi etika alapjai: Bevezetés a bioetikába (The Basis of Modern Medical Ethics: Introduction to Bioethics)*. Budapest: Medicina Publishing.

Kovacs, Maria M. 1985. "Aesculapius Militans." *Valosag*. 28: 69–82.

Kraut, Alan. 1994. *Silent Travelers: Germs, Genes, and the "Immigrant Menace"*. New York: Basic Books.

Krawietz, Birgit. 1990. *Die Hurma: Schariatrechtlicher Schutz vor Eingriffen in die körperliche Unversehrtheit nach arabischen Fatwas des 20. Jahrhunderts*. Berlin: Duncker und Humboldt.

Krawietz, Birgit. 1991. *Die Hurma*. Berlin: Duncker and Humblot.

Krawietz, Birgit. 1999. "Ethical versus Medical Values according to Contemporary Islamic Law." *Recht van de Islam*. 16: 1–26.

Kröner, Hans-Peter. 1989. "Die Emigration deutschsprachiger Mediziner im Nationalsozialismus." *Berichte zur Wissenschaftsgeschichte*. 12: 1–37.

Kudlien, Fridolf. 1985. *Ärzte im Nationalsozialismus*. Cologne: Kiepenheuer und Witsch.

Kühl, Stefan. 1994. *The Nazi Connection: Eugenics, American Racism, and German National Socialism*. New York: Oxford University Press.

Kühn, Carl Gottlob, ed. [1964] 1821–33. *Claudii Galeni Opera Omnia*. 22 vols. in 20. [Hildesheim: Georg Olms]. Reprint. Leipzig: Karl Knoblauch Verlag.

Kuhn, Thomas S. 1962. *The Structure of Scientific Revolutions*. Chicago: University of Chicago Press.

Kuhn, Thomas S. 1970. *The Structure of Scientific Revolutions*. 2nd ed. Chicago: University of Chicago Press.

Kümmel, Werner Friedrich. 2001. "'Dem Arzt nötig oder nützlich'? Legitimierungsstrategien der Medizingeschichte im 19. Jahrhundert." In *Die Institutionalisierung der Medizinhistoriographie. Entwicklungslinien vom 19. ins 20. Jahrhundert*, edited by Andreas Frewer and Volker Roelcke, 75–89. Stuttgart: Franz Steiner Verlag.

Kurihara, Keisuke. 1986. *Kokyo, Shinsyaku Kanbun Taikei (The Teaching of Filial Piety, The New Interpretaion of Chinese Compendium of Classic)*. Tokyo: Meiji Shoin.

Kuti, Éva. 1984. "Az orvosi hálapénzről – a következmények fényében (On the tipping of physicians – in the light of consequences)." *Valóság (Reality)*. 3: 62–70.

Kuzmin, Mikhail K. 1984. "O proiskhozhdenii Prisjagi vracha Sovetskogo Soyuza." *Sovetskaya Meditsyna*. 8:117–9.

Kyaw, David. 1999. "Issues of Ethics in Health Care: A Myanmar Perspective." In *Health Ethics in Six SEAR Countries*, edited by Nimal Kasturiaratchi, Reidar Lie, and Jens Seeberg, 59–63. New Delhi: WHO-SEAR, World Health Organization, Regional Office for South-East Asia.

Labisch, Alfons. 1997. "From Traditional Individualism to Collective Professionalism: State, Patient, Compulsory Health Insurance, and the Panel Doctor Question in Germany, 1883–1931." In *Medicine and Modernity: Public Health and Medical Care in Nineteenth- and Twentieth-Century Germany*, edited by Manfred Berg and Geoffrey Cocks, 35–54. Cambridge UK: Cambridge University Press.

Labouvie, Eva. 1998. *Andere Umstände: Eine Kulturgeschichte der Geburt*. Köln/Weimar/Wien: Böhlau.

Lachmund, Jens, and Gunnar Stollberg. 1995. *Patientenwelten: Krankheit und Medizin vom späten 18. bis zum frühen 20. Jahrhundert im Spiegel von Autobiographien*. Opladen: Leske & Budrich.

LaFleur, William A. 1990. "Contestation and Confrontation: The Morality of Abortion in Japan." *Philosophy East and West*. 40: 529–42.

LaFleur, William A. 1992. *Liquid Life: Abortion and Buddhism in Japan*. Princeton NJ: Princeton University Press.

LaFleur, William A. 1995. "Silences and Censures: Abortion, History and Buddhism in Japan: A Rejoinder to George Tanabe." *Japanese Journal of Religious Studies*. 22: 185–96.

LaFleur, William A. 1999. "Abortion in Japan: Towards a Middle Way for the West?" In *Buddhism and Abortion*, edited by Damien Keown, 67–92. Honolulu HI: University of Hawaii Press.

Laín Entralgo, Pedro. 1969a. *El médico y el enfermo*. Madrid: Ediciones Guadarrama.

Laín Entralgo, Pedro. 1969b. *Doctor and Patient*, translated from Spanish by Frances Partridge. New York: McGraw-Hill (World University Library).

Lake, Kirsopp, trans. 1965. "The Didache." In *The Apostolic Fathers*. 1: 303–33. Cambridge MA: Harvard University Press.

Lakhtin, Mikhail G. 1903. "Russkaia Meditsyna do 16 Veka." *Vestnik Sankt-Peterburgskogo Vrachebnogo Obshestva Vzaimnoi Pomoshi*. 8: 445–51.

Lakhtin, Mikhail. n.d. *Vrachebnaya Taina*. Reprint. Moscow: State Medical Library of Moscow.

Lalonde, Marc. 1974. *A New Perspective on the Health of Canadians*. Ottawa: Department of National Health and Welfare.

Lamanna, Alessandro, Giovanni Moro, and Melody Ross, eds. 2005. *Citizens Report on the Implementation of the European Charter on Patients' Rights (Working Paper, February 2005)*. Active Citizenship Network. www.activecitizenship.net/projects/project_europe_chart.htm (visited October 28, 2007).

Lamb, David. 1985. *Death, Brain Death and Ethics*. Albany NY: State University of New York Press.

La Mettrie, Julian Offray de. [1748] 1994. *Man a Machine*. Indianapolis IN: Hackett Publication Co.

Lammers, Stephen E., and Allen Verhey, eds. 1998. *On Moral Medicine: Theological Perspectives in Medical Ethics*. 2nd ed. Grand Rapids MI: Eerdmans.

Landa, Fray Diego de. [1560] 1973. "Ordenanzas de Tomás López." In *Relación de las cosas de Yucatán*. 10th ed., edited by Angel María Garibay K., 203–19. México: Porrúa.

Lang, Lany T. 1990. "Aspects of the Cambodian Death and Dying Process." In *Social Work Practice with the Terminally Ill: The Transcultural Perspective*, edited by Joan K. Parry, 205–11. Springfield IL: Charles C. Thomas.

Langer, William. 1974. "Infanticide: A Historical Survey." *History of Childhood Quarterly*. 1: 353–66.

Langius, Johannes. 1589. *Epistolarum Medicinalium*. Frankfurt: Apud heredes Andreae Wecheli, Claudium Marnium & Joann Aubrium.

Langstaff, John Brett. 1942. *Doctor Bard of Hyde Park*. New York: E. P. Dutton.

Lanning, J. T. 1985. *The Royal Protomedicato: The Regulation of the Medical Profession in the Spanish Empire*. Durham NC: Duke University Press.

Lansang, M., and F. P. Crawley. 2000. "The Ethics of International Biomedical Research." *British Medical Journal*. 321: 777–8.

Lansbury, Coral. 1985. *The Old Brown Dog: Women, Workers, and Vivisection in Edwardian England*. Madison WI: University of Wisconsin Press.

Lapie, Paul. 1905. "La Hiérarchie des Professions." *Revue de Paris*. 5 (September 15): 390–410.

Laqueur, Thomas W. 2003. *Solitary Sex: A Cultural History of Masturbation*. New York: Zone Books.

Larson, Edward J. 1995. *Sex, Race, and Science: Eugenics in the Deep South*. Baltimore: Johns Hopkins University Press.

Larson, Edward J., and Darrel W. Amundsen. 1998. *A Different Death: Euthanasia and the Christian Tradition*. Downers Grove IL: InterVarsity Press.

Las Casas, Fray Bartolomé de. [1552] 1977. *Brevísima relación de la destrucción de Indias*, facsimile edition, edited by Manuel Ballesteros Gaibrois. Madrid: Fundación Universitaria Española.

Lassen, H. C. A. 1953. "A Preliminary Report on the 1952 Epidemic of Poliomyelitis in Copenhagen with Special Reference to the Treatment of Respiratory Insufficiency." *The Lancet*. 1.1: 37–41.

Last, Murray. 1986. "The Professionalization of African Medicine: Ambiguities and Definitions." In *The Professionalization of African Medicine*, edited by Murray Last and G. L. Chavunduka, 1–19. Manchester: Manchester University Press, International African Institute.

Laurence, Jeremy. 2000. "Total of Doctors Facing Misconduct Charges Doubles." *The Independent*, May 23.

Lawrence, Susan. 1993. "Medical Education." In *Companion Encyclopedia of the History of Medicine*, edited by William F. Bynum and Roy Porter, 1151–79. London/New York: Routledge.

Lawrence, Susan. 1996. *Charitable Knowledge: Hospital Pupils and Practitioners in Eighteenth-Century London*. Cambridge UK: Cambridge University Press.

Leake, Chauncey, ed. 1927. *Percival's Medical Ethics*. Baltimore: Williams and Wilkins.

Leakey, Louis Seymour Bazett. 1977. *The Southern Kikuyu Before 1903*. London and New York: Academic Press.

Leavitt, Judith Walzer. 1986. *Brought to Bed: Childbearing in America, 1750–1950*. New York: Oxford University Press.

Leavitt, Judith Walzer. 1996. *Typhoid Mary: Captive to the Public's Health*. Boston: Beacon Press.

Leavitt, Judith Walzer, and Ronald L. Numbers. 1978. "Sickness and Health in America: An Overview." In *Sickness and Health in America: Readings in the History of Medicine and Public Health*, edited by Judith Walzer Leavitt and Ronald L. Numbers, 3–10. Madison WI: University of Wisconsin Press.

Leavitt, Yeruham Frank. 2001. "Is Asian Bioethics at Fault? Commentary on Tsuchiya, Morioka and Nie." *Eubios Journal of Asian and International Bioethics*. 11: 7–8.

Leavitt, Yeruham Frank. 2003. "Let's Stop Bashing Japan: Commentary on Tsuchiya, Sass, Thomas and Nie." *Eubios Journal of Asian and International Bioethics*. 13: 134–5.

Lebacqz, Karen. 1983. *Genetics, Ethics, and Parenthood*. New York: Pilgrim.

Lecaldano, Eugenio. 1999. *Bioetica: Le Scelte Morali*. Rome: Laterza.

Lecky, William. 1905. *History of European Morals: From Augustus to Charlemagne*. London: Longmans, Green, and Co.

Lederer, Susan E. 1984. "'The Right and Wrong Way of Making Experiments on Human Beings': Udo J. Wylie and Syphilis 1916." *Bulletin of the History of Medicine*. 58: 380–97.

Lederer, Susan E. 1985. "Hideyo Noguchi's Luetin Experiment and the Antivivisectionists." *Isis*. 76: 31–48.

Lederer, Susan E. 1992. "Political Animals: The Shaping of Biomedical Research Literature in Twentieth-Century America." *Isis*. 83: 61–79.

Lederer, Susan E. 1995. *Subjected to Science: Human Experimentation in America before the Second World War*. Baltimore: Johns Hopkins University Press.

Lederer, Susan E. 1999. "Cannon, Walter Bradford." In *American National Biography*, edited by John A. Garraty and Mark C. Carnes, vol. 4, 338–40. New York: Oxford University Press.

Lederer, Susan E. 2004. "Research without Borders: The Origins of the Declaration of Helsinki." In *Twentieth-Century Ethics of Human Subjects Research: Historical Perspectives on Values, Practices, and Regulations*, edited by Volker Roelcke and Giovanni Maio, 199–218. Stuttgart: Steiner Verlag.

Lederer, Susan E. 2008. "Hollywood and Human Experimentation: Representing Medical Research in Popular Film." In *Medicine's Moving Pictures: Medicine Health and Bodies in American Film and Television*, edited by Paula Treichler, Nancy Tomes, and Leslie Reagan, 282–306. Rochester NY: University of Rochester Press

Lee, Tao. 1943. "Medical Ethics in Ancient China." *Bulletin of the History of Medicine*. 13: 268–77.

Lefèbvre, Bruno. 1991. "L'Argent et le Secret: Dégradations et Recompositions." In *L'Honneur: L'Image de Soi ou Don de Soi*, edited by Marie Gautheron, 142–7. Paris: Editions Autremont.

Leflar, Robert B. 1996. "Informed Consent and Patients' Rights in Japan." *Houston Law Review*. 33: 1–112.

Legge, James, trans. 1970. *Mencius*. New York: Dover Publications Inc.

Legge, James, trans. 1971. *Analects, the Great Learning, & the Doctrine of the Mean*. New York: Dover Publications Inc.

Lehrman, Sally. 1997. "Berkeley Employee Fight Ruling on Gene Tests without Consent." *Biotechnology Newswatch*, May 5.

Leichter, Howard M. 1999. "Oregon's Bold Experiment: Whatever Happened to Rationing?" *Journal of Health Politics, Policy, and Law*. 24: 147–60.

Leiser, Gary. 1983. "Medical Education in Islamic Lands from the Seventh to the Fourteenth Century." *Journal of the History of Medicine and Allied Sciences*. 38: 48–75.

Lennox, James G. 1995. "Health as an Objective Value." *Journal of Medicine and Philosophy*. 20: 499–511.

Lenz, Fritz. [1917] 1933. *Die Rasse als Wertprinzip Zur Erneuerung der Ethik*. Reprint. Munich: J. F. Lehmann.

Leo XIII. 1884. *Humanum Genus*. www.papalencyclicals.net.

Leo XIII. 1888. *Libertas Praestantissimum*. www.papalencyclicals.net.

Leo XIII. 1896. *Satis Cognitum*. www.papalencyclicals.net.

Léonard, Jacques. 1981a. "Le Corps Médicale au Début de la IIIe République." In *Médecine et Philosophie à la fin du XIXe Siècle*, edited by J. Poirier and J.-L. Poirier, 11–21. Paris: Institut de Recherche Universitaire.

Léonard, Jacques. 1981b. *Le Médecine entre les Pouvoirs et les Savoirs*. Paris: Aubier.

León C., Augusto. 1978. "Medical Ethics: Latin America in the Twentieth Century." In *Encyclopedia of Bioethics*, edited by Warren T. Reich, 1005–7. New York: Macmillan.

Leopold, Nathan. 1958. *Life Plus Ninety-Nine Years*. Garden City NY: Doubleday.

Lepukaln, N. 1927. "O tak nazyvaemykh 'spetsakh'." *Vestnik Sovremennoi Meditsyny*, no. 6: 377–80.

Lerner, Barron H. 1998. *Contagion and Confinement: Controlling Tuberculosis Along the Skid Row*. Baltimore: Johns Hopkins University Press.

Lerner, Barron H. 1999. "Catching Patients: Tuberculosis and Detention in the 1990s." *Chest*. 115: 236–41.

Lerner, Barron H. 2000. "From Laennec to Lobotomy: Teaching Medical History at Academic Medical Centers." *American Journal of the Medical Sciences*. 319: 279–84.

Lesch, John E. 1984. *Science and Medicine in France: The Emergence of Experimental Physiology*. Cambridge MA: Harvard University Press.

Lescouflair, Edric. 2004. *Walter Bradford Cannon: Experimental Physiologist 1871–1945*. www.harvardsquarelibrary. org/unitarians/cannon_walter.html (visited October 28, 2007).

Lesky, Erna. 1976. *A System of Complete Medical Police: Selections from Johann Peter Frank*. Baltimore: Johns Hopkins University Press.

Leslie, Charles. 1978. "Pluralism and Integration in the Indian and Chinese Medical Systems." In *Culture and Healing in Asian Societies: Anthropological, Psychiatric and Public Health Studies*, edited by Arthur Kleinman, Peter Kunstader, E. Russell Alexander, and James L. Gate, 235–52. Cambridge MA: Schenkman Publishing Company.

Leslie, Charles. 1984. "Interpretations of Illness: Syncretism in Modern Āyurveda." In *History of Diagnostics: Proceedings of the 9th International Symposium* on the *Comparative History of Medicine – East and West*, 7–42. Susono-shi, Shizuoka, Japan: Division of Medical History, Taniguchi Foundation.

Letamendi, José de. 1894. *Curso de clínica general*. T. 1. Madrid: Imprenta de los sucesores de Cuesta.

Leven, Karl-Heinz. 1987. *Medizinisches bei Eusedios von Kaisareia*. Düsseldork: Triltsch Verlag.

Leven, Karl-Heinz. 1994. "Hippokrates im 20. Jahrhundert: Ärztliches Selbstbild, Idealbild und Zerrbild." In *Selbstbilder des Arztes im 20. Jahrhundert*, edited by Karl-Heinz Leven and Cay-Rüdiger Prüll, 39–96. Freiburg im Breisgau: Hans Ferdinand Schulz Verlag.

Leven, Karl-Heinz. 1997. "Der Hippokratische Eid im 20. Jahrhundert." In *Geschichte und Ethik in der Medizin*, edited by R. Toellner and U. Wiesing, 111–29. Jena: Fischer.

Leven, Karl-Heinz. 1998. "The Invention of Hippocrates: Oath, Letters and Hippocratic Corpus." In *Ethics Codes in Medicine: Foundations and Achievements of Codification since 1947*, edited by Ulrich Tröhler, Stella Reiter-Theil, and Eckhard Herych, 2–23. Aldershot: Ashgate.

Levey, Martin. 1963. "Fourteenth-Century Muslim Medicine and the Ḥisba." *Medical History*. 7: 176–82.

Levey, Martin. 1971. "Preventive Medicine in Ninth-Century Persia." *Studies in Islam*. 8: 8–16.

Levine, Edwin Burton. 1971. *Hippocrates*. New York: Twayne Publishers.

Levine, Robert J. 1999. "The Need to Revise the Declaration of Helsinki." *New England Journal of Medicine*. 341: 531–4.

Levinsky, Norman G. 1999. "Quality and Equity in Dialysis and Renal Transplantation." *New England Journal of Medicine*. 341:1691–93.

Lewis, C. S. 1962. *The Problem of Pain*. New York: Macmillan.

Lewis, Sinclair. [1925] 1976. *Arrowsmith*. Cutchogue NY: Buccaneer Books.

Lewis, Thornton Todd. 1994. "A Modern Guide for Mahàyàna Buddhist Life-Cycle Rites: The Nepàl Jana Jīvan Kriyā Paddhati." *Indo-Iranian Journal*. 37: 1–46.

Li, Shizhen. [1592] 1988. *Bencao Gangmu (The Great Pharmacopeias)*. Beijing: Chinese Bookstore.

Liang, J. 1995. *Zhongguo Gudai Yizheng Shilue (A Short History of Chinese Medical System)*. China: Inner Mongolia People's Press.

Liao, Y., F. Fu, and J. Zheng. 1998. *Zhongguo Kexue Jishu Shi: Yixue Juan (A History of Chinese Science and Technology: Medicine)*. Beijing: Science Press.

Liao, Yuqun. 1993. *Qihuang Yidao (The Way of Chinese Medicine)*. Taipei: Hongye Wenhua Shiye Youxiangongsi.

Lichtenthaeler, Charles. 1984. *Der Eid des Hippokrates: Ursprung und Bedeutung (XII. Hippokratische Studie)*. Cologne: Deutscher Arzte-Verlag.

Lieber, Elinor. 1984. "*Asaf's Book of Medicines*: A Hebrew Encyclopedia of Greek and Jewish Medicine, possibly compiled in Byzantium on an Indian model." *Dumbarton Oaks Papers*. 20: 233–49.

Lifton, Robert J. 1986. *The Nazi Doctors: Medical Killing and the Psychology of Genocide*. New York: Basic Books.

Light, Donald W., and Glenn McGee. 1998. "On the Social Embededness of Bioethics." In *Bioethics and Society: Constructing the Ethical Enterprise*, edited by Raymond De Vries and Janaedan Subedi, 1–15. Upper Saddle River NJ: Prentice Hall.

Liguori, Alphonsus. [1785] 1905–1912. *Theologia Moralis*, edited by P. Leondardi Gaudé. Rome: Ex Typographia Vaticana.

Lin, Yu-Sheng. 1979. *The Crisis of Chinese Consciousness: Radical Antitraditionism in the May Fourth Era*. Madison WI: University of Wisconsin Press.

Lincoln, W. Bruce. 1978. *Nicolas I: Emperor and Autocrat of All the Russias*. London: Bloomington.

Lindbeck, Violette. 1984. "Thailand: Buddhism Meets the Western Model." *Hastings Center Report*. 14: 24–6.

Lindemann, Mary. 1996. *Health and Healing in Eighteenth-Century Germany*. Baltimore: Johns Hopkins University Press.

Lipner, Julius J. 1989. "The Classical Hindu View on Abortion and the Moral Status of the Unborn." In H. C. Coward, Julius J. Lipner, and Katherine Young, *Hindu Ethics: Purity, Abortion, and Euthanasia*, 41–69. Albany NY: State University of New York Press.

Lippman, Abby. 1991. "Prenatal Genetic Testing and Screening: Constructing Needs and Reinforcing Inequities." *American Journal of Law & Medicine*. 17: 15–50.

Little, David, and Sumner B. Twiss. 1978. *Comparative Religious Ethics*. San Francisco CA: Harper & Row Publishers.

Littré, Emile, ed. and trans. 1839–1861. *Oeuvres complètes d'Hippocrate*. 10 vols. Paris: J. B. Baillière.

Littré, Emile, ed. [1839–1861] 1962. *Oeuvres complètes d'Hippocrate*. 10 vols. Reprint. Amsterdam: Hakkert.

Litvinenko, Yury G. e.a. 1977. "Nekotorye voprosy deontolopgii v onkologicheskoi practike." In *Problemy Vrachebnoi Etiki i Meditsynskoi Deontologii*, edited by Yu. D. Ryzhkov et al., 93–4. Postov-on-Don: Rostovsky gosudarstvennyi meditsynskii institut.

Liu, Yanchi. 1988. *The Essential Book of Traditional Chinese Medicine: Volume I: Theory*, translated by Fang Tingyu and Chen Laidi. New York: Columbia University Press.

Live Organ Donor Consensus Group. 2000. "Consensus Statement on the Live Organ Donor." *Journal of the American Medical Association*. 284: 2919–26.

Lo, P. 1998. "Confucian Values of Life and Death and Euthanasia." *Chinese and International Philosophy of Medicine*. 1: 35–73 [Chinese].

Lobanov, S. V. 1912. *Vrach I Meditsyna v Prioisvedeniyakh L. N. Tolstogo*. Tomsk.

Lock, Margaret. 1999. "Genetic Diversity and the Politics of Difference." *Chicago-Kent Law Review*. 75: 83–111.

Locke, John. [1690] 1980. *Concerning Civil Government, Second Essay: An Essay Concerning The True Original Extent And End Of Civil Government*, edited by C. B. McPherson. Indianapolis IN: Hackett Publishing Company.

Loewy, Erich H. 1989. *Textbook of Medical Ethics*. New York/London: Plenum Medical Book Company.

Loewy, Erich H. 1995. *Ethische Fragen in der Medizin*. Wien/New York: Springer.

Loewy, Erich H. 2002. "Bioethics: Past, Present, and an Open Future." *Cambridge Quarterly of Healthcare Ethics*. 11: 388–97.

Lohlker, Rüdiger. 1996. "Scharia und Moderne: Diskussionen zum Schwangerschaftsabbruch, zur Versicherung und zum Zinswesen." *Abhandlungen für die Kunde des Morgenlandes*. 51: 7–156.

Lolas Stepke, Fernando. 1994. "El discurso bioético: Una anécdota personal." *Quirón*. 25: 28–30.

Lolas Stepke, Fernando. 1998. *Bioética*. Santiago de Chile: Editorial Universitaria, S.A.

Lolas Stepke, Fernando. 2000a. *Bioética y Antropología Médica*. Santiago de Chile: Mediterráneo.

Lolas Stepke, Fernando. 2000b. "Bioethics and the Culture of Life: A Contribution to Peace." *Bioética Informa*. 6: 8–11. Programa Regional de Bioética. OPS/OMS.

Loncke, Yvette, and Jean Laroze. 1987. *Le Syndicalisme Médical, 1945–1947*. Cahier Georges Valingot # 1.

López, Piñero, and José María. 1964. "El saber médico en la sociedad española del siglo XIX." In *Medicina y sociedad en la España del siglo XIX*. Madrid: Moneda y Crédito.

Lorsch Book of Drugs. 1989. *Lorscher Arzneibuch*. 2 vols., edited by Ulrich Stoll and Gundolf Keil. Stuttgart: Wissenschaftliche Verlagsgesellschaft.

Losonczi, Agnes. 1986. *Anatomy of Defencelessness in the Health Care System*. Budapest: Magveto Publisher [Hungarian].

Loudon, Irvine. 1986a. "Deaths in Childbed from the Eighteenth Century to 1935." *Medical History*. 30: 1–41.

Loudon, Irvine. 1986b. *Medical Care and the General Practitioner, 1750–1850*. Oxford: Oxford University Press.

Loudon, Irvine. 1993 "Childbirth." In *Companion Encyclopedia of the History of Medicine*, edited by William F. Bynum and Roy Porter, 1072–91. London/New York: Routledge.

Lovejoy, Arthur O. 1964. *The Great Chain of Being: A Study of the History of an Idea*. Cambridge MA: Harvard University Press.

Lowell, Charles. 1825. *Report of the Trial of an Action, Charles Lowell against John Faxon and Micajab Hawks, Doctors of Medicine, Defendants, for Malpractice in the Capacity of Physicians and Surgeons, at the Supreme Judicial Court of Maine*. Portland ME.

Lublinsky, P. I. 1930. "Vrachebnaya taina s pravovoi i eticheskoi tochki zrenuja." In *Vrachebnaya Taina i Vrachebnaya Etika. Rechi i Stat'i*, edited by V. I. Voyachek and V. P. Osipov, 41–69. Leningrad: Krasnaya Gazeta.

Lucas, James. 1800. *A Candid Inquiry into the Education, Qualifications, and Office of the Surgeon-Apothecary*. Bath: S. Hazard.

Ludger, Wess, ed. 1998. *Die Träume der Genetik – Gentechnische Utopien vom sozialen Fortschritt*. Frankfurt: Mabuse Verlag.

Luk, Bernard H. 1977. "Abortion in Chinese Law." *The American Journal of Comparative Law*. 25: 372–90.

Luker, Kristin. 1984. *Abortion and the Politics of Motherhood*. Berkeley CA: University of California Press.

Luo, W. 1999. "Establishing Basic Health Care in China's Poverty-Stricken Rural Areas." *Chinese and International Philosophy of Medicine*. 2: 139–52 [Chinese].

Lurie, Peter, and Sidney M. Wolfe. 1997. "Unethical Trials of Interventions to Reduce Perinatal Transmission of the Human Immmunodeficiency Virus in Developing Countries." *New England Journal of Medicine*. 337: 853–6.

Lusthaus, Daniel. 1998. "Sāṅkhya." In *Routledge Encyclopedia of Philosophy. Vol. 8*, edited by Edward Craig, 461–7. London: Routledge.

Lyons, Malcolm C. 1961. "The Kitāb al-Nāfiᶜ of ᶜAlī ibn Riddwān." *Islamic Quarterly*. 6: 65–71.

Lyons, Malcolm C., and B. Towers, eds. 1962. *Galen on Anatomical Procedures: The Later Books*, translated by W. L. H. Duckworth. Cambridge UK: Cambridge University Press.

Ma, Boyin. 1993. *The History of Chinese Medical Culture*. Shanghai: Shanghai People's Press.

Ma, Kanwen. 1986. "Physicians in History." *Chinese Journal of Medical History*. 16: 1–11.

Macbride, David. 1764. *Experimental Essays*. London: Millar.

Macdonald, Duncan B. 1903. *Development of Muslim Theology, Jurisprudence, and Constitutional Theory*. New York: Charles Scribner's Sons.

MacKinney, Loren C. 1952. "Medical Ethics and Etiquette in the Early Middle Ages: The Persistence of Hippocratic Ideals." *Bulletin of the History of Medicine*. 26: 1–31.

Macklin, Ruth. 2003. "Dignity is a Useless Concept." *British Medical Journal*. 327: 1419–20.

Macklin, Ruth, and Florencia Luna. 1996. "Bioethics in Argentina: A Country Report." *Bioethics*. 10: 140–53.

MacLean, Una. 1971. *Magical Medicine: A Nigerian Case-Study*. London: Allen Lane.

Maehle, Andreas-Holger. 1990a. "Präventivmedizin als wissenschaftliches und gesellschaftliches Problem: Der Streit über das Reichsimpfgesetz von 1874." *Medizin, Gesellschaft, und Geschichte.* 9: 127–48.

Maehle, Andreas-Holger. 1990b. "Literary Responses to Animal Experimentation in Seventeenth- and Eighteenth-Century Britain." *Medical History.* 34: 27–51.

Maehle, Andreas-Holger. 1992. *Kritik und Verteidigung des Tierversuchs: Die Anfänge der Diskussion im 17. und 18. Jahrhundert.* Stuttgart: Franz Steiner Verlag.

Maehle, Andreas-Holger. 1993. "The Ethical Discourse on Animal Experimentation, 1650–1900." In *Doctors and Ethics: The Earlier Historical Setting of Professional Ethics,* edited by Andrew Wear, Johanna Geyer-Kordesch, and Roger French, 203–51. Amsterdam: Rodopi.

Maehle, Andreas-Holger. 1996. "Organisierte Tierversuchsgegner: Gründe und Grenzen ihrer gesellschaftlichen Wirkung, 1879–1933." In *Medizinkritische Bewegungen im Deutschen Reich (ca. 1870 – ca. 1933),* edited by Martin Dinges, 109–25. Stuttgart: F. Steiner Verlag.

Maehle, Andreas-Holger. 1999a. *Drugs on Trial: Experimental Pharmacology and Therapeutic Innovation in the Eighteenth Century.* Amsterdam/Atlanta GA: Rodopi.

Maehle, Andreas-Holger. 1999b. "Professional Ethics and Discipline: The Prussian Medical Courts of Honour, 1899–1920." *Medizinhistorisches Journal.* 34: 309–38.

Maehle, Andreas-Holger. 2000. "Assault and Battery, or Legitimate Treatment? German Legal Debates on the Status of Medical Interventions without Consent, c. 1890–1914." *Gesnerus.* 57: 206–21.

Maehle, Andreas-Holger. 2001. "Zwischen medizinischem Paternalismus und Patientenautonomie: Albert Molls 'Ärztliche Ethik' (1902) im historischen Kontext." In *Medizingeschichte und Medizinethik: Kontroversen und Begründungsansätze, 1900–1950,* edited by Andreas Frewer and Josef N. Neumann, 44–56. Frankfurt: Campus Verlag.

Maehle, Andreas-Holger. 2002. "The Emergence of Medical Professional Ethics in Germany." In *Historical and Philosophical Perspectives on Biomedical Ethics: From Paternalism to Autonomy?* edited by Andreas-Holger Maehle and Johanna Geyer-Kordesch, 37–48. Aldershot: Ashgate.

Maehle, Andreas-Holger. 2003. "Protecting Patient Privacy or Serving Public Interests? Challenges to Medical Confidentiality in Imperial Germany." *Social History of Medicine.* 16: 383–401.

Maehle, Andreas-Holger, and Johanna Gaya-Kordisch, eds. 2002. *Historical and Philosphical Perspectives on Biomedical Ethics: From Paternalism to Autonomy?* Aldershot: Ashgate.

Maehle, Andreas-Holger, and Ulrich Tröhler. 1990. "Animal Experimentation from Antiquity to the End of the Eighteenth Century: Attitudes and Arguments." In *Vivisection in Historical Perspective,* edited by Nicolaas A. Rupke, 14–47. London/New York: Routledge.

Maguire, Daniel C. 1974. *Death by Choice.* Garden City NY: Doubleday.

Magyar, Közlöny. 1997. "Patients' Rights and Obligations." *Health Act of 1997.* Budapest: Hungarian Law.

Magyar, Laszlo A. 1997. "Medical Honoraria in the Seventeenth Century." *Vesalius.* 3: 91–4.

Mahmood, Tahir. 1977. *Family Planning: The Muslim Viewpoint.* New Delhi: Vikas Publishing House.

Mahmud, Abd al-Halim. 1986. *Fatawa.* Cairo: Dar al-Maᵓarif.

Mahmud, 'Abd al-Munsif. 7. 3. 1996. *Al-Liwa' al-Islami.* 7.

Mahnke, C. B. 2000. "The Growth and Development of a Specialty: The History of Pediatrics." *Clinical Pediatrics.* 39.12: 705–14.

Mahoney, John. 1987. *The Making of Moral Theology: A Study of the Roman Catholic Tradition.* Oxford: Clarendon Press.

Maimonides, Moses. 1963–1968. *Commentary on the Mishnah,* translated from Arabic by Joseph Kappah. [Hebrew]

Maimonides, Moses. 1964. *The Guide of the Perplexed,* translated by Shlomo Pines. Chicago: University of Chicago Press.

Mainetti, José A. 1987. "Bioethical Problems in the Developing World: A View from Latin America." *Unitas: A Quarterly for the Arts and Sciences.* 60: 238–48.

Mainetti, José A. 1990. "Out of America: The Scholastic and Mundane Bioethical Scene in Argentina." From the symposium "Transcultural Dimensions of Medical Ethics" cosponsored by the Fidia Research Foundation and Georgetown University Center for the Advanced Study of Ethics, National Academy of Sciences, Washington DC, April 26–27.

Mainetti, José A. 1995. "History of Medical Ethics: V. The Americas: D. Latin America." In *Encyclopedia of Bioethics.* 2nd ed., edited by Warren T. Reich, 1639–44. New York: Simon & Schuster Macmillan.

Mainetti, José A. 1996. "In Search of Bioethics: A Personal Postscript." *Journal of Medicine and Philosophy.* 21: 671–9.

Mainetti, José A., Gustavo Pis Diez, and Juan Carlos Tealdi. 1992. "Bioethics in Latin America." In *Bioethics Yearbook: Regional Development in Bioethics, 1989–1991,* vol. 2, edited by B. Andrew Lustig, 83–96. Dordrecht: Kluwer Academic Publishers.

Maio, Giovanni. 1996. "Das Humanexperiment vor und nach Nürnberg: Überlegungen zum Menschenversuch und zum Einwilligungsbegriff in der französischen Diskussion des 19. und 20. Jahrhunderts." In *Medizin und Ethik im Zeichen von Auschwitz: 50 Jahre Nürnberger Ärzteprozeß,* edited by

Claudia Wiesemann and Andreas Frewer, 45–78. Erlangen/Jena: Palm & Enke.

Maio, Giovanni. 1999. "Is Etiquette Relevant to Medical Ethics? Ethics and Aesthetics in the Works of John Gregory (1724–1773)." *Medicine, Health Care, and Philosophy*. 2: 181–7.

Maio, Giovanni. 2000. "Ärztliche Ethik als Politikum: Zur französischen Diskussion um das Humanexperiment nach 1945." *Medizinisches Journal*. 35: 35–80.

Maio, Giovanni. 2002a. *Ethik der Forschung am Menschen: Zur Begründung der Moral in ihrer historischen Bedingtheit*. Stuttgart: Frommann-Holzboog.

Maio, Giovanni. 2002b. "Medizinhistorische Überlegungen zur Medizinethik 1900–1950: Das Humanexperiment in Deutschland und Frankreich." In *Medizingeschichte und Medizinethik: Kontroversen und Begründungsansätze, 1900–1950*, edited by Andreas Frewer and Josef N. Neumann, 374–84. Frankfurt/New York: Campus Verlag.

Majūsī, ʿAlī ibn al-ʿAbbās al-. 1877. *Kitāb Kāmil al-ṣināʿa al-ṭibbiyya (Exhaustive Description of the Medical Art)*. 2 vols. Būlāq.

Makhluf, Hasanayn Muhammad. 1952. *Fatawa Shar'iyya waBuhuth Islamiyya (Legal Fatwas and Islamic Research)*. Cairo: Dar al-Katib al-Arabi.

Makshantseva, N. V. 2001. "Russkoe, Sobornost." In *Mezhkul'turnaya Kommunikatsija*, edited by Valery Zusman, 103–19. Nizhnii Novgorod: Dekom.

Malis, Yury G. 1904. "Vrachebnoe vmeshatel'stvo i otvetstvennost' vracha pered ugolovnym zakonom." *Vestnik Sankt-Peterburgskogo Vrachebnogo Obshestva Vzaimnoi Pomoshi*, no. 9–10: 54–5.

Maluf, N. S. 1954. "History of Blood Transfusion." *Journal of the History of Medicine and Allied Sciences*. 9: 59–107.

Manetti, Daniela, and Amneris Roselli. 1994. "Galeno commentatore di Ippocrate." In *Aufstieg und Niedergang der römischen Welt*. II, 37.2, edited by Wolfgang Haase and Hildegard Temporini, 1529–1635. Berlin/New York: Walter De Grutyer.

Mangan, Joseph T. 1949. "An Historical Analysis of the Principle of Double Effect." *Theological Studies*. 10: 41–61.

Mann, Jonathan, et al. 1994. "Health and Human Rights." *Health and Human Rights*. 1: 6–23.

Mann, Jonathan M., et al., eds. 1999. *Health and Human Rights*. New York/London: Routledge.

Manna', Hasan Murad. 1990. *Fatawa waTawjihat (Fatwas and Instructions)*. Cairo: Dar al-Safwa.

Manning, Aubrey, and James Serpell, eds. 1994. *Animals and Human Society: Changing Perspectives*. London: Routledge.

Marañón, Gregorio. 1947. *Vocación y ética y otros ensayos*. 3rd ed. Revisada y aumentada. Madrid: Espasa-Calpe.

March Noguera, Joan. 2001. *Jaume Salvà i Munar i el mallorquinis me cientific*. Ajuntament d'Algaida: Edicions Pere Capellà.

Marchionne di Coppo. 1903. "Cronaca Fiorentina." In *Rerum Italicarum Scriptores: Raccolta degli Storici Italiani dal Cinquecento al Millecinquecento 30*, edited by Gosuè Carducci and Vittorio Fiorini, 230–2. Città di Castello: Casa Edizione Lapi.

Markel, Howard. 1997. *Quarantine! East European Jewish Immigrants and the New York City Epidemics of 1882*. Baltimore: Johns Hopkins University Press.

Markowitz, Gerald, and David Rosner. 2002. *Deceit and Denial: The Deadly Politics of Industrial Pollution*. Berkeley CA: Milbank/University of California Press.

Marks, Jonathan. 1995. *Human Biodiversity, Race, and History*. New York: Aldine de Gruyter.

Marmion, V. J. 2002. "The Death of Claudius." *Journal of the Royal Society of Medicine*. 95 (5): 260–1.

Marmoy, C. F. A. 1958. "The Auto-Icon of Jeremy Bentham at University College London." *Medical History*. 2: 77–86.

Marrus, Michael R. 1999. "The Nuremberg Doctors' Trial in Historical Context." *Bulletin for the History of Medicine*. 73: 106–23.

Marshall, Barry, ed. 2002. *Helicobacter Pioneers: Firsthand Accounts from the Scientists who Discovered Helicobacters, 1892–1982*. Victoria, Australia/Malden MA: Blackwell.

Marshall, P. A., David C. Thomasma, and J. Bergsma. 1998 "Intercultural Reasoning: The Challenge for Intercultural Bioethics." In *Health Care Ethics*, edited by J. F. Monagle and David C. Thomasma, 584–93. Gaithersburg MD: Aspen Publishers.

Martensen, Robert. 2001. "The History of Bioethics: An Essay Review." *Journal of the History of Medicine and Allied Sciences*. 56: 168–75.

Martinez, Martin. 1730. *Philosophia Sceptica: extracto de la physica antigua, y moderna, recopilada en dialogos, entre un Aristotelico, Cartesiano, Gasendista, y Sceptico, para instruccion de la curiosidad española*. Madrid: publisher unknown.

Martínez, Martín. 1748a. *Medicina sceptica y cirugia moderna con un tratado de operaciones chirurgicas, tomo primero, que llaman tentativa medica*. Segunda impresión. Madrid: Imprenta Real.

Martínez, Martín. 1748b. *Tomo segundo: primera parte: apologema, en favor de los medicos scepticos. Segunda parte: apomathema, contra los medicos dogmaticos, en que se contiene todo el acto de fiebres*. Madrid: Imprenta Real.

Martyn, S., R. Wright, and L. Clark. 1988. "Required Request for Organ Donation: Moral, Clinical, and Legal Problems." *Hastings Center Report*. 18: 27–34.

Marx, Karl Friedrich Heinrich. [1826] 1952. "Medical Euthanasia; a Paper Published in Latin in 1826, Translated and Reintroduced to the Medical

Profession." *Journal of the History of Medicine and Allied Sciences*, translated by Walter Cane. 7: 401–16.

Marx, Karl Friedrich Heinrich. 1874. *Gegen nicht zu billigende Angewöhnungen und Richtungen der jetzigen Aerzte*. Göttingen: Dieterichsche Verlagsbuchhandlung.

Marx, Karl Friedrich Heinrich. 1876. *Ärztlicher Katechismus: Über die Anforderungen an die Ärzte*. Stuttgart: Verlag von F. Enke.

Maryland Session Laws. 1972. ch. 693.

Masters, W. H., and V. E. Johnson. 1966. *Human Sexual Response*. Philadephia: Lippincott Williams & Wilkins Publishers.

Masters, W. H., and V. E. Johnson. 1970. *Human Sexual Inadequacy*. Boston: Little Brown.

Mastroianni, Anna C., Ruth R. Faden, and Daniel Federman, eds. 1994. *Women and Health Research: Ethical and Legal Issues in Including Women in Clinical Studies*. Washington DC: National Academy Press.

Masud, Muhammad Khalid, Brinkley Messick, and David S. Powers, eds. 1996. *Islamic Legal Interpretation: Muftis and their Fatwas*. Cambridge MA: Harvard University Press.

Mata, Pedro. 1859. *Hipócrates y las escuelas hipocráticas: Discurso de apertura de las sesiones del año de 1859 en la Real Academia de Medicina de Madrid*. Madrid: Manuel Rojas.

Mata, Pedro. 1860. *Doctrina medico-filosofica española: Sostenida durante la gran discusión sobre Hipócrates y las escuelas hipocráticas en la Academia de Medicina y Cirugía de Madrie y en la prensa médica*. Madrid: Carlos Bailly-Bailliere.

Mata, Pedro. 1868. *De la libertad moral o libre albedrío: Cuestiones fisio-psicológicas sobre este tema y otros relativos al mismo con aplicación a la distinción fundamental de los actos de los locos y de los de los apasionados o personas responsables*. Madrid: Carlos Bailly-Bailliere.

Mather, Cotton. 1702. *Magnalia Christi Americana*. London: Printed for T. Parkhurst.

Mather, Cotton. [1710] 1966. *Bonifacius: An Essay upon the Good*, edited by David Levin. Cambridge MA: Belknap Press.

Mather, Cotton. 1972. *The Angel of Bethesda: An Essay Upon the Common Maladies of Mankind*, edited by Gordon W. Jones. Barre MA: American Antiquarian Society and Barre Publishers.

Mathieu, Bertrand. 1998. "Ethical "Norms" and the Law: Legitimacy of "Experts" or Democratic Legitimacy." In *Ethics Codes in Medicine: Foundations and Achievements of Codification since 1947*, edited by Ulrich Tröhler and Stella Reiter-Theil, 163–84. Aldershot/Brookfield/Singapore/Sydney: Ashgate.

Matilal, Bimal Krishna. 1989. "Moral Dilemmas: Insights from the Indian Epics." In *Moral Dilemmas in the Mahàbbàrata*, edited by Bimal Krishna Matilal. Delhi: Motilal Banarsidass.

Mauss, Marcel. 1954. *The Gift: Forms and Functions of Exchange in Archaic Societies*, translated by Ian Cunnison. Glencoe IL: Free Press.

Mautner, Thomas, ed. 1999. *Penguin Dictionary of Philosophy*. London: Penguin Books.

Maximilian, Constantin. 1991. "Bioethics in Romania." *Bulletin of Medical Ethics*. 72: 22–3.

May, William F. 1983. *The Physician's Covenant: Images of the Healer in Medical Ethics*. Philadelphia: Westminster Press.

Mbiti, John. 1969. *African Religions & Philosophy*. Nairobi/Ibadan/London: Heinemann.

McCarthy, Charles R. 1994. "Historical Background of Clinical Trials Involving Women and Minorities." *Academic Medicine*. 69: 695–8.

McCarthy, Colman. 1979. "Head of Ethics Institute Thrived on Clash of Ideas." *Washington Post*, 12 May 1979, A24.

McClory, Robert. 1995. *Turning Point: The Inside Story of the Papal Birth Control Commission, and How Humanae Vitae Changed the Life of Patty Crowley and the Future of the Church*. New York: Crossroad.

McCormick, Richard A. 1973. *Ambiguity in Moral Choice*. Milwaukee: Marquette University Press.

McCormick, Richard A. 1979a. "André Hellegers Dies: In Memoriam." *National Catholic Reporter*. 15 (30): 5.

McCormick, Richard A. 1979b. "He Was a Bridge Builder." *Kennedy Institute Quarterly Report*. 5 (1).

McCormick, Richard A. 1981. *How Brave a New World: Dilemas in Bioethics*. Garden City NY: Doubleday.

McCormick, Richard A. 1983. "The Ethical Matrix of Medicine." *European Journal of Obstetrics, Gynecology and Reproductive Biology*. 14 (5): 283–7.

McCormick, Richard A. 1984. *Health and Medicine in the Catholic Tradition: Tradition in Transition*. New York: Crossroad.

McCormick, Richard A. 1985. *How Brave a New World*. Garden City NY: Doubleday.

McCormick, Richard A. 1993a. "Killing the Patient." *The Tablet*. 247: 1410–2.

McCormick, Richard A. 1993b "Veritatis Splendor and Moral Theology." *America*. 169.13 (October 30): 8–11.

McCormick, Richard A. 1994. "Some Early Reactions to *Veritatis Splendor*." *Theological Studies*. 55: 481–506.

McCormick, Richard A. 1995. "The Gospel of Life." *America*. 172.15 (April 29): 10–7.

McCullough, Laurence B. 1998a. *John Gregory and the Invention of Professional Medical Ethics and the Profession of Medicine*. Dordrecht: Kluwer Academic Publishers.

McCullough, Laurence B., ed. 1998b. *John Gregory's Writings on Medical Ethics and Philosophy of Medicine*. Dordrecht: Kluwer Academic Publishers.

McCullough, Laurence B. 1999. "Hume's Influence on John Gregory and the History of Medical Ethics." *Journal of Medicine and Philosophy*. 24: 376–95.

McCullough, Laurence B. 2000. "Holding the Present and Future Accountable to the Past: History and the Maturation of Clinical Ethics as a Field of the

Humanities." *Journal of Medicine and Philosophy*. 25: 5–11.

McCullough, Laurence B. 2002. "The Accidental Bioethicist" *CQ: Cambridge Quarterly of Healthcare Ethics*. 11 (4): 359–68.

McDermott, James P. 1999. "Abortion in the Pàli Canon and Early Buddhist Thought." In *Buddhism and Abortion*, edited by Damien Keown, 157–82. Honolulu HI: University of Hawaii Press.

McFadden, Charles J. 1949. *Reference Manual for Medical Ethics*. Philadelphia: F. A. Davis.

McFadden, Charles J. 1976. *The Dignity of Life: Moral Values in a Changing Society*. Huntington IN: Our Sunday Visitor.

McFarland-Icke, Bronwyn Rebekah. 1999. *Nurses in Nazi Germany: Moral Choice in History*. Princeton NJ: Princeton University Press.

McGeary, Johanna. 2001. "Death Stalks A Continent." *Time*. www.time.com/time/2001/aidsinafrica/cover.html (visited October 14, 2007).

McKeown, Thomas. 1976. *The Role of Medicine: Dream, Mirage, or Nemesis?* London: Nuffield Provincial Hospitals Trust.

McKinney, Loren. [1952] 1977. "Medical Ethics and Etiquette in the Early Middle Ages: The Persistence of Hippocratic Ideals." [*Bulletin of the History of Medicine*. 26: 1–31]. Reprinted in *Legacies in Ethics and Medicine*, edited by Chester R. Burns, 173–203. New York: Science History Publications.

McLean, Charles. 1817–1818. *Results of an Investigation Respecting Epidemic and Pestilential Diseases*. London: Underwood.

McManners, John. 1981. *Death and the Enlightenment*. Oxford: Clarendon Press.

McNamara, Anne. 1994. "Vote Yes; 40-Cent Per Pack Will Discourage Smoking." *Phoenix Gazette*. October 20: B5.

McNeill, John T., and Helena M. Gamer. 1938. *Medieval Handbooks of Penance: A Translation of the Principal Libri Poenitentiales and Selections from Related Documents*. New York: Columbia University Press.

McNeill, Paul. 1993. *The Ethics and Politics of Human Experimentation*. Cambridge UK: Cambridge University Press.

Medical Council of India. 2000. "Code of Medical Ethics." http://www.medclik.com/his/mci.asp (visited January 30, 2008).

"Medical Ethics Workshop in Peradeniya." n.d. www.hf.uib.no/i/Filosofisk/ethica/peradeni.html (visited October 14, 2007): 1–2.

Medical Research Council. 1953. Draft Statement (revised) on Clinical Investigations, 9 October 1953, signed by H. F. Hinsworth. Public Record Office. Manuscript MRC.53/518/B.

Medical Society of the State of New York. 1823. *System of Medical Ethics*. New York: William Grattan.

Medical Society of the State of New York. 1882. *Transactions of the Medical Society of New York*.

Medico-Chirurgical Society of Baltimore. 1832. *A System of Medical Ethics, Adopted by the Medico-Chirurgical Society of Baltimore being the Report of the Committee on Ethics and published by the Order of the Society*. Baltimore: Medico-Chirurgical Society of Baltimore, printed by James Lucas and E. K. Deaver.

Meditsynskii Rabotnik. 1961. No. 21, March 14.

Mellanby, Kenneth. 1945. *Human Guinea Pigs*. London: Victor Gollancz.

Mellanby, Kenneth. 1947. "Medical Experiments on Human Beings in Concentration Camps in Nazi Germany." *British Medical Journal*. 4490: 148–50.

Meltzer, Ewald. 1925. *Das Problem der Abküzung 'lebensunwerten' Lebens (The Problem of the Curtailment of Life 'Unworthy' of Life)*. Halle: Marhold.

Menière, M. P., and M. C. Brouchoud. 1860. *De La Noblesse des Médecins et Les Avocats en France Jusqu'au Dix-Huitième Siècle*. Paris: n.p.

Mercurio, Girolamo (Scipione). 1603. *De Gli Errori Popolari d'Italia*. Venetia, Gio: Battista Ciotti.

Merrison, A. W. 1975. *Report of the Committee of Inquiry into the Regulation of the Medical Profession*. London: Her Majesty's Stationary Office Cmnd. 6018.

Merton, Robert K. 1957. "Priorities in Scientific Discovery: A Chapter in the Sociology of Science." *American Sociological Review*. 22: 635–59.

Meulanbelt, Gerrit Jan. 1999. *History of Indian Medical Literature*. Groningen: E. Forsten.

Meyerhof, Max. [1935] 1984a. "Thirty-Three Clinical Observations by Rhazes (c. 900 AD)." [*Isis*. 23: 321–56, and 14 pp. in Arabic]. Reprinted in Max Meyerhof, *Studies in Medieval Arabic Medicine: Theory and Practice*, no. V, edited by Penelope Johnstone. London: Variorum.

Meyerhof, Max. [1938] 1984b. "Mediaeval Jewish Physicians in the Near East, from Arabic Sources." [*Isis*. 28: 434–60]. Reprinted in Max Meyerhof, *Studies in Medieval Arabic Medicine: Theory and Practice*, no. VII, edited by Penelope Johnstone. London: Variorum.

Meyerhof, Max. [1944] 1984c. "La surveillance des professions médicales et para-médicales chez les arabes." [*Bulletin de l'Institut d'Égypte*. 26: 119–34]. Reprinted in Max Meyerhof, *Studies in Medieval Arabic Medicine: Theory and Practice*, no. XI, edited by Penelope Johnstone. London: Variorum.

Michalczyk, John J., ed. 1994. *Medicine, Ethics, and the Third Reich: Historical and Contemporary Issues*. Kansas City MO: Sheed & Ward.

Micheau, Françoise. 1993. "Les traités sur 'l'examen du médecin' dans le monde arabe médiéval." In *Maladies, Médecines et Sociétés: Approches Historiques pour le Présent*. Actes du VIᵉ Colloque d'Histoire au Présent, 2: 117–28. Paris: L'Harmattan et Histoire au Présent.

Midrash Rabbah. 1939. Translated into English with notes, glossary and indices under the editorship of H. Freedman and Maurice Simon. London: Soncino Press.

Milbank Memorial Fund. 1998. *Enhancing the Accountability of Alternative Medicine.* New York: Milbank Memorial Fund.

Miles, S. 2004. *The Hippocratic Oath and the Ethics of Medicine.* New York: Oxford University Press.

Miller, Timothy. 1985. *The Birth of the Hospital in the Byzantine Empire.* Baltimore: Johns Hopkins University Press.

Minister der Geistlichen, Unterrichts- und Medizinal-Angelegenheiten. [1900] 1901. "Anweisung an die Vorsteher der Kliniken, Polikliniken und sonstigen Krankenanstalten." *Centralblatt für die gesamte Unterrichts-Verwaltung in Preußen*, 188–9. December 29, 1900.

Minnen, Peter van. 1995. "Medical Care in Late Antiquity." In *Ancient Medicine in its Socio- Cultural Context*, edited by Philip J. van der Eijk et al., 153–69. Amsterdam: Rodopi.

Minor Tractates, Semahoth, The. 2nd ed. 1971. Translated by A. Cohen. London: Soncino Press.

Minot, Francis. 1881. "Hints in Ethics and Hygiene." *Medical Correspondence of the Massachusetts Medical Society.* 12: 137–59.

Misra, G. S. P. 1984. *Development of Buddhist Ethics.* New Dehli: Munshiram Manoharlal.

Mitchill, Samuel L., et al., eds. 1821. "Editorial letter to Doctors William Gedney of Milton, John Barnes & Thomas Cooper of Poughkeepsie, and Barnabas Benton & Adna Heaton of Plattekill." In *The Medical Repository of Original Essays and Intelligence, Relative to Physick, surgery, chemistry, and natural history, With a Critical analysis of Recent Publications on These Department of Knowledge, and their Auxiliary Branches*, 94. New York: Van Winkle, Wiley, & Co.

Mitscherlich, Alexander, and Fred Mielke. 1949. *Doctors of Infamy: The Story of the Nazi Medical Crimes.* New York: Henry Schuman.

Mitscherlich, Alexander, and Fred Mielke. 1960. *Medizin ohne Menschlichkeit.* Frankfurt: S. Fischer.

Mitscherlich, Alexander, and Fred Mielke, eds. 1962. *Medizin ohne Menschlichkeit: Dokumente des Nürnberger Ärzteprozesses.* Frankfurt/Main: Fischer Bücherei.

Mohr, James C. 1978. *Abortion in America: The Origins and Evolution of National Policy, 1800–1900.* New York: Oxford University Press.

Mohr, James C. 1993. *Doctors and the Law: Medical Jurisprudence in Nineteenth-Century America.* Baltimore: Johns Hopkins University Press.

Mohr, James C. 2000. "American Medical Malpractice Litigation in Historical Perspective." *Journal of the American Medical Association.* 283: 1731–7.

Moll, Albert. 1902. *Ärztliche Ethik. Die Pflichten des Arztes in allen Beziehungen seiner Thätigkeit (Doctor's Ethics: The Duties of the Doctor with Regard to All his Activities).* Stuttgart: Verlag von F. Enke.

Moll, Albert. 1903. *Vrachebnaya Etika: Obyazannosti Vracha vo Vsekh Otraslyakh Ego Deyatelnosti. Dlya Vrachei i Publiki. Perevod s Nemetskogo i Primechaniya Ya. I. Levinsona.* Saint-Petersburg: A. F. Marks.

Moll, Albert. 1904. *Vrachebnaya Etika: Obyazannosti Vracha vo Vsekh Proyavlenuyakh Ego Deyatel'nosti. Perevod s Nemetskogo pod Redaktsiei i s Predisloviem V. Veresaeva.* Moscow: Magazin "Knizhnoe Delo."

Mollaret, Pierre, and M. Coulon. 1959. "Le Coma Depasse." *Revue Neurologique.* 101: 5–15.

Mondeville, Henri de. 1892. *Die Chirurgie von Heinrich von Mondeville nach Berliner, Erfurter und Pariser Codices zum ersten Mal herausgegeben.* Berlin: Hirschwald.

Mondeville, Henri de. [1897–98] 1964–1965. *La Chirurgie de Maitre Henri de Mondeville. Traduction contemporaine de l'auteur*, edited by Alphonse Bos (Société des Anciens Textes Francais 41), I-II. Reprint. [London/New York: Johnson (only with the first two tracts)]. Paris: Didot.

Monk of St. Tikhon's Monastery, trans. 1987. *Book of Needs.* South Canaan PA: St. Tikhon's Seminary Press.

Mookerji, Radha Kumud. [1947] 1989. *Ancient Indian Education.* 2nd ed. Delhi: Motilal Banarsidass.

Moore, Francis D. 1968. "Medical Responsibility for the Prolongation of Life." *Journal of the American Medical Association.* 206: 384–6.

Moore, Josiah. 1947. "The Office of the Treasurer." In Morris Fishbein, *A History of the American Medical Association 1847–1947*, 846–51. Philadelphia: W. B. Saunders.

Morache, Georges. 1901. *La Profession Médicale: Ses Devoirs, Ses Droits.* Paris: Alcan.

Moran, Bruce. 1990. "Prince-Practitioning and the Direction of Medical Roles at the German Court: Maurice of Hesse-kassel and his Physicians." In *Medicine at the Courts of Europe 1500–1837*, edited by Vivian Nutton, 95–116. London: Routledge.

More, Ellen. 1994. "'Empathy' Enters the Profession of Medicine." In *The Empathic Practitioner: Empathy, Gender, and Medicine*, edited by Ellen More and Mary Milligan, 19–39. New Brunswick NJ: Rutgers University Press.

Moreno, Jonathan D. 2000. *Undue Risk: Secret State Experiments on Humans.* New York: W. H. Freeman.

Moreno, Jonathan D. 2001. *Undue Risk: Secret State Experiments on Humans.* New York: Routledge.

Moreno, Jonathan D., and Ronald Bayer. 1985. "The Limits of the Ledger in Public Health Promotion." *Hastings Center Report.* 15: 37–41.

Morgenstern, Leon. 2002. "Dr. Isaac Hays and Dr. Isaac Israel Hayes: Their Adventure in Two Worlds." *Journal of Medical Biography*. 10:125–28.

Morimura, Seiichi. [1981, 1982] 1985. *Akuma no Hoshoku (Devils' Gluttony)*. [Vol. 1, Vol. 2. Tokyo: Kobunsha]. Reprint. Vol. 3. Tokyo: Kadokawa Shoten.

Morioka, Masahiro. 2000. "Commentary on Tsuchiya." *Eubios Journal of Asian and International Bioethics*. 10: 180–1.

Morison, Robert. 1971. "Death: Process or Event?" *Science*. 173: 694–702.

Morrice, Andrew A. G. 2002. "'Honour and Interests': Medical Ethics and the British Medical Association." In *Historical and Philosophical Perspectives on Biomedical Ethics: From Paternalism to Autonomy?*, edited by Andreas-Holger Maehle and Johanan Geyer-Kordesch, 11–36. Aldershot Ashgate.

Morus, Thomas. 1981. *Utopia*, translated by A. Hartmann. Basel: Diogenes.

Moses, Julius. 1928. "Arbeiterkinder als Versuchskaninchen: 20 Proletarierkinder gleich 100 Raten." *Volkswacht (Bielefeld)*. March 8.

Moses, Julius. 1930. *Der Totentanz von Lübeck*. Radebeul: Madaus.

Moskowitz, Marc L. 2001. *The Haunting Fetus: Abortion, Sexuality, and the Spirit World in Taiwan*. Honolulu HI: University of Hawaii Press.

Mosse, George L. 1964. *The Crisis of German Ideology: Intellectual Origins of the Third Reich*. New York: Grosset and Dunlap.

Mosse, Werner Eugen. [1958] 1995. *Alexander II and the Modernization of Russia*. Reprint. London and New York: I. B. Tauris.

Motzki, Harald. 1991. "Die Anfänge der islamischen Jurisprudenz." *Abhandlungen für die Kunde des Morgenlandes*. 50: 1–292.

Mudrov, Matvei Ya. 1814. *Slovo o Blagochestii I Nravstvennykh Kachestvakh Gippokratova Vracha, na Obnovlenie v Imperatorskom Moskovskom Universitete Meditsynskogo Fakul'teta v torzhestvennom Ego Sobranii 1813 Goda Oktyabrya 13-go Dnya Proiznesennoe Dekanom Vrachebnogo Otdelenija ... Matfiem Mudrovym*. Moscow: V Universitetskoi Typografii.

Mudry, Phillippe. 1997. "Ethique et medecine a Rome: La Preface de Scribonius Largus ou l'affirmation d'une singularite." In *Médecine et Morale dans l'Antiquité (Entretiens sur l'antiquite classique XLIII)*, edited by Hellmut Flashar and Jacques Jouanna, 297–336. Vandoeuvres, Geneva: Fondation Hardt.

Müller, Gerhard. 1967. "Arzt, Kranker und Krankheit bei Ambrosius von Mailand (334–397)." *Sudhoffs Archiv*. 51: 193–216.

Müller-Hill, Benno. 1988. *Murderous Science: Elimination by Scientific Selection of Jews, Gypsies, and Others, Germany 1933–1945*, translated by George R. Fraser. Oxford: Oxford University Press.

Munk, William. 1887. *Euthanasia: or, Medical Treatment in Aid of An Easy Death*. London/New York: Longmans, Green, and Co.

Muntendam, P. 1972. *Euthanasie*. Leiden: Ned Bibliotheek voor de Geneeskunde.

Murano, Senchu. [1974] 1991. *The Lotus Sutra: The Sutra of the Lotus Flower of the Wonderful Dharma*. Tokyo: Nichiren Shu Headquarters.

Murray, Charles. 1984. *Losing Ground: American Social Policy, 1950–1980*. New York: Basic Books.

Murti, Vasu, and Mary Krane Deer. 1998. "Abortion is Bad Karma: Hindu Perspectives." *Feminism and Nonviolence Studies: An Interdisciplinary Journal*. http://www.fnsa.org/fall98/murti1.html (visited January 30, 2008)

Musallam, Basim F. 1983. *Sex and Society in Islam: Birth Control Before the Nineteenth Century*. Cambridge UK: Cambridge University Press.

Musallam, Basim F. 1990. "The Human Embryo in Arabic Scientific and Religious Thought." In *The Human Embryo: Aristotle and the Arabic and European Traditions*, edited by G. R. Dunstan, 32–46. Exeter: University of Exeter Press.

Muslim, Abū al-Ḥusain Muslim b. al-Ḥaǧǧāǧ al-Qušairī al-Nisābūrī. n.d. *Al-Ǧāmi' al-Ṣaḥīḥ*. 4 vols. Bairūt: Dār al-Fikr.

Musto, David F. 1984. "Worthington Hooker (1806–1867): Physician and Educator." *Connecticut Medicine*. 48 (9): 569–74.

Musto, David F. 1986. "Quarantine and the Problem of AIDS." *Milbank Quarterly*. 64. Supplement. 1: 97–117.

Muteau, Charles. 1870. *Du Secret Professionnel de son Étendue de la Responsabilité Qu'il Entraine d'Après la Loi et la Jurisprudence*. Paris: Maresq Aîné.

Myers, G., K. MacInnes, and B. Korber. 1992. "The Emergence of Simian/Human Immunodeficiency Viruses." *AIDS Research and Human Retroviruses*. 8.3: 373–86.

Myers, S. H. 1990. *The Bluestocking Circle: Women, Friendship, and the Life of the Mind in Eighteenth-Century England*. Oxford: Clarendon Press.

Myerson, Abraham, et. al. 1936. *Eugenical sterilization; a reorientation of the problem, by the Committee of the American Neurological Association for the investigation of eugenical sterilization*. New York: Macmillan Company.

Nagel, Tilman. 1978. "Das Leben nach dem Tod in islamischer Sicht." In *Tod und Jenseits im Glauben der Völker*, edited by Hans-Joachim Klimkeit, 130–44. Wiesbaden: Harrassowitz.

Nahmanides, Moses. 1963–64. *Kitve Rabenu Moshe ben Nahman*, edited by C. B. Chavelle. Jerusalem: Mossad Harav Kook [Hebrew].

Nakasone, Ronald Y. 1990. *Ethics of Enlightenment: Essays and Sermons in Search of a Buddhist Ethic.* Fremont CA: Dharma Cloud Publishers.

Nakayama, Shigeru. 1976–1977. "Ways of Thinking of Japanese Physicians." In *History of Traditional Medicine: Proceedings of the 1st and 2nd International Symposia on the Comparative History of Medicine – East and West,* edited by Teizo Ogawa. Division of Medical History, Taniguchi Foundation.

Ñāṇamoli, Bhikkhu, trans. and ed. [1956] 1975. *The Path of Purification (Visuddhimagga).* Kandy: Buddhist Publication Society.

Nanji, Azim A. 1988. "Medical Ethics and the Islamic Tradition." *Journal of Medicine and Philosophy.* 13: 257–75.

Nanjing Zhongyi Xueyuan (Nanjing College of Chinese Medicine). 1981. *Huandi Neijing Suwen Yishi (Suwen of The Yellow Emperor's Classic of Medicine: Text, Translation, and Annotation).* Shanghai: Shanghai Science and Technology Press [Modern Chinese].

Nanjing Zhongyi Xueyuan (Nanjing College of Chinese Medicine). 1986. *Huandi Neijing Lingshu Yishi (Lingshu of The Yellow Emperor's Classic of Medicine: Text, Translation, and Annotation).* Shanghai: Shanghai Science and Technology Press [Modern Chinese].

Nardi, Enzo. 1971. *Procurato Aborto Nel Mondo Greco-Romano.* Milan: A. Guiffre.

Nascher, Ignatz Leo. 1914. *Geriatrics; the diseases of old age and their treatment, including physiological old age, home and institutional care, and medico-legal relations, with an introduction by A. Jacobi, M.D. With 50 plates containing 81 illustrations.* Philadelphia: Blakiston.

Nasr, Seyyed H. 1976. *Islamic Science.* Westerham: Kent.

Nassar, Seraphim, ed. 1979. *Divine Prayers and Services of the Catholic Orthodox Church of Christ.* Englewood NJ: Antiochian Orthodox Christian Archdiocese.

National Academy of Sciences. 1993. *Veterans at Risk: The Health Effects of Mustard Gas and Lewisite.* Washington DC: National Academy Press.

National Bioethics Advisory Commission. 2001. *Ethical and Policy Issues in International Research: Clinical Trials in Developing Countries,* vol. 1. Bethesda MD: U.S. Dept. of Commerce, Technology Administration, National Technical Information Service.

National Commission for the Protection of Human Subjects of Biomedical and Behavioral Research. 1979. *The Belmont Report: Ethical Princples and Guidelines for the Protection of Human Subjects of Research.* DHEW (OS) 78–0012. Washington DC: U.S. Government Printing Office.

National Commission for the Protection of Human Subjects of Biomedical and Behavioral Research. [1979] 1998. *The Belmont Report: Code of Federal Regulations.* In *Source Book in Bioethics: A Documentary History,* edited by Albert R. Jonsen, Robert M. Veatch, and LeRoy Walters, 22–8. Washington DC: Georgetown University Press.

National Hospice and Palliative Care Organization. 2003. *Hospice Facts.* National Hospice and Palliative Care Organization, Alexandria Virginia.

National Research Council. 1997. *Evaluating Genetic Diversity.* 19–20. Washington DC: National Academy Press.

Navarro, Vicente. 1975. "The Political Economy of Health Care." *The International Journal of Health Services.* 5: 65–94.

Navarro, Vicente. [1976] 1978. *La medicina bajo el capitalismo. [Medicine Under Capitalism.* New York: Neale Watson Academic Publications]. Reprint. Barcelona: Editorial Crítica.

Navarrus (Azpilcueta, Martin). 1574. *Enchiridion sive Manuale Confessariorum et Poenitentium.* Lyons: Rouillius.

Ndinya-Achola, Jecknoniah. 1995. "History of Medical Ethics: II. Africa: A. Sub-Saharan Countires." In *Encyclopedia of Bioethics.* 2nd ed., edited by Warren T. Reich, 1460–5. New York: Simon & Schuster Macmillan.

Needham, Joseph. [1956] 1980. *Science and Technology in China, Volume II: History of Scientific Thought.* Cambridge UK: Cambridge University Press.

Needham, Joseph. 1970. *Clerks and Craftsmen in China and the West.* Cambridge UK: Cambridge University Press.

Needham, Joseph. 2000. *Science and Technology in China, Volume VI, Part 6: Medicine.* Cambridge UK: Cambridge University Press.

Nelkin, Dorothy, and Mark Michaels. 1998. "Biological Categories and Border Controls." *International Journal of Sociology and Social Policy.* 16: 33–59.

Nelkin, Dorothy, and Laurance Tancredi. 1995. *Dangerous Diagnostic: The Social Power of Biological Information.* Chicago: University of Chicago Press.

Neuburger, Max. 1911. *Geschichte der Medizin.* 2 vols. Stuttgart: Ferdinand Enke.

Neuhaus, John Richard. 1995. "Moral Theology at its Pique." *First Things.* 49 (January): 88–92.

Neumann, Josef N. 1991. "Christoph Wilhelm Hufeland (1762–1836)." In *Klassiker der Medizin,* edited by Dietrich von Engelhardt and Fritz Hartmann, vol. 1, 339–59. München: Beck.

Neuschel, Kristen. 1989. *Word of Honor: Interpreting Noble Culture in Sixteenth-Century France.* Ithaca NY: Cornell University Press.

New Hampshire Medical Society. 1822. *The Charter, by-laws, regulations, and police, of the New-Hampshire Medical Society.* Concord NH: New Hampshire Medical Society.

New Jersey Medical Society. 1766. *Instruments of Association and Constitution of the New Jersey Medical Society.*

"New Jersey Declaration of Death Act." 1991. *Kennedy Institute of Ethics Journal.* 1.4: 289–92.

Newman, Louis E. 1998. *Past Imperatives: Studies in the History and Theory of Jewish Ethics*. Albany NY: State University of New York Press.

Newmyer, Stephen T. 1989. "The Oath of Asaph and its Hippocratic Original." *Newsletter of the Society for Ancient Medicine and Pharmacy*. 17: 10.

Newmyer, Stephen T. 1996. "Talmudic Medicine and Greco-Roman Science: Crosscurrents and Resistance." In *Aufstieg und Niedergang der Römischen Welt II*. 37.3, edited by Wolfgang Haase, 2895–911. Berlin: Walter de Gruyter.

Ni, Peimin. 1999. "Confucian Virtues and Personal Health." In *Confucian Bioethics*, edited by Ruiping Fan, 27–44. Dordrecht: Kluwer Academic Publishers.

Nickens, Herbert. 1996. "The Genome Project and Health Services for Minority Populations." In *The Human Genome Project and the Future of Health Care*, edited by Thomas Murray, Mark A. Rothstein, and Robert Murray. Bloomington IN: University of Indiana Press.

Nie, Jing-Bao. 1996. "The Physician as General." *Journal of American Medical Association*. 276: 1099.

Nie, Jing-Bao. 1999a. "'Human Drugs' in Chinese Medicine and the Confucian View: An Interpretive Study." In *Confucian Bioethics*, edited by Ruiping Fan, 167–206. Dordrecht: Kluwer Academic Publishers.

Nie, Jing-Bao. 1999b. "The Myth of the Chinese Culture, the Myth of the Chinese Medical Ethics." *Bioethics Examiner*. 3: 1, 2, 5.

Nie, Jing-Bao. 1999c. "The Problem of Coerced Abortion in China and Related Ethical Issues." *Cambridge Quarterly of Healthcare Ethics*. 8: 463–79.

Nie, Jing-Bao. 2000. "The Plurality of Chinese and American Medical Moralities: Toward an Interpretative Cross-Cultural Bioethics." *Kennedy Institute of Ethics Journal*. 10: 239–60.

Nie, Jing-Bao. 2001a. "Challenges of Japanese Doctors' Human Experimentation in China for East-Asian and Chinese Bioethics." *Eubios Journal of Asian and International Bioethics*. 11: 3–7.

Nie, Jing-Bao. 2001b. "Is Informed Consent Not Applicable in China? Intellectual Flaws of the Cultural Difference Argument." *Formosan Journal of Medical Humanities*. 2: 67–74.

Nie, Jing-Bao. 2001c. "'So Bitter That No Words Can Describe It': Mainland Chinese Women's Moral Experiences and Narratives of Abortion." In *Globalizing Feminist Bioethics: Crosscultural Perspectives*, edited by Rosemarie Tong, Aida Santos, and Gwen Anderson, 151–64. Boulder CO: Westview Press.

Nie, Jing-Bao. 2002a. "Chinese Moral Perspectives on Abortion and Foetal Life: An Historical Account." *New Zealand Bioethics Journal*. 3: 15–31.

Nie, Jing-Bao. 2002b. "Foreign Lenses and Native Concerns: Significance of Western Feminism for Bioethics in China." *Ethics and Society*. 9: 2–16. Newsletter for the Centre for Applied Ethics, Hong Kong Baptist University.

Nie, Jing-Bao. 2002c. "Japanese Doctors' Experimentation in Wartime China." *The Lancet*. 360: s5–s6.

Nie, Jing-Bao. 2002d. "Mainland Chinese People's Moral Views and Experiences of Abortion: A Brief Report." In *Advances in Chinese Medical Ethics: Chinese and International Perspectives*, edited by Ole Döring and Chen Renbiao, 279–89. Hamburg: Institute for Asian Studies.

Nie, Jing-Bao. 2002e. "Truth-Telling in Chinese Medical Ethics Tradition: Some Misconceptions and Misuses of Culture in Bioethics." Paper presented at the 6th annual meeting of American Society for Bioethics and Humanities, October 25, 2002.

Nie, Jing-Bao. 2003a. "Japanese Doctors' Experimentation in Wartime China against East Asian Morality: Medicine as the Art of Humanity and Universality of the Informed Consent Principle." Paper presented at the 9th annual conference of the Australasian Bioethics Association held in Queenstown, New Zealand, July 3, 2003.

Nie, Jing-Bao. 2003b. "Let's Never Stop Bashing Inhumanity: A Reply to Frank Leavitt and an Appeal for Further Ethical Studies on Japanese Doctors' Wartime Experimentation." *Eubios Journal of Asian and International Bioethics*. 13: 162–6.

Nie, Jing-Bao. 2004a. "Feminist Bioethics and its Language of Human Rights in the Chinese Context." In *Linking Visions: Feminist Bioethics, Human Rights and the Developing World*, edited by Rosemarie Tong, Anne Donchin and Susan Dodds, 73–88. Boulder CO: Rowman & Littlefield Publishers.

Nie, Jing-Bao. 2004b. "State Violence in Twentieth-Century China: Some Shared Features of Japanese Army's Atrocities and the Cultural Revolution's Terror." Paper prepared for the research project *Human Rights, Cultures, and Violence: Perspectives of Intercultural Ethics* of the Center for European Integration Studies (ZEI), Bonn University, Germany.

Nie, Jing-Bao. 2004c. *Voices Behind the Silence: Chinese Views and Experiences of Abortion*. Boulder CO: Rowman & Littlefield.

Nieto de Piña, Cristóbal. 1779. *Discurso Medico Moral: Los que usan leche medicinal deben considerease entre los dispensados al Fasting Eclesiastico Sevilla*. Manuel Nicolás Vazquez.

Nieto Serrano, Matías. 1860. *Ensayo de medicina general, o sea de filosofía médica*. Madrid: Imprenta de Manuel de Rojas.

Nieto Serrano, Matías. 1869. *La libertad moral (Réplica a un libro del Sr. D. Pedro Mata)*. Madrid: Imprenta de P. G. y Orga.

Nietzsche, Friedrich. [1883, 1885] 1964a. *Thus Spake Zarathustra*. In *The Complete Works of Friedrich Nietzsche: First*

Complete and Authorised English Translation, edited by Oscar Levy, translated by Anthony M. Ludovici. New York: Russell & Russell.

Nietzsche, Friedrich. [1887] 1964b. *The Geneaology of Morals.* In *The Complete Works of Friedrich Nietzsche: First Complete and Authorised English Translation*, edited by Oscar Levy, translated by Anthony M. Ludovici. New York: Russell & Russell.

Nietzsche, Friedrich. [1888] 1964c. *The Twighlight of the Idols: Or, How to Philosophise with the Hammer.* In *The Complete Works of Friedrich Nietzsche: First Complete and Authorised English Translation*, edited by Oscar Levy, translated by Anthony M. Ludovici. New York: Russell & Russell.

Nietzsche, Friedrich. [1901, 1906] 1968. *Der Wille zur Macht (Will to Power)*, translated by Walter Kaufman and R. J. Hollingdale. New York: Vintage Books.

NIH/DOE Task Force on the Ethical, Legal, and Social Implications of Genetic Testing. 1997. Baltimore MD.

Nikitina, E. V. 1966. "Nekotorye Voprosy Vrachebnoi Etiki v Svete Moral'nogo Kodeksa Stroitelja Kommunizma." Avtoreferat. Diss... Kand. Filosof. Nauk. Dushanbe.

Nilges, Richard G. 1984. "The Ethics of Brain Death: Thoughts of a Neurosurgeon Considering Retirement." *The Pharos of Alpha Omega Alpha-Honor Medical Society.* 47: 34–5.

Nolan, Martin. 1968. "The Principle of Totality in Moral Theology." In *Absolutes in Moral Theology*, edited by Charles E. Curran, 232–48. Washington DC: Corpus Books.

Nolte, Winfried. 1981. "Der hippokratische Eid und der Abschlusseide der früheren und jetzigen deutschsprachigen Hochschulen." M.D. diss., University of Bochum.

"Non-Heart-Beating Donor Protocols to Increase Organ Donation." 1993. *Kennedy Institute of Ethics Journal.* 23: 1–262. Special Issue: Papers from the October 10, 1992, University of Pittsburgh conference.

Noorda, Sijbolt. 1979. "Illness and Sin, Forgiving and Healing: The Connection of Medical Treatment and Religious Beliefs in Ben Sira. 38: 1–15." In *Studies in Hellenistic Religions*, edited by M. J. Vermaseren, 215–24. Leiden: E. J. Brill.

Norheim, O. F. 1995. "The Norwegian Welfare State in Transition: Rationing and Plurality of Values as Ethical Challenges for the Health Care System." *Journal of Medicine and Philosophy.* 20: 639–55.

Norman Bloodsaw v. Lawrence Berkeley Laboratory. No. C-95–3220-VWR (N.D. Cal., June 10, 1996). "Case Law," *Employment Testing – Law and Policy Reporter.* 138 (September 1996).

Novak, David. 1985. "Judaism and Contemporary Bioethics." In *Halakha in a Theological Dimension*, edited by David Novak, 82–101. Chico: CA: Scholars Press.

Novak, William J. 1996. *The People's Welfare: Law and Regulation in Nineteenth-Century America.* Chapel Hill NC: University of North Carolina Press.

Nudeshima, Jiro. 1989. "The Need to Go Beyond a Traditional Framework in Doctor-Patient Relationships: Movement Toward Alternative Medical Relationships in Japan During the 80's." In *History of the Doctor-Patient Relationship: Proceedings of the 14th International Symposium on the Comparative History of Medicine – East and West*, edited by Yosio Kawakita, Shizu Sakai, and Yasuo Otsuka. Susono-shi, Shizuoka, Japan: Ishiyaku EuroAmerica Inc., Publishers.

Nudeshima, Jiro. 1991. "Obstacles to Brain Death and Organ Transplantation in Japan." *The Lancet.* 338: 1063–4.

Nudeshima, Jiro. 1997. "Biomedical Ethics in Japan: An Imperative." *NIRA Review.* (Spring): 3–5. Also see www.nira.go.jp.

Nudeshima, Jiro. 2001. "Human Cloning Legislation in Japan." *Eubios Journal of Asian and International Bioethics.* 11: 2.

Nuffield Council on Bioethics. 2001. *The Ethics of Research Related to Health Care in Developing Countries.* http://www.nuffieldbioethics.org/go/ourwork/developingcountries/publication_309.html (visited January 30, 2008).

Nuland, Sherwin. 2003. *The Doctors' Plague: Germs, Childbed Fever, and the Strange Story of Ignác Semmelweis.* New York: W. W. Norton & Co. Inc.

Numbers, Ronald L., ed. 1987. *Medicine in the New World: New Spain, New France, and New England.* Knoxville TN: University of Tennessee Press.

Numbers, Ronald L., and Darrel W. Amundsen, eds. [1986] 1998. *Caring and Curing: Health in the Western Religious Traditions.* [New York: Macmillan]. Reprint. Baltimore: Johns Hopkins University Press.

Núñez, Toribio. 1820. *Sistema de la Ciencia social ideado por Jeremías Bentham y puesto en ejecución conforme a los principios del autor.* Salamanca: Bernardo Martín.

Nutton, Vivian. 1985a. "From Galen to Alexander: Aspects of Medicine and Medical Practice in Late Antiquity." In *Symposium on Byzantine Medicine*, edited by John Scarborough, 1–14. Washington DC: Dumbarton Oaks Library and Collection.

Nutton, Vivian. 1985b. "Humanist Surgery." In *The Medical Renaissance of the Sixteenth Century*, edited by Andrew Wear, Roger French, and Iain Lonie, 75–99. Cambridge UK: Cambridge University Press.

Nutton, Vivian. 1993. "Beyond the Hippocratic Oath." In *Doctors and Ethics: The Earlier Historical Setting of Professional Ethics*, edited by Andrew Wear, Johanna Geyer-Kordesch, and Roger French, 10–37. Amsterdam: Rodopi.

Nutton, Vivian. 1995. "What's in an Oath?" *Journal of the Royal College of Physicians of London.* 29.6: 518–24.

Nutton, Vivian. 1996a. "Hippocratic Morality and Modern Medicine." In *Médecine et Morale dans l'Antiquité (Entretiens sur l'antiquite classique XLII)*, edited by Hellmut Flashar and Jacques Jouanna, 31–64. Vandoeuvres, Geneva: Fondation Hardt.

Nutton, Vivian. 1996b. "Idle Old Trots, Coblers and Costardmongers: Pieter van Foreest on Quackery." In *Petrus Forestus Medicus*, edited by Henriette A. Bosman-Jelgersma, 243–56. Amsterdam: Stichting A D & L.

Nye, Robert A. 1993. *Masculinity and Male Codes of Honor in Modern France.* New York: Oxford University Press.

Nye, Robert A. 1995. "Honor Codes and Medical Ethics in Modern France." *Bulletin of the History of Medicine.* 69: 91–111.

Oberndörfer, Johann. 1600. *De Veri et Falsi Medici Agnitione Tractatus Brevis, in Theorematum Forma Conscriptus.* Lavingae: Ex officina typographica Leonhardi Reinmichaelii.

Oberndörfer, Johann. [1600] 1602. *The Anatomyes of the True Physition, and Counterfeit Mountebanke: wherein both of them are graphically described, and set out in their Right, and Orient Colours*, translated by Francis Herring. London: Printed for Arthur Johnson.

Obeyesekere, Gananath. 1976. "The Impact of Ayurvedic Ideas on the Culture and the Individual in Sri Lanka." In *Asian Medical Systems: A Comparative Study*, edited by Charles Leslie, 201–26. Berkeley CA: University of California Press.

Obeyesekere, Gananath. 1978. "Illness, Culture, and Meaning: Some Comments on the Nature of Traditional Medicine." In *Culture and Healing in Asian Societies: Anthropological, Psychiatric and Public Health Studies*, edited by Arthur Kleinman, et al., 253–64. Cambridge: Schenkman Publishing Company.

Objazannosti i Prava Vrachei. Eticheskie Pravila, Prinyatye Varshavskim Obshestvom Vrachei. 1884. *Vrach.* 29: 497–9.

Obshestvo Vrachei Volynskoi Gubernii (Society of Physicians of Volynsk Region). 1886. "Pravila dlya Vzaimnykh Otnoshenii Vrachei u Posteli Bol'nogo, Vyrabottannye Obshestvom Vrachei Volynskoi Gubernii v 1885 Godu." Prilozhenija k Protokolan Obshestva Vrachei Volynskoi Gubernii. Zhitomir.

O'Connell, Marvin R. [1986] 1998. "The Roman Catholic Tradition Since 1545." In *Caring and Curing: Health and Medicine in the Western Religious Traditions*, edited by Ronald L. Numbers and Darrel W. Amundsen, 108–45. [New York: Macmillan]. Reprint. Baltimore: Johns Hopkins University Press.

O'Donnell, Thomas J. 1956. *Morals in Medicine.* Westminster MD: Newman Press.

O'Donnell, Thomas J. 1976. *Medicine and Christian Morality.* New York: Alba House.

Office of the Inspector General, U.S. Department of Health and Human Services. 2001. "The Globalization of Clinical Trials." OEI 01–00–00190.

Ohno, Yasumaro. [712] 1958. *Kojiki (Records of Ancient Matters)*, translated by Kenji Kurano and Yukichi Takeda. Tokyo: Iwanami Shoten.

O'Meara, Edmund. 1665. *Examen Diatribae Thomae Willisii . . . de febribus.* London: Pulleyn jun.

Omran, Abdel-Rahim. 1980. *Population in the Arab World.* New York: Croom Helm Ltd.

Omran, Abdel-Rahim. 1992. *Family Planning in the Legacy of Islam.* London: Routledge.

Ongaro, Giuseppe. 1981. "La Medicina nello Studio di Padova e nel Veneto." In *Storia della Cultura Veneta 3/III (Dal primo Quattrocento al Concilio di Trento)*, 75–134. Vicenza: Neri Pozza.

Ordre National des Médecins. 1983. *Guide d'Exercice Professional.* 13th ed. Paris: Masson.

Oregon Department of Health Services, Office of Disease Prevention and Epidemiology. 2005. *Seventh Annual Report on Oregon's Death With Dignity Act.* Eugene, OR.

Orhonlu, Cengiz. 1993. "Sünnet Düğünü." In *Islam Ansiklopedisi.* 11, 245–7. Istanbul: M. E. B.

Origenes. 1968. *Origène, Contre Celse*, vol. 2 (livre 3–4), edited by M. Borret. Paris: Edition du Cerf.

Ortí y Lara, Juan Manuel. 1853. *Ética o Principios de filosofía moral.* Madrid: Imprenta de las Escuelas Pías.

Osgood, Robert S., and Robert W. Tucker. 1967. *Force, Order, and Justice.* Baltimore: Johns Hopkins University Press.

Oshima, Tomoo. 1983. "The Japanese-German System of Medical Education in the Meiji and Taisho Eras, 1868–1926." In *The History of Medical Education: Proceedings of the 6th International Symposium on the Comparative History of Medicine-East and West*, edited by Teizo Ogawa, 211–36. Tokyo: Saikon Publishing Co. Ltd.

Osler, William. 1905. *Science and Immortality.* Boston: Houghton.

Otsuka, Yasuo. 1984. "Chinese Traditional Medicine in Japan." In *Asian Medical Systems: A Comparative Study*, edited by Charles Leslie, 322–40. Berkeley/Los Angeles CA: University of California Press.

Owoahene-Acheampong, Stephen. 1998. *Inculturation and African Religion: Indigenous and Western Approaches to Medical Practice.* New York: Peter Lang.

Oxea, Fernando. 1777. *Disertación médica de la sinplicidad i sencillez con que se debe egercer la medicina.* Santiago: Ignacio Aguayo i Aldemunde.

O. Z. 2002. "Three quarter of the Hungarian suicides are men." *Nepszabadsag*, July 18.

Packard, Frances R. [1901] 1963. *History of Medicine in the United States.* [Philadelphia: Lippincott]. Reprint. New York: Hafner.

Padfield, Peter. 1995. *Himmler: Reichsführer SS*. London: Papermac.

Pagel, Julius Leopold, ed. 1892. *Die Chirurgie des Heinrich von Mondeville (Hermondaville) nach Berliner, Erfurter und Pariser Codices zum ersten Mal herausgegeben*. Berlin: Hirschwald.

Pagel, Julius Leopold. 1897. *Medicinische Deontologie: Ein kleiner Katechismus für angehende Praktiker (Medical Deontology: A Brief Catechism for Future Practitioners)*. Berlin: Verlag von O. Coblentz.

Pagel, Walter. 1944. "The Religious and Philosophical Aspects of van Helmont's Science and Medicine." *Supplement to the Bulletin of the History of Medicine*. 2.

Pagel, Walter. 1951. "Julius Pagel and the Significance of Medical History for Medicine." *Bulletin of the History of Medicine*. 25: 207–25.

Pagel, Walter. 1958. *Paracelsus*. Basel: Karger.

Pagel, Walter. 1982. *Joan Baptista van Helmont: Reformer of Science and Medicine*. Cambridge UK: Cambridge University Press.

Palazzini, Pietro. 1962. "Alphonsus." In *Dictionary of Moral Theology*. 2nd ed., translated by Henry J. Yamnone, edited by Francesco Roberti and Pietro Palazzini, 59–62. London: Burns and Oates.

Palely, William. 1785. *The Moral and Political Philosophy*. London: R. Faulder.

Paley, William. [1795] 1985. *The Principles of Moral and Political Philosophy*. In William Paley, *The Works of William Paley, D. D.*, Vol. 4, edited by Edmund Paley. London: C. and J. Rivington.

Paley, William. [1802, 1809] 1998. *Natural Theology: or, Evidences of the Existence and Attributes of the Deity, Collected from the Appearances of Nature*. London: J. Faulder. http://darwin-online.org.uk/content/frameset?itemID=A142&viewtype=text&pageseq=1 (visited January 30, 2008).

Pallis, Christopher. 1982a. "ABC of Brain Stem Death: Diagnosis of Brain Stem Death – I." *British Medical Journal*. 285: 1558–60.

Pallis, Christopher. 1982b. "ABC of Brain Stem Death: Diagnosis of Brain Stem Death – II." *British Medical Journal*. 285: 1641–4.

Pandya, Sunil K. 1999. "The Importance of Love in Ancient Indian Biomedical Ethics." *Eubios Journal of Asian and International Bioethics*. 9: 42–3.

Papal Teachings: The Human Body. 1960. Boston: St. Paul Editions.

Pappworth, Maurice H. 1967a. *Human Guinea Pigs: Experimentation on Man*. London: Routledge & Kegan Paul.

Pappworth, Maurice H. 1967b. *Human Guinea Pigs: Experimentation on Man*. Boston: Beacon Press.

Paracelsus. 1965–68. *Theophrastus Paracelsus Werke*. Bd. 1–5. Besorgt von Will-Erich Peuckert. Basel/Stuttgart: Schwabe.

Parascandola, John. 1992. *The Development of American Pharmacology: John J. Abel and the Shaping of a Discipline*. Baltimore: Johns Hopkins University Press.

Paré, Ambroise. 1963. *Rechtfertigung und Bericht über meine Reisen in verschiedene Orte*, edited by E. Ackerknecht. Bern/Stuttgart: Huber.

Paret, Rudi, trans. 1993. *Der Koran*. Stuttgart: Kohlhammer.

Parikh, Firuza. 1998. "Sex Selection by IVF: Detrimental to Indian Women." *International Journal of Medical Ethics* 6:2 http://www.ijme.in/062de055.html (visited January 30, 2008).

Park, Catherine. 1985. *Doctors and Medicine in Early Renaissance Florence*. Princeton NJ: Princeton University Press.

Park, Catherine. 1992. "Medicine and Society in Medieval Europe." In *Medicine in Society*, edited by Andrew Wear, 59–90. Cambridge UK: Cambridge University Press.

Parker, Robert. 1983. *Miasma: Pollution and Purification in Early Greek Religion*. Oxford: Clarendon Press.

Parker, Samuel. 1715. *An Essay Upon the Duty of Physicians and Patients, The Dignity of Medicine, And the Prudentials of Practice in Two Dialogues*. London: National Library of Medicine, NLM UI 2721761R.

Parsons, Talcott. 1951. *The Social System*. London: Routledge & Kegan Paul.

Pascal, Blais. 1987. *Les Provinciales ou Les Lettres écrites par Louis de Montalte à un provincial de ses amis et aux RR. PP. Jésuites sur le sujet de la morale et de la politique de ces Pères*. Paris: Gallimard.

Pascual, Prudencia María. 1821. *Sistema de la moral o La teoría de los deberes*. Valencia: Oficina de José Ferrer de Orga.

Passmore, John. 1975. "The Treatment of Animals." *Journal of the History of Ideas*. 36: 195–218.

Pasteur, Louis. 1879. "Septicémie puerpérale." *Bulletin de l'Académie de médecine Paris*. 2nd série, 8: 505–8.

"Patient-centred Healthcare." 2002. *The Sunday Times: The Daily Mirror Online*. http://www.dailymirror.lk/2002/11/13/editorial.html (visited October 13, 2007): 1–2.

Paton, William, Sir. 1993. *Man and Mouse: Animals in Medical Research*. 2nd ed. Oxford: Oxford University Press.

Pattison, F. L. M. 1987. *Granville Sharp Pattison: Anatomist and Antagonist, 1791–1851*. Edinburgh: Canongate.

Paul VI. 1968. *Humanae Vitae*. www.papalencyclicals.net.

Paulina, Éva, and Dr. Jánosi Gábor. 1991. *Pénzt vagy életet? (Your Money or Your Life?)* Budapest: Hungaprint Kiadó és Nyomda (Hunga-print Publisher and Printing Office).

Pauser, Josef. 1998. "Sektion als Strafe?" In *Körper ohne Leben – Begegnung und Umgang mit Toten*, edited by N. Stefenelli, 527–35. Wien/Köln/Weimar: Böhlau.

Pease, Arthur Stanley. 1914. "Medical Allusions in the Works of St. Jerome." *Harvard Studies in Classical Philology*. 25: 73–86.

Pechura, Constance M., and David P. Rall, eds. 1993. *Veterans At Risk: The Health Effects of Mustard Gas and Lewisite*. Washington DC: National Academy Press.

Peiffer, Jürgen. 1991. "Neuropathology in the Third Reich: Memorial to those Victims of National-Socialist Atrocities in Germany who were Used by Medical Science." *Brain Pathology*. 1: 125–31.

Peiffer, Jürgen, ed. 1992. *Menschenverachtung und Opportunismus: Zur Medizin im Dritten Reich*. Tübingen: Attempto.

Peiffer, Jürgen. 1997. *Hirnforschung im Zwielicht: Beispiele verführbarer Wissenschaft aus der Zeit des Nationalsozialismus: Julius Hallervorden – H. J. Scherer – Berthold Ostertag*. Husum: Matthiesen.

Peiffer, Jürgen. 1999. "Assessing Neuropathological Research carried out on Victims of the 'Euthanasia' Programme." *Medizinhistorisches Journal*. 34: 339–55.

Peinador, Antonio. 1962. *Tratado de moral profesional*. Madrid: La editorial católica.

Peinard, Dr. 1894. *La Profession de Médecine*. Paris: Société des Editions Scientifiques.

Peiró, Francisco. 1944. *Manual de deontología médica*. Madrid: Estades.

Pebley, A. R., A. I. Hermalin, and J. Knodel. 1991. "Birth Spacing and Infant Mortality: Evidence for Eighteenth and Nineteenth Century German Villages." *Journal of Biosocial Science*. 23: 445–59.

Pellegrino, Edmund D. 1979. *Humanism and the Physician*. Knoxville TN: University of Tennessee Press.

Pellegrino, Edmund D. 1985. "Thomas Percival's Ethics: The Ethics Beneath the Etiquette." In *Medical Ethics: Or, A Code of Institutes and Precepts, Adapted to the Professional Conduct of Physicians and Surgeons, by Thomas Percival, M.D.*, edited by Edmund D. Pellegrino, 1–52. Birmingham AL: The Classics of Medicine Library.

Pellegrino, Edmund D. 1986. "Percival's Medical Ethics: The Moral Philosophy of an 18th- Century English Gentleman." *Archives of Internal Medicine*. 146: 2265–9.

Pellegrino, Edmund D., and Alice H. Pellegrino. 1988. "Humanism and ethics in Roman medicine: Translation and Commentary on a Text of Scribonius Largus." *Literature and Medicine*. 7: 22–38.

Pellegrino, Edmund D., and David C. Thomasma. 1981. *A Philosophical Basis of Medical Practice: Toward a Philosophy and Ethics of the Healing Professions*. New York: Oxford University Press.

Pellegrino, Edmund D., and David C. Thomasma. 1988. *For the Patient's Good: The Restoration of Beneficence in Health Care*. New York: Oxford University Press.

Pellegrino, Edmund D., and David C. Thomasma. 1993. *The Virtues in Medical Practice*. New York: Oxford University Press.

Pelling, Margaret. 1987. "Medical Practice in Early Modern England: Trade or Profession?" In *The Professions in Early Modern England*, edited by Wilfrid Prest, 90–128. London: Croom Helm.

Pence, Gregory. 1990. *Classic Cases in Medical Ethics: Accounts of Cases that Have Shaped Medical Ethics With Philosophical, Legal and Historical Backgrounds*. New York: McGraw-Hill.

Pence, Gregory E. 1995. *Classic Cases in Medical Ethics: Accounts of Cases that Have Shaped Medical Ethics With Philosophical, Legal and Historical Backgrounds*. 2nd ed. New York: McGraw-Hill.

Pence, Gregory E. 2000. *Classic Cases in Medical Ethics: Accounts of Cases that Have Shaped Medical Ethics With Philosophical, Legal and Historical Backgrounds*. 3rd ed. Boston: McGraw-Hill.

Pence, Gregory E. 2004. *Classic Cases in Medical Ethics: Accounts of Cases that Have Shaped Medical Ethics With Philosophical, Legal and Historical Backgrounds*. 4th ed. Boston: McGraw-Hill.

Percival, Thomas. 1768. *On The Disadvantages Which Attend The Inoculation Of Children In Early Infancy*. London: J. Johnson & T. Cadell.

Percival, Thomas. 1769, 1772, 1773, 1788–1789. *Essays Medical And Experimental*. London: J. Johnson.

Percival, Thomas. 1775, 1777, 1803a. *A Father's Instructions to His Children: Consisting of Tales, Fables, and Reflections; Designed to Promote the Love of Virtue, a Taste for Knowledge, and an Early Acquaintance with the Works of Nature*. London. J. Johnson.

Percival, Thomas. 1775? *Tables Shewing the Number of Deaths Occasioned by the Small-Pox in the Several Periods of Life, and Different Seasons of the Year: Together with Its Comparative Fatality to Males and Females: Extracted from the Register of the Collegiate or Parish Church in Manchester, and from Other Bills of Mortality by Dr. Percival*. Manchester.

Percival, Thomas. 1781. *A Socratic Discourse on Truth and Faithfulness: In Which the Nature, Extent, and Obligation, Together with the Various Branches and Subordinations of These Moral Duties Are Explained, Illustrated, and Enforced by Examples: Being the Sequel to a Father's Instructions*. Warrington: W. Ashton.

Percival, Thomas. 1784, 1789. *Moral and Literary Dissertations, on the Following Subjects: 1. On Truth and Faithfulness. 2. On Habit and Association. 3. On Inconsistency of Expectation in Literary Pursuits. 4. On a Taste for the General Beauties of Nature. 5. On a Taste for the Fine Arts. 6. On the Alliance of Natural History, and Philosophy, with Poetry. To Which Are Added a Tribute to the Memory of Charles de Polier, Esq. and an Appendix*. Warrington: J. Johnson.

Percival, Thomas. 1794. *Medical Jurisprudence: Or a Code of Ethics and Institutes, Adapted to the Professions of Physic and Surgery*. Manchester UK.

Percival, Thomas. 1803b. *Medical Ethics: Or a Code of Institutes and Precepts, Adapted to the Professional Conduct of*

Physicians and Surgeons. London: J. Johnson & R. Bickerstaff.

Percival, Thomas. [1803a] 1849. *Medical Ethics; or, A Code of Institutes and Precepts, Adapted to the Professional Conduct of Physicians and Surgeons by the Late Thomas Percival, M.D., F. R. S.,* edited by William Alexander Greenhill, M.D. Oxford: John Henry Parker; London: John Churchill.

Percival, Thomas. [1803b] 1975. *Medical Ethics: A Code of Institutes and Precepts, Adapted to the Professional Conduct of Physicians and Surgeons,* edited by Chester R. Burns. Huntington NY: Robert E. Krieger Publishing Company.

Percival, Thomas. [1803c] 1985. *Medical Ethics: A Code of Institutes and Precepts, Adapted to the Professional Conduct of Physicians and Surgeons by Thomas Percival, M.D.,* edited by Edmund Pellegrino. Birmingham AL: Classics of Medicine Library.

Percival, Thomas. [1803d] 1927. *Percival's Medical Ethics,* edited by Chauncey D. Leake. Baltimore: Williams & Wilkins.

Percival, Thomas. 1807. *The Works, Literary, Moral, and Medical of Thomas Percival, M.D., To Which are Prefixed Memoirs of His Life and Writings and A Selection From His Literary Correspondence,* edited by Edward Percival. London: Printed by Cruttwell for Johnson.

Perez de Escobar, Antonio. 1788. *Medicina Patria ó Elementos de la Medicina práctica de Madrid: Puede servir de aparato a la Historia Natural y Médica de España.* Madrid: Imprenta de D. Antonio Muñoz.

Perkins, Honorable Frances. 1940. *Proceedings.* The Tri-State Conference on Silicosis, April 23. National Archives, Record Group 1000, 7–0–4 (3).

Perley, Sharon, et al. 1992. "The Nuremberg Code: An International Overview." In *The Nazi Doctors and the Nuremberg Code: Human Rights in Human Experimentation,* edited by George J. Annas, and Michael A. Grodin, 149–73. New York/Oxford: Oxford University Press.

Pernick, Martin S. 1982. "The Patient's Role in Medical Decisionmaking: A Social History of Informed Consent in Medical Therapy." In *Making Health Care Decisions: Appendices, Studies on the Foundations of Informed Consent,* edited by the President's Commission for the Study of Ethical Problems in Medicine and Biomedical and Behavioral Research. 3: 1–35. Washington DC: Government Printing Office.

Pernick, Martin S. 1985. *A Calculus of Suffering: Pain, Professionalism, and Anesthesia in Nineteenth-Century America.* New York: Columbia University Press.

Pernick, Martin S. 1996. *The Black Stork: Eugenics and the Death of "Defective" Babies in American Medicine and Motion Pictures Since 1915.* New York: Oxford University Press.

Pernick, Martin S. 1999. "Brain Death in a Cultural Context: The Reconstruction of Death 1967–1981."

In *The Definition of Death: Contemporary Controversies,* edited by Stuart J. Youngner, Robert M. Arnold, and Renie Schapiro, 3–33. Baltimore: Johns Hopkins University Press.

Perreau, E. H. 1905. *Éléments de Jurisprudence Médicale à l'Usage des Médecins.* Paris: Librairie de Droit.

Peset, Mariano, and José Luis Peset. 1974. *La Universidad Española: Siglos XVIII y XIX.* Madrid: Taurus.

Peter, Jürgen. 1994. *Der Nürnberger Ärzteprozeß im Spiegel seiner Aufarbeitung anhand der drei Dokumentensammlungen von Alexander Mitscherlich und Fred Mielke.* Münster: Lit.

Peter, Saint. 1983. "The 15 Canons of our Father among Saints Peter, Archbishop (Pope, fl. 304) of Alexandria and a Martyr." In *The Rudder of the Orthodox Catholic Church,* edited by Sts. Nicodemus and Agapius, translated by D. Cummings, 740–56. New York: Luna Printing.

Peters, Ted. 1997. *Playing God? Genetic Determination and Human Freedom.* New York: Routledge.

Petrarca, Francesco. 1978. *Invectiva contra medicum quendam: Testo Latino e volgarizzamento di Ser Domenico Silvestri,* edited by Pier Giorgio Ricci. Roma: Edizioni di Storia e letteratura.

Petrov, Boris D. 1970. "Deontologija v Istorii Otechestvennoi Meditsyny." In *Pervaja Vsesoyuznaya Konferentsija po Problemam Meditsynskoi Deontologii: Moscow, January 28–29, 1969,* edited by A. F. Bilibin, et al., 11–27. Moscow: Meditsyna.

Petrov, F. A. 1998. *Rossiiskie Universitety v Pervoi Polovine XIX veka. Formirovanie Sistemy Universitetskogo Obrazovanija. Kniga 1: Zarozhdenie Systemy Universitetskogo Obrazovanija v Rossii. Kniga 2: Stanovlenie Systemy Universitetskogo Obrazovanija v Rossii v Pervye Desjatiletija XIX veka.* Moscow: Gosudarstvenny Istoricheskii Muzei.

Petrov, Nikolai N. 1956. *Voprosy Khirurgicheskoi Deontologii.* Leningrad: Meditsyna.

Petrovski, Boris V., ed. 1988. *Deontologija v Meditsyne,* vols. 1–2. Moscow: Meditsyna.

Petschnig, Mária. 1983. "Az orvosi hálapénzről – nem etikai alapon (On the tipping of physicians – not on an ethical basis)." *Valóság (Reality).* 11: 82–93.

Pfeifer, Klaus. 2000. *Medizin der Goethezeit: Christoph Wilhelm Hufeland und die Heilkunst des 18. Jahrhunderts.* Köln: Böhlau.

Phillips, E. D. 1973. *Greek Medicine.* London: Thames and Hudson.

Philipsborn, Alexandre. 1950. "La compagnie d'ambulanciers 'paralalani' d'Alexandrie." *Byzantion.* 20: 185–90.

Physicians for Human Rights. 2000. *The Problem of Dual Loyalty: Standards of Conduct for the Health Professions.* Washington DC: Physicians for Human Rights.

Pickstone, John V. 1993. "Thomas Percival and the Production of *Medical Ethics.*" In *The Codification of Medical Morality: Historical and Philosophical Studies of the Formalization of Western Medical Morality in the Eighteenth and Nineteenth Centuries: Volume One: Medical Ethics and Etiquette in the Eighteenth Century*, edited by Robert Baker, Dorothy Porter, and Roy Porter, 161–78. Dordrecht: Kluwer Academic Publishers.

Pickstone, John V., and S. V. F. Butler. 1984. "The Politics of Medicine in Manchester 1788–1792: Hospital Reform and Public Health Services in the Early Industrial City." *Medical History*. 28: 227–49.

Pickthall, Mohammed M., trans. 1930. *The Meaning of the Glorious Qur³ān*. Hyderabad: Ta-Ha Publishers.

Pigeaud, Jackie. 1997. "Les fondements philosophiques de l'ethique medicale: le cas de Rome." In *Médecine et Morale dans l'Antiquité (Entretiens sur l'anitquite classique XLII)*, edited by Hellmut Flashar and Jacques Jouanna, 225–96. Vandoeuvres, Geneva: Fondation Hardt.

Pinault, Jody Rubin. 1992. *Hippocratic Lives and Legends*. Leiden: E. J. Brill.

Piquer, Andrés. 1755. *Philosophia Moral para la juventud española*. 2 vols. Madrid: Joachin Ibarra.

Piquer, Andrés. 1771. *Lógica*. Madrid: Joachin de Ibarra.

Pirumova, Natalja A., Boris S. Itenberg, and Vadim S. Antonov. 1990. *Russia and the West: 19th Century*, translated from Russian by Vitalii Bskakov et al. Moscow: Progress.

Pius IX. 1864. *Syllabus of Errors*. www.papalencyclicals.net.

Pius XI. 1930. *Casti Connubii*. www.papalencyclicals.net.

Pius XII. 1939. *Summi Pontificatus*. www.papalencyclicals.net.

Pius XII. 1943. *Divino Afflante Spiritu*. www.papalencyclicals.net.

Pius XII. 1950. *Humani Generis*. www.papalencyclicals.net.

Pius XII. 1952. "The Moral Limits of Medical Research and Treatment." www.papalencyclicals.net.

Pius XII. 1957a. "Address of February 24, 1957." *Acta Apostolicae Sedis*. 47: 147.

Pius XII. 1957b. "Address to an International Congress of Anesthesiologists." http://www.lifeissues.net/writers/doc/doc_31resuscitation.html (visited October 13, 2007).

Pius XII. 1958. "Address of November 24, 1957." *Der Anaesthesist*. 7: 242–43.

Placzek, Siegfried. 1909. *Das Berufsgeheimnis des Arztes*. 3rd ed. Leipzig: Verlag von G. Thieme.

Platen-Hallermund, Alice. [1948] 1998. *Die Tötung Geisteskranker in Deutschland*. Reprint. Frankfurt: Psychiatrie Verlag.

Plato. 1968. *The Last Days of Socrates*, translated by Hugh Tredennick. London: Penguin Books.

Plato. 1945. *Republic*, translated by F. M. Cornford. New York: Oxford University Press.

Pleadwell, Frank Lester. [1950] 1977. "Samuel Sorbière and His Advice to a Young Physician." [*Bulletin of the History of Medicine*. 24: 264–86]. Reprinted in *Legacies in Ethics and Medicine*, edited by Chester R. Burns, 237–69. New York: Science History Publications.

Plessner, Martin. 1974. "The Natural Sciences and Medicine." In *The Legacy of Islam*. 2nd ed., edited by Joseph Schacht, 423–60. New York: Oxford University Press.

Ploetz, Alfred. 1895a. "Ableitung einer Rassenhygiene und ihre Beziehung zur Ethik." *Vierteljahrsschrift für wissenschaftliche Philosophie*, no. 19: 368–76.

Ploetz, Alfred. 1895b. *Die Tüchtigkeit unsrer Rasse und der Schutz der Schwachen. Ein Versuch über Rassenhygiene und ihr Verhältnis zu den humanen Idealen, besonders zum Socialismus*. Berlin: S. Fischer.

Ploetz, Alfred. 1911. "Die Begriffe Rasse und Gesellschaft und einige damit zusammenhängende Probleme." *Schriften der deutschen Gesellschaft für Soziologie*, no. 1, reprinted in Archiv für Gesellschafts- und Rassenbiologie, no. 23 (1934): 415–37.

Ploetz, Alfred. 1911. "Ziele und Aufgabe der Rassenhygiene." *Deutsche Vierteljahrsschrift für öffentliche Gesundheitspflege*, no. 43: 164–92.

Polievktov, Mikhail A. 1918. *Nikolai I. Biografia i Obzor Tsarstrovanija*. Moscow: M. i S. Sabashnikovy.

Pollock, Linda. 1993. *With Faith and Physick: The Life of a Tudor Gentlewoman Lady Grace Mildmay, 1552–1620*. London: Collins & Brown.

Pomata, Gianna. 1998. *Contracting a Cure: Patients, Healers, and the Law in Early Modern Bologna*, translated by the author with the assistance of Rosemarie Foy and Anna Taraboletti-Segre. Baltimore and London: Johns Hopkins University Press.

Porter, Dorothy. 1995. "The Mission of the Social History of Medicine: An Historical Overview." *Social History of Medicine*. 8: 345–59.

Porter, Dorothy. 1999. *Health, Civilization, and the State: A History of Public Health from Ancient to Modern Times*. New York: Routledge.

Porter, Dorothy, and Roy Porter. 1988. "The Enforcement of Health: The British Debate." In *AIDS: The Burdens of History*, edited by Elizabeth Fee and Aaniel M. Fox, 97–120. Berkeley CA: University of California Press.

Porter, Dorothy, and Roy Porter. 1989. *Patient's Progress: Doctors and Doctoring in Eighteenth-Century England*. Palo Alto CA: Stanford University Press.

Porter, Roy. 1987. "A Touch of Danger: The Man-Midwife as Sexual Predator." In *Sexual Underworlds of the Enlightenment*, edited by G. S. Rousseau and Roy Porter, 206–32. Manchester: Manchester University Press.

Porter, Roy. 1989. "Death and Doctors in Georgian England." In *Death, Ritual, and Bereavement*, edited by Ralph Houlbrooke, 77–94. London: Routledge.

Porter, Roy. 1990a. *The Enlightenment*. London: Macmillan.

Porter, Roy. 1990b. *Mind-Forg'd Manacles: A History of Madness in England from the Restoration to the Regency*. London: Penguin Books.

Porter, Roy. 1993a. "Plutus of Hygeia? Thomas Beddoes and the Crisis of Medical Ethics in Britain at the Turn of the Nineteenth Century." In *The Codification of Medical Morality: Historical and Philosophical Studies of the Formalization of Western Medical Morality in the Eighteenth and Nineteenth Centuries: Volume One: Medical Ethics and Etiquette in the Eighteenth Century*, edited by Robert Baker, Dorothy Porter, and Roy Porter, 73–91. Dordrecht: Kluwer Academic Publishers.

Porter, Roy. 1993b. "Thomas Gisborne: Physicians, Christians and Gentleman." In *Doctors and Ethics: The Earlier Historical Setting of Professional Ethics*, edited by Andrew Wear, Johanna Geyer-Kordesch, and Roger French, 252–73. Amsterdam: Rodopi.

Porter, Roy. 1995. "Medical Ethics, History of Nineteenth Century Great Britain." In *Encyclopedia of Bioethics*. 2nd ed., edited by Warren T. Reich, 1550–4. New York: Simon and Schuster Macmillan.

Porter, Roy. 1997. *The Greatest Benefit to Mankind: A Medical History of Humanity from Antiquity to the Present*. London: Harper Collins.

Porter, Roy. 2000. *Enlightement: Britain and the Creation of the Modern World*. London: Penguin Books.

Porter, Roy, and Miklas Teich, eds. 1981. *The Enlightenment in National Context*. Cambridge UK: Cambridge University Press.

Portes, Louis. 1954. *À la Recherche d'Une Éthique Médicale*. Paris: Presses Universitaires de France.

Post, Alfred Charles. 1883. *An Ethical Symposium: Being a Series of Papers Concerning Medical Ethics and Etiquette from a Liberal Standpoint*. New York: G. P. Putnam's Sons.

Post, Stephen, ed. 2004. *Encyclopedia of Bioethics*. 3rd ed. New York: Thompson/Gale.

Postell, William Dosite. 1958. "Medical Education and Medical Schools in Colonial America." In *History of American Medicine: A Symposium*, edited by Felix Marti-Ibanez, 48–54. New York: MD Publications Inc.

Potter, Van Rensselaer. 1970. "Bioethics, the Science of Survival." *Perspectives in Biology and Medicine*. 14: 127–53.

Potter, Van Rensselaer. 1971. *Bioethics: Bridge to the Future*. Englewood Cliffs NJ: Prentice Hall.

Poussin, Louis de La Vallée. 1961. "Suicide (Buddhist)." In *Encyclopedia of Religion and Ethics*, edited by James Hastings, John A. Selbie, and Louis H. Gray, 12: 24–26. New York: Charles Scribner's Sons.

Powderly, Kathleen E. 2000. "Patient Consent and Negotiation in the Brooklyn Gynecological Practice of Alexander J. C. Skene: 1863–1900." *Journal of Medicine and Philosophy*. 25: 12–27.

Powell, James M. 1971. *The Liber Augustalis or Constitutions of Melfi: Promulgated by the Emperor Frederick II for the Kingdom of Sicily in 1231*. Syracuse NY: Syracuse University Press.

Powell, John W. 1981. "Japan's Biological Weapons, 1930–1945: A Hidden Chapter in History." *Bulletin of the Atomic Scientists*. (October): 41–5.

Pozdnyakova, S. A. 1965. "Filosofskie Problemy Vrachebnoi Etiki." Avtoreferat. Diss. Kand. Filosof. Nauk. Minsk.

Pravila dlya Vzaimnykh Otnoshenii Vrachei u Posteli Bol'nogo, Vyrabottannye Obshestvom Vrachei Volynskoi Gubernii v 1885 Godu. 1886. Prilozhenija k Protokolan Obshestva Vrachei Volynskoi Gubernii. Zhitomir.

Prebish, Charles S., and Kenneth K. Tanaka, eds. 1998. *The Faces of Buddhism in America*. Berkeley CA: University of California Press.

Preobrazhenskii V. N. 1928. "Mozhno li govorit' bol'nomu pravdu?" *Vestnik Sovremennoi Meditsyny*, no. 5: 311–13.

President's Commission for the Study of Ethical Problems in Medicine and Biomedical and Behavioral Research. 1981. *Defining Death: Medical, Legal and Ethical Issues in the Definition of Death*. Washington DC: U.S. Government Printing Office.

President's Commission for the Study of Ethical Problems in Medicine and in Biomedical and Behavioral Research. [1981] 1998a. "Defining Death: A Report on the Medical, Legal, and Ethical Issues in the Definition of Death." Washington DC: U.S. Government Printing Office. In *Source Book in Bioethics: A Documentary History*, edited by Albert R. Jonsen, Robert M. Veatch, and LeRoy Walters, 118–41. Washington DC: Georgetown University Press.

President's Commission for the Study of Ethical Problems in Medicine and in Biomedical and Behavioral Research. [1982] 1998b. "Splicing Life." Washington DC: U. S. Government Printing Office. In *Source Book in Bioethics: A Documentary History*, edited by Albert R. Jonsen, Robert M. Veatch, and LeRoy Walters, 299–313. Washington DC: Georgetown University Press.

President's Commission for the Study of Ethical Problems in Medicine and Biomedical and Behavioral Research. 1983. *Summing Up: Final Report on Studies of the Ethical and Legal Problems in Medicine and Biomedical and Behavioral Research*. Washington DC: U.S. Government Printing Office.

President's Commission for the Study of Ethical Problems in Medicine and in Biomedical and Behavioral Research. [1983] 1998c. "Screening and Counseling for Genetic Conditions." Washington DC: U.S. Government Printing Office. In *Source Book in Bioethics: A Documentary History*, edited by Albert R. Jonsen, Robert M. Veatch, and LeRoy Walters, 263–87. Washington DC: Georgetown University Press.

Preußischer Ehrengerichtshof für Ärzte. 1908–34. *Entscheidungen*. 5 vols. Berlin: Verlagsbuchhandlung von R. Schoetz.

Proctor, Robert N. 1988. *Racial Hygiene: Medicine Under the Nazis*. Cambridge MA: Harvard University Press.

Proctor, Robert N. 1991. *Value-Free Science*. Cambridge MA: Harvard University Press.

Proctor, Robert N. 1992. "Nazi Doctors, Racial Medicine, and Human Experimentation." In *The Nazi Doctors and the Nuremberg Code: Human Rights in Human Experimentation*, edited by George J. Annas and Michael A. Grodin, 17–31. New York/Oxford: Oxford University Press.

Proctor, Robert N. 1999. *The Nazi War on Cancer*. Princeton NJ: Princeton University Press.

Program in Applied Ethics and Biotechnology and the Canadian Program on Genomics and Global Health. 2002. *Top 10 Biotechnologies for Improving Health in Developing Countries*. University of Toronto Joint Center for Bioethics.

Programa Regional de Bioética OPS/OMS. 2000. "Instituciones y Centros especializados en Bioética en América Latina y el Caribe." Santiago de Chile.

Pross, Christian. 1992a. "Nazi Doctors, German Medicine, and Historical Truth." In *The Nazi Doctors and the Nuremberg Code: Human Rights in Human Experimentation*, edited by George J. Annas and Michael A. Grodin, 32–52. New York/Oxford: Oxford University Press.

Pross, Christian. 1992b. "Nazi Physicians: Criminals, Charlatans, or Pioneers? The Commentaries of the Allied Experts at the Nuremberg Medical Trial." In *Medical Science without Compassion: Past and Present*, edited by Charles Roland, Henry Friedlander, and Benno Müller-Hill. Hamburg: Hamburger Stiftung für Sozialgeschichte des 20. Jahrhunderts.

Pross, Christian, and Götz Aly, eds. 1989. *Der Wert des Menschen: Medizin in Deutschland, 1918–1945*. Berlin: Edition Hentrich.

Prüll, Cay-Rüdiger. 2000. "No Law, No Rights? Autopsy in Germany since 1800." In *Coping with Sickness: Medicine, Law and Human Rights – Historical Perspectives*, edited by John Woodward and Robert Jütte, 29–53. Sheffield: EAHMH Publications.

Prüll, Cay-Rüdiger. 2004. *Medizin am Toten oder am Lebenden? Pathologie in Berlin und in London 1900 bis 1945*. Basle: Schwabe.

Prüll, Cay-Rüdiger, and Marianne Sinn. 2002. "Problems of Consent to Surgical Procedures and Autopsies in Twentieth-Century Germany." In *Historical and Philosophical Perspectives on Biomedical Ethics: From Paternalism to Autonomy?* edited by Andreas-Holger Maehle and Johanna Geyer-Kordesch, 73–93. Aldershot: Ashgate.

Pufendorf, Samuel von. 1744. *De jure naturae et gentium*. 2 vols., edited by G. Mascovius. Frankfurt: Ex Officina Knochiana.

al-Qaradawi, Yusuf. 1984. *The Lawful and the Prohibited in Islam, Al-Halal Wal Haram Fil Islam*, translated by Kamal El-Helbawy et al. Delhi: Hindustan Publications.

Qaradawi, Yusuf al-. 1987. *Fatawa Mu'asira (Contemporary Fatwas)*. Kuweit: Dar al-Qalam.

Qian, Mu. 1987. *Huang Di (Yellow Emperor)*. Taipei: Dongda Tushu Gongsi.

Qiu, Hongzhong. 1993. *Yixue yu Renlei Wenhua (Medicine and Human Culture)*. Changsa: Hunan Science and Technology Press.

Qiu, Hongzhong. 1999. "To Face Life Through Death: Traditional Chinese Medicine's Perspective on Death." *Chinese & International Philosophy of Medicine*. 2: 29–44.

Qiu, Ren-Zhong. 1988a. *Bioethics*. Shanghai: Shanghai People's Press [Chinese].

Qiu, Ren-Zhong. 1988b. "Medicine – The Art of Humaneness: On Ethics of Traditional Chinese Medicine." *Journal of Medicine and Philosophy*. 13: 277–300.

Qiu, Ren-Zhong, X. Zhuo, and J. Feng. 1996. *The Rights of the Patient*. Beijing: The Press of Beijing Medical University and Beijing Union Medical University [Chinese].

Qiu, Xiangxing, ed. 1999. *Yixue Lunlixue (Medical Ethics)*. Beijing: People's Health Press.

Quasten, Johannes. 1950–1986. *Patrology*. 4 vols. Westminster MD: Christian Classics.

Quinisext Council. 1983. "The 102 Canons of the Holy and Ecumenical Sixth Council." In *The Rudder of the Orthodox Catholic Church*, edited by Sts. Nicodemus and Agapius, translated by D. Cummings, 290–412. New York: Luna Printing.

Quinlan, Joseph, Julia Quinlan, and Phyliss Battelle. 1977. *Karen Ann: The Quinlan's Tell Their Story*. New York: Doubleday Anchor.

Quinn, T., et al. 1986. "AIDS in Africa: An Epidemiologic Paradigm." *Science*. 234: 955–63.

The Qur'ān. 1939. 2 vols., translated by Richard Bell. Edinburgh: T & T Clark.

R. v. Adams. Crim LR 365. (1957).

R. v. Arthur. 12 BMLR 1. (1981).

R. v. Bourne. 3 All ER 615; [1939] 1 KB 687. (1938).

R. v. Cox. 12 BMLR 38. (1992).

Rabban aṭ-Ṭabari, ʿAlī b. Sahl. 1928. *Firdaus al-ḥikma fiʾt-tibb*, edited by M. Z. Siddiqi. Berlin: Sonne.

Rabi, Barbara. 2002. *Ärztliche Ethik – Eine Frage der Ehre? Die Prozesse und Urteile der ärztlichen Ehrengerichtshöfe in Preußen und Sachsen 1918–1933*. Frankfurt/Main: P. Lang.

Rafal'kes, S. 1928. "V pokhod!" *Vrachebnoe Delo*, no. 2: 147–48.

Rafter, Nicole Hahn. 1997. *Creating Born Criminals*. Chicago: University of Illinois Press.

Ragab, M. Ismail. 1981. "Islam and the Unwanted Pregnancy." In *Abortion and Sterilization: Medical and Social Aspects*, edited by Jane E. Hodgson. London: Academic Press.

Rahman, Fazlur. 1985. "Law and Ethics in Islam." In *Ethics in Islam*, edited by Richard G. Hovannisian, 3–15. Malibu CA: Undena Publications.

Rahman, Fazlur. 1987. *Health and Medicine in the Islamic Tradition*. New York: Crossroad.

Rahula, Wapola. [1959] 1962. *What the Buddha Taught*. New York: Grove Press.

Raja, Asad J., and Daniel Wikler. 2001. "Developing Bioethics in Developing Countries." *Journal of Health Population and Nutrition*. 19.1: 4–5.

Rajan, V. G. Julie. 1996. "Will India's Ban on Prenatal Sex Determination Slow Abortion of Girls?" *Hinduism Today*. www.hinduism-today.com/1996/4/.

Rajan, V. G. Julie. 1998. "Welcome the New Healers." *Hinduism Today*. January. www.hinduismtoday.com/archives/1998/1/1998-1-09.shtml (visited October 13, 2007): 1–9.

Ramsey, Matthew. 1988. *Professional and Popular Medicine in France, 1780–1830: The Social World of Medical Practice*. Cambridge UK: Cambridge University Press.

Ramsey, Matthew. 1999. "Alternative Medicine in Modern France." *Medical History*. 43: 286–322.

Ramsey, Paul. 1970a. *Fabricated Man: The Ethics of Genetic Control*. New Haven CT: Yale University Press. .

Ramsey, Paul. 1970b. *The Patient as Person: Explorations in Medical Ethics*. New Haven CT: Yale University Press.

Ramsey, Paul. 1978. *Ethics at the Edges of Life: Medical and Legal Intersections*. New Haven CT: Yale University Press.

Ramu, G. N. 1988. *Family Structure and Fertility: Emerging Patterns in an Indian City*. New Dehli: Sage Publications.

Rapalski, Adam J. 1953. United States Armed Forces Epidemiological Board. Memorandum to Colin MacCleod, President, Armed Forces Epidemiological Board, 2 March.

Raskin, Naomi. 1961. "Doctors Afield: Vikenti Vikentievich Veresaev (Smidovich) 1867–1945." *New England Journal of Medicine*. 265: 1154–5.

Rasslan, Wassel. 1934. "Mohammed und die Medizin nach den Ueberlieferungen." *Abhandlungen zur Geschichte der Medizin und der Naturwissenschaften*. 1: 4–51.

Ratanakul, Pinit. 1988. "Bioethics in Thailand: The Struggle for Buddhist Solutions." *Journal of Medicine and Philosophy*. 13: 301–12.

Ratanakul, Pinit. 1999. "Socio-Medical Aspects of Abortion." In *Buddhism and Abortion*, edited by Damien Keown, 53–66. Honolulu HI: University of Hawaii Press.

Ratzinger, Joseph. 2002. "Current Doctrinal Relevance of the *Catechism of the Catholic Church*." www.vatican.va/roman_curia/congregations/cfaith/documents/rc_con_cfaith_doc_20021009_ratzinger-catechetical-congress_en.html (visited October 13, 2007).

Rawls, John. [1971] 1999. *A Theory of Justice*. Cambridge MA: Belknap Press.

Razetti, Luis. [1916] 1963. "Código Venezolano de Moral Médica." In *Obras Completas*. I: 111–35. Caracas: Ministerio de Sanidad y Asistencia Social.

Rāzī, Abū Bakr Muḥammad ibn Zakariyyāʾ al-. 1987. *Al-Kitāb al-Manṣūrī fī l-ṭibb (The Book on Medicine Dedicated to al-Manṣūr)*, edited by Ḥāzim al-Bakrī al-Ṣidīdqī. Kuwait: Institute of Arab Manuscripts.

Reagan, Leslie J. 1997. *When Abortion was a Crime: Women, Medicine, and Law in the United States, 1867–1973*. Berkeley CA: University of California Press.

Recep, Ömer. 1969. "Ṭibb an-Nabī." Ph.D. diss., Philipps-Universität, Marburg.

Records of the United States Nürnberg War Crimes Trials. 1946–1947. *United States of America v. Karl Brandt et al (Case 1)*. November 21, 1946–August 20, 1947. National Archives Washington. Microfilm Publication M887 (47 reels).

Reddy, Sita. 2002. "Asian Medicine in America: The Ayurvedic Case." *Amercian Academy of Political and Social Sciences*. 583: 97–121.

Reddy, William M. 1997. *The Invisible Code: Honor and Sentiment in Postrevolutionary France, 1814–1848*. Berkeley CA: University of California Press.

Regan, Tom. 1983. *The Case for Animal Rights*. Berkeley CA: University of California Press.

Regula, Benedicti. 1992. *Regula Benedicti – Die Benediktusregel: Lateinisch-Deutsch*. Beuron: Beuroner Kunstverlag.

Reich, Warren T. 1974. "Medical Ethics in a Catholic Perspective: Some Present-Day Trends." In *Pastoral Care of the Sick: A Practical Guide for the Catholic Chaplain in Health Care Facilities*, edited by the National Association of Catholic Chaplains, 173–200. Washington DC: United States Catholic Conference.

Reich, Warren T., ed. 1978. *The Encyclopedia of Bioethics*. New York: Macmillan.

Reich, Warren T. 1994. "The Word "Bioethics": Its Birth and the Legacies of Those Who Shaped It." *Kennedy Institute of Ethics Journal*. 4: 319–35.

Reich, Warren T., ed. 1995a. *The Encyclopedia of Bioethics*. 2nd ed. New York: Simon & Schuster Macmillan.

Reich, Warren T., ed. 1995b. "Introduction." In *The Encyclopedia of Bioethics (Revised Edition)*, edited by Warren T. Reich, xix–xxxii. New York: Simon & Schuster Macmillan.

Reich, Warren T. 1995c. "The Word "Bioethics": The Struggle Over Its Earliest Meanings." *Kennedy Institute of Ethics Journal*. 5: 19–34.

Reich, Warren T. 1996. "Revisiting the Launching of the Kennedy Institute: Re-Visioning the Origins of Bioethics." *Kennedy Institute of Ethics Journal*. 6: 323–7.

Reich, Warren T. 2001. "The Care-Based Ethic of Nazi Medicine and the Moral Importance of What

We Care About." *American Journal of Bioethics*. 1: 64–74.

Reich, Warren T. 2003. "Shaping and Mirroring the Field: The Encyclopedia of Bioethics." In *The Story of Bioethics: From Seminal Works to Contemporary Explorations*, edited by Jennifer K. Walter and Eran P. Klein, 165–96. Washington DC: Georgetown University Press.

Reichsgericht. 1894. "Von welchen rechtlichen Voraussetzungen hängt die Strafbarkeit oder Straflosigkeit von Körperverletzungen ab, welche zum Zwecke des Heilverfahrens von Ärzten bei operativen Eingriffen begangen werden?" *Entscheidungen des Reichsgerichts in Strafsachen*. 25: 375–89 (decision of 31 May 1894).

Reichsgericht. 1912. "1. Ist der Arzt verpflichtet, den Kranken auf die nachteiligen Folgen aufmerksam zu machen, die möglicherweise bei einer beabsichtigten Operation entstehen können? 2. Zur Frage der Beweislast beim Eintritte schädlicher Folgen einer Operation." *Entscheidungen des Reichsgerichts in Zivilsachen. Neue Folge*. 28: 432–6 (decision of 1 March 1912).

Reichsminister des Innern. 1931. "Rundschreiben . . . betr. Richtlinien für neuartige Heilbehandlung und für die Vornahme wissenschaftlicher Versuche am Menschen." *Reichsgesundheitsblatt*. 6: 174–5 (dated 28 February 1931).

Reinert, Benedikt. 1968. *Die Lehre vom tawakkul in der klassischen Sufik*. Berlin: Walter De Gruyter.

Reiser, Stanley J. 1977. "The Dilemma of Euthanasia in Modern Medical History: The English and American Experience." In *Ethics in Medicine: Historical Perspectives and Contemporary Concerns*, edited by Stanley J. Reiser, Arthur J. Dyck, and William J. Curran, eds., 488–94. Cambridge MA: MIT Press.

Reiser, Stanley J., Arthur J. Dyck, and William J. Curran, eds. 1977. *Ethics in Medicine: Historical Perspectives and Contemporary Concerns*. Cambridge MA: MIT Press.

Reiss, Oscar. 2000. *Medicine in Colonial America*. New York: University Press of America.

Renan, Ernest. 1852. *Averroes et l'averroisme. Essai Historique*. Paris: Durand.

Renaud, Henri Paul Joseph. 1935. "Un chirurgien musulman du royaume de Grenade: Muḥammad aš-Šafra." *Hespéris*. 20: 1–20.

Report of the Committee on Order No. 5 of the Surgeon General. 1863. *Transactions of the American Medical Association*. 14: 29–33.

Republic of Kenya. 1979. *Development Plan, 1979–1983*. Nairobi: Government Printer.

Rescher, Nicholas. 1969. "The Allocation of Exotic Medical Lifesaving Therapy." *Ethics*. 79: 173–86.

Reuchlin, Johannes. 1512. *Hippocrates De praeparatione hominis ad ptolemaeum regem, nuper e greco in latinum traductus . . .* Tuebingen: Thomas Anshelm.

Reusser, Ruth. 2002. "Das Konzept des Übereinkommens über Menschenrechte und Biomedizin (ÜMB)." In *Das Menschenrechtsübereinkommen zur Biomedizin des Europarates: taugliches Vorbild für eine weltweit geltende Regelung?* hrsg. Jochen Taupitz, 49–62. Berlin: Springer.

Reverby, Susan, ed. 2000. *Tuskegee's Truths: Rethinking the Tuskegee Syphilis Study*. Chapel Hill NC: University of North Carolina Press.

Reverby, Susan, and David Roser. 1979. "Beyond 'the Great Doctors.'" In *Health Care in America: Essays in Social History*, edited by Susan Reverby and David Rosner, 3–16. Philadelphia: Temple University Press.

Rhodes, Rosamond, ed. 1999. "Special Issue: Minorities in Medicine" *Mount Sinai Journal of Medicine*. 66.

Rice, Thurman. 1929. *Radical Hygiene: A Practical Discussion of Eugenics and Race Culture*. New York: Macmillan.

Richardson, E. 1990. "Julius Hallervorden." In *The Founders of Child Neurology*, edited by S. Ashwal, 506–12. San Francisco CA: Norman

Richter, Christian Friederich. 1705. *Kurtzer und deutlicher Unterricht Von Dem Leibe und natürliche Leben des Menschen: Woraus ein jelicher/ auch Ungelehrte erkennen kan/ Was die Gesundheit ist*. Halle: Waysenhause.

Rida, Muhammad Rashid. 1970–1971. *Fatawa Rashid Rida (The Fatwas of Rashid Rida)*. Beirut: Dar al-Kitab al-Jadid.

Riddle, John M. 1992. *Contraception and Abortion from the Ancient World to the Renaissance*. Cambridge MA/London: Harvard University Press.

Ridwan, Ali B. 1984. *Medieval Islamic Medicine*. Berkeley CA: University of California Press.

Riera, Juan. 1973. *Idealisme i positivisme en la medicina catalana del segle XIX*. Barcelona: Institut d'Estudis Catalans.

Riesco Le-Grand, Inocencio María. 1848. *Tratado de embriología sagrada*. Madrid: Tipografía Grego-Latina.

Rigdon, Susan M. 1996. "Abortion Law and Practice in China: An Overview with Comparisons to the United States." *Social Sciences & Medicine*. 42: 543–60.

Riis, Povl. 2000. "Perspectives on the Fifth Revision of the Declaration of Helsinki." *Journal of the American Medical Association* 284: 3045–6.

Ring, G. C. 1958. "Walter Bradford Cannon, born October 19, 1871, died October 1, 1945." *Physiologist*. 1 (5): 37–42.

Riolan, Jean Jun. 1653. *Opuscula nova anatomica*. 2nd part. Paris: Dupuis.

Riquelme U., Horacio. 1995. *Entre la obediencia y la oposición: Los médicos y la ética profesional bajo la dictadura militar*. Caracas: Nueva Sociedad.

Risa, Nuri Bey. 1906. "Studie über die rituale Beschneidung vornehmlich im Osmanischen Reiche." *Sammlung klinischer Vorträge*. 438: 585–626.

Rispler-Chaim, Vardit. 1993. *Islamic Medical Ethics in the Twentieth Century*. Leiden: E. J. Brill.

Rispler-Chaim, Vardit. 1996. "Postmortem Examinations in Egypt." In *Islamic Legal Interpertation: Muftis and their Fatwas*, edited by Muhammad Khalid Masud, Brinkley Messicle, and David S. Pavers, 278–85. Cambridge MA: Harvard University Press.

Rispler-Chaim, Vardit. 1998. "Genetic Engineering in Contemporary Islamic Thought." *Science in Context*. 11: 567–73.

Rispler-Chaim, Vardit. 1999. "The Right Not to Be Born." *The Muslim World*. 89 (April): 130–43.

Risse, Gunther B. 1986. *Hospital Life in Enlightenment Scotland: Care and Teaching at the Royal Infirmary of Edinburgh*. Cambridge UK: Cambridge University Press.

Rist, John M. 1982. *Human Value: A Study in Ancient Philosophical Ethics*. Leiden: E. J. Brill.

Ritvo, Harriet. 1987. *The Animal Estate: The English and Other Creatures in the Victorian Age*. Cambridge MA: Harvard University Press.

Ritzmann, Iris. 1999. "Der Verhaltenskodex des 'Savoir faire' als Deckmantel Ärztlicher Hilflosigkeit? Ein Beitrag zur Arzt-Patient-Beziehung im 18. Jahrhundert." *Gesnerus*. 56: 197–219.

Robert, Jean-Noel, Nippon Bukkyo no nakano. 1998. "Sei, Ro, Shi (Living, Aging and Death in the Japanese Buddhism)." In *Ojyoko-Nipponjin no Sei, Ro, Shi*, edited by Noboru Miyata and Takanori Shintani. Tokyo: Shogakukan.

Robertson, John. 1999. "The Dead Donor Rule." *Hastings Center Report*. 29: 6–14.

Robinson, H. W. 1940. *Suffering: Human and Divine*. London: Student Christian Movement Press.

Robinson, James C. 1999. *The Corporate Practice of Medicine*. Berkeley CA and London: Milbank Memorial Fund and the University of California Press.

Robinson, Richard H., and Willard L. Johnson. [1970] 1977. *The Buddhist Religion: A Historical Introduction*. 2nd ed. Encino CA: Dickenson Publishing Company.

Rodríguez, Antonio José. 1734–1754. *Palestra critico-medica: en que se trata introducir la verdadera medicina, y desaloxar la tyrana intrusa del reyno de la naturaleza*. Tomo I, Pamplona: Joseph Joachin Martinez. Tomo II, Zaragoza: Francisco Moreno [s.a.]; Tomo III, Zaragoza: Francisco Moreno. Tomo IV, Zaragoza: Francisco Moreno. Tomo V, Zaragoza: Facinco Moreno. Tomo VI, Zaragoza: Francisco Moreno.

Rodriguez, Antonio José. 1742–1760. *Nuevo aspecto de theologia medico-moral y ambos derechos o paradoxas physico-theologico legales: obra critica, provechosa a parrocos confessores y professores de ambos drechos*. Tomo primero. Zaragoza: Francisco Moreno. Tomo segundo. Zaragoza: Francisco Moreno. Tomo tercero. Zaragoza, Francisco Moreno. Tomo cuarto. Madrid: Eliseo Sánchez.

Rodriguez, Antonio José. 1748. *Reflexiones theologico-canonico-medicas, sobre el fasting eclesiastico: Que establecen su practica despues de los breves de nuestro santissimo padre Benedicto XIV: Dividida en dos partes, la primera apothemata en favor de su observancia, la segunda apologema contra la sarcophagia*. Madrid: Manuel de Moya.

Roe v. Wade. 410 US 113. (1973).

Rolfinck, Werner. 1656. *Dissertationes anatomicae methodo synthetica exaratae*. Nuremberg: Endter.

Rollin, Bernard E. 1995. *The Frankenstein Syndrome: Ethical and Social Issues in the Engineering of Animals*. Cambridge UK: Cambridge University Press.

Romanovsky, G. B. 2003. "Pravo na abort: Otechestvenny i zarubezhny opyt." *Chelovek*, no. 6: 141–5.

Rose, Nikolas. 1985. *The Psychological Complex*. London: Routledge and Kegan Paul.

Rose, Nikolas. 1998. "Governing Risky Individuals." *Psychiatry, Psychology and the Law*. 5: 177–95.

Rose, Steven. 1995. "The Rise of Neurogenetic Determinism." *Nature*. 373: 380–2.

Rosen, George. 1946a. "Fees and Fee Bills: Some Economic Aspects of Medical Practice in Nineteenth-Century America." *Bulletin of the History of Medicine*, no. 6 (Supplement). Baltimore: Johns Hopkins University Press.

Rosen, George. 1946b. "The Philosophy of Ideology and the Emergence of Modern Medicine in France." *Bulletin of the History of Medicine*. 20: 328–39.

Rosen, George. 1993. *A History of Public Health*, expanded edition. Baltimore: Johns Hopkins University Press.

Rosenberg, Charles E. 1962. *The Cholera Years*. Chicago: University of Chicago Press.

Rosenberg, Charles E. 1979. "The Therapeutic Revolution: Medicine, Meaning, and Social Change in Nineteenth-Century America." In *The Therapeutic Revolution*, edited by Morris J. Vogel and Charles E. Rosenberg, 3–25. Philadelphia: University of Pennsylvania Press.

Rosenberg, Charles E. 1987. *The Care of Strangers: The Rise of America's Hospital System*. New York: Basic Books.

Rosenberg, Charles E. 1992. "Framing Disease: Illness, Society, and History." In *Framing Disease: Studies in Cultural History*, edited by Charles E. Rosenberg and Janet Golden, xii–xxvi. New Brunswick NJ: Rutgers University Press.

Rosenberg, Charles E. 1999a. "Codes Visible and Invisible: The Twentieth-Century Fate of a Nineteenth-Century Code." In *The American Medical Ethics Revolution: How the AMA's Code of Ethics Has Transformed Physicians' Relationships to Patients, Professionals, and Society*, edited by Robert Baker et al., 207–17. Baltimore: Johns Hopkins University Press.

Rosenberg, Charles E. 1999b. "Meanings, Policies, and Medicine: On the Bioethical Enterprise and History." *Daedalus*. 128: 27–46.

Rosenberg, Charles E., and Janet Golden, eds. 1992. *Framing Disease: Studies in Cultural History*. New Brunswick NJ: Rutgers University Press.

Rosenberg, Charles E., and Carroll S. Rosenberg. 1968. "Pietism and the Origins of the American Public Health Movement: A Note on John H. Griscom and Robert M. Hartley." *Journal of the History of Medicine and Allied Sciences*. 23: 16–35.

Rosenblatt, Roger. 1992. *Life Itself: Abortion in the American Mind*. New York: Random House.

Rosenkrantz, Barbara. 1972. *Public Health and the State: Changing Views in Massachusetts, 1842–1936*. Cambridge MA: Harvard University Press.

Rosenthal, Franz. 1956. "An Ancient Commentary on the Hippocratic Oath." *Bulletin of the History of Medicine*. 30: 52–87.

Rosenthal, Franz. [1956] 1990a. "An Ancient Commentary on the Hippocratic Oath." [*Bulletin of the History of Medicine*. 30: 52–87]. Reprinted in Franz Rosenthal, *Science and Medicine in Islam: A Collection of Essays*, no. III. Aldershot: Variorum.

Rosenthal, Franz. [1969] 1990b. "The Defense of Medicine in the Medieval Muslim World." [*Bulletin of the History of Medicine*. 43: 519–32]. Reprinted in Franz Rosenthal, *Science and Medicine in Islam: A Collection of Essays*, no. IX. Aldershot: Variorum.

Rosenthal, Franz. 1975. *The Classical Heritage in Islam*, translated by Emile Marmorstein and Jenny Marmorstein. London: Routledge & Kegan Paul.

Rosenthal, Franz. [1978] 1990c. "The Physician in Medieval Muslim Society." [*Bulletin of the History of Medicine*. 52: 475–91]. Reprinted in Franz Rosenthal, *Science and Medicine in Islam: A Collection of Essays*, no. XI. Aldershot: Variorum.

Rosén von Rosenstein, Nils. 1766. *Anweisung zur Kenntniss und Cur der Kinderkrankheiten / aus dem Schwedischen übersetzt und mit Anmerkungen erläutert von Johann Andreas Murray*. Gotha, Göttingen: Bey Johann Christian Dieterich.

Rosner, David, and Gerald Markowitz. 1987. *Dying for Work: Workers Safety and Health in Twentieth-Century America*. Bloomington IN: University of Indiana Press.

Rosner, David, and Gerald Markowitz. 1991. *Deadly Dust: Silicosis and the Politics of Occupational Disease in Twentieth-Century America*. Princeton NJ: Princeton University Press.

Rosner, Fred. 1972. *Modern Medicine and Jewish Law*. New York: Yeshiva University.

Rosner, Fred. [1986] 1991. *Modern Medicine and Jewish Ethics*. 2nd revised and augmented edition. Hoboken NJ/Ktav NY: Yeshiva University Press.

Rosner, Fred. 2001. "Lord Immanuel Jakobovits: Grandfather of Jewish Medical Ethics." *Israel Medical Association Journal*. 3: 304–10.

Rosner, Fred, and Moses D. Tendler. 1980. *Practical Medical Halacha*. 2nd ed. Jerusalem/New York: Rephael Society.

Ross, Andrew, ed. 1996. *Science Wars*. Durham NC: Duke University Press.

Rost, Karl L. 1987. *Sterilisation und Euthanasie im Film des 'Dritten Reiches'*. Husum: Matthiesen.

Roth, Karl-Heinz. 1985. "Filmpropaganda für die Vernichtung der Geisteskranken und Behinderten im 'Dritten Reich'." In *Reform und Gewissen: 'Euthanasie' im Dienst des Fortschritts*, edited by Götz Aly et al., 125–93. Berlin: Rotbuch.

Roth, Karl-Heinz, Ulf Schmidt, and Paul Weindling. 1999. "Origins and Consequences of the Nuremberg Doctors' Trial: Documents and Materials." In *The Nuremberg Doctors' Trial 1946/47*, edited by Klaus Dörner and Angelika Ebbinghaus Fiche, 285–320. Munich: K. G. Sauer. Mikrofiche.

Rothberg, Donald. 1998. "Responding to the Cries of the World: Socially Engaged Buddhism in North America." In *The Faces of Buddhism in America*, edited by Charles S. Prebish and Kenneth K. Tanaka, 266–86. Berkeley CA: University of California Press.

Rothmaler, Christiane. 1991. *Sterilisation nach dem "Gesetz zur Verhütung erbkranken Nachwuchses" vom 14. Juli 1933: Eine Untersuchung des Erbgesundheitsgerichts und zur Durchführung des Gesetzes in Hamburg in der Zeit zwischen 1934 und 1944*. Husum: Matthiesen.

Rothman, David J. 1991. *Strangers at the Bedside: A History of How Law and Bioethics Have Transformed Medical Decision Making*. New York: Basic Books.

Rothman, David J. 1995. "Research, Human: Historical Aspects." In *Encyclopedia of Bioethics*. 2nd ed., edited by Warren T. Reich, 2248–58. New York: Simon & Schuster Macmillan.

Rothman, David J. 1997. *Beginnings Count: The Technological Imperative in American Health Care*. New York: Oxford University Press.

Rothman, David J. 1998. "The Nuremberg Code in Light of Previous Principles and Practices in Human Experimentation." In *Ethics Codes in Medicine: Foundations and Achievements of Codification since 1947*, edited by Ulrich Tröhler and Stella Reiter-Theil, 50–59. Aldershot, Brookfield, Singapore, and Sydney: Ashgate.

Rothman, David J., Steven Marcus, and Stephanie Kiceluk. 1995. *Medicine and Western Civilization*. New Brunswick NJ: Rutgers University Press.

Rothman, Sheila M. 1994. *Living in the Shadow of Death: Tuberculosis and the Social Experience of Illness in American History*. New York: Basic Books.

Rothstein, Mark A. 1983. "Employee Selection Based on Susceptibility on Occupational Illness." *Michigan Law Review*. 81: 1379–1496.

Rothstein, William G. 1985. *American Physicians in the 19th Century: From Sects to Science.* Baltimore: Johns Hopkins University Press.

Roux, L. [1841] 1982. *Les Gens de Médecine.* Paris: Les Editions Errance.

Roy, David J., and John R. Williams. 1995. "History of Medical Ethics: V. The Americas: C. Canada." In *The Encyclopedia of Bioethics.* 2nd ed., edited by Warren T. Reich, 1632-38. New York: Simon and Schuster Macmillan.

Royal College of Physicians. 1772. *Statuta Moralia Collegii Regalis MEDICORUM LONDINENSIUM.* London.

Rüdin, Ernst. 1940. "Alfred Ploetz zum Gedächtnis." In *Archiv für Rassen- und Gesellschaftsbiologie,* 1–3.

Ruhāwī, Isḥāq ibn ʿAlī al-. Ruhāwī, Isḥāq b. ʿAlī al-. [1347] 1985. *Adab aḥ ṭ-ḥ Ṭabīb,* facsimilie edition. Frankfurt/M.: Ernst Klett.

al-Ruhāwī, Isḥāq ibn ʿAlī. Ruhāwī, Isḥāq b. ʿAlī al-. 1967a. "Medical Ethics of Medieval Islam with special reference to al-Ruhāwī's "Practical Ethics of the Physician." Translation of the book *Adab aḥ ṭ-ḥ Ṭabīb* by Isḥāq b. ʿAlī al-Ruhāwī by Martin Levey." *Transactions of the American Philosophical Society.* 57: 1–100.

al-Ruhāwī, Isḥāq ibn ʿAlī. 1967b. *Medical Ethics of Medieval Islam with Special Reference to al-Ruhāwī's "Practical Ethics of the Physician",* translated by Martin Levey. Philadelphia PA: Philadelphia: The American Philosophical Society.

al-Ruhāwī, Isḥāq ibn ʿAlī. 1992. *Adab al-tabīb (The Practical Ethics of the Physician),* edited by M. ʿAsīrī. Riyad: King Faisal Centre of Islamic Research and Studies.

Rupke, Nicolaas A., ed. 1987. *Vivisection in Historical Perspective.* London: Croom Helm.

Rupke, Nicolaas A. 1990a. "Pro-Vivisection in England in the Early 1880s: Arguments and Motives." In *Vivisection in Historical Perspective.* 2nd ed., edited by Nicolaas A. Rupke, 188–208. London: Routledge.

Rupke, Nicolaas A., ed. 1990b. *Vivisection in Historical Perspective.* 2nd ed. London: Routledge.

Rush, Benjamin. 1805. *Observations on the Duties of a Physician, and the Methods of Improving Medicine. Accommodated to the Present State of Society and Manners in the United States.* In Benjamin Rush, *Medical Inquiries and Observations.* 2nd ed., Vol. I, 345–408. Philadelphia: J. Conrad & Co.

Rush, Benjamin. 1811. *Sixteen Introductory Lectures, to Courses of Lectures upon the Institutes and Practice of Medicine: with a Syllabus of the Latter, to which are Added, Two Lectures upon the Pleasures of the Senses and of the Mind, with an Inquiry into their Proximate Cause, delivered in the University of Pennsylvania.* Philadelphia: Bradford and Innskeep.

Rush, Benjamin. 1818. *Medical Inquiries and Observations.* Philadelphia: M. Carey & Son.

Rush, Benjamin. 1948. *The Autobiography of Benjamin Rush,* edited by George W. Corner. Princeton NJ: Princeton University Press.

Rushton, J. Phillipe. 1995. *Race, Evolution, and Behavior.* New Brunswick NJ: Transaction Publishers.

Rusnock, Andrea. 2002. *Vital Accounts: Quantifying Health and Population in Eighteenth-Century England and France.* Cambridge MA: Cambridge University Press.

Russell, Colin A. 1998. "Objections to Anaesthesia: The Case of James Young Simpson." In *Gases in Medicine: Anaesthesia,* edited by E. B. Smith and S. Daniels, 173–87. Cambridge UK: Royal Society of Chemistry.

Rutherford, John. 1750. "Clinical Lectures Delivered in the Royal Infirmary of Edinburgh 1750–1756." Student notes, author unknown. Royal College of Physicians and Surgeons of Glasgow MS 1/9/3.

Rütten, Thomas. 1993. *Hippokrates im Gespräch.* Münster: Universitäts- und Landesbibliothek.

Rütten, Thomas. 1994. *Geschichten vom hippokratischen Eid.* Unpublished Habilitationschrift. Munster.

Rütten, Thomas. 1996a. "Medizinethische Themen in den deontologischen Schriften des Corpus Hoppocraticum." In *Médecine et Morale dans l'Antiquité,* edited by Hellmut Flashar and Jacques Jouanna, 65–111. Vandoeuvres, Geneva: Fondation Hardt.

Rütten, Thomas. 1996b. "Receptions of the Hippocratic Oath in the Renaissance: The Prohibition of Abortion as a Case Study in Reception." *Journal of the History of Medicine and Allied Sciences.* 51: 456–83.

Rütten, Thomas. 1996c. "Die Herausbildung der ärztlichen Ethik: Der Eid des Hippokrates." In *Meilensteine der Medizin,* edited by Heinz Schott, 57–66. Dortmund: Harenberg.

Rütten, Thomas. 1997. "Medizinische Themen in den deontologischen Schriften des Corpus Hippocraticum." In *Médecine et Morale dans l'Antiquité (Entretiens sur l'antiquite classique XLIII),* edited by Hellmut Flashar and Jacques Jouanna, 65–120. Vandoeuvres Geneva: Fondation Hardt.

Rütten, Thomas, and Leonie von Reppert-Bismarck. 1996. "Receptions of the Hippocratic Oath in the Renaissance: The Prohibition of Abortion as a Case Study in Reception." *Journal of the History of Medicine and Allied Sciences.* 51 (4): 456–83.

Rutherford, John. 1750. "Clinical Lectures Delivered in the Royal Infirmary of Edinburgh 1750–1756." Student notes, author unknown. Glasgow: Royal College of Physicians and Surgeons of Glasgow MS 1/9/3.

Ryan, Michael. 1831a. "Letter From Dr. Ryan." *The Lancet.* 1, 1831–1832. (November 5): 222–24.

Ryan, Michael. 1831b. *A Manual of Jurisprudence, Compiled from the Best Medical and Legal Works: comprising an account of: I. The Ethics of the Medical Association; II. The Charter and Statutes Relating to the Faculty; and III. All Medico-Legal Questions, with the Latest Discussions. Being an Analysis of a Course of Lectures on Forensic Medicine Annually Delivered in*

London and Intended as a Compendium for the Use of Barristers, Solicitors, Magistrates, Coroners, and Medical Practitioners. London: Rensaw and Rush.

Ryan, Michael. 1832. *A Manual of Medical Jurisprudence, Compiled from the best Medical and Legal works; being an Analysis of a Course of Lectures on Forensic Medicine, annually delivered in London.* 2nd ed. Philadelphia: Carrey and Lea.

Ryerson, James. 2000. "The Outrageous Pragmatism of Judge Richard Posner." *Lingua Franca.* 2000: 27–34.

Sachedina, Abdulaziz. 2002. "'Right to Die?': Muslim Views about End of Life Decisions." www.people.virginia.edu/~aas/article/article3.htm (visited September 21, 2002).

Saddhatissa, Hammalawa. 1970. *Buddhist Ethics: Essence of Buddhism.* London: George Allen & Unwin Ltd.

Sadler, Alfred, Jr., Blair Sadler, and E. Blythe Stason. 1968. "The Uniform Anatomical Gift Act: A Model for Reform." *JAMA: Journal of the American Medical Association.* 206: 2505–6.

Sahagún, Fray Bernardino de. [1582] 1975. *Historia General de las Cosas de Nueva España.* 3rd ed., edited by Angel María Garibay K. México: Porrúa.

Ṣāʿid ibn al-Ḥasan. [c.1072] 1968a. *Kitāb at-Tašwīq aṭ-Ṭibbī,* edited by Otto Spies. Bonn: Bonner Orientalische Studien.

Ṣāʿid ibn al-Ḥasan. 1968b. *Das Buch At-Tašwīq aṭ-ṭibbī (Book on the Arousal of Desire for Medicine) des Ṣāʿid ibn al-Ḥasan: Ein arabisches Adab-Werk über die Bildung des Arztes.* Herausgegeben und bearbeitet von Otto Spies. Bonn: Orientalisches Seminar der Universität Bonn.

Ṣāʿid ibn al-Ḥasan. 1968c. *Übersetzung und Bearbeitung des Kitāb at-Tašwīq aṭ-ṭibbī des Ṣāʿid ibn al-Ḥasan: Ein medizinisches Adabwerk aus dem 11. Jahrhundert.* (Von) Schah Ekram Taschkandi. Bonn: Orientalisches Seminar der Universität Bonn.

Sakai, Shizu. 1984. "Chinese Traditional Medicine and Dutch Medicine in Japan." In *One Thousand Years of Ishimpo – Dawning of Japanese Medicine,* edited by the One Thousand Year Anniversary Committee of Ishinpom, 94–99. Tokyo: Ishimpo Issennen Kinenkai.

Sakai, Shizu. 1986. *Nippon no Iryoshi (History of Japanese Medical Service).* Tokyo: Tokyo Shoseki Kabushiki Kaisha.

Sakai, Shizu. 1993. *Nippon Ekibyoshi (History of Japanese Epidemics).* Tokyo: Hoso Daigaku Kyoiku Shinkokai.

Sakai, Shizu. 1998. "Translation and the Origins of Western Science in Japan." In *The Introduction of Modern Science and Technology to Turkey and Japan,* edited by Feza Günergun and Shigehisa Kuriyama, 137–57. Kyoto: International Research Center for Japanese Studies.

Sakai, Shizu. 1999a. "Kagawa Ryu Sanka (Obstetrics of Kagawa School)." *The Family Patient.* 12: 28–29.

Sakai, Shizu. 1999b. "Humane Medical Care in the History of Medical Science." *Asian Medical Journal.* 42: 314–20.

Sakai, Shizu. 2002. *Yamaiga kataru Nihonshi (Disease Tells us the History of Japan).* Tokyo: Kodansha.

Sakai, Shizu. 2003. *Edo no Yamai to Yojo (Disease and the Care for Life in Edo).* Tokyo: Kosansha.

Salam, Abdus. 1981. "The Renaissance of Sciences in Arab and Islamic Lands." *Islamic Quarterly.* 25: 86–99.

Salama, Muhammad Sayyid. 1997. "Al-Istinsakh al-Bayuluji waHimayat Huquq al-Insan (Biological cloning and the protection of human rights)." *Majallat al-Azhar.* 8: 1249–53.

Salmon, William. 1796. *The works of Aristotle: In four parts. Containing I. his Complete master-piece; displaying the secrets of nature in the generation of man. To which is added, The family physician . . . II. his Experienced midwife . . . III. his Book of problems . . . IV. His Last legacy; unfolding the secrets of nature respecting the generation of man.* London: Printed for, and sold by all the booksellers.

Salmon, William. [1694–1776] 1986. *Aristotle's master-piece; Aristotle,s compleate master piece; Aristotle's book of problems; Aristotle's last legacy.* Reprint of works originally published 1694–1776. New York: Garland.

Salt, Henry. 1894. *Animals' Rights Considered in Relation to Social Progress.* New York: Macmillan.

Šaltūt, Mahmūd. 1965. *Al-Islām, ʿAqīda wa Šarīʾa.* Cairo: Dār al-Qalam.

Salvá, Jaime. 1844. *Lecciones de moral médica dadas en la Universidad de Barcelona, en 1844.* Manuscript. Papeles de Salvá. Madrid: Biblioteca de la Facultad de Medicina de la Universidad Complutense.

Samiullah, Mohammad. 1983. "Islam and Birth Control." *Universal Message (Karachi).* 5: 15–19.

SAMS (Swiss Academy of Medical Sciences). 2001. *Ethische Richtlinien/Ethics Guidelines and Recommendations.* www.samw.ch/ (visited February 8, 2004).

Sánchez-Albornoz, Nicolás. [1973] 1977. *La población de América Latina: Desde los tiempos precolombinos al año 2000.* 2nd ed. Madrid: Alianza Editorial.

Sanders, David, and Jesse Dukeminier. 1968. "Medical Advance and Legal Lag: Hemodialysis and Kidney Transplantation." *UCLA Law Review.* 15: 357–413.

Sándor, Judit. 1992. *Abortusz és és jog (Abortion and Law).* Budapest: Literatura Medica.

Sándor Judit. 1997. *Gyógyítás és ítélkezés (Treatment and Judgment).* Budapest: Medicina Publishing.

Sankt-Peterburgskoe Vrachebnoe Obshestvo Vzaimnoi Pomoshi, Tverskoe Otdelenie (Tver Branch of the St. Petersburg Physicians' Society for Mutual Aid). 1903. "Otchet o Deyatel'nosti Pravlenija Tverskogo Otdelenija za 1902 g." *Vestnik Sankt-Peterburgskogo Vrachebnogo Obshestva Vzaimnoi Pomoshi.* 6: 232–34.

Santero, Tomás. 1859. *Defensa de Hipócrates, de las escuelas hipocráticas y del vitalismo.* Madrid: Imp. De Manuel de Rojas.

Sapp, Jan. 1990. "The Nine Lives of Gregor Mendel." In *Experimental Inquiries: Historical, Philosophical and Social*

Studies of Experimentation in Science, edited by Homer E. Le Grand, 137–66. Dordrecht: Reidel.

Saqr, Atiyya. May-June 1994. In: *Minbar al-Islam*, 84; July 1994. In: *Minbar al-Islam*, 106; 15 July 1996. In: *Mayu*, 4; 22 August 1996. In: *Al-Liwa' al-Islami*; November 1999. In: *Minbar al-Islam*, 134.

SARETI. 2002. www.up.ac.za/academic/medicine/shsph/sareti.htm (visited December 10, 2002).

Sargent, Frederick, II. 1982. *Hippocratic Heritage: A history of Ideas About Weather and Human Health*. New York: Pergamon Press.

Sarmiento, Domingo Faustino. [1845] 1969. *Facundo*. Reprint. Madrid: EDAF.

Sass, Hans-Martin. 1983. "Reichsrundschrieben 1931: Pre-Nuremberg German Regulations Concerning New Therapy and Human Experimentation." *Journal of Medicine and Philosophy*. 8: 99–111.

Sass, Hans-Martin. 2003. "Ambiguities in Judging Cruel Human Experimentation: Arbitrary American Responses to German and Japanese Experiments." *Eubios Journal of Asian and International Bioethics*. 13: 102–4.

Sauerteig, Lutz. 2000. "Ethische Richtlinien, Patientenrechte und ärztliches Verhalten bei der Arzneimittelerprobung (1892–1931)." *Medizinhistorisches Journal*. 35: 303–34.

Sauerteig, Lutz. 2002. "Health Costs and the Ethics of the German Sickness Insurance System." In *Historical and Philosophical Perspectives on Biomedical Ethics: From Paternalism to Autonomy?*, edited by Andreas-Holger Maehle and Johanna Geyer-Kordesch, 49–72. Aldershot: Ashgate.

Saundby, Robert. 1902. *Medical Ethics: A Guide to Professional Conduct*. Bristol: John Wright; London: Simpkin, Marshall, Hamilton, Kent.

Saundby, Robert. 1907. *Medical Ethics: A Guide to Professional Conduct*. London: Charles Griffin; Philadelphia: Lippincott.

Savignano, Armando. 1995. *Bioética mediterránea: Etica della virtù e della felicità*. Pisa: Edizioni ETS.

Savitt, Todd L. 1978. *Medicine and Slavery: The Diseases and Health Care of Blacks in Antebellum Virginia*. Urbana IL: University of Illinois Press.

Savitt, Todd L. 1982. "The Use of Blacks for Medical Experimentation and Demonstration in the Old South." *Journal of Southern History*. 48: 331–48.

Sayılı, Aydın. 1965. "Gondēshāpūr." In *The Encyclopaedia of Islam*. 2: 1119–20. Leiden: E. J. Brill.

Schacht, Joseph. 1964. *An Introduction to Islamic Law*. Oxford: Clarendon Press.

Schacht, Joseph. 1975. *The Origins of Muhammadan Jurisprudence*. Oxford: Clarendon Press.

Schacht, Joseph, and Max Meyerhof. 1937. *The Medico-Philosophical Controversy between Ibn Butlān of Baghdad and Ibn Ridwān of Cairo: A Contribution to the History of Greek Learning among the Arabs*. Cairo: Barbey.

Schadewaldt, H. 1965. "Die Apologie der Heilkunst bei den Kirchenvätern." *Veröffentlichungen Internat: Geseleschaft Geschichte Pharmazie*. 26: 115–30.

Schaff, Philip, and Henry Wace, eds. 1994. *Nicene and Post-Nicene Fathers*, second series. Peabody MA: Hendrickson Publishers.

Scharfe, Hartmut. 1999. "The Doctrine of the Three Humors in Traditional Indian Medicine and the Alleged Antiquity of Tamil Siddha Medicine." *Journal of the American Oriental Society*. 119: 609–29.

Schaupp, Walter. 1993. *Der Ethische Gehalt der Helsinki Deklaration*. Frankfurt: P. Lang.

Schenker, Joseph G. 1992. "Religious Views Regarding Treatment of Infertility by Assisted Reproductive Technologies." *Journal of Assisted Reproduction and Genetics*. 9: 3–8.

Scherz, Gustav. 1963. "Pionier der Wissenschaft: Niels Stensen in seinen Schriften.1." *Acta Historica Scientiarum Naturalium et Medicinalium*. 18. Copenhagen: Munksgaard.

Schiebinger, Londa. 2003. "Human Experimentation in the Eighteenth Century: Natural Boundaries and Valid Testing." In *The Moral Authority of Nature*, edited by Lorraine Daston and Fernando Vidal, 384–408. Chicago: University of Chicago Press.

Schifferli, Pat. 1979. "A Community of Responsible Adults." *Kennedy Institute Quarterly Report*. 5 (1).

Schiller, Joseph. 1967. "Claude Bernard and Vivisection." *Journal of the History of Medicine and Allied Sciences*. 22 (3): 246–60.

Schimmel, Annemarie. 1989. *Islamic Names*. Edinburgh: Edinburgh University Press.

Schipperges, Heinrich. 1965. "Zur Tradition des 'Christus Medicus' in frühen Christentum und in der älteren Heilkunde." *Arzt und Christ*. 11: 12–20.

Schleiner, Winfried. 1995. *Medical Ethics in the Renaissance*. Washington DC: Georgetown University Press.

Schmidt, Ulf. 1997. "German Medical War Crimes, Medical Ethics and Post-War Justice: A Symposium held at the University of Oxford to Mark the 50th Anniversary of the Nuremberg Medical Trial, 14 March 1997." *German History*. 15.3: 385–91.

Schmidt, Ulf. 1998. "Reform Psychiatry and Society Between Imperial and Nazi Germany: Review of Anstaltsärzte zwischen Kaiserreich und Bundesrepublik (Kersting) and Psychiatrie und Gesellschaft in der Moderne (Walter)." *Social History of Medicine*. 11.2: 336–37.

Schmidt, Ulf. 1999a. "The History of the Kaiser Wilhelm Society During National Socialism: Observations on a Three-Day Working Conference organised by the Max Planck Society in Berlin, 10–13 March 1999." *German History*. 17.4: 551–57.

Schmidt, Ulf. 1999b. "Reassessing the Beginning of the 'Euthanasia' Programme." *German History*. 17.4: 543–50.

Schmidt, Ulf. 2000a. "Kriegsausbruch und 'Euthanasie': Neue Forschungsergebnisse zum 'Knauer Kind' im Jahre 1939." In *"Euthanasie" und die aktuelle Sterbehilfe-Debatte: Die historischen Hintergründe medizinischer Ethik*, edited by Andreas Frewer and Clemens Eickhoff, 113–29. Göttingen: Campus.

Schmidt, Ulf. 2000b. "Sozialhygienische Filme und Propaganda in der Weimarer Republik." In *Gesundheitskommunikation: Medieninhalte und Mediennutzung aus Sicht der Public Health-Forschung*, edited by Ditmar Jasbinski, 53–82. Wiesbaden: Westdeutscher Verlag.

Schmidt, Ulf. 2001a. "Der Ärzteprozeß als moralische Instanz? – Der Nürnberger Kodex und das Problem 'Zeitloser Medizinethik'." In *Medizingeschichte und Medizinethik 1900–1950*, edited by Andreas Frewer and Josef N. Neumann, 333–76. Göttingen: Campus.

Schmidt, Ulf. 2001b. "Lebensläufe: Biographien und Motive der Angeklagte aus der Perspektive des medizinischen Sachverständigen, Dr. Leo Alexander, 1945–1947." In *Vernichten und Heilen: Der Nürnberger Ärzteprozeß und seine Folgen*, edited by Klaus Dörner and Angelika Ebbinghaus, 374–404. Berlin: Aufbau.

Schmidt, Ulf. 2001c. "Discussing Slave Labourers in Nazi Germany: Topography of Research or Politics of Memory?" *German History*. 19.3: 408–17.

Schmidt, Ulf. 2002. *Medical Films: Ethics and Euthanasie in Nazi Germany*. Husum: Matthiesen.

Schmidt, Ulf. 2004. *Justice at Nuremberg: Leo Alexander and the Nazi Doctors' Trial*. London: Palgrave Macmillan.

Schmidt, Ulf. 2005. "The Scars of Ravensbrück: Medical Experiments and British War Crimes Policy, 1945–1950." *German History*. 23.1: 20–49.

Schmidt. Ulf. 2007. *Karl Brandt: The Nazi Doctor, Medicine, and Power in the Third Reich*. London: Hambledon Continuum.

Schmuhl, Hans-Walter. 1987. *Rassenhygiene, Nationalsozialismus, Euthanasie: Von der Verhütung zur Vernichtung 'lebensunwerten Lebens', 1890–1945*. Göttingen: Vandenhoeck & Ruprecht.

Schmuhl, Hans-Walter. 1992. *Rassenhygiene, Nationalsozialismus, Euthanasie. Von der Verhütung zur Vernichtung "lebensunwerten Lebens."* 2nd ed. Göttingen: Vandenhoeck & Ruprecht.

Schmuhl, Hans-Walter. 1997. "Eugenik und Euthanasie' – Zwei Paar Schuhe? Eine Antwort auf Michael Schwartz." *Westfälische Forschungen*. 47: 757–62.

Schneck, Peter. 1995. "Christoph Wilhelm Hufeland." In *Ärztelexikon. Von der Antike bis zum 20. Jahrhundert*, edited by Wolfgang U. Eckart and Christoph Gradmann, 200–201. München: Beck.

Schneck, Peter. 1997. "Hufeland, Christoph Wilhelm." In *Deutsche Biographische Enzyklopädie (DBE)*, edited by Walther Killy and Rudolf Vierhaus, vol. 5, 215. Darmstadt: Wissenschaftliche Buchgesellschaft.

Scholle Connor, Susan, and Hernán Fuenzalida. 1990. *Bioethics: Issues and Perspectives*. Washington DC: Pan American Health Organization.

Scholle Connor, Susan, and Hernán Fuenzalida-Puelma, eds. 1991. "Bioethics: Special Number." *Bulletin of the Pan American Health Organization*. 25: 1.

Schomerus, Georg. 2001. *Ein Ideal und sein Nutzen: Aerztliche Ethik in England und Deutschland, 1902–1933*. Frankfurt/Main: Peter Lang.

Schöne-Seifert, Bettina. 1999. "Defining Death in Germany." In *The Definition of Death: Contemporary Controversies*, edited by Stuart J. Youngner, Robert M. Arnold, and Renie Schapiro, 257–71. Baltimore MD and London: Johns Hopkins University Press.

Schopenhauer, Arthur. 1947–50. *Sämtliche Werke*. 2nd ed., 7 vols., edited by A. Hübscher. Wiesbaden: Brockhaus.

Schultz, Julius Henri. 1986. *Albert Molls Ärztliche Ethik*. Zurich: Juris Druck & Verlag.

Schultz, Karoly. 1992. "Treating Defective Neonates in Hungary." *Bulletin of Medical Ethics*. 78: 20–21.

Schuster, Evelyne. 1997. "Fifty Years Later: The Significance of the Nuremberg Code." *New England Journal of Medicine*. 337: 1436–40.

Schwartz, Michael. 1996. "Rassenhygiene, Nationalsozialismus, Euthanasie? Kritische Anfragen an eine These Hans-Walter Schmuhls." *Westfälische Forschungen*. 46: 604–22.

Schwartz, Michael. 1998. "'Euthanasie' – Debatten in Deutschland." *Vierteljahreshefte für Zeitgeschichte*. 4: 617–65.

Sconocchia, Sergio, ed. 1983. *Scriboni Largi Compositiones*. Leipzig: B. G. Teubner.

Securis, John. 1566. *A Detection and Querimonie of the Daily Enormities and Abuses Committed in Physick*. London: T. Marsh.

Segota, Ivan. 1999. "The First Bioethics Committees in Croatia." *HEC Forum*. 11.3: 258–62.

Seidler, Eduard. 1991. *Die medizinische Fakultät der Albert-Ludwigs-Universität Freiburg im Breisgau. Grundlagen und Entwicklungen*. Berlin: Springer-Verlag.

Semashko, Nikolai A. 1945. "Ob etike sovetskogo vracha." *Gigiena i Sanitarija*, no. 1–2: 9–15.

Semashko, Nikolai A. 1954. *Izbrannye Proizvedenija*. Moscow: Medgiz.

Semmelweis, I. P. 1861. *Die Aetiologie, der Begriff und die Prophylaxis des Kindbettfiebers*. Pest-Wien-Leipzig: Hartleben.

Sen, Amartya. 1992. *Inequality Reexamined*. Cambridge MA: Harvard University Press.

Seneca. 1962. *Ad Lucilium Epistulae Morales (Moral Epistles)*, translated by Richard M. Gummere. Loeb Classical Library. Cambridge MA: Harvard University Press.

Şentürk, Lütfi, and Seyfettin Yazıcı. 1998. *Diyanet İslâm İlmihali*. Ankara: Diyanet İşleri Başkanlığı Yayınları.

Serour, Gamal I. 1994. "Islam and the Four Principles." In *Principles of Health Care Ethics*, edited by Raanan Gillon. Chichester: John Wiley & Sons Ltd.

Severino, Marco Aurelio. 1645. *Zootomia Democritaea*. Nuremberg: Endter.

"Sexual Health Exchange no. 2000–1: Sri Lanka." 2000. www.kit.nl/information_servides/exchange_content/ html/20001_sri_lanka_hiv_rep (visited January 3, 2003): 1.

Seybold, Klaus, and Ulrich B. Mueller. 1981. *Sickness and Healing*, translated by Douglas W. Stott. Nashville TN: Abingdon.

Sgreccia, Msgr. Elio. 1999. *Manuale de Bioetica*, vol. 1. Milano: Vita e Pensiero.

Sgreccia, Msgr. Elio. 2002. *Manuale de Bioetica*, vol. 2. Milano: Vita e Pensiero.

Shaham, Ron. 1997. *Family and the Courts in Modern Egypt: A Study Based on Decisions by the Shari'a Courts, 1900–1955*. Leiden: E. J. Brill.

Shaltut, Mahmud. 1966. *Al-Fatawa (The Fatwas)*. Cairo: Dar al-Qalam.

Shanks, Robert A. 1966. "Granville Pattison and the Uses of History." *Scottish Medical Journal*. 11: 267–76.

Sha'rawi, Muhammad Mutawalli al-. 1981. *Al-Fatawa (The Fatwas)*. Cairo: Maktabat al-Qur'an.

Sharma, Arvind, ed. 1993. *Our Religions*. San Francisco CA: Harper, SanFrancisco.

Sharma, Arvind. 1995. *The Philosophy of Religion: A Buddhist Perspective*. Delhi: Oxford University Press.

Sharma, Arvind. 2002. *The Hindu Tradition: Religious Beliefs and Healthcare Decisions*. Chicago: The Park Ridge Center for the Study of Health, Faith, and Ethics.

Sharma, Arvind and Katherine Young. 1990. "The meaning of *ātmahano janāḥ* in *Īśā Upaniṣad* 3." *Journal of the American Oriental Society*. 110.4 (October–December): 595–602.

Sharma, Priya Vrat. 1972. *Indian Medicine in the Classical Age*. Varanasi: Chowkhamba Sanskrit Series Office.

Sharma, Ram Karan, and Vaidya Bhagwan Dash, eds. and trans. 1976–77. *Caraka Samhità: Text with English Translation and Critical Exposition Based on Cakrapàni Datta's âyurveda Dāpikà: Vols. 1–2*. Varanasi: Chowkhamba Sanskrit Series Office.

Sharpe, Virginia A., and Alan I. Faden. 1998. *Medical Harm: Historical, Conceptual, and Ethical Dimensions of Iatrogenic Illness*. Cambridge UK: Cambridge University Press.

Shayzarī, 'Abdalraḥmān ibn Naṣr al-. 1946. *Kitāb Nihāyat al-rutba fī talab al-ḥisba (The Highest Degree of Aspiring after the Office of the Market Inspector)*, edited by al-Sayyid al-Bāz al-'Arīnī. Cairo.

Sheehan, Bernard W. 1985. "The Problem of Moral Judgments in History." *South Atlantic Quarterly*. 84: 37–50.

Sheldon, T. 1994. "Europe Backs New Declaration on Patients' Rights." *British Medical Journal*. 308: 997.

Shevell, Michael I. 1996. "Neurology's Witness to History: The Combined Intelligence Operative Sub-Committee Reports of Leo Alexander." *Neurology*. 47 (4): 1096–1103.

Shevell, Michael I. 1998. "Neurology's Witness to History: Part II. Leo Alexander's Contributions to the Nuremberg Code (1946 to 1947)." *Neurology*. 50 (1): 274–78.

Shields, Christopher. 1999. *Order in Multiplicity: Homonymy in the Philosophy of Aristotle*. Oxford: Clarendon Press.

Shorter, Edward. 1997. *A History of Psychiatry: From the Era of the Asylum to the Age of Prozac*. New York: John Wiley & Sons.

Shotter, E. F., ed. 1970. *Matters of Life and Death*. London: Darton, Longman & Todd.

Shotter, E. F., ed. 1975a. *The London Medical Group – The First Ten Years*. London: London Medical Group.

Shotter, E. F. 1975b. "London Medical Group Annual Report 1972–1973." In *The London Medical Group – The First Ten Years*, edited by E. F. Shotter, 1–4. London: London Medical Group.

Shotter, E. F. 1988. *Twenty-Five Years of Medical Ethics*. London: Institute of Medical Ethics.

Showalter, Elaine. 1985. *The Female Malady: Women, Madness, and Culture in England 1830–1898*. New York: Pantheon.

Shriver, Sargent. 1979. "Knowledge for Service." *Kennedy Institute Quarterly Report*. 5 (1).

Shryock, Richard Harrison. [1929] 1970. *Letters of Richard D. Arnold, M.D. 1808–1876*. New York: AMS Press.

Shryock, Richard Harrison. 1960. *Medicine and Society in America: 1660–1860*. Ithaca NY: Great Seal Books.

Shryock, Richard Harrison. 1967. *Medical Licensing in America, 1650–1965*. Baltimore: Johns Hopkins University Press.

Shulman, Stanford T. 2004. "The History of Pediatric Infectious Diseases." *Pediatric Research*. 55.1: 163–76.

Shuster, Evelyne. 1997. "Fifty Years Later: The Significance of the Nuremberg Code." *New England Journal of Medicine*. 337: 1436–40.

Shuster, Evelyne. 1998. "The Nuremberg Code: Hippocratic Ethics and Human Rights." *Lancet*. 351: 974–77.

Siccus, Joannes Antonius. 1551. *De optimo Medico . . . Caput primum libri primi de antiqua medicina ejusdem auctoris*. Venice.

Siddiqi, Muhammad I. 1986. *The Family Laws of Islam*. New Delhi: International Islamic Publishers.

Sidgwick, Henry. 1898. *Practical Ethics*. London: Swan Sonnenschein & Co.

Siegler, Mark. 1999. "Medical Ethics as a Medical Matter." In *The American Medical Ethics Revolution: How the*

AMA's Code of Ethics Has Transformed Physicians' Relationships to Patients, Professionals, and Society, edited by Robert Baker, et al., 171–79. Baltimore: Johns Hopkins University Press.

Siemen, Hans-Ludwig. 1993. "Die Reformpsychiatrie der Weimarer Republik: Subjektive Ansprüche und die Macht des Faktischen." In *Nach Hadamar: Zum Verhältnis von Psychiatrie und Gesellschaft im 20. Jahrhundert*, edited by Franz-Werner Kersting, Karl Teppe, and Bernd Walter, 98–108. Paderborn: Ferdinand Schöningh.

Sigerist, Henry E. 1940. "The Social History of Medicine." *Western Journal of Surgery, Obstetrics & Gynecology*. 48.12: 715–22.

Sigerist, Henry E. 1943. *Civilization and Disease*. Ithaca NY: Cornell University Press.

Sigerist, Henry E. 1946. "Bedside Manners in the Middle Ages: The Treatise "De cautelis medicorum" attributed to Arnald of Villanova." In *Quarterly Bulletin of the North-Western University Medical School*. 20: 136–43.

Sigerist, Henry E. 1956. *Landmarks in the History of Hygiene*. London: Oxford University Press.

Silverman, Kenneth. 1984. *The Life and Times of Cotton Mather*. New York: Harper & Row.

Simek, Jiri, et al. 2000. "Ethics Committees in the Czech Republic." In *Ethics Committees in Central and Eastern Europe*, edited by Jozef Glasa, 125–31. Bratislava: Charis-IMEB FDN.

Simon, Maxmilien. 1845. *Déontologie Médicale ou les Devoirs et les Droits des Médecins dans l'État Actuel de la Civilisation*. Paris: Baillière.

Simon, Rita J. 1998. *Abortion: Statutes, Policies, and Public Attitudes the World Over*. Westport CT: Praeger.

Sims, J. Marion. 1876. "Address of J. Marion Sims, M.D., President of the Association." *Transactions of the American Medical Association*. 27: 91–99.

Sims, J. Marion. [1884] 1968. *The Story of My Life*. New York: DaCapo Press.

Sinclair, Daniel B. 1989. *Tradition and the Biological Revolution*. Edinburgh: Edinburgh University Press.

Sindiga, Isaac, Chacha Nyaigotti-Chacha, and Mary Peter Kanunah, eds. 1995. *Traditional Medicine in Africa*. Nairobi: East African Educational Publishers.

Singer, Charles, ed. 1956. *Galen on Anatomical Procedures*. London: Oxford University Press.

Singer, Peter. 1975. *Animal Liberation: A New Ethics for Our Treatment of Animals*. New York Review/Random House.

Singer, Peter. 1976. *Animal Liberation: A New Ethics for Our Treatment of Animals*. London: J. Cape.

Singer, Peter. 1993. "On Being Silenced in Germany." In *Practical Ethics*. 2nd ed., edited by Peter Singer, 337–57. Cambridge UK: Cambridge University Press.

Siraisi, Nancy G. 1981. *Taddeo Alderotti and his Pupils: Two Generations of Medical Learning*. Princeton NJ: Princeton University Press.

Siraisi, Nancy G. 1990. *Medieval and Early Renaissance Medicine: An Introduction to Knowledge and Practice*. Chicago: University of Chicago Press.

Skinner v. Oklahoma ex rel. Williamson. 316 US 535. (1942).

Slavskii, K. G. 1911. "O Chastnoi Praktike Zemskikh Vrachei." *Obshestvennyi Vrach*. 2: 43–49.

Sleeboom-Faulkner, Margaret. 2006. "The Chinese Concept of Euthanasia and Health Care." *Bioethics*. 20 (4): 203–12.

Sloan, Douglas. 1971. *The Scottish Enlightenment and the American College Ideal*. New York: Teachers College Press.

Smith, Dale C. 1996. "The Hippocratic Oath and Modern Medicine." *Journal of the History of Medicine and Allied Sciences*. 51 (4): 484–500.

Smith, Richard M. 1993. "Demography and Medicine." In *Companion Encyclopedia of the History of Medicine*, edited by William F. Bynum and Roy Porter, 1663–92. London and New York: Routledge.

Smith, Russell G. 1994. *Medical Discipline: The Professional Conduct Jurisdiction of the General Medical Council, 1858–1990*. Oxford and London: Clarendon Press.

Smith, Russell G. 1995. "Legal Precedent and Medical Ethics: Some Problems Encountered by the General Medical Council in Relying upon Precedent when Declaring Acceptable Standards of Professional Conduct." In *The Codification of Medical Morality: Historical and Philosophical Studies of the Formalization of Western Medical Morality in the Eighteenth and Nineteenth Centuries: Volume Two: Anglo-American Medical Ethics and Medical Jurisprudence in the Nineteenth Century*, edited by Robert Baker, 205–18. Boston: Kluwer Academic Publishers.

Smith, T. Southwood. 1827. *Use of the Dead to the Living*. Albany NY: Websters & Skinners.

Smith, Wesley D. 1979. *The Hippocratic Tradition*. Ithaca NY and London: Cornell University Press.

Smith, Wilson. 1956. *Professors & Public Ethics Studies of Northern Moral Philosophers before the Civil War*. Ithaca NY: Cornell University Press.

Smyth, D. H. 1978. *Alternatives to Animal Experiments*. London: Scolar Press.

Snell, A. M. 1952. "Retirement of Dr. Andrew C. Ivy." *Gastroenterology*. 22 (2): 227–28.

Snow, Charles Percy. 1961. *Two Cultures and the Scientific Revolution*. New York: Cambridge University Press.

Snow, Charles Percy. 1964. *The Two Cultures, and a Second Look*. Cambridge UK: Cambridge University Press.

Sobradillo, Agapito de. 1950. *Enquiridion de deontología médica*. Madrid: Ediciones Studium de Cultura.

Society of Kiev Physicians. 1889. *Proekt Eticheskikh Pravil, Sostavlennyi Komissiei, Izbrannoi Obshestvom Kievskikh Vrachei*. Kiev.

Soda, Hajime. 1989. *Zusetsu Nippon Iryo Bunkashi (The Cultural History of Japanese Medical Services with Photography and Illustrations)*. Kyoto: Shibunkaku Shuppan.

Solomon, Howard. 1972. *Public Welfare, Science and Propaganda in Seventeenth-Century France: The Innovations of Théophraste Renandot*. Princeton NJ: Princeton University Press.

Somerville, Margaret A. 2000. *The Ethical Canary: Science, Society and the Human Spirit*. Toronto: Penguin Books Canada.

Song, Guobin. 1933. *Yiye Lunlixue (Professional Ethics of Medicine)*. Shanghai: Guoguang Bookstore.

Song, Guobin. 1993. *Ethics of Medical Practice*. Shanghai: Gouguang Bookstore.

Sorbiere, Samuel. 1672. *Avis a un ieune medecin, sur la maniere dont il se doit comporter en la pratique de la medecine, . . .* Lyon: Antoine Offray.

South African Medical Services. 1997. *Submission to the Truth and Reconciliation Commission of South Africa*. Truth and Reconciliation Commission of South Africa Archive. Government Archives, South African Library, Cape Town.

Specter, Michael. 2001. "India's Plague." *The New Yorker*, December 17, 74–85.

Spencer, W. G., ed. and trans. 1935–1938. *Celsus: De Medicina*. 3 vols. Loeb Classical Library. Cambridge MA: Harvard University Press.

Spenlen, Jeannette. 1994. *Sexualethik und Familienplanung im muslimischen und christlichen Ägypten*. Frankfurt/M.: Peter Lang.

Spicer, Carol Mason. 1995a. "Appendix: Nature and Role of Codes, and Other Ethics Directives." In *Encyclopedia of Bioethics*. 2nd ed., edited by Warren T. Reich, 2605–12. New York: Simon & Schuster Macmillan.

Spicer, Carol Mason, ed. 1995b. "Appendix: Section II: Oath of Initiation (Caraka Samhita)." In *Encyclopedia of Bioethics*. 2nd ed., edited by Warren T. Reich, 2632–33. New York: Simon & Schuster Macmillan.

Spinsanti, Sandro. 1992. "Obtaining Consent from the Family: A Horizon for Clinical Ethics." *Journal of Clinical Ethics*. 3: 188–92.

Spinsanti, Sandro. 1995. *La Bioetica: Biografie per una disciplina*. Milano: Franco Angeli.

Spiro, H. 1993. "What is Empathy and Can It be Taught?" In *Empathy and the Practice of Medicine*, edited by H. Spiro, et al., 7–14. New Haven CT: Yale University Press.

Spitz, Vivien. 2005. *Doctors From Hell: The Horrific Account Of Nazi Experiments On Humans*. Boulder CO: Sentient Publications.

Sprott, S. E. 1961. *The English Debate on Suicide from Donne to Hume*. LaSalle IL: Open Court.

"Sri Lanka: Asia's Health Leader Faces 21st Century." 1997. http://kafula.msrc.sunysb.edu/~sbarrkum/newsgroups/sl.health (visited January 17, 2003): 1–2.

Stacey, Margaret. 1992. *Regulating British Medicine*. Chichester: John Wiley & Sons.

Stannard, David E. 1977. *The Puritan Way of Death*. New York: Oxford University Press.

Starr, Douglas. 1998. *Blood: An Epic History of Medicine and Commerce*. New York: A. Knopf.

Starr, Paul. 1982. *The Social Transformation of American Medicine*. New York: Basic Books.

Stefanelli, Norbert. 1998. *Körper ohne Leben – Begegnung und Umgang mit Toten*, edited by Norbert Stefenelli. Wien-Koeln-Weimar: Böhlau.

Steinberg, Abraham. 1988. *Encyclopedia of Medicine and Jewish Law*. Jerusalem: Schlesinger Institute [Hebrew].

Steinberg, Avraham. 2003. *Encyclopedia of Jewish Medical Ethics: A Compilation of Jewish Medical Law on All Topics of Medical Interest*, translated by Fred Rosner. Nanuet NY: Feldheim Publishers.

Steinschneider, Moritz. 1866. "Wissenschaft und Charlatanerie unter den Arabern im neunten Jahrhundert: Nach der hebräischen Übersetzung eines Schriftchens von Rhases." *Virchows Archiv*. 36: 570–86.

Stendahl, Krister, ed. 1965. *Immortality and Resurrection: Four Essays by Oscar Cullman, Harry A. Wolfson, Werner Jaeger, and Henry J. Cadbury*. New York: Macmillan.

Stern, Samuel M. 1962. "A Collection of Treatises by ʿAbd al-Laṭīf al-Baghdādī." *Islamic Studies*. 1: 53–70.

Stevens, M. L. Tina. 2000. *Bioethics in America: Origins and Cultural Politics*. Baltimore: Johns Hopkins University Press.

Stevens, Rosemary A. 1998. *American Medicine and the Public Interest: A History of Specialization*, revised edition. Berkeley CA: University of California Press.

Stevens, Rosemary A. 1999. "The Challenge of Specialism in the 1900s." In *The American Medical Ethics Revolution: How the AMA's Code of Ethics Has Transformed Physicians' Relationships to Patients, Professionals, and Society*, edited by Robert Baker, et al., 70–90. Baltimore: Johns Hopkins University Press.

Stewart, Agnes G. 1901. *The Academic Gregories*. Edinburgh: Oliphant Anderson & Ferrier.

Stillé, Alfred. 1880. "Memoir of Issac Hays, M.D." *Transactions of the College of Physicians of Philadelphia*. 3rd series. 5:1, xxvii–cxv.

Stolberg, Sheryl. 1995. "Fear Clouds Search for Genetic Roots of Violence." *Los Angeles Times*, Dec. 23, A1.

Stookey, Byron. 1962. *A History of Colonial Medical Education: In the Province of New York, with its Subsequent Development (1767–1830)*. Springfield IL: Charles C. Thomas.

Storer, Horatio Robinson. 1860. *On Criminal Abortion in America*. Philadelphia: Lippincott.

Storer, Horatio Robinson. 1866a. "The Criminality and Evils of Forced Abortions: Being the Prize Essay To Which the American Medical Association Awarded the Gold Medal for MDCCCLXV." *Transactions of the American Medical Association.* 16: 709–45.

Storer, Horatio Robinson. 1866b. *Why Not? A Book for Every Woman.* Boston: Lee and Shepard.

Stover, Eric. 1987. *The Open Secret: Torture and the Medical Profession in Chile.* Washington DC: American Association for the Advancement of Science.

Stover, Eric, and Elena O. Nightingale. 1985. *The Breaking of Bodies and Minds: Torture, Psychiatric Abuse, and the Health Professions.* New York: WH Freeman and Company.

Strashun, Il'ja D. 1937. *Sovetskii Vrach.* Moscow: Profizdat.

Strätling, Meinolfus. 1997. "John Gregory (1724–1773) and his Lectures on the Duties and Qualifications of a Physician Establishing Modern Medical Ethics on the Base of the Moral Philosophy and the Theory of Science of the Empiric British Enlightenment." *Medicina Nei Secoli.* 9: 455–75.

Strätling, Meinolfus. 1998. *Die Begründung der neuzeitlichen Medizinethik in Praxis, Lehre und Forschung: John Gregory (1724–1773) und seine Lectures on the Duties and Qualifications of a Physician.* Frankfurt am Main: P. Lang.

Strohmaier, Gotthard. 1974. "Hunayn ibn Ishāq et le Serment hippocratique." *Arabica.* 21: 318–23.

Strottman, Nissa M. 1999. "Public Health and Private Medicine: Regulation in Colonial and Early National America." *Hastings Law Journal.* 50: 383–406.

Styrap, Jukes de. 1878, 1886, 1899, 1895. *A Code of Medical Ethics: with Remarks on the Duties of Practitioners to their Patients, etc.* London: J. and A. Churchill, H. K. Lewis.

Styrap, Jukes de. [1878] 1995. *A Code of Medical Ethics.* In *The Codification of Medical Morality: Historical and Philosophical Studies of the Formalization of Western Medical Morality in the Eighteenth and Nineteenth Centuries: Volume Two: Anglo-American Medical Ethics and Medical Jurisprudence in the Nineteenth Century,* edited by Robert Baker, 149–71. Dordrecht: Kluwer Academic Publishers.

Suárez de Rivera, Francisco. 1729. *Theatro chyrurgico anatomico del cuerpo del hombre viviente, objeto de la cirugía y medicina.* Madrid: Francisco del Hierro.

Subatto, Ajahn Chah. 1997. "Our Real Home." *Tricycle: The Buddhist Review,* May 24–26.

Sudhoff, Karl. 1912. "Pestschriften aus den ersten 150 Jahren nach der Epidemie des Schwarzen Todes 1348." *Archiv Geschichte der Medizin.* 5: 36–87.

Sudhoff Karl. 1916. "Antipocras. Streitschrift für mystische Heilkunde in Versen des Magisters Nicolaus von Polen." *Sudhoffs Archiv.* 9: 31–52.

Sugimoto, Tsutomu. 1992. *Edo Ranpol kara no Messeiji (The Message from Dutch School Physicians in Edo Era).* Tokyo: Perikansha.

Sugitatsu, Yishikazu. 1984. "The Scrolls and Printed Versions of the 'Ishimpo.'" In *One Thousand Years of Ishimpo-Dawning of Japanese Medicine,* edited by the One Thousand Year Anniversary Committee of Ishinpo, 108–14. Tokyo: Ishimpo Issennen Kinenkai.

Sugunasiri, S. H. J. 1990. "The Buddhist View Concerning the Dead Body." *Transplantation Proceedings.* 22: 947–49.

Sulima, K. P. 1903. "K voprosu o vrachebnoi taine." *Vestnik Sank-Peterburgskogo Vrachebnogo Obshestva Vzaimnoi Pomoshi,* no. 8: 433–44.

Sullivan, Francis A. 1983. *Magisterium: Teaching Authority in the Catholic Church.* New York: Paulist Press.

Support Principal Investigators. 1995. "A Controlled Trial to Improve Care for Seriously Ill Hospitalized Patients." *JAMA: Journal of the American Medical Association.* 274: 1951–58.

Surty, Muhammad I. 1996. *Muslim's Contribution to the Development of Hospitals.* Birmingham: QAF.

Sussman, George. 1977. "The Glut of Doctors in Mid-Nineteenth Century France." *Comparative Studies in Society and History.* 19: 287–304.

Suyematsu, Kencho. 1905. *The Risen Sun.* London: Archibald Constable & Co. Ltd.

Suzuki, Daisetsu. 1972. *Japanese Spirituality,* translated by Norman Waddell. Tokyo: Japan Society for the Promotion of Science.

Svod Zakonov Rossiiskoi Imperii. n.d. *Kniga. 5, Tom XV. Ulozhenie o Nakazaniyakh Ugolovnykh i Ispravitel'nykh.* Saint-Petersburg.

"Swami, Bill Clinton Has a Question: The President is Asking All Faiths, Including Hinduism, about the Ethics of Human Cloning." 1997. *Hinduism Today.* www.hinduism-today.com/1997/6/.

Sydenham, Diane. 1978. "Practitioner and Patient: The Practice of Medicine in Eighteenth-Century South Carolina." Ph.D. diss., Johns Hopkins University, Maryland.

Sydenham, Thomas. 1676. *Observationes medicae circa morborum acutorum historiam et curationem.* Londoni: G. Kettilby.

Syndicat Médical de Lille et de la Région. 1903. *Oeuvres de Défense et de Prévoyance Professionelles.* Lille.

Szasz, Thomas S. 1963. *Law, Liberty, and Psychiatry.* New York: Collier Books.

Szasz, Thomas S. 1996. "Routine Neonatal Circumcision: Symbol of the Birth of the Therapeutic State." *Journal of Medicine and Philosophy.* 21: 137–48.

Szawarski, Zbigniew. 1987. "Poland: Biomedical Ethics in a Socialist State." *Hastings Center Report.* 17: S27–S29.

Szawarski, Zbigniew. 1992. "Research Ethics in Eastern Europe." *Bulletin of Medical Ethics.* 82: 13–18.

Szilard, Janos. 1973. *Medical Ethics.* Szeged: University Publisher.

Tachibana, Shundo. 1993. *The Ethics of Buddhism*. Surrey: Curzon Paperbacks.

Takahashi, Bonsen. 1936. *Datai Mabiki no Kenkyu (The Studies on Abortion and Mabiki)*. Chuo Shakai Jigyo Kyokai: Shakai Jigyo Kenkyujyo.

"Talking Across Disciplines: Joining History and Bioethics." 1999. The Third John Conley Conference on Medical Ethics, New York Presbyterian Hospital, February 26, 1999.

Tanaka, Yuki. 1996. *Hidden Horrors: Japanese War Crimes in World War II*. Boulder CO: Westerview.

Tanba, Yasuyori. [1984] 1991. *Ishinpo (Medicine's Heart and Method)*. Kokuho Nakaraike Hon Ishinpo. Tokyo: Oriento Syuppan.

Tangwa, G. B. 1999. "Is Bioethics Love of Life? An African View-Point." *IAB News*. 9: 4–6.

Taniguchi, Shoyo. 1987. "Biomedical Ethics from a Buddhist Perspective." *Pacific World*. 3: 75–83.

Taniguchi, Shoyo. 1994. "Methodology of Buddhist Biomedical Ethics." In *Religious Methods and Resources in Bioethics*, edited by Paul F. Camenisch, 31–65. Chicago: Kluwer Academic Press.

Tanneberger, Stephan. 1989. "Ethical Responsibility in the German Democratic Republic." *Hastings Center Report*. 19: S9–S10.

Tannenbaum, Cara, Nancy Mayo, and Francine Ducharme. 2005. "Older Women's Health Priorities and Perceptions of Care Delivery: Results of the WOW Health Survey." *Canadian Medical Association Journal*. 173: 153–59.

Tanner, Norman P., ed. 1990. *Decrees of the Ecumenical Councils*. Washington DC: Georgetown University Press.

Tantawi, Muhammad Sayyid. 1996. "Tanzim al-usra kahall limushkilat al-infijar al-sukkani (Family planning as a solution to the problem of population explosion)." *Al-Liwa' al-Islami*, August 22, 13.

Taschkandi, S. Ekram. 1968. *Übersetzung und Bearbeitung des Kitāb at-Tašwīq aṭ-Ṭibbī des Ṣaʾid ibn al-Ḥasan: Ein medizinisches Adabwerk aus dem 11. Jahrhundert*, translation and analysis by S. Ekram Taschkandi. Bonn: Bonner Orientalische Studien.

Tashiro, Elke. 1991. *Die Waage der Venus: Venerologische Versuche am Menschen zwischen Fortschritt und Moral*. Husum. Matthiesen.

Task Force on Death and Dying. Institute of Society, Ethics, and the Life Sciences. 1972. "Refinements in Criteria for the Definition of Death: An Appraisal." *JAMA: Journal of the American Medical Association*. 221: 48–53.

Task Force on Organ Transplantation. U.S. Department of Health and Human Services. 1986. *Organ Transplantation: Issues and Recommendations*. In *Source Book in Bioethics: A Documentary History*, edited by Albert R. Jonsen, Robert M. Veatch, and LeRoy Walters, 418–47. Washington DC: Georgetown University Press.

Tatz, Mark, ed. 1986. *Asanga's Chapter on Ethics with the Commentary of Tsong-Kha-Pa: The Basic Path to Awakening, The Complete Bodhisattva*. Lewiston NY: Edwin Mellon Press.

Tauber, Conrad. 1979. "Asking the Right Questions." *Kennedy Institute Quarterly Report*. 5 (1).

Taylor, A. S. 1844. *A Manual of Medical Jurisprudence*. London: John Churchill.

Taylor, A. S. 1984. *Taylor's Principles and Practice of Medical Jurisprudence*, edited by K. Mant. Edinburgh: Churchill Livingston.

Taylor, Angus. 1999. *Magpies, Monkeys, and Morals: What Philosophers Say about Animal Liberation*. Peterborough: Broadview Press.

Taylor, Frederick Winslow. [1911] 1985. *The Principles of Scientific Management*. Easton PA: Hive Publishing Company.

Taylor, Jeremy. [1651] 1873. *The Rule and Exercises of Holy Dying*. Reprint. London: Bickers and Son.

Taylor, John. 1759. *An Examination of the Scheme of Morality Advanced by Dr. Hutcheson*. London: n. p.

Taylor, Telford. 1992. *The Anatomy of the Nuremberg Trials: A Personal Memoir*. New York: Knopf.

Tealdi, Juan Carlos. 1993. "Bioethical Concerns in Environmental Problems in Latin American Countries." In *International Bioethics Symposium*, series 6.7, edited by Kazumasa Hoshino, 36–64. Tokyo: Sokyusha Publishers.

Tealdi, Juan Carlos, Gustavo Pis Diez, and Oscar M. Esquisabel. 1995. "Bioethics in Latin America: 1991–1993." In *Bioethics Yearbook: Volume 4. Regional Development in Bioethics: 1991–1993*, edited by B. Andrew Lustig, 113–35. Dordrecht: Kluwer Academic Publishers.

Teleky, Ludwig. 1948. *History of Factory and Mine Hygiene*. New York: Columbia University Press.

Temkin, Owsei. 1956. *Soranus' Gynecology*. Baltimore and London: Johns Hopkins University Press.

Temkin, Owsei. 1991. *Hippocrates in a World of Pagans and Christians*. Baltimore: Johns Hopkins University Press.

Temme, L. A. 2003. "Ethics in Human Experimentation: The Two Military Physicians Who Helped Develop the Nuremberg Code." *Aviation Space Environmental Medicine*. 74 (12): 1297–1300.

ten Have, Henk A. M. J. 1998. "Philosophy of Medicine and Health Care – European Perspectives." *Medicine, Health Care, and Philosophy*. 1: 1–3.

Tentler, Thomas N. 1977. *Sin and Confession on the Eve of the Reformation*. Princeton NJ: Princeton University Press.

Tertullian. 1961. *Tertullien, Apologétique*. 2nd ed., edited by J. P. Waltzing. Paris: Les belles letters.

Tesh, Sylvia. 1988. *Hidden Arguments*. New Brunswick NJ: Rutgers University Press.

Thamin, R., and Paul Lapie. 1903. *Extraites des Auteurs Anciens et Modernes*. Paris: Hachette.

Thane, Pat. 1993. "Geriatrics." In *Companion Encyclopedia of the History of Medicine*, edited by William F. Bynum and Roy Porter, 1092–1115. London and New York: Routledge.

Tharien, A. K. 1995. "Euthanasia in India." *Eubios Journal of Asian and International Bioethics*. 5: 33–35.

Tharien, A. K. 1996. "Organ Transplantation in India." *Eubios Journal of Asian and International Bioethics*. 6: 168–9.

Thau, Christian, and Alexandru Popescu-Prahovara. 1992. "Romanian Psychiatry in Turmoil." *Bulletin of Medical Ethics*. 78: 13–16.

Thielicke, Helmut. 1966. *Theological Ethics*, Vol. 1, edited by William H. Lazareth. Philadelphia: Fortress Press.

Thiery, Joachim, and Ulrich Tröhler. 1987. "Doubt about Progress, but Trust in Compassion. Wagner the Anti-Vivisectionist: His Motives and His Contemporaries' Reactions." In *'Parsifal' Programmheft II*, edited by Wolfgang Wagner, 65–101. Bayreuth: Bayreuther Festspiele.

Thom, Achim, and Genadij I. Caregorodcev, eds. 1989. *Medizin unterm Hakenkreuz*. Berlin: Volk und Gesundheit.

Thomas, Keith. 1971. *Religion and the Decline of Magic*. New York: Scribner.

Thomas, Keith. 1983. *Man and the Natural World: A History of the Modern Sensibility*. New York: Pantheon Books.

Thomas, Michael. 2003a. "Ethics Lessons of the Failure to Bring the Japanese Doctors to Justice." *Eubios Journal of Asian and International Bioethics*. 13: 104–6.

Thomas, Michael. 2003b. "Let's Deal with the Issue: Commentary on Leavitt." *Eubios Journal of Asian and International Bioethics*. 13: 166–67.

Thomas Aquinas, Saint. 1951–1952. *Summa Theologiae*. 5 vols. Madrid: Biblioteca de Autores Cristianos.

Thomas Aquinas, Saint. 1984. *Summe der Theologia*. 3rd ed., 3 vols., edited by Joseph Bernhart. Stuttgart: Kröner.

Thomasma, David C., et al., eds. 1998. *Asking to Die: Inside the Dutch Debate about Euthanasia*. Dordrecht: Kluwer Academic Publishers.

Thompson, I. E., ed. 1979. *Dilemmas of Dying*. Edinburgh: Edinburgh University Press.

Thomsen, O. O., et al. 1993. "What do Gastroenterologists in Europe Tell Cancer Patients?" *The Lancet*. 20: 473–76.

Thomson, Judith J. 1971. "A Defence of Abortion." *Philosophy and Public Affairs*. 1: 47–66.

Thouvenin, Dominique. 1982. *Le Secret Médical et L'Information de Malade*. Lyon: Presses Universitaires de Lyon.

Tichtchenko, Pavel, and Boris Yudin. 1992. "Towards a Bioethics in the New Russia." *Bulletin of Medical Ethics*. 78: 32–33.

Tikk, Arvo, and V. Parve. 2000. "Ethics Committees in the Czech Republic." In *Ethics Committees in Central and Eastern Europe*, edited by Jozef Glasa, 173–78. Bratislava: Charis-IMEB FDN.

Tikriti, Raji Abbas al-. 1981. *Al-Suluk al-Mihni lilAtibba' (The Professional Ethics of Physicians)*. Beirut: Dar al-Andalus.

Tilak, Shrinivas. 1989. *Religion and Aging in the Indian Tradition*. Albany NY: State University of New York Press.

Tirmiḏī, Abū ʿĪsā Muḥammad b. ʿĪsā b. Šura. 1994. *Sunan at-Tirmīḏī*. 5 vols., edited by Ṣ. M. Ğamīl al-ʾAṭṭār. Bairūt: Dār al-Fikr.

Tissot, Samuel Auguste. 1761. *Avis au peuple sur sa santé*. Lausanne: J. Zimmerli.

Tissot, Simon-Auguste-Andre-David. 1767. *Onanism: Or, a Treatise upon the Disorders produced by Masturbation*. 3rd ed., translated by A. Hume. London: W. Wilkinson.

Titmuss, Richard M. 1970. *The Gift Relationship*. London: George Allen & Unwin.

Tokat, Y., et al. 1995. "Posttransplant Problems Requiring Regrafting: An Analysis of 72 Patients with 96 Liver Retransplants." *Transplantation Proceedings*. 27: 1264–5.

Tolle, S. W., et al. 2004. "Characteristics and Proportion of Dying Oregonians who Personally Consider Physician-Assisted Suicide." *Journal of Clinical Ethics*. 15: 111–8.

Tollemache, Lionel. 1873. "The New Cure for Incurables." *Fortnightly Review*. 218–30.

Tong, Rosemarie. 1993. *Feminine and Feminist Ethics*. Belmont CA: Wadsworth Publishing Company.

Tooley, Michael. 1983. *Abortion and Infanticide*. Oxford: The Clarendon Press.

Toorawa, Shawkat M. 1994. "The Dhimmī in Medieval Islamic Society: Non-Muslim Physicians of Iraq in Ibn Abī Uṣaybiʿah's ʿUyūn al-anbāʾ fī ṭabakāt al-aṭibbāʾ." *Fides et Historia*. 26.1: 10–21.

Tournier, Paul. 1985. *Creative Suffering*. London: SCM Press.

Toyka, Klaus V. 1998. "Neurology's Witness to History: Leo Alexander [letter]." *Neurology*. 51 (6): 1772.

Trevor-Roper, Hugh. 1990. "The Court Physician and Paracelsianism." In *Medicine at the Courts of Europe 1500–1837*, edited by Vivian Nutton, 79–94. London: Routledge.

Tribe, Laurence H. 1971. "Trial by Mathematics: Precision and Ritural in the Legal Process." *Harvard Law Review*. 84: 1329–93.

Tröhler, Ulrich. 1993. "Surgery (modern)." In *Companion Encyclopedia of the History of Medicine*, edited by William F. Bynum and Roy Porter, 984–1028. London and New York: Routledge.

Tröhler, Ulrich. 1998. "From Rehn's Risky Cardiac Suture (1896) to Routine Cardiac Transplantation (1996): Historical and Ethical Perspectives." *The Journal of Cardiovascular Surgery.* 39. Suppl. 1 to No. 2: 7–22.

Tröhler, Ulrich. 1999. "Das ärztliche Ethos und die Kodifizierung von Ethik in der Medizin." In *Medizinische Ethik im ärztlichen Alltag,* edited by A. Bondolfi and H. Müller, 39–61. Basle-Bern: EMH: Schweiz. Ärzteverlag.

Tröhler, Ulrich. 2000a. "Asilomar-Konferenz zu Sicherheit in der Molekularbiologie von 1975: Rückschau und Ausblick." *Schweizerische Ärztezeitung.* 28: 1585–87.

Tröhler, Ulrich. 2000b. *To Improve the Evidence of Medicine: The 18th Century British Origins of a Critical Approach.* Edinburgh: Royal College of Physicians.

Tröhler, Ulrich. 2002. "Human Research: From Ethos to Law, From National to International Regulations. In *Historical and Philosophical Perspectives on Biomedical Ethics: From Paternalism to Autonomy?,* edited by Andreas-Holger Maehle and Johanna Geyer-Kordesch, 95–117. Aldershot, Burlington, and Singapore: Ashgate.

Tröhler, Ulrich, and Andreas-Holger Maehle. 1987. "Anti-Vivisection in Nineteenth-Century Germany and Switzerland: Motives and Methods." In *Vivisection in Historical Perspective,* edited by Nicolaas A. Rupke, 149–87. London: Croom Helm.

Tröhler, Ulrich, and Andreas-Holger Maehle. 1990. "Anti-Vivisection in Nineteenth-Century Germany and Switzerland: Motives and Methods." In *Vivisection in Historical Perspective.* 2nd ed., edited by Nicolaas A. Rupke, 149–87. London: Routledge.

Tröhler, Ulrich, and Stella Reiter-Theil. 1997. *Ethik und Medizin: 1947–1997, Was leistet de Kodification von Ethik?.* Göttingen: Wallstein Verlag.

Tröhler, Ulrich, and Stella Reiter-Theil. 1998. *Ethics Codes in Medicine: Foundations and Achievements of Codification since 1947.* Aldershot: Ashgate.

Trontelj, J. 2000. "Ethics Committees in Slovenia." In *Ethics Committees in Central and Eastern Europe,* edited by Jozef Glasa, 239–50. Bratislava: Charis-IMEB FDN.

Trubuhovich, R. V. 2004. "August 26th 1952 at Copenhagen: 'Bjorn Ibsen's Day'; a significant event for Anaesthesia." *Acta Anaesthesiology Scandinavia.* 48.3: 272–77.

Trucco, T. 1989. "Sales of Kidneys Prompt New Laws and Debate." *New York Times,* Aug. 1, C1, C6.

Truog, R. D., and John C. Fletcher. 1989. "Anencephalic Newborns: Can Organs Be Transplanted Before Brain Death?" *New England Journal of Medicine.* 321: 388–91.

Truth and Reconciliation Commission of South Africa. 1998a. *Truth and Reconciliation Commission of South Africa Report.* Cape Town: Juta and Co. Ltd.

Truth and Reconciliation Commission of South Africa. 1998b. *Transcript of Chemical and Biological Warfare Hearings.* www.trc.org.za/special/cbw/ (visited May 11, 2000).

Tsomo, Karma Lekshe. 1996. *Sisters in Solitude: Two Traditions of Buddhist Monastic Ethics for Women.* Albany NY: State University of New York Press.

Tsuchiya, Takashi. 2000. "Why Japanese Doctors Performed Human Experiments in China, 1933–1945." *Eubios Journal of Asian and International Bioethics.* 10: 179–80.

Tsuchiya, Takashi. 2003. "In the Shadow of the Past Atrocities: Research Ethics with Human Subjects in Contemporary Japan." *Eubios Journal of Asian and International Bioethics.* 13: 100–102.

Tsuneishi, Keiichi. 1981. *Kieta Saikinsen Butai: Kantongun Dai 731 Butai (The Germ Warfare Unit That Disappeared).* Tokyo: Kaimeisha.

Tsuneishi, Keiichi. 1994. *Igakusha Tachi no Soshiki Hanzai (The Conspiracy of Medical Researchers).* Tokyo: Asahi Shimbun.

Tsuneishi, Keiichi. 1995. *731 Butai (Unit 731).* Tokyo: Kodansha.

Tu, Wei-Ming. 1997. "Destructive Will and Ideological Holocaust: Maoism as a Source of Social Suffering in China." In *Social Suffering,* edited by Arthur Kleinman, Veena Das, and Margaret Lock, 149–180. Berkeley CA: University of California Press.

Tucker, Robert C., ed. 1972. *The Marx-Engels Reader.* New York NY and London: W. W. Norton & Company.

Turner, James C. 1980. *Reckoning with the Beast: Animals, Pain, and Humanity in the Victorian Mind.* Baltimore: Johns Hopkins University Press.

Tworkov, Helen. 1997. "In Light of Death: An Interview with Rick Fields on Living With Cancer." *Tricycle: The Buddhist Review.* May. 24–26, 44–48, 100–105.

Ubel, Peter A. 2000. *Pricing Life: Why It's Time for Health Care Rationing.* Cambridge MA and London: The MIT Press.

Uden, K. F. 1783. *Medizinische Politik.* Leipzig: Weygansche Buchhandlung.

Ui, Hakujuyu. 1943. *Bukkyo Shiso Kenkyu (The Studies on Buddhist Thoughts).* Tokyo: Iwanami Shoten.

Ulman, H. L. 1990. *The Minutes of the Aberdeen Philosophical Society.* Aberdeen: Aberdeen University Press.

Ullmann, Manfred. 1970. *Die Medizin im Islam.* Leiden: E. J. Brill.

Ullmann, Manfred. 1978. *Islamic Medicine.* Edinburgh: Edingurgh University Press.

Ulrich, Laurel Thatcher. 1990. *A Midwife's Tale: The Life of Martha Ballard, Based on Her Diary, 1785–1812.* New York: Vintage Books.

Umri, Jalaluddin. 1987. "Suicide or Termination of Life." *Islamic and Comparative Law Quarterly.* 7: 136–44.

UNAIDS/UNFPA. 2001. "Strategic Options for HIV/AIDS Advocacy in Africa." www.unfpa.org/tpd/publications/advoafr.pdf (visited November 12, 2002).

United Nations. 1992. "Rio Declaration." In *Yearbook of the United Nations*. 46: 670–72. Dordrecht: Martinus Nijhoff Publishers.

United Nations Development Program. 1994. *The Dakar Declaration*. www.undp.org/hiv/policies/dakare.htm (visited August 27, 2002).

United Nations Development Program. 1998. *Report on Human Social Development in Lithuania*. Vilnius: 61 [Lithuanian].

United Nations Environmental Program. 1992. *Convention on Biological Diversity*. www.biodiv.org/convention/articles.asp (visited August 27, 2002).

United Nations Organization, United Nations General Assembly. 1952. *Protocol for the Prohibition of the Use in War of Asphyxiating, Poisonous or Other Gases, and of Bacteriological Methods of Warfare*. www.unog.ch/frames/disarm/distreat/bac_28.pdf (visited June 8, 2000).

United Nations Organization, United Nations General Assembly. 1972. *Convention on the Prohibition of the Development, Production and Stockpiling of Bacteriological (Biological) and Toxin Weapons and on their Destruction*. www.unog.ch/frames/disarm/distreat/bac_72.htm (visited June 8, 2000).

United Nations Organization, United Nations General Assembly. 1993. *Convention on the Prohibition of the Development, Production, Stockpiling and Use of Chemical Weapons and on their Destruction*. www.unog.ch/frames/disarm/distreat/chemical.htm (visited June 8, 2000).

United Nations War Crimes Commission. 1948. *History of the United Nations War Crimes Commission and the Development of the Laws of War*. London: HMSO.

United Nations War Crimes Commission. 1949. *German Medical War Crimes: A Summary of Information*. London: British Medical Association House.

United States Catholic Bishops Conference, the National Conference of Catholic Bishops. 1983. *The Challenge of Peace: Promise and Our Response*. Washington DC.

United States Congress, Office of Technology Assessment. 1990. *Genetic Monitoring and Screening in the Workplace*. 22.

United States Department of the Army. 1990. Regulation 70–25, "Use of Volunteers as Subjects of Research." 25 January.

United States Department of the Army. 1999. Regulation 600–20, "Army Command Policy." 15 July.

United States Department of the Army, Office of the Inspector General. 1975. *Use of Volunteers in Chemical Agent Research*. Washington DC: General Printing Office.

United States Department of Health, Education, and Welfare. 1957. *Healthy People: The Surgeon General's Report on Health Promotion and Disease Prevention*. Washington DC: DHEW.

United States Department of Health and Human Services. 1998. "Organ Procurement and Transplantation Network; Final Rule [42 CFR Part 121]." *Federal Register*. 63 (2 April): 16296.

United States Department of Justice. National Institute of Justice, Commission on the Future of DNA Evidence. 1998. *Minutes of Meeting*. Washington DC, July 20, 1998.

United States House of Representatives Subcommittee on Energy Conservation and Power of the Committee on Energy and Commerce. 1986. *American Nuclear Guinea Pigs: Three Decades of Radiation Experiments on U.S. Citizens*. Washington DC: U.S. Government Printing Office.

United States v. Karl Brandt, et al. 1947. "The Medical Case, Trials of War Criminals before the Nuremberg Military Tribunal under Control Council Law No. 10."

Unschuld, Paul U. 1979. *Medical Ethics in Imperial China: A Study of Historical Anthropology*. Berkeley CA: University of California Press.

Unschuld, Paul U. 1985. *Medicine in China: A History of Ideas*. Berkeley CA: University of California Press.

Unschuld, Paul U. 1990. *Forgotten Traditions of Ancient Chinese Medicine*. Brookline MA: Paradigm Publications.

Unschuld, Paul. 2001. "Chinese Medical Ethics and the Role of Medical History." *Acta Medica Nagaskiensia*. 46. Supplement: Ethical Problems of Modern Medicine in the East and West. English: 14–18; Japanese: 46–50.

Usborne, Cornelie. 1992. *The Politics of the Body in Weimar Germany: Women's Reproductive Rights and Duties*. Ann Arbor MI: University of Michigan Press.

'Uthaymin, Muhammad al-Salih al-. 1995. *Fatawa al-Mar'a Al-Muslima (Fatwas of the Muslim Woman)*. Riyad: Maktabat al-Tabariyya.

Uvarov, M. S. 1903. "Polozhenie Vrachei, Rabotayuschikh v Oblasti Obschestvennoi Meditsiny." In *A. Moll. Vrachebnaya Etika. Obyazannosti Vracha vo Vsekh Otraslyakh Ego Deyatelnosti. Dlya Vrachei i Publiki*, 143–55. Saint-Petersburg.

Van Buitenen, J. A. B., ed. 1973. *Mahābhārata: The Book of the Beginning*. Chicago, University of Chicago Press.

Van der Maas, Paul J., et al. 1996a. "Euthanasia, Physician-Assisted Suicide, and Other Medical Practices Involving the End of Life in the Netherlands, 1990–1995." *New England Journal of Medicine*. 335:1699–1705

Van der Mass, Paul J., et al. 1996b. "Evaluation of the Notification Procedure for Physician-Assisted Death." *New England Journal of Medicine*. 335: 1706–12.

Van der Poel, Cornelius. 1968. "The Principle of Double Effect." In *Absolutes in Moral Theology*, edited by Charles E. Curran, 186–210. Washington DC: Corpus.

Van der Wal, Gerrit, and Robert J. M. Dillmann. 1994. "Euthanasia in the Netherlands." *British Medical Journal*. 308: 1346–49

Van der Zeijden, Albert. 2000. "Citizens and Patients as Partners in Decision-Making and Implementation." *Issues in Eureopean Health Policy*. 3: 8.

Van Ingen, Philip. 1949. *The New York Academy of Medicine: Its First Hundred Years*. New York: Columbia University Press.

Van Minnen, Peter. 1995. "Medical Care in Late Antiquity." In *Ancient Medicine in its Socio-Cultural Context*, edited by Philip J. van der Eijk, et al., 153–69. Amsterdam: Rodopi.

Van Till-d'Aulnis de Bourouill, Adrienne. 1975. "How Dead Can You Be?" *Medical Science and Law*. 15: 133–47.

Varshavskoe Obshestvo Vrachei (Warsaw Physicians' Society). 1884. "Objazannosti i Prava Vrachei: Eticheskie Pravila, Prinyatye Varshavskim Obshestvom Vrachei." *Vrach*. 29: 497–9.

Vaux, Kenneth L., and Stanley G. Schade. 1988. *The Search for Universality in the Ethics of Human Research: Andrew C. Ivy, Henry K. Beecher, and the Legacy of Nuremberg*. Boston: Kluwer Academic Publishers.

Veatch, Robert M. 1975. "The Whole-Brain Oriented Concept of Death: An Outmoded Philosophical Formulation." *Journal of Thanatology*. 3: 13–30.

Veatch, Robert M. 1976. *Death, Dying, and the Biological Revolution: Our Last Quest for Responsibility*. New Haven CT: Yale University Press.

Veatch, Robert M. 1981. *A Theory of Medical Ethics*. New York: Basic Books.

Veatch, Robert M. 1989a. "Introduction." In *Cross Cultural Perspectives in Medical Ethics: Readings*, edited by Robert M. Veach, 4–5. Boston: Jones and Barlett Publishers.

Veatch, Robert M., ed. 1989b. *Medical Ethics*. Boston: Jones and Bartlett.

Veatch, Robert M. 1995a. "Diverging Traditions: Professional and Religious Medical Ethics of the Nineteenth Century." In *The Codification of Medical Morality: Historical and Philosophical Studies of the Formalization of Western Medical Morality in the Eighteenth and Nineteenth Centuries: Volume Two: Anglo-American Medical Ethics and Medical Jurisprudence in the Nineteenth Century*, edited by Robert Baker, 121–32. Boston: Kluwer Academic Publishers.

Veatch, Robert M. 1995b. "Medical Codes and Oaths: II. Ethical Analysis." In *The Encyclopedia of Bioethics*, edited by Warren T. Reich, 1427–35. New York: Simon & Schuster Macmillan.

Veatch, Robert M., ed. 1997. *Medical Ethics*. 2nd ed. Sudbury MA: Jones and Bartlett.

Veatch, Robert M. 1999. "The Conscience Clause: How Much Individual Choice in Defining Death Can Our Society Tolerate?" In *The Definition of Death: Contemporary Controversies*, edited by Stuart J. Youngner, Robert M. Arnold, and Renie Schapiro, 137–60. Baltimore: Johns Hopkins University Press.

Veatch, Robert M. 2002. "The Birth of Bioethics: Autobiographical Reflections of a Patient Person." *Cambridge Quarterly of Healthcare Ethics*. 10: 344–52.

Veatch, Robert M. 2005. *Disrupted Dialogue: Medical Ethics and the Collapse of Physician-Humanist Communication (1770–1980)*. New York: Oxford University Press.

Velshtein, E. P. 1911. "Ugolovnaya Otvetstvennost' Vrachei." *Obshestvennyi Vrach*. 3: 57–67.

Vel'yaminov, Nikolai A. 1901. "Rech' na Godovom Zasedanii Peterburgskogo Mediko-khirurgicheskogo Obshestva." *Vach*. 49: 1529–30.

Veresaev, Vikenty V. 1903. *Po Povodu "Zapisok Vracha": Otvet Moim Kritikam*. Saint-Petersburg: Elektopechatnja N.Nikitenko.

Veresaev, Vikenty V. 1904. "Predislovie." In *Albert Moll (1904): Vrachebnaya Etika. Obyazannosti Vracha vo Vsekh Proyavlenuyakh Ego Deyatel'nosti*, vii–viii. Moscow: Magazin "Knizhnoe delo."

Veresaev, Vikenty V. 1948. *Sochinenija v Chetyrekh Tomakh*. T.1: 461–649. Moscow: Goslitizdat.

Verhey, Allen. 1995. "Protestantism." In *The Encyclopedia of Bioethics*. 2nd ed., edited by Warren T. Reich, 2117–26. New York: Simon & Schuster Macmillan.

Verhey, Allan, and Stephen Lammers, eds. 1993. *Theological Voices in Medical Ethics*. Grand Rapids MI: Eerdmans.

Verma, K. K. 1997. "Case of the First Test Tube Baby in India." *Eubios Journal of Asian and International Bioethics*. 7: 66–7.

Verma, Kusum, et al. 1999. "Ethics Perspectives from India." In *Health Ethics in Six SEAR Countries*, edited by Nimal Kasturiaratchi, Reidar Lie, and Jens Seeberg, 19–48. New Delhi: WHO-SEAR, World Health Organization, Regional Office for South-East Asia.

Vesalius, Andreas. [1543] 1964. *De humani corporis fabrica libri septem*. Reprint. Brussels: Culture et Civilisation.

Villey, Raymond. 1986. *Histoire du Secret Médical*. Paris: Seghers.

Vines, Gail. 1995. "Genes in Black and White." *New Scientist*. July 8.

Virgil. 1965. *Vergil, Aeneis: Lateinisch-Deutsch*. 2nd ed., edited by Johannes Götte. München: Heimeran.

Vitoria, Francisco de. [1539] 1974. *Relecciones del Estado, de los Indios, y del derecho de la Guerra*, edited by Antonio Gómez Robledo. México: Porrúa.

Vogel, Morris J., and Charles E. Rosenberg. 1979. *The Therapeutic Revolution: Essays in the Social History of American Medicine*. Philadelphia: University of Pennsylvania Press.

Vogel, Samuel Gottlieb. 1793. *Das Kranken-Examen: Oder allgemeine philosophische medicinische Untersuchung zur Erforschung der Krankheiten des menschlichen Körpers.* Stendal: D. C. Franze & Grosse.

Vogel, Virgil J. 1970. *American Indian Medicine.* Norman OK: University of Oklahoma Press.

Vogt, A. 1948. "Die Allgemein Sterbelichkeit . . . ," quoted in *History of Factory and Mine Hygiene,* by Ludwig Teleky, 199. New York: Columbia University Press.

Vollmann, Jochen, and Rolf Winau. 1996. "Informed Consent in Human Experimentation before the Nuremberg Code." *British Medical Journal.* 313: 1445–7.

Vom Brocke, Rüdiger. 2001. "Pagel, Julius Leopold." In *Ärzte Lexikon. Von der Antike bis zur Gegenwart.* 2nd ed., edited by Wolfgang U. Eckart and Christoph Gradmann, 238–9. Berlin: Springer.

Von Hebra, Ferdinand. 1847. "Höchst wichtige Erfahrungen über die Aetiologie der in Gebäranstalten epidemischen Puerperalfieber." *Zeitschrift der kaiserlich-königlichen Gesellschaft der Ärzte zu Wien.* 4, pt. 2: 242–4.

Von Hebra, Ferdinand. 1849. "Letter: Zeitschrift der kaiserlich-königlichen Gesellschaft der Ärzte zu Wien." 5: 64–5.

Von Staden, Heinrich. 1989. *Herophilus: The Art of Medicine in Early Alexandria: Edition, Translation and Essays.* Cambridge UK: Cambridge University Press.

Von Staden, Heinrich. 1990. "Incurability and Hopelessness: The Hippocratic Corpus." In *La Maladie et les maladies dans la Collection hippocratique: Actes du IV Colloque international hippocratique,* edited by Paul Potter, Gilles Maloney, and Jacques Desautels, 77–112. Quebec: Editions du Sphinx.

Von Staden, Heinrich. 1992a. "The Discovery of the Body: Human Dissection and its Cultural Contexts in Ancient Greece." *Yale Journal of Biology and Medicine.* 65: 223–41.

Von Staden, Heinrich. 1992b. "Women and Dirt." *Helios.* 19: 7–30.

Von Staden, Heinrich. 1996a. "In a Pure and Holy Way': Personal and Professional Conduct in the Hippocratic Oath?" *Journal of the History of Medicine and Allied Sciences.* 51 (4): 404–37.

Von Staden, Heinrich. 1996b. "Liminal Perils: Early Roman Receptions of Greek Medicine." In *Tradition, Transmission, Transformation,* edited by F. Jamil Ragep and Sally G. Ragep with Steven Livesey, 369–418. Leiden: E. J. Brill.

Von Staden, Heinrich. 1997. "Character and Competence: Personal and Professionl Conduct in Greek Medicine." In *Médecine et Morale dans l'Antiquité (Entretiens sur l'antiquite classique XLIII),* edited by Hellmut Flashar and Jacques Jouanna, 157–210. Vandoeuvres Geneva: Fondation Hardt.

Vovelle, Michel. 1983. *La Mort et l'Occident de 1300 à Nos Jours.* Paris: Gallimard.

Vrachebnaya, Etika (Polozhenija, Vyrabotannye Obshestvom Umanskikh Vrachei). 1903. *Vestnik Sankt-Peterburgskogo Vrachebnogo Obshestva Vzaimnoi Pomoshi.* 8: 485–8.

Wachter, Maurice de. 1979. "Des Andes à la Bioéthique [Interview with André E. Hellegers]." *Cahiers de Bioéthique, 1. La Bioéthique,* 11–9. Québec: Les Presses de l'Université Laval.

Waddington, Ivan. 1975. "The Development of Medical Ethics – A Sociological Analysis." *Medical History.* 19: 36–51.

Waddington, Ivan. 1984. *The Medical Profession in the Industrial Revolution.* Dublin: Gill & Macmilan.

Waite, Gloria Martha. 1993. *A History of Traditional Medicine and Health Care in Pre-Colonial East-Central Africa.* Lewiston NY: E. Mellen Press.

Wallace-Hadrill, J. M. 1951. "The Work of Gregory of Tours in the Light of Modern Research." In *Transactions of the Royal Historical Society.* 5th series. 1: 25–45.

Wallis, Patrick. 2006. "Plagues, Morality and the Place of Medicine in Early Modern England." *English Historical Review,* vol. CXXI, no. 490: 1–24.

Walsh, James J. 1907. *History of the Medical Society of the State of New York.* New York: Medical Society of the State of New York.

Walter, Bernd. 1996. *Psychiatrie und Gesellschaft in der Moderne: Geisteskrankenfürsorge in der Provinz Westfalen zwischen Kaiserreich und NS-Regime.* Paderborn: Ferdinand Schöningh.

Walters, LeRoy, ed. 1972-. *Bibliography of Bioethics.* Washington DC: Kennedy Institute of Ethics.

Walters, LeRoy. 1974. "Medical Ethics." In *New Catholic Encyclopedia,* volume XVI (Supplement 1967–1974), 290–1. New York: McGraw-Hill Book Company.

Walters, LeRoy. 1985. "Religion and the Renaissance of Medical Ethics in the United States: 1965–1975." In *Theology and Bioethics: Exploring the Foundations and Frontiers,* edited by Earl E. Shelp, 3–16. Boston: D. Reidel.

Walters, LeRoy. 2003. "The Birth and Youth of the Kennedy Institute of Ethics." In *The Story of Bioethics: From Seminal Works to Contemporary Explorations,* edited by Jennifer K. Walter and Eran P. Klein, 215–31. Washington DC: Georgetown University Press.

Walton, Michael T. 1983. "The Advisory Jury and Malpractice in 15th Century London: The Case of William Forest." *Journal of the History of Medicine and Allied Sciences.* 40: 478–80.

Walton, Michael T., Robert M. Fineman, and Phyllis J. Walton. 1993. "Of Monsters and Prodigies: The Interpretation of Birth Defects in the Sixteenth Century." *American Journal of Medical Genetics.* 47.1 (August): 7–13.

Walzer, Michael. 1977. *Just and Unjust Wars.* New York: Basic Books.

Walzer, Michael, et al., eds. 2003. *The Jewish Political Tradition: Volume 2: Membership*. New Haven CT: Yale University Press.

Wang, Maohe, ed. 1995. *Taiyu Xuanji (The Mystery of Child-Bearing and Child-Raising)*. Zhengzhou: Zhongzhou Guji Press.

Ward, P. S. 1984. "'Who Will Bell the Cat?' Andrew C. Ivy and Krebiozen." *Bulletin of the History of Medicine*. 58 (1): 28–52.

Warfield, Benjamin B. [1918] 1972. *Counterfeit Miracles*. London: Banner of Truth Trust.

Warner, John Harley. 1986. *The Therapeutic Perspective: Medical Practice, Knowledge, and Identity in America, 1820–1885*. Cambridge MA: Harvard University Press.

Warner, John Harley. 1991. "Ideals of Science and Their Discontents in Late Nineteenth-Century American Medicine." *Isis*. 82: 454–78.

Warner, John Harley. 1999. "The 1880's Rebellion Against the AMA Code of Ethics: Scientific Democracy and the Dissolution of Orthodoxy." In *The American Medical Ethics Revolution: How the AMA's Code of Ethics Has Transformed Physicians' Relationships to Patients, Professionals, and Society*, edited by Robert Baker et al., 52–69. Baltimore: Johns Hopkins University Press.

Warren, Mary Anne. [1973] 1997. "On the Moral and Legal Status of Abortion." [*The Monist*. 57: 43–61]. Reprinted in *The Problem of Abortion*. 3rd ed., edited by Susan Dwyer and Joel Feinberg, 59–74. Belmont CA: Wadsworth.

Warren, Stafford L. 1947. United States Atomic Energy Commission. Report of the Meeting of the Interim Medical Committee, 23–24 January.

Wasil, Nasr Farid. 1998. "Al-Mujtama mulzam bi'iadat al-bikara ila al-mughtasabat (Society is obliged to restore virginity to raped women)." *Ruz al-Yusuf*. (October 26): 146–9.

Wasunna, Angela. 2000a. "Averting a Clash Between Culture, Law and Science: An Examination of the Effects of New Reproductive Technologies in Kenya." Unpublished LL. M. diss., McGill University, Montreal.

Wasunna, Angela. 2000b. "Towards Redirecting the Female Circumcision Debate." *McGill Journal of Medicine*. 49: 5.

Watson, Patricia Ann. 1991. *The Angelical Conjunction: The Preacher-Physicians of Colonial New England*. Knoxville TN: The University of Tennessee Press.

Watt, Montgomery W. 1948. *Free Will and Predestination in Early Islam*. London: Luzac.

Wayman, Alex. 1982. "The Religious Meaning of Concrete Death in Buddhism." *Studia Missionalia*. 31: 273–95.

Wear, Andrew. 1985. "Puritan Perceptions of Illness in Seventeenth-Century England." In *Patients and Practitioners: Lay Perceptions of Medicine in Pre-Industrial Society*, edited by Roy Porter, 55–99. Cambridge UK: Cambridge University Press.

Wear, Andrew. 1987. "Interfaces: Perceptions of Health and Illness in Early Modern England." In *Problems and Methods in the History of Medicine*, edited by Roy Porter and Andrew Wear, 230–55. London: Croom Helm.

Wear, Andrew. 1993. "Medical Ethics in Early Modern England." In *Doctors and Ethics: The Earlier Historical Setting of Professional Ethics*, edited by Andrew Wear, Johanna Geyer-Kordesch, and Roger French, 98–130. Amsterdam: Rodopi.

Wear, Andrew. 1996. "Religious Beliefs in Medicine in Early Modern England." In *The Task of Healing: Medicine, Religion and Gender in England and the Netherlands, 1450–1800*, edited by Hilary Marland and Margaret Pelling, 145–69. Rotterdam: Erasmus Publishing.

Wear, Andrew. 2000. *Knowledge and Practice in English Medicine, 1550–1680*. Cambridge UK: Cambridge University Press.

Wear, Andrew, Johanna Geyer-Kordesch, and Roger French, eds. 1993 *Doctors and Ethics: The Earlier Historical Setting of Professional Ethics*. Amsterdam: Rodopi.

Weatherall, David. 2000. "Academia and Industry: Increasingly Uneasy Bedfellows." *The Lancet*. 355: 1574.

Weatherall, Miles. 1990. *In Search of a Cure: A History of Pharmaceutical Discovery*. Oxford: Oxford University Press.

Weber, Matthias M. 1993. *Ernst Rüdin: Eine kritische Biographie*. Munich: Springer.

Webster, Charles. 1975. *The Great Instauration: Science, Medicine and Reform, 1626–1660*. London: Duckworth.

Webster, Charles. 1983. "The Historiography of Medicine." In *Information Sources for the History of Science and Medicine*, edited by P. Corsi and P. J. Weindling, 29–42. London/Boston: Butterworth Scientific.

Webster, Charles. 1993. "Paracelsus: Medicine as Popular Protest." In *Medicine and the Reformation*, edited by Ole Peter Grell and Andrew Cunningham, 57–77. London: Routledge.

Wei, Z., and L. Nie. 1994. *Zhongyi Zhongyao Shi (History of Traditional Chinese Medicine)*. Taipei: Wenjin Press.

Weigel, George. 1999. *Witness to Hope: The Biography of Pope John Paul II*. New York: Cliff Street Books.

Weikart, Richard. 2004. *From Darwin to Hitler: Evolutionary Ethics, Eugenics, and Racism in Germany*. New York: Palgrave Macmillan.

Weindling, Paul J. 1981. "Theories of the Cell State in Imperial Germany." In *Biology, Medicine and Society, 1840–1940*, edited by Charles Webster, 99–155. Cambridge UK and New York: Cambridge University Press.

Weindling, Paul J. 1985. "Weimar Eugenics: The Kaiser Wilhelm Institute for Anthropology, Human Heredity and Eugenics in Social Context." *Annals of Science*. 42: 303–18.

Weindling, Paul J. 1989. *Health, Race, and German Politics Between National Unification and Nazism, 1870–1945*. Cambridge and New York: Cambridge University Press.

Weindling, Paul J. 1996a. "Ärzte als Richter: Internationale Reaktionen auf die medizinischen Verbrechen während des Nürnberger Ärzteprozesses im Jahre 1946–47." In *Medizin und Ethik im Zeichen von Auschwitz: 50 Jahre Nürnberger Ärzteprozeß*, edited by Claudia Wiesemann and Andreas Frewer, 31–44. Erlangen/Jena: Palm & Enke.

Weindling, Paul J. 1996b. "Human Guinea Pigs and the Ethics of Experimentation: The BMJ's Correspondent at the Nuremberg Medical Trial." *British Medical Journal*. 313: 1467–70.

Weindling, Paul J. 2000. *Epidemics and Genocide in Eastern Europe, 1890–1945*. Oxford/New York: Oxford University Press.

Weindling, Paul J. 2001. "The Origins of Informed Consent: The International Scientific Commission on Medical War Crimes and the Nuremberg Code." *Bulletin of the History of Medicine*. 75: 37–71.

Weindling, Paul J. 2004. *Nazi Medicine and the Nuremberg Trials: From Medical War Crimes to Informed Consent*. New York: Palgrave Macmillan.

Weiner, Sigrid. 1985. *Maschallah, Islam und Alltag in der Türkei*. Donauwörth: Auer.

Weingart, Peter, Jürgen Kroll, and Kurt Bayertz. 1988. *Rasse, Blut und Gene: Geschichte der Eugenik und Rassenpflege in Deutschland*. Frankfurt a.M.: Suhrkamp.

Weinhart, Ferdinand Karl. 1703. *Medicus Officiosus*. Innsbruck: n. p.

Weiss, Sheila F. 1987. *Race Hygiene and National Efficiency: The Eugenics of Wilhelm Schallmayer*. Berkeley CA/London: University of California Press.

Weisser, Ursula. 1983. *Zeugung und Vererbung und pränatale Entwicklung in der Medizin des arabisch-islamischen Mittelalters*. Erlangen: Verlagsbuchhandlung Hannelore Lüling.

Weisser, Ursula. 1991. "Unter den Künsten die nützlichste: Aspekte des ärztlichen Berufs im arabisch-islamischen Mittelalter." *Medizinhistorisches Journal*. 26: 3–25.

Weisser, Ursula. 1997. "Zur Tradition der ärztlichen Deontologie im Islam: Überlegungen zum Verhältnis arabischer Ärztespiegel zum antiken Erbe." *Medicina nei Secoli*. N. S. 9: 403–33.

Weisz, George. 1979. "The Politics of Medical Professionalization in France, 1845–1848." *Journal of Social History*. 12: 3–30.

Weisz, George. 1990. "The Origins of Medical Ethics in France: The International Congress of Morale Médicale of 1955." In *Social Science Perspectives on Medical Ethics*, edited by George Weisz, 145–61. Dordrecht: Kluwer Academic Publishers.

Weisz, George. 1995. *The Medical Mandarins: The French Academy of Medicine in the Nineteenth and Early Twentieth Centuries*. New York: Oxford University Press.

Weisz, George. 2003. "The Emergence of Medical Specialization in the Nineteenth Century." *Bulletin of the History of Medicine*. 77: 536–75.

Welborn, Mary Catherine. 1938. "The Long Tradition: A Study in Fourteenth-Century Medical Deontology." In *Medieval and Historiographical Essays in Honor of James Westfall Thompson*, edited by James Lea Cate and Eugene N. Anderson, 344–57. Chicago: University of Chicago Press.

Welborn, Mary Catherine. [1938] 1977. "The Long Tradition: A Study in Fourteenth-Century Medical Deontology." [*Medieval and Historiographical Essays in Honor of James Westfall Thompson*. Chicago: University of Chicago Press]. Reprinted in *Legacies in Ethics and Medicines*, edited by Chester R. Burns, 204–17. New York: Sciences History Publications.

Welch, C. E. 1976. "Henry K. Beecher (obituary)." *New England Journal of Medicine*. 295: 730.

Welsome, Eileen. 1999. *The Plutonium Files: America's Secret Medical Experiments in the Cold War*. New York: Dell.

Wenkebach, Ernst, ed. 1932–1933. "Der hippokratische Arzt als das Ideal Galens." *Quellen und Studien zur Geschichte der Naturwissenschaften und der Medizin*. 3: 155–75.

Wenkebach, Ernst, and Franz Pfaff, ed. 1934. *Galeni In Hippocratis Epidemiarum Libros I et II (Corpus Medicorum Graecorum V 10, 1)*. Leipzig and Berlin: B. G. Teubner.

Wenkebach, Ernst, and Franz Pfaff, eds. 1946. *Galeni In Hippocratis Epidemiarum Librum VI Commentaria I–VIII. (Corpus Medicorum Graecorum V 10, 2, 2)*. 2nd ed. Berlin: Akademie der Wissenschaften.

Wepfer, Johann Jakob. 1695. *Cicutae aquaticae historia et noxae*. Basle: J. R. König.

Wertz, Dorothy C. 1998. "Eugenics is Alive and Well: A Survey of Genetic Professionals around the World." *Science in Context*. 11: 493–510.

Wertz, Richard M., and Dorothy C. Wertz. 1989. *Lying-In: A History of Childbirth in America*. New Haven CT: Yale University Press.

Wesley, John. 1747. *Primitve Physick: or, An Easy and Natural Method of Curing Most Diseases*. London: n. p.

Westermark, Edward. 1912. *The Origin and Development of the Moral Ideas*. 2nd ed. London: Macmillan.

Westphalen, Daniela. 1989. *Karl Binding (1841–1920). Materialien zur Biographie eines Strafrechtsgelehrten.*

(Frankfurter kriminalwissenschaftliche Studien 26). Frankfurt am Main.

White (Whytt), Robert. n.d. "Clinical Lectures by Doctor Robert White." Student notes, author unknown. Royal College of Physicians and Surgeons of Glasgow. MS 1/9/4.

Wiesemann, Claudia, and Andreas Frewer, eds. 1996. *Medizin und Ethik im Zeichen von Auschwitz: 50 Jahre Nürnberger Ärzteprozeß*. Erlangen/Jena: Palm & Enke.

Wiesner-Hanks, Merry E. 1993. "The Midwives of South Germany and the Public/Private Dichotomy." In *The Art of Midwifery: Early Modern Midwives in Europe*, edited by Hilary Marland, 77–94. London: Routledge.

Wikler, Daniel. 1991. "What Has Bioethics to Offer Health Policy?" *Milbank Quarterly*. 69: 233–51.

Wiley, Harry R. 1904. *A Treatise on Pharmacal Jurisprudence*. San Francisco CA: The Hicks-Judd Company.

Wilkie, Tom, and Elizabeth Graham. 1998. "Power without Responsibility: Media Portrayals of Dolly and Science." *Cambridge Quarterly of Healthcare Ethics*. 7: 150–9.

Wilkins, Ernest Hatch. 1961. *Life of Petrarch*. Chicago: University of Chicago Press.

Willems, Dick L., et al. 2000. "Attitudes and Practices Concerning the End of Life: A Comparison Between Physicians From the United States and From the Netherlands." *Archives of Internal Medicine*. 160: 63–8.

Williams, P., and D. Wallace. 1989. *Unit 731: The Japanese Army's Secret of Secrets*. London: Hodder & Stoughten.

Williams, Samuel D., Jr. 1870. "Euthanasia." In Samuel D. Williams, *Essays of the Birmingham Liberal Club*. Birmingham, United Kingdom.

Williams, Samuel D., Jr. 1872. *Euthanasia*. London: Williams and Norgate.

Williamson, G. 1969. "The Libertine Donne." In *Seventeenth Century Contexts*, 42–62. Revised ed. Chicago: University of Chicago Press.

Willis, Thomas. 1664. *Cerebri anatome*. London: Martyn and Allestry.

Wilson, Carroll L. 1947a. United States Atomic Energy Commission. Letter to Stafford Warren, Dean of Medical School at the University of California, Los Angeles, 30 April.

Wilson, Carroll L. 1947b. United States Atomic Energy Commission. Letter to Robert Stone, 5 November.

Wilson, Charles E. 1953. United States Department of Defense. Memorandum to the Secretaries of the Army, Navy and Air Force, 26 February.

Wiltshire, Martin G. 1983. "The Suicide Problem in the Pàli Canon." *Journal of International Association of Buddhist Studies*. 6: 124–40.

Winau, Rolf. 1996. "Medizin und Menschenversuch: Zur Geschichte des 'informed consent.'" In *Medizin und*

Ethik im Zeichen von Auschwitz: 50 Jahre Nürnberger Ärzteprozeß, edited by Claudia Wiesemann and Andreas Frewer, 13–29. Erlangen/Jena: Palm & Enke.

Winkler, Johann Heinrich, ed. 1743. *Die verschiedenen Meynungen einiger Weltweisen von der Existenz der Seelen der Thiere in einer Gesellschaft guter Freunde untersucht*. 3rd ed. Leipzig: Breitkopf.

Winslade, William J., and Todd L. Krause. 1998. "The Nuremberg Code Turns Fifty." In *Ethics Codes in Medicine: Foundations and Achievements of Codification since 1947*, edited by Ulrich Tröhler and Stella Reiter-Theil, 140–62. Aldershot/Brookfield/Singapore/Sydney: Ashgate.

Withington, Edward Theodore. 1924. "Roger Bacon and the Errors of Physicians." In *Essays on the History of Medicine Presented to Karl Sudhoff*, edited by Charles Singer and Henri E. Sigerist, 139–57. London/Zürich. Oxford University Press.

Wittgenstein, Ludwig. [1922] 1961. *Tractatus Logico-Philosophicus*, new translation by D. F. Pears and B. F. McGuiness. London: Allen and Unwin.

Wolf, Ursula. 1988. "Haben wir moralische Verpflichtungen gegen Tiere?" *Zeitschrift für philosophische Forschung*. 42: 222–46.

Wolff, Christian Sigismund. 1709. *Disputatio philosophica de moralitate anatomes circa animalia viva occupatae*. Leipzig: Fleischer.

Wolpe, Paul Root. 1999. "Alternative Medicine and the AMA." In *The American Medical Ethics Revolution: How the AMA's Code of Ethics Has Transformed Physicians' Relationships to Patients, Professionals, and Society*, edited by Robert Baker, et al., 218–39. Baltimore: Johns Hopkins University Press.

Wolstenholme, G. E. W., and M. O'Connor, eds. 1966. *Ethics in Medical Progress With Special Reference to Transplantation*. Boston: Little Brown.

Wood, William M. 1849. "Thoughts on Suits for Malpractice, suggested by Certain Judicial Proceedings in Erie County, Pennsylvania." *American Journal of Medical Sciences*. n. s.: 395.

Woodard, S., et al. 2003. "Older Women with Breast Carcinoma are Less Likely to Receive Adjuvant Chemotherapy: Evidence of possible age bias?" *Cancer*. 98.6 (September): 1141–9.

Worboys, Michael. 2000. *Spreading Germs: Disease Theories and Medical Practice in Britain, 1865–1900*. Cambridge UK: Cambridge University Press.

World Bank. 1993. *World Development Report 1993*. New York: Oxford University Press.

World Bank. 1999. "Intensifying Action Against HIV/AIDS in Africa: Responding to a Development Crisis." Washington DC: World Bank, Africa Region.

World Health Organization, World Health Assembly. 1970. *The Rapid Prohibition of Chemical and Bacteriological (Biological) Weapons.* Geneva: The World Health Organization.

World Medical Association. [1948] 1995a. "Declaration of Geneva." In *Encyclopedia of Bioethics.* 2nd ed., edited by Warren T. Reich, 2646–7. New York: Simon & Schuster Macmillan.

World Medical Association. [1949] 1995b. "International Code of Medical Ethics." In *Encyclopedia of Bioethics.* 2nd ed., edited by Warren T. Reich, 2647–8. New York: Simon & Schuster Macmillan.

World Medical Association. 1949a. "Serment de Geneve, Declaration of Geneva, Declaracion en Gemebra." *World Medical Association Bulletin.* 1.2: 35–7.

World Medical Association. 1949b. "Proceedings." *World Medical Association Bulletin.* 1.1: 7.

World Medical Association. [1954] 1995c. "Principles for Those in Research and Experimentation." In *Encyclopedia of Bioethics.* 2nd ed., edited by Warren T. Reich, 2764. New York: Simon & Schuster Macmillan.

World Medical Association. 1964. *The Declaration of Helsinki.* http://www.cirp.org/library/ethics/helsinki/ (visited January 30, 2008).

World Medical Association. 2000. "The Declaration of Helsinki (revised version adopted October 3 in Edinburgh)." *Bulletin of Medical Ethics.* (October): 8–11.

"World Medical Association Declaration of Helsinki: Ethical Principles for Medical Research Involving Human Subjects." 2000. *Journal of the American Medical Assoication.* 284: 3043–5.

World Medical Association, 2nd General Assembly of the World Medical Association. 1948. *Declaration of Geneva.* http://www.cirp.org/library/ethics/geneva/ (visited January 30, 2008).

World Medical Association, 3rd General Assembly of the World Medical Association. 1949. *International Code of Medical Ethics.* http://www.cirp.org/library/ethics/intlcode/ (visited January 30, 2008).

World Medical Association, 10th World Medical Assembly. 1956. *Regulations in Time of Armed Conflict.* http://www.wma.net/e/policy/a20.htm (visited January 30, 2008).

World Medical Association, 38th World Medical Assembly. 1986a. *Declaration on Physician Independence and Professional Freedom.* http://www.wma.net/e/policy/f9.htm (visited January 30, 2008).

World Medical Association, 42nd World Medical Assembly. 1986b. *Declaration on Chemical and Biological Weapons.* http://www.wma.net/e/policy/b1.htm (visited January 30, 2008).

Wu, Tien-Wei. "A Preliminary Review of Studies of Japanese Biological Warfare and Unit 731 in the United States." www.centurychina.com/wiihist/germwar/731rev.htm (visited October 25, 2007).

Wu, Zeng (Song). 1984. *Nengaizai Manlu (Informal Records of Nenguizai).* Shanghai: Shanghai Classics Press.

Wujastyk, Dominik. 1998. *The Roots of Ayurveda.* New Delhi: Penguin Books India.

Wulff, H. R. 1998. "Contemporary Trends in Health Care Ethics." In *Consensus Formation in Health Care Ethics,* edited by Henk A. M. J. ten Have and H.-M. Sass, 63–72. Dordrecht: Kluwer Academic Publishers.

Xiao-Jing (The Classic of Filial Piety). 1995. Shanghai: Shanghai Classics Press.

Xue, Gongceng, ed. 1999. *Lun Yi Zhong Ru Shi Dao (On Confucianism, Daoism and Buddhism in Chinese Medicine).* Beijing: Chinese Medical Classics Press.

Xunzi. For an English translation, see John Knoblock, *Xunzi: A Translation and Study of the Complete Works.* 1990. Palo Alto CA: Stanford University Press.

Yanakita, Kunio. 1970. *About Our Ancestors: The Japanese Family System,* translated by F. H. Mayer and Y. Ishiwara. Tokyo: Japan Society for the Promotion of Science.

Yano, Michio. 1976–1977. "A Comparative Study of the Sustrasthānas Caraka, Suśruta, and Vāgbhaṇa." *History of Traditional Medicine: Proceedings of the 1st and 2nd International Symposia on the Comparative History of Medicine – East and West.* Susuno-shi, Shizuoka, Japan: Division of Medical History, Taniguchi Foundation.

Yates, John. 1987. *Why Are We Waiting? An Analysis of Hospital Waiting Lists.* Oxford: Oxford University Press.

Yazır, Elmalılı H. 1971. *Hak Dini Kur'an Dili.* 10 vols. Istanbul: Eser.

Yediyıldız, Bahaeddin. 1993. "Vakıf." In *İslâm Ansiklopedisi.* 13: 153–72. Istanbul: Millî Eğitim Basımevi.

Yonemoto, Shohei. 1988. *Advanced Medical Technologies and Revolution in Medicine.* Tokyo: Chuou Kouronsha Publishers [Japanese].

Young, A. T. 1890. *The Annals of the Barber-Surgeons of London.* London: East and Blades.

Young, James. 1980. "The Foolmaster Who Fooled Them." *Yale Journal of Biology and Medicine.* 53 (6): 555–66.

Young, Katherine K. 1994a. "A Cross-Cultural Historical Case against Planned Self-Willed Death and Assisted Suicide." *McGill Law Journal.* 39: 657–707.

Young, Katherine K. 1994b. "Hindu Bioethics." In *Religious Methods and Resources in Bioethics,* edited by Paul F. Camenisch, 3–30. Chicago: Kluwer Academic Publishers.

Young, Katherine K. 1995. "Death: Eastern Thought." In *Encyclopedia of Bioethics.* 2nd ed., edited by Warren T. Reich, 487–97. New York: Simon and Schuster Macmillan.

Young, Robert M. 1971. "Evolutionary Biology and Ideology: Then and Now." *Science Studies*. 1: 177–206.

Young, Thomas. 1798. *An Essay on Humanity to Animals*. London: Cadwell Jun. & Davies.

Youngner, Stuart J., Robert M. Arnold, and Michael DeVita. 1999. "When is 'Dead'?" *Hastings Center Report*. 29: 14–21.

Youngner, Stuart J., Robert M. Arnold, and Renie Schapiro, eds. 1999. *The Definition of Death: Contemporary Controversies*. Baltimore: Johns Hopkins University Press.

Yu, Lin, and Dapu Shi. 1998. "Euthanasia Should Be Legalized in China." *Chinese and International Philosophy of Medicine*. 1: 159–75 [Chinese].

Yudin, Boris. 1992. "Bioethics for the New Russia." *Hastings Center Report*. 22: 5–6.

Zacchia, Paolo. 1621–1625. *Quaestiones medico-legales: In quibus omnes eae materiae medicae, quae ad legales facultates videntur pertinere, proponuntur, pertractantur, resoluuntur: opus ipsis iurisperitis apprimè necessarium, medicis perutile, caeteris non iniucundum*. 7 vols. Romae: Andreae Brugiotti/Iacobum Mascardum.

Zacchia, Paolo. 1621–1625. *Questiones Medical-Legales*. Romae: A. Brugiotti for J. Mascardus.

Zacchia, Paolo. 1621, 1701. *Quaestiones Medico-Legales*. Lyons: Anisson and Joannis Posuel.

Zacchiae, Pauli. [1621–1635] 1651. *Quaestiones Medico-Legales*. 3rd ed. Amsterdam: Joannis Blaev.

Zaidān, ʿAbd-al-Karīm. 1976. *Al-Madhal li-dirāsat aš-Šariʾa al-islāmīya*. Bairūt: Maktabat al-Quds.

Zalba, Marcelino, and Jorge Bozal. 1955. *El magisterio eclesiástico y la medicina*. Madrid: Fax.

Zancariis, Albertus de. 1914. *Die Schrift des Albertus de Zancariis aus Bologna: De cautelis medicorum habendis. Nach Leipziger und Pariser Handschriften*, edited by Manuel Morris. Medical diss. Leipzig: Peter.

Zapata, Diego Mateo. 1733. *Dissertacion medico-theologica y carta responsoria al eruditissimo Doct. D. Francisco Criado y Balboa*. Madrid: Gabriel del Barrio.

Zarqaʾ, Mustafa al-. 1999. *Fatawa Mustafa al-Zarqaʾ (The Fatwas of Mustafa al-Zarqaʾ)*. Damascus: Dar al-Qalam.

Zayyin, Samih ʿAtif al-. 1991. *ʿIlm al-Nafs (Psychology)*. Beirut: Dar al-Kitab al-Lubnani.

Zemer, Moshe. 1998. *Evolving Halakhah: A Progressive Approach to Traditional Jewish Law*. Woodstock VT: Jewish Lights.

Zerbi, Gabriele de. 1495. *Opus perutile de cautelis medicorum*. Biblioteca Palatina IV 586. Venedig: Biblioteca Palatina.

Zerbi, Gabriel de. 1528. *Opus Perutile de Cautelis Medicorum, in Pillularium Omnibus Medicis Necessarium Clarissimi Doctoris Magistri Panthaleonis*. Lyons: Antonium Blanchard.

Zerbi, Gabriele. 1988. *Gerontocomia: On the care of the aged*, translated from the Latin by L. R. Lind (American Philosophical Society; Memoirs 182). Philadelphia.

Zeyst, H. Van. 1961. "Abortion." In *Encyclopedia of Buddhism*, edited by G. P. Malalasekera, 137–8. Ceylon: Government of Ceylon.

Zhang, Daqing, and Zhifan Cheng. 2000. "Medicine is a Humane Art: The Basic Principles of Professional Ethics in Chinese Medicine." *Hastings Center Report*. 30: S8–S12.

Zhang, Z. 1996. "Organ Transplantation Should be Voluntary and Transparent." *Medicine and Philosophy*. 17: 151–2 [Chinese].

Zhbankov, D. N. 1903. *O Vrachakh*. Moscow: Izdanie S. Dorovatovskogo i A. Charushnikova.

Zhbankov, D. N. 1911. "Zemskaya Meditsyna i Chastnaya Praktika." *Obshestvennyi Vrach*. 8: 14–28.

Zhbankov, D. N. 1927. "Otnoshenie naselenija k vracham i meditsynskomu personalu." *Vrachebnoe Delo*, no. 1: 61–62.

Zhbankov, D. N. 1928. "Smertnost' vrachei v 1924–1927gg." *Acta Medica*. 19: 60–7.

Zhen, Zhiya, ed. 1997. *Zhongguo Yixueshi (The History of Chinese Medicine)*, revised edition. Shangshai: Shanghai Science and Technology Press.

Zhou, Yimou. 1983. *Lidai Mingyi Lun Yide (Ancient well-known Chinese Physicians on Medical Morality)*. Changsha: Hunan Science and Technology Press.

Ziegler, Philip. 1969. *The Black Death*. London: Collins.

Ziemssen, Oswald. 1899. *Die Ethik des Arztes als medicinischer Lehrgegenstand*. Leipzig: Verlag von G. Thieme.

Zil'ber, Anatolii P. 1998. *Traktat ob Evtanazii*. Petrozavodsk: Izdatel'stvo Petrozavodskogo gosudarstavennogo universiteta.

Zohar, Noam J. 1997. *Alternatives in Jewish Bioethics*. Albany NY: State University of New York Press.

Zoloth-Dorfman, Laurie. 1999. *Health Care and the Ethics of Encounter: A Jewish Discussion of Social Justice*. Chapel Hill NC: University of North Carolina Press.

Zubayr, Al-Zayn Yaʾqub al-. 1991. *Mawqif al-Shariʾa al-Islamiyya min Tanzim al-Nasl (The Position of Islamic Law on Family Planning)*. Beirut: Dar al-Jil.

Zuckerman, Connie. 1999. *End of Life Care and Hospital Legal Counsel: Current Involvement and Opportunities for the Future*. New York: Milbank Memorial Fund and United Hospital Fund.

Zuhayli, Wahba al-. 1989. *Al-Fiqh al-Islami waAdillatuhu (Islamic Law and its Guidelines)*. Damascus: Dar al-Fikr.

Zylicz, Z. 1993. "The Story Behind the Blank Spot: Hospice in Holland." *American Journal of Hospice and Palliative Care*. 10.4: 30–4.

Zysk, Kenneth G. 1985. *Religious Healing in the Veda: With Translations and Annotations of Medical Hymns in the Ṛgveda and the Atharvaveda from the Corresponding Ritual Texts*. Vol. 75. 7. Philadelphia: American Philosophical Society.

Zysk, Kenneth G. [1985] 1996. *Medicine in the Veda*. Delhi: Motilal Banarsidass Publishers.

Zysk, Kenneth G. 1991. *Asceticism and Healing in Ancient India: Medicine in the Buddhist Monastery*. New York: Oxford University Press.

INDEX